Medical Radiology

Diagnostic Imaging

For further volumes:
http://www.springer.com/series/4354

Regina G. H. Beets-Tan • Wim J. G. Oyen
Vincenzo Valentini
Editors

Imaging and Interventional Radiology for Radiation Oncology

Springer

Editors
Regina G. H. Beets-Tan
Department of Radiology
The Netherlands Cancer Institute
Amsterdam, The Netherlands

Vincenzo Valentini
Department of Radiology, Radiation
Oncology and Hematology Fondazione
Policlinico Universitario A.Gemelli
IRCCS
Università Cattolica del Sacro Cuore
Rome, Italy

Wim J. G. Oyen
Humanitas University and Humanitas
Clinical and Research Center
Milan, Italy

Department of Radiology and Nuclear
Medicine
Rijnstate Hospital
Arnhem, The Netherlands

ISSN 0942-5373 ISSN 2197-4187 (electronic)
Medical Radiology
ISBN 978-3-030-38263-6 ISBN 978-3-030-38261-2 (eBook)
https://doi.org/10.1007/978-3-030-38261-2

This Springer imprint is published by the registered company Springer Nature Switzerland AG
The registered company address is: Gewerbestrasse 11, 6330 Cham, Switzerland

Contents

Part I Imaging in Oncology: From Diagnosis to Outcomes (Vincenzo Valentini, Regina G. H. Beets-Tan, Wim J. G. Oyen)

Theragnostics in Modern Oncology: The Role of Imaging 3
Nicolò Gennaro, Margarita Kirienko, and Arturo Chiti

The Role of a Radiologist and Nuclear Medicine Physician in a Multidisciplinary Tumour Board 13
Cristina Grippo, Maria Cristina Cortese, and Riccardo Manfredi

Part II From Simulation to Delivery Guided by Imaging: Technical Aspects (Vincenzo Valentini, Uulke van der Heide)

Optimal CT Protocols for CT-Guided Planning Preparation in Radiotherapy 27
Alessandra Bolsi and Lorenzo Placidi

Management of Respiratory-Induced Tumour Motion for Tailoring Target Volumes during Radiation Therapy 47
Willem Grootjans, Jennifer Dhont, Bas Gobets, and Dirk Verellen

Principles and Constraints of Nonrigid Registration 69
Zoi Giavri, Durval C. Costa, and Nickolas Papanikolaou

Radiotherapy Target Volume Definition Based on PET/CT Imaging Data 81
Daniela Thorwarth

CT in Room Gating During Radiotherapy 91
Mariangela Massaccesi

High-Field MRI In-Room Guidance for Radiotherapy Adaptation 107
Martin F. Fast and Markus Glitzner

Low Tesla MRI in-Room Gating during Radiotherapy 129
Davide Cusumano and Francesco Cellini

Endoluminal Brachytherapy: Technicalities and Main Clinical Evidences 137
G. C. Mattiucci, L. Tagliaferri, R. Autorino, and G. Kovacs

Part III Imaging for Tumor Staging and Volume Definition (Wim J. G. Oyen, Monique Maas, Ursula Nestle)

Staging and Target Volume Definition by Imaging in CNS Tumors . . . 151
Bas Jasperse and Gerben Borst

T-Staging and Target Volume Definition by Imaging in Head and Neck Tumors . . . 169
Ivan Platzek, Linda Agolli, Bettina Beuthien-Baumann, and Esther G. C. Troost

T-Staging and Target Volume Definition by Imaging in Breast Tumours . . . 183
Roberto C. Delgado Bolton, Adriana K. Calapaquí Terán, and Philip Poortmans

T-Staging and Target Volume Definition by Imaging in GI Tumors . . . 203
Maria Isabel Morales, Feyza Sen, Bülent Polat, Philip Kleine, and Andreas Buck

T Staging and Target Volume Definition by Imaging in GU Tumors . . . 221
Paolo Castelluci, Stefano Fanti, Stefano Bracci, Valeria Panebianco, Alessio Giuseppe Morganti, and Rezarta Frakulli

T-Staging and Target Volume Definition by Imaging in GYN Tumors . . . 255
A. Alessi, B. Pappalardi, A. Cerrotta, G. Calareso, and F. Crippa

N-stage Challenges . . . 275
Jasenko Krdzalic, Michelle Versleijen, and Monique Maas

Tumor Biology Characterization by Imaging in Laboratory . . . 293
Alberto Conficoni, Antonio Poerio, Eleonora Farina, and Alessio G. Morganti

Tumour Biology Characterisation by Imaging in Clinic . . . 325
Aravind S. Ravi Kumar, W. Phillip. Law, Craig Wilson, Shankar Siva, and Michael S. Hofman

Imaging-Based Prediction Models . . . 361
Luca Boldrini, Carlotta Masciocchi, and Lucia Leccisotti

Part IV Response Evaluation and Follow-Up by Imaging (Regina G. H. Beets-Tan, Daniel Zips, Roberto C. Delgado Bolton)

Response Evaluation and Follow-Up by Imaging in Brain Tumours . . . 381
R. Gahrmann, J. Arbizu, A. Laprie, M. Morales, and M. Smits

Response Assessment and Follow-Up by Imaging in Head and Neck Tumours 405
Vincent Vandecaveye, Sandra Nuyts, and Roberto C. Delgado Bolton

Response Assessment and Follow-Up by Imaging in Lung Tumours 417
Anna Rita Larici, Alessandra Farchione, Giuseppe Cicchetti, Annemilia del Ciello, Giovanna Mantini, Adriana K. Calapaquí Terán, and Roberto C. Delgado Bolton

Response Assessment and Follow-Up by Imaging in Breast Tumors 451
Mireille van Goethem, Angelo Castello, Marc B. I. Lobbes, Fiorenza De Rose, Marta Scorsetti, and Egesta Lopci

Response Assessment and Follow-Up by Imaging in Gastrointestinal Tumours 475
Doenja M. J. Lambregts and Francesco Giammarile

Response Assessment and Follow-Up by Imaging in GU Tumours 495
Cédric Draulans, Ivo G. Schoots, Bernd J. Krause, Sofie Isebaert, Stijn W. T. P. J. Heijmink, Sascha Nitsch, Karin Haustermans, and Sarah M. Schwarzenböck

Response Assessment and Follow-Up by Imaging in GYN Tumours 517
Andrea Rockall, Maximilian P. Schmid, and Judit A. Adam

Part I

Imaging in Oncology: From Diagnosis to Outcomes (Vincenzo Valentini, Regina G. H. Beets-Tan, Wim J. G. Oyen)

Theragnostics in Modern Oncology: The Role of Imaging

Nicolò Gennaro, Margarita Kirienko, and Arturo Chiti

Contents

1 **Theragnostics Applications in Oncology** 4
2 **The Role of Imaging** 5
3 **Which Imaging in Oncology** 5
4 **Interventional Radiology in Oncology** 10
5 **Conclusions** 10
References 10

N. Gennaro · M. Kirienko
Humanitas University, Milan, Italy

A. Chiti (✉)
Humanitas University, Milan, Italy

Humanitas Clinical and Research Hospital, Milan, Italy
e-mail: arturo.chiti@hunimed.eu

Abstract

Theragnostics in modern medicine is defined as a treatment strategy for individual patients, which associates both a diagnostic test that identifies patients most likely to be helped or harmed by a new medication and targeted drug therapy based on the test results. The strategy combines therapeutics with diagnostics, and this is where the term theragnostics comes from. Theragnostics covers a wide range of topics that include predictive medicine, personalized medicine, and pharmacodiagnostics. Precision medicine aims to use multiple types of data to classify patients into groups that will most likely respond to a given treatment. These data are derived from genetics, proteomics, and diagnostic tools used to study an individual patient or a group of individuals with similar characteristics related to their disease. Applications of theragnostics exist in several fields of modern medicine. In general, they require a four-step approach to be implemented:

Efficacy: identification of subgroups of patients presenting a profile likely to give a positive response to a targeted treatment.

Safety: identification of subgroups of patients at risk of aggravated side effects during treatment.

Response: monitoring the response to a particular treatment.

R. G. H. Beets-Tan et al. (eds.), *Imaging and Interventional Radiology for Radiation Oncology*, Medical Radiology, Diagnostic Imaging, https://doi.org/10.1007/978-3-030-38261-2_1

Development: development of a particular drug or therapeutic intervention.

This chapter will briefly introduce how theragnostics concepts are applied in radiation-related oncology fields.

1 Theragnostics Applications in Oncology

The strong commitment in oncology to promote therapies that reflect the uniqueness of each single patient has its cornerstone in the optimization of the diagnostic workup, as either laboratory tests, genomic analysis, biomarker profiling, or imaging techniques. The complex and univocal characterization of the oncologic patient, and the consequent appropriate collocation in the right subset of patients with common features, appears as the only way to deliver treatment with the highest risk-benefit balance.

A wide variety of young but rapidly expanding disciplines like functional genomics, pharmacogenomics, proteomics, and molecular imaging represent today valuable tools to play a seminal role across the different levels of the therapeutic process, which starts with the selection of the most appropriate diagnostic approach.

New diagnostic tools are now responsible to validate different treatment solutions, to guide therapy in real time, and to monitor treatment response. A proper use of these diagnostic methods influences directly the overall quality of the therapy, providing sensitive data about the patient prognosis and reinforcing the safety profile. Carefully selected patients will only benefit from previously well-validated therapy.

It is straightforward to realize that diagnosis and therapy are two sides of the patient care, intrinsically bound together throughout the entire care process, even in the right moment of the therapy delivery (Fig. 1). In fact, the need for a new target to dispose of dedicated diagnostic technologies has brought diagnosis and therapy so close that they can coincide in the same medical act, like in the case of isotope-labeled or ferromagnetic nanoparticles detectable

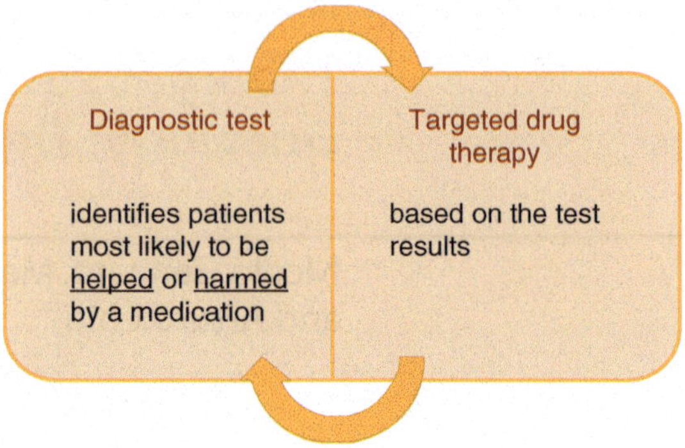

Fig. 1 The theragnostics concept

respectively by immuno-positron emission tomography (PET) or magnetic resonance imaging (MRI). Thus, these separate but intimate moments of the patient care can be framed in one comprehensive approach, and from this concept of interdependence and simultaneity, the term "theragnostics" or "theranostics" was born, as a synthesis of the words "diagnosis" and "therapy."

This term also represents a sustainable and cost-effective model for the drug industry: it is no coincidence that the first to introduce it in 1998 was John Funkhouser, CEO of *PharmaNetics*, who tried to resume in just one visionary term the concepts of diagnosis, treatment, and follow-up. In the setting of an optimization of the resources, cost-cutting measures have been taken by the industry toward the development of diagnostic test with high specificity for precise therapeutic programs, like the diagnostic test "*HercepTest*" and "*PathVysion*" for validation of trastuzumab therapy or "*DakoCytomation EGFR pharmDx test*" for validation of cetuximab-imatinib therapies. This patient-centered approach represents a switching paradigm from the trial-and-error medicine to a healthcare based on prediction and prevention. Theragnostics is clearly the direction modern oncology is moving toward and arguably represents today's most complete lexical portrayal of what the so-called personalized medicine wants to be: an innovative methodological approach that considers diagnostic exams as companion tests for targeted therapies, reaching its complete expression in the deployment of bimodal agents, with either diagnostic or therapeutic roles.

2 The Role of Imaging

Diagnostic oncologic assessment is a multidisciplinary effort where imaging plays a pivotal role providing anatomical and functional information. An oncologic patient is by definition a complex patient to approach, and the correct characterization is critical for the treatment's success. Cancer screening, staging, and treatment require imaging technologies to first identify and then to adequately characterize even small tumors, which is still a strenuous challenge for imaging modalities that still have resolution thresholds that limit their performance. The valuable information coming from the tridimensional features of tumors, essential in radiation oncology, are even more difficult to achieve if the dimensions are particularly small or technically impossible when malignant cells occupy just a few voxels of the imaging study. The increasing availability of PET scanners and particular MRI sequences has added precise functional information to implement patient's characterization profile, and recent advances in molecular imaging have opened new perspectives in how imaging can contribute to patient selection, prediction of adverse reactions, and response monitoring. Also in drug development, a significant foothold has already been gained, as the ability to perform receptor occupancy studies (like dose finding in phase I trials) allows to investigate the pharmacokinetics, pharmacodynamics, and metabolism of new drugs.

In the theragnostics era, it is ought to remember that medical imaging had already brought close diagnostic and therapeutic moments when nuclear medicine first introduced thyroid studies using radioactive iodine to select patients eligible for iodine-131 therapy. Moreover, nuclear medicine has already availed of specific receptors to selectively transport radionuclides, like in the case of somatostatin or noradrenaline receptors for the treatment of neuroendocrine tumors or neuroblastoma. Molecular imaging projects itself as a high-sensible and specific technology able to fill the gap with traditional imaging (X-rays, CT, MRI) beyond the macroscopic features of the neoplasia (vascularization, dimensions, texture, draining lymph node).

3 Which Imaging in Oncology

Nowadays, the two main imaging modalities that can give functional key information about the tumors are positron emission tomography (PET) and magnetic resonance imaging (MRI) that includes functional MRI (fMRI), diffusion MRI (DWI, ADC, DTI), perfusion MRI (PWI), and pharmacological MRI (PhMRI). fMRI is a broad area of intense research that allows to image physiological and molecular metabolism alterations before they become macroscopically visible with morphologic imaging methods, like MRI or CT (Higgins and Pomper 2011). Cell metabolism, angiogenesis, and cellularity are the parameters that can be assessed through spectroscopy, perfusion, and diffusion imaging, respectively. Magnetic resonance spectroscopy quantifies the distribution and the levels of various metabolites inside the lesion and resulted in a useful tool in the assessment of brain, prostate, and breast cancers. Increased levels of choline (a cell proliferation marker) with simultaneous decreased levels of N-acetylaspartate and creatine (a marker of energetic processes) are found in brain cancers. Once again in breast cancer, choline levels have been demonstrated to increase, and in prostate cancer, particular attention is focused on choline-creatine-citrate ratio and polyamine levels. Perfusion imaging is based on the deployment of exogenous contrast medium, usually gadolinium-based agents, and the sequential acquisition at different times of the tissue in order to study the dynamics of its contrast enhancement. Signal intensity/time curves are thus created to quantitatively or qualitatively analyze tissue perfusion, especially in breast, brain, and rectum cancers. This type of assessment not only allows for faster diagnosis but also represents a prognostic factor in the evaluation of recurrent disease. Other perfusion techniques are being studied, like arterial spin labeling techniques, that do not request an infusion of exogenous contrast agents. Gadobenate or gadoxetic acid, due to their longer permanence inside the vessels and their selective uptake by the hepatocytes, represents MRI contrast agents that can give further information about liver lesions. Finally, DWI-MRI has become a standard imaging technique capable of providing both qualitative and quantitative valuable information to improve cancer detection, to assess the cellularity of the tissue with no need of contrast medium or invasive procedures, and to evaluate tumor response to treatment. Currently, DWI is under evaluation as a source of predictive or prognostic information (Guimaraes et al. 2014). DWI's efficacy in cancer detection has been well-demonstrated in prostate cancer (where it proved to be superior to morphologic MRI sequences for the detection of disease recurrences after radiation therapy), but also application in bladder tumors, lymphomas, renal tumors, gynecologic tumors, and peritoneal disease has been explored and exported in clinical practice. Recent attempts to correlate DWI information with standardized uptake value (SUV) measurements with PET/MR hybrid imaging systems are very interesting, especially for lymph node assessment, where multi-parametric MRI does not achieve high sensitivity alone (Koh et al. 2016). The deployment of specific PET radiopharmaceuticals, like prostate-specific antigen for prostate cancer, has further improved diagnostic accuracy and the understanding of tumor biology.

In fact, every molecule can be technically imaged if appropriately bound to a radioisotope or magnetic particles. Today, even though PET [^{18}F]FDG, using a glucose analogue, is still the most deployed technique to reflect tumor metabolism, many other different molecules are used to provide relevant information in addition to the evaluation of glucose uptake like hexokinase and AKT, which trigger the upregulation of glucose transporters, or molecular target of rapamycin (mTOR), also involved in glucose metabolism (Rosenkrantz et al. 2016). Some of these radiopharmaceuticals are already introduced in the clinical practice in some countries, although many others are under evaluation in clinical trials. For instance, radiopharmaceuticals like gallium-labeled prostate-specific membrane antigen (PSMA) have been introduced for prostate cancer imaging. Others, like [^{18}F]fluorodeoxythymidine ([^{18}F]FLT), are markers of increased synthesis of DNA/thymidine kinase 1 in tumors and can be deployed in the evaluation of platinum-based doublet chemotherapy for early-stage non-small-cell lung cancers. Another example is [^{18}F]fluoromisonidazole ([^{18}F]FMISO) that can be used as a sensitive and specific marker for hypoxic tumor cells (Sai et al. 2017).

This additional information about tumor biology, complemented by the current morphologic evaluation in terms of change in tumor size, allows to properly investigate drug effects at a cellular level, reaching high sensitivity and specificity in detecting tumor modifications. These efforts in providing new markers in oncologic imaging represent the first step toward the substitution of the imaging radiopharmaceuticals with a therapeutic agent, usually beta- or alpha-emitter particles (Fig. 2). Let us consider, for instance, the prostate cancer imaging agent gallium-68 PSMA, used to detect the presence of disease with PET imaging. Positron-emitting gallium-68 can be replaced with beta-emitting lutetium-177, or even actinium-225, an alpha-emitter, in order to deliver effective and specific target therapy (Kratochwil et al. 2016). A more consolidated approach uses ^{68}Ga-DOTA-TOC to define the distribution of somatostatin receptors in patients affected by neuroendocrine tumors of the gastroenteropancreatic tract. After demonstration of receptors in patients affected by these diseases, they can be successfully treated with a lutetium-177-labeled peptide (Figs. 3 and 4).

PET imaging proved to be a successful technique also to monitor treatment response early after initiation of therapy, to display residual masses after completion of treatment, and to assess changes in metabolism, directly linked with the reduction of viable tumor cells. This is particularly true for [^{18}F]FDG-PET in monitoring treatment response of GIST and sarcomas treated with imatinib. This task benefits from surrogate metrics usually expressed in terms of response rate, progression-free survival, or time to tumor progression. Many tools have been introduced in clinical practice to monitor treatment response, like the World Health Organization (WHO) criteria (1979), the Response Evaluation Criteria in Solid Tumor (RECIST) (2000), and the RECIST 1.1 (2009). Recently, a new method called

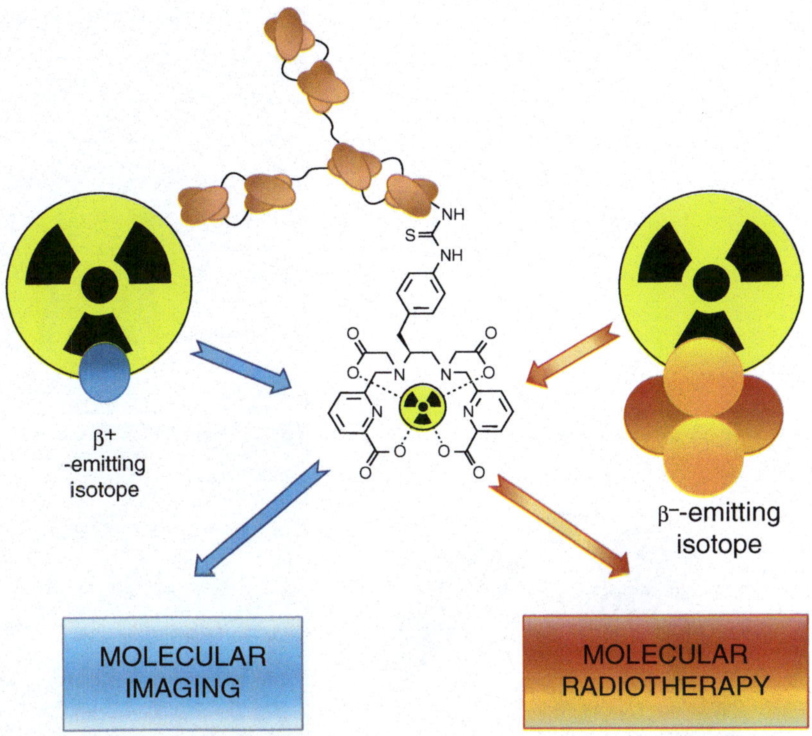

Fig. 2 The theragnostics model in radiation therapy

PERCIST 1.0 has been proposed, with a particular focus on the evaluation of the standardized uptake value (SUV) over time (Wahl et al. 2009).

The so-called immuno-PET promises a revolution in diagnostic oncologic imaging, using PET technology to track and quantify monoclonal antibodies (MAb) and to monitor MAb target therapy. This field is producing exciting results in non-Hodgkin lymphoma imaging, where, after the initial introduction of copper-64 rituximab to display CD20 receptors, zirconium-89 rituximab is obtaining excellent results in imaging b-cell NHL (Jauw et al. 2016). The same agent once labeled with trastuzumab has also been successfully deployed in breast cancer imaging to display HER2-positive metastases, which show lower [^{18}F]FDG uptake than ER-positive tumors. The HER2/neu expression in breast cancer has been imaged via both single-photon emission computed tomography (SPECT) and PET, thanks to the deployment of monoclonal antibodies radiolabeled with iodine-131, indium-111, and technetium-99 m for SPECT and iodine-124, ittrium-86, bromine-76, and zirconium-89 for PET imaging.

These PET studies demonstrated which metastases from HER2-positive primitive tumor are likely to respond to treatment, but also that even HER2-negative breast tumors can produce unsuspected HER2+ metastases (Ulaner et al. 2016).

Radiation therapy is receiving major benefits from imaging techniques: the incorporation of MR imaging along with CT has improved the target delineation by assessing with great precision soft tissues. PET imaging is also consolidating its role in optimizing treatment protocols. Data gathered by monitoring or restaging PET can be used to adjust the target volume in a careful re-treatment planning. Patient selection, volume selection, delineation, and isodose distribution can therefore be reprogrammed. Response assessment can then be visualized as a decreased area of PET uptake. Moreover, by acquiring simultaneous DCE-MR imaging and [^{18}F]FDG-PET imaging, a correlation between dynamic changes of tracer uptake and tumor perfusion dynamics has been proposed. The incorporation of DCE-MR imaging into the PET tracer kinetic

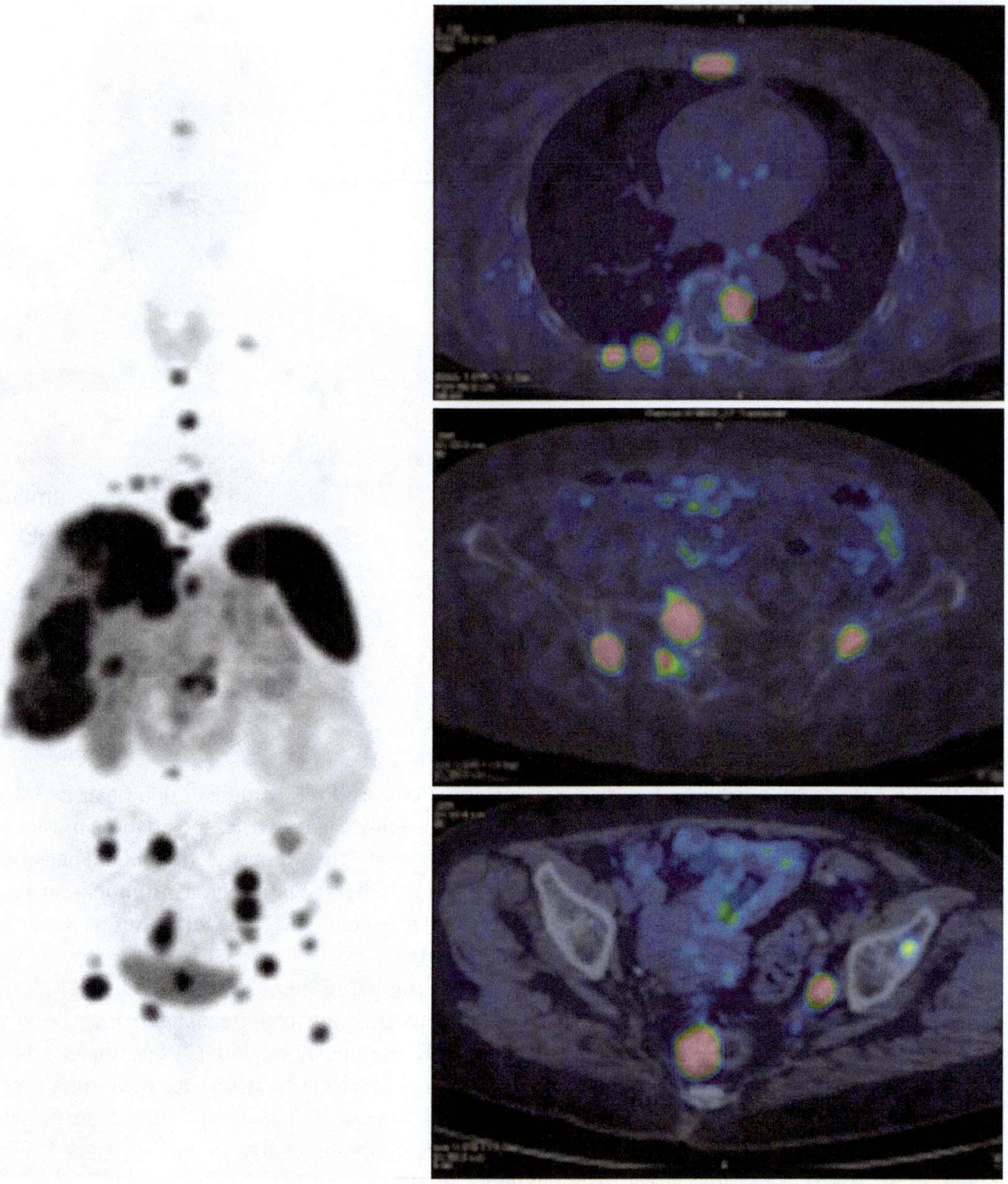

Fig. 3 Neuroendocrine tumor of the rectum. Progression of disease after multiple treatments: evaluation for peptide receptor therapy eligibility. Pre-therapy ^{68}Ga-DOTA-TOC PET/CT shows high uptake of primary tumor and multiple metastases (the liver, bones, lymph nodes). Courtesy of Dr. Annibale Versari, IRCCS Arcispedale Santa Maria Nuova, Reggio Emilia, Italy

model represents a further step in the evolution of PET imaging (Citrin 2017).

PET scanners and functional MRI sequences are just two of the diagnostic tools used in medical imaging to provide diagnosis, prognosis, and guide treatment. In the era of big data, texture analysis and radiomics can give a critical contribution to stratify patients and provide predictive data about treatment response. In particular, texture features can differentiate between adenocarcinoma and squamous cellular carcinoma, not only aiding the diagnostic process but

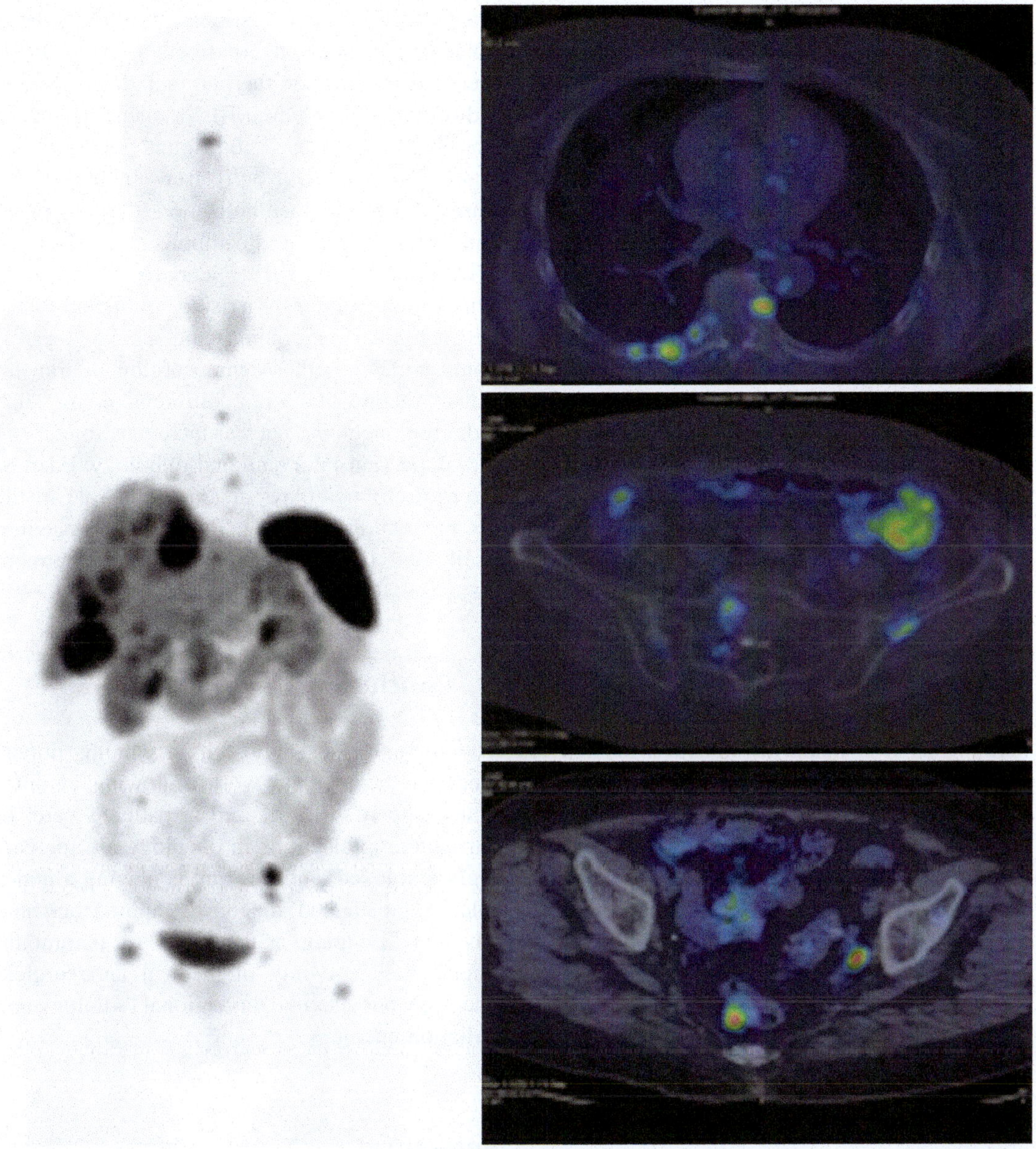

Fig. 4 Neuroendocrine tumor of the rectum. The patient entered a clinical trial and was treated with six cycles of 177Lu/90Y-DOTA-TOC. Post-therapy 68Ga-DOTA-TOC PET/CT reveals partial response to treatment. Courtesy of Dr. Annibale Versari, IRCCS Arcispedale Santa Maria Nuova, Reggio Emilia, Italy

also helping to differentiate malignant and benign pulmonary nodules through the analysis of the heterogeneity of the radiological appearance in CT imaging. Intra-tumor heterogeneity also appeared to be a strong independent outcome predictor after radiotherapy. Radiomics is expected to play a major role even in predicting treatment success, as shown in cervical and NSCL cancers (Gillies et al. 2016).

After validating the radiomic approach (Park et al. 2019), efforts in pairing radiomics with genomics have been carried out, with promising results (Pinker et al. 2017; Bodalal et al. 2019).

Finally, hybrid imaging provides synergistic data from different modalities, representing a concrete proof of shared efforts from nuclear medicine and radiology by pulling together the molecular sensitivity of nuclear imaging with the anatomic specificity of the morphologic imaging modalities, CT and T1w-T2w-MRI sequences. After the introduction of PET/CT and SPECT/CT in the early 2000s, PET/RM has increasingly been introduced in research centers and clinical institutes thanks to the advent of solid-state PET detectors compatible with MRI's strong magnetic fields (Bailey et al. 2017).

4 Interventional Radiology in Oncology

Another point that deserves particular attention is the raising importance earned by interventional radiology (IR) in oncologic patient care. Interventional radiology can be the element that closes the theragnostics circle by calling the same radiologists who made the diagnosis to deliver therapy (Abi-Jaoudeh et al. 2013). IR's main contribution to personalized medicine currently consists in tissue procurement. This delicate operation can be superbly guided with the optimal deployment of the entire imaging apparatus available in the imaging department. In fact, new techniques to perform high-precision biopsy are daily practice in most centers. Hybrid imaging represents one of these valuable tools for interventional radiologists. It's becoming more and more popular that PET/CT hybrid systems, when conventional radiologic investigations cannot identify pathologic findings, are used first to characterize the lesion, then to serve as a guiding tool to perform percutaneous biopsy right in the area of increased PET activity, and finally to assess the success of the procedure (Imperiale et al. 2015; Mauri et al. 2019). Image-guided biopsy can play an interesting role not just in the diagnosis but also in the monitoring of drug therapy. Serial biopsies before and after drug therapy have been performed during vandetanib chemotherapy targeting fEGFR, VEGFR2, and RET in cases of ovarian cancers. In addition to biopsy, interventional radiologists can perform a wide range of procedures to contribute to cancer treatment: percutaneous thermal ablations include radiofrequency ablation (RFA), microwave ablation (MWA), focused ultrasound (fUS), cryogenic ablation (CA) and laser ablation (LA), transarterial chemoembolization (TACE)/DEB, and transarterial radioembolization (TARE) (Filippiadis et al. 2019; Gennaro et al. 2019). This last one represents a rising option mainly for hepatocellular carcinoma and cholangiocarcinoma and is another demonstration of translational therapy between different areas such radiation oncology, nuclear medicine, diagnostic radiology, and interventional radiology. Each of these disciplines plays an important role in the pre-procedural planning, during the procedure itself, and in the assessment of the treatment response (Tong et al. 2016).

5 Conclusions

The theragnostics approach is gaining importance in the medical world, allowing an integrated approach to be used in patient's care. In particular, applications in oncology are increasingly employed, and imaging is playing a major role. Sophisticated diagnostic approaches and advanced imaging analysis are of paramount importance, not only in medical and surgical oncology but also in interventional radiology and radiation oncology.

References

Abi-Jaoudeh N, Duffy AG, Greten TF et al (2013) Personalized oncology in interventional radiology. J Vasc Interv Radiol 24:1083–1092. https://doi.org/10.1016/j.jvir.2013.04.019

Bailey DL, Pichler BJ, Gückel B, Antoch G, Barthel H, Bhujwalla ZM, Biskup S, Biswal S, Bitzer M, Boellaard R, Braren RF, Brendle C, Brindle K, Chiti A, la Fougère C, Gillies R, Goh V, Goyen M, Hacker M, Heukamp L, Knudsen GM, Krackhardt AM, Law I, Morris JC, Nikolaou K, Nuyts J, Ordonez AA, Pantel K, Quick HH, Riklund K, Sabri O, Sattler B, Troost EGC, Zaiss M, Zender L, Beyer T (2017) Combined PET/MRI: Global Warming-Summary Report of the

6th International Workshop on PET/MRI, March 27–29, 2017, Tübingen, Germany. Mol Imaging Biol. https://doi.org/10.1007/s11307-017-1123-5
Bodalal Z, Trebeschi S, Nguyen-Kim TDL, Schats W, Beets-Tan R (2019) Radiogenomics: bridging imaging and genomics. Abdom Radiol 44(6):1960–1984
Citrin DE (2017) Recent developments in radiotherapy. N Engl J Med 377(11):1065–1075. https://doi.org/10.1056/NEJMra1608986
Filippiadis D, Mauri G, Marra P, Charalampopoulos G, Gennaro N, De Cobelli F (2019) Percutaneous ablation techniques for renal cell carcinoma: current status and future trends. Int J Hyperther 36(2):21–30
Gennaro N, Mauri G, Varano GM, Monfardini L, Pedicini V, Poretti D, Solbiati LA (2019) Thermal ablations for colorectal liver metastases. Digest Dis Intervent 03(02):117–125
Gillies RJ, Kinahan PE, Radiomics HH (2016) Images are more than pictures, they are data. Radiology 278(2):563–577. https://doi.org/10.1148/radiol.2015151169. Epub 2015 Nov 18
Guimaraes MD, Schuch A, Hochhegger B, Gross JL, Chojniak R, Marchiori E (2014) Functional magnetic resonance imaging in oncology: state of the art. Radiol Bras 47(2):101–111
Higgins LJ, Pomper MG (2011) The evolution of imaging in cancer: current state and future challenges. Semin Oncol 38:3–15. https://doi.org/10.1053/j.seminoncol.2010.11.010
Imperiale A, Garnon J, Bachellier P et al (2015) Simultaneous (18)F-FDOPA PET/CT-guided biopsy and radiofrequency ablation of recurrent neuroendocrine hepatic metastasis: further step toward a theranostic approach. Clin Nucl Med 40:e334–e335. https://doi.org/10.1097/RLU.0000000000000765
Jauw YW, Menke-van der Houven van Oordt CW, Hoekstra OS, Hendrikse NH, Vugts DJ, Zijlstra JM, Huisman MC, van Dongen GA (2016) Immuno-positron emission tomography with Zirconium-89-Labeled monoclonal antibodies in oncology: what can we learn from initial clinical trials? Front Pharmacol 7:131. https://doi.org/10.3389/fphar.2016.00131
Koh D-M, Lee J-M, Bittencourt LK et al (2016) Body diffusion-weighted MR imaging in oncology: imaging at 3 T. Magn Reson Imaging Clin N Am 24:31–44. https://doi.org/10.1016/j.mric.2015.08.007
Kratochwil C, Bruchertseifer F, Giesel FL et al (2016) 225Ac-PSMA-617 for PSMA-targeted α-radiation therapy of metastatic castration-resistant prostate cancer. J Nucl Med 57:1941–1944. https://doi.org/10.2967/jnumed.116.178673
Mauri G, Gennaro N, De Beni S, Ierace T, Goldberg SN, Rodari M, Solbiati LA (2019) Real-time US-^{18}FDG-PET/CT Image fusion for guidance of thermal ablation of ^{18}FDG-PET-positive liver metastases: the added value of contrast enhancement. Cardiovasc Intervent Radiol 42(1):60–68
Park JE, Park SY, Kim HJ, Kim HS (2019) Reproducibility and generalizability in radiomics modeling: possible strategies in radiologic and statistical perspectives. Korean J Radiol 20(7):1124
Pinker K, Shitano F, Sala E, Do RK, Young RJ, Wibmer AG, Hricak H, Sutton EJ, Morris EA (2017) Background, current role, and potential applications of radiogenomics. J Magn Reson Imaging. https://doi.org/10.1002/jmri.25870
Rosenkrantz AB, Friedman K, Chandarana H et al (2016) Current status of hybrid PET/MRI in oncologic imaging. AJR Am J Roentgenol 206:162–172. https://doi.org/10.2214/AJR.15.14968
Sai KKS, Zachar Z, Bingham PM, Mintz A (2017) Metabolic PET imaging in oncology. AJR Am J Roentgenol 209(2):270–276. https://doi.org/10.2214/AJR.17.18112. Epub 2017 May 2. Review
Tong AK, Kao YH, Too CW, Chin KF, Ng DC, Chow PK (2016) Yttrium-90 hepatic radioembolization: clinical review and current techniques in interventional radiology and personalized dosimetry. Br J Radiol 89(1062):20150943. https://doi.org/10.1259/bjr.20150943. https://www.ncbi.nlm.nih.gov/pmc/articles/PMC5258157/.
Ulaner GA, Hyman DM, Ross DS et al (2016) Detection of HER2-positive metastases in patients with HER2-negative primary breast cancer using 89Zr-Trastuzumab PET/CT. J Nucl Med 57:1523–1528. https://doi.org/10.2967/jnumed.115.172031
Wahl RL, Jacene H, Kasamon Y, Lodge MA (2009) From RECIST to PERCIST: evolving considerations for PET response criteria in solid tumors. J Nucl Med 50(Suppl 1):122S–150S. https://doi.org/10.2967/jnumed.108.057307

The Role of a Radiologist and Nuclear Medicine Physician in a Multidisciplinary Tumour Board

Cristina Grippo, Maria Cristina Cortese, and Riccardo Manfredi

Contents

1 **Multidisciplinary Tumour Board: How It Improves the Quality of Cancer Care** 13

2 **Why Should Radiologists and Nuclear Medicine Physicians Reserve a Seat on an MTB?** 16

2.1 Diagnosis 16

2.2 Tissue Biopsy 17

2.3 Staging 18

2.4 Response Evaluation 19

2.5 Posttreatment Surveillance 19

3 **Examples of Tumours Whose Course Is Significantly Modified by MTB** 19

3.1 Breast Cancer 19

3.2 Lung Cancer 22

3.3 Head and Neck Cancer 22

References 23

Abstract

Multidisciplinary Tumour Boards (MTBs) are nowadays integral part of comprehensive oncological care provision in order to improve diagnostic accuracy, adherence to clinical practice guidelines, and some clinical outcomes.

These meetings typically involve core groups of medical oncologists, radiation oncologists, surgeons, radiologists, nuclear medicine and pathologists, as well as other healthcare professionals. MTBs are an opportunity for radiologists to demonstrate their value to referring clinicians, the hospital, and patients. The role of physicians dedicated to diagnostic imaging is vital to ensure patient quality and safety in each of these steps: diagnosis, tissue biopsy, staging/preoperative planning, response evaluation and posttreatment surveillance. Personalised medicine in oncology care is a trend that requires an immense amount of knowledge and MTBs are the working environment to gather all particular subspecialty skills.

1 Multidisciplinary Tumour Board: How It Improves the Quality of Cancer Care

During the past three decades, multidisciplinary clinics (MDCs) have played an increasingly prominent role in the care of patients with cancer in both the community and in academic cancer

C. Grippo (✉) · M. C. Cortese · R. Manfredi
Dipartimento di Diagnostica per Immagini, Radioterapia Oncologica ed Ematologia, Istituto di Radiologia, Fondazione Policlinico Universitario "A. Gemelli"—IRCCS, Università Cattolica del Sacro Cuore, Rome, Italy
e-mail: c.grippo@idi.it; riccardo.manfredi@unicatt.it

R. G. H. Beets-Tan et al. (eds.), *Imaging and Interventional Radiology for Radiation Oncology*, Medical Radiology, Diagnostic Imaging, https://doi.org/10.1007/978-3-030-38261-2_2

centres. Their development has been promoted in healthcare management literature and by the National Cancer Institute. Intuitively, a multidisciplinary approach provides a rational and coordinated mechanism for evaluation and treatment of patients with complex diseases by bringing healthcare providers in the surgical, medical and radiation oncology disciplines together (Bunnell et al. 2010). Multidisciplinary Tumour Boards (MTBs) are a direct extension of the multidisciplinary care model: quite simply, it can be defined as a regularly scheduled formal meeting between physicians who manage cancer patients; the goal is to expedite patient care and ensure that the highest level of care is maintained (Lesslie and Parikh 2017). Such meetings are considered integral part of comprehensive oncological care provision, since nowadays the fact that cancer patient management is not a single person's job is undeniable (Abdulrahman Jr 2011).

The US National Guideline Clearinghouse lists over 2700 clinical practice guidelines, and more than 25,000 new clinical trials are published each year. It is not only difficult for one person to absorb this amount of information, but it is potentially harmful to treat patients without the adequate amount of knowledge. For this reason, care teams have been created for cancer care as well as other aspects of medicine (Keating et al. 2013).

Moreover, a large number of genetic mutations are being identified for each cancer type that change the cancer's susceptibility or response to current therapeutics. Examples include oestrogen receptor or HER2-positive breast cancer (BC), non-small cell lung cancer (NSCLC) with epidermal growth factor (EGF)-activating mutations, colorectal cancer with KRAS mutations and malignant gliomas with hyper-methylation of the methyl guanine methyl transferase (MGMT) gene. This rapidly growing field of knowledge in tumour biology and patient pharmacokinetics will change the paradigms of treatment for individual cancer patients. It will be even more important going forward that physicians work together as part of teams to reconcile this growing fund of knowledge to offer the best and most effective treatment to their patients.

MTBs generally consist of oncologists, surgeons, pathologists, diagnostic radiologists, interventional radiologists and radiation oncologists. Each of these specialists adds knowledge from their specialty-specific literature to come to a consensus management on a patient-specific basis (Hoffman et al. 1997).

Generally, MTBs meet weekly for 60–90 min, depending on how many cases physicians bring to the table. Cases are presented for a number of reasons. An MTB may want to see results of patients who have undergone treatment, to assess what worked and what did not. Other times, the purpose is to seek colleagues' opinions on how to proceed with a case. Sometimes, other members of the MTB may endorse what you say, so you have more ammunition to go back to the patient with 'This is what the group thought'.

All types of cases are discussed: previously untreated 'new' cancer cases; recurrent cancer cases; cases suspicious for cancer, in need of further diagnostic steps; cases treated surgically, for pathologic review to determine the need for postoperative adjuvant therapy; and cases treated nonsurgically, to determine the type of response and need for other intervention. If the decision-making is not straightforward, patients appreciate that all the heads are in the room at the same time. The emphasis is placed on confirming that all the pertinent data accrued in the patient evaluation are known to the physicians involved in the patient's care (Adam and Kenny 2015).

According to the relevance of the cancer institute, it is possible to find MTBs specialising in hepatobiliary, colorectal, pancreatic, lung and musculoskeletal malignancies that are attended by subspecialised interventional radiologists, oncologists, pathologists, surgeons, radiation oncologists and diagnostic radiologists. All of the members of the care team are encouraged to submit patients for discussion in advance. The physician who submitted the case typically presents a brief history and course of treatment for each patient followed by a discussion of the patient's imaging by the diagnostic radiologist.

Following identification of findings, a plan of care is determined by the team directing the patient to the appropriate member of the team for that management (Lesslie and Parikh 2017). Medical and radiation oncologists, pathologist, oncological surgeons, radiologist and nuclear physicians are the integral part of the MTB: they meet regularly to weigh in on complex cancer cases and recommend treatment plans for patients. The board helps determine the type of tumour, the extent of disease, the risk for progression and a recommended course of treatment (Abdulrahman Jr 2011).

The pathologist-radiologist correlation helps in better tumour staging, whereas surgeon-oncologist correlation results in improved treatment plan. With the advent of hybrid imaging like positron emission tomography (PET)-computed tomography (CT) and PET-MR, the role of imaging has considerably increased. In fact, these hybrid imaging are considered as standard of care in management of many tumour like lymphoma. Hybrid imaging undeniably contributes in staging, restaging, response evaluation, prognostication and early detection of tumour recurrence. It is a known fact that based on findings of hybrid imaging, down- or upstaging in tumour has been observed in a sizeable portion of patients, which indeed helps to modify the treatment strategies accordingly. Their role has also become more important in response evaluation due to introduction of many tumouristatic therapies where metabolic response is the harbinger of response as compared to tumouricidal treatment where a change in anatomic size is the response evaluation parameter. Physicians involved in diagnostic imaging now also have better liaison with radiation oncologists by providing information about metabolic tumour volume and image-guided radiation therapy (IGRT). A large body of data have concluded that these meetings significantly contribute to the better treatment outcomes for patients. Obviously, we must be aware of the fact that success of such meetings is integrated with sincere and invaluable participation from all stakeholders (Adam and Kenny 2015).

Undeniably, nowadays, the interventional radiology plays an important role in the management of many malignancies, such as the hepatocellular carcinoma, where it offers many chances in cases not suitable for surgery. Other examples of how the interventional oncologist is an important member of the care team include the growing utility of ablation in patients with primary and metastatic lung malignancy as well as ablation of bone tumours for palliation of pain.

Patients who benefit most from multidisciplinary decision-making are patients who do not have a clear option for treatment based on marginal indication for surgery, poor theoretical success of systemic therapies and potential treatment with unproven therapeutic options. Minimally invasive therapies by interventional radiology frequently arise in these situations, and it is important that interventional radiology be a part of this team to explain how interventional oncology techniques complement traditional medical, radiation and surgical options. As cancer's therapeutic options continue to change, interventional radiology will be central in both the diagnostic and therapeutic aspects of targeted and personalised therapy (Urbański 2012).

Along with significant benefits to patients, collaboration on MTBs also helps develop relationships among physicians. When perceived as part of a multidisciplinary team, for example, interventional radiologists are more likely to receive patient referrals from medical, surgical and radiation oncologists.

To summarise, MTBs play a very important role in defining a better treatment of the cancer patients in many cases.

In addition, other fundamental goals achievable by the MTBs are as follows:

- Aggregating all pertinent diagnostic material regarding individual cases to permit review.
- Assigning a recommended management plan and offering reasonable alternatives.
- Assigning definitive staging; creating an interactive environment to foster communication between specialties.
- Teaching to the participating staff, fellow and resident physicians.
- Providing a forum whereby second opinions are routinely offered.
- Developing a detailed database.

All of this is possible because members from different specialties augment each other's interpretations. Discussing increased number of cases with more attendance improves the outcome of these meetings. In the current era, the role of radiologists and nuclear physicians has considerably increased due to availability of hybrid imaging like PET-CT and PET-MR. It is therefore recommended that all tumour cases be discussed in MTBs regardless of site, staging and grading. It will also play a beneficial role in improving academics and research work.

2 Why Should Radiologists and Nuclear Medicine Physicians Reserve a Seat on an MTB?

MTB is a growing area of physician collaboration designed to allow for evidence-based and patient-centred management in specialised cases. Working as part of a multidisciplinary team to plan patient care is part of the larger movement towards personalised medicine in which radiologists and nuclear medicine physicians should play a critical role (Knechtges and Carlos 2007).

In the last two decades, many physicians involved in diagnostic imaging were satisfied with and well compensated for their work producing high volumes of radiology reports in quiet, dark reading rooms. That outdated paradigm of the fee-for-service model of reimbursement resulted in limited interaction with patients, referring clinicians and administrators. Radiologists traditionally could be described as image interpreters who thrived in the model that rewarded radiologists based on volume. However, the eventual fragmentation of imaging services and the advent of teleradiology led to radiologists becoming almost invisible. A new age of medicine has evolved as radiology moves from a fee-for-service model centred on volume to a patient-centric, value-based model. This cultural transformation demands that radiologists expand their role in the healthcare system to that of expert diagnostic imaging consultants. Instead of focusing on volume, value is prioritised, which is essentially determined by referring healthcare providers and patients as consumers (Kherlopian et al. 2008).

So how do radiologists and nuclear medicine physicians step away from the reading room and demonstrate their value as members of the healthcare team in this new era of healthcare? One answer is by actively participating in MTBs.

Patients discussed in these meetings predominantly have newly diagnosed cancer but also may include patients with complex management questions, such as discordance in biopsy results, restaging after neoadjuvant therapy or suspected recurrence.

The role of physicians dedicated to diagnostic imaging is vital to ensure patient quality and safety in each of these steps:

- Diagnosis.
- Tissue biopsy.
- Staging/preoperative planning.
- Response evaluation.
- Posttreatment surveillance.

2.1 Diagnosis

There are various ways to detect cancer using imaging methods. Cancer may be detected incidentally, when an examination is carried out for other reasons, or there may be clear symptoms and the patient may undergo imaging to confirm, locate and determine the extent of the disease. In any of these cases, imaging plays a major role in cancer care. Nowadays, imaging is not only defining the abnormal anatomy of pathologic conditions but also about providing detailed information about structural or cancer-related changes. Emerging methods of molecular imaging, which combine traditional imaging technology and nuclear medicine techniques, can also be used to obtain more detailed information about abnormalities, including their distinct metabolism. Molecular imaging differs from traditional imaging because take advantage of biomarker probes to target specific areas or suspicious findings (Wallace 2014). One of the most promising molecular imaging techniques is positron emission tomography (PET), which is most often combined with CT (PET-CT) and used to track probes in order to detect metastatic disease. When it comes to the characterisation of a finding or the differentiation between a malignant or benign abnormality, it is sometimes difficult to reach a final diagnosis (Fig. 1).

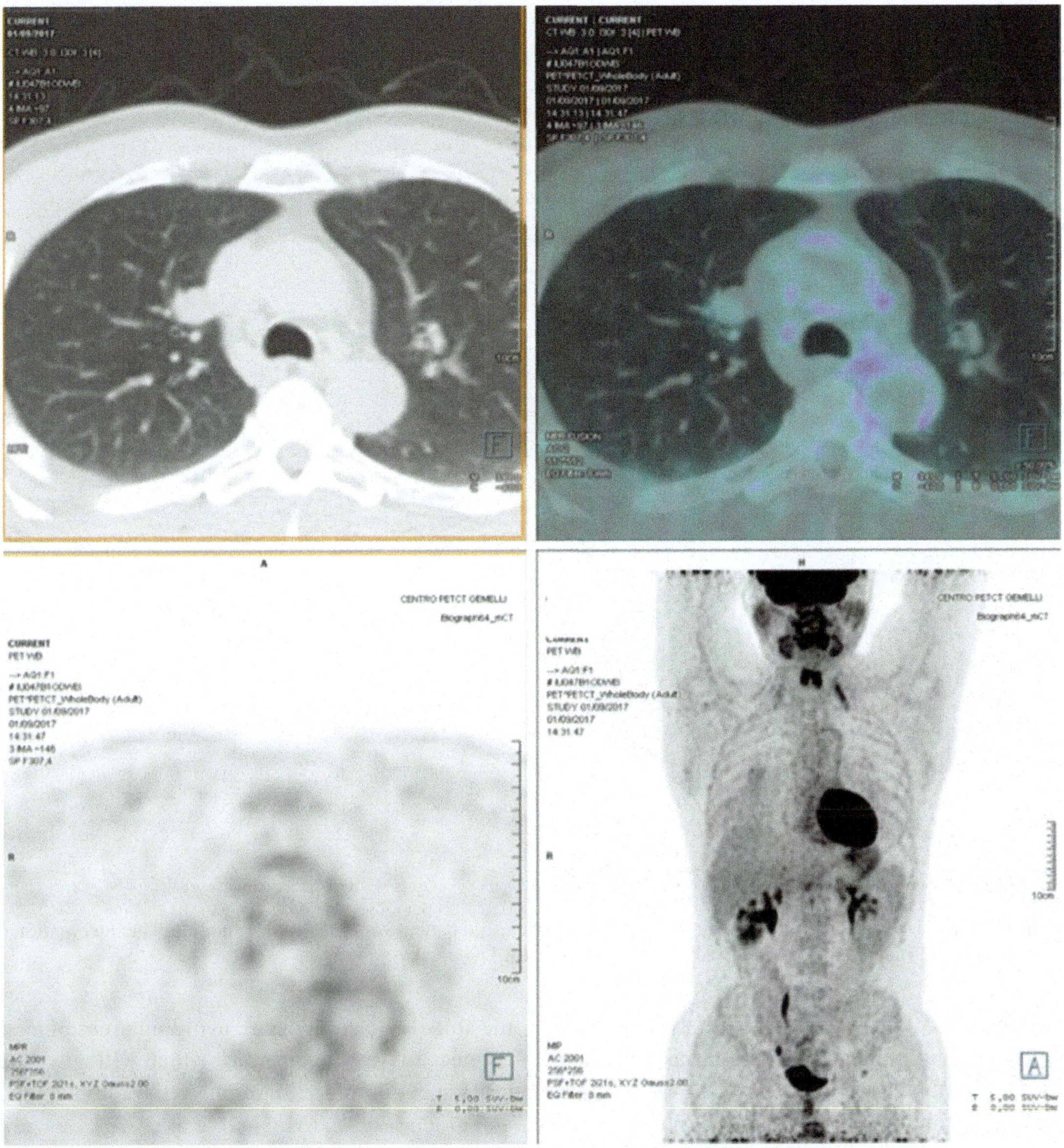

Fig. 1 PET-CT of a 72-year-old patient with a suspect pulmonary nodule detected at chest X-ray. The absence of [^{18}F] FDG uptake, matched with the presence of intralesional fat, confirmed the diagnosis of pulmonary hamartoma

To avoid unnecessary invasive procedures and save the patient further discomfort, a comparison of various images, often obtained through different methods, is the first step towards a final diagnosis. If a definite diagnosis still cannot be made, imaging techniques could be used to perform a biopsy, where small parts of the abnormality are collected for tissue examination.

2.2 Tissue Biopsy

A preoperative tissue diagnosis is often essential to determine treatment. Nowadays, imaging-guided biopsies are performed in several different ways in any part of the body. Tissue samples can be obtained by placing a needle through the skin (percutaneously) into the area of

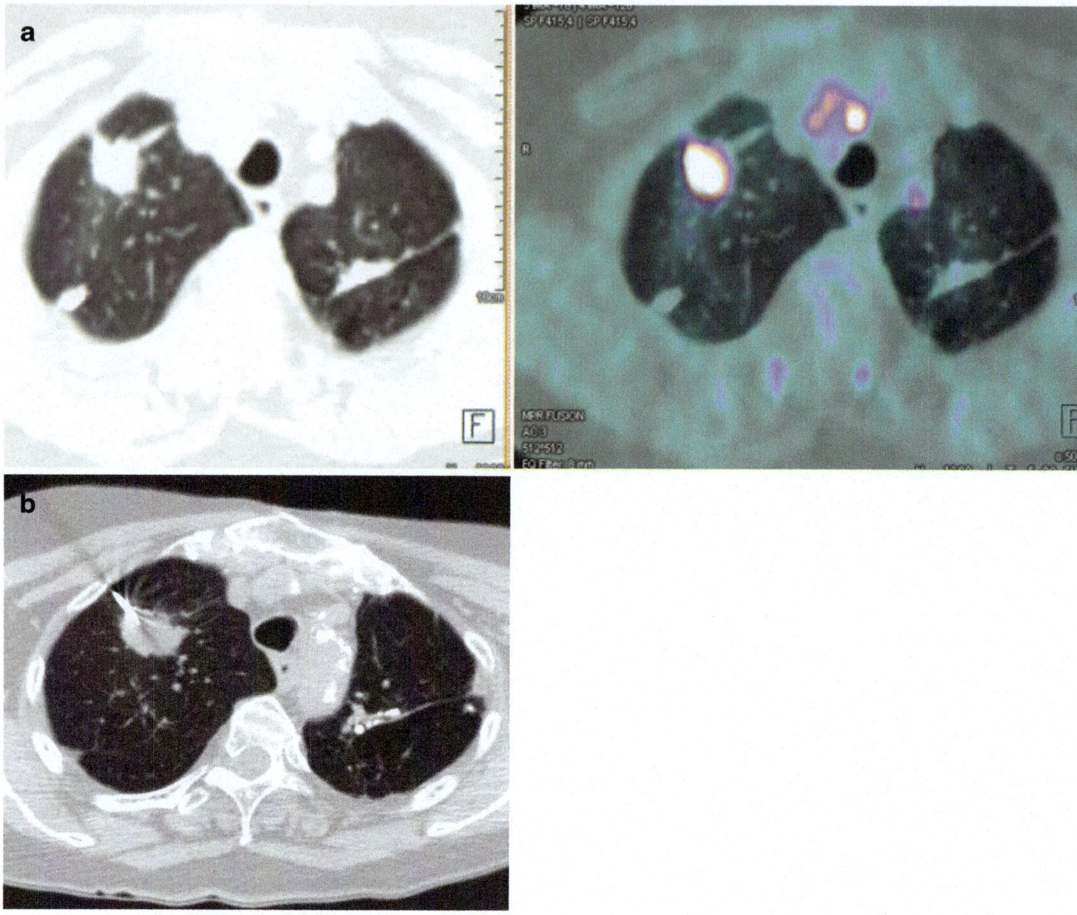

Fig. 2 PET-CT (**a**) and CT-guided lung biopsy (**b**) of a 65-year-old patient with a pulmonary nodule. The interventional radiology performed the biopsy in the area of maximum [^{18}F]FDG uptake

abnormality. Biopsies can be safely performed with imaging guidance such as ultrasound (US), X-ray, computed tomography (CT), or magnetic resonance imaging (MRI). Imaging-guided, minimally invasive procedures, such as needle biopsies, are most often performed by a specially trained radiologist, an interventional radiologist or a neuro-radiologist. Compared to open and closed surgical biopsies, needle biopsy is less invasive and expensive (Wu et al. 2008). Careful biopsy planning is critical to the success of the procedures. MTBs are the most suitable circumstances to allow for high diagnostic yield, by discussing together. Radiologists, together with surgical oncologists, carefully review preoperative imaging and selectively target the most aggressive-appearing portion of the lesion (e.g., the soft-tissue component, avoiding areas of cystic necrosis or degeneration) that will give the most accurate representation of the tumour type and grade (Fig. 2) (Mitchell et al. 2013).

2.3 Staging

As the previously explained, radiology provides vital tools for detecting and characterising tumours, but it is also extremely useful in taking the next step. Once a histologic diagnosis is made, imaging is the key diagnostic tool used to stage the cancer, which is to determine exactly where the primary tumour is located and how far the cancer has spread. For some tumours, imaging findings are still supplemented by findings from surgery, but with the continuous advancement of cross-sectional imaging and the development of molecular imaging, staging laparotomy is becoming obsolete.

Accurate staging is essential in order to select the appropriate treatment. Imaging is by far the most effective method to accurately stage cancer, and this is where the radiologist's skill, and experience of medical images, plays a very important part. Thus, by staging cancer, radiologists and other imaging specialists significantly influence cancer care.

The radiologist's expert analysis will be an integral factor in the decision about the course of action to be taken, but the decisions are usually made by a multidisciplinary team, responsible for the management of each cancer patient. Images obtained in the examinations will be presented and commented on by the radiologist, before being discussed by the team, usually including oncologists and pathologists. Frequently, new questions may be raised, due to new events or biological findings, and very commonly, the radiologist will return to previous examinations with the same or another imaging tool, in order to characterise images or to ensure that nothing was missed (Disselhorst et al. 2014).

2.4 Response Evaluation

Once cancer has been localised and staged, doctors can proceed with treatment. Here, as in every stage of oncologic care, imaging is of fundamental importance. Imaging techniques can be used to monitor therapy, which allows doctors to gauge the success of the therapeutic plan from the beginning. Being able to check the effectiveness of a treatment early on means a change in course can be made as soon as it becomes necessary, which is crucial and time-saving. Conventional imaging, such as X-ray, US, CT and MRI, utilise measurements to assess response or progression. The role of hybrid imaging techniques (like PET-CT or PET-MR) has also become more important in response evaluation due to introduction of many tumouristatic therapies where metabolic response is the harbinger of response as compared to tumouricidal treatment where a change in anatomic size is the response evaluation parameter (Falcon et al. 2017).

2.5 Posttreatment Surveillance

Medical imaging is vitally important to monitoring therapy response and follow-up care of cancer patients. The radiologist is responsible for interpreting the images acquired through a range of techniques and then communicating their analysis to the patient's physician. This means the radiologist needs to understand more than just images; they must be familiar with oncologic medicine in order to distinguish the appearance of cancer from other diseases or anomalies. Given the radiologist's knowledge and experience of the imaging features of cancer and its recurrence, they are often the first to spot the early signs of cancer recurrence, making their role pivotal to the effectiveness of follow-up care (Fig. 3).

Again, as is the case of earlier stages of cancer care, the radiologist operates as part of a medical team to give patients the best follow-up care and to ensure prompt detection of any possible complications or recurrence. The radiologist works behind the scenes to provide treating physicians with indispensable information, helping them to make crucial decisions on further treatment or tests.

3 Examples of Tumours Whose Course Is Significantly Modified by MTB

The following paragraphs will provide peculiar aspects of some cancer types MTB; these, in addition to the others described until now, can significantly modify their course.

3.1 Breast Cancer

In a breast cancer (BC) MTB, first of all, the radiologist has the opportunity to inform and

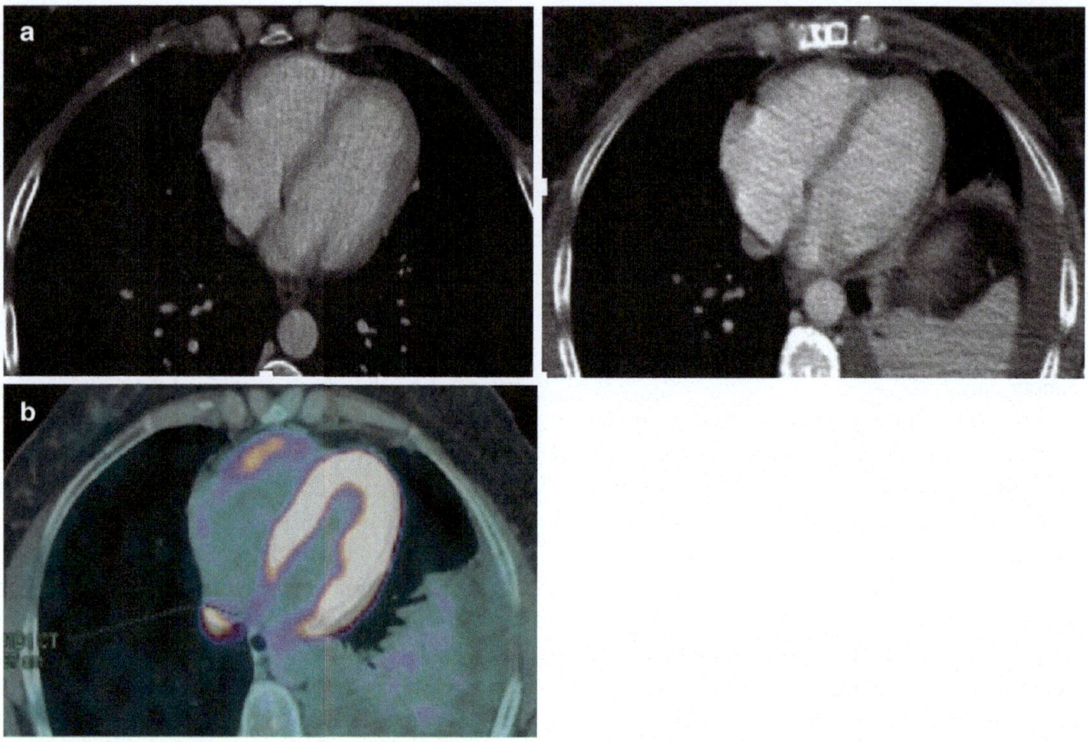

Fig. 3 Follow-up CT scans (**a**) of a 45-year-old patient who underwent thymectomy for thymic carcinoma revealed small pleural thickening progressively increasing. PET-CT (**b**) showed increased [^{18}F]FDG uptake of the pleural thickening, confirming the suspect of recurrence

educate members of other disciplines about relevant data regarding screening mammography, including data from randomised control trials demonstrating reduced mortality rates with screening, scientific analyses demonstrating the maximum number of lives saved owing to annual screening, statistics demonstrating that skipping a mammogram every other year would miss up to 30% of cancers and studies revealing reduced treatment morbidity with screening (Wu et al. 2008).

In MTBs, radiologists can also help advocate for capital investment that can enhance patient care: for example, the use of three-dimensional digital breast tomosynthesis in the community radiology setting has resulted in a reduction in screening recall rates combined with a higher cancer detection rate when compared to two-dimensional digital mammography alone; therefore, a radiologist can advocate for the use of three-dimensional digital breast tomosynthesis by informing clinicians of its proven benefits in the captured audience in an MTB in a community hospital, and the multidisciplinary team can support and help advocate for the purchase of this equipment by a community hospital.

Radiologists can take a number of proactive steps to reduce the cost and waste associated with unnecessary imaging studies and procedures.

The common goals are the optimisation of the length of time from BC screening to diagnosis (achievable by decreasing the time from the diagnosis of breast cancer to surgery), the improvement of the rate of breast-conserving surgery and the decrease of pathologic core biopsy turnaround time.

In MTBs, the radiologist can directly assist in the selection of the best diagnostic imaging examination based on a cancer patient's unique clinical circumstances in accordance with the ACR Appropriateness Criteria. Additional imaging procedures that may not alter staging or treatment may result in unnecessary radiation exposure, expense and anxiety for the patient. Radiologists are direct advocates for their patients by assisting in the selection of appropriate imaging studies in the setting of shared decision-making with other consulting physicians. For example, performance of a routine radionuclide bone scan to evaluate osseous metastatic disease is not useful for patients with stage I BC owing to its low yield and lack of proven benefit regarding disease management and survival (Lesslie and Parikh 2017). Furthermore, in MTBs, radiologists can demonstrate value by advocating for appropriate biopsies for cancer patients. For example, core needle biopsy not only is an acceptable alternative to surgical excisional biopsy but also is now considered the optimal method of tissue acquisition for image-detected breast abnormalities, even because of its several advantages over surgical excisional biopsy (lower cost, lower complication rates and less cosmetic deformity). Multidisciplinary breast centres can achieve a higher rate of cancer diagnosis using percutaneous core biopsy than open surgical biopsy. By advocating for the appropriate type of biopsy, radiologists demonstrate commitment to cost-effective, high-value cancer care (Feigenberg et al. 2012).

In some institutions, patients are seen on the same day in the multidisciplinary clinic held immediately after the conference by the three primary cancer specialists (surgical oncology, medical oncology and radiation oncology). The preliminary work-up and treatment recommendations are then made the same day; the benefit of seeing newly diagnosed breast cancer patients on the same day of the MTB is that the team can rapidly implement recommendations for further work-up if deemed necessary. In addition, the benefit to the patients is that they are seen by the three primary cancer specialists on 1 day and do not have to make several trips to be re-evaluated. Often, patients are not aware that the management of breast cancer may require treatments after surgery with radiation to the breast, hormonal therapy and/or chemotherapy. These basic concepts of management of early-stage breast cancer can also be introduced to the patients during their first visit to the multidisciplinary clinic (Margenthaler et al. 2006).

Radiologists can assist in accurately staging breast cancer. Additional suspicious radiological findings may be found, potentially revealing additional sites of disease. Imaging findings that may alter breast cancer staging, prognosis or treatment include tumour size, tumour number, total span of the disease, regional lymph node status (such as axillary, internal mammary or infraclavicular involvement), loco-regional spread (involvement of the chest wall, skin or nipple) and presence of distant metastasis.

Radiological findings are increasingly integrated into clinical staging, which helps in choosing between breast conservation surgery and mastectomy and between sentinel lymph node biopsy (SLNB) and axillary lymph node dissection, as well as in determining the need for adjuvant chemotherapy or radiation therapy. A study at the University of Michigan in 2006 demonstrated that MTBs changed the BC diagnosis in 45% of cases and changed the surgical management in 11% of them. In addition, a team from the University of Pennsylvania found that MTBs at their institutions changed the treatment of BC for 43% of referred patients. Open communication between radiologists and pathologists in an MTB can assist in the evaluation of imaging and histologic correlations in percutaneous image-guided breast biopsy results. Discordance between imaging and histologic findings indicates that a lesion submitted to biopsy analysis may not have been adequately sampled. Such discordance is an indication for repeat biopsy or surgical excision to potentially reduce any delays in breast cancer diagnosis. Conversely, concordance between histology and percutaneous image-guided core biopsy results for patients with benign or high-risk benign breast lesions can reduce the number of unnecessary excisional biopsies (Gagan and Van Allen 2015).

Furthermore, personalised medicine in oncology care is a trend that requires an immense amount of knowledge about the cancers being treated that can only be attained by specialists in that particular subspecialty. A large number of genetic mutations are being identified for each cancer type that change the cancer's susceptibility or response to current therapeutics. Examples include oestrogen receptor or HER2-positive breast cancer (Lesslie and Parikh 2017).

In an MTB, the interdisciplinary team can perform a root cause analysis in such cases and determine subsequent management, including an immediate postoperative mammogram.

3.2 Lung Cancer

In the case of lung cancer (LC), as in so many other tumours, a common type of case under discussion may involve stage 3: team members would assess whether the tumour responded to chemotherapy and radiation therapy and has become operable or determine if the patient would be an appropriate candidate for clinical trials (Feigenberg et al. 2012).

Another field of application that makes the MTB protagonist is the one in which it is necessary to illuminate concern of false positive results caused by radiation pneumonitis (AL-Jahdali et al. 2012).

As a matter of fact, fluorodeoxyglucose ([^{18}F]FDG) PET-CT is increasingly employed in radiotherapy planning, prediction of prognosis in terms of tumour response to neoadjuvant, radiation and chemotherapy treatment (Feigenberg et al. 2012). [^{18}F]FDG PET-CT has also many other uses: it is a useful adjunct in the characterisation of indeterminate solitary lung nodules and pretreatment staging of non-small cell lung cancer (NSCLC); it has the ability to assess locoregional lymph node spread more precisely than CT, to detect metastatic lesions that would have been missed on conventional imaging or are located in difficult areas and to help in the differentiation of lesions that are equivocal after conventional imaging.

Sometimes, it could happen that at the post-therapy PET registered after a treatment with stereotactic body radiotherapy (SBRT), in a patient with a NSCLC who couldn't undergo surgery, an increase in the size of the neoplastic pulmonary nodule is apparently visible as well as increased intensity of [^{18}F]FDG uptake in the area, suggesting that there has been no significant response to radiation therapy with progression of tumour growth. In these situations, only an accurate review of the imaging exams can clarify the meaning of the imaging findings (an asymptomatic radiation pneumonitis, not as suspicious as the report indicated). This example besides emphasises the importance of pre-SBRT PET values, post-SBRT PET values and changes in PET values over the course of therapy (Adam and Kenny 2015).

As said before, the trend of personalised medicine in oncology care requires wide knowledge about the cancers being treated that can only be attained by specialists in that particular subspecialty, for example, the large number of genetic mutations identified for each cancer type, such as the epidermal growth factor (EGF)-activating mutations in some NSCLC types (Wheless et al. 2010).

3.3 Head and Neck Cancer

Head and neck cancer is a challenging topic, given the wide variety of treatment options available, the complexity of the anatomy and the dependence of the treatment plan on imaging information.

The training in the interpretation of the head and neck cancer imaging is a small fraction of the residency program of diagnostic radiology, so that many radiologists have difficulty in interpreting these scans at the end of the training program. A subset of radiologists, approximately 10–20%, pursue one or 2 years of fellowship training in diagnostic neuroradiology, which includes head and neck imaging and brain and spine imaging. Radiologists with this fellowship training should be sought for staffing of MTBs and for the interpretation of imaging studies in patients with known or suspected head and neck cancer.

Some authors recommend identifying at least two radiologists to share the MTB staffing responsibilities, so that gaps in coverage can be minimised. In many academic centres, there is often a subset of the group of diagnostic neuroradiologists who have additional training, interest or experience in head and neck imaging. Ideally, these individuals should be identified and specifically recruited to participate in head and neck MTB. Radiologists with this added level of subspecialisation are able to contribute more degrees of nuances and better identify subtle findings that can dramatically alter treatment plans. These radiologists are more likely to be abreast of the current literature in the field and contribute to improving and evolving the clinical practice.

As the management of head and neck tumours has expanded to include many complex treatment modalities, the multidisciplinary team approach has become critical in optimising treatment planning and patient outcomes. In fact, many argue that MTBs represent a new standard of care (Natt et al. 2010).

Obviously, it appears that MTB has a greater impact on the management of malignant tumours than benign tumours. The statistically significant difference in the rate of treatment changes between the two groups is due to the expanding role of multi-modality treatment. As cases of malignancy are more likely to benefit from multimodality approaches, when these cases are presented for review, treatment plans are more often augmented. In these discussions, experts from radiation oncology, medical oncology, radiology and pathology work with the otolaryngologist to design an optimal treatment plan, in accordance with 'best practice' standards (Pillay et al. 2016).

Regarding the effect of the multidisciplinary team on care decisions, some studies identified that MTBs resulted in a change in care management in 2–52% of patient cases. This was reflected by a change in the patient's pathologic diagnosis, staging and use of chemotherapy (Essaihi et al. 2003).

References

Abdulrahman GO Jr (2011) The effect of multidisciplinary team care on cancer management. Pan Afr Med J 9:20. https://doi.org/10.4314/pamj.v9i1.71195

Adam A, Kenny LM (2015) Interventional oncology in multidisciplinary cancer treatment in the 21(st) century. Nat Rev Clin Oncol 12(2):105–113. https://doi.org/10.1038/nrclinonc.2014.211

AL-Jahdali H, Khan AN, Loutfi S, Al-Harbi AS (2012) Guidelines for the role of FDG-PET/CT in lung cancer management. J Infect Public Health 5(5 Suppl 1). https://doi.org/10.1016/j.jiph.2012.09.003

Bunnell CA, Weingart SN, Swanson S, Mamon HJ, Shulman LN (2010) Models of multidisciplinary cancer care: physician and patient perceptions in a comprehensive cancer center. J Oncol Pract 6(6):283–288. https://doi.org/10.1200/JOP.2010.000138

Disselhorst JA, Bezrukov I, Kolb A, Parl C, Pichler BJ (2014) Principles of PET/MR imaging. J Nucl Med 55:2–10. https://doi.org/10.2967/jnumed.113.129098

Essaihi A, Michel G, Shiffman RN (2003) Comprehensive categorization of guideline recommendations: creating an action palette for implementers. AMIA Annu Symp Proc:220–224. http://eutils.ncbi.nlm.nih.gov/entrez/eutils/elink.fcgi?dbfrom=pubmed&id=14728166&retmode=ref&cmd=prlinks%5Cnpapers2://publication/uuid/0CD48B3B-D1CB-4932-A7A1-57A98220E6A6

Falcon S, Williams A, Weinfurtner J, Drukteinis J (2017) Imaging management of breast density, a controversial risk factor for breast cancer. Cancer Control 24(2):125–136. http://www.embase.com/search/results?subaction=viewrecord&from=export&id=L615786352

Feigenberg S, Campassi C, Sharma N, Kesmodel SB, Tkaczuk K, Yu JQ (2012) Integration of modern imaging into the multidisciplinary setting: the radiation oncology perspective. Appl Radiol 41(3):24–30

Gagan J, Van Allen EM (2015) Next-generation sequencing to guide cancer therapy. Genome Med 7(1):80. https://doi.org/10.1186/s13073-015-0203-x

Hoffman HT, McCulloch T, Gustin D, Karnell LH (1997) Organ preservation therapy for advanced-stage laryngeal carcinoma. Otolaryngol Clin N Am 30(1):113–130

Keating NL, Landrum MB, Lamont EB, Bozeman SR, Shulman LN, McNeil BJ (2013) Tumor boards and the quality of cancer care. J Natl Cancer Inst 105(2):113–121. https://doi.org/10.1093/jnci/djs502

Kherlopian AR, Song T, Duan Q et al (2008) A review of imaging techniques for systems biology. BMC Syst Biol 2(1):74. https://doi.org/10.1186/1752-0509-2-74

Knechtges PM, Carlos RC (2007) The evolving role of radiologists within the Health Care System. J Am Coll Radiol 4(9):626–635. https://doi.org/10.1016/j.jacr.2007.05.014

Lesslie MD, Parikh JR (2017) Multidisciplinary tumor boards: an opportunity for radiologists to demonstrate value. Acad Radiol 24(1):107–110. https://doi.org/10.1016/j.acra.2016.09.006

Margenthaler JA, Duke D, Monsees BS, Barton PT, Clark C, Dietz JR (2006) Correlation between core biopsy and excisional biopsy in breast high-risk lesions. Am J Surg 192(4):534–537. https://doi.org/10.1016/j.amjsurg.2006.06.003

Mitchell DG, Javitt MC, Glanc P et al (2013) ACR appropriateness criteria staging and follow-up of ovarian cancer. J Am Coll Radiol 10(11):822–827. https://doi.org/10.1016/j.jacr.2013.07.017

Natt R, Karkos PD, Karkanevatos A (2010) Influence of audit on clinical practice: multidisciplinary team data documentation for cutaneous head and neck malignancy. Am J Otolaryngol – Head Neck Med Surg 31(4):261–265. https://doi.org/10.1016/j.amjoto.2009.03.001

Pillay B, Wootten AC, Crowe H et al (2016) The impact of multidisciplinary team meetings on patient assessment, management and outcomes in oncology settings: a systematic review of the literature. Cancer Treat Rev 42:56–72. https://doi.org/10.1016/j.ctrv.2015.11.007

Urbański B (2012) The future of radiation oncology: considerations of young medical doctor. Rep Pract Oncol Radiother 17(5):288–293. https://doi.org/10.1016/j.rpor.2012.09.002

Wallace MJ (2014) Image-guided interventions in oncology. Surg Oncol Clin N Am 23(4):937–955. https://doi.org/10.1016/j.soc.2014.06.004

Wheless SA, McKinney KA, Zanation AM (2010) A prospective study of the clinical impact of a multidisciplinary head and neck tumor board. Otolaryngol – Head Neck Surg 143(5):650–654. https://doi.org/10.1016/j.otohns.2010.07.020

Wu JS, Goldsmith JD, Horwich PJ, Shetty SK, Hochman MG (2008) Bone and soft-tissue lesions: what factors affect diagnostic yield of image-guided Core-needle biopsy? Radiology 248(3):962–970. https://doi.org/10.1148/radiol.2483071742

Part II

From Simulation to Delivery Guided by Imaging: Technical Aspects (Vincenzo Valentini, Uulke van der Heide)

Optimal CT Protocols for CT-Guided Planning Preparation in Radiotherapy

Alessandra Bolsi and Lorenzo Placidi

Contents

1 **Simulation Methods** 28

2 **Specification and Relevant Parameters of CT Simulation** 32

3 **Factors Driving the Definition of the Protocols: Image Quality and Dose Calculation Accuracy** 34

4 **QA in CT Simulation** 39

5 **CT Simulation Tomorrow** 40
5.1 Dual-Energy CT (DECT) 41
5.2 Imaging Methods for Adaptation 41
5.3 Substitute CT 42

6 **Conclusion** 43

References 43

A. Bolsi (✉)
Center for Proton Therapy, Paul Scherrer Institute, ETH Domain, Villigen, Switzerland
e-mail: alessandra.bolsi@psi.ch

L. Placidi (✉)
Dipartimento di Scienze Radiologiche, Radioterapiche ed Ematologiche, Istituto di Radiologia, Fondazione Policlinico Universitario A. Gemelli IRCCS—Università Cattolica Sacro Cuore, Roma, Italy
e-mail: lorenzo.placidi@policlinicogemelli.it

Abstract

The invention of the computed tomography (CT) in 1972 by Cormack and Hounsfield allowed for the very first time the acquisition of 3D images. CT scans taken for radiotherapy treatment planning usually differ from those taken for diagnostic use, since those are optimized to perform a three-dimensional dose calculation inside the patient. Radiation dose is of less concern than in diagnostic imaging, even though it should be always minimized. Image quality (IQ) has indeed relevant importance as it affects the accuracy of the treatment planning (par. 2). In order to correctly simulate a radiation treatment condition, several requirements are suggested: it is essentially the identification of the optimal CT acquisition parameter settings (CT scanner protocols), considering the special requirements of CT simulation (par. 3).

For CT scanners used as a simulator for radiotherapy treatment, the quality assurance (QA) needs to be very comprehensive as it includes two important aspects: imaging CT and treatment planning, as it provides input for the TPS (par. 4).

Improvements in the CT simulations are also a topic of recent research. In particular, the use of dual-energy CT (DECT) and cone beam CT (CBCT) as CT simulators is described in paragraph 5. Another area of research, which is now being transferred into clinical operation, is the one related to

R. G. H. Beets-Tan et al. (eds.), *Imaging and Interventional Radiology for Radiation Oncology*, Medical Radiology, Diagnostic Imaging, https://doi.org/10.1007/978-3-030-38261-2_3

MRI-based delivery systems. This growing technology allows acquisition of online MRI images which present with the major advantages as compared to CT images: high soft tissue contrast and radiation-free (par. 5).

1 Simulation Methods

The invention of the computed tomography (CT) in 1972 by Cormack and Hounsfield allowed for the very first time the acquisition of 3D images, which could then be used to perform a three-dimensional dose calculation inside the patient. This led to several advantages in radiation therapy, especially in improving the accuracy of the dose distribution calculation and dose optimization. All these achievements were possible since CT images can be used to identify both the position of the tumor volumes and of the organs at risk and attenuation coefficients of the tissues. Therefore, calculation and optimization of the dose distribution can be performed to achieve the prescribed dose in the target volume while sparing the surrounding healthy tissue. Moreover, the acquisition of a CT dataset allowed the possibility of generating digitally reconstructed radiographs or DDR (Fig. 1) for patient positioning verification at the time of treatment, using the Linac onboard imaging system.

Considering all those factors, it is clear how CT scanners' development and use have revolutionized the concept of radiotherapy, especially in the planning stage.

Treatment simulation is a crucial process of the radiotherapy workflow, through which the most appropriate way to irradiate the patient is optimized. It is a key point in order to achieve the three-dimensional (3D) patient anatomy visualization and target definition that enables planning to conform the dose to the target volume avoiding the critical organs. Even though less and less common in clinical practice, the verification simulation approach could be still in use in some centers. In this process, the CT images of the patients are acquired, and it is possible to visualize on them radiopaque markers, useful for the volume of interest delineation. Once the treatment planning is completed, the plan verification is performed on a radiographic simulator. A simulator is an isocentrically mounted diagnostic X-ray machine with an image intensifier, but it duplicates the radiotherapy treatment unit in terms of its geometric, mechanical, and optical proprieties (McCullough 1990; McCullough and Earl 1979).

Currently there are two main approaches to perform a treatment simulation:

- CT simulation process: the simulation is performed on a CT scanner via special computer software that provides a full 3D patient representation in the treatment planning position. Then, a complete treatment planning strategy can be designed, a process referred to as vir-

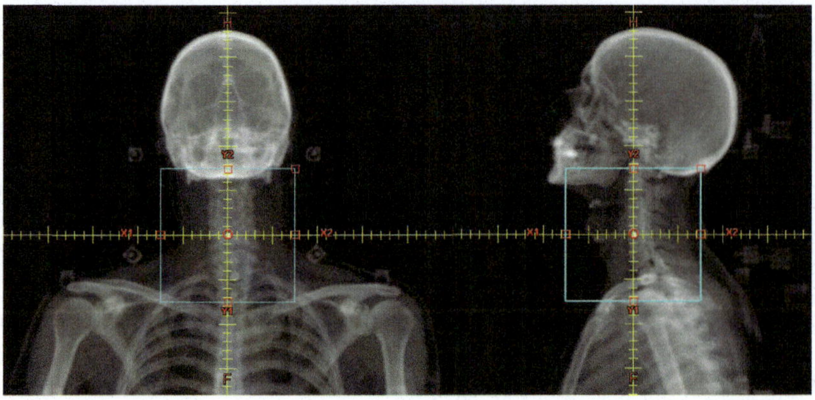

Fig. 1 Creation of digital reconstructed radiographs or DRRs from CT

tual simulation (Sherouse et al. 1990a; Sherouse 1998).

– 4D CT simulation process: when the anatomy that is imaged is mobile, the image data are subject to motion artifacts that can impact not only on the image quality but also on the accuracy of the calculated dose in treatment planning. 4D CT scanning protocols achieve the goal of capturing the temporal position of the tumor in the imaging study.

The CT simulation process is summarized in Fig. 2. 4D CT simulation process is described and discussed later in this session.

CT scans taken for radiotherapy treatment planning usually differ from those taken for diagnostic use. Ideally, planning CT scans is taken on a dedicated radiotherapy CT scanner by a radiographer trained in radiotherapy. The patient is positioned using supporting aids and immobilization devices and aligned using tattoos and midline and lateral laser lights identical to those used for subsequent radiotherapy treatment. A tattoo is made on the skin over an immobile bony landmark nearest to the center of the target volume. It is marked with radiopaque material such as a catheter or barium paste for visualization on the CT image. Additional lateral tattoos are used to prevent lateral rotation of the patient and are aligned using horizontal lasers. Multi-slice CT

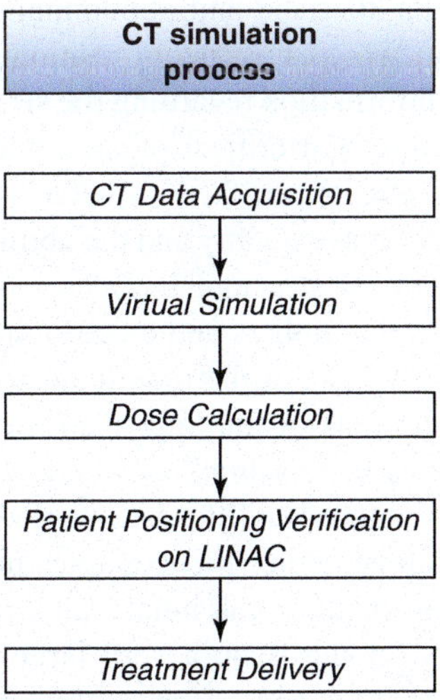

Fig. 2 CT simulation process

scanners perform a scan of the entire chest or abdomen in a few seconds with the patient breathing normally. DRRs are produced from CT density information and are compared with electronic portal images (EPIs).

The transfer of planning information (reference marks, field entry point, etc.) from CT simulation, to the planning system, to the treatment unit is the most critical step. Without an accurate and reliable method of doing this, the usefulness of CT planning is greatly reduced and, indeed, may introduce error. The practice of virtual simulation relies on this concept being realizable. The two main elements of virtual simulation for accurate patient's treatment are transfer of coordinates (marks identifying beam centers, field edges, block position, etc. as necessary) and reconstruction of digitally reconstructed radiographs (DRR). Goitein et al. (1983) developed the concept of beam's eye view following the idea of McShan et al. (1979) and recognized the importance of projecting through CT section to produce an image for verification purposes. It was Sherouse et al. (1987) and Sherouse and Chaney (1991) who first used the terms virtual simulation and virtual simulator, and the concept of the DRR was further developed by Sherouse et al. (1990b). The DDR traces rays from the X-ray source through a three-dimensional model of the patient made up of voxel determined from CT scans. This particular DRR software separated photoelectron and Compton components in order to compute either a DRR similar to a verification image on the simulator or a DRR that looked more like the high-energy portal radiograph images are produced using different image processing technique in the modern virtual simulator. In addition, more information can be visualized than in conventional radiography, even if some detail is lost in the digital nature of the image with its finite number of pixel (typically 512 × 512). In general, DRR is superior to a conventional radiograph, particularly if bones overlie with the region of interest. A key factor to the efficient use of CT simulation is the speed of the reconstruction of DRR (nowadays almost in real time). Another feature of CT planning and virtual simulation (as described below) is the use of noncoplanar beams (Mohan 1988).

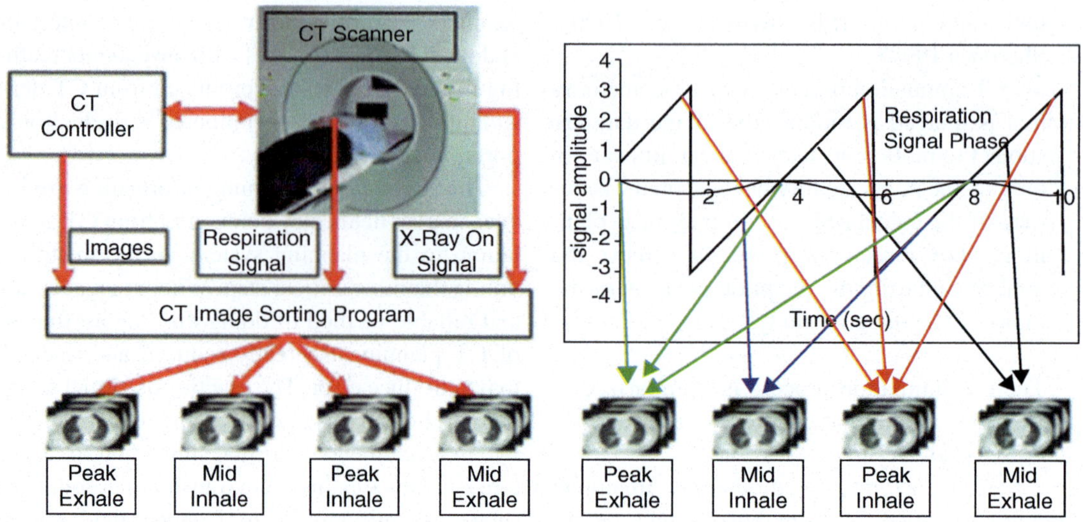

Fig. 3 4D CT phase-sorting process: CT images, breathing taking signal, and "X-ray on" signal form the input data stream. The breathing cycle is divided into distinct bin (e.g., peak exhale, mid-inhale, peak inhale, mid-exhale). Images are sorted into those image bins depending on the phase of the breathing cycle in which they were acquired (Vedam et al. 2003)

Verification of these beams (already in use to treat patients) was not often possible because the size of the image intensifier on the simulator often prevented positioning of the beam with the correct geometry with respect to the target and the patient. With virtual simulation, the image interpretation became possible since not only it could be processed to improve image quality but also it was possible to see the various organs and structures covered by the beam.

It could be summarized that CT simulation is associated with "virtual simulation," a term coined by Sherouse et al. (1987), which refers to the process on a computer, using a 3D CT patient dataset, that allows full simulation and verification of radiotherapy treatment.

CT is the gold standard 3D method, which is most widely used for treatment planning. The images are represented in terms of CT number, the so-called Hounsfield units, which represent the attenuation coefficient of the specific tissue. From those units, it is possible to derive mass attenuation coefficient or attenuation characteristics for high-energy photon, X-ray, and gamma ray and relative stopping power for heavy particles and therefore compute an accurate dose calculation, even in presence of tissues heterogeneity. Moreover, the 3D CT images present with a high level of geometric accuracy, as they are not subject to geometric distortion, which can easily occur for MRI images. Additionally, with modern CT scanners, the acquisition time of 3D CT images is much shorter as compared to MR or PET, thus implying that CT can be used also to assess organ/tumor motion (Li and Xiao 2013).

Four-dimensional CT (4D CT) is another and recent development used to quantify respiratory and organ motion. Normally, the 4D CT is acquired for thoracic and abdominal regions of interest, in which respiratory motion can cause incorrect information regarding the size and position of tumor and critical organs, that can also cause significant artifacts. Artifacts not only degrade the image quality and the ability to delineate anatomical structure but also can result in erroneous CT numbers and electron density values in the vicinity of the mobile anatomy. A 4D CT scan consists of multiple scans obtained for each location (oversampling) whereby the organ motion is captured at different sampled phases of the respiratory cycle, for example, in the peak exhale, mid-inhale, peak inhale, and mid-exhale. At the end of the scan, a very large set of 3D images are produced corresponding to each of the phases in which the breathing cycle was sampled (Fig. 3). The collection of those 3D CT

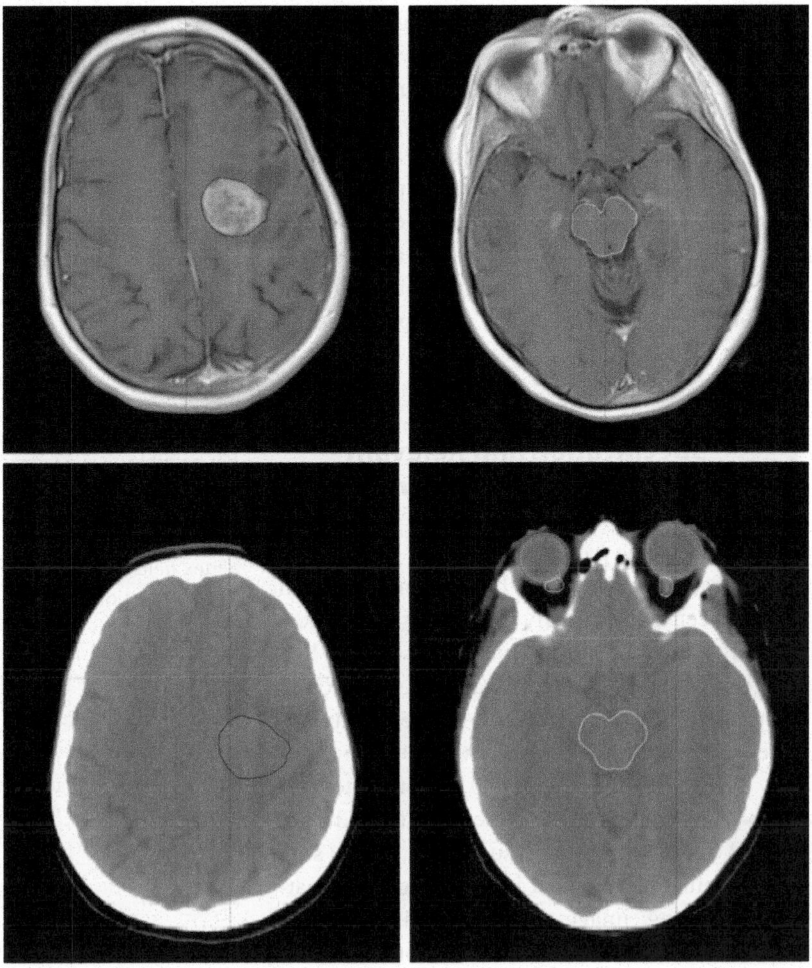

Fig. 4 Differences in the soft tissue contrast from two images: T1-weighted MR with contrast (top) and CT image (bottom). The ROIs show on the left the clinical target volume (CTV) in red and on the right the brain stem and the optical nerves (yellow color) and the eyes (pink color)

scans constitutes the 4D CT study for this patient. This method is also known as retrospective image reconstruction. 4D CT simulation allows to segment the target and organ volumes with high specificity resulting in not only a more educated decision on margin selection but also accurate dose calculation during treatment planning.

The primary disadvantage of CT for treatment planning is the low tissue contrast which can result in the tumor definition varying significantly from physician to physician. For this reason, in contemporary radiation therapy, as already mentioned, MRI and PET are often used to complement CT for tumor delineation and normal tissue identification (Fig. 4), although only CT images are used for dose calculation.

Therefore, the ability to accurately co-register these various image sets is one of the most powerful tools for radiation therapy planning. Most radiation treatment planning systems (TPS) support image registration and fusion, with several algorithms available. The most common is a geometric transformation (rigid and nonrigid) that can be point-based, intensity-based, or based on the tissue contrast. Unfortunately, registration algorithms are very complex and can create undesirable image artifacts, thus causing errors in the tumor and normal tissue localization. In order to minimize potential issues using software-based registration, it is desirable to position patients as similarly as possible for the acquisitions in the different modalities and to use the software to refine the results.

This can be achieved if the same immobilization devices are used for all the different imaging devices (CT, MRI, PET) and if they are equipped with flat tabletops, which match the geometry of the treatment couch.

Nevertheless, the process of fusing multiple image techniques in radiation oncology is labor-intensive and requires manual verification of the quality of registration by qualified experts. Other disadvantages (most of them have now reduced thanks to technical developments) and advantages of the CT simulation approach are summarized in Table 1, based on the table proposed by Conway and Robinson (1997).

2 Specification and Relevant Parameters of CT Simulation

Since most of the patient undergoing CT simulation in radiation oncology have been diagnosed with cancer and generally only one scan is used for CT simulation, the radiation dose is of less concern than in diagnostic imaging, even though it should be always minimized. Image quality has indeed relevant importance as it affects the accuracy of the treatment planning. In order to correctly simulate a radiation treatment condition, several requirements are suggested (e.g., skin surface must be included in the image for treatment planning: image truncation is intolerable). The main parameters and specifications of a general CT scanner for CT simulation are listed below (Table 2).

Liu et al. (2008) evaluated the image quality of five different multichannel CT scanners using helical scan mode, by two CT phantoms. In particular, they compared the effects of various pitches, detector configuration, rotation time parameters on image artifacts, and spatial and contrast resolution. Some further consideration of some parameters is discussed below.

The detector pitch is defined as table distance travelled in one 360° gantry rotation divided by beam collimation. Choice of pitch affects both image quality and patient dose:

- $P = 1.0$: X-ray beams are contiguous for adjacent rotation.
- $P > 1.0$: X-ray beams are not contiguous for adjacent rotations, i.e., there are gaps in

Table 1 Advantages and disadvantage of the CT simulation for treatment planning

Advantages	Disadvantages	Disadvantages: comment
Full 3D simulation allowing unique verification of beam coverage and avoidance in three dimensions	A large number of CT slices are often required at <3 mm thickness, for optimal DRR resolution	Now easily and quickly achievable. Sometimes 5 mm slices are unavoidable where large volumes are to be scanned
Beams can be simulated and verified that are not possible with conventional simulation, e.g., vertex fields	State-of-the-art hardware is required for interactive capabilities	Now achieved
The verification images, DRRs, can contain more information than conventional simulation and can be manipulated to enhance tumor visualization	DRRs do not provide information about patient movement or anatomical movement that may be necessary for accurate field coverage	This can be resolved partially by multiple fast scans that can be registered at different breath hold positions or slow scanning to blur movements and registration with fast scans
There is a much closer connection to diagnostic information with CT Sim, allowing integration of multimodality images	DRR resolution is unlikely to equal radiographic film resolution	Resolution now entirely acceptable for most uses
	Field portal visualization on the patient's skin not available	Now available on many systems using room's eye view
	Patients may have to be immobilized for extended periods during the virtual simulation procedure	Scan times are now very much shorter, and planning methods can be adapted to reduce the requirement for the patient's physical presence

Table 1 (continued)

Advantages	Disadvantages	Disadvantages: comment
	The radiotherapist needs to be present for extended periods to mark target volume	Still true but procedure is now speeded up with effective editing systems. Markup can be done post-scan and utilize reference marking only
	Correcting (shifts) to the marked isocenter may be required before the plan is finalized	Still true and still a concern in terms of the potential for error. Portal imaging on the treatment set provides final check; this step becomes more important
	Some patient positions may not be possible	Still true but dedicated CT scanners with large apertures may eliminate this problem

between the X-ray beams and tissue is not irradiated.

- $P < 1.0$: there is X-ray beam overlap, i.e., a volume of tissue is irradiated more than once per scan.

CT noise, which is described by the fluctuation (standard deviation) of the pixel values for images on the homogeneous phantom, is a key parameter, especially for the image quality. Noise is also included in the signal-to-noise ratio (SNR) where the level of the desired signal (photons) is compared to the level of background noise (pixel deviation from normal). The higher the ratio, the less noise is present on the image. The following factors affect noise (and consequently SNR):

- mAs (tube current x exposure time, related to the dose of a CT scan): it has a direct relationship with the number of photons utilized in the examination. A useful stat to keep in mind is 2 × mAs = 40% increase SNR. Increasing the dose of the scan will decrease the amount of noise and hence improve the contrast resolution of the image.
- Slice thickness: the number of photons available to generate an image has a linear relationship to the slice thickness. The thicker the slice, the more photons available, the better SNR (increasing the slice thickness will also decrease the spatial resolution in the *z*-axis).
- Patient size: larger patient will absorb more radiation than smaller ones; meaning fewer photons will reach the detector hence reducing the SNR.

Table 2 Main features of a typical CT scanner

Parameter	Specification[a]
Aperture	At least 80/85 cm
Number of detectors	>750 per row
X-ray tube	80–130 kV, 250–500 mA (depending on kV)
Detector pitch	0.7–1.5
Heat capacity	6–7 MHU
Anode heat cooling	700–900 kHU min^{-1}
Minimum slice width	1 mm
Patient support	Tabletop identical to that used on treatment machine
Spatial resolution	High contrast better than 13 lines pairs cm^{-1} (at 0% MTF). Low contrast: 5 mm at 3% resolution
Acquisition time	1–2 slice/rev s^{-1} (multi-slice: Four or eight slice/rec s^{-1}), covering a width of 20–32 mm at isocenter
Reconstruction time	Few seconds up to 60 s total time to end of 30 mm range
DRR calculation	Few seconds (tolerable), sub-second (desirable)
Capacity to store	12,000–60,000 uncompressed images on hard disc
Laser accuracy	±1 mm
Accuracy of slice location	<1 mm

DRR digitally reconstructed radiograph, *MHU* mega heat units, *MTF* modulation transfer function
[a]Specification can differ slightly from different scanner's model

Another relevant parameter is the scanner acquisition speed, which could typically be between 3 and 15 s for 50 cm scan range. This can be achieved by multi-slice scanners, which have totally replaced traditional single-slice ones. Fast scan times are advantageous in reducing motion artifacts, but only one of the breathing phases (not easy to determine) will be represented in the scans. Even if faster scanners, which are now available in more and more centers, present with advantages in dealing with motion, the implementation of 4D CT scanner is moving to a different approach based on different breathing phases selection.

In the CT simulation process, the comfort and reproducibility of the patient positioning are essential to guarantee accurate radiotherapic treatment, as the position at simulation needs to be accurately reproduced in daily treatments. Therefore, as mentioned above, it is very advantageous to have the same tabletop for CT simulation and treatment. The CT therapy couch top should also be designed to take the usual accessories needed to position the patient, for example, breast boards and headrests. These accessories significantly enhance positioning accuracy and patient comfort and reduce patient setup time.

The importance of efficient and accurate connectivity between CT simulation and radiotherapy treatment planning system cannot be overemphasized. Standards such as Digital Imaging and Communications in Medicine (DICOMv3) and the standard image transfer protocol for radiotherapy (DICOM-RT) enable export of radiotherapy images, treatment plans, and structure sets (contours). Transfer protocols should be fully tested for all condition and any inconsistencies reported.

3 Factors Driving the Definition of the Protocols: Image Quality and Dose Calculation Accuracy

As it has been previously mentioned, the CT simulation in radiation therapy is the procedure which leads to accurate geometric patient representation and accurate determination of the mass attenuation coefficient for high-energy photons and X-rays. Those aspects are crucial for accurate dose calculation.

As regards the definition of the protocols, it is important to distinguish CT scanner simulators from diagnostic CT scanners, as their implementation is different. For radiation oncology CT scanners, regular practice in diagnostic such as contrast injection, variable image thickness, and gantry tilt is discouraged. The use of contrast will affect the accuracy of the HU representation of the material absorbing the medium. This is critical especially for particle therapy as a modified tissue HU will result in an incorrect particle range estimation.

CT scanner protocols should be defined and optimized to guarantee accurate image quality and minimal artifacts.

For accurate dose calculation, patient surface should be included in the CT images for treatment planning as image truncation is not acceptable (patient tissue will be considered as air for beam passing through it). For patients treated in the head and neck region, the shoulders should be included in the scan area as they will affect the daily positioning.

For both of those reasons, the field of view (FoV) should be as large as possible (i.e., the body or large FoV, between 50 and 65 cm), for all the scan area. For CT scanners and simulators, it is extremely advantageous that the aperture of the scanner is larger than the standard 70 cm, thus reaching 80 or 85 cm. In case part of the patient is outside of the scan FoV, the lack of data can be corrected and compensated outside the FoV, but the accuracy of the HU values in this area is limited to typically ±50 HU.

Slice spacing normally required in CT simulation is between 2 and 3 mm, which is a compromise of accurate geometric patient representation and the effort required from the clinician to contour the volume of interest on each slice.

Generally, those acquisitions parameters should be evaluated for each scanner and each protocol available for the CT scanners used in radio oncology. Catphan phantom (The Phantom Laboratory, Salem, New York) has been designed for those purposes (The Phantom Laboratory Inc 2002). Normally, higher image quality (IQ) is

Table 3 CT radiation dose parameters

Dose parameter	Definition	Effects on radiation dose	Unit
Tube potential or voltage	X-ray beam energy	Proportional to square of tube voltage change	kV
Product of tube current and time	Photon fluence; number of photons in defined exposure time	Directly proportional to radiation dose	mAs
Pitch	Ratio of table feed per gantry rotation to nominal width of beam collimation	Inversely proportional to radiation dose	–
CTDIw	Average radiation dose in scan volume measured in standard CT phantoms; 1/3 CTDI center +2/3 CTDI periphery	Directly proportional to radiation dose in unit volume, influenced By pitch factor	mGy
CTDIvol	CTDIw/pitch	Directly proportional to radiation dose in unit volume, irrespective of pitch factor	mGy
Dose length product	CTDIvol × scan length (cm)	Directly proportional to total scanned radiation dose	mGy cm
Effective dose	Overall risk-related radiation exposure; ΣW_T (tissue weighting factor) × H_T (tissue equivalent dose)	Directly proportional to total scanned radiation dose and overall risk of irradiated tissue	mSv

CTDIvol volume CT dose index, *CTDIw* weighted CT dose index

reached for smaller detector configurations and pitch, which results in slightly higher dose (Goo 2012). For those reasons, the best compromise should be found measuring both IQ and radiation dosimetry, usually described by CT dose index (CTDI) and dose length product (DLP) quantities as described in the report from AAPM (McNitt-Gray 2002).

The effects of different parameters for dose optimization are summarized in the following table (Table 3).

The goal of dose optimization is to minimize radiation dose while obtaining sufficient CT simulation images quality. Therefore, the protocols should be defined to get good-quality images with proper dose optimization. The four fundamental elements determining CT image quality consist of image noise, image contrast, spatial resolution, and artifacts (Table 4). In principle, the radiation dose is inversely proportional to the square of the image noise. Image contrast is significantly increased by the use of a contrast agent and is influenced by tube potential in some materials with high atomic numbers such as iodine due to the different photoelectric interaction. The required image quality of CT differs somewhat among different diagnostic tasks. Therefore, the required CT radiation dose is also fairly diverse and thus should be tailored according to clinical indications.

To be compliant with the so-called "as low as reasonably achievable (ALARA)" principle, it is imperative to justify CT examinations beforehand. Obviously, several differences between diagnostic CT and CT scans taken for radiotherapy treatment planning drive the way to apply the ALARA principle. Nevertheless, it should make every effort to reduce the radiation dose of CT examinations while maintaining diagnostic quality when planning CT is acquired. A checklist for CT dose optimization is described in Table 5.

Body-size-adapted CT protocol is a fundamental part of CT dose optimization because the minimal radiation dose required for diagnostic image quality would be varied even at the same diagnostic task depending on body size and habitus. Therefore, the optimal tube voltage and current should be determined for the adapted radiation dose. One of the common misconceptions is that lowering the tube voltage at the same tube current is a good strategy for low-dose CT. Actually, a higher tube current should be used at a lower tube potential to compensate for the increased image noise. Another misconception is that tube current modulation can automatically adapt the CT radiation dose to different

Table 4 CT image quality parameters

Image quality parameter	Definition	Relationships with radiation dose parameters	Calculation method
Image noise	Random variation of CT numbers	Inversely proportional to square root of radiation dose, inversely proportional to tube voltage, inversely proportional to fourth power of spatial resolution, influenced by section thickness and reconstruction algorithm	Standard deviation of measured CT numbers
Contrast-to-noise resolution	Ability to distinguish between different CT numbers	Not significantly changed at different tube voltages in most of materials except for some with high atomic numbers such as iodine (increased at low tube voltage); low contrast resolution greatly influenced by image noise level	$(S_A - S_B) / \sigma$, where S_A and S_B are CT attenuation measured in structures A and B and σ is measured image noise
Spatial resolution	Ability to distinguish small details of object	Inversely proportional to focal spot size, detector collimation; influenced by reconstruction algorithm	Voxel size, line pairs per centimeter, point or line spread function, modulation transfer function
Artifacts	Unwanted structures degrading CT image quality	Photon starvation artifacts, inversely proportional to radiation dose; physiologic motion artifacts, inversely proportional to temporal resolution; other artifacts, no direct relationships with radiation dose parameters	

body sizes and anatomical regions and therefore allows a constant image quality. However, this is erroneous, and a user-defined target image quality considering patient size should be determined for each anatomical region and each tube voltage. In general, a CT protocol derived from a best-fit equation is generally preferred to a classic CT dose table or chart for more accurate dose adaptation and better compliance.

Tube current modulation greatly contributes to CT dose optimization by reducing CT dose according to body size, shape, and attenuation without degrading image quality. CT dose reduction achieved by tube current modulation has been reported to be up to 26–50% in children and adults (Goo 2011; Goo and Suh 2006). Other factors influencing tube current modulation include tube voltage, maximum tube current, scan speed, and scan direction (Lee et al. 2008; Israel et al. 2008). With thicker or denser body parts, the tube current saturation occurs earlier. Since image quality is subject to deterioration resulting from the increased image noise at region scanned at a saturated tube current, the use of a higher tube voltage, slower scan speed (either slower gantry rotation time or a lower pitch), or a combination of both should be considered as a remedy for this potential pitfall. Tube current is not truly automatic: the experience on how we can determine this target image quality index for tube current modulation is very limited (Irie and Inoue 2005; Prakash et al. 2010).

The CT images calibration, from Hounsfield unit to electron density (Seco and Evans 2006) when importing them in the treatment planning system, is an extremely important and essential step in the CT simulation process.

This conversion can be affected, even if not dramatically (<2%), by the peak voltage (kVp) and mAs as described by Guan et al. (2002). A comprehensive analysis and overview of the CT protocol used for radiotherapy scans have been recently reported (Davis et al. 2017). This study evaluated multiple CT scans and came to the conclusion that HU stability (within ±20HU for soft tissue and ±50 HU for the lung and soft tissue) is essential to restrict dose changes in treatment plans <1%.

This applies for photon radiotherapy, while for proton and heavy ions, the calibration curve represents the relationship between HU and proton stopping power. This can be obtained essentially by two methods, the stoichiometric one (Schneider et al. 1996), which has been validated also for biological samples (Pedroni and Shaffner

Table 5 Recommendations for dose reduction in the planning CT acquisition

Checkup items	Recommendations
Body-size-adapted CT protocol	• Traditionally based on body weight or body mass index • Based on cross-sectional dimensions and/or body attenuation for better dose adaptation to individually varied body habitus • Use best-fit equation rather than dose table or chart
Tube current modulation	• Always turn on if applicable • Set up appropriate reference image quality index • Check how much modulated tube current reaches to maximal limits ("tube current saturation"), and adjust parameters such as tube voltage and scan speed to obtain maximal dose reduction by tube current modulation
Optimal tube voltage at Equivalent radiation dose	• Select most dose-efficient tube voltage • Consider lower tube voltages for contrast-enhanced examination, higher tube voltages for examinations requiring lower noise (e.g., unenhanced brain CT) and for examinations detecting low-contrast lesions (e.g., microabscesses in the liver or ground-glass opacity in the lung)
Longitudinal scan range	• Adjust to minimal range as required for planning indications, desirably by using clear anatomical landmarks
Repeated scanning	• Reduce number of repeated scanning • Omit precontrast examination if possible
Noise-reducing image Reconstruction algorithms	• Use noise-reducing, spatial resolution-preserving algorithms (e.g., iterative reconstruction algorithms) at lower radiation dose

1998), and the mass density one (Soukup et al. 2005), which uses the mass density as a dependent variable, and the calibration curve links directly HU to mass density.

CT scans acquisition parameters can significantly influence (>2%) the relative proton stopping power derived by the calibration curve.

The most critical ones are the kVp and the detector configuration as it is visible in Fig. 5.

Therefore, it is essential to restrict CT scans acquisition to the well-defined parameters, which have been used for the CT calibration. Average curves related to different regions (such as the head and body) could be used depending on the numbers of calibration curves supported or introduced in the TPS. Value of 120 kVp represents a good compromise between dose and image quality to well-defined bony structures and accuracy of the stoichiometric calibration. Detector configuration needs to be defined for the calibration procedure as it has an effect on the slope of the curve and on both signal-to-noise ratio and dose to the patient. Optimization of the current (mAs value) considering the specific tissue attenuation has shown no significant differences in the HU values, but low mAs values result in an increased images noise, therefore a reduction of the IQ (as described in Table 4).

Different reconstruction algorithms are available for the same CT acquisitions, and those also should be fixed when reconstructing the images for the TPS, even if their effect is significant in case of specific algorithms used to visualize cardiac or lung structures, or to segment metallic structures.

Those reconstruction algorithms are a crucial part of the process of generating CT images from raw data. The mathematical problem that CT image reconstruction is trying to solve is to compute the attenuation coefficients of different X-ray absorption paths (ray sum) that are obtained as a set of data (projection). Some of the more common algorithms utilized in commercially available CT today are described below:

- Iterative algorithms without statistical modelling:
  - Used originally by Hounsfield however not commercially used due to computer limitations.
  - Will use an assumption, and will compare to the assumption with its measured data. Then, will continue with iterations until the two datasets are in agreement.

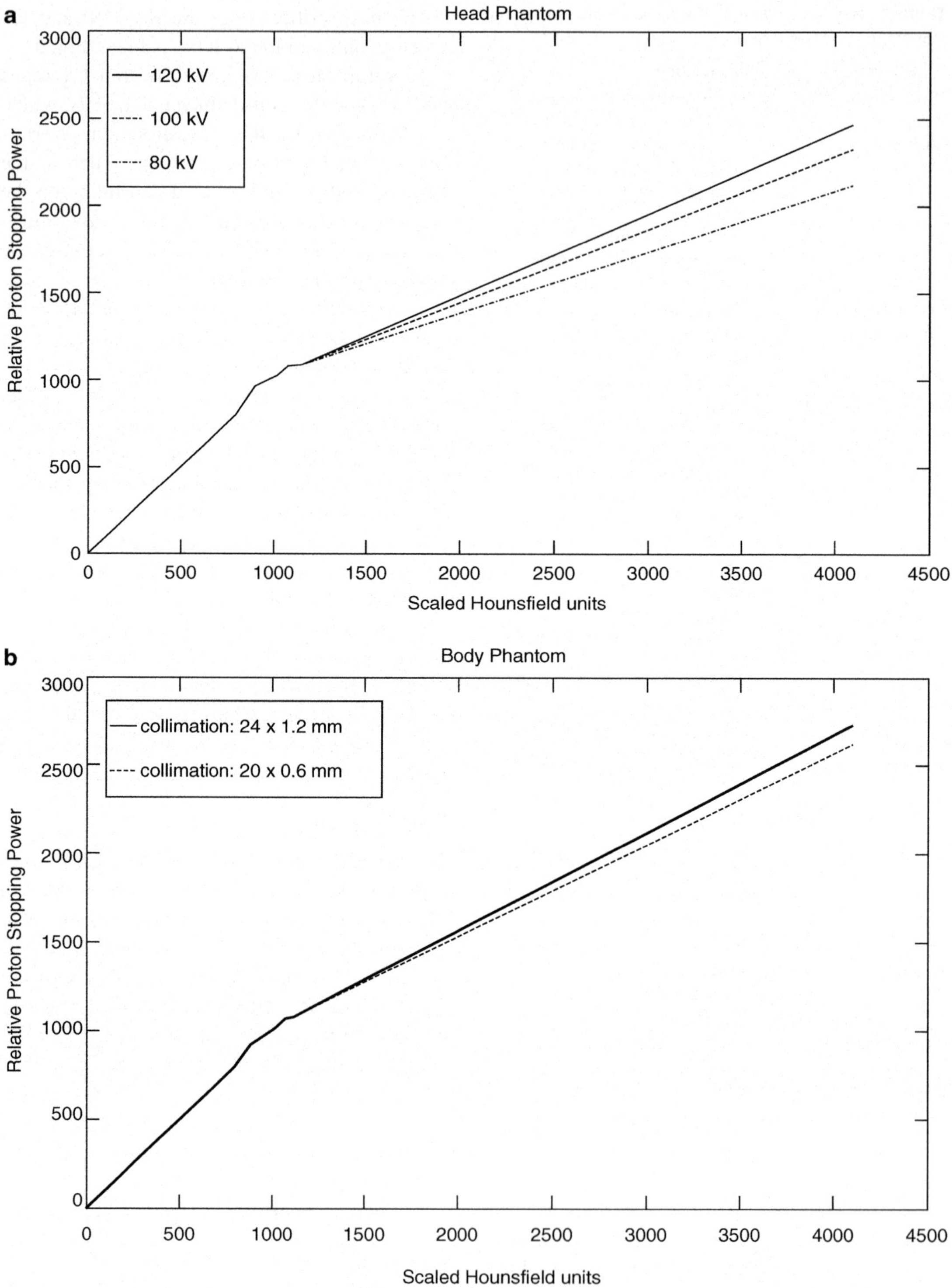

Fig. 5 CT calibration curves of the head phantom obtained with different tube voltages. Scaled HU are computed as 1000 + HU nominal values

- Iterative algorithms with statistical modelling:
  - Iterative reconstruction with statistical modelling that takes into account either:
    - Optics (X-ray source, image voxels, and detector),
    - Noise (photon statistics),
    - Physics (data acquisition),
    - Object (radiation attenuation),
- Back projection:
  - Not used in the clinical setting, as it is unable to produce sharp images.
  - Known for its distinctive artifact that resembles a star.
- Filtered back projection (convolution method):
  - Still widely used in CT today.
  - Utilizes a convolution filter to alleviate the blurring associated with back projection.
  - Fast, however has several limitations including noise and artifact creation.

Additionally, most of the recent scanners provide metal artifacts correction algorithms, which mitigate the streak artifacts, thus resulting in better quality images. Those algorithms can be used with no restrictions for CT scanners dedicated to photon therapy departments, as the HU changes derived by them are very limited. In order to use them for CT image improvements in proton therapy, a careful evaluation of the HU in all the tissues (and not only in the artifacts regions) is strongly recommend, as manufacturers do not guarantee the consistency of the values in case those algorithms are used.

4 QA in CT Simulation

As described above, CT simulators are CT scanners equipped with specialized software, which allows treatment planning on volumetric patient CT scans. They are generally located in a radiation oncology department, and regular quality assurance (QA) program needs to be performed on such machines from the therapy medical physicist.

The QA of CT scanners used as simulator needs to be very comprehensive including two important aspects: imaging CT and treatment planning, as it provides input for the TPS.

The goals of such QA program are explained and detailed in the report of AAPM (Mutic et al. 2003) where multiple goals are listed:

1. Patient, public, and staff safety.
2. Accurate target localization and treatment simulation.

As regards safety, radiation protection measurements are mandatory for CT simulators, and they should comply with standard CT limits. As regards accurate target localization and simulation, the CT scanners must provide high-quality images with accurate geometry. This needs to apply also for CT-on-rails scanners (see par. below), which have been designed for surgical rooms, but they are installed in multiple proton therapy centers.

CT scanners QA should include therefore regular image quality tests and test on the accuracy of the image geometry, which is dependent also on the linearity of the movements either of the tables (for traditional CT) or of the CT scanner (for on-rails devices).

CT scanner QA program should also include accuracy and reproducibility of HU values and constancy of the calibration curve (either to electron density for photon therapy or to proton stopping power, for proton therapy).

As the CT images acquired during the simulation process and used for therapy planning are transferred to the TPS, the transfer process needs to be checked regularly by a proper QA program which needs to guarantee that the accuracy of the geometry and HU values have been preserved in the transfer. Those CT data are also used, via digital reconstructed radiography (DRR) generation, as reference images for the regular (daily or weekly) patient positioning. Therefore, the accuracy of the CT data transfer between the different software used in the clinical workflow has to be guaranteed.

A detailed QA program should therefore include various aspects:

1. CT dosimetry, based on CT dose index (CTDI), regular dose measurements, and measurements of the dose length product (DLP). This should be performed for the specific protocols used during CT simulation.
2. Image quality parameters (i.e., spatial resolution, contrast, contrast resolution) as they are described for diagnostic CT scanners in the AAPM Diagnostic X-Ray Imaging Committee Task Group 2 report (Lin et al. 1993) (see par. 2).
3. Radiation profile and sensitivity to check the collimation as reported in Report 39 of the AAPM.
4. Specific CT simulator checks for gantry tilt, lasers, and couch top. Gantry tilt is a useful feature for diagnostic CT scanners, but normally not used for planning CT acquisitions. If used, the accuracy and reproducibility of the tilt angle and of the reference zero tilt should be tested by the QA program. For accurate patient positioning, both at the simulation and at the therapy, lasers are used in combination with positioning marks on patient skin. Room lasers and CT gantry lasers should be regularly checked as they define the reproducibility of the patient positioning for CT scanner to treatment machine. An alignment tool or a specific phantom is used to check the laser geometry and accuracy.

   CT scanners used for CT simulations are equipped with a specific flat couch top to mimic the treatment couch. To guarantee an accurate daily patient positioning during therapy, the geometric accuracy of the couch top and of the indexing system is necessary; therefore, it should be checked regularly (i.e., flatness of the couch top, accurate and reproducible vertical and longitudinal motion, correct indexing, absence of screws or other devices which could generate artifacts)
5. HU values derived from planning CT will be used for dose calculation in the TPS. Therefore, the accuracy of those CT numbers should be regularly tested with tissue substitute phantoms. The relationship of HU values to electron density (or proton stopping power) is scanner-specific. If multiple scanners are present in the same department, their consistency should also be checked. More details on those checks specific to radiotherapy are presented in the report of the AAPM Radiation Therapy Committee Task Group 53 (Fraas et al. 1998).

5 CT Simulation Tomorrow

Significant advances in radiation oncology have been happening in the last two decades with the introduction of techniques such as intensity-modulated radiation therapy (IMRT), arc therapy, and online image guidance. Improvements on the CT simulations are also a topic of recent research that aims at reducing the uncertainties in the tissue properties determination from the HU values.

Indeed, electron density is the most important tissue property influencing photon and ion dose distributions in radiotherapy patients. Dual-energy computed tomography (DECT) enables the determination of electron density by combining the information on photon attenuation obtained at two different effective X-ray energy spectra (van Elmpt et al. 2016).

Research is also focused on the use of cone beam CT not only for image guidance but also to perform dose calculations as part of daily adaptive radiotherapy. The problem with CBCT-based dose calculation is that planning CT and CBCT imaging differs in how they are influenced by scatter radiation and artifacts, as well as in HU values between them (Islam et al. 2006; Arai et al. 2017).

Use of DECT and CBCT as CT simulators is described in paragraph (5a and 5b). Another area of research, which is now being transferred into clinical operation, is the one related to MRI-based delivery systems. This growing technology allows acquisition of online MRI images which present with the major advantages as compared to CT images: high soft tissue contrast and radiation-free. This will be described in paragraph 5c.

5.1 Dual-Energy CT (DECT)

Dual-energy CT scanners development is not a recent idea, as already in the early days of CT imaging DE techniques were described (Hounsfield 1973). In recent years, DECT imaging has gained attention in radiology departments, and new strategies for the use of DECT in radiation therapy are being investigated (van Elmpt et al. 2016).

Those DECT scans present advantages as they can improve dose calculation accuracy in proton therapy, metal artifact reductions, and normal tissue characterization. Multiple modalities to acquire DECT images are now available: the simplest one is the rotate-rotate DE which acquires two different scans with two different kVp settings sequentially. In this case, the disadvantage is the time differences between the two scans, which might be influenced by patient breathing and motion. Another approach is based on the use of two orthogonal X-rays tubes, which are operated at two different kVp settings. A third technology is based on the fast switch of kV of the single X-rays tube. Alternatively, there are dual-energy layers detectors, which allow the detection of high- and low-energy photons coming from the same tube. The most recent solution is based on the splitting of the X-rays beam into two energy spectra at the kV source, using dedicated filters.

As a result of DE image acquisitions, there are attenuation coefficients calculated for two different energies. Based on the dependence of attenuation coefficient on energy, it is possible to get the material decomposition.

For photon therapy, new calibration schemes using a linear combination of the high- and low-energy scans have resulted in a more accurate estimation of the electron density, thus reducing the dose uncertainties from 11% to 1% for specific geometries (Tsukihara et al. 2015).

As regards proton therapy, DECT has the potential to improve the estimation of the proton stopping power ratio (medium to water, SPR), which is required by pencil beam algorithms to determine the proton range. DECT images can be converted in Rho and *Z* images, which can be directly converted in SPR. A few studies have been published on this topic, and research in this area is very promising (Yang et al. 2010; Saito 2012; van Abbema et al. 2015; Schwahofer et al. 2015). A comprehensive summary of the accuracy of different methods and algorithms is reported in the work of Bär et al. (2017).

DECT is a very interesting technique to reduce metal artifacts, in case of streak artifacts caused by the presence of metal implants. For simulation CT scans, those artifacts compromise accurate imaging, structure delineation electron density, SPR quantification (proton therapy), and consequently the accuracy of the dose calculation. Two studies (Bamberg et al. 2011; Zhou et al. 2011) showed superior image quality compared to standard imaging in the presence of metallic implants.

DECT could also be interesting to improve image quality in the tumor characterization as various tumors present with low contrast on CT imaging which could be improved by the acquisition of CT images at different kVp values of the X-rays tube. Still, no literature has shown increase of delineation accuracy in radiotherapy planning.

5.2 Imaging Methods for Adaptation

Radiation therapy accuracy can be severely impaired by foreseen or not foreseen anatomical changes, which could occur during the entire course of the treatment. Those could derive spontaneously (i.e., weight changes if not impairment of feeding is present) or as a consequence of the therapy (i.e., shrinkage of neck nodes for head and neck cancer patients). Ideally, radiation therapy planning should be updated and adapted in a very short time to take into account such variations. This is particularly true for ions therapy where anatomical changes could dramatically affect range accuracy (Albertini et al. 2008; Placidi et al. 2017).

Ideally, the adaptive planning procedure, based on CT simulations, should be executed daily: this will enable to deliver accurate dose distributions considering the daily anatomy and patient positioning. CT scanners used for planning CT acquisitions should then be located in the room, allowing CT scans performed just before the delivery. Fast dose calculation and QA should be provided as well to complete the radiotherapy planning sequence before delivery.

Linac accelerators are equipped with X-ray sources which can be used to reconstruct CT images, the so-called cone beam computed tomography (CBCT) images. The image quality of CBCT is limited by severe shading artifacts, hindering its quantitative applications in radiation therapy. Compared to conventional CT scanners, cone beam CT image suffers from an increased contribution of scattered radiation (Siewerdsen and Jaffraay 2001). In addition, this contribution is largely dependent on patient geometry. As a result, the CT values of a CBCT cannot simply be converted to electron densities and directly used for dose calculation as this will lead to errors up to 5% for photon radiotherapy, and even larger for proton. Histogram matching algorithms are a current research topic as they allow HU modification between original planning CT and cone beam CT. As a result of this modification, CBCT could be used as planning CT for daily adaptation (van Zijtveld et al. 2007; Onozato et al. 2014). For proton therapy, this conversion and modification are even more critical due to variation of RPSP as a function of HU values. Nevertheless, a recent study has shown that actually this method could potentially be valid also for proton dose calculation (Arai et al. 2016).

As the accuracy of HU evaluation from CT is a well-known problem affecting range accuracy for proton, some institutions have decided to install in-room CT-on-rails. Those systems present the advantage that the patient is in treatment position on the proton-specific treatment couch during image guidance and afterward when driven to the gantry for the delivery. Those CT scanners, as compared to CBCT, present with better image quality, and they can be used as CT simulators in the treatment area, without compromising the HU accuracy. For image guidance protocols, it is instead essential that the evaluation and setup of specific acquisition protocols minimize the CT dose to patients. This choice has also been shared by photon center where soft tissue image guidance and accurate dose recalculation and daily dose adaptation were the main focus (Liu et al. 2014).

5.3 Substitute CT

MR-based delivery system is a growing technology. Several MRI-Linac systems are nowadays under clinical operation. These hybrid machines are designed to acquire online MR images and to track the treatment delivery by stopping the beam radiation when the target structure results outside a boundary set by the user. In the image-guided radiotherapy (IGRT) context, these systems can acquire a daily volumetric magnetic resonance image (MRI) by scanning the patient before starting the treatment session. Therefore, the treatment planning system can then predict the relative dose distribution on the acquired image. Once the dose distribution has been predicted, a treatment plan re-optimization is possible in order to satisfy the required dose constraint, according to the modern vision of adaptive radiotherapy. The electron density (ED) information necessary to calculate dose distribution on MRI are provided by the CT scan acquired during the CT simulation scan. The ED assigned MRI scan is commonly named as substitute CT (sCT) or synthetic CT. In particular, the TPS co-register the CT simulation image on the MRI by rigid and deformable registration, and then, it transfers the ED map from CT to MRI. Obviously one major challenge of performing dose calculations on MRI is the lack of correspondence between the voxel intensity and the associated attenuation property of the tissue, unlike CT images, where the voxel intensity directly reflects the radiological characteristics of the tissue; MRI intensities rather correlate with tissue proton density and the magnetic relaxation. This leads to voxel ambiguity for tissues such as bone and air which both appear dark on MRI although they have very different attenuation coefficient. A complete review of this topic has been performed by Edmund and Nyholm (2017). Further challenges constitute scanner-induced geometric distortion arising from gradient nonlinearity and magnet inhomogeneities and patient-induced artifacts such as susceptibility and chemical shifts (Nyholm et al. 2009). In particular, converting the MRI signal into a CT number further constitutes normalization of absolute signal intensities and data correction strategies such as bias field correction.

6 Conclusion

The identification of the optimal CT acquisition parameter settings (CT scanner protocols), considering the special requirements of CT simulation, is a key factor in order to correctly simulate a radiation treatment condition.

As reported by Davis et al. (2017), the impact of scan parameters in radiotherapy CT is not well-detailed in the literature. Nevertheless, several publications investigate and support the optimization of the scan protocol settings to achieve a significant image quality, considering the radiation dose delivered from CT imaging and tailoring the scan protocols also for the specific disease sites. Optimal parameter settings selection should ensure good-quality imaging with careful assessment of the dosimetric impact for clinical treatment condition.

In the near future, several changes and potential improvements are foreseen for CT scanners used as radiotherapy simulators. First of all, the use of DECT as CT simulators is already starting to be a standard clinical procedure, especially to increase the accuracy of the determination of ED map. CBCT as CT simulators is approaching to be a generalized clinical procedure, in particular to perform dose calculations as part of daily adaptive radiotherapy respectively. Another promising research is to obtain the ED map by MR imaging, above all in the MRI-Linac system. This approach could lead to a radiotherapy MRI-only workflow, removing at all the concept of planning CT, even though several issues have to be assessed before its clinical implementation.

Based on the mentioned topics, the selection of the optimal CT protocol for CT-guided planning preparation is still an essential step to guarantee a high-performance radiotherapy treatments.

References

Albertini F, Bolsi A, Lomax AJ, Rutz HP, Timmerman B, Goitein G (2008) Sensitivity of intensity modulated proton therapy plans to changes in patient weight. Radiother Oncol 86(2):187–194

Arai K, Kadoya N, Kato T, Endo H, Komori S, Abe Y, Nakamura T, Wada H, Kikuchi Y, Takai Y, Jingu K (2017) Feasibility of CBCT-based proton dose calculation using a histogram-matching algorithm in proton beam therapy. Phys Med 33:68–76

Arai K et al (2016) Feasibility of CBCT-based proton dose calculation using a histogram-matching algorithm in proton beam therapy. Phys Med 33:68–76

Bamberg F, Dierks A, Nikolaou K, Reiser MF, Becker CR, Johnson TR (2011) Metal artifact reduction by dual energy computed tomography using monoenergetic extrapolation. Eur Radiol 21:1424 1429

Bär E, Lalonde A, Royle G, Lu HM, Bouchard H (2017) The potential of dual-energy CT to reduce proton beam range uncertainties. Med Phys 44(6):2332–2344. https://doi.org/10.1002/mp.12215. Epub 2017 Apr 21

Conway J, Robinson MH (1997) CT virtual simulation. Br J Radiol 70(Suppl):S106–S118

Davis AT, Palmer AL, Nisbet A (2017) Can CT scan protocols used for radiotherapy treatment planning be adjusted to optimize image quality and patient dose? A systematic review. Br J Radiol 90(1076):20160406

Edmund JM, Nyholm T (2017) A review of substitute CT generation for MRI-only radiation therapy. Radiat Oncol 12:28., Published online 2017 Jan 26. https://doi.org/10.1186/s13014-016-0747-y

Fraas B et al (1998) American Association of Physicists in Medicine Radiation Therapy Committee Task Group 53: quality assurance for clinical radiotherapy treatment planning. Med Phys 25:1773–1829

Goitein M, Abrams M, Rowell D, Pollari H, Wiles J (1983) Multi-dimensional treatment planning: II. Beam's eye view, back projection, and projection through CT sections. Int J Radiat Oncol Biol Phys 9:789–797

Goo HW (2011) Individualized volume CT dose index determined by cross-sectional area and mean density of the body to achieve uniform image noise of contrast-enhanced pediatric chest CT obtained at variable kV levels and with combined tube current modulation. Pediatr Radiol 41:839–847

Goo HW, Suh DS (2006) Tube current reduction in pediatric non-ECG-gated heart CT by combined tube current modulation. Pediatr Radiol 36:344–351

Goo HW (2012) CT radiation dose optimisation and estimation: an update for radiologists. Korean J Radiol 13(1):1–11

Guan H, Yin FF, Kim JH (2002) Accuracy of inhomogeneity correction in photon radiotherapy from CT scans with different settings. Phys Med Biol 47(17):N223–N231

Hounsfield GN (1973) Computerized transverse axial scanning (tomography). 1. Description of system. Br J Radiol 46:1016–1022

Irie T, Inoue H (2005) Individual modulation of the tube current-seconds to achieve similar levels of image noise in contrast-enhanced abdominal CT. AJR Am J Roentgenol 184:1514–1518
Islam MK, Purdie TG, Norrlinger BD et al (2006) Patient dose from kilovoltage cone beam computed tomography imaging in radiation therapy. Med Phys 33:1573–1582
Israel GM, Herlihy S, Rubinowitz AN, Cornfeld D, Brink J (2008) Does a combination of dose modulation with fast gantry rotation time limit CT image quality? AJR Am J Roentgenol 191:140–144
Lee CH, Goo JM, Ye HJ, Ye SJ, Park CM, Chun EJ et al (2008) Radiation dose modulation techniques in the multidetector CT era: from basics to practice. Radiographics 28:1451–1459
Li J, Xiao Y (2013) Application of FDG-PET/CT in radiation oncology. Front Oncol 3:1–6
Lin P., Beck T., Borras C., Cohen G, Jucius R.A., Kriz R.J., Nickoloff E.L., Rothenberg L.N., Strauss K.J., Villafana T. et al. (1993) Specification and acceptance testing of computed tomography scanners. AAPM Report no. 39 of AAPM Task Group 2
Liu F, Ahunbay E, Lawton C, Li XA (2014) Assessment and management of interfractional variations in daily diagnostic-quality-CT guided prostate-bed irradiation after prostatectomy. Med Phys. 41(3):031710
Liu RR, Prado KL, Cody D (2008) Optimal acquisition parameter selection for CT simulators in radiation oncology. JACMP 9(4):2878
McCullough EC (1990) Radiotherapy treatment simulators. AAPM Monograph No 19, 491–499
McCullough EC, Earl JD (1979) The selection, acceptance testing and quality control of radiotherapy treatment simulators. Radiology 131:221–230
McNitt-Gray MF (2002) AAPM/RSNA physics tutorial for residents: topics in CT. Radiation dose in CT. Radiographics 22(6):1541–1553. Review
McShan DL, Silverman A, Lanza D, Reinstein L, Glicksman A (1979) Three dimensional radiation treatment planning and dose display utilizing interactive color graphics. Br J Radiol 52:478–481
Mohan R (1988) 3-D radiation treatment planning. Int J Radiat Oncol Biol Phys 15:481–495
Mutic S, Palta J, Das I et al (2003) Quality assurance for computed-tomography simulators and the computed-tomography simulation process: report of the AAPM radiation therapy committee task group no. 66. Med Phys 30(10):2762–2792
Nyholm T, Nyberg M, Karlsson MG, Karlsson M (2009) Systematization of spatial uncertainties for comparison between a MR and a CT-based radiotherapy workflow for prostate treatments. Radiat Oncol 4:54. https://doi.org/10.1186/1748-717X-4-54
Onozato Y, Kadoya N, Fujita Y, Arai K, Dobashi S, Takeda K, Kishi K, Umezawa R, Matsushita H, Jingu K (2014) Evaluation of on-board kV cone beam computed tomography-based dose calculation with deformable image registration using Hounsfield unit modifications. Int J Radiat Oncol Biol Phys 89(2):416–423
Pedroni E, Shaffner B (1998) The precision of proton range calculations in proton radiotherapy treatment planning: experimental verification of the relation between CT-HU and proton stopping power. Phys Med Biol 43(6):1579–1592
Placidi L, Bolsi A, Lomax AJ, Schneider RA, Malyapa R, Weber DC, Albertini F (2017) Effect of anatomic changes on pencil beam scanned proton dose distributions for cranial and extracranial tumours. Int J Radiat Oncol Biol Phys 97(3):616–623
Prakash P, Kalra MK, Gilman MD, Shepard JA, Digumarthy SR (2010) Is weight-based adjustment of automatic exposure control necessary for the reduction of chest CT radiation dose? Korean J Radiol 11: 46–53
Saito M (2012) Potential of dual-energy subtraction for converting CT numbers to electron density based on a single linear relationship. Med Phys 39:2021–2030
Schneider U, Pedroni E, Lomax A (1996) The calibration of CT Hounsfield unit for radiotherapy treatment planning. Phys Med Biol 41:111–124
Schwahofer A, Bar E, Kuchenbecker S, Grossmann JG, Kachelriess M, Sterzing F (2015) The application of metal artifact reduction (MAR) in CT scans for radiation oncology by monoenergetic extrapolation with a DECT scanner. Z Med Phys 25:314
Seco J, Evans PM (2006) Assessing the effect of electron density in photon dose calculations. Med Phys 33(2):540–552
Sherouse GW (1998) Radiotherapy treatment simulators. In: Khan FM, Potish R (eds) Treatment planning in radiation oncology. Williams & Wilkins, Baltiore, MD, pp 39–53
Sherouse GW, Bourland JD, Reynolds K et al (1990a) Virtual simulation in the clinical setting: some practical consideration. Int J Radiat Oncol Biol Phys 19:1059–1065
Sherouse GW, Chaney EL (1991) The portable virtual simulator. Int J Radiat Oncol Biol Phys 21:475–481
Sherouse GW, Mosher CE, Novins KL, Rosenmann JG, Chaney EL (1987) Virtual simulation: concept and implementation. In: Bruinvis IAD, van der Giessen PH, van Kleffens HJ, Wittkamper FW (eds) Ninth International Conference on the Use of Computers in Radiation Therapy. North Holland Publishing Co., Amsterdam, The Netherlands, pp 433–436
Sherouse GW, Novins KL, Chaney EL (1990b) Computation of digitally reconstructed radiographs for use in radiotherapy treatment design. Int J Radiat Oncol Biol Phys 18:651–658
Siewerdsen JH, Jaffraay DA (2001) Cone-beam computed tomography with a flat-panel imager: magnitude and effects of X rays scatter. Med Phys 28:220–231
Soukup M, Fippel M, Alber M (2005) A pencil beam algorithm for intensity modulated proton therapy derived from Monte Carlo simulations. Phys Med Biol 50(21):5089–5104

The Phantom Laboratory Inc (2002) Catphan manual. The Phantom Laboratory Inc., Salem, New York

Tsukihara M, Noto Y, Sasamoto R, Hayakawa T, Saito M (2015) Initial implementation of the conversion from the energy-subtracted CT number to electron density in tissue inhomogeneity corrections: an anthropomorphic phantom study of radiotherapy treatment planning. Med Phys 42:1378

van Abbema JK, van Goethem MJ, Greuter MJ, van der Schaaf A, Brandenburg S, van der Graaf ER (2015) Relative electron density determination using a physics based parameterization of photon interactions in medical DECT. Phys Med Biol 60(9):3825–3846

van Elmpt W, Landry G, Das M, Verhaegen F (2016) Dual energy CT in radiotherapy: Current applications and future outlook. Radiother Oncol 119(1):137–144. https://doi.org/10.1016/j.radonc.2016.02.026. Epub 2016 Mar 11. Review

van Zijtveld M, Dirkx M, Heijmen B (2007) Correction of cone beam CT values using a planning CT for derivation of the "dose of the day". Radiother Oncol 85(2):195–200

Vedam SS, Keal PK, Kini VR et al (2003) Acquiring a four-dimensional computed tomography dataset using an external respiratory signal. Phys Med Biol 48:45–62

Yang M et al (2010) Theoretical variance analysis of single- and dual-energy computed tomography methods for calculating proton stopping power ratios of biological tissues. Phys Med Biol 55:1343–1362

Zhou C, Zhao YE, Luo S, Shi H, Li L, Zheng L et al (2011) Monoenergetic imaging of dual-energy CT reduces artifacts from implanted metal orthopedic devices in patients with factures. Acad Radiol 18:1252–1257

Management of Respiratory-Induced Tumour Motion for Tailoring Target Volumes during Radiation Therapy

Willem Grootjans, Jennifer Dhont, Bas Gobets, and Dirk Verellen

Contents

1 **Management of Respiratory-Induced Tumour Motion in the Era of High-Precision Radiotherapy** ... 48

2 **The Radiotherapy Workflow** ... 49
2.1 Pretreatment Imaging for Radiotherapy Planning ... 49
2.2 Target Delineation ... 50
2.3 Radiotherapy Planning ... 50
2.4 Position Verification and Treatment Delivery ... 51

3 **Radiotherapy of Mobile Target Lesions** ... 51
3.1 Respiratory Motion Artefacts in Pretreatment Imaging ... 51
3.2 Radiotherapy Planning of Mobile Target Lesions ... 53
3.3 Radiotherapy Techniques for Mobile Target Lesions ... 56
3.4 Real-Time Tumour Tracking Using the Linear Accelerator ... 59
3.5 Multi-Leaf Collimator and Couch Tracking ... 61

4 **Inter-Fraction Geometrical Uncertainties and the Promise of Adaptive Radiotherapy** ... 62

5 **Future Prospects** ... 62

References ... 64

E pur si muove: *Galileo Galilei (1564–1642).*

W. Grootjans (✉)
Department of Radiology, Leiden University Medical Center, Leiden, The Netherlands
e-mail: W.Grootjans@lumc.nl

J. Dhont
Department of Radiotherapy, Universitair Ziekenhuis Brussel, Vrije Universiteit Brussel, Brussel, Belgium

B. Gobets
Department of Radiation Oncology, Leiden University Medical Center, Leiden, The Netherlands

D. Verellen
Department of Radiotherapy, Iridium Kankernetwerk, University of Antwerp, Faculty of Medicine and Health Sciences, Antwerp, Belgium

Faculty of Medicine and Pharmacy, Vrije Universiteit Brussel, Brussels, Belgium

Abstract

Radiotherapy is one of the main treatment modalities in modern day's oncology practice and is used to treat tumours in up to 50% of all cancer patients. The key to successful delivery of a high radiation dose to the tumour without causing unacceptable toxicity of normal tissues is the use of treatment fractionation. During fractionated radiotherapy, it is of importance to reduce inter- and intra-fraction geometrical uncertainties in order to ensure adequate dose delivery to the tumour and preventing unnecessary irradiation of normal tissues. Geometrical uncertainties can be the result of many different factors, including patient set-up, mechanical errors, patient or organ motion, and anatomical changes during

R. G. H. Beets-Tan et al. (eds.), *Imaging and Interventional Radiology for Radiation Oncology*,
Medical Radiology, Diagnostic Imaging, https://doi.org/10.1007/978-3-030-38261-2_4

the course of treatment. Of these factors, respiratory induced organ motion significantly contributes to geometrical uncertainties during radiotherapy. Therefore, adequate management of moving targets during radiotherapy contributes to the reduction of geometrical uncertainties in radiotherapy planning and improves accuracy of dose delivery. Many technological solutions have been developed for management of respiratory motion during radiotherapy. These include the use of different planning methods in combination with conventional radiotherapy techniques, respiratory gated radiotherapy, and real-time tumour tracking approaches. This chapter will provide an overview of the most important radiotherapy strategies to account for organ motion due to patient respiration. Different technical considerations and solutions regarding respiratory motion management during all the steps of radiotherapy workflow will be discussed.

1 Management of Respiratory-Induced Tumour Motion in the Era of High-Precision Radiotherapy

Radiotherapy is one of the main treatment modalities in modern day's oncology practice and is used to treat tumours in up to 50% of all cancer patients (Rosenblatt et al. 2013; Borras et al. 2015). The sole purpose of radiotherapy in this setting is to control malignant cell growth by means of delivering a high dose of ionizing radiation to cancerous tissues whilst sparing normal healthy tissues around the tumour as much as possible. The primary mechanism by which ionizing radiation will damage tissue is through ionization of molecular structures, particularly deoxyribonucleic acid (DNA), resulting in direct killing of cells (Baskar et al. 2014). Furthermore, generation of free radicals by excitation of water molecules in cells can cause indirect damage to these cellular structures (Baskar et al. 2014). The key to successful delivery of a high radiation dose to the tumour without causing unacceptable toxicity of normal tissues is the use of treatment fractionation (Baskar et al. 2014). It is observed that when the total radiation dose is divided into several smaller fractions over a period of several days, healthy cells have the ability to recover whilst cancerous cells tend to accumulate damage due to intrinsic genetic instability and deregulation of molecular pathways. Depending on the cancer type, radiotherapy is typically delivered in up to 35 fractions.

During fractionated radiotherapy, it is of importance to reduce inter- and intra-fraction geometrical uncertainties. Geometrical uncertainties arise due to the fact that the position and shape of the target lesion during treatment delivery can deviate from the position and shape during treatment planning, which can eventually result in errors in dose delivery to the target volume (Ekberg et al. 1998; Urie et al. 1991). Error in dose delivery in this setting is defined as the difference between planned and the actual delivered dose to the target volume and healthy surrounding tissues (van Herk 2004). This can be the result of many different factors, including patient set-up, mechanical errors, patient or organ motion and anatomical changes during the course of treatment. Geometrical uncertainties can be modelled as systematic and random errors. Systematic errors can be interpreted as the average set-up error over all fractions, whilst random errors are all variations that occur during a single fraction or between successive fractions (de Boer et al. 2001).

In view of advances in radiotherapy techniques over the last decade, such as intensity-modulated radiotherapy (IMRT) and volumetric-modulated arc therapy (VMAT), which made it possible to create dose distributions with steep dose fall-off around the target volume, the reduction of geometrical uncertainties is an important aspect to ensure an adequate dose coverage of designated target volumes and to avoid irradiation of normal tissues (Connell and Hellman 2009). This is particularly important in hypofractionated radiotherapy, such as stereotactic body radiotherapy (SBRT), where the radiation dose is delivered in fewer fractions at a higher dose per fraction (Giraud et al. 2011). The most important factors contributing to geometrical uncertainties are anatomical shifts resulting in baseline variation in anatomy (e.g. bladder filling) (Chen et al. 2016), organ motion due to patient physiology (e.g. respiration, cardiac motion) (van Herk 2004; Korreman 2012), intra-fraction patient movement, uncertainties in target lesion delineation and patient set-up. In this setting, random uncertainties will cause blurring of the planned dose around the target, whilst systematic uncertainties cause a shift of the delivered dose with respect to the planned dose (Engelsman et al. 2001).

Reduction of geometrical uncertainties in radiotherapy starts with accurately delineating the target volume and performing adequate patient positioning before each radiotherapy fraction (Urie et al. 1991; van Herk 2004). Both steps require the use of appropriate medical imaging modalities before and during radiotherapy, which will be discussed in more detail later in this chapter. Furthermore, organ motion can be a significant source of uncertainty in radiotherapy (Bortfeld et al. 2002). Different radiotherapy strategies have been developed in an attempt to adequately manage the effects of organ motion during radiotherapy. Of the various sources of organ motion, respiratory motion will generally result in the largest organ movement. Therefore, many technological solutions have been developed for the management of respiratory motion during radiotherapy, often making use of its inherent periodic nature. In a number of cases, organ motion due to patient respiration can result in the requirement for large planning margins to ensure adequate coverage of the target volume and the delivery of a high radiation dose to normal tissues. Furthermore, organ motion may interfere with the dynamics of the modern radiotherapy treatment itself, as parameters such as field shape and dose rate are varied continuously on a timescale comparable with that of organ motion, resulting in inaccuracies in the dose delivery (Korreman 2012). The specific errors in dose delivery due to these interplay effects are difficult to estimate and will strongly depend on the specific frequencies, directions and amplitudes of all dynamic processes involved. Although such interplay effects on errors in dose delivery are predictable in conventional radiotherapy fractionation schemes where radiotherapy is delivered over many fractions, causing blurring of the planned dose, the result of interplay effects in case of hypofractionation is more unpredictable (Bortfeld et al. 2004; Hubley and Pierce 2017).

Therefore, adequate management of moving targets during radiotherapy can significantly contribute to the reduction of geometrical uncertainties in radiotherapy planning and improve accuracy of dose delivery. This chapter will provide an overview of the most important radiotherapy strategies to account for organ motion due to patient respiration. The chapter will start with a brief overview of the radiotherapy workflow, given that motion management strategies are typically involved throughout the entire radiotherapy process. Subsequently, different technical considerations and solutions regarding respiratory motion management during all the steps of radiotherapy workflow will be discussed. The chapter will conclude with a short discussion on considerations for management of interfraction uncertainties.

2 The Radiotherapy Workflow

2.1 Pretreatment Imaging for Radiotherapy Planning

Although specific requirements for radiotherapy will vary between different patients and cancer types, all radiotherapy protocols adhere to the same basic workflow, starting with pretreatment imaging for the purpose of treatment planning. Traditionally, X-ray computed tomography (CT) imaging is the most important imaging modality used in radiotherapy, as discussed in Chap. 3. The CT images provide the radiation oncologist and dosimetrist with valuable information regarding both the anatomy and spatial distribution of tissue densities within the patients. The latter is an important prerequisite for accurate dose calculations. Figure 1 depicts such a dose distribution of a radiotherapy plan projected over a CT image for a patient treated for non-small-cell lung cancer (NSCLC).

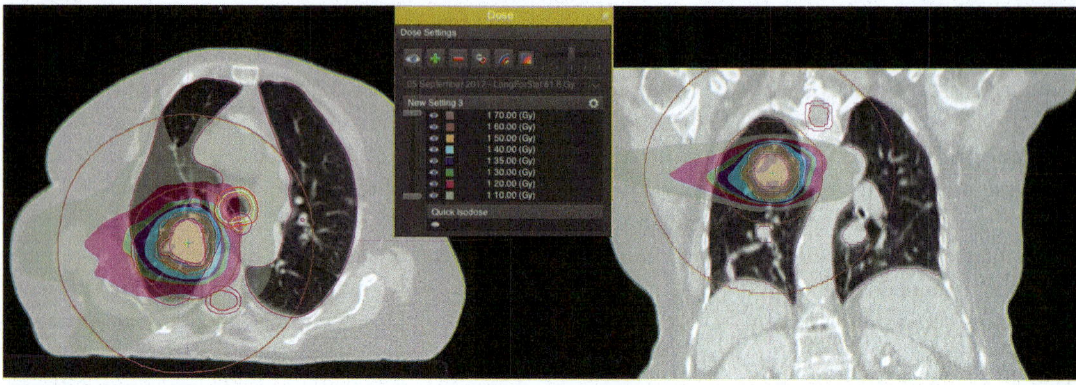

Fig. 1 Planned dose distribution of a patient treated for non-small-cell lung cancer with intensity-modulated radiotherapy, projected over the maximum exhale phase of the 4DCT. On the pretreatment 4DCT, target motion of 0.5 cm could be observed. An internal target volume (ITV) approach, explained later in this chapter, was applied in the context of motion management

2.2 Target Delineation

After pretreatment CT imaging, it is of importance to identify and delineate target lesions on these images. The CT images are being used by the radiation oncologist to (semiautomatically) delineate the correct target volumes and nearby organs at risk (OARs). Delineation of the target volumes on medical images results in generation of a gross tumour volume (GTV). Usually, the GTV will be expanded to cover subclinical disease that is not readily depicted by imaging, yielding a clinical target volume (CTV).

In this setting, careful delineation of the GTV using medical images is of great importance, since error in GTV delineation is currently considered to be one of the major sources of systematic uncertainty (Guckenberger et al. 2017). Furthermore, there are a number of other inter- and intra-fraction variabilities, as mentioned in the introduction of this chapter, that have to be taken into account. This is performed by creating a planning target volume (PTV), ensuring that the prescribed dose will be delivered to the entire CTV with a clinically acceptable probability given these uncertainties. The PTV is created by adding a safety margin to the CTV, taking all relevant (geometrical) uncertainties into account that arise during radiotherapy and compromise adequate dose delivery (Burnet et al. 2004).

Whilst CT is the imaging modality of choice for EBRT planning and dosimetry, delineation of GTVs can be challenging due to limited soft tissue contrast CT images provide. In numerous situations, cancer lesions and metastatic lymph nodes have a density similar to normal tissues, rendering accurate depiction of the tumour on CT images challenging (Njeh 2008). These difficulties associated with target delineation can be resolved through addition of other imaging modalities during radiotherapy planning, such as positron emission tomography (PET) (Grootjans et al. 2016) and magnetic resonance (MR) imaging. Indeed, modern treatment planning systems provide tools for multimodality image registration and target lesion delineation. Additionally, the advantage of using different imaging modalities is that additional information regarding tumour biology can be considered, facilitating in treatment choice and the creation of a more personalized treatment plan, such as molecularly imaging-based dose painting techniques (Bentzen and Gregoire 2011; Grootjans et al. 2015). Furthermore, with improved depiction of the target lesions, intra- and interobserver variability regarding target delineation can be considerably reduced (van Baardwijk et al. 2007).

2.3 Radiotherapy Planning

In the radiotherapy planning stage, all parameters of the radiation delivery are optimized for the specific geometry of the patient and choice of treatment. For this purpose, CT images are used to create a virtual patient. Based on this virtual patient, the positions and intensity of the external radiation beams are optimized for the specific geometry of the patient. The Hounsfield units on CT images can be used to calculate the attenuation of the megavolt (MV) photons used for treatment and generate a planned dose distribution within the patient. The radiotherapy plan will be evaluated for dose coverage of the PTV and whether the dose to the OARs does not exceed the predefined dose constraints.

2.4 Position Verification and Treatment Delivery

In current clinical practice, dose delivery during the course of treatment will generally be performed according to a single pretreatment radiotherapy plan. Therefore, accurate and reproducible set-up of the patient between radiotherapy fractions is of importance to ensure adequate coverage of the CTV and prevent unnecessary irradiation of normal tissues. Generally, errors in set-up can be divided in mechanical and geometrical errors. Mechanical errors are minimized by performing regular quality assurance and acceptance testing. Geometrical errors are minimized by using skin markers in combination with laser positioning systems and immobilization devices. Furthermore, after patient alignment using external markers, position verification of internal anatomy is of great importance. In this regard, in-room image guidance is an essential part for adequate patient set-up. Current in-room imaging modalities include planar X-ray imaging, electronic portal imaging device (EPID) using the megavolt (MV) treatment beam, cone-beam CT (CBCT) and, to a lesser extent, ultrasound imaging (Verellen et al. 2007). Furthermore, in-room MR image guidance is also increasingly being implemented in clinical theatres. Using image guidance, the position of the target lesion can be verified any time during treatment, making it possible to compensate for errors in dose delivery due to shifts in anatomy with respect to the original radiotherapy plan. However, different imaging modalities have varying accuracies regarding position verification of the target lesion, and remaining uncertainties should always be incorporated in the PTV. Furthermore, when imaging relies on the use of ionizing radiation, a balance should be found between delivery accuracy and imaging dose to the patient.

3 Radiotherapy of Mobile Target Lesions

3.1 Respiratory Motion Artefacts in Pretreatment Imaging

3.1.1 X-Ray Computed Tomography Imaging

Management of organ motion due to patient respiration in radiotherapy starts with adequate depiction of the target lesion using medical imaging. If not corrected for, respiratory motion during free-breathing CT imaging will result in distortion of local anatomy during image acquisition (Barrett and Keat 2004). The root cause of these artefacts is the dynamic interaction between image acquisition and the asynchronous motion of local anatomy (Rietzel et al. 2005). These artefacts typically consist of blurring, slice shuffling or discontinuity artefacts, depending on the exact nature and speed of the shift in local anatomy (Rietzel et al. 2005; Hertanto et al. 2012; Lu et al. 2005).

Organ motion due to the respiratory cycle is complex, consisting of translations, rotations, deformations and possible hysteresis (Seppenwoolde et al. 2002). In order to ensure adequate dose coverage of the CTV, without geographical misses and exceeding radiation dose limits to normal tissues, recording the trajectory of the target lesion during the respiratory cycle is of great importance. Several techniques have been developed to capture movement of target lesions due to the respiratory cycle of the patient. However, the imaging technique chosen for treatment planning is closely linked to the radiotherapy technique that is being used. In this regard, slow CT scanning techniques, in which the tube rotation time and pitch are considerably reduced, have been reported to capture all possible positions of the patient's anatomy in the respiratory cycle in a single acquisition (Lagerwaard et al. 2001). These time-averaged blurred images are then used for target delineation and radiotherapy planning. These slow CT scanning techniques are typically being used to generate internal target volumes (ITVs) during radiotherapy planning, as discussed in the radiotherapy planning section of this chapter. Alternatively to slow CT scanning, monitoring of the tumour trajectory can be performed using respiration-correlated 4DCT imaging (De Ruysscher et al. 2010).

As discussed in Chap. 3, a 4DCT scan consists of a series of 3DCT scans representing different moments in the breathing cycle, adding a fourth dimension, time, to the CT scan. This provides the radiation oncologist with important information regarding the internal displacement of anatomy during a respiratory cycle (Rietzel et al. 2005). This can be accomplished by recording a respiratory surrogate signal simultaneously with the CT data (van der Geld et al. 2008; Underberg et al. 2004). The respiratory surrogate signal essentially tracks the respiration of the patient during image acquisition using respiratory tracking sensors. Respiratory tracking sensors include pressure sensors, thermocouples, spirometers and fiducial markers used in combination with video tracking (Korreman 2012). These sensors measure different physiological parameters, such as thoracic wall excursions, temperature of breathed air, airflow and volume, that are correlated with respiration of the patient.

The respiratory surrogate signal is then used to sort the acquired imaging data to specific respiratory phases, generating static images depicting the position of anatomy at these different respiratory phases. Methods that have been used to correct images for respiratory motion artefacts are collectively referred to as respiratory gating. Removal of respiratory motion artefacts from the CT images improves shape fidelity of the depicted anatomy and delineation of target lesions. Respiratory gating can be generally categorized as prospective and retrospective respiratory gating approaches. Prospective and retrospective respiratory gating typically rely on acquisition of a respiratory surrogate signal that is correlated with patient respiration using external markers or sensors (Korreman 2012). During retrospective gating, these surrogate signals are used to sort acquired imaging data that has already been acquired. This differs from prospective gating strategies, where imaging data will only be acquired prospectively when the respiratory signal falls within the set gating level (Nehmeh et al. 2011). For 4DCT imaging, both prospective and retrospective respiratory gating methods are employed by different manufacturers.

Depending on the respiratory gating method, sorting of imaging data into different bins can be performed with respect to time (phase-based binning) or amplitude (amplitude-based binning) of the respiratory surrogate signal (Abdelnour et al. 2007; Jani et al. 2013; Dawood et al. 2007). During phase-based binning, each bin represents an equal percentage of the period of the respiratory waveform. In radiotherapy, phase-based binning is often used and can be exploited to calculate the delivered radiation dose over the entire breathing cycle by summation of the dose in each 4DCT frame. However, in case of retrospective binning, misalignments and artefacts easily arise due to irregularities in the breathing pattern (Li et al. 2012), while prospective respiratory gating techniques can result in unacceptable lengthening of image acquisition time. Therefore, care should be taken by appropriately perform patient setup and instruct the patient before image acquisition. The second binning approach is amplitude-based, where each bin represents a percentage of the inhale or exhale amplitude of the respiratory waveform. Although this method is less prone to imaging artefacts, it still suffers from breath-to-breath amplitude variations and does not contain information directly related to time. Given that a typical 4DCT scan is acquired over multiple breathing cycles, it is implicitly assumed that the internal displacement of anatomy is constant between the different breathing cycles. Typically, a number of 10–12 bins are used to capture tumour motion during the respiratory cycle. Figure 2 depicts an amplitude-based reconstructed 4DCT image set of a patient with a NSCLC lesion in the right lower lung lobe.

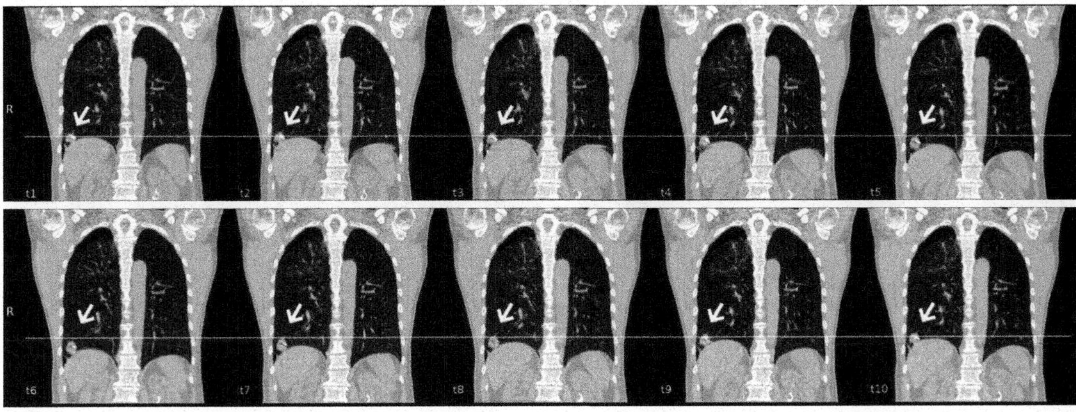

Fig. 2 Amplitude-based reconstructed 4DCT set consisting of 10 breathing phases of a patient with a non-small-cell lung cancer lesion in the right lower lung lobe (white arrow). A high-contrast implanted marker is visible within the target lesion. The horizontal white line serves as a reference to illustrate the cranio-caudal motion of the lesion throughout the breathing cycle. It can also be observed that the patient suffered from mild pneumothorax due to the implantation of the fiducial marker

The advantage of 4DCT imaging is that these images more accurately depict the patient's anatomy at different respiratory phases, whereas the blurred slow CT images inadequately depict the true size and shape of anatomical structures, particularly for the target lesion. If not taken into account, this can potentially result in inadequate dose coverage or a substantial increase of the target volumes.

3.1.2 Respiratory Gating in Other Imaging Modalities

Similar to CT imaging, MR and PET images suffer from respiratory motion artefacts. Due to the relatively long acquisition times, particularly for PET images, respiratory motion during image acquisition results mostly in blurring of anatomy due to averaging of imaging data over multiple respiratory cycles (Grootjans et al. 2014). Given that PET and MR imaging provide important information for target delineation, these images should be ideally matched directly to the pretreatment CT images. Similar strategies have been proposed to perform respiratory gating for PET and MRI images, where the simultaneous recording of a respiratory surrogate signal is used to sort imaging data into different respiratory phases (Chang et al. 2010). Figure 3 depicts a standard free-breathing (non-gated) and optimally respiratory-gated (ORG) $[^{18}F]$fluorodeoxyglucose ($[^{18}F]$FDG) PET image of a patient with a NSCLC lesion in the left lower lung lobe, demonstrating the effects of respiratory motion artefacts on morphological appearance and image quantification. If images from MRI and PET are to be used in radiotherapy planning, respiratory gating and adequate spatial mating of these images with the acquired CT images is essential.

3.2 Radiotherapy Planning of Mobile Target Lesions

3.2.1 The Internal Target Volume and Mid-Ventilation Concept

In case of tumour motion during radiotherapy, delineation of GTVs and subsequent generation of CTVs and PTVs can be performed in different ways. Commonly, the concept of the ITV is used to treat mobile target lesions. Delineation of the ITV is typically performed by using a blurred slow 3DCT or creating a maximum intensity projection (MIP) from the 4DCT image set. The MIP images are created by selecting the maximum voxel value at each image position in the entire 4DCT image set. The resulting ITV is a volume which encompasses all possible positions that the target lesions can occupy during the respiratory cycle and is essentially a composite CTV repre-

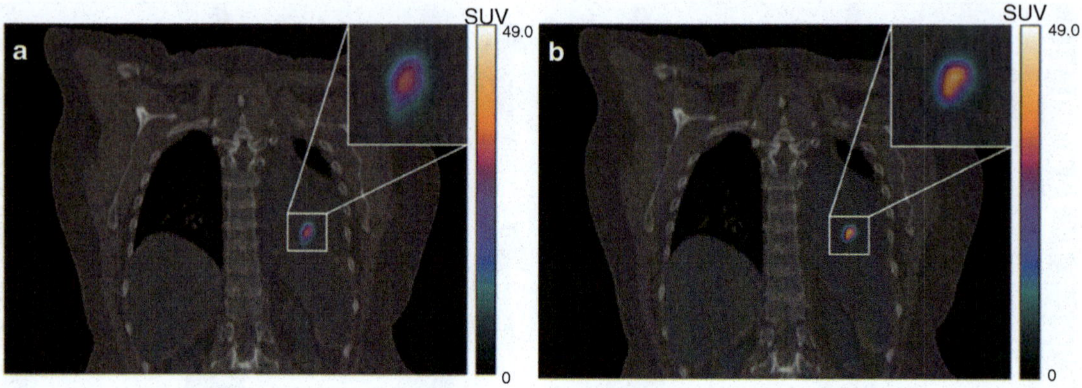

Fig. 3 Coronal non-gated and optimally respiratory-gated (ORG) positron emission tomography (PET) images of a patient with a non-small-cell lung cancer (NSCLC) lesion in the left lower lobe fused with low dose CT (LDCT) images. (**a**) Non-gated PET image fused with an LDCT image; (**b**) ORG PET image reconstructed with a 35% duty cycle fused with a LDCT image. The PET and CT images are displayed with equal window-level settings. In addition to a different morphological appearance of the lesion between the non-gated and ORG PET images, there is a considerable increase in mean standardized uptake value (SUV) of 31.9% and a decrease in volume of 23.0% (Adapted from Grootjans et al. 2014)

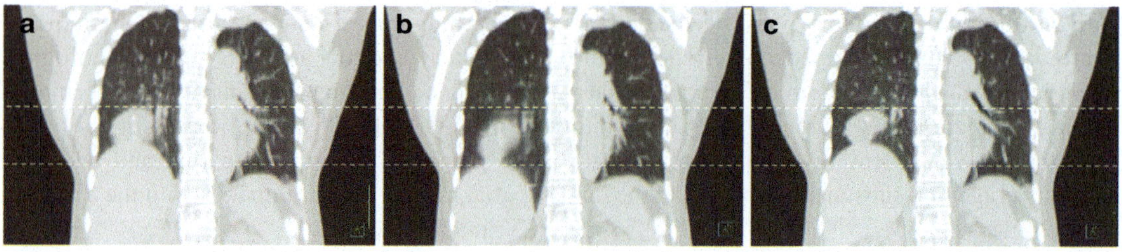

Fig. 4 Maximum intensity projection (MIP) (**a**) and 0% (**b**) and 50% (**c**) phase images of the 4DCT of a stage III non-small-cell lung cancer (NSCLC) patient. The volume encompassing the motion path of the tumour is underestimated using only the MIP, since part of the tumour trajectory is hidden behind the MIP of the diaphragm. An internal target volume (ITV) delineated using the maximum intensity projection (MIP) should therefore always be verified, and extended when necessary, using the phase images. The white dashed lines indicate the real range of the cranio-caudal motion obtained from the phase images

sented at different phases of the respiratory cycle (Shih et al. 2004). In case delineation is performed using the 4DCT MIP image, individual images of the respiratory phases will still need to be checked to determine whether the tumour is sufficiently covered. Particularly if the lesion is situated near other moving anatomical structures, the MIP image can mask a part of the tumour trajectory, as depicted in Fig. 4.

Given that the ITV will cover the entire trajectory of the lesion, lesion motion is effectively treated as if it was a single stationary target (Peulen et al. 2014). Although the ITV approach is a valid strategy for appropriate dose coverage of the entire target lesion, with high reported local control rates (Lagerwaard et al. 2008) for patients with lesions that demonstrate considerable motion during therapy, the ITV will increase considerably. This results in increased exposure of normal tissues to high radiation doses and subsequently higher normal tissue complication probabilities (NTCP), limiting the possibility to perform dose escalation. Given that the ITV will cover the entire tumour trajectory, the ITV methods result in the largest, and thus most suboptimal, target volume.

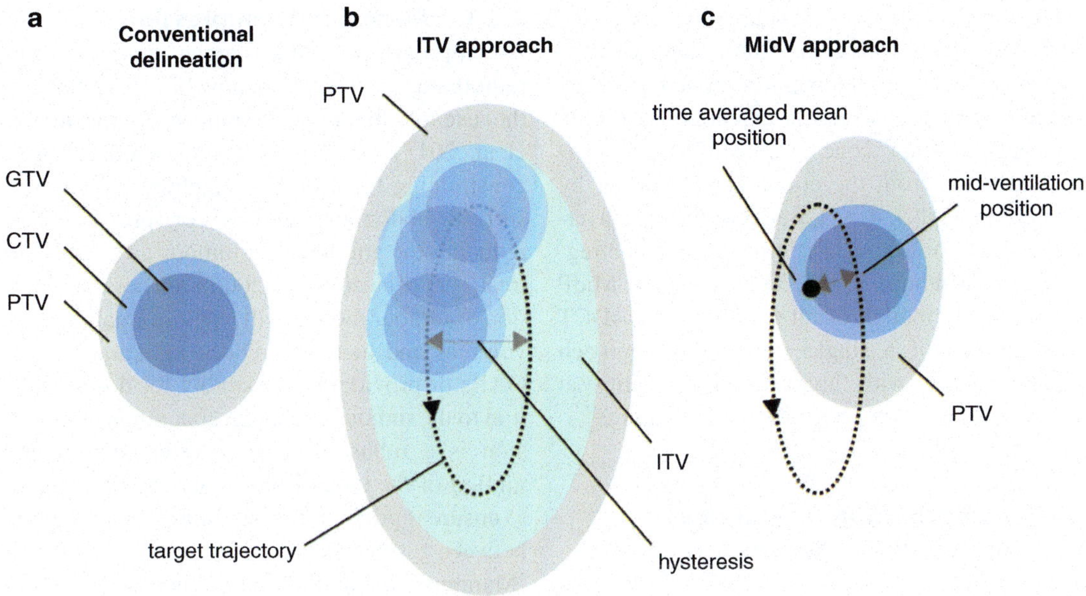

Fig. 5 Definition of target volume in external beam radiotherapy (EBRT). During conventional EBRT (**a**), a gross tumour volume (GTV) is defined to be the gross disease extent depicted by medical images. The GTV will be expanded to cover subclinical disease that is not readily depicted by imaging, yielding a clinical target volume (CTV). Subsequently, the CTV is expanded with a safety margin to create the PTV, which takes relevant geometrical uncertainties that arise during EBRT into account. The internal target volume (ITV) concept (**b**), which is essentially a composite of CTVs at different phases of the respiratory cycle, can be used for mobile target lesions. The ITV envelops the entire trajectory of the target lesion, treating motion as a systematic error. The mid-ventilation (MidV) (**c**) concept relies on finding a 3D time-weighted position on 4DCT imaging. Motion of the target lesion from this position is treated as a random geometrical uncertainty covered by the PTV margin

For this reason, other delineation strategies have been proposed that take advantage of the cyclic nature of respiratory motion, restricting the CTV to the area where the target is most often located during the breathing cycle and boosting the dose to this region (Peulen et al. 2014). One of these approaches is the mid-ventilation (MidV) approach, which relies on finding a 3D time-weighted mean position of the target lesion. The mean 3D time-weighted position of the target lesion is typically derived from 4DCT imaging data, depicting the trajectory of the target lesion. Subsequently, a 3D MidV CT scan is reconstructed using the 4DCT sinogram data of the respiratory phase that most closely represents the target lesion in its mean position (Wolthaus et al. 2006). Motion of the target lesion from this position is treated as a random geometrical uncertainty covered by the PTV margin (Wolthaus et al. 2006). It has been shown that the size of PTVs can be considerably reduced using the MidV approach in radiotherapy of target lesions situated in the thorax and upper abdomen (Peulen et al. 2014; Lens et al. 2015). Fig. 5 depicts the different types of target volumes used during radiotherapy.

Successful employment of the MidV concept relies on the amplitude of the motion, size of the target lesion and shape of the target lesion's trajectory (Wanet et al. 2014). Particularly in presence of hysteresis, where the trajectory during the inspiratory and expiratory phase differ, essentially forming a closed loop, the time-averaged mean position is not necessarily situated on the trajectory of the target lesion, resulting in a remaining systematic geometrical error (Wolthaus et al. 2008). Furthermore, artefacts residing in the reconstructed 3D MidV CT images can hinder accurate target delineation. These include motion artefacts due to irregular patient breathing and higher noise content due to suboptimal use of the 4DCT data (Wolthaus et al. 2008). These difficulties inspired the development of the mid-position (MidP) approach, which is essentially a refinement of the MidV concept. A MidP CT scan is reconstructed from the entire 4DCT dataset by transforming each 4DCT frame to the time-averaged mean position using deformable image registration (Wolthaus et al. 2008). Since the MidP CT uses information of all frames of the 4DCT scan instead of a single frame, this approach yields images with higher image quality at reduced patient exposure during CT imaging.

3.3 Radiotherapy Techniques for Mobile Target Lesions

The advantage of the ITV, MidV and MidP planning is that these can be used in conjunction with conventional radiotherapy techniques, without considering specific motion of the tumour during actual dose delivery. As described in the previous section, 4DCT imaging techniques can be used to generate such target volumes. The benefit of these approaches is that the actual external beam radiotherapy (EBRT) technique does not deviate from that of a stationary lesion and can be implemented in almost all clinical arenas without additional equipment or technical modifications to in-room imaging devices or to the linear accelerators (LINACs). Furthermore, treatment is not necessarily prolonged or more demanding for the patient. These radiotherapy techniques have found widespread implementation in clinical practice and are typically used when treating mobile target lesions. However, by relying on a single pretreatment 4DCT image set for motion management, day-to-day variability in patient respiration is not taken into account, which can result in significant geometrical uncertainties (Ge et al. 2013; Dhont et al. 2018). Therefore, radiotherapy strategies have been developed that interact with motion of the target lesion by restraining the patient or rely on monitoring the patient's respiratory cycle and making real-time adjustments during dose delivery. These techniques will be discussed in the following sections.

3.3.1 Abdominal Compression

An approach to reduce organ motion during radiotherapy is forced shallow breathing through the use of abdominal compression (Mampuya et al. 2013). Abdominal compression relies on constraining the patient's breathing with a pressurized abdominal cushion or pressure pad, reducing the amplitude of tumour motion during treatment (Tewatia et al. 2006). Successful reduction of tumour motion will result in smaller target volumes and therefore reduce radiation dose to OARs or provide the possibility for dose escalation to the tumour. Although abdominal compression is a robust method to effectively reduce motion of the target lesion, care should be taken to ensure reproducible restraining of target lesion between subsequent radiotherapy fractions (Mampuya et al. 2013; Bouilhol et al. 2013). Therefore, strategies for target matching are required to correct and minimize the inter-fraction variation regarding the position of the target lesion. Minimization of inter-fraction variation is typically being achieved by using position verification techniques using in-room imaging devices. However, use of abdominal compression can cause considerable patient discomfort, which might limit successful employment of such strategies for patients with co-morbidities and reduced performance status (Heinzerling et al. 2008).

3.3.2 Free-Breathing Respiratory-Gated Radiotherapy

During free-breathing respiratory-gated radiotherapy, the target lesion will be intermittently irradiated based on the position of the target lesion with respect to the treatment area. After appropriate patient set-up using in-room imaging, a respiratory surrogate signal is acquired in order to track the patient's respiratory cycle (Berson et al. 2004). When the target lesion moves into the treatment area, the beam will be switched on. As soon as the target lesion leaves the treatment area, the beam will be switched off. During free-breathing respiratory-gated radiotherapy, the patient will continue to breathe normally. The respiratory gating computer will acquire the respiratory signal and compare this to the gating level set for the beam-on condition. When the respiratory signal meets the criterion for a beam-on condition, the computer will communicate with the LINAC control, and the beam will be automatically switched on. Similarly, when the respiratory signal stops fulfilling the set gating criterion, the beam will be switched off. Figure 6a depicts such a respiratory surrogate signal together with the beam-on and beam-off conditions during free-breathing respiratory-gated radiotherapy.

The duty cycle, defined as the percentage of the respiratory cycle in which the beam is switched on, during free-breathing respiratory-gated radiotherapy typically ranges from 20% to 30% (Berson et al. 2004). This means that treatment time of free-breathing gated radiotherapy is inevitably longer than that of non-gated radiotherapy. In addition to increasing patient discomfort due to longer treatment times, the probability of intra-fraction motion and drifting of anatomy is also increased which can in turn compromise delivery accuracy (Murphy et al. 2003).

3.3.3 Breath-Hold Radiotherapy

Breath-hold radiotherapy is essentially a modification of free-breathing gated radiotherapy and relies on providing breathing instructions to the patient. In this setting, patients perform breath-hold manoeuvres for adequate dose delivery. Breath-hold radiotherapy is a commonly employed technique to separate the target lesion from the OARs, resulting in sparing of dose to the heart and lungs (Nissen and Appelt 2013). Furthermore, breath-hold radiotherapy has also been used in the context of motion management of target lesions. The breath-hold manoeuvres result in fixation of the target lesion into the treatment area during dose delivery. The advantage of breath-hold radiotherapy is that the PTVs can be considerably reduced compared to the ITV, MidV and MidP approaches. Furthermore, the target lesion is fixated during dose delivery, preventing the complex interplay effects due to the dynamic interaction between the LINAC components and motion of the target lesion, reducing the blurring effects of the dose distribution.

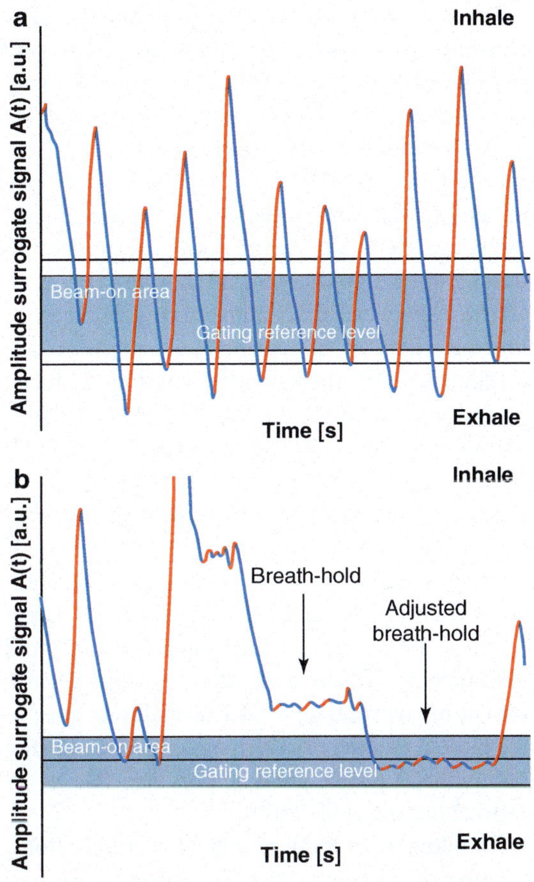

Fig. 6 Respiratory surrogate signals together with beam-on conditions during free-breathing respiratory-gated radiotherapy (**a**), and breath-hold radiotherapy. During free-breathing respiratory-gated radiotherapy, the patient will continue to breathe freely during dose delivery. When the respiratory signal meets the specified respiratory gating criteria, the radiation beam will be switched on. Similarly, when the signal stops fulfilling the respiratory gating criteria, the radiation beam will be switched off. With breath-hold radiotherapy (**b**), the patient is instructed to perform breath-hold manoeuvres at the specified gating level. When the amplitude of the respiratory gating signal falls within the set gating level, the beam will be switched on for the duration of the breath-hold manoeuvre

However, successful employment of breath-hold radiotherapy requires that the patient is able to perform breath-hold manoeuvres for prolonged time intervals. Many studies, particularly for thoracic target lesions, involve deep inspiration breath-hold (DIBH) radiotherapy (Scherman Rydhög et al. 2017; Boda-Heggemann et al. 2016). In addition to immobilization of the target lesion, the use of DIBH radiotherapy causes lung tissue to inflate and expand, resulting in movement of a relatively large part of normal lung tissue to move outside of the treatment area (Hanley et al. 1999). Furthermore, DIBH has shown to improve image quality and reduce registration uncertainty of CBCT data during patient set-up before treatment (Josipovic et al. 2016; Ottosson et al. 2016). However, DIBH manoeuvres require significant effort of the patient and might be too difficult to perform in patients with a reduced performance status. Adaptations to DIBH radiotherapy, such as moderate DIBH (mDIBH) radiotherapy, have been introduced for patients that are unable to perform DIBH manoeuvres for prolonged time intervals (Gong et al. 2013).

Reproducibility of the breath-hold manoeuvres to ensure adequate coverage of the target lesion is an important aspect during breath-hold radiotherapy (Takao et al. 2016). In this regard, providing appropriate visual or auditory ques to the patient and the use of image guidance during radiotherapy are of great importance (He et al. 2016; Linthout et al. 2009).

In addition to these technical considerations, training is an essential part during preparation of the patient for breath-hold therapy. These training sessions are used both to test whether the patient is capable to reproducibly perform the breath-hold manoeuvres and to familiarize the patient with the procedure ahead of the actual treatment (Keall et al. 2006). In addition, the patient can be assisted by active breathing control devices during breath-hold radiotherapy, which help the patient to reproducibly perform breath-hold manoeuvres during dose delivery (Eccles et al. 2006; Panakis et al. 2008).

A common strategy to instruct the patient for breath-hold manoeuvres is to display the patient's breathing simultaneously with the appropriate gating level visually on a monitor. The patient is then instructed to hold his or her breath at the level indicated on the monitor, as depicted by Fig. 6b. Similar to free-breathing gated radiotherapy, external markers or sensors will be used to track the patient's respiratory cycle. If the respiratory surrogate signal reaches the required gating level, the radiotherapy beam will be switched on, and the target will be irradiated.

3.3.4 Position Monitoring of the Target Lesion

The success of free-breathing radiotherapy and breath-hold radiotherapy relies on adequate monitoring the position of internal anatomy. This can be performed either directly, by imaging fiducial markers implanted near the target, or indirectly by measuring a respiratory surrogate signal using external markers. Although percutaneous marker implantation can be used to track the target lesion using in-room imaging, implantation of such markers under image guidance is invasive and associated with risk of complication, compromising the otherwise non-invasive character of radiotherapy. Complications of such marker placement include the occurrence of pneumothorax and haemorrhaging (Bhagat et al. 2010; Yousefi et al. 2007; Mongeon et al. 2017). Although different solutions have been advocated to improve lesion accessibility and reduce complication rate, for example, marker placement by bronchoscopy in case of lung cancer, markers are often placed further away from the lesion, resulting in different movement patterns of the marker than the lesion itself. Furthermore, positional stability of the markers during the course of treatment can be an issue, with reports of markers being expelled from the patient due to coughing (Roman et al. 2012; Persson et al. 2013).

In this regard, the use of indirect measurements, using external markers or sensors, for the purpose of monitoring the position of internal anatomy have been proposed. Several technologies, including mechanical surface tracking sensors, magnetic distance sensors, infrared- and laser-based surface motion tracking, spirometer-based breathing control, radiofrequency (RF) transponder-based surface tracking and mixed modality KV-IR fusion systems, have been developed for tracking the patient's respiratory cycle (Kalet et al. 2019). However, external markers and sensors used for tracking respiratory motion are known to have variable accuracy for accurately estimating the internal shift of anatomy. This is emphasized by several imaging studies, which have shown that there can be considerable discordance between anatomical shift and observed thoracic wall excursions (van der Vos et al. 2015; Koch et al. 2004). Furthermore, whilst there might be a correlation between the respiratory surrogate signal and the internal position anatomy at the beginning of treatment, this correlation might deteriorate over the course of the treatment (Poels et al. 2014a). Therefore, image guidance plays an important role in the verification of these correlations during patient set-up as well as over the course of treatment. In this regard, there is much interest in strategies that rely on near real-time tracking of internal anatomical displacement using in-room imaging. Examples include the use of a patient-controlled respiratory gating system using near real-time cine MR imaging for visual guidance of the breath-hold manoeuvres (Kim et al. 2017). Although such strategies are technically feasible, they have not found widespread use in clinical practice and are still under active development. Another approach is the use of fast imaging in combination with fast treatment delivery protocols. In a study conducted by Arns et al., such ultrafast imaging protocols were investigated (Arns et al. 2019). The authors emphasize that such ultrafast imaging in combination with fast treatment delivery could be used for treatment within a single breath-hold phase.

3.3.5 Real-Time Tumour Tracking

In parallel to breath-hold and respiratory-gated radiotherapy, other active motion management strategies, collectively known as real-time tumour tracking (RTTT), were developed. With RTTT, the goal is to keep the treatment beam aligned with the target during delivery of radiation dose. In order to accomplish this, the position of the target is monitored in real time, and treatment delivery is adapted accordingly. If successfully employed, these RTTT techniques permit adequate dose coverage of moving targets whilst keeping the PTV relatively small when compared to conventional motion management approaches (Colvill et al. 2016). Due to hardware limitations, the first clinical applications of RTTT were limited to slow and only occasionally moving targets, such as the prostate. These RTTT approaches typically consisted of periodic imaging and repositioning the patient when necessary. However, with technological advances over the years, RTTT techniques have evolved and became applicable for the management of relatively fast-moving lesions with larger motion amplitudes. In particular, technical improvements made continuous real-time monitoring and adaptation of the treatment beam possible, which subsequently resulted in development of respiratory tracking applications that can be used for tracking target lesions that are subjected to motion due to the patient's respiration. Real-time alignment of the treatment beam and target lesion can be accomplished in several ways, though clinical applications have largely been limited to two different approaches, moving the treatment beam by moving the entire linear accelerator or by moving the treatment couch or multi-leaf collimators (MLCs) (Sayeh et al. 2007; Haas et al. 2012; Depuydt et al. 2014; Booth et al. 2016).

3.4 Real-Time Tumour Tracking Using the Linear Accelerator

Employment of RTTT by moving the entire linear accelerator is limited to dedicated RTTT machines of which there are only two clinically in use: the CyberKnife Robotic Radiosurgery system (*Accuray*, Sunnyvale, CA, USA) and Vero SBRT system (*Mitsubishi Heavy Industries*, Ltd., *Tokyo*, Japan, and *BrainlAB* AG, *Feldkirchen*, Germany) (Hoogeman et al. 2009; Depuydt et al. 2011). The CyberKnife Robotic Radiosurgery system consists of a 6 MV linear accelerator mounted on a six degree-of-freedom (DOF) Keller und Knappich Augsburg (KUKA) industrial robot (Sayeh et al. 2007). The advantage of this configuration is that it permits many different possibilities (degrees of freedom) regarding the treatment angles that can be used when compared to conventional LINACs, with the potential to further optimize dose delivery to the patient. The system offers various ways to locate and track target lesions in different anatomical regions using a combination of external and internal

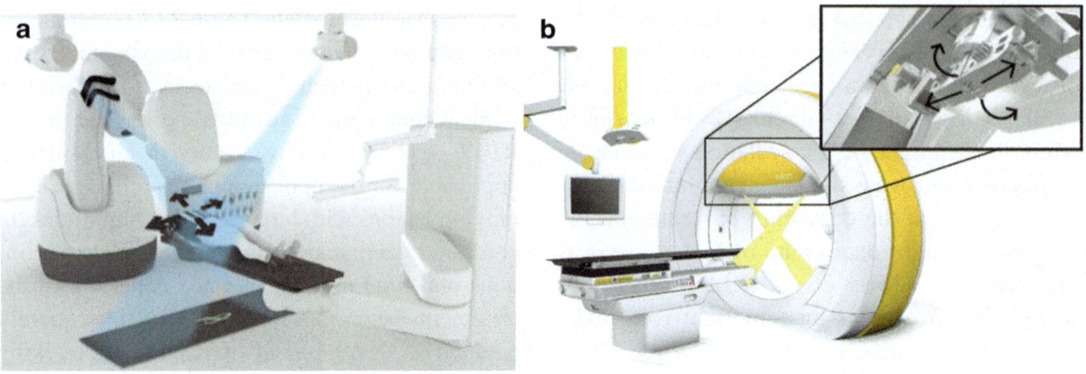

Fig. 7 Real-time tumour tracking (RTTT) using the CyberKnife Robotic Radiosurgery system with orthogonal kilovolt (kV) imager systems on the ceiling and floor (**a**) and Vero stereotactic body radiotherapy (SBRT) system with on-board orthogonal kV imager systems (**b**). Both systems are equipped with a camera pointed towards the couch to capture the external breathing signal positioned on the moving chest of the patient

markers for the purpose of position verification. Internal markers used in this setting are typically fiducial gold markers that are implanted in the target lesion, whereas external markers consist of light-emitting diodes (LED) that are placed on the exterior surface of the patient. Tracking of the internal and external markers will be performed by two orthogonal planar X-ray imaging systems and a video tracking system, respectively.

The Vero SBRT system has a design that significantly differs from the CyberKnife Robotic Radiosurgery system and consists of a 6 MV C-band LINAC mounted on two orthogonal gimbals incorporated in an O-ring gantry (Depuydt et al. 2014; Kamino et al. 2007). Tracking of the target lesion is performed by using pan and tilt motions of the LINAC. Furthermore, a stereoscopic dual-source kV X-ray imaging system is incorporated into the O-ring gantry for fluoroscopy image guidance during target tracking (Depuydt et al. 2014, 2013). This configuration permits the acquisition of a cone-beam CT and orthogonal X-ray images. An integrated automated infrared optical tracking device is used for both pre-positioning of the patient and acquisition of a respiratory surrogate signal (Depuydt et al. 2013). Furthermore, the presence of an EPID imaging device allows direct verification of the alignment between the beam and target (Poels et al. 2014b). Figure 7 depicts RTTT with the CyberKnife Robotic Radiosurgery and Vero SBRT systems.

Though the CyberKnife Robotic Radiosurgery and Vero SBRT systems have a considerably different design, the RTTT workflow of both systems is remarkably similar. Both systems use positional data of the external markers to monitor patient respiration (Ernst et al. 2012; Akimoto et al. 2013). This respiratory surrogate signal is correlated to the internal target motion at the beginning of each fraction using orthogonal kV fluoroscopy imaging. Synchronization of the respiratory surrogate signal with internal target motion is then performed by fitting a mathematical model that permits prediction of internal motion from this respiratory surrogate signal (Cho et al. 2008). During treatment, the surrogate signal is used as input for the correlation model to estimate the position of the target lesion, whilst forward prediction is used to overcome system latencies induced by delay in mechanical response. Both systems verify the accuracy of the correlation model during treatment through periodic X-ray imaging and comparison of the real and predicted location of the target lesion. When the model becomes inaccurate, for example, due to baseline drifts, change in breathing frequency or pattern, the correlation model can be updated or completely rebuild (Poels et al. 2014a).

Although modelling internal motion of the target volume using a respiratory surrogate signal might be less accurate than direct tracking through continuous imaging, it significantly reduces system latency and radiation exposure to the patient due to frequent imaging. Another disadvantage of both systems is the requirement to implant fiducial markers in the target lesion for fast and reliable automated localization of the target lesion on fluoroscopy images. This limits the application of RTTT to lesions that are accessible for marker implantation. In order to circumvent the requirement for marker implantation, the CyberKnife has been equipped with a 'markerless' software tool, allowing the target to be localized without requiring implantation of fiducial markers (Fu et al. 2007). Using digitally reconstructed radiographs obtained from the planning CT, the target can be located automatically on real-time images. However, the method still requires a certain degree of tumour visibility, limiting the applicability to lesions having high contrast on X-ray images (Bahig et al. 2013).

3.5 Multi-Leaf Collimator and Couch Tracking

Although LINAC based tracking techniques have a high accuracy for dynamic tracking of target lesions which can result in significant reduction of PTVs, these systems are highly specialized and not widespread in clinical use (Toftegaard et al. 2017). In this regard, other tracking strategies that can be performed using conventional LINACs, including MLC and couch tracking, have been proposed. During MLC tracking, as first proposed by Keall et al. (2001), the MLC aperture is shifted according to internal motion of the target lesion. Alternatively, the treatment couch can be used to counteract motion of the target lesion during radiotherapy. This concept is also known as couch tracking and was first proposed by D'Souza et al. (2005). Although vendors of conventional LINACs currently support dynamic tracking only in research mode on these devices, MLC tracking has been successfully employed in a number of clinical applications, including prostate (Colvill et al. 2014, 2015) and lung cancers (Caillet et al. 2017). The extent in which the MLCs can be used to simultaneously perform beam shaping and tracking of the target lesion is currently being investigated. However, it is expected that there will be limits with respect to plan complexity that can be achieved whilst simultaneously safeguarding accurate tumour tracking (Pommer et al. 2013).

Contrary to the implantation of radio-opaque fiducial markers and fluoroscopy in LINAC-based RTTT, implanted electromagnetic (EM) transponders were used to track the target lesion, omitting the requirement for recording an external respiratory surrogate signal and establishing a correlation model (Ravkilde et al. 2011). However, similar to the fiducial markers used in LINAC-based RTTT, this approach suffers the same issues pertinent to marker placement, including marker instability during the course of the treatment and risk of complications during implantation. Whilst MLC tracking has the potential to improve dose delivery to mobile target lesions, tracking latency and limits of system dynamics (finite collimator leaf speeds, collimator leaf localization and fitting errors) can still yield dosimetric errors (Poulsen et al. 2012). Furthermore, a major limitation of MLC tracking is its inability to accurately adapt to target shifts perpendicular to the MLC leaves due to the finite width of the collimator leaves.

Alternatively, synchronized movement of the treatment couch has been used to counteract motion of the target lesion. Although these couch tracking techniques have a good accuracy for tracking of target lesions, the dynamics of this tracking is relatively slow and has not been used in clinical practice so far (Toftegaard et al. 2017). Large couch movements may also reduce patient comfort or lead to the patient reacting to the movement, reducing the accuracy of dose delivery (Toftegaard et al. 2017). Recent developments regarding MLC- and couch-based RTTT involve the combination of these two techniques (Toftegaard et al. 2017; Podder et al. 2008). Such hybrid tracking approaches, where MLC- and couch-based RTTT are used in parallel, have the potential to further improve tracking dynamics and accuracy of RTTT using conventional LINACs (Toftegaard et al. 2017).

Despite many technological advances in RTTT, accurate real-time visualization of the target lesion using kV fluoroscopy remains the main obstacle, preventing successful widespread employment of such techniques in clinical practice. Although different markerless approaches have been suggested, such strategies are not suitable for every patient due to limited contrast of target lesions on these images (Poels et al. 2014b; Rottmann et al. 2013; Dhont et al. 2015; Shieh et al. 2017). Therefore, it is expected that utilization of near real-time in-room imaging, such as MR imaging, will significantly contribute to an improved accuracy of RTTT, making it possible to extend the clinical indications for the use of such techniques.

4 Inter-Fraction Geometrical Uncertainties and the Promise of Adaptive Radiotherapy

The previous sections emphasized the importance of motion management for reducing intra-fraction geometrical uncertainties in order to ensure adequate dose delivery during radiotherapy. In current clinical practice, dose delivery will typically be performed using a single pretreatment radiotherapy plan. Although such a plan is representative for the patient at the time of pretreatment imaging, the position and shape of internal anatomy can change due to treatment effects during the course of radiotherapy (Grootjans et al. 2018). These effects, including tumour regression, the emergence of pleural effusion or ascites and dissolving atelectasis, can result in a differential baseline shift of the primary tumour and lymph nodes, contributing to increasing geometrical uncertainties (Grootjans et al. 2015). These geometrical uncertainties can, to some extent, be accounted for by using in-room image guidance before each radiotherapy fraction. In this setting, in-room imaging, typically consisting of fluoroscopy or (4D)CBCT imaging, is used for the purpose of position verification and monitoring the trajectory of the target lesion before radiotherapy. This information can be used to make adjustments to patient positioning to ensure adequate coverage of the target lesion (Ge et al. 2013; Minn et al. 2009).

However, there are limitations regarding the adaptations that can be achieved with external repositioning of the patients, particularly in the presence of non-rigid deformations of anatomy. In order to more accurately account for internal long-term variations, imaging and replanning can be performed during the course of treatment. This concept is known as image-guided adaptive radiotherapy (IGART), the relevance of which was emphasized by Guckenberger et al. (2011) who reported continuous tumour regression of approximately 1.2% per day, as measured by CT, with a total mean GTV reduction of 50% after 6 weeks of treatment. The decrease in tumour volume observed in this study emphasizes the opportunity to modify target volumes to spare normal tissues from radiation dose and indicates the possibility to perform dose escalation to the tumour. Figure 8 illustrates the concept of IGART using sequential [^{18}F]FDG-PET–CT imaging in a patient with stage IIIB NSCLC.

The IGART approach permits to adapt the radiotherapy plan during the course of treatment, with the purpose of redistribution of the radiation dose. This includes dose escalation to high-risk areas, with suspected residual disease, and dose de-escalation to low-risk areas that have a good response to therapy. Although IGART has the potential to personalize radiotherapy to the individual, it can be logistically difficult to implement in a busy clinical practice. Furthermore, it introduces several new uncertainties into the workflow, such as registration and dose accumulation errors. Patient benefit of such approaches in terms of local control and long-term survival is currently being investigated.

5 Future Prospects

In this chapter, the importance of managing intra- and inter-fraction geometrical uncertainties in the era of high-precision radiotherapy was discussed. In particular, different strategies for managing uncertainties that arise from organ

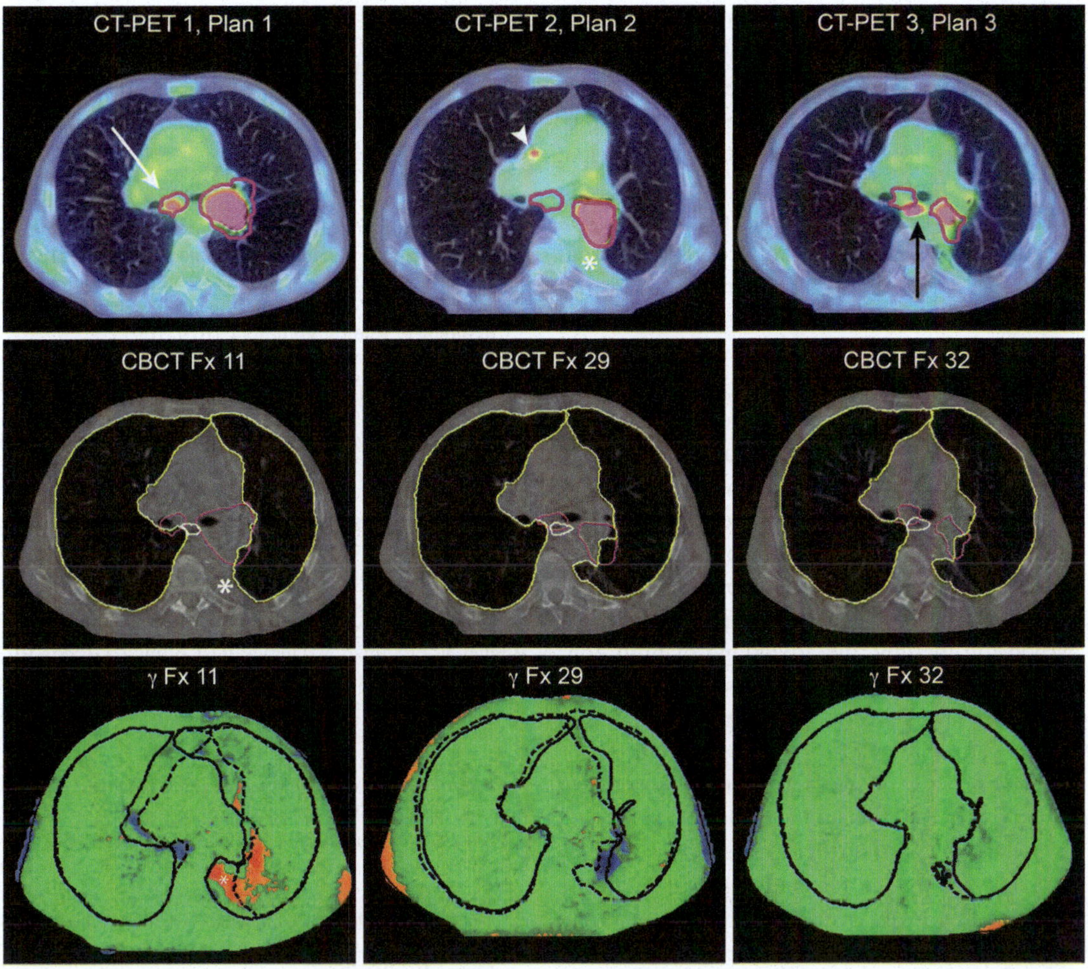

Fig. 8 Adaptive radiotherapy planning using serial [^{18}F] fluorodeoxyglucose ([^{18}F]FDG) positron emission tomography (PET) CT imaging in a patient with stage IIIB non-small cell lung cancer (NSCLC). The initial radiotherapy plan was adapted twice because of changes in dose coverage observed during the course of treatment. The first column of images (plan 1) depicts the initial plan, with the clinical target volume (CTV) (magenta contour) of the primary tumour in the left lung and mediastinal metastatic lymph node (white arrow) overlaid on the pretreatment [^{18}F]FDG-PET–CT image (top row). During treatment, an atelectasis developed (white asterisks) displacing the mediastinum to the left, visualized by cone beam CT (CBCT) imaging at fraction 11 (Fx 11; middle row). In addition to the CTV (magenta contour), the oesophagus (white contour) is delineated in the CBCT images. The resulting dose difference between planned and delivered dose is illustrated in the γ-evaluation (dose difference/distance to agreement: 3%/3 mm, γ Fx 11; bottom row) showing overdosage in the left lower lobe (red) and underdosage in the CTV of the lymph node metastasis (blue), necessitating an [^{18}F]FDG-PET–CT-based treatment adaptation. The second column (plan 2) shows the respective images with target volumes adapted to avoid overdosage of normal tissue (mediastinum and lung) and underdosage of metastatic lymph node as detected by the aforementioned γ-evaluation. Note that the additional 'hotspot' on the [^{18}F]FDG-PET–CT (white arrowhead) corresponds to the myocardium. Upon resolution of the atelectasis after 29 fractions of treatment, which resulted in underdosing of the primary tumour at this time point (blue region in γ Fx 29 image; bottom row), a third treatment plan was generated (magenta contour; third column, top row); note the focal [^{18}F]FDG uptake in the oesophagus (black arrow) due to treatment-induced inflammation. Respective CBCT and γ-evaluation images of this treatment plan (plan 3) at treatment fraction 32 are presented in the third column. Beyond this time point, no further treatment adaptation was necessary (Adapted from Grootjans et al. 2015)

motion due to patient respiration have been elaborated. Although there have been numerous technological advances in the field of radiotherapy and medical imaging, adequate management of such intra- and inter-fraction geometrical uncertainties remains a topic of active research. Whilst many technological solutions have been developed for specific patient groups or clinical situations, there is a requirement to further develop these techniques in order to make widespread use in clinical routine possible. The use of motion management techniques becomes increasingly important for generating patient-specific margins in dose escalation strategies, where reduction in PTVs provide the possibility to increase radiation dose to the target tissues. Furthermore, reduction of geometrical errors is essential in conjunction with particle therapy. During particle therapy, such as proton or heavy carbon ion therapy, the advantage of high conformity and steep dose gradients due to the specific absorption profile of charged particles in tissues can rapidly turn into a significant disadvantage in case of inadequate management of target motion (Engelsman et al. 2013). Target motion during particle therapy results in changes in density along the ray path, especially in the lung, leading to differences in beam range and significant deviations from the planned dose distribution (Engelsman and Kooy 2005; Jakobi et al. 2018). Although similar motion management strategies have been developed for proton therapy (Kanehira et al. 2017; De Ruysscher et al. 2015; Engelsman et al. 2006) many of these techniques are currently being researched regarding their robustness and accuracy in a particle therapy setting.

References

Abdelnour AF, Nehmeh SA, T P, Humm JL, Vernon P, Schöder H et al (2007) Phase and amplitude binning for 4D-CT imaging. Phys Med Biol 52:3515

Akimoto M, Nakamura M, Mukumoto N, Tanabe H, Yamada M, Matsuo Y et al (2013) Predictive uncertainty in infrared marker-based dynamic tumor tracking with Vero4DRTa. Med Phys 40:091705

Arns A, Wertz H, Boda-Heggemann J, Schneider F, Blessing M, Abo-Madyan Y et al (2019) Ultrafast single breath-hold cone-beam CT lung cancer imaging with faster linac gantry rotation. Radiother Oncol 135:78–85

Bahig H, Campeau M-P, Vu T, Doucet R, Béliveau Nadeau D, Fortin B et al (2013) Predictive parameters of CyberKnife fiducial-less (XSight lung) applicability for treatment of early non-small cell lung cancer: a single-center experience. Int J Radiat Oncol Biol Phys 87:583–589

Barrett JF, Keat N (2004) Artifacts in CT: recognition and avoidance. Radiographics 24:1679–1691

Baskar R, Dai J, Wenlong N, Yeo R, Yeoh K-W (2014) Biological response of cancer cells to radiation treatment. Front Mol Biosci 1:24

Bentzen SM, Gregoire V (2011) Molecular imaging based dose painting: a novel paradigm for radiation therapy prescription. Semin Radiat Oncol 21:101–110

Berson AM, Emery R, Rodriguez L, Richards GM, Ng T, Sanghavi S et al (2004) Clinical experience using respiratory gated radiation therapy: comparison of free-breathing and breath-hold techniques. Int J Radiat Oncol Biol Phys 60:419–426

Bhagat N, Fidelman N, Durack JC, Collins J, Gordon RL, LaBerge JM et al (2010) Complications associated with the percutaneous insertion of fiducial markers in the thorax. Cardiovasc Intervent Radiol 33:1186–1191

Boda-Heggemann J, Knopf A-C, Simeonova-Chergou A, Wertz H, Stieler F, Jahnke A et al (2016) Deep inspiration breath hold—based radiation therapy: a clinical review. Int J Radiat Oncol Biol Phys 94:478–492

Booth JT, Caillet V, Hardcastle N, O'Brien R, Szymura K, Crasta C et al (2016) The first patient treatment of electromagnetic-guided real time adaptive radiotherapy using MLC tracking for lung SABR. Radiother Oncol 121:19–25

Borras JM, Lievens Y, Dunscombe P, Coffey M, Malicki J, Corral J et al (2015) The optimal utilization proportion of external beam radiotherapy in European countries: an ESTRO-HERO analysis. Radiother Oncol 116:38–44

Bortfeld T, Jiang SB, Rietzel E (2004) Effects of motion on the total dose distribution. Semin Radiat Oncol 14:41–51

Bortfeld T, Jokivarsi K, Goitein M, Kung J, Jiang SB (2002) Effects of intra-fraction motion on IMRT dose delivery: statistical analysis and simulation. Phys Med Biol 47:2203

Bouilhol G, Ayadi M, Rit S, Thengumpallil S, Schaerer J, Vandemeulebroucke J et al (2013) Is abdominal compression useful in lung stereotactic body radiation therapy? A 4DCT and dosimetric lobe-dependent study. Phys Med 29:333–340

Burnet NG, Thomas SJ, Burton KE, Jefferies SJ (2004) Defining the tumour and target volumes for radiotherapy. Cancer Imaging 4:153–161

Caillet V, Keall PJ, Colvill E, Hardcastle N, O'Brien R, Szymura K et al (2017) MLC tracking for lung SABR

reduces planning target volumes and dose to organs at risk. Radiother Oncol 124:18–24
Chang G, Chang T, Pan T, Clark JW, Mawlawi OR (2010) Implementation of an automated respiratory amplitude gating technique for PET/CT: clinical evaluation. J Nucl Med 51:16–24
Chen Z, Yang Z, Wang J, Hu W (2016) Dosimetric impact of different bladder and rectum filling during prostate cancer radiotherapy. Radiat Oncol 11:103
Cho B, Suh Y, Dieterich S, Keall PJ (2008) A monoscopic method for real-time tumour tracking using combined occasional x-ray imaging and continuous respiratory monitoring. Phys Med Biol 53:2837
Colvill E, Booth J, Nill S, Fast M, Bedford J, Oelfke U et al (2016) A dosimetric comparison of real-time adaptive and non-adaptive radiotherapy: a multi-institutional study encompassing robotic, gimbaled, multileaf collimator and couch tracking. Radiother Oncol 119:159–165
Colvill E, Booth JT, O'Brien RT, Eade TN, Kneebone AB, Poulsen PR et al (2015) Multileaf collimator tracking improves dose delivery for prostate Cancer radiation therapy: results of the first clinical trial. Int J Radiat Oncol Biol Phys 92:1141–1147
Colvill E, Poulsen PR, Booth JT, O'Brien RT, Ng JA, Keall PJ (2014) DMLC tracking and gating can improve dose coverage for prostate VMAT. *Med Phys* **41**:091705
Connell PP, Hellman S (2009) Advances in radiotherapy and implications for the next century: a historical perspective. Cancer Res 69:383–392
Dawood M, Büther F, Lang N, Schober O, Schäfers KP (2007) Respiratory gating in positron emission tomography: a quantitative comparison of different gating schemes. Med Phys 34:3067–3076
de Boer HCJ, Van Sörnsen de Koste JR, Senan S, Visser AG, Heijmen BJM (2001) Analysis and reduction of 3D systematic and random setup errors during the simulation and treatment of lung cancer patients with CT-based external beam radiotherapy dose planning. Int J Radiat Oncol Biol Phys 49:857–868
De Ruysscher D, Faivre-Finn C, Nestle U, Hurkmans CW, Le Péchoux C, Price A et al (2010) European Organisation for Research and Treatment of Cancer recommendations for planning and delivery of high-dose, high-precision radiotherapy for lung Cancer. J Clin Oncol 28:5301–5310
De Ruysscher D, Sterpin E, Haustermans K, Depuydt T (2015) Tumour movement in proton therapy: solutions and remaining questions: a review. Cancers (Basel) 7:1143–1153
Depuydt T, Poels K, Verellen D, Engels B, Collen C, Buleteanu M et al (2014) Treating patients with real-time tumor tracking using the Vero gimbaled linac system: implementation and first review. Radiother Oncol 112:343–351
Depuydt T, Poels K, Verellen D, Engels B, Collen C, Haverbeke C et al (2013) Initial assessment of tumor tracking with a gimbaled linac system in clinical circumstances: a patient simulation study. Radiother Oncol 106:236–240
Depuydt T, Verellen D, Haas O, Gevaert T, Linthout N, Duchateau M et al (2011) Geometric accuracy of a novel gimbals based radiation therapy tumor tracking system. Radiother Oncol 98:365–372
Dhont J, Vandemeulebroucke J, Burghelea M, Poels K, Depuydt T, Van Den Begin R et al (2018) The long- and short-term variability of breathing induced tumor motion in lung and liver over the course of a radiotherapy treatment. Radiother Oncol 126:339–346
Dhont J, Verellen D, Poels K, Tournel K, Burghelea M, Gevaert T et al (2015) Feasibility of markerless tumor tracking by sequential dual-energy fluoroscopy on a clinical tumor tracking system. Radiother Oncol 117:487–490
D'Souza WD, Naqvi SA, Yu CX (2005) Real-time intra-fraction-motion tracking using the treatment couch: a feasibility study. Phys Med Biol 50:4021
Eccles C, Brock KK, Bissonnette J-P, Hawkins M, Dawson LA (2006) Reproducibility of liver position using active breathing coordinator for liver cancer radiotherapy. Int J Radiat Oncol Biol Phys 64:751–759
Ekberg L, Holmberg O, Wittgren L, Bjelkengren G, Landberg T (1998) What margins should be added to the clinical target volume in radiotherapy treatment planning for lung cancer? Radiother Oncol 48:71–77
Engelsman M, Damen EMF, De Jaeger K, van Ingen KM, Mijnheer BJ (2001) The effect of breathing and set-up errors on the cumulative dose to a lung tumor. Radiother Oncol 60:95–105
Engelsman M, Kooy HM (2005) Target volume dose considerations in proton beam treatment planning for lung tumors. Med Phys 32:3549–3557
Engelsman M, Rietzel E, Kooy HM (2006) Four-dimensional proton treatment planning for lung tumors. Int J Radiat Oncol Biol Phys 64:1589–1595
Engelsman M, Schwarz M, Dong L (2013) Physics controversies in proton therapy. Semin Radiat Oncol 23:88–96
Ernst F, Bruder R, Schlaefer A, Schweikard A (2012) Correlation between external and internal respiratory motion: a validation study. Int J Comput Assist Radiol Surg 7:483–492
Fu D, Kahn R, Wang B, Wang H, Mu Z, Park JM et al (2007) Xsight lung tracking system: a fiducial-less method for respiratory motion tracking. In: Urschel HC (ed) Treating tumors that move with respiration. Springer, pp 226–282
Ge J, Santanam L, Noel C, Parikh PJ (2013) Planning 4-dimensional computed tomography (4DCT) cannot adequately represent daily Intrafractional motion of abdominal tumors. Int J Radiat Oncol Biol Phys 85:999–1005
Giraud P, Morvan E, Claude L, Mornex F, Le Pechoux C, Bachaud J-M et al (2011) Respiratory gating techniques for optimization of lung Cancer radiotherapy. J Thorac Oncol 6:2058–2068

Gong G, Wang R, Guo Y, Zhai D, Liu T, Lu J et al (2013) Reduced lung dose during radiotherapy for thoracic esophageal carcinoma: VMAT combined with active breathing control for moderate DIBH. Radiat Oncol 8:291–291

Grootjans W, De Geus-Oei L-F, Bussink J (2018) Image-guided adaptive radiotherapy in patients with locally advanced non-small cell lung cancer: the art of PET. Q J Nucl Med Mol Imaging 62:369–384

Grootjans W, de Geus-Oei L-F, Meeuwis APW, van der Vos CS, Gotthardt M, Oyen WJG et al (2014) Amplitude-based optimal respiratory gating in positron emission tomography in patients with primary lung cancer. Eur Radiol 24:3242–3250

Grootjans W, de Geus-Oei L-F, Troost EGC, Visser EP, Oyen WJG, Bussink J (2015) PET in the management of locally advanced and metastatic NSCLC. Nat Rev Clin Oncol 12:395–407

Grootjans W, Usmanij EA, Oyen WJG, van der Heijden EHFM, Visser EP, Visvikis D et al (2016) Performance of automatic image segmentation algorithms for calculating total lesion glycolysis for early response monitoring in non-small cell lung cancer patients during concomitant chemoradiotherapy. Radiother Oncol 119:473–479

Guckenberger M, Andratschke N, Dieckmann K, Hoogeman MS, Hoyer M, Hurkmans C et al (2017) ESTRO ACROP consensus guideline on implementation and practice of stereotactic body radiotherapy for peripherally located early stage non-small cell lung cancer. Radiother Oncol 124:11–17

Guckenberger M, Wilbert J, Richter A, Baier K, Flentje M (2011) Potential of adaptive radiotherapy to escalate the radiation dose in combined Radiochemotherapy for locally advanced non–small cell lung Cancer. Int J Radiat Oncol Biol Phys 79:901–908

Haas OCL, Skworcow P, Paluszczyszyn D, Sahih A, Ruta M, Mills JA (2012) Couch-based motion compensation: modelling, simulation and real-time experiments. Phys Med Biol 57:5787

Hanley J, Debois MM, Mah D, Mageras GS, Raben A, Rosenzweig K et al (1999) Deep inspiration breath-hold technique for lung tumors: the potential value of target immobilization and reduced lung density in dose escalation. Int J Radiat Oncol Biol Phys 45:603–611

He P, Li Q, Zhao T, Liu X, Dai Z, Ma Y (2016) Effectiveness of respiratory-gated radiotherapy with audio-visual biofeedback for synchrotron-based scanned heavy-ion beam delivery. Phys Med Biol 61:8541

Heinzerling JH, Anderson JF, Papiez L, Boike T, Chien S, Zhang G et al (2008) Four-dimensional computed tomography scan analysis of tumor and organ motion at varying levels of abdominal compression during stereotactic treatment of lung and liver. Int J Radiat Oncol Biol Phys 70:1571–1578

Hertanto A, Zhang Q, Hu Y-C, Dzyubak O, Rimner A, Mageras GS (2012) Reduction of irregular breathing artifacts in respiration-correlated CT images using a respiratory motion model. Med Phys 39:3070–3079

Hoogeman M, Prévost J-B, Nuyttens J, Pöll J, Levendag P, Heijmen B (2009) Clinical accuracy of the respiratory tumor tracking system of the CyberKnife: assessment by analysis of log files. Int J Radiat Oncol Biol Phys 74:297–303

Hubley E, Pierce G (2017) The influence of plan modulation on the interplay effect in VMAT liver SBRT treatments. Phys Med 40:115–121

Jakobi A, Perrin R, Knopf A, Richter C (2018) Feasibility of proton pencil beam scanning treatment of free-breathing lung cancer patients. Acta Oncol 57:203–210

Jani SS, Robinson CG, Dahlbom M, White BM, Thomas DH, Gaudio S et al (2013) A comparison of amplitude-based and phase-based positron emission tomography gating algorithms for segmentation of internal target volumes of tumors subject to respiratory motion. Int J Radiat Oncol Biol Phys 87:562–569

Josipovic M, Persson GF, Bangsgaard JP, Specht L, Aznar MC (2016) Deep inspiration breath-hold radiotherapy for lung cancer: impact on image quality and registration uncertainty in cone beam CT image guidance. Br J Radiol 89:20160544

Kalet AM, Cao N, Smith WP, Young L, Wootton L, Stewart RD et al (2019) Accuracy and stability of deep inspiration breath hold in gated breast radiotherapy – a comparison of two tracking and guidance systems. Phys Med 60:174–181

Kamino Y, Miura S, Kokubo M, Yamashita I, Hirai E, Hiraoka M et al (2007) Development of an ultrasmall C-band linear accelerator guide for a four-dimensional image-guided radiotherapy system with a gimbaled x-ray head. Med Phys 34:1797–1808

Kanehira T, Matsuura T, Takao S, Matsuzaki Y, Fujii Y, Fujii T et al (2017) Impact of real-time image gating on spot scanning proton therapy for lung tumors: a simulation study. Int J Radiat Oncol Biol Phys 97:173–181

Keall PJ, Kini VR, Vedam SS, Mohan R (2001) Motion adaptive x-ray therapy: a feasibility study. Phys Med Biol 46(1):1

Keall PJ, Mageras GS, Balter JM, Emery RS, Forster KM, Jiang SB et al (2006) The management of respiratory motion in radiation oncology report of AAPM Task Group 76a. Med Phys 33:3874–3900

Kim JI, Lee H, Wu HG, Chie EK, Kang HC, Park JM (2017) Development of patient-controlled respiratory gating system based on visual guidance for magnetic-resonance image-guided radiation therapy. Med Phys 44:4838–4846

Koch N, Liu HH, Starkschall G, Jacobson M, Forster K, Liao Z et al (2004) Evaluation of internal lung motion for respiratory-gated radiotherapy using MRI: part I—correlating internal lung motion with skin fiducial motion. Int J Radiat Oncol Biol Phys 60:1459–1472

Korreman SS (2012) Motion in radiotherapy: photon therapy. Phys Med Biol 57:R161

Lagerwaard FJ, Van Sornsen de Koste JR, Nijssen-Visser MRJ, Schuchhard-Schipper RH, Oei SS, Munne A et al (2001) Multiple "slow" CT scans for incorporating lung tumor mobility in radiotherapy planning. Int J Radiat Oncol Biol Phys 51:932–937

Lagerwaard FJ, Haasbeek CJA, Smit EF, Slotman BJ, Senan S (2008) Outcomes of risk-adapted fractionated stereotactic radiotherapy for stage I non–small-cell lung Cancer. Int J Radiat Oncol Biol Phys 70:685–692

Lens E, van der Horst A, Versteijne E, van Tienhoven G, Bel A (2015) Dosimetric advantages of midventilation compared with internal target volume for radiation therapy of pancreatic cancer. Int J Radiat Oncol Biol Phys 92:675–682

Li H, Noel C, Garcia-Ramirez J, Low D, Bradley J, Robinson C et al (2012) Clinical evaluations of an amplitude-based binning algorithm for 4DCT reconstruction in radiation therapy. Med Phys 39:922–932

Linthout N, Bral S, Van de Vondel I, Verellen D, Tournel K, Gevaert T et al (2009) Treatment delivery time optimization of respiratory gated radiation therapy by application of audio-visual feedback. Radiother Oncol 91:330–335

Lu W, Parikh PJ, Hubenschmidt JP, Politte DG, Whiting BR, Bradley JD et al (2005) Reduction of motion blurring artifacts using respiratory gated CT in sinogram space: a quantitative evaluation. Med Phys 32:3295–3304

Mampuya WA, Nakamura M, Matsuo Y, Ueki N, Iizuka Y, Fujimoto T et al (2013) Interfraction variation in lung tumor position with abdominal compression during stereotactic body radiotherapy. Med Phys 40:091718

Minn AY, Schellenberg D, Maxim P, Suh Y, McKenna S, Cox B et al (2009) Pancreatic tumor motion on a single planning 4D-CT does not correlate with Intrafraction tumor motion during treatment. Am J Clin Oncol 32:364–368

Mongeon M, Thibault F, Chartrand-Lefebvre C, Gorgos A-B, Soulez G, Filion E et al (2017) Safety and efficacy of endovascular fiducial marker insertion for CyberKnife stereotactic radiation therapy planning in early-stage lung Cancer. J Vasc Interv Radiol 28:1090–1097

Murphy MJ, Chang SD, Gibbs IC, Le Q-T, Hai J, Kim D et al (2003) Patterns of patient movement during frameless image-guided radiosurgery. Int J Radiat Oncol Biol Phys 55:1400–1408

Nehmeh SA, Haj-Ali AA, Qing C, Stearns C, Kalaigian H, Kohlmyer S et al (2011) A novel respiratory tracking system for smart-gated PET acquisition. Med Phys 38:531–538

Nissen HD, Appelt AL (2013) Improved heart, lung and target dose with deep inspiration breath hold in a large clinical series of breast cancer patients. Radiother Oncol 106:28–32

Njeh CF (2008) Tumor delineation: the weakest link in the search for accuracy in radiotherapy. J Med Phys 33:136–140

Ottosson W, Rahma F, Sjöström D, Behrens CF, Sibolt P (2016) The advantage of deep-inspiration breath-hold and cone-beam CT based soft-tissue registration for locally advanced lung cancer radiotherapy. Radiother Oncol 119:432–437

Panakis N, McNair HA, Christian JA, Mendes R, Symonds-Tayler JRN, Knowles C et al (2008) Defining the margins in the radical radiotherapy of non-small cell lung cancer (NSCLC) with active breathing control (ABC) and the effect on physical lung parameters. Radiother Oncol 87:65–73

Persson GF, Josipovic M, von der Recke P, Aznar MC, Juhler-Nøttrup T, Munck af Rosenschöld P et al (2013) Stability of percutaneously implanted markers for lung stereotactic radiotherapy. J Appl Clin Med Phys 14:187–195

Peulen H, Belderbos J, Rossi M, Sonke J-J (2014) Mid-ventilation based PTV margins in stereotactic body radiotherapy (SBRT): a clinical evaluation. Radiother Oncol 110:511–516

Podder TK, Buzurovic I, Galvin JM, Yu Y (eds) Dynamics-based decentralized control of robotic couch and multi-leaf collimators for tracking tumor motion. 2008 IEEE International Conference on Robotics and Automation; 2008 19–23 May 2008

Poels K, Depuydt T, Verellen D, Gevaert T, Dhont J, Duchateau M et al (2014a) Improving the intra-fraction update efficiency of a correlation model used for internal motion estimation during real-time tumor tracking for SBRT patients: Fast update or no update? Radiother Oncol 112:352–359

Poels K, Verellen D, Van de Vondel I, El Mazghari R, Depuydt T, De Ridder M (2014b) Fiducial marker and marker-less soft-tissue detection using fast MV fluoroscopy on a new generation EPID: Investigating the influence of pulsing artifacts and artifact suppression techniques. *Med Phys* **41**:101911

Pommer T, Falk M, Poulsen PR, Keall PJ, O'Brien RT, Munck af Rosenschöld P (2013) The impact of leaf width and plan complexity on DMLC tracking of prostate intensity modulated arc therapy. Med Phys 40:111717

Poulsen PR, Fledelius W, Cho B, Keall P (2012) Image-based dynamic multileaf collimator tracking of moving targets during intensity-modulated arc therapy. Int J Radiat Oncol Biol Phys 83:e265–e271

Ravkilde T, Keall PJ, Højbjerre K, Fledelius W, Worm E, Poulsen PR (2011) Geometric accuracy of dynamic MLC tracking with an implantable wired electromagnetic transponder. Acta Oncol 50:944–951

Rietzel E, Pan T, Chen GTY (2005) Four-dimensional computed tomography: image formation and clinical protocol. Med Phys 32:874–889

Roman NO, Shepherd W, Mukhopadhyay N, Hugo GD, Weiss E (2012) Interfractional positional variability of fiducial markers and primary tumors in locally advanced non-small-cell lung Cancer during audiovisual biofeedback radiotherapy. Int J Radiat Oncol Biol Phys 83:1566–1572

Rosenblatt E, Izewska J, Anacak Y, Pynda Y, Scalliet P, Boniol M et al (2013) Radiotherapy capacity in European countries: an analysis of the directory of radiotherapy Centres (DIRAC) database. Lancet Oncol 14:e79–e86

Rottmann J, Keall P, Berbeco R (2013) Markerless EPID image guided dynamic multi-leaf collimator tracking for lung tumors. Phys Med Biol 58:4195

Sayeh S, Wang WT, Kilby W, Maurer CR (2007) Respiratory motion tracking for robotic radiosurgery.

In: Urschel HC (ed) Treating tumors that move with respiration. Springer-Verlag, Berlin Heidelberg
Scherman Rydhög J, Riisgaard de Blanck S, Josipovic M, Irming Jølck R, Larsen KR, Clementsen P et al (2017) Target position uncertainty during visually guided deep-inspiration breath-hold radiotherapy in locally advanced lung cancer. Radiother Oncol 123:78–84
Seppenwoolde Y, Shirato H, Kitamura K, Shimizu S, van Herk M, Lebesque JV et al (2002) Precise and real-time measurement of 3D tumor motion in lung due to breathing and heartbeat, measured during radiotherapy. Int J Radiat Oncol Biol Phys 53:822–834
Shieh C-C, Caillet V, Dunbar M, Keall PJ, Booth JT, Hardcastle N et al (2017) A Bayesian approach for three-dimensional markerless tumor tracking using kV imaging during lung radiotherapy. *Phys Med Biol* 62:3065
Shih HA, Jiang SB, Aljarrah KM, Doppke KP, Choi NC (2004) Internal target volume determined with expansion margins beyond composite gross tumor volume in three-dimensional conformal radiotherapy for lung cancer. Int J Radiat Oncol Biol Phys 60:613–622
Takao S, Miyamoto N, Matsuura T, Onimaru R, Katoh N, Inoue T et al (2016) Intrafractional baseline shift or drift of lung tumor motion during gated radiation therapy with a real-time tumor-tracking system. Int J Radiat Oncol Biol Phys 94:172–180
Tewatia D, Zhang T, Tome W, Paliwal B, Metha M (2006) Clinical implementation of target tracking by breathing synchronized delivery. Med Phys 33:4330–4336
Toftegaard J, Hansen R, Ravkilde T, Macek K, Poulsen PR (2017) An experimentally validated couch and MLC tracking simulator used to investigate hybrid couch-MLC tracking. Med Phys 44:798–809
Underberg RWM, Lagerwaard FJ, Cuijpers JP, Slotman BJ, Van Sörnsen de Koste JR, Senan S (2004) Four-dimensional CT scans for treatment planning in stereotactic radiotherapy for stage I lung cancer. Int J Radiat Oncol Biol Phys 60:1283–1290
Urie MM, Goitein M, Doppke K, Kutcher JG, LoSasso T, Mohan R et al (1991) The role of uncertainty analysis in treatment planning. Int J Radiat Oncol Biol Phys 21:91–107
van Baardwijk A, Bosmans G, Boersma L, Buijsen J, Wanders S, Hochstenbag M et al (2007) PET-CT–based auto-contouring in non–small-cell lung Cancer correlates with pathology and reduces Interobserver variability in the delineation of the primary tumor and involved nodal volumes. Int J Radiat Oncol Biol Phys 68:771–778
van der Geld YG, van Triest B, Verbakel WFAR, van Sörnsen de Koste JR, Senan S, Slotman BJ et al (2008) Evaluation of four-dimensional computed tomography-based intensity-modulated and respiratory-gated radiotherapy techniques for pancreatic carcinoma. Int J Radiat Oncol Biol Phys 72:1215–1220
van der Vos CS, Grootjans W, Osborne DR, Meeuwis APW, Hamill JJ, Acuff S et al (2015) Improving the spatial alignment in PET/CT using amplitude-based respiration-gated PET and respiration-triggered CT. J Nucl Med 56:1817–1822
van Herk M (2004) Errors and margins in radiotherapy. Semin Radiat Oncol 14:52–64
Verellen D, Ridder MD, Linthout N, Tournel K, Soete G, Storme G (2007) Innovations in image-guided radiotherapy. Nat Rev Cancer 7:949–960
Wanet M, Sterpin E, Janssens G, Delor A, Lee JA, Geets X (2014) Validation of the mid-position strategy for lung tumors in helical TomoTherapy. Radiother Oncol 110:529–537
Wolthaus JWH, Schneider C, Sonke J-J, van Herk M, Belderbos JSA, Rossi MMG et al (2006) Mid-ventilation CT scan construction from four-dimensional respiration-correlated CT scans for radiotherapy planning of lung cancer patients. Int J Radiat Oncol Biol Phys 65:1560–1571
Wolthaus JWH, Sonke JJ, van Herk M, Damen EMF (2008) Reconstruction of a time-averaged midposition CT scan for radiotherapy planning of lung cancer patients using deformable registration. Med Phys 35:3998–4011
Yousefi S, Collins BT, Reichner CA, Anderson ED, Jamis-Dow C, Gagnon G et al (2007) Complications of thoracic computed tomography–guided fiducial placement for the purpose of stereotactic body radiation therapy. Clin Lung Cancer 8:252–256

Principles and Constraints of Nonrigid Registration

Zoi Giavri, Durval C. Costa, and Nickolas Papanikolaou

Contents

1 **Similarity Measure** 70
2 **Transformation Model** 74
3 **Optimization and Interpolation** 76
3.1 Validation 77
References 79

Abstract

Medical image registration refers to the process of determining the correspondence of anatomical or functional features between two or more images collected at different time points (serial image registration) or acquired as part of different sequences or imaging modalities (multi-modal image registration). Registration and fusion applications are proved to be of great help to the medical experts due to their contribution to the diagnostic procedure. The aim of this paper is to provide a solid theoretical review of the principles and constraints around non-rigid registration methodologies that are implemented in the medical field. The core components of these methodologies such as the similarity measures, the transformation models and the optimisation, interpolation and validation techniques are introduced and described.

Medical image registration refers to the process of determining the correspondence of anatomical or functional features between two or more images collected at different time points (serial image registration) or acquired as part of different sequences or imaging modalities (multi-modal image registration) (El-Baz et al. 2011). The aforementioned correspondence can be used to transform one image so that it more closely resembles the appearance of another in order for the pair to be directly compared, fused, and processed. According to the nature of the

Z. Giavri
Research and Development, Advantis Medical Imaging, Eindhoven, Netherlands

D. C. Costa
Nuclear Medicine Department, Centre for the Unknown, Champalimaud Foundation, Lisbon, Portugal

N. Papanikolaou (✉)
Computational Clinical Imaging Group, Lisbon, Portugal
e-mail: nickolas.papanikolaou@research.fchampalimaud.org

R. G. H. Beets-Tan et al. (eds.), *Imaging and Interventional Radiology for Radiation Oncology*, Medical Radiology, Diagnostic Imaging, https://doi.org/10.1007/978-3-030-38261-2_5

transformation, the registration methodologies are classified into two categories: the rigid (global) and the nonrigid (elastic/deformable) registration methods (Maintz and Viergever 1998).

The rigid methods (Mani 2013) are mainly applied in the cases where the images to be aligned contain small changes in the object shape, and they simply need to be rotated and translated to achieve correspondence. They consist a widely used tool in clinical practice mainly due to the rigid body constraints, which lead to a good approximation for a large number of medical imaging modalities. What should also be highlighted is that rigid methods are often extended to include affine registration (scale factors and shears) and can partially correct for calibration differences or differences in scale among the images. However, although this class of methods includes few parameters to be determined, the images of most of the human body organs have spatially variant geometric differences, requiring more sophisticated methodologies to accomplish the registration process. Thus, the scientific community has focused more on the development and improvement of nonrigid approaches.

According to literature, nonrigid registration methodologies are proved to lead to more accurate results than the rigid ones, especially in the cases where deformable soft tissue is involved (Rueckert et al. 1999). In nonrigid registration, the basic aim is to define the optimal geometric transformations that are capable of locally warping the target image to align with the reference image. Therefore, the algorithms that apply to this category consist of the components mentioned and analyzed below (Crum et al. 2004):

- *A similarity measure or registration basis*, which quantifies the level of alignment between the two images.
- *A transformation model*, which specifies a geometric transformation in order for the source image to be changed and match the target.
- *An optimization method* that varies the parameters of the aforementioned transformation model in order to maximize the matching criterion, which in this case is the similarity measure.

Listed as a final component should always be the *validation* of the registration accuracy, a measure not trivial to be calculated mainly due to the absence of a gold standard regarding the clinical practice.

1 Similarity Measure

Similarity measure is the step where the input images are compared to each other in order to measure the similarity between them. The effective measurement should resist noise and background changes. Using medical image content as a criterion, registration approaches can be divided into geometric and intensity ones.

In the case of the geometric or feature-based approaches (Pennec et al. 1998), the identifiable anatomical features of each image are used to build explicit models. Those features typically include point landmarks, edges, functionally important surfaces, or, in some cases, even the distances between corresponding features (Rohr 2001). Those corresponding point landmarks can be defined either anatomically or geometrically (Franz et al. 2006), given that they can be reliably identified in both images, by noticing the changes of the pixel/voxel intensity across the image. In the case when landmarks are identified manually, it is of high importance to use measures of location accuracy in the registration process. Once the explicit correspondence models between the pairs of point landmarks are established, interpolation is used to deduce correspondence throughout the rest of the image in a consistent way. In order to ensure the high quality of the results, several approaches have been used in the pre-interpolation step, according to literature, in which the local orientation of contours at landmark points has been used to further constrain the registration or other linear features called ridges or crest lines are extracted directly from three-dimensional (3D) images and matched with the target in a nonrigid way (Maintz et al. 1996). Given that point and line matching is a quite light process from a computational perspective, there is ground for a large number of solutions and potential

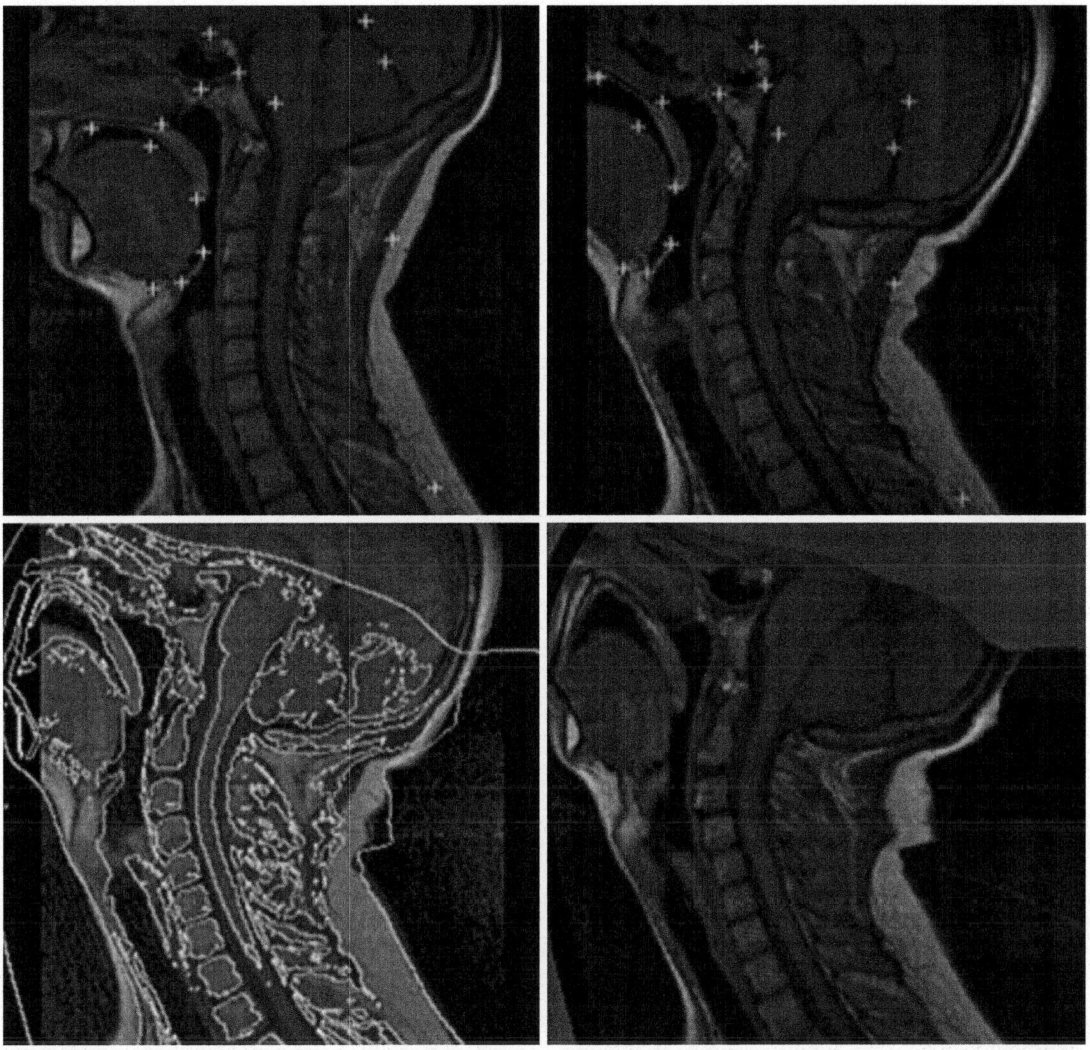

Fig. 1 The top pair of images shows sagittal MR slices of a volunteer's head scanned in two very different positions. Landmarks used to constrain the deformation are also shown. The bottom right image shows the result of deforming the top left image to match the top right, while the bottom left image shows an edge map of the deformed image superimposed on the top right image (Hawkes 1998)

correspondences to be explored. In Fig. 1 (Hawkes 1998), a reference of an example image that has undergone deformation using a modified radial basis function (Little and Hawkes 1997) is presented.

However, although geometric/feature-based approaches have the advantages of working efficiently on both single- and multi-modality registration and ensuring that the mapping is characterized by biological validity as it is based on structural information, any error during the manual or automated feature extraction process will ruin the registration and can hardly be recovered at a later stage. Those kinds of errors are avoided with the second category of registration approaches, based on image content, the intensity-based ones (Godin et al. 1994). In the intensity approaches, there is no need for feature extraction as they match intensity patterns in each image using mathematical or statistical criteria (Melbourne et al. 2010; Ulysses and Conci 2010). They rely on voxel-based similarity as they define a measure of intensity similarity between the moving/source and the target image and adjust the transformation until the similarity is maximized. Even though those approaches are simple for mono-modality and more complex for multi-modality registration, they tend to be highly robust and accurate, and this is mainly the reason why, over the past years, they have become the most widely chosen method for measuring image alignment.

The simplest statistical similarity measure is the squared sum of intensity differences (SSD) between the images I_A and I_B, as described in Eq. 1 below:

$$I_{\mathrm{SSD}} = -\frac{\Sigma\left(I_{\mathrm{A}}(x) - I_{\mathrm{B}}(T(x))\right)^2}{n} \quad (1)$$

where x is a position in image I_{A}, $I_{\mathrm{A}}(x)$ is the intensity of the position x in image I_{A}, $I_{\mathrm{B}}(T(x))$ is the intensity at the corresponding point given by the current estimate of the transformation $T(x)$, and n is the number of voxels in the overlap region. This measure is based on the assumption that the registered images are identical except for the (Gaussian) noise, and thus, it is restricted to mono-modal image registration. Moreover, it is proven to be sensitive to small number of voxels that have very large intensity differences (Goshtasby 2012).

In order to overcome the restriction, which is posed from the aforementioned assumption of identical imaging modalities, a more general approach can be used, which assumes that corresponding image intensities are related in a linear way. This approach is expressed through the normalized cross-correlation coefficient (NCCC), as described in Eq. 2 below:

$$I_{\mathrm{NCCC}} = \frac{\Sigma\left(I_{\mathrm{A}}(x) - \overline{I_{\mathrm{A}}}\right)\left(I_{\mathrm{B}}(T(x)) - \overline{I_{\mathrm{B}}}\right)}{\sqrt{\left(\Sigma I_{\mathrm{A}}(x) - \overline{I_{\mathrm{A}}}\right)^2 \left(\Sigma I_{\mathrm{B}}(T(x)) - \overline{I_{\mathrm{B}}}\right)^2}} \quad (2)$$

where I_A and I_B stand for the average voxel intensities in images A and B correspondingly. Even though it is more flexible than SSD, NCCC is again restricted to mono-modal registration where the images do not differ significantly in terms of their intensity characteristics (Andronache et al. 2008). It should also be highlighted that in the case of NCCC, segmentation of interesting features is often necessary (Andronache et al. 2008).

In the case of multi-modal registration, the approaches that have been developed and implemented over the past years suggest similarity measures, which define weaker relationships between intensities to reflect the different intensity characteristics of various imaging modalities. One of those approaches is the correlation ratio (CR) (Roche et al. 1998) that assumes a functional relationship between intensities. The correlation ratio is defined in terms of sums and sums of squares of source voxels that correspond to a number of N_i iso-intense voxels in the target image I_{B} and is described as follows in Eq. 3:

$$I_{\mathrm{CR}} = 1 - \frac{1}{N\sigma^2} \sum_i N_i \sigma_j^2 \quad (3)$$

where

$$\sigma^2 = \frac{1}{N} \sum_{\text{overlaps}} I_{\mathrm{B}}(x)^2 - \left(\frac{1}{N} \sum_{\text{overlaps}} I_{\mathrm{B}}(x)\right)^2$$

and

$$\sigma_{\mathrm{i}}^2 = \frac{1}{N_i} \sum_{x\gamma(x)=i} I_{\mathrm{B}}(x)^2 - \left(\frac{1}{N_i} \sum_{x\gamma(x)=i} I_{\mathrm{B}}(x)\right)^2$$

Being based on the information content or entropy, a number of approaches regarding the measures of alignment have been developed. The most important component of those approaches is the feature space of the image intensities, which may be interpreted as a joint probability distribution and, thus, visualized as a two-dimensional histogram of the image intensities' co-occurrences for each trial alignment. Through the process of changing the degree to which the images are aligned, it can be proved that each image pair has a unique feature space signature at alignment and that feature space disperses when misalignment increases (Hawkes 1998). In an information-theoretic framework, the Shannon-Wiener entropy corresponds to the information content of images I_A and I_B and is described correspondingly by Eqs. 4 and 5:

$$H(I_{\mathrm{A}}) = -\sum_a p(a) \log p(a) \quad (4)$$

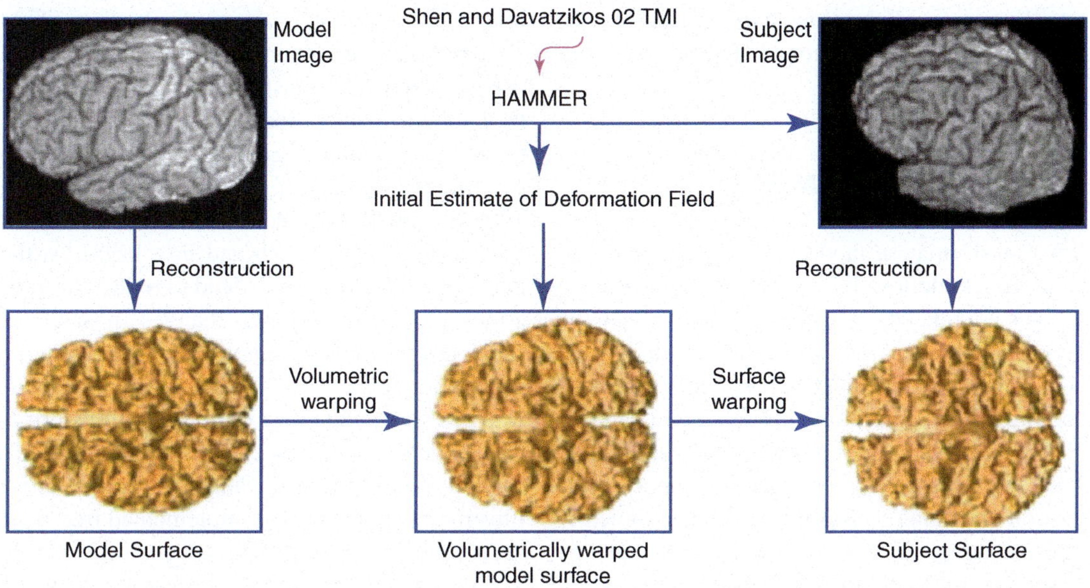

Fig. 2 As indicated in the flowchart, initially, HAMMER registers the model and subject images and produces an initial estimate of the deformation field. Afterward, the cortical surfaces are reconstructed from the volume images of both model and subject, and the model cortical surface is warped into subject space using the deformation field provided by the HAMMER algorithm. Finally, a surface warping method is used to refine the results of volumetric warping (Liu et al. 2004)

$$H(I_B) = -\sum_{b} p(b)\log p(b) \qquad (5)$$

where $p(a)$ and $p(b)$ are the probabilities of occurrence for intensities a and b in images I_A and I_B correspondingly. The joint entropy $H(I_A, I_B)$ of the overlapping region between the images I_A and I_B can be described by Eq. 6:

$$H(I_A, I_B) = -\sum_{a}\sum_{b} p(a,b)\log p(a,b) \qquad (6)$$

where $p(a,b)$ is the joint probability that a voxel in the overlapping region of the image pair has intensity values a and b, respectively. A widely used similarity measure, which belongs to the aforementioned category of information-theoretic multi-modality measures, is the mutual information (Maes et al. 1997; Viola and Wells III 1997). Mutual information, which should be maximized at alignment, is defined in terms of entropies of the intensity distribution as follows:

$$I_{MI} = H(I_A) + H(I_B) - H(I_A, I_B) \qquad (7)$$

In order to overcome the fact that mutual information measure can occasionally be affected by the degree of overlapping between the two images (Studholme et al. 1999), the use of the normalized mutual information (NMI) as a similarity measure was proposed. The normalized mutual information can be described by Eq. 8 as follows:

$$I_{NMI} = \frac{H(I_A) + H(I_n)}{H(I_A, I_B)} \qquad (8)$$

Summing up, as also mentioned above, the intensity-based similarity measures compare intensity patterns over the image but do not incorporate anatomical information. On the other hand, feature-based approaches make use of anatomical knowledge, but the latter one is usually sparsely distributed throughout the images. Hybrid algorithmic approaches are thus preferable in order to establish more accurate correspondences between the image pairs to be coregistered, as they combine model-based criteria with intensity features and are already proven more robust in difficult registration problems (Hellier and Barillot 2003; Liu et al. 2004). In Fig. 2 (Liu et al. 2004), presented is an illustration of the flowchart of HAMMER, one of the aforementioned hybrid warping methods.

2 Transformation Model

The transformation model used for the registration process defines how the coordinates of two images are related, characterizing in this way the type and number of possible deformations that will be needed. The most well-known example is the rigid body or affine transformation (Van den Elsen et al. 1993). This, for a pair of images and, is often expressed as a single coordinate transformation that maps each point into an anatomically corresponding location in image. It can be described by between 6 parameters (3 translations and 3 rotations) and 12 parameters (3 translations, 3 rotations, 3 zooms/scaling, and 3 shears) for the overall shape and size of the image (Ashburner and Friston 2001) (Fig. 3). These parameters are applied to a vector locating a point in an image to estimate its new location in another image.

Although rigid methods can be useful for the registration in the presence of rigid bodies, various body organs show spatially variant geometric differences that require more adaptable methods to successfully fulfill the registration task. This is the case of nonrigid transformations (Zagorchev and Goshtasby 2006), where there is an absence of a global linear model applied to the entire image, and a spatially varying displacement field is optimized to express the transformation (Fig. 4). Nonrigid transformations are characterized by their smoothness and invertibility and range from smooth regional variation described by a limited number of parameters (Woods et al. 1998) to dense displacement fields defined at each voxel (Freeborough and Fox 1998). At the majority of the cases, they tend to reflect the variations in anatomy where changes in size and shape are far more common than changes in the general topology.

There is a wide range of nonrigid transformation models that have an established role in medical image registration nowadays. A representative illustration are the widely implemented free-form deformations (FFDs) (Sederberg and Parry 1986), which were initially developed inside the computer graphics and computer-aided design communities. An FFD is a geometric technique used to model simple deformations of rigid objects, based on the idea of enclosing an object within a cube or another hull object and transforming the object within the hull as the latter one is deformed (Yahya et al. 2006). Deformation of the hull is based on the concept of so-called hyper-patches, which are three-dimensional analogs of parametric curves such as Bézier curves, B-splines, or Non-Uniform Rational B-splines. The technique was first described by Sederberg and Parry (1986) and is based on an earlier technique by Barr (1984). It was extended by Coquillart to a technique described as extended

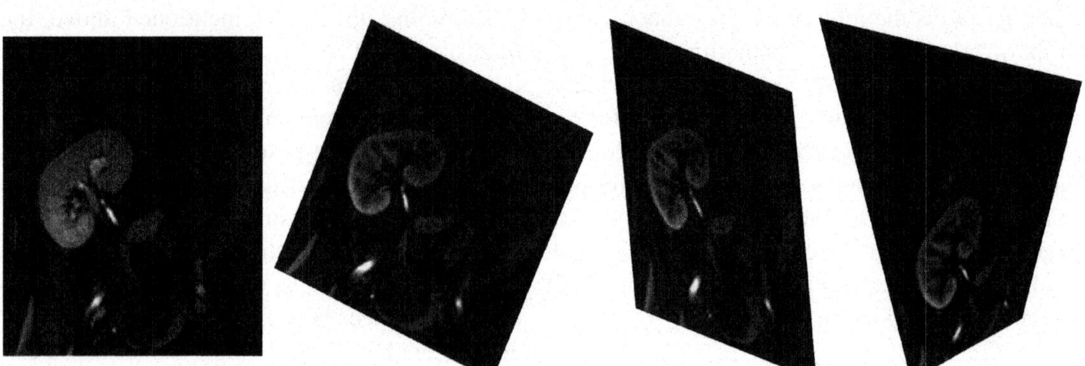

Fig. 3 Types of rigid transformations: from left to right—the reference image and similarity, affine, and projective transformations of the target image (Khalifa et al. 2011)

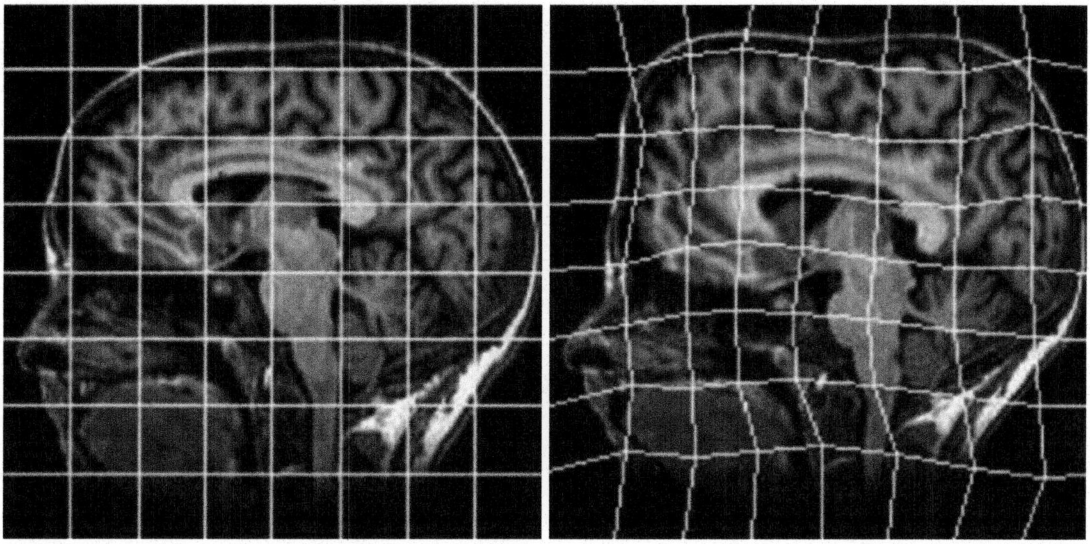

Fig. 4 Nonrigid (local) deformation example (Duy 2009)

free-form deformation, which refines the hull object by introducing additional geometry or by using different hull objects such as cylinders and prisms (Coquillart 1990).

More explicitly, an FFD is defined by a set of vectors associated with the points of a discrete 3D lattice. A blend of the vectors is used to define the displacement at a general location in the image with nearer neighbors having a greater influence. The blending weights are determined by a weighting function, and to this direction, spline functions, such as B-splines, are often used (Schwarz 2007). B-spline-based nonrigid registration techniques are widely used due to their generic applicability, transparency, and efficiency in terms of computation (Rueckert et al. 1999; Cheung and Constantinides 2003). However, they bare the disadvantage of requiring additional measures to prevent folding of the deformation field, which may be more difficult to enforce at finer resolutions (Cheung and Constantinides 2003). As mentioned previously, FFDs are classified as parametric transformations and geometric in their construction, but transformations from more physical models, such as diffusion, elastic deformation of fluid flow can possibly be derived. This nature of small deformation modeling makes them suitable for application to cases where a gradual change in anatomy is noticed. However, in cases of wide deformations, as the ones noticed in the cardiac muscle, a flow field-derived large deformation model could lead to more accurate results (Schwarz 2007).

In the case of flow-based nonparametric transformation models (Kessler 2006), the deformation field can be estimated by applying spatial and temporal smoothness constraints, additionally to the maximization of the similarity measure. Instead of seeking to optimize the displacements at each location, the optical flow has been widely used to estimate a velocity field describing the movement of corresponding features (Pai et al. 2015). The corresponding points represent the start and end points of a flow determined by the velocity. The main assumption of this methodology is that point intensities remain constant through time, and as previously mentioned, their temporal flow trajectory reflects the deformation of images. The displacement fields can be computed at any time within the temporal interval using the estimated velocity. Preferring velocity to displacement to solve for bears the advantage of restraining the transformation function with temporal consistency. However, the optimization can be a challenge, given that the velocity field can experience temporal and spatial variations.

3 Optimization and Interpolation

As mentioned above, the similarity measure can be perceived as an n-dimensional function, where n corresponds to the degrees of freedom of the transformation implemented. The optimum of this function when adjusted is linked to the transformation that appropriately registers the initial input images. The aim of the optimization algorithm is the search of the maximum or minimum value of the similarity measure previously used. In the majority of the cases, the structure of the similarity measures is such that the optimal registration is accomplished when their value is minimized.

In general, a good optimizer is considered to be the one that concludes to the best transformation in the most efficient way in terms of time and reliability. Its choice demands a deep understanding of the registration problem and the constraints that can be applied as well as knowledge of the numerical analysis. This choice, in the case of nonrigid registration, can be difficult considering that the increase of the flexibility (nonrigidity) degree in the transformation model is accompanied by an increase in the number of the parameters needed in order to describe it. Thus, the time required to make a parameter choice increases, and so does the probability of this choice to result to a good image match, but not the best one (the "local minima" problem). Another problem rising refers to the fact that, even though the transformation parameter choice leads to a good match between the initial input images or feature similarity, the result may lack physical meaning. An example of the aforementioned regards the cases when there is a prior belief that the registration should be diffeomorphic, meaning that in the case of the transformation's application to a real physical object, there would be an absence of tearing effects. The problem is that in a large number of cases like serial MR brain registration in diffuse atrophy, tearing or folding often results in a transformation that makes images more similar but lacks physical validity, and thus, they should not be required to secure a good match. In general, tearing is a result of correspondence problems. As examples, we can mention the cases of intersubject brain registration where one of the subjects has a large extrinsic tumour or abdominal registration where fluid- and gas-filled spaces appear and disappear between scans. Here, correspondence is not well defined, and tearing or folding may be necessary to describe the underlying physical transformation. Another constraint regards the choice of the transformation model in order to be in accordance with the behavior of the deforming elastic body. Thus, the optimization methodology should secure balancing between application-specific constraints and the discovery of the best set of correspondences.

From an algorithmic point of view, in deformable image registration, the similarity measure implemented is frequently addressed as the energy functional. Thus, the aim of the registration process is to detect the displacement field that represents the minimal energy functional used. The latter problem is usually translated in a problem of solving a set of partial differential equations. For this purpose, specific methodologies such as finite difference method (Lu et al. 2004), finite element method (Brock et al. 2005), variational method (Hermosillo et al. 2002), and Green's function-based methods (Marsland and Twining 2004) can be implemented. In cases where the optimization problem is translated in a set of linear equations that have to be solved simultaneously, other methodologies like singular value decomposition (Zhilkin and Alexander 2000) or least squares (Friston et al. 1995) can be considered. Support vector machine technique has also been reported to be used in image registration protocols (Zhang et al. 2005). Those algorithms are usually based on prior knowledge obtained from the joint intensity distribution between two or more registered images. This prior knowledge is integrated in the registration procedure to obtain an estimation for the similarity measure in terms of the geometric transformation. Support vector machine technique is supposed to be very efficient in computational time due to the fact that in this case the optimization is a sparse problem.

In general, the similarity measure contains a large number of local extremes, and thus, it is considered not to be smooth. A fraction of those extremes appear due to interpolation imperfections and lack of robustness in the similarity measure, while others do represent local best solutions. The iterative optimization algorithms usually include a pyramidal strategy using a coarse-to-fine approach. The whole process initiates by down-sampling the target and moving/source images through a pair of image pyramids that has been priorly defined. Afterward, the registration starts from the lower to the higher resolution images. In each step, the transformation generated is used as the new initial registration for the next step. Relative to the methodologies that just make use of the original images, this approach bears the advantage of higher convergence radius and is faster and more robust to local optimums. In the case of point correspondence-based registration algorithms, the optimal transformation between the target and the moving/source image can directly be derived based on the established matching. A well-known example of such minimization strategies is the Procrustes method (Hill et al. 2001). Similar solutions are those that are based on the least squares techniques.

A characteristic of many registration approaches is their asymmetric expression. The common practice applied for the estimation of the similarity measure is that the algorithm loops over the voxels of the target image, identifying the corresponding locations in the moving/source image under the current transformation estimate. From the overall process, each target-source intensity pair is afterward used for the similarity estimation. However, the exact correspondence between the locations of the target and the source voxel is highly unlikely, as in the majority of the cases the target voxel corresponds to an intermediate location within the source voxel lattice. This phenomenon necessitates the implementation of interpolation in the source image in order to estimate the intensity at the new position.

The interpolation solution used can affect the accuracy and speed of the registration process. For example, in the cases when a nearest neighbor or linear interpolation scheme is applied, the source image undergoes a low-passing filtering resulting in loss of detail that can affect the registration (Thévenaz et al. 2000). However, such effects are mainly small especially when the aforementioned pyramidal strategy is applied. More complex interpolation approaches (Tsao 2003), such as windowed sinc interpolators or cubic B-spline, can be used, but attention should be paid to the heavy computational load that may lead to severe decrease of the overall speed. In cases when the similarity measure's smoothness or robustness is highly affected by side effects of the interpolation, a superior interpolation is recommended to be implemented during the optimization step.

3.1 Validation

A very important step of the overall medical image registration process regards the evaluation of the algorithms that are selected to be implemented, given that registration's value lowers significantly if it fails in establishing correspondence between the input images or, even worse, if its accuracy cannot be evaluated. One should take into consideration that the process of validating the registration performance is often affected by the lack of knowledge regarding patient's movement and the extent to which the latter has affected the clinical usefulness of the data. Thus, in order to ensure the maintenance of the clinical usefulness, it is of major importance to ensure the success of the registration.

There are two approaches in validating a registration process, the qualitative and the quantitative one. In the majority of the cases, an initial visual inspection aids in the qualitative assessment of registration accuracy, followed by quantitative tests regarding the robustness and the consistency of the methodology implemented. In the absence of a ground truth correspondence estimate, robustness checks measure the accuracy by testing the bias and sensitivity, after an event of adding noise or choosing different starting estimates, while consistency checks evaluate the capability of a registration methodology to detect circular transformations based on a registration circuit (Chui and Rangarajan 2003). However, we should note that, even though consistency checks have been successfully implemented in cases of intra-modality rigid body registration applications, they are proved to be sensitive to bias and may not be suitable for noninvertible transformations generated by nonrigid registration approaches (West et al. 1997). In terms of the qualitative assessment, the methods that can be used from a trained professional to perform visual assessment of registration performance include the inspection of anatomical landmarks, contour or segmentation overlays, or alternate voxel displays. The aforementioned approaches mainly regard the inspection of results derived from application of rigid registration methodologies, but by the time they involve the inspection of an image pair's entire volume domain, they can be extended to nonrigid registration approaches. However, in the case of nonrigid registration, locally implausible deformations that cannot be detected through visual assessment yet remain a significant challenge.

Regarding the quantitative assessment, since the image registration problem is perceived as an optimization problem, the image similarity measure optimization can serve as an accuracy measure. However, the problem in this case is that most similarity measures have no geometric or physical significance. To solve the issue of the absence of a ground truth transformation, a simple approach is to apply a transformation to an image and then implement the registration algorithm to realign both images (D'agostino et al. 2003). In this case, the applied transformation can be regarded as ground truth. A similar approach is based on generating medical image artificial/synthetic datasets and evaluating the registration algorithm on the data that have been produced. Schnabel et al. (2003) introduced a biomechanical motion simulator, modeling physically plausible tissue deformations of the breast for clinically realistic motion scenarios.

More reliable solutions are still considered the ones that involve the manual identification of a set of corresponding points in input images and their use to assess the registration accuracy (Mattes et al. 2003). The target registration error, which evaluates the registration performance based on point correspondence, is an important measure of the accuracy of the performed registration. However, even though the fact that its value reflects the Euclidean distance between the corresponding points and, thus, it has an immediate physical meaning, its drawback remains the dependency on fiducial localization error (FLE). Another probabilistic approach that was proposed (Hub et al. 2009) regarded the distinction between areas where the mono-modal B-spline-based registration performs well from those in which the accuracy of the results is lower. Moreover, another evaluation (Schnabel et al. 2003) on the performance of B-spline-based registration approach includes the use of synthetic images deformed by the finite element method. The Dice similarity coefficient has also been implemented (Alterovitz et al. 2006) to assess the registration accuracy through the quantification of the amount of overlapping regions. Finally, it is known that the segmentation process can provide a measurement of surface distance prior to and after segmentation but does not provide any information regarding the registration performance within the structure or along its outline. However, if the goal of the registration includes the automation of the segmentation process, segmentation quality can serve as a substitute measurement (Klein et al. 2009).

At any case, given that, as mentioned previously, the image registration process is mainly perceived as an optimization problem with a multiple set of tunable parameters, it is clear that its performance can highly be affected by the selection of those parameters. In the majority of the cases, those parameters tend to be adjusted manually through the observation of the registration results and thus not securing that the best combination is selected. Yeo et al. (2010) proposed a machine learning-based solution to this problem through presenting a principled framework for learning thousands of parameters of registration cost functions, such as a spatially varying trade-off between the image dissimilarity and regularization terms.

References

Alterovitz R, Goldberg K, Pouliot J, Hsu I, Joe C, Kim Y, Noworolski SM, Kurhanewicz J (2006) Registration of MR prostate images with biomechanical modeling and nonlinear parameter estimation. Med Phys 33(2):446–454

Andronache A, von Siebenthal M, Székely G, Cattin P (2008) Non-rigid registration of multi-modal images using both mutual information and cross-correlation. Med Image Anal 12(1):3–15

Ashburner JT and Friston KJ, (2001) Computational neuroanatomy (Doctoral dissertation, University of London)

Barr AH (1984) Global and local deformations of solid primitives. In ACM Siggraph Computer Graphics (Vol. 18, No. 3, pp. 21–30). ACM

Brock KK, Sharpe MB, Dawson LA, Kim SM, Jaffray DA (2005) Accuracy of finite element model-based multi-organ deformable image registration. Med Phys 32(6):1647–1659

Cheung PY and Constantinides GA (2003) Field-programmable logic and applications: 13th International Conference, FPL 2003, Lisbon, Portugal, September 1–3, 2003, Proceedings (Vol. 2778). Springer Science & Business Media

Chui H, Rangarajan A (2003) A new point matching algorithm for non-rigid registration. Comput Vis Image Underst 89(2):114–141

Coquillart S (1990) Extended free-form deformation: a sculpturing tool for 3D geometric modeling (Vol. 24, no. 4, pp. 187-196). ACM

Crum WR, Hartkens T, Hill DLG (2004) Non-rigid image registration: theory and practice. Br J Radiol 77(suppl_2):S140–S153

D'agostino E, Maes F, Vandermeulen D, Suetens P (2003) A viscous fluid model for multimodal non-rigid image registration using mutual information. Med Image Anal 7(4):565–575

Duy LVN (2009) Review and enhancement optimization methods in image registration. MEng. Computing, Department of Computing, Imperial College London

El-Baz AS, Acharya R, Mirmehdi M, Suri JS (2011) Multi modality state-of-the-art medical image segmentation and registration methodologies (Vol. 1). Springer Science & Business Media

Franz A and Carlsen IC, Koninklijke Philips Electronics, NV (2006). Adaptive Point-Based Elastic Image Registration US Patent Application 12/097,530

Freeborough PA, Fox NC (1998) Modeling brain deformations in Alzheimer disease by fluid registration of serial 3D MR images. J Comput Assist Tomogr 22(5):838–843

Friston K, Ashburner J, Frith CD, Poline JB, Heather JD, Frackowiak RS (1995) Spatial registration and normalization of images. Hum Brain Mapp 3(3):165–189

Godin G, Rioux M and Baribeau R (1994) Three-dimensional registration using range and intensity information. In: Proceedings of SPIE videometric III (Vol. 2350, pp. 279–290)

Goshtasby AA (2012) Image registration: principles, tools and methods. Springer Science & Business Media

Hawkes DJ (1998) Algorithms for radiological image registration and their clinical application. J Anat 193(3):347–361

Hellier P, Barillot C (2003) Coupling dense and landmark-based approaches for nonrigid registration. IEEE Trans Med Imaging 22(2):217–227

Hermosillo G, Chefd'Hotel C, Faugeras O (2002) Variational methods for multimodal image matching. Int J Comput Vis 50(3):329–343

Hill DL, Batchelor PG, Holden M, Hawkes DJ (2001) Medical image registration. Phys Med Biol 46(3):R1

Hub M, Kessler ML, Karger CP (2009) A stochastic approach to estimate the uncertainty involved in b-spline image registration. IEEE Trans Med Imaging 28(11):1708–1716

Kessler ML (2006) Image registration and data fusion in radiation therapy. Br J Radiol 79(special_issue_1):S99–S108

Khalifa F, Beache GM, Gimel'farb G, Suri JS and El-Baz AS (2011) State-of-the-art medical image registration methodologies: a survey. In Multi modality state-of-the-art medical image segmentation and registration methodologies (pp. 235–280). Springer US

Klein A, Andersson J, Ardekani BA, Ashburner J, Avants B, Chiang MC, Christensen GE, Collins DL, Gee J, Hellier P, Song JH (2009) Evaluation of 14 nonlinear deformation algorithms applied to human brain MRI registration. NeuroImage 46(3):786–802

Little JA, Hawkes DJ (1997) The registration of multiple medical images acquired from a single subject: why, how, what next? Stat Methods Med Res 6(3): 239–265

Liu T, Shen D, Davatzikos C (2004) Deformable registration of cortical structures via hybrid volumetric and surface warping. NeuroImage 22(4):1790–1801

Lu W, Chen ML, Olivera GH, Ruchala KJ, Mackie TR (2004) Fast free-form deformable registration via calculus of variations. Phys Med Biol 49(14):3067

Maes F, Collignon A, Vandermeulen D, Marchal G, Suetens P (1997) Multimodality image registration by maximization of mutual information. IEEE Trans Med Imaging 16(2):187–198

Maintz JA, Viergever MA (1998) A survey of medical image registration. Med Image Anal 2(1):1–36

Maintz JBA, van den Elsen PA, Viergever MA (1996) Evaluation of ridge seeking operators for multimodality medical image matching. IEEE Trans Pattern Anal Mach Intell 18(4):353–365

Mani VRS (2013) Survey of medical image registration. J Biomed Eng Technol 1(2):8–25

Marsland S, Twining CJ (2004) Constructing diffeomorphic representations for the groupwise analysis of nonrigid registrations of medical images. IEEE Trans Med Imaging 23(8):1006–1020

Mattes D, Haynor DR, Vesselle H, Lewellen TK, Eubank W (2003) PET-CT image registration in the chest

using free-form deformations. IEEE Trans Med Imaging 22(1):120–128
Melbourne A, Ridgway G and Hawkes DJ (2010) Image similarity metrics in image registration. SPIE-The International Society for Optical Engineering
Pai A, Sommer S, Sørensen L, Darkner S, Sporring J and Nielsen M (2015) Image registration using stationary velocity fields parameterized by norm-minimizing Wendland kernel. In Medical Imaging: Image Processing (p. 941335)
Pennec X, Guttmann CR, Thirion JP (1998) Feature-based registration of medical images: estimation and validation of the pose accuracy. In: International Conference on Medical Image Computing and Computer-Assisted Intervention. Springer, Berlin, Heidelberg, pp 1107–1114
Roche A, Malandain G, Pennec X and Ayache N (1998) The correlation ratio as a new similarity measure for multimodal image registration. Medical Image Computing and Computer-Assisted Intervention—MICCAI '98, pp. 1115–1124
Rohr K (2001) Landmark-based image analysis: using geometric and intensity models (Vol. 21). Springer Science & Business Media
Rueckert D, Sonoda LI, Hayes C, Hill DL, Leach MO, Hawkes DJ (1999) Nonrigid registration using free-form deformations: application to breast MR images. IEEE Trans Med Imaging 18(8):712–721
Schnabel JA, Tanner C, Castellano-Smith AD, Degenhard A, Leach MO, Hose DR, Hill DL, Hawkes DJ (2003) Validation of nonrigid image registration using finite-element methods: application to breast MR images. IEEE Trans Med Imaging 22(2): 238–247
Schwarz LA (2007) Non-rigid registration using free-form deformations. In Ph. D. dissertation, Dept. Comput. Sci., Tech. Univ. Munchen
Sederberg TW and Parry SR, (1986) Free-form deformation of solid geometric models. ACM SIGGRAPH computer graphics, 20(4), pp.151–160
Studholme C, Hill DL, Hawkes DJ (1999) An overlap invariant entropy measure of 3D medical image alignment. Pattern Recogn 32(1):71–86
Thévenaz P, Blu T, Unser M (2000) Interpolation revisited [medical images application]. IEEE Trans Med Imaging 19(7):739–758
Tsao J (2003) Interpolation artifacts in multimodality image registration based on maximization of mutual information. IEEE Trans Med Imaging 22(7):854–864
Ulysses JN and Conci A (2010) Measuring similarity in medical registration. In IWSSIP 17th International Conference on Systems, Signals and Image Processing
Van den Elsen PA, Pol EJ, Viergever MA (1993) Medical image matching-a review with classification. IEEE Eng Med Biol Mag 12(1):26–39
Viola P, Wells WM III (1997) Alignment by maximization of mutual information. Int J Comput Vis 24(2):137–154
West J, Fitzpatrick JM, Wang MY, Dawant BM, Maurer CR Jr, Kessler RM, Maciunas RJ, Barillot C, Lemoine D, Collignon A, Maes F (1997) Comparison and evaluation of retrospective intermodality brain image registration techniques. J Comput Assist Tomogr 21(4):554–568
Woods RP, Grafton ST, Watson JD, Sicotte NL, Mazziotta JC (1998) Automated image registration: II. Intersubject validation of linear and nonlinear models. J Comput Assist Tomogr 22(1):153–165
Yahya SN, Suaib NM, Bade A and Shamsuddin SMH (2006) Solid deformation modeling techniques. In Computing & Informatics, 2006. ICOCI '06. International Conference on (pp. 1–14). IEEE
Yeo BT, Sabuncu MR, Vercauteren T, Holt DJ, Amunts K, Zilles K, Golland P, Fischl B (2010) Learning task-optimal registration cost functions for localizing cytoarchitecture and function in the cerebral cortex. IEEE Trans Med Imaging 29(7):1424–1441
Zagorchev L, Goshtasby A (2006) A comparative study of transformation functions for nonrigid image registration. IEEE Trans Image Process 15(3):529–538
Zhang HH, Ahn J, Lin X, Park C (2005) Gene selection using support vector machines with non-convex penalty. Bioinformatics 22(1):88–95
Zhilkin P, Alexander ME (2000) 3D image registration using a fast noniterative algorithm. Magn Reson Imaging 18(9):1143–1150

Radiotherapy Target Volume Definition Based on PET/CT Imaging Data

Daniela Thorwarth

Contents

1 **Introduction** ... 82

2 **PET/CT Acquisition and Tracers for RT Target Volume Definition** ... 82

3 **PET/CT Image Registration for RT Treatment Planning** ... 83

4 **Methods for PET-Based Target Volume Definition** ... 84

4.1 Relative Thresholding ... 84

4.2 Absolute Thresholding ... 85

4.3 Iterative Thresholding ... 85

4.4 Source-to-Background Algorithms ... 86

4.5 Gradient-Based Auto-Contouring ... 86

4.6 Advanced Algorithms ... 86

5 **Definition of Biological Target Volumes Using PET** ... **86**

6 **Conclusion** ... 87

References ... 87

Abstract

To enable high-precision radiotherapy (RT), accurate target volume delineation (TVD) is a major prerequisite. Today, positron emission tomography (PET) allows to visualize the metabolism of tumors with a high sensitivity and specificity. Therefore, [^{18}F]-fluorodeoxyglucose ([^{18}F]FDG) PET imaging is an ideal tool to segment gross tumor volumes (GTV) for RT treatment planning.

This chapter summarizes the main steps to be considered for PET-based RT TVD including patient positioning during PET acquisition as well as registration algorithms for the fusion of PET data to computed tomography (CT) scan dedicated to RT treatment planning. Furthermore, a number of automatic and semiautomatic algorithms that were proposed in the past for PET-based RT TVD are described in detail and compared to each other. In a last paragraph, the definition of biological target volumes (BTV) based on PET using different radiotracers is discussed.

D. Thorwarth (✉)
Section for Biomedical Physics, Department of Radiation Oncology, University of Tübingen, Tübingen, Germany
e-mail: daniela.thorwarth@med.uni-tuebingen.de

R. G. H. Beets-Tan et al. (eds.), *Imaging and Interventional Radiology for Radiation Oncology*, Medical Radiology, Diagnostic Imaging, https://doi.org/10.1007/978-3-030-38261-2_6

1 Introduction

In the era of high-precision radiotherapy (RT) applications, precise and accurate target volume delineation (TVD) is a major prerequisite for a robust treatment planning procedure. For more than two decades, computed tomography (CT) imaging has been the main imaging modality to base RT treatment planning on. This is due to its high spatial resolution and to the fact that CT intrinsically measures electron densities of the tissue, which are required for accurate RT dose calculation (Ahnesjo and Aspradakis 1999). However, CT substantially lacks soft tissue contrast; therefore, it may be difficult to delineate the geometric outline of a tumor region with high accuracy. Furthermore, CT imaging does not contain any information about biological and functional properties of the underlying tumor tissue, such as the clonogenic cell density, metabolic activity, cellular proliferation, or tumor hypoxia. In contrast, these functional and biological properties can be assessed using positron emission tomography (PET) with a high sensitivity and specificity (Hicks et al. 2001; Jeraj et al. 2015; Troost et al. 2010a; Zips et al. 2012). Consequently, it seems highly beneficial to use either combined PET/CT imaging data only for RT treatment planning or in addition to a dedicated planning CT to improve the accuracy of TVD (Nestle et al. 2006; Troost et al. 2010b). Several studies have shown in the past the advantage of using functional PET/CT data for improved target volume delineation in non-small-cell lung cancer (NSCLC) (Bayne et al. 2010; Fleckenstein et al. 2011; Hanna et al. 2010), head and neck cancer (HNC) (Gregoire et al. 2018; Wang et al. 2013; Wu et al. 2016), and other tumor entities (Jeraj et al. 2015). Moreover, dedicated recommendations on the use of PET/CT for accurate TVD were published recently (Konert et al. 2015; Macmanus et al. 2009). Several studies also point out that the full potential of using PET/CT data for improved RT treatment planning can only be explored in a collaborative setting where nuclear medicine and radiation oncology specialists work closely together (Doll et al. 2014; Hanna et al. 2010; Thorwarth et al. 2012).

This chapter will discuss the technical requirements in terms of image acquisition, reconstruction, and analysis as well as pitfalls of using PET/CT data for RT TVD. Furthermore, in addition to some details on image registration, different methods for semiautomatic and automatic PET-based TVD will be introduced and discussed. In the last part of this chapter, methods for the definition of biological target volumes (BTV) encompassing regions of, e.g., increased tumor hypoxia will be discussed.

2 PET/CT Acquisition and Tracers for RT Target Volume Definition

The most used PET tracer for RT planning and TVD is [^{18}F]-fluorodeoxyglucose ([^{18}F]FDG), a radioactively marked glucose analogue, which visualizes glucose metabolism in tissue and can therefore be used for accurate tumor detection and volume definition.

However, there are a number of technical challenges when using PET for TVD, which may affect the resulting target contours significantly. First, the image acquisition procedure directly influences the measured data as [^{18}F]FDG retention is depending on different factors such as the amount of activity injected, the time delay between tracer injection and image acquisition, the image acquisition protocol used, and individual, patient-specific physiological factors (Cheebsumon et al. 2011a, b; Lee 2010; Thorwarth et al. 2012). Furthermore, for image reconstruction, a number of different algorithms exist. Several studies have shown that PET-based TVD results may change when using different reconstruction algorithms for the same set of raw data (Knausl et al. 2013; Knudtsen et al. 2014). Figure 1 shows differences in target contours delineated with the same automatic contouring algorithm on image data sets that were reconstructed from the same raw data using different algorithms.

Despite its high sensitivity, PET suffers from a low spatial resolution. Clinical PET scanners today reach a geometric resolution of approximately 6–8 mm. Consequently, PET-based TVD can only be applied to larger tumor volumes. Due to the low geometric resolution, PET imaging is not able to

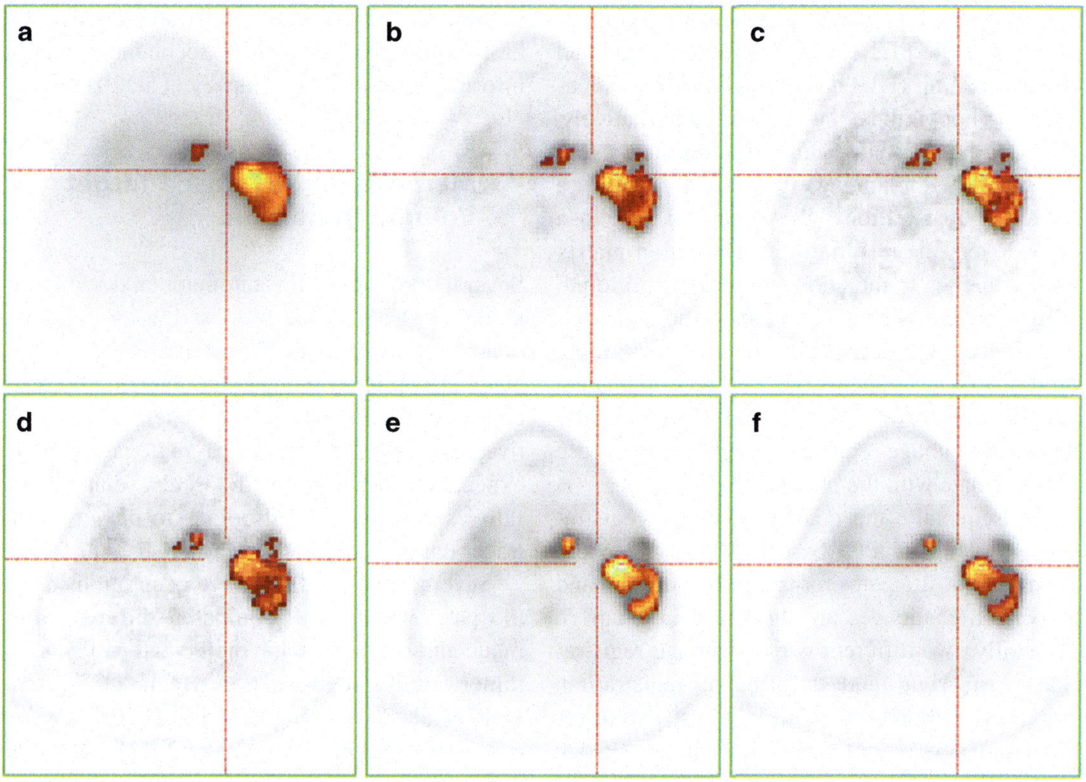

Fig. 1 [^{18}F]FDG PET imaging data of a patient with head and neck cancer reconstructed using six different methods, followed by automatic target volume delineation using a 40% SUV_{max} technique. (**a**) OSEM 2i4s, (**b**) OSEM 4i8s, (**c**) OSEM 2i24s, (**d**) time-of-flight (TOF) reconstruction, (**e**) resolution modeling (RM) reconstruction, (**f**) TOF + RM

display fine biological and functional structures (Cheebsumon et al. 2011a, b; Knausl et al. 2013; Lee 2010; Thorwarth et al. 2012, 2010).

However, in recent years, PET imaging experienced many hardware- and software-based advances which improved cancer imaging significantly (Van Der Vos et al. 2017). Nevertheless, reproducible PET-based TVD for RT requires standardized PET image data acquisition as input. To achieve this, procedures for PET scanner harmonization and standardization were proposed which especially in multicenter trails guarantee the comparability of data between different institutions and scanners (Boellaard et al. 2015, 2010). A study comparing different RT contouring methods and different PET reconstruction settings demonstrated that automatic contouring of lung tumors after PET scanner harmonization was an accurate means of overcoming reconstruction variability in PET-based TVD (Lasnon et al. 2017).

Hence, for robust and reproducible PET-derived RT target volumes, standardized procedures in terms of imaging protocols, tracer injection, and reconstruction settings are required. For multicenter comparability of the data including RT volumes, a certified harmonization of the PET scanner is recommended.

3 PET/CT Image Registration for RT Treatment Planning

RT treatment planning based on PET/CT imaging data can either be done by using the PET/CT scanner directly for simulation. This implies that patients are positioned during PET/CT acquisition in RT treatment position. Additionally, a laser bridge for external patient marking is required at the PET/CT scanner and a validated Hounsfield unit (HU) calibration for dose calculation (Thorwarth et al. 2012). Alternatively, PET/CT data may be acquired additionally to a dedicated RT planning CT. In this case, a CT-to-CT registration will be carried out. In a second step, the resulting transformation matrix will be applied to the PET data for registration to the RT planning data. To obtain sufficient registration accuracy, RT-specific patient positioning during PET/CT acquisition is recommended. Alternatively, or in addition, one might consider deformable image registration techniques to fuse PET/CT data with the planning CT.

Consequently, the quality of image registration is crucial for PET-based TVD in RT. More details about strategies for image registration and associated challenges are discussed in Chap. 5. Generally, two different ways of image registration exist: rigid and deformable registration. Rigid registration is much more robust, as a lower number of degrees of freedom is used here (Brock et al. 2017). However, often, patient positioning and/or patient anatomy and volume are not identical from the day of CT simulation to PET/CT. This applies especially to situations where PET/CT data during or after therapy are registered to a pre-treatment CT. Here, deformable registration can significantly improve registration results. However, several mathematical approaches to perform deformable registration exist (Leibfarth et al. 2013; Teske et al. 2017; Vasquez Osorio et al. 2015). Often, it is extremely challenging to assess and validate registration accuracy, robustness, and errors of the method in a general way (Brock et al. 2017; Castadot et al. 2008). Hence, there are risks of considerable misregistrations when using deformable registration algorithms (Fortunati et al. 2015). Visual approval of the registration result by experts is recommended. Therefore, a strategy to deal with this issue in clinical practice is to position patients for functional imaging intended to guide TVD in RT treatment position, i.e., with flat tabletop, vacuum cushion, and thermoplastic mask in order to achieve better results during deformable image registration. Recent studies have shown that combining both strategies, RT-specific patient positioning plus deformable registration, yields the best results for integrating secondary imaging information into TVD (Hanvey et al. 2013).

4 Methods for PET-Based Target Volume Definition

Several approaches for automatic and semiautomatic TVD have been proposed in the literature (Thorwarth and Schaefer 2010; Zaidi and El Naqa 2010). Even though automatic methods for contouring of PET data seem beneficial as objective, user-independent tumor regions are to be expected, automated methods also contain pitfalls especially when it comes to physiological tracer uptake, e.g., in the heart.

Several investigations have been published in the past, which have compared different automatic and semiautomatic methods for PET-based tumor volume segmentation (Bayne et al. 2010; Doll et al. 2014; Shepherd et al. 2012; Wanet et al. 2011; Werner-Wasik et al. 2012). Also standardized manual delineation approaches have shown to result in very accurate and reproducible contouring results (Bayne et al. 2010; Doll et al. 2014). However, this requires highly standardized imaging and delineation protocols (Bayne et al. 2010) as well as experienced staff for delineation (Doll et al. 2014).

For algorithm validation and benchmarking, it is difficult to define valid and accessible gold standards. In general, only phantom experiments with spherical lesions can be used for quality assurance and validation of automatic segmentation approaches. However, automatic PET-based segmentation methods are strongly dependent on image contrast, noise, and also imaging protocols as well as reconstruction algorithms.

4.1 Relative Thresholding

The most used automatic contouring approach is relative thresholding (cf. Fig. 2a). This method aims at creating a tumor contour at a certain cutoff value in terms of standardized uptake value (SUV) which is defined relative to the maximum tracer uptake SUV_{max} in the tumor region.

Therefore, image voxels with intensities I higher or equal than this threshold are considered in the tumor region of interest (ROI), with:

$$I_{\text{tumor}} \geq r \cdot \text{SUV}_{\text{max}}$$

where r is the relative cutoff value. Calibration of r can be done using phantom experiments and was shown to be in the range r = 40–50% (Erdi et al. 1997). A number of multicenter studies and initiatives have recently decided to use relative thresholding to automatically segment tumor ROIs based on [^{18}F]FDG PET data as this approach is simple to implement and yields robust results (Van Elmpt et al. 2012). Care should be taken to identify the maximum uptake in the tumor lesion and not to apply this approach in areas close to regions with physiological tracer uptake. To ensure this, a lot of software implementations ask to identify a subregion (e.g., a mask) inside the PET data set containing the tumor.

4.2 Absolute Thresholding

Similar to relative thresholding, also during absolute thresholding (cf. Fig. 2b), PET voxels belonging to the tumor ROI are identified by signal intensities above an absolute activity threshold R:

$$I_{\text{tumor}} \geq R$$

Most studies used values of R = 2.5–3 in units of SUV here (Hellwig et al. 2007). Main difficulty when using absolute thresholding is that absolute SUVs are subject to inter-patient variation depending on individual physiological factors.

4.3 Iterative Thresholding

Iterative thresholding also uses a threshold value to distinguish cancerous from noncancerous tissue. In contrast to the previous methods, the cut-

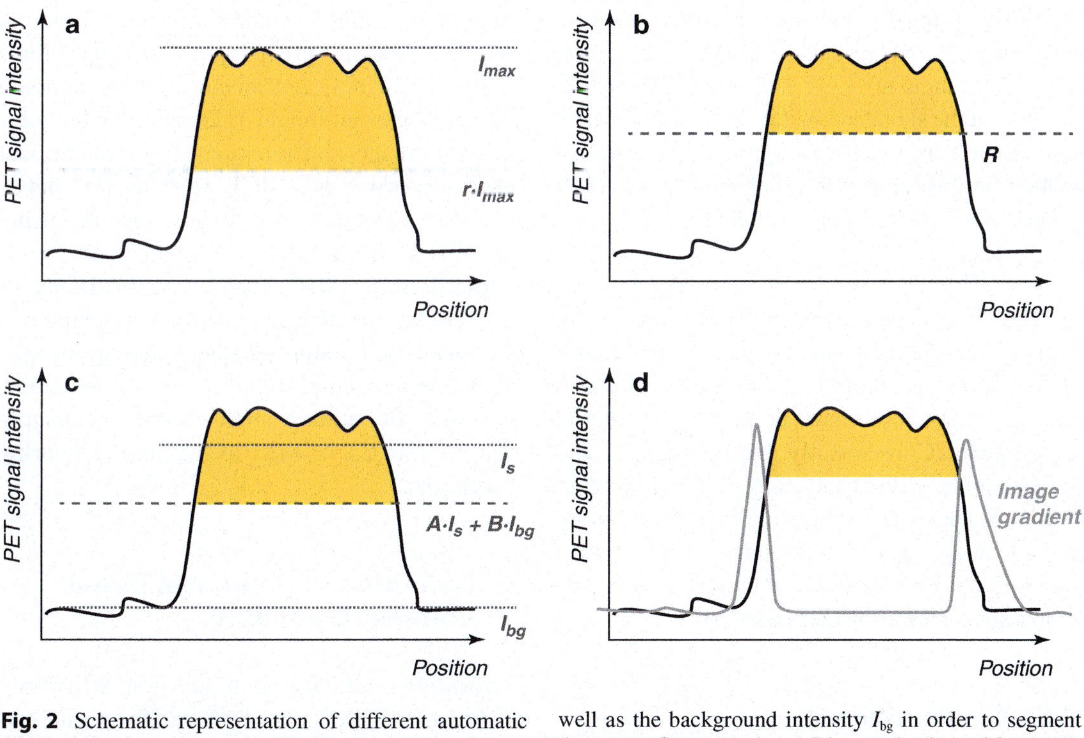

Fig. 2 Schematic representation of different automatic PET-based contouring methods frequently used in RT treatment planning. (**a**) Relative thresholding using a certain cutoff r relative to the maximum PET intensity I_{max}. (**b**) Absolute thresholding applies a fixed cutoff value R to segment the data. (**c**) Source-to-background algorithms take into account the PET intensity inside the source I_s as well as the background intensity I_{bg} in order to segment the tumor. Constants A and B have to be derived from calibration measurements. (**d**) Gradient-based segmentation requires first the calculation of a gradient image, which is then used to segment the tumor where gradients of the original PET image take maximum values

off value used for segmentation is not fixed a priori. This cutoff value is determined in an iterative process in order to find an optimal border of the tumor. The threshold is iteratively varied as long as it falls into a segment of signal intensities where the thresholded volume would maximally change with respect to the cutoff value, i.e., into a region with a mean maximum signal gradient:

$$I_{\text{tumor}} \geq t \cdot \text{SUV}_{\max}$$

Here, t is a relative threshold value applied to the maximum SUV, which has been determined iteratively.

4.4 Source-to-Background Algorithms

Source-to-background (SB) algorithms were proposed in the past by different research groups (Daisne et al. 2003; Schaefer et al. 2008). In general, SB algorithms use the fact that the PET signal inside a tumor lesion may be surrounded by physiological background uptake. Therefore, those algorithms not only derive a segmentation on basis of the signal intensities in the high-uptake region but also use the background signal information for this (cf. Fig. 2c). Schaefer et al. (2008) proposed to use the following SB algorithm:

$$I_{\text{tumor}} \geq A \cdot I_{\text{s}} + B \cdot I_{\text{bg}}$$

where I_S and I_{BG} are the PET intensities in the source, i.e., the high-uptake part of the tumor lesion and the background, respectively. A and B are calibration constants defined by phantom experiments. Consequently, the constants A and B are scanner specific and can vary from center to center. Schaefer et al. have used SB-based auto-segmentation in a multicenter trial, which required calibration of the method in each participating center (Schaefer et al. 2012).

4.5 Gradient-Based Auto-Contouring

Inspired by the fact that most thresholding algorithms for PET-based tumor segmentation have considerable limitations when it comes to small tumor lesions or to heterogeneous tracer uptake inside the lesion, Geets et al. (2007) have developed a gradient-based algorithm to automatically segment [^{18}F]FDG PET data. Basically, this algorithm uses a two-step segmentation approach where in the first step the PET image is edge-enhanced and smoothed. The second step then consists of detecting the gradients present in the image domain in order to use the positions where the steepest gradients can be detected as tumor outlines (cf. Fig.2d). A study published by Wanet et al. (2011) confirmed that gradient-based segmentation is more robust and accurate compared to thresholding techniques especially when tumor volumes are small.

4.6 Advanced Algorithms

Recently, a number of advanced automatic segmentation algorithms were proposed using, e.g., machine learning or other modern computing methods. Several groups proposed algorithms which do not only use advanced computational strategies for automatic segmentation but also include image information from additional sources compared to PET, such as CT and/or MRI data available from hybrid imaging using PET/CT or PET/MRI (Berthon et al. 2017; Leibfarth et al. 2015; Yang et al. 2015). All of these studies nicely show that the low spatial resolution of PET compromising accuracy of segmentation techniques based on PET only can be improved by adding high-resolution imaging data such as CT or MRI to the auto-contouring algorithms.

5 Definition of Biological Target Volumes Using PET

Depending on the research question, other tracers than [^{18}F]FDG may be used for segmentation purposes in clinical trials. In contrast to [^{18}F]FDG, which is able to visualize metabolism and thus geometric extension of the gross tumor volume (GTV), other tracers may be needed to visualize different biological properties of a tumor such as hypoxia or proliferation. It has been shown before that functional tracers such as [^{18}F]-fluoromisonidazole (FMISO) (Lock et al. 2017; Thorwarth et al. 2007; Welz et al. 2017; Zips et al. 2012) or [^{18}F]-fluorothymidine (FLT) (Troost et al. 2010a), which can be used to image hypoxia or proliferation, respectively, can potentially be used for the definition of a biological target volume (BTV). The definition of a BTV includes areas with higher or worse biological activity compared to the normal state. Studies have shown that the definition of such BTV based on functional PET tracers different from [^{18}F]FDG may be quite challenging due to the low signal-to-noise ratio that those tracers present with frequently (Monnich et al. 2015). Hence, different methods for PET-based BTV delineation have to be applied. Several groups propose to use a tumor-to-muscle ratio (TMR) or a tumor-to-background ratio (TBR) above a certain threshold to segment BTVs (Mortensen et al. 2012; Zips et al. 2012). Therefore, robust and reproducible automatic contouring of BTV based on experimental tracers is challenging especially in multicenter settings. Even though several approaches have been discussed and compared in literature, so far no consensus has been reached on this. Quantitative imaging is a major prerequisite for accurate definition of a BTV. Therefore, quantitative functional PET, including also dynamic PET imaging data analyzed via pharmacokinetic models, seem to be a promising alternative for automatic PET-based definition of biological target volumes (Grkovski et al. 2017a, b; Welz et al. 2017).

6 Conclusion

PET imaging is a powerful and highly sensitive as well as specific imaging modality, which makes it well-suited for RT purposes, especially for PET-based target volume delineation. Consequently, when acquiring PET image data in RT-specific positioning and using adequate image registration tools, highly accurate segmentation of the GTV can be performed to guide RT treatment planning.

References

Ahnesjo A, Aspradakis MM (1999) Dose calculations for external photon beams in radiotherapy. Phys Med Biol 44.:R:99–155

Bayne M, Hicks RJ, Everitt S et al (2010) Reproducibility of "intelligent" contouring of gross tumor volume in non-small-cell lung cancer on PET/CT images using a standardized visual method. Int J Radiat Oncol Biol Phys 77:1151–1157

Berthon B, Evans M, Marshall C et al (2017) Head and neck target delineation using a novel PET automatic segmentation algorithm. Radiother Oncol 122:242–247

Boellaard R, O'doherty MJ, Weber WA et al (2010) FDG PET and PET/CT: EANM procedure guidelines for tumour PET imaging: version 1.0. Eur J Nucl Med Mol Imaging 37:181–200

Boellaard R, Delgado-Bolton R, Oyen WJ et al (2015) FDG PET/CT: EANM procedure guidelines for tumour imaging: version 2.0. Eur J Nucl Med Mol Imaging 42:328–354

Brock KK, Mutic S, Mcnutt TR et al (2017) Use of image registration and fusion algorithms and techniques in radiotherapy: report of the AAPM Radiation Therapy Committee Task Group No. 132. Med Phys 44:e43–e76

Castadot P, Lee JA, Parraga A et al (2008) Comparison of 12 deformable registration strategies in adaptive radiation therapy for the treatment of head and neck tumors. Radiother Oncol 89:1–12

Cheebsumon P, Van Velden FH, Yaqub M et al (2011a) Effects of image characteristics on performance of tumor delineation methods: a test-retest assessment. J Nucl Med 52:1550–1558

Cheebsumon P, Yaqub M, Van Velden FH et al (2011b) Impact of [(1)(8)F]FDG PET imaging parameters on automatic tumour delineation: need for improved tumour delineation methodology. Eur J Nucl Med Mol Imaging 38:2136–2144

Daisne JF, Sibomana M, Bol A et al (2003) Tri-dimensional automatic segmentation of PET volumes based on measured source-to-background ratios: influence of reconstruction algorithms. Radiother Oncol 69:247–250

Doll C, Duncker-Rohr V, Rucker G et al (2014) Influence of experience and qualification on PET-based target volume delineation. When there is no expert – ask your colleague. Strahlenther Onkol 190:555–562

Erdi YE, Mawlawi O, Larson SM et al (1997) Segmentation of lung lesion volume by adaptive positron emission tomography image thresholding. Cancer 80:2505–2509

Fleckenstein J, Hellwig D, Kremp S et al (2011) F-18-FDG-PET confined radiotherapy of locally advanced NSCLC with concomitant chemotherapy: results of the PET-PLAN pilot trial. Int J Radiat Oncol Biol Phys 81:e283–e289

Fortunati V, Verhaart RF, Verduijn GM et al (2015) MRI integration into treatment planning of head and neck

tumors: can patient immobilization be avoided? Radiother Oncol 115:191–194
Geets X, Lee JA, Bol A et al (2007) A gradient-based method for segmenting FDG-PET images: methodology and validation. Eur J Nucl Med Mol Imaging 34:1427–1438
Gregoire V, Thorwarth D, Lee JA (2018) Molecular imaging-guided radiotherapy for the treatment of head-and-neck squamous cell carcinoma: does it fulfill the promises? Semin Radiat Oncol 28:35–45
Grkovski M, Lee NY, Schoder H et al (2017a) Monitoring early response to chemoradiotherapy with (18) F-FMISO dynamic PET in head and neck cancer. Eur J Nucl Med Mol Imaging 44:1682–1691
Grkovski M, Schoder H, Lee NY et al (2017b) Multiparametric imaging of tumor hypoxia and perfusion with (18)F-Fluoromisonidazole dynamic PET in head and neck cancer. J Nucl Med 58:1072–1080
Hanna GG, Carson KJ, Lynch T et al (2010) 18F-fluorodeoxyglucose positron emission tomography/computed tomography-based radiotherapy target volume definition in non-small-cell lung cancer: delineation by radiation oncologists vs. joint outlining with a PET radiologist? Int J Radiat Oncol Biol Phys 78:1040–1051
Hanvey S, Mcjury M, Tho LM et al (2013) The influence of MRI scan position on patients with oropharyngeal cancer undergoing radical radiotherapy. Radiat Oncol 8:129
Hellwig D, Graeter TP, Ukena D et al (2007) 18F-FDG PET for mediastinal staging of lung cancer: which SUV threshold makes sense? J Nucl Med 48:1761–1766
Hicks RJ, Kalff V, Macmanus MP et al (2001) (18)F-FDG PET provides high-impact and powerful prognostic stratification in staging newly diagnosed non-small cell lung cancer. J Nucl Med 42:1596–1604
Jeraj R, Bradshaw T, Simoncic U (2015) Molecular imaging to Plan radiotherapy and evaluate its efficacy. J Nucl Med 56:1752–1765
Knausl B, Rausch IF, Bergmann H et al (2013) Influence of PET reconstruction parameters on the TrueX algorithm. A combined phantom and patient study. Nuklearmedizin 52:28–35
Knudtsen IS, Van Elmpt W, Ollers M et al (2014) Impact of PET reconstruction algorithm and threshold on dose painting of non-small cell lung cancer. Radiother Oncol 113:210–214
Konert T, Vogel W, Macmanus MP et al (2015) PET/CT imaging for target volume delineation in curative intent radiotherapy of non-small cell lung cancer: IAEA consensus report 2014. Radiother Oncol 116:27–34
Lasnon C, Enilorac B, Popotte H et al (2017) Impact of the EARL harmonization program on automatic delineation of metabolic active tumour volumes (MATVs). EJNMMI Res 7:30
Lee JA (2010) Segmentation of positron emission tomography images: some recommendations for target delineation in radiation oncology. Radiother Oncol 96:302–307
Leibfarth S, Monnich D, Welz S et al (2013) A strategy for multimodal deformable image registration to integrate PET/MR into radiotherapy treatment planning. Acta Oncol 52:1353–1359
Leibfarth S, Eckert F, Welz S et al (2015) Automatic delineation of tumor volumes by co-segmentation of combined PET/MR data. Phys Med Biol 60:5399–5412
Lock S, Perrin R, Seidlitz A et al (2017) Residual tumour hypoxia in head-and-neck cancer patients undergoing primary radiochemotherapy, final results of a prospective trial on repeat FMISO-PET imaging. Radiother Oncol 124:533–540
Macmanus M, Nestle U, Rosenzweig KE et al (2009) Use of PET and PET/CT for radiation therapy planning: IAEA expert report 2006-2007. Radiother Oncol 91:85–94
Monnich D, Welz S, Thorwarth D et al (2015) Robustness of quantitative hypoxia PET image analysis for predicting local tumor control. Acta Oncol 54:1364–1369
Mortensen LS, Johansen J, Kallehauge J et al (2012) FAZA PET/CT hypoxia imaging in patients with squamous cell carcinoma of the head and neck treated with radiotherapy: results from the DAHANCA 24 trial. Radiother Oncol 105:14–20
Nestle U, Kremp S, Grosu AL (2006) Practical integration of [18F]-FDG-PET and PET-CT in the planning of radiotherapy for non-small cell lung cancer (NSCLC): the technical basis, ICRU-target volumes, problems, perspectives. Radiother Oncol 81:209–225
Schaefer A, Kremp S, Hellwig D et al (2008) A contrast-oriented algorithm for FDG-PET-based delineation of tumour volumes for the radiotherapy of lung cancer: derivation from phantom measurements and validation in patient data. Eur J Nucl Med Mol Imaging 35:1989–1999
Schaefer A, Nestle U, Kremp S et al (2012) Multi-Centre calibration of an adaptive thresholding method for PET-based delineation of tumour volumes in radiotherapy planning of lung cancer. Nuklearmedizin 51:101–110
Shepherd T, Teras M, Beichel RR et al (2012) Comparative study with new accuracy metrics for target volume contouring in PET image guided radiation therapy. IEEE Trans Med Imaging 31:2006–2024
Teske H, Bartelheimer K, Meis J et al (2017) Construction of a biomechanical head and neck motion model as a guide to evaluation of deformable image registration. Phys Med Biol 62:N271–N284
Thorwarth D, Schaefer A (2010) Functional target volume delineation for radiation therapy on the basis of positron emission tomography and the correlation with histopathology. Q J Nucl Med Mol Imaging 54:490–499
Thorwarth D, Eschmann SM, Paulsen F et al (2007) Hypoxia dose painting by numbers: a planning study. Int J Radiat Oncol Biol Phys 68:291–300
Thorwarth D, Geets X, Paiusco M (2010) Physical radiotherapy treatment planning based on functional PET/CT data. Radiother Oncol 96:317–324
Thorwarth D, Beyer T, Boellaard R et al (2012) Integration of FDG-PET/CT into external beam radiation therapy

planning: technical aspects and recommendations on methodological approaches. Nuklearmedizin 51:140–153
Troost EG, Bussink J, Hoffmann AL et al (2010a) 18F-FLT PET/CT for early response monitoring and dose escalation in oropharyngeal tumors. J Nucl Med 51:866–874
Troost EG, Schinagl DA, Bussink J et al (2010b) Innovations in radiotherapy planning of head and neck cancers: role of PET. J Nucl Med 51:66–76
Van Der Vos CS, Koopman D, Rijnsdorp S et al (2017) Quantification, improvement, and harmonization of small lesion detection with state-of-the-art PET. Eur J Nucl Med Mol Imaging 44:4–16
Van Elmpt W, De Ruysscher D, Van Der Salm A et al (2012) The PET-boost randomised phase II dose-escalation trial in non-small cell lung cancer. Radiother Oncol 104:67–71
Vasquez Osorio EM, Kolkman-Deurloo IK, Schuring-Pereira M et al (2015) Improving anatomical mapping of complexly deformed anatomy for external beam radiotherapy and brachytherapy dose accumulation in cervical cancer. Med Phys 42:206–220
Wanet M, Lee JA, Weynand B et al (2011) Gradient-based delineation of the primary GTV on FDG-PET in non-small cell lung cancer: a comparison with threshold-based approaches, CT and surgical specimens. Radiother Oncol 98:117–125
Wang K, Heron DE, Clump DA et al (2013) Target delineation in stereotactic body radiation therapy for recurrent head and neck cancer: a retrospective analysis of the impact of margins and automated PET-CT segmentation. Radiother Oncol 106:90–95
Welz S, Monnich D, Pfannenberg C et al (2017) Prognostic value of dynamic hypoxia PET in head and neck cancer: results from a planned interim analysis of a randomized phase II hypoxia-image guided dose escalation trial. Radiother Oncol 124:526–532
Werner-Wasik M, Nelson AD, Choi W et al (2012) What is the best way to contour lung tumors on PET scans? Multiobserver validation of a gradient-based method using a NSCLC digital PET phantom. Int J Radiat Oncol Biol Phys 82:1164–1171
Wu VW, Leung WS, Wong KL et al (2016) The impact of positron emission tomography on primary tumour delineation and dosimetric outcome in intensity modulated radiotherapy of early T-stage nasopharyngeal carcinoma. Radiat Oncol 11:109
Yang J, Beadle BM, Garden AS et al (2015) A multimodality segmentation framework for automatic target delineation in head and neck radiotherapy. Med Phys 42:5310–5320
Zaidi H, El Naqa I (2010) PET-guided delineation of radiation therapy treatment volumes: a survey of image segmentation techniques. Eur J Nucl Med Mol Imaging 37:2165–2187
Zips D, Zophel K, Abolmaali N et al (2012) Exploratory prospective trial of hypoxia-specific PET imaging during radiochemotherapy in patients with locally advanced head-and-neck cancer. Radiother Oncol 105:21–28

CT in Room Gating During Radiotherapy

Mariangela Massaccesi

Contents

1 **Introduction** 92

2 **Sources of Geometric Uncertainty for Tumors that Move with Respiration** 92

2.1 Target Delineation Errors 93

2.2 Phantom Transfer Errors 93

2.3 Setup Errors 93

2.4 Respiratory Motion 93

2.5 PTV Margin Recipes 95

2.6 Traditional Two-Dimensional (2D) Image Guidance Strategies 95

3 **Motion Management Strategies** 96

3.1 Motion-Encompassing Strategies and "Mid-Position" Approaches 96

3.2 Volumetric Image Guidance 97

4 **Conclusions** 102

References 103

M. Massaccesi (✉)
Radiation Oncology Department, Gemelli ART, Fondazione Policlinico Universitario Agostino Gemelli, Rome, Italy
e-mail: mariangela.massaccesi@policlinicogemelli.it

Abstract

Respiratory motion is a major source of geometric uncertainty in radiotherapy, accounting for a variable part of the safety margin needed to ensure an adequate dose coverage to the tumor (margin for planning target volume, PTV), depending on both the amplitude of tumor motion (TM) and the strategies used for treatment planning and delivery. Respiration typically determines a random intra-fractional movement of the target around a mean position. Nevertheless, the mean target position may vary relatively to bony structures between simulation and treatment due to planning error and/or variation in the breathing pattern. Volumetric image guidance, particularly online cone-beam computed tomography (CBCT) scan and soft-tissue match on tumor, offers the opportunity of reducing the PTV margin as compared to conventional two-dimensional image guidance strategies. Indeed, online CBCT scan enables the correction of both the systematic and random components of inter-fractional uncertainties due to patient setup and baseline tumor shifts, potentially allowing for PTV margin of 5 mm for TM amplitude up to 15 mm (delineation errors not considered). For larger TM, other strategies that are more complex can be used to restrain, or virtually eliminate, the TM during irradiation (e.g., breath hold, respiratory gating and tracking strategies). Technological refinements of CBCT image guidance include respiratory-correlated four-dimensional (4D)

R. G. H. Beets-Tan et al. (eds.), *Imaging and Interventional Radiology for Radiation Oncology*, Medical Radiology, Diagnostic Imaging, https://doi.org/10.1007/978-3-030-38261-2_7

CBCT, faster CBCT acquisition methods, and CBCT scan during treatment delivery. This chapter will provide an overview of the different methods for breathing motion management in radiotherapy with a particular focus on the possibilities and limitations offered by image guidance with in-room CT.

1 Introduction

Several sources of geometric uncertainties exist in the radiotherapy process. Therefore, a safety margin has to be added around the clinical target volume (CTV) to obtain the planning target volume (PTV), to ensure an adequate coverage of the tumor with the intended dose. Increasing the accuracy of the treatment allows for reduced treatment volumes with a potential for reduced toxicity and dose escalation. A major source of uncertainty is tumor motion (TM) due to internal organ movement such as respiration, cardiac function, peristaltic activity, and organ filling and emptying. Particularly, respiratory-induced tumor motion up to 2 cm is common in the lung and upper abdomen, and even larger excursions can occur (Chen et al. 2001).

Various methods exist to deal with respiratory motion in radiotherapy including motion-encompassing strategies, reducing or eliminating breathing motion (e.g., abdominal compression or breath hold (BH)), gating the treatment delivery to a specific phase of the breathing cycle, or tracking the tumor motion (TM) with the treatment beam.

In order to increase the geometric accuracy of the treatment, thus maintaining reasonable PTV margins, the American Association of Physicists in Medicine Task Group on the management of respiratory motion in radiation oncology (TG-76) recommends considering motion management strategies for breathing motion exceeding 5 mm (Keall et al. 2006). Therefore, the measurement of the three-dimensional (3D) extent of the respiratory-induced TM is the first step to select the patients who can benefit from motion management strategies. Regardless of the technique used, tumor motion must be managed similarly during both simulation and treatment (e.g., breath hold or free breathing), and patient-specific CTV-PTV margins should be defined in order to compensate for residual uncorrected inter- and intra-fractional tumor shifts.

The use of image guidance for radiotherapy has improved as technology has become available. Megavoltage (MV) treatment beams were initially used to align the spine and high contrast anatomy, such as the diaphragm, or implanted fiducial markers. The integration of kilovoltage (kV) imaging, ultrasound, and volumetric imaging (both kV and MV) has improved the visualization of the tumor and surrounding anatomy and the ability to use these structures for accurate image guidance. Since large inter-fractional baseline shifts with respect to the bony anatomy may occur when irradiating moving tumors, patient positioning using volumetric image with soft-tissue matching on the tumor is the preferred image guidance method whenever high precision is required.

This chapter will provide an overview of the different methods for breathing motion management in radiotherapy with a particular focus on the possibilities and limitations offered by image guidance with in-room CT.

2 Sources of Geometric Uncertainty for Tumors that Move with Respiration

Uncertainties in target localization can occur either in the pre-treatment stage and systematically reproduced during treatment or in the delivery stage varying on a daily basis.

Systematic errors are consistent errors, occurring in the same direction and of similar magnitude over the course of treatment. Random errors vary in direction and magnitude from day-to-day and are represented by the range of different positions for each delivered treatment fraction.

Target delineation, phantom transfer errors, patient setup errors, and internal organ motion/

deformation are the main sources of geometric uncertainty (Korreman et al. 2010).

2.1 Target Delineation Errors

Tumor delineation errors are an important source of a systematic error, being often above 3 mm (Rasch et al. 2005; Liang et al. 2014). Inter- and intra-observer variability, as well as the quality of imaging, can affect the tumor volume identification. Particularly, inter-observer variability represents the largest uncertainty in the radiotherapy process for most tumor sites (Segedin and Petric 2016). A variety of methods can be used to quantify inter-observer variability, as the ratio of the largest and the smallest delineated volume (V_{max}/V_{min}), concordance measures (i.e., conformity, concordance or similarity index, Dice-Jaccard coefficient, percent overlap, ratio of encompassing and common volume, geographical miss index) (Fotina et al. 2012), and methods for local inter-observer variation assessment (i.e., local standard deviation (SD), inter-delineation distance, or radial line measurement variation).

2.2 Phantom Transfer Errors

Phantom transfer errors can occur when transferring image data from initial localization through the treatment-planning system to the linear accelerator and are due to limitations in the accuracy of manufacturing that result in minor differences between the simulator and treatment machine. The transfer error can be measured using a rigid phantom and is generally within 1 mm (Falco et al. 2011) with currently commercially available devices.

2.3 Setup Errors

Setup errors occur when the position and the anatomy of the patient (bony anatomy) at the planning CT are not reproduced accurately during treatment and can have both a systematic and random component. Setup errors can occur on a daily basis, thus affecting the inter-fractional reproducibility of the treatment (changes between simulation and treatment and between different fractions) and during each fraction (intra-fractional changes). The body habitus, the immobilization device, and the duration of the treatment can all affect the extent of such error (Sio et al. 2014). Even without any immobilization device, intra-fractional variation of bony anatomy position can be negligible (<1 mm) if treatment duration is short (Cuijpers et al. 2017). In a series of 24 patients treated with stereotactic body frame, Guckenberger did not observed any significant systematic 3D patient motion during treatment (<0.1 mm) (Guckenberger et al. 2007a, b). The SD of patient motion ranged between 1.3 mm (superior–inferior (SI) and anterior–posterior (AP)) and 1.7 mm (left–right (LR)).

2.4 Respiratory Motion

Breathing-induced motion of tumors located in the thorax and the upper abdomen determines positional variation of the target and organs at risk (OARs) with respect to the bony anatomy. Like setup errors, errors due to internal organ motion can be due to either systematic or random and inter- or intra-fractional changes.

Respiratory-induced TM can be modeled by an asymmetrical periodic function where more time is spent at exhale than inhale (Seppenwoolde et al. 2002). Typical motion magnitudes vary depending on the location of the tumor. Lung tumor movements are generally larger in the superior–inferior (SI) direction, and the motion amplitude in this direction increased for tumors located in the middle and lower parts of the lungs. Motions in left–right (LR) or anterior–posterior (AP) direction show no such relation (Sarudis et al. 2017).

In a large series including 145 lung cancer patients treated with stereotactic radiotherapy, motion amplitudes >8 mm in the SI direction were observed only in the lower half of the lungs. Motion amplitudes >15 mm were observed only in the lower quarter of the lungs. Motion amplitudes >5 mm were not observed in the upper geometric third of the lungs (Knybel et al. 2016). In the series by Seppenwoolde et al. (2002), the majority of patients had TM (78%) of less than a 1 cm amplitude.

Generally, abdominal organ motion is in the SI direction, with no more than a 2 mm displacement in the AP and lateral directions (Korin et al. 1992; Davies et al. 1994).

van Herk et al. (2003) suggests to treat respiration with a peak–peak amplitude of less than 1 cm the same as random errors (the corresponding SD of respiration motion is about 0.3 A) and use a nonuniform margin of 0.25–0.45 A when the respiration exceeds 1 cm in association with the use of a mid-position (MidP) of the tumor as reference.

A typical respiratory cycle takes about 4 s, while the radiation treatment is typically delivered in a longer period (multiple fractions, each lasting for several seconds) meaning that many respiratory cycles take place during treatment delivery. Conventional CT scans as commonly used for treatment planning can include severe motion artifacts that result from interplay effects between the advancing scan plane and object motion (Rietzel et al. 2005). Planning 3D CT scans are commonly obtain with fast multi-slice CT scanner, representing actually a snapshot of the anatomy in an arbitrary breathing phase. Therefore, the target centroid position relative to the bony structures in CT planning images may have an undefined displacement with respect to its mean position during treatment, thus constituting a localization error in planning imaging (systematic error). Systematic (and random) errors due to respiratory motion can be estimated using the standard deviation (SD) of the TM (approximately one-third of the peak-to-peak amplitude) (van Herk et al. 2003). Furthermore, tumor shape deformation in 3D CT image may occur depending on scanner velocity with faster scans having smaller shape distortion than slower scans (Wink et al. 2005). MacKenzie and colleagues observed that the margin necessary for shape changes is similar to that needed for displacement errors (McKenzie 2004). Considering the fact that a fast scan has a large displacement uncertainty and vice versa for a slow scan, it can be approximated that the combination of tumor displacement errors and shape changes is constant (independent of tumor size and scan speed). The "combined" systematic motion error can be therefore estimated by the SD of the TM (Wolthaus et al. 2008).

The breathing pattern (frequency, amplitude, period, and tumor trajectory) may vary from day to day and even from breath to breath, thus potentially determining both inter- and intra-fractional variations in the centroid tumor position. In a large series of patient treated with stereotactic radiotherapy for lung cancer, Knybel et al. (2016) found that mean inter-fractional amplitude variability was low in all directions. The mean inter-fractional amplitude variability was 1.1 ± 0.9, 0.9 ± 0.9, and 1.0 ± 0.9 mm for the SI, LL, and AP directions, respectively. However, 9% of patients demonstrated inter-fractional amplitude variability >3 mm in one of the directions, which could be affected by contact with surrounding structures, such as the diaphragm, the parietal pleura, and the mediastinum. Furthermore, there was a significant difference between the upper and lower halves of the lungs for inter-fractional amplitude variability in the SI direction. High mean motion variation was mainly found in women with metastatic lesions.

Both inter-fractional and intra-fractional changes correlated to intra-fractional motion or peak-to-peak motion. Baseline changes >3 mm are observed almost exclusively in the lower third of the lung (Knybel et al. 2016).

In a series of 24 lung cancer patients (27 lesions) treated with stereotactic body radiation therapy (SBRT) and image guidance with CBCT, Guckenberger et al. (2007a, b) observed that changes of the tumor position due to patient motion and due to drifts independently from the bony anatomy were of similar magnitude. No systematic intra-fractional patient motion in any direction during treatment was observed (<0.5 mm). The SD of patient motion ranged between 1.3 mm (SI and AP) and 1.7 mm (LR). A small systematic tumor drift in posterior direction was observed with 1.3 mm. The SD of the tumor drift was largest in AP direction with 1.9 mm and smallest in SI direction with 1.5 mm.

In patients treated with volumetric-modulated arc stereotactic radiotherapy for lung cancer using a customized vacuum immobilization device, Mathieu et al. (2017) reported systematic intra-fractional shifts of 0.9, 0.7, and 0.6 and random shifts of 1.5, 1.1, and 1.0 mm in the AP, IS, and RL directions, respectively, after a mean treatment time of about 20 min.

Table 1 shows reported values for mean intra-fractional vector motion in lung stereotactic radiotherapy.

2.5 PTV Margin Recipes

Several margin recipes have been published to compute the margin needed to achieve adequate dose coverage of the tumor. The margin recipe of van Herk et al. (2000, 2003) can be used to compute the margin needed to deliver a dose of at least 95% of the prescribed dose to the CTV (for 90% of the population) for conventionally fractionated treatments as follows:

$$M_{\mathrm{PTV}} = 2.5\Sigma + 1.64\sqrt{\sigma^2 + \sigma_{\mathrm{p}}^2} - 1.64\sigma_{\mathrm{p}}(\mathrm{mm})$$

In the formula, Σ and σ represent the standard deviations (SDs) of the systematic and random errors, respectively, and σ_{p} denotes the SD of the dose gradient or "penumbra," which may vary for different tissues and techniques of irradiation (Witte et al. 2004).

If dose prescription is at 80% isodose instead of 95%:

$$M_{\mathrm{PTV}} = 2.5\Sigma + 0.84\sqrt{\sigma^2 + \sigma_{\mathrm{p}}^2} - 0.84\sigma_{\mathrm{p}}(\mathrm{mm})$$

The final PTV margin results from the quadratic sum of the various components of the systematic and random uncertainties, which amplitude may vary depending on several factors.

Table 2 summarizes the major sources of geometric uncertainties for tumors that move because of respiration as well as main determining factors.

2.6 Traditional Two-Dimensional (2D) Image Guidance Strategies

Image guidance strategies aim at reducing geometric uncertainty by evaluating the patient geometry at treatment and either altering the patient position or adapting the treatment plan with respect to anatomical changes that occur during the radiotherapy treatment course. Two main image guidance strategies exist, off-line and

Table 1 Intra-fractional motion in lung stereotactic radiotherapy

Study	Number of lesions treated/number of fractions	PTV definition method	Immobilization device	Time interval	Mean intra-fractional vector
Guckenberger et al. (2007a, b)	27	ITV, on exhale–inhale 3D CT	Stereotactic body frame	21 min	2.8 ± 1.6 mm
Shah et al. (2013)	409/1337		Several immobilization devices	24 min 28 s	3.1 ± 2.0 mm
			Body frame		2.3 ± 1.4 mm
			Hybrid device		2.7 ± 1.6 mm
			Alpha cradle		3.0 ± 1.7 mm
			Body fix		3.0 ± 2.5 mm
			Wing board		3.3 ± 1.7 mm
			No immobilization		3.3 ± 2.2 mm
Siva et al. (2014)	18/19		Vacuum immobilization	24 min	1.5 ± 1.7 mm
Mathieu et al. (2017)	96/367		Customized dual vacuum immobilization device	22 min 58 s	1.5 ± 1.4 mm

Table 2 Sources of geometric uncertainties for tumors moving with respiration

Source of uncertainty	Determining factors
Delineation errors	• Image quality/contrast resolution • Tumor site • Radiation oncologist experience
Phantom transfer errors	• Accuracy of manufacturing
Patient repositioning errors	• Immobilization device • Patient habitus (i.e., weight)
Respiratory motion	• Motion amplitude (which depends in turn on tumor location, lung function, proximity/infiltration of mediastinum, chest, vertebras, or abdominal wall)
Intra-fractional motion (patient and tumor shifts)	• Immobilization device • Patient habitus (i.e., weight, performance status) • Respiratory motion amplitude • Lung function

online. In the off-line strategy, the images are acquired prior to treatment; however, the analysis is performed off-line. Often 3–5 images are obtained during the initial part of the treatment and then are used to determine a systematic and random error; afterward the systematic error can be corrected, and the random error can be accounted for in the PTV (Yan et al. 1997) for the remaining fractions. In the online strategy, the images are acquired and evaluated prior to treatment delivery potentially allowing for the correction of both random and systematic setup errors.

Two-dimensional imaging techniques, such as electronic portal images or planar radiographs for bony anatomy setup, may lack in accuracy whenever there is no stable relationship between bony anatomy and tumor position. This is mostly the case of thoracic and abdominopelvic tumors. Indeed, inter-fractional baseline variations of the mean tumor position relative to the bony structures are well-documented and represent a major source of uncertainty. Therefore, unless radiopaque markers are implanted within the tumor to be used as surrogates of tumor position during treatment delivery, image guidance protocols based on bony structure match only allow the correction for the component of uncertainty due to setup error. Particularly, off-line protocols with image match on bony structures, which are commonly used for conventionally fractionated treatments, only enable a partial correction of the systematic component of the setup error, resulting in large margins needed to ensure adequate dose coverage of the CTV.

3 Motion Management Strategies

Several approaches for treatment planning and delivery can be used to ensure that tumors moving with the breathing cycle receive the intended dose with different possibilities of enabling a reduction of the PTV margin, as compared with conventional treatment. Some methods allow treating the patient while breathing normally (motion-encompassing methods, mid-ventilation (MidV) approaches, respiratory gating and tracking techniques); other strategies aim to restrict the breathing motion extent by coaching the patient to shallow breathing, limiting the diaphragmatic excursion through abdominal compression, or treating the patient during breath hold.

3.1 Motion-Encompassing Strategies and "Mid-Position" Approaches

The simplest solution to deal with respiratory motion is treating the patient while breathing normally, targeting the internal target volume (ITV) which encompasses the target volume at each phase of the respiratory cycle as described in the Report 62 of the International Commission on Radiation Units and Measurements (1999) (ICRU 622009). The ITV can be determined by simply summing the gross target volumes (GTV) drawn in each of two 3D CT scans taken at exhale and inhale. While widely used, the ITV solution is probably the most unfavorable choice to make; indeed, it can result in very large PTV in case of large tumor motion amplitude. Furthermore, the trajectory of the tumor from inhale to exhale varies compared to exhale to inhale, resulting in a 3D elliptical tumor trajectory instead of a line (phenomenon termed hysteresis) (Vedam et al. 2003).

Time-correlated four-dimensional (4D) CT images can overcome these limitations by depicting the full extent of TM during normal respiration. The common underlying principle in these approaches has been to acquire axial/helical tomographic images while simultaneously recording the respiratory breathing pattern. CT data acquisition is oversampled at each slice for the duration of the patient's respiratory cycle (plus the time needed for a full CT gantry rotation). These data are then reorganized (resorted) to generate multiple spatiotemporally coherent anatomical dataset scans. (Rietzel et al. 2005). On 4D CT images, the ITV can be derived by merging the GTVs contoured on each CT datasets corresponding to each individual breathing phase. To reduce the workload of contouring multiple target volumes in 4D CT, post-processing tools can be used, including maximum intensity projection (MIP) or minimum intensity projection (MinIP) reconstructions for hyperdense or hypodense tumors, respectively (Underberg et al. 2004; Cuijpers et al. 2010; Bradley et al. 2006).

MIPs and MinIPs provide a 3D CT scan whose voxel values are the greatest voxel and least intensity values, respectively, throughout the 4D CT dataset. However, the ITV solution overestimates the PTV since motion amplitude is linearly added to the CTV as a systematic component of uncertainty, while respiration actually induces a random motion of the tumor around a mean position.

The average intensity projection (AIP) CT represents the mean intensity of each voxel over the breathing cycle (Bradley et al. 2006). AIP comprises not only the tumor motion extent but also the probability that the tumor is present. However, the averaging process blurred the GTV edges as a result of tumor motion and partial volume effect, making the GTV difficult to contour. In a series of patients with lung cancer, Bradly and colleagues observed that AI-defined gross target volume (GTV) was significantly smaller than the MIP-defined GTV, while the spatial isocenter coordinates for each tumor were not altered significantly by the imaging methods (Bradley et al. 2006).

In the last decade, a method termed "mid-ventilation" approach has gained growing consensus. In this solution, the mid-ventilation phase is identified by analyzing the trajectory of the target in the 4D CT dataset, as the single 3D CT frame in which the target is closest to its "time-weighted" average position during the breathing cycle (mid-ventilation CT scan) (Wolthaus et al. 2006). The MidV scan eliminates the risk of planning the treatment at a tumor position that is far away from the tumor mean position during the respiratory cycle, thus permitting a reduction of the treatment margin. Furthermore, the MidV scan also reduces the problem of tumor shape distortion of conventional FB 3D CT scan that is mostly due to the interplay effect of tumor motion and progression of the scan acquisition. However, a small systematic geometric error with respect to the mean position can be introduced owing to hysteresis in the TM. As a solution, the mid-position (MidP) concept has been developed, which reconstructs a new CT scan from the 4D CT dataset representing all the internal structures, including the tumor, in their exact time-weighted mean position of the respiratory motion. While MIP, MinIP, and AIP reconstructions generate composite images with moving structures resulting as blurred objects, mid-ventilation and mid-position CT scans represent a single 3D CT frame. Importantly, although the MidP looks like a single 3D image, it is entirely artificial as the tumor in most cases doesn't come in MidP ever.

3.2 Volumetric Image Guidance

Radiation therapy evolved from 2D to 3D in the treatment-planning process, in the same way a similar evolution can be observed in image guidance. Volumetric imaging techniques nowadays provide the soft-tissue contrast required for daily positioning, providing online information concerning organs at risk as well as tumors and identifying anatomical changes during the course of radiotherapy. There are four commercially available distinct solutions widely used: kilovoltage fan-beam CT (kV CT-on-rails) (Aoki et al. 1987), kilovoltage cone-beam CT (kV CBCT) (Jaffray et al. 2002), megavoltage cone-beam CT (MV CBCT) (Herman et al. 2001), and megavoltage fan-beam CT (MV CT, commercially available as the integrated TomoTherapy solution).

In 2010, the European Society of Therapeutic Radiology and Oncology–European Institute of Radiotherapy (ESTRO–EIR) published a practical and technical review on the use of 3D in room image guidance (Korreman et al. 2010). In this report, a list of issues contributing to the workflow of CT-based image guidance is discussed. Particularly, the report focuses on several issues concerning image acquisition (i.e., field of view extent, CT acquisition time, possibility to stop and resume the CT acquisition, etc.) and image quality and processing (i.e., choice of energy within the kV spectrum and the tube current, image registration and setup evaluation, and general factors such as data handling, dose and QA, and clinical implementation).

The main advantage of 3D kV imaging to 3D in-room MV imaging techniques is an enhanced image contrast for soft-tissues achievable with low-to-moderate imaging doses.

There are two categories of 3D kV imaging solutions currently used in clinical radiation therapy: the so-called CT-on-rails technology, which consists of a standard diagnostic CT gantry mounted in the treatment room, and linac-integrated kV imaging equipment, consisting of a diagnostic X-ray source and a flat panel electronic imaging device. A concern of the CT-on-rails technology is that minor undetectable setup errors might be caused by the required movement of the patient between imaging and treatment.

Image guidance with kV CBCT scan partially overcomes such limitations. Indeed, simple quality assurance measures guarantee a very precise geometric co-registration of the kV CBCT with the treatment isocenter (Bissonnette et al. 2008). However, based on its hardware components, the achievable image quality is compromised in comparison with diagnostic CT images. Furthermore, motion artifacts caused by breathing or peristalsis during the enhanced scanning times can degrade image quality.

The acquisition of CBCT scan takes between 1 and 2 min; therefore, it spans several breathing cycles; therefore, a mobile tumor will result as a blurred object, which roughly represents the tumor in its time-weighted average position.

Using different CT datasets for image registration with free breathing (FB) CBCTs can result in different 3D couch shifts. Furthermore, manual registrations achieve partly different 3D shifts than automatic registrations, and inter-observer variability may exist. In a series by Oechsner et al. (2016), AIP-CTs yielded the smallest shift differences as compared with slow planning CT, maximum intensity projection (MIP), and mid-ventilation CTs (MidV) as reference images; therefore, the authors concluded that AIP CT might be the most appropriate CT dataset for registration with 3D FB-CBCTs (Oechsner et al. 2016).

AIP CT datasets can be used for OAR contouring and dose calculations (Han et al. 2010). AIP is particularly recommended as the reference image for registration to FB-CBCT when target alignment is performed in the presence of asymmetrical respiratory motion, whereas MIP causes systematic target positioning error (Shirai et al. 2014).

Together, AIP planning and online CBCT with soft-tissue match on tumor can virtually correct for any systematic and random inter-fractional errors due to patient (setup errors) and respiratory motion (error due to TM artifacts in planning 3D CT, baseline tumor shift). However, when obtaining data for validating PTV margins from online CBCT image guidance, it is essential to account for measurement and system inaccuracies (Cuijpers et al. 2017). Shift differences increase with increasing 3D tumor motion and decrease image quality of the 3D CBCT (Oechsner 2017) as in small and mobile tumors and in tumors located immediately superior to the diaphragm (Sweeney et al. 2012).

Respiration-correlated 4D CBCT can improve the accuracy of image guidance by more precise target localization in the presence of breathing-induced target motion and by reduced inter-observer variability compared to 3D CBCT (Sweeney et al. 2012). In 4D CBCT acquisition, similarly to respiratory-correlated CT (4D CT), the images are retrospectively binned according to the respiratory phase (usually 10 phases are reconstructed). 4D CBCT substantially reduces respiration-induced motion blurring artifacts in three-dimension (3D), thus ensuring a reasonable dose and better image quality when moving targets are involved compared to 3D CBCT (Thengumpallil et al. 2016). The technique is shown to be applicable to abdominal sites, where image contrast of soft tissues is low (Kincaid Jr et al. 2013). The accuracy of localizing the moving target with 4D CBCT is generally within 2 mm. The main challenge in 4D CBCT reconstruction is the limited number of projections at each phase. Indeed, small scan angles and low number of projections are used to provide fast low-dose 4D target verification, which result in a reconstruction full of noise and streak artifacts with the conventional analytical algorithms. Therefore, the image quality of 4D CBCT is significantly degraded which may affect its accuracy in localizing a mobile tumor for high-precision IGRT. To address this problem, several approaches have been proposed (Zhang et al. 2017a, b, Park et al. 2017, Harris et al. 2017, Zhang et al. 2017b). Particularly, changing the gantry speed changes the number of projections used for reconstruction, affecting both image quality and imaging dose if X-ray tube current is held constant. From the results of a study by Santoso et al. (2016), a gantry speed between 2 and 3°/s was optimal when considering image quality, dose, and reconstruction time.

Respiratory-correlated simulation CT and CBCT scans enable the correction of both the systematic and random components of inter-fractional uncertainties due to patient and tumor shifts. However, the breathing pattern (frequency, amplitude, period, and duration of each phase) may vary from day to day and even from breath to breath. Therefore, a single simulation 4D CT scan may be not fully representative of breathing motion during therapy, as well as a single CBCT before fraction delivery (Guckenberger et al. 2007a, b; Worm et al. 2013; Park et al. 2012; Chan et al. 2013; Ge et al. 2013). Moreover, the larger is the tumor motion amplitude, the higher the intra-fractional amplitude variability observed (Knybel et al. 2016).

Limiting (or nearly eliminating) breathing motion during irradiation might represent a convenient solution particularly for tumors with large breathing excursions.

3.2.1 Voluntary Shallow Breathing

A simple solution is coaching the patient to keep his breath shallow during the treatment. However, this is dependent on the patient being compliant and understanding the importance of maintaining the modified breathing throughout the treatment. Visual biofeedback devices can be helpful to ensure patient compliance through monitoring over the course of treatment (Masselli et al. 2009).

3.2.2 Abdominal Compression

Another method is using abdominal compression to limit diaphragmatic excursion during breathing. Particularly, the abdominal compression of the subxiphoid area has been found to effectively limit liver motion during respiration (Hu et al. 2016). In a recent study including 19 patients with abdominal tumors and breath constrained by pneumatic compression, tumor motion exceeded 7.5 mm in only 7.6% of patients (Yorke et al. 2016). Nevertheless, for thoracic cancer treatment, abdominal compression has been shown to be beneficial only for lower-lobe tumors and have no effect or even a negative effect on middle- and upper-lobe tumors (Bouilhol et al. 2013). Furthermore, patient compliance to abdominal compression might be reduced due to comorbid conditions (i.e., abdominal aneurism, surgical intervention, chronic obstructive pulmonary disease) (Mampuya et al. 2013). Moreover, despite reducing lung tumor motion, the use of abdominal compression may increase the inter-fractional variation in tumor position. Therefore, target matching is required to correct or minimize the inter-fractional variation (Mampuya et al. 2013).

3.2.3 Breath Hold Approaches

Assisted or voluntary breath hold (BH) can allow marked reduction in the PTV in patients with large breathing excursions. Several recent developments in linear accelerator-based radiation therapy such as fast multi-leaf collimators, volumetric-modulated arc therapy, and flattening filter-free (FFF) high-dose-rate therapy have dramatically shortened the duration of treatment fractions (Boda-Heggemann et al. 2013), possibly enabling treatment in breath hold in a large proportion of patients. BH can be achieved by repeated voluntary breath hold or be assisted with computer-controlled commercially available devices that usually automatically trigger treatments based on breath hold gating signals.

Voluntary deep inspiration breath hold (DIBH) seems acceptable for breast tangential radiotherapy allowing for significant lung, heart, and liver sparing (Prabhakar et al. 2007; Bartlett et al. 2014; Pedersen et al. 2004). The depth of breath hold can be verified by checking the distance between the room lasers and the skin markers. With DIBH, acceptable precision data in chest wall repositioning has been found with 2D imaging methods (Bartlett et al. 2013; Betgen et al. 2013). However, almost no information on reproducibility of the internal anatomy are still available, demanding for further evaluation before being used in the context of radiotherapy to the lung and liver.

Computer-assisted breath hold can be performed by either breathing volume-based approaches through quantifying the inspiration volume with a spirometer or using optical surface systems through monitoring the excursion of the body surface during respiration.

Volume-based approaches such as the ABC system (Elekta) allow for acceptable intra-fractional and inter-fractional reproducibility (1.7 and 3.7 mm, respectively) (Chan et al. 2013; Dawson et al. 2005). Nevertheless, since different breathing maneuvers (chest vs abdominal breathing) can lead to variations in chest wall position even if inspiration volume is the same, optical surface monitoring system might allow for a greater reproducibility (Mittauer et al. 2015).

Optical surface monitoring can be performed indirectly by monitoring the movements of reflectors that are placed on the surface of the patient. Commercially available devices are the RPM (Varian, Palo Alto, CA), ExacTrac (BrainLab, Feldkirchen, Germany), and Synchrony (Accuray, Morges, Switzerland) systems.

More recently, markerless systems that project visible light on the patient to detect the body surface and the surface movements caused by respiration (AlignRT produced by Vision RT, London, the United Kingdom, or Catalyst produced by C-RAD, Uppsala, Sweden) have been shown to offer an opportunity for accurate positioning and intra-fractional monitoring, particularly in breast tangential radiotherapy (Fassi et al. 2014; Tang et al. 2014, 2015; Tanguturi et al. 2015; Gierga et al. 2012).

While intra-breath-hold precision of BH techniques has been reported to be generally excellent, inter-breath-hold positional variations tend to be larger, demanding for image guidance to ensure positioning of the tumor at the time of each fraction (Dawson et al. 2001; Eccles et al. 2006). Furthermore, during DIBH, large misalignments of the tumor to the spine can be observed due to the fact that the patients may tend to arch their back in order to compensate for insufficient compliance to reach the patient-specific breath hold amplitude level (Ottosson et al. 2016). Markerless lung tumor motion monitoring using kV projection images has proven to be technically challenging due to limited visibility of the lung tumors on such images, especially for small, low-density, or centrally located tumors (van Sörnsen de Koste et al. 2015). Invasively implanted fiducial markers are available which can be inserted into or next to the tumor and then imaged during irradiation, but they are associated with additional risks, costs, and the requirement for expertise that limit their use.

The diaphragm can also be used with 2D imaging as surrogate for liver or lung (lower-lobe) lesions. However, 2D imaging does not provide information about the position of organs at risks.

Volumetric image guidance may enable markerless tumor and organ-at-risk visualization. As compared to FB-CBCT, DIBH CBCT can improve image quality and reduced registration uncertainty in image-guided RT of locally advanced lung cancer (Josipovic et al. 2016).

Standard linac-mounted CBCTs require >180° gantry rotation; therefore, multiple breath holds are often needed before such a CBCT can be reconstructed (usually three breath holds each of 20 s) so that inter-breath-hold variations may result in blurring of the tumor.

A faster method to verify the position of tumor and organ at risk before treatment delivery would be desirable. Combined kV–MV cone-beam CT (CBCT) is a promising approach to accelerate imaging for patients with lung tumors treated with deep inspiration breath hold. During a single breath hold (15 s), a 3D kV–MV CBCT can be acquired, thus minimizing motion artifacts and increasing patient comfort (Arns et al. 2016).

Nevertheless, inter-breath-hold variability cannot be completely addressed or at least quantified, unless image guidance is used during actual treatment delivery.

For breath hold lung SBRT, variations in tumor position typically occur in the superior–inferior direction due to inter-breath-hold differences. Therefore, the ability to verify whether the tumor is inside the PTV during each breath hold is valuable. Cine megavoltage (MV) images can be obtained with the electronic portal image device (EPID) to verify the maintenance of the breath hold during the beam delivery (Shiinoki et al. 2017). Fluoroscopic kV imaging can also serve to confirm breathing motion and breath hold stability, usually coupled with fiducial markers (Bedos et al. 2017). However, both methods, as previously stated, in most cases do not allow for a direct visualization of the tumor.

New developments are currently undergoing final refinement before clinical testing, such as combined kV–MV imaging (Blessing et al. 2010; Wertz et al. 2010) or limited-arc KV CBCT that offers both the possibilities to acquire a full 3D dataset during one breath hold (<15 s) with excellent positioning precision, just before treatment delivery, and to image the tumor position during the actual treatment delivery. Particularly, CBCT scan during irradiation would represent a substantial improvement on what is currently available, by allowing for correcting large geometric discrepancies whenever needed, increasing treatment efficiency when multiple arcs are used (by eliminating the need for a scan between the arcs), and assessing dose distribution on the actual treatment anatomy (Hazelaar et al. 2017).

Breath hold methods require optimal patient collaboration and longer treatment time as compared with non-gated treatment. Although, with the advent of fast multi-leaf collimators, VMAT, and particularly the FFF technology, the prolongation of treatment time has been considerably reduced allowing for better patient compliance (Boda-Heggemann et al. 2016), still a number of patients cannot adequately maintain the breath hold.

3.2.4 Gating and Tracking Strategies

An alternative but more complex method is to synchronize the radiation delivery with the normal respiratory cycles of the patient by either turning the treatment beam on when the tumor is within a limited pre-defined window of the breathing trajectory (gating) or tracking the tumor with the radiation beam. Gating minimizes the treatment margin by irradiating the tumor only when it is in a given location, but the inherent duty cycle of 30–50% (Keall et al. 2006) markedly extends treatment time. Tumor tracking follows the tumor motion, thus potentially allowing for a 100% duty cycle and a more time efficient delivery.

Treatment plans for both tumor gating and tracking techniques are tailored to specific patient respiratory motions given by 4D CT data. Thus, during treatment delivery, the patient must breathe in a similar fashion as during planning 4D CT. Tumor motion would need to be modeled to achieve a regular and reproducible respiratory pattern (Low et al. 2005; McClelland et al. 2006), and audiovisual respiratory guidance would be required during the radiation delivery (George et al. 2005; Venkat et al. 2008).

Both methods require a technology link between detection of the tumor position during the breathing cycle and the linear accelerator. Variations in the correlation between tumor movements and surrogate signals can lead to uncertainties resulting in a poor treatment outcome. Especially in gated treatment with external respiration monitoring, the lack of correct

-internal information on which to gate may lead to underestimation of the geometric errors so that respiratory-gated beam delivery cannot result in margin reduction without respiratory-correlated image guidance (Korreman et al. 2008).

Current real-time tumor tracking technologies rely on radiopaque fiducial or electromagnetic transponder beacons. However, marker or beacon implantation is an invasive, expensive, time-consuming procedure and is not available at every radiotherapy clinic. Existing markerless tracking methods rely on the tumors to be consistently visible on kV projection images. Three-dimensional tumor localization with digital tomosynthesis (DTS) has been proposed by several authors to improve tumor visibility. However, currently DTS is only used for pre-treatment imaging and has not yet been implemented for real-time guidance.

Recently, Shieh and colleagues proposed a markerless lung tumor tracking method based on short kV imaging arcs and 4D CBCT prior knowledge (short-arc tumor tracking, SATT). The drawback of SATT is the trade-off in time resolution (1.5–9 s depending on gantry speed) due to the short-arc nature and the computation time needed to process multiple projections and anatomy subtraction (Shieh et al. 2015, 2017). Further prospective evaluation and clinical implementation of SATT are needed before this technique is introduced in clinical practice.

4 Conclusions

It is still a matter of debate which motion management strategy to use for which patients. The PTV margin reduction required for high-precision delivery of high-focused radiation dose is generally accomplished at the expense of increased complexity of treatment and/or technological demand and/or decreased patient comfort (i.e., increased treatment time and/or breath hold requirement). At departmental level, many different strategies could be available. The choice should be personalized in each single case, based on patient-related factors (i.e., the ability to maintain the breath hold), tumor-related factors (i.e., motion amplitude, proximity to normal structures with serial architecture, tumor volume relative to normal structures with parallel organization), and treatment-related factors (i.e., workload, workflow complexity, resources, and technological requirements).

Widely used ITV concept is the least favorable approach, and pretty much all alternatives are better, particularly in cases of large tumor motion amplitude.

The use of the mid-ventilation approach with in-room CT image guidance is very convenient for clinical use for several reasons. Treatment is delivered during normal respiration and through the entire breathing cycle; therefore, neither prolonged breath hold nor extra time is required to complete the fraction, without any adjunctive patient compliance issues as compared to conventional treatment. Moreover, there is no need to deal with the problem of synchronizing the treatment with respiration. According to Korreman et al. (2012), this could be the most important motion management strategy for motion magnitudes less than approximately 15 mm. In a large sample of lung cancer patients, the maximum TM amplitude observed was 8.8 and 6.3 mm, in the anterior–posterior and latero-lateral direction, respectively (Knybel et al. 2016). Motion amplitude >15 mm in the superior–inferior direction was observed only in the lower quarter of the lungs. Therefore, only a minority of patients are likely to benefit from more complex motion management strategies. In patients with large TM, trying to limit the TM extent through voluntary shallow breathing and audiovisual feedback might be a convenient solution.

Assisted or voluntary breath hold (BH) can allow marked reduction in the PTV in patients with large breathing excursions. With the advent of fast multi-leaf collimators, VMAT, and particularly the flattening filter-free technology, the prolongation of treatment time has been considerably reduced allowing for better patient compliance. Nevertheless, inter-breath-hold variability cannot be completely addressed unless image guidance is used during the actual treatment delivery. New developments are currently undergoing final refinement before clinical testing, such as combined kV–MV imaging or limited-arc KV CBCT that offers the possibilities to acquire a full 3D dataset during one breath hold (<15 s) with excellent markerless positioning precision.

An alternative but more complex method is to synchronize the radiation delivery with the normal respiratory cycles of the patient by either turning the treatment beam on when the tumor is within a limited pre-defined window of the breathing trajectory (gating) or tracking the tumor with the radiation beam. However, respiratory-gated beam delivery cannot result in margin reduction without respiratory-correlated image guidance. Current real-time tumor tracking technologies rely on radiopaque fiducial or electromagnetic transponder beacons. Markerless tracking methods are under development; however, they require tumors to be consistently visible on kV projection images.

References

Aoki Y, Akanuma A, Karasawa K et al (1987) An integrated radiotherapy treatment system and its clinical application. Radiat Med 5:131–141

Arns A, Blessing M, Fleckenstein J et al (2016) Towards clinical implementation of ultrafast combined kV-MV CBCT for IGRT of lung cancer: evaluation of registration accuracy based on phantom study. Strahlenther Onkol 192:312–321

Bartlett FR, Colgan RM, Carr K et al (2013) The UK HeartSpare study: randomised evaluation of voluntary deep-inspiratory breath-hold in women undergoing breast radiotherapy. Radiother Oncol 108:242–247

Bartlett FR, Colgan RM, Donovan EM et al (2014) Voluntary breath-hold technique for reducing heart dose in left breast radiotherapy. J Vis Exp (89). https://doi.org/10.3791/51578

Bedos L, Riou O, Aillères N et al (2017) Evaluation of reproducibility of tumor repositioning during multiple breathing cycles for liver stereotactic body radiotherapy treatment. Rep Pract Oncol Radiother 22:132–140

Betgen A, Alderliesten T, Sonke JJ et al (2013) Assessment of set-up variability during deep inspiration breath hold radiotherapy for breast cancer patients by 3D-surface imaging. Radiother Oncol 106:225–230

Bissonnette JP, Moseley DJ, Jaffray DA (2008) A quality assurance program for image quality of cone-beam CT guidance in radiation therapy. Med Phys 35:1807–1815

Blessing M, Stsepankou D, Wertz H et al (2010) Breath-hold target localization with simultaneous kilovoltage/megavoltage cone-beam computed tomography and fast reconstruction. Int J Radiat Oncol Biol Phys 78:1219–1226

Boda-Heggemann J, Knopf AC, Simeonova-Chergou A et al (2016) Deep inspiration breath hold-based radiation therapy: a clinical review. Int J Radiat Oncol Biol Phys 94:478–492

Boda-Heggemann J, Mai S, Fleckenstein J et al (2013) Flattening-filter-free intensity modulated breath-hold image-guided SABR (Stereotactic ABlative Radiotherapy) can be applied in a 15-min treatment slot. Radiother Oncol 109:505–509

Bouilhol G, Ayadi M, Rit S et al (2013) Is abdominal compression useful in lung stereotactic body radiation therapy? A 4DCT and dosimetric lobe-dependent study. Phys Med 29:333–340

Bradley JD, Nofal AN, El Naqa IM et al (2006) Comparison of helical, maximum intensity projection (MIP), and averaged intensity (AI) 4D CT imaging for stereotactic body radiation therapy (SBRT) planning in lung cancer. Radiother Oncol 81:264–268

Chan MK, Kwong DL, Tam E et al (2013) Quantifying variability of intrafractional target motion in stereotactic body radiotherapy for lung cancers. J Appl Clin Med Phys 14:140–152

Chen MS, Weinhous FC, Deibel JP et al (2001) Fluoroscopic study of tumor motion due to breathing: facilitating precise radiation therapy for lung cancer patients. Med Phys 28:1850–1856

Cuijpers JP, Dahele M, Jonker M et al (2017) Analysis of components of variance determining probability of setup errors in CBCT-guided stereotactic radiotherapy of lung tumors. Med Phys 44:382–388

Cuijpers JP, Verbakel WFAR, Slotman BJ et al (2010) A novel simple approach for incorporation of respiratory motion in stereotactic treatments of lung tumors. Radiother Oncol 97:443–448

Davies SC, Hill AL, Holmes RB et al (1994) Ultrasound quantitation of respiratory organ motion in the upper abdomen. Br J Radiol 67:1096–1102

Dawson LA, Brock KK, Kazanjian S et al (2001) The reproducibility of organ position using active breathing control (ABC) during liver radiotherapy. Int J Radiat Oncol Biol Phys 51:1410–1421

Dawson LA, Eccles C, Bissonnette JP et al (2005) Accuracy of daily image guidance for hypofractionated liver radiotherapy with active breathing control. Int J Radiat Oncol Biol Phys 62:1247–1252

Eccles C, Brock KK, Bissonnette JP et al (2006) Reproducibility of liver position using active breathing coordinator for liver cancer radiotherapy. Int J Radiat Oncol Biol Phys 64:751–759

Falco MD, Fontanarosa D, Miceli R et al (2011) Preliminary studies for a CBCT imaging protocol for offline organ motion analysis: registration software validation and CTDI measurements. Med Dosim 36:91–101

Fassi A, Ivaldi GB, Meaglia I et al (2014) Reproducibility of the external surface position in left-breast DIBH radiotherapy with spirometer based monitoring. J Appl Clin Med Phys 15:4494

Fotina I, Lütgendorf-Caucig C, Stock M et al (2012) Critical discussion of evaluation parameters for inter-observer variability in target definition for radiation therapy. Strahlenther Onkol 188:160–167

Ge J, Santanam L, Noel C et al (2013) Planning 4-dimensional computed tomography (4DCT) cannot adequately represent daily intrafractional motion of abdominal tumors. Int J Radiat Oncol Biol Phys 85:999–1005
George R, Vedam SS, Chung TD, Ramakrishnan V et al (2005) The application of the sinusoidal model to lung cancer patient respiratory motion. Med Phys 32:2850–2861
Gierga DP, Turcotte JC, Sharp GC et al (2012) A voluntary breath-hold treatment technique for the left breast with unfavorable cardiac anatomy using surface imaging. Int J Radiat Oncol Biol Phys 84:e663–e668
Guckenberger M, Meyer J, Wilbert J et al (2007a) Intrafractional uncertainties in cone-beam CT based image-guided radiotherapy (IGRT) of pulmonary tumors. Radiother Oncol 83:57–64
Guckenberger M, Wilbert J, Meyer J et al (2007b) Is a single respiratory correlated 4D-CT study sufficient for evaluation of breathing motion? Int J Radiat Oncol Biol Phys 67:1352–1359
Han K, Basran PS, Cheung P (2010) Comparison of helical and average computed tomography for stereotactic body radiation treatment planning and normal tissue contouring in lung cancer. Clin Oncol (R Coll Radiol) 22:862–867
Harris W, Zhang Y, Yin FF et al (2017) Estimating 4D-CBCT from prior information and extremely limited angle projections using structural PCA and weighted free-form deformation for lung radiotherapy. Med Phys 44:1089–1104
Hazelaar C, Dahele M, Scheib S et al (2017) Verifying tumor position during stereotactic body radiation therapy delivery using (limited-arc) cone beam computed tomography imaging. Radiother Oncol 123:355–362
Herman MG, Balter JM, Jaffray DA et al (2001) Clinical use of electronic portal imaging: report of AAPM Radiation Therapy Committee Task Group 58. Med Phys 28:712–737
Hu Y, Zhou YK, Chen YX et al (2016) 4D-CT scans reveal reduced magnitude of respiratory liver motion achieved by different abdominal compression plate positions in patients with intrahepatic tumors undergoing helical tomotherapy. Med Phys 43:4335
International Commission on Radiation Units and Measurements (1999) ICRU report 62. Prescribing recording and reporting photon beam therapy. ICRU, Bethesda, MD
Jaffray DA, Siewerdsen JH, Wong JW, Martinez AA (2002) Flat-panel cone-beam computed tomography for image-guided radiation therapy. Int J Radiat Oncol Biol Phys 53:1337–1349
Josipovic M, Persson GF, Bangsgaard JP et al (2016) Deep inspiration breath-hold radiotherapy for lung cancer: impact on image quality and registration uncertainty in cone beam CT image guidance. Br J Radiol 89:20160544
Keall PJ, Mageras GS, Balter JM et al (2006) The management of respiratory motion in radiation oncology report of AAPM Task Group 76. Med Phys 33:3874–3900
Kincaid RE Jr, Yorke ED, Goodman KA et al (2013) Investigation of gated cone-beam CT to reduce respiratory motion blurring. Med Phys 40:041717
Knybel L, Cvek J, Molenda L et al (2016) Analysis of lung tumor motion in a large sample: patterns and factors influencing precise delineation of internal target volume. Int J Radiat Oncol Biol Phys 96:751–758
Korin HW, Ehman RL, Riederer SJ et al (1992) Respiratory kinematics of the upper abdominal organs: a quantitative study. Magn Reson Med 23:172–178
Korreman S, Juhler-Nottrup T, Boyer A (2008) Respiratory gated beam delivery cannot facilitate margin reduction, unless combined with respiratory correlated image guidance. Radiat Oncol 84:S87
Korreman S, Persson G, Nygaard D et al (2012) Respiration-correlated image guidance is the most important radiotherapy motion management strategy for most lung cancer patients. Int J Radiat Oncol Biol Phys 83:1338–1343
Korreman S, Rasch C, McNair H et al (2010) The European Society of Therapeutic Radiology and Oncology-European Institute of Radiotherapy (ESTRO-EIR) report on 3D CT-based in-room image guidance systems: a practical and technical review and guide. Radiother Oncol 94:129–144
Liang J, Li M, Zhang T et al (2014) The effect of image-guided radiation therapy on the margin between the clinical target volume and planning target volume in lung cancer. J Med Radiat Sci 61:30–37
Low DA, Parikh PJ, Lu W et al (2005) Novel breathing motion model for radiotherapy. Int J Radiat Oncol Biol Phys 63:921–929
Mampuya WA, Nakamura M, Matsuo Y et al (2013) Interfraction variation in lung tumor position with abdominal compression during stereotactic body radiotherapy. Med Phys 40:091718
Masselli GM, Silvestri S, Ramella S et al (2009) Design and evaluation of a methodology to perform personalized visual biofeedback for reducing respiratory amplitude in radiation treatment. Med Phys 36:1467–1472
Mathieu D, Campeau MP, Bedwani S et al (2017) The impacts of mid-treatment CBCT-guided patient repositioning on target coverage during lung VMAT. J Med Imaging Radiat Oncol 61:543–549
McClelland JR, Blackall JM, Tarte S et al (2006) A continuous 4D motion model from multiple respiratory cycles for use in lung radiotherapy. Med Phys 33:3348–3358
McKenzie A (2004) Defining the PTV and PRV – new ideas about old problems. Radiat Oncol 73:203
Mittauer KE, Deraniyagala R, Li JG et al (2015) Monitoring ABC-assisted deep inspiration breath hold for left-sided breast radiotherapy with an optical tracking system. Med Phys 42:134
Oechsner M, Chizzali B, Devecka M et al (2016) Registration uncertainties between 3D cone beam computed tomography and different reference CT datasets in lung stereotactic body radiation therapy. Radiat Oncol 11:142

Oechsner M, Chizzali B, Devecka M, et al (2017) Interobserver variability of patient positioning using four different CT datasets for image registration in lung stereotactic body radiotherapy. Strahlenther Onkol 193:831–839
Ottosson W, Rahma F, Sjöström D et al (2016) The advantage of deep-inspiration breath-hold and cone-beam CT based soft-tissue registration for locally advanced lung cancer radiotherapy. Radiother Oncol 119:432–437
Park JC, Park SH, Kim JH et al (2012) Liver motion during cone beam computed tomography guided stereotactic body radiation therapy. Med Phys 39:6431–6442
Park S, Kim S, Yi B et al (2017) A novel method of cone beam ct projection binning based on image registration. IEEE Trans Med Imaging 36:1733–1745. [Epub ahead of print]
Pedersen AN, Korreman S, Nystrom H et al (2004) Breathing adapted radiotherapy of breast cancer: reduction of cardiac and pulmonary doses using voluntary inspiration breath-hold. Radiother Oncol 72:53–60
Prabhakar R, Tharmar G, Julka PK et al (2007) Impact of different breathing conditions on the dose to surrounding normal structures in tangential field breast radiotherapy. J Med Phys 32:24–28
Rasch C, Steenbakkers R, van Herk M (2005) Target definition in prostate, head, and neck. Semin Radiat Oncol 15:136–145
Rietzel E, Pan T, Chen GT (2005) Four-dimensional computed tomography: image formation and clinical protocol. Med Phys 32:874–889
Santoso AP, Song KH, Qin Y et al (2016) Evaluation of gantry speed on image quality and imaging dose for 4D cone-beam CT acquisition. Radiat Oncol 11:98
Sarudis S, Karlsson Hauer A et al (2017) Systematic evaluation of lung tumor motion using four-dimensional computed tomography. Acta Oncol 56:525–530
Segedin B, Petric P (2016) Uncertainties in target volume delineation in radiotherapy – are they relevant and what can we do about them? Radiol Oncol 50:254–262
Seppenwoolde Y, Shirato H, Kitamura K et al (2002) Precise and real-time measurement of 3D tumor motion in lung due to breathing and heartbeat, measured during radiotherapy. Int J Radiat Oncol Biol Phys 53(4):822–834
Shah C, Kestin LL, Hope AJ et al (2013) Required target margins for image-guided lung SBRT: assessment of target position intrafraction and correction residuals. Pract Radiat Oncol 3:67–73
Shieh CC, Caillet V, Dunbar M et al (2017) A Bayesian approach for three-dimensional markerless tumor tracking using kV imaging during lung radiotherapy. Phys Med Biol 62:3065–3080
Shieh CC, Keall PJ, Kuncic Z (2015) Markerless tumor tracking using short kilovoltage imaging arcs for lung image-guided radiotherapy. Phys Med Biol 60:9437–9454
Shiinoki T, Hanazawa H, Yuasa Y et al (2017) Verification of respiratory-gated radiotherapy with new real-time tumour-tracking radiotherapy system using cine EPID images and a log file. Phys Med Biol 62:1585–1599
Shirai K, Nishiyama K, Katsuda T et al (2014) Phantom and clinical study of differences in cone beam computed tomographic registration when aligned to maximum and average intensity projection. Int J Radiat Oncol Biol Phys 88:189–194
Sio TT, Jensen AR, Miller RC et al (2014) Influence of patient's physiologic factors and immobilization choice with stereotactic body radiotherapy for upper lung tumors. J Appl Clin Med Phys 15:4931
Siva S, Devereux T, Kron T et al (2014) Vacuum immobilisation reduces tumour excursion and minimises intrafraction error in a cohort study of stereotactic ablative body radiotherapy for pulmonary metastases. J Med Imaging Radiat Oncol 58:244–252
Sweeney RA, Seubert B, Stark S et al (2012) Accuracy and inter-observer variability of 3D versus 4D cone-beam CT based image-guidance in SBRT for lung tumors. Radiat Oncol 7:81
Tang X, Cullip T, Dooley J et al (2015) Dosimetric effect due to the motion during deep inspiration breath hold for left-sided breast cancer radiotherapy. J Appl Clin Med Phys 16:91–99
Tang X, Zagar TM, Bair E et al (2014) Clinical experience with 3-dimensional surface matching-based deep inspiration breath hold for left-sided breast cancer radiation therapy. Pract Radiat Oncol 4:e151–e158
Tanguturi SK, Lyatskaya Y, Chen Y et al (2015) Prospective assessment of deep inspiration breath-hold using 3-dimensional surface tracking for irradiation of left-sided breast cancer. Pract Radiat Oncol 5: 358–365
Thengumpallil S, Smith K, Monnin P et al (2016) Difference in performance between 3D and 4D CBCT for lung imaging: a dose and image quality analysis. J Appl Clin Med Phys 17:6459
Underberg RW, Lagerwaard FJ, Cuijpers JP et al (2004) Four-dimensional CT scans for treatment planning in stereotactic radiotherapy for stage I lung cancer. Int J Radiat Oncol Biol Phys 60:1283–1290
van Herk M, Remeijer P, Rasch C et al (2000) The probability of correct target dosage: dose-population histograms for deriving treatment margins in radiotherapy. Int J Radiat Oncol Biol Phys 47:1121–1135
van Herk M, Witte M, van der Geer J et al (2003) Biological and physical fractionation effects of random geometrical errors. Int J Radiat Oncol Biol Phys 57:1460–1471
van Sörnsen de Koste JR, Dahele M, Mostafavi H et al (2015) Markerless tracking of small lung tumors for stereotactic radiotherapy. Med Phys 42:1640–1652
Vedam SS, Keall PJ, Kini VR et al (2003) Acquiring a four-dimensional computed tomography dataset using an external respiratory signal. Phys Med Biol 48:45–62
Venkat RB, Sawant A, Suh Y et al (2008) Development and preliminary evaluation of a prototype audio-

visual biofeedback device incorporating a patient-specific guiding waveform. Phys Med Biol 53:N197–N208

Wertz H, Stsepankou D, Blessing M et al (2010) Fast kilovoltage/megavoltage (kVMV) breathhold cone-beam CT for image-guided radiotherapy of lung cancer. Phys Med Biol 55:4203–4217

Wink NM, McNitt-Gray MF, Solberg TD (2005) Optimization of multi-slice helical respiration-correlated CT: the effects of table speed and rotation time. Phys Med Biol 50:5717–5729

Witte MG, van der Geer J, Schneider C et al (2004) The effects of target size and tissue density on the minimum margin required for random errors. Med Phys 31:3068–3079

Wolthaus JW, Schneider C, Sonke JJ et al (2006) Mid-ventilation CT scan construction from four-dimensional respiration-correlated CT scans for radiotherapy planning of lung cancer patients. Int J Radiat Oncol Biol Phys 65:1560–1571

Wolthaus JW, Sonke JJ, van Herk M et al (2008) Comparison of different strategies to use four-dimensional computed tomography in treatment planning for lung cancer patients. Int J Radiat Oncol Biol Phys 70:1229–1238

Worm ES, Hoyer M, Fledelius W et al (2013) Variations in magnitude and directionality of respiratory target motion throughout full treatment courses of stereotactic body radiotherapy for tumors in the liver. Acta Oncol 52:1437–1444

Yan D, Wong J, Vicini F et al (1997) Adaptive modification of treatment planning to minimize the deleterious effects of treatment setup errors. Int J Radiat Oncol Biol Phys 38:197–206

Yorke E, Xiong Y, Han Q et al (2016) Kilovoltage imaging of implanted fiducials to monitor intrafraction motion with abdominal compression during stereotactic body radiation therapy for gastrointestinal tumors. Int J Radiat Oncol Biol Phys 95:1042–1049

Zhang H, Kruis M, Sonke JJ (2017b) Directional sinogram interpolation for motion weighted 4D cone-beam CT reconstruction. Phys Med Biol 62:2254–2275

Zhang H, Ma J, Bian Z et al (2017a) High quality 4D cone-beam CT reconstruction using motion-compensated total variation regularization. Phys Med Biol 62:3313–3329

High-Field MRI In-Room Guidance for Radiotherapy Adaptation

Martin F. Fast and Markus Glitzner

Contents

1	**Introduction**	108
1.1	Motion Characterization and Motion Management	108
1.2	Current In-Room Guidance Systems and Limitations	109
1.3	Advantages of High-Field MRI-Based In-Room Guidance	110
1.4	Clinical Rationale for In-Room MRI Guidance	111
1.5	High-Field In-Room Guidance Systems	113
2	**MR Imaging Techniques for Radiotherapy Adaptations**	114
2.1	Anatomic Imaging	114
2.2	Dynamic 2D Cine MRI	115
2.3	4D MRI	116
2.4	Motion Estimation and Contour Propagation for On-Line MRI	118
3	**Inter-Fractional Treatment Adaptations**	119
3.1	Rigid Aperture Morphing	120
3.2	Warm-Start Optimization	120
3.3	Full Re-planning	120
4	**Intra-Fractional Treatment Adaptations**	120
4.1	Respiratory Gating	121
4.2	Dynamic Tumour Tracking	121
4.3	Impact of Imaging in Real-Time Applications	122
4.4	Real-Time Dose Accumulation and Intra-Fractional Re-planning	123
5	**Conclusions and Outlook**	125
References		125

M. F. Fast (✉) · M. Glitzner
Department of Radiotherapy, University Medical Center Utrecht (UMCU),
Utrecht, The Netherlands
e-mail: M.F.Fast@umcutrecht.nl

Abstract

Intra-fractional motion is the main source of uncertainty when targeting treatment sites in the thorax and upper abdomen. Predominately periodic respiratory and cardiac-induced motion, and irregular gastrointestinal activity displace and deform targets and healthy organs compared to their observed position during treatment planning. Adapting treatment to this complex motion pattern requires precise and frequent on-board imaging. Current X-ray based in-room imaging techniques induce additional radiation exposure, suffer from poor soft-tissue contrast in the 2D projection images, and usually require implanted fiducial markers for guidance. In comparison, high field magnetic resonance imaging (MRI) offers customizable, diagnostic-quality soft-tissue contrast and much greater flexibility in selecting the appropriate image dimension for detecting anatomical motion.

In this chapter we will first introduce the clinical rationale for in-room guidance based on MRI. A survey will highlight existing technical implementations while focussing on the Elekta Unity MR-linac. We will then identify suitable MRI techniques for radiotherapy adaptations. This will include an overview of typical sequences used for anatomical imaging. Several possible image dimensions, ranging from real-time 2D cine imaging to retrospectively sorted 4D motion models will be presented in detail. The resulting increase in observer confidence due to the higher image

R. G. H. Beets-Tan et al. (eds.), *Imaging and Interventional Radiology for Radiation Oncology*, Medical Radiology, Diagnostic Imaging, https://doi.org/10.1007/978-3-030-38261-2_8

quality is complemented with an array of suitable inter-fractional and intra-fractional treatment adaptations based on on-line MRI. We will emphasize the benefits and challenges of several motion mitigation techniques including beam gating, dynamic tumour tracking, and intra-fractional re-planning based on online accumulated dose.

1 Introduction

1.1 Motion Characterization and Motion Management

The radiotherapy process typically begins with imaging. A computed tomography (CT) scan is acquired for treatment planning to capture the unique anatomy of each patient. Next, therapy-relevant structures including the target and organ at risks (OARs) are delineated using the volumetric images. Furthermore, the CT is used to obtain a physical description of the patient anatomy in the form of an electron density (ED) distribution, which is required for performing dose calculations in the treatment planning system (TPS).

This *snapshot* CT acquisition is then used throughout the course of treatment which can take up to 7 weeks. During this period, the anatomy in and around the target site experiences morphological changes as shown in Fig. 1. The changes occurring between fractions are termed *inter-fractional* variations and are caused by gradual weight loss, tumour regression/progression and filling of internal organs on a day-to-day basis. Geometric variations due to respiration (Fig. 2), peristalsis in the stomach, bowel and rectum and bladder filling are imposed on a shorter time scale (seconds to minutes) and are therefore termed *intra-fractional* variations.

Prior to the arrival of in-room imaging, changes in the internal anatomy were completely hidden, as the matching of the planning- and treatment coordinate system (positioning) was performed according to superficial markers, e.g. on the skin. Consequently, target volumes were expanded using generous treatment margins, creating a (geometrical, non-clinical) planning target volume (PTV), which includes all likely target volume positions. Once in-room imaging became available, target positions could be determined in and during each fraction. In addition to position verification, the spatial distribution of target positions (Kotte et al. 2007; van der Heide et al. 2007) and the according calculation of treatment margins (van Herk et al. 2000) were studied extensively. The use of geometric, population-based margin concepts inherently sacrifices surrounding healthy tissues and OARs for target coverage. Depending on the sensitivity to radiation of these structures, this can lead to acute toxicities and long-term side effects.

As a consequence of *inter-fractional* and *intra-fractional* anatomical variations, active motion management became a prerequisite for modern radiotherapy. Increased dose conformity is the main goal of image-guided radiation therapy (IGRT). This is especially important for hypo-fractionated treatment regimes where increased doses per fraction require an improved sparing of surrounding OAR and thus increased conformity to the actual target. By using imaging devices, which are integrated into the treatment machine, the patient anatomy can be sampled when it matters most—at the time of treatment. This allows for precise and frequent estimations of the actual target position, facilitating margin reduction and thus sparing of healthy tissue. For each fraction, the current target position can act as a reference to set up the patient with respect to the treatment device, reducing systematic and random positioning uncertainties. Furthermore, during treatment, continuously incoming target positions can be fed into active motion compensation systems such as beam gating and beam steering/tracking to reduce *intra-fractional* uncertainties.

The recent arrival of high-field MRI in-room guidance facilitates a drastic improvement for IGRT going far beyond better image quality. The different treatment sites, motion characteristics (amplitude, frequency) and types (spontaneous, periodic) pose different requirements to the required imaging modality. For MRI,

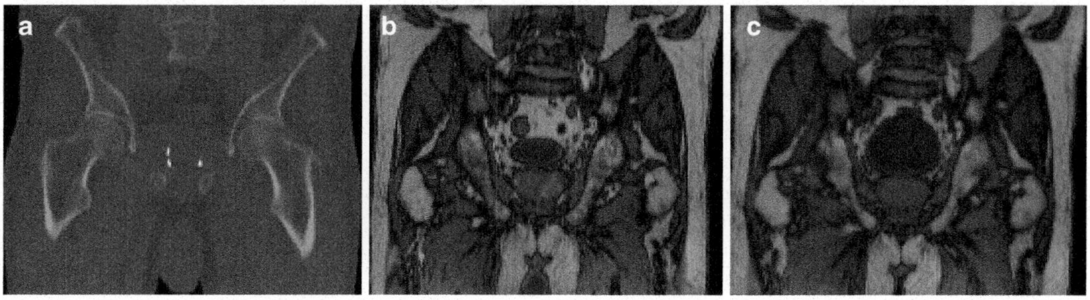

Fig. 1 *Inter-fractional* variation during the treatment course: bladder filling causes the prostate to migrate away from the planned position. (**a**) Planning CT. (**b**) Planning MRI. (**c**) Fraction MRI

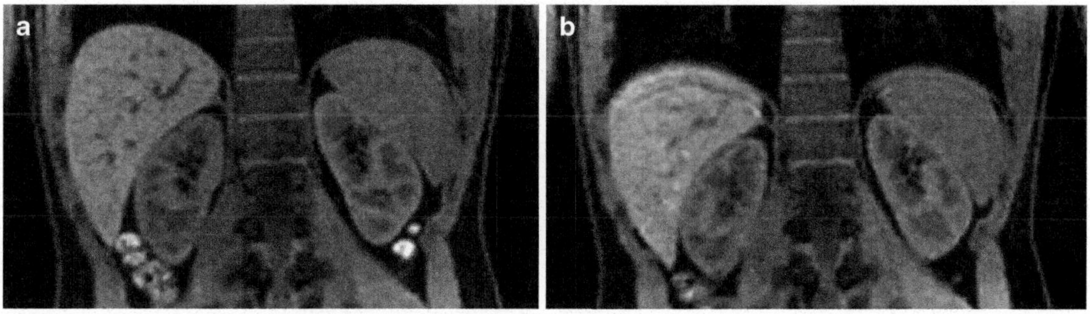

Fig. 2 *Intra-fractional* variation during a respiratory cycle: breathing continuously changes the positions of all organs in the thorax and upper abdomen. (**a**) Exhalation MRI. (**b**) Inhalation MRI

spatio-temporal resolution and dimensionality are merely a matter of parametrization. Therefore, image acquisition schemes for a variety of applications can be implemented, ranging from high-resolution position sequences to fast, real-time target tracking. At the same time, a superior quality image containing excellent soft-tissue contrast and a high level of signal-to-noise ratio (SNR) en par with diagnostic imaging is maintained. This also aligns IGRT with the increasing use of MRI for radiotherapy planning and follow-ups.

1.2 Current In-Room Guidance Systems and Limitations

Non-MRI in-room guidance systems are widely available and their use is considered mandatory when using highly conformal treatment techniques such as intensity modulated radiation therapy (IMRT) or volumetric modulated arc therapy (VMAT) (Moran et al. 2011; Jaffray et al. 2013). Table 1 lists the most commonly used in-room guidance systems. Note that Chap. 7 contains a detailed description of X-ray based in-room image guidance.

Electromagnetic target localization and often also X-ray based imaging rely on implanted markers. The implantation procedure poses an additional burden for the patient and can lead to complications. Using markers instead of directly monitoring the anatomy also assumes that there is no differential motion between target and markers. The same assumption of correlation needs to be made for surface based imaging systems. These systems need to be used with caution as external motion can misrepresent internal motion (Gierga et al. 2005). Only ultrasound (US) and cone-beam computed tomography

Table 1 System characteristics of the currently used (non-MRI) in-room guidance systems

System	Principle	Invasive	Ionizing	Dimension	Real-time	Anatomical sites	Soft-tissue contrast
Electromagnetic	Passive implanted transponders + antenna array	Yes	No	3D + *t*	Yes	Prostate, cervix, lung	No
Surface-based	Optical or infra-red surface sensor	No	No	1D/2D + *t*	Yes	Thorax, abdomen	No
Ultrasound	Sound propagation in tissue	No	No	2D/3D + *t*	Yes	Abdomen, pelvis	Limited
X-ray	Projection imaging	No/ Yes[a]	Yes	2D + *t*	Yes	Most	Poor
	Cross-sectional imaging (CBCT)	No/ Yes[a]	Yes	3D (+ *t*)	No	Most	Poor (kV), No (MV)

[a] Usually used in combination with implanted markers

(CBCT) imaging offer direct target and OAR visualization. Current US systems are somewhat limited in their utility for moving anatomy as the ultrasound waves cannot penetrate bone (e.g. ribs). Maintaining a close contact between US probe and patient is crucial to ensure consistent image quality, but also challenging especially in case of transabdominal ultrasound. Robotic arms are needed to keep the US transducer in place during irradiation (Schlosser et al. 2010).

CBCT imaging is widely available and has proven very useful for patient set-up verification. A limiting factor is the additional dose exposure to the patient, although this is less of a concern for hypo-fractionated treatments with few fractions. Image quality on linear accelerators, however, is worse than on diagnostic CT scanners especially with regard to soft-tissue differentiation. CBCT captures the motion of the patient before and\or after treatment (with some limited exceptions such as concurrent VMAT irradiation and CBCT imaging in lung SBRT). As the image reconstruction requires 2D projection images from a 200–360° gantry rotation, CBCT cannot provide a real-time signal of the patient anatomy during treatment.

A very important consideration when evaluating the capabilities of in-room guidance systems is the dimensionality of the problem. Anatomical motion is a four-dimensional problem. 4D motion can include translation, rotations and also deformations, all evolving over time. This complexity is difficult to capture with today's in-room guidance systems. Instead, complexity is reduced by limiting the number of dimensions or averaging motion. 4D CBCT, for example, generates an average (synthetic) representation of respiratory motion but does not provide true temporal resolution. Even greater simplicity in the case of point-like motion surrogates comes at the cost of precision and accuracy.

1.3 Advantages of High-Field MRI-Based In-Room Guidance

In-room guidance is especially relevant for target sites that undergo substantial intra-fractional motion and that present a challenge for current IGRT technologies due to, for example, poor tumour visibility. Using on-board MRI allows to acquire images of the patient in treatment position and in diagnostic quality. This greatly simplifies comparing and registering the in-room images with pre-treatment planning magnetic resonance (MR) images.

The main specification of MRI scanners, both technically and commercially, is the strength of the main magnetic field B_0. Increasing B_0 not only leads to increases in SNR, translating into improvements in spatial or temporal resolution, but also magnifies susceptibility-induced field inhomogeneities that can, e.g., negatively affect lung MRI. While no single field strength can be considered *optimal* for all image acquisition techniques (Rutt et al. 1996; Maubon et al.

1999), the absence of variable field-strength scanners requires a pragmatic choice. Over the last years there has been a clear trend towards higher field strengths for diagnostic imaging. Next to the increased SNR figures, higher B_0 facilitates spectral fat suppression and fast Dixon-based water-fat separation techniques, leading to an improved diagnostic contrasts (Bley et al. 2010). Today, 1.5 T MRI scanners represent the state-of-the-art in diagnostic MRI, with medical staff trained on the contrasts generated from such field strength. For radiotherapy workflows, MRI scanners with 1.5 or 3 T meet most of the requirements (Paulson et al. 2016). Another relevant hardware performance characteristic is the strength and slew rate of the imaging gradients $G_{x,y,z}$, determining the capability to perform fast, real-time imaging.

In the future, in-room MRI guidance is anticipated to move beyond morphological imaging towards quantitative functional imaging. This is expected to start an era of biologically guided treatments where changes in, e.g., tumour density or oxygenation inform the decision to adapt therapy (van der Heide et al. 2012). Especially for functional MRI applications, employing high-field systems is beneficial, as examinations are sped up significantly due to the higher SNR per unit time compared to low-field strength scanners.

1.4 Clinical Rationale for In-Room MRI Guidance

In radiation treatments, intra-fractional anatomical motion is the main source of targeting uncertainty for treatment sites in the thorax and upper abdomen (Keall et al. 2006). Motion induced by respiration, the heartbeat and gastrointestinal activity easily exceeds 1 cm (c.f. Fig. 3). For many of the treatment sites affected by motion, 5-year relative survival is below 40% for local disease (Howlader et al. 2016), highlighting the need for more precise and effective radiotherapy. Without claiming completeness, this section will discuss several potential target sites that could benefit from in-room MRI guidance.

With today's technologies, stereotactic body radiation therapy (SBRT) treatments for early stage lung cancer result in excellent local control rates in case of peripheral tumours (defined as being more than 2 cm away from the proximal bronchial tree, major vessels and other mediastinal structures). For central tumours, the proximity of mediastinal OARs often limits the ability to hypo-fractionate treatments due to motion and shallow dose gradients. Central tumours are therefore expected to benefit from in-room MRI-guidance (Menten et al. 2017). For locally advanced lung cancer, it is expected that MRI will help resolve the differential motion of involved mediastinal and hilar lymph nodes relative to the primary tumour (Poulsen et al. 2016), resulting in future opportunities for treatment adaptations.

Another potentially interesting application for MRI-guidance is hepatocellular carcinoma (liver cancer) and metastatic liver disease. In recent years, SBRT has become increasingly important for patients with unresectable liver lesions. Aggressive fractionation schemes (e.g. 3×20 Gy) have resulted in high local control (>90%) but patient selection is crucial to avoid excessive toxicities. Extensive liver motion (Kirilova et al. 2008) in combination with passive SBRT delivery techniques (internal target volume (ITV) or mid-ventilation approaches) results in a relatively large PTV. MRI has been reported to provide excellent visualization of liver lesions.

The rationale for escalating the dose is not yet established in oesophageal cancer patients treated with definitive chemoradiation but prospective dose escalation studies are awaited. Retrospective studies indicate that a majority of recurrences occur in the gross tumour volume (GTV), indicating that current dose levels (~50 Gy) are insufficient (Welsh et al. 2012). However, the ability to escalate dose is limited by adjacent OARs, especially the heart and lungs. Tumour motion in the lower oesophagus near the gastrointestinal junction may exceed 1 cm (Lever et al. 2014), further challenging conventional treatment approaches.

Pancreatic cancer is also a challenging type of tumour. For unresectable tumours, SBRT

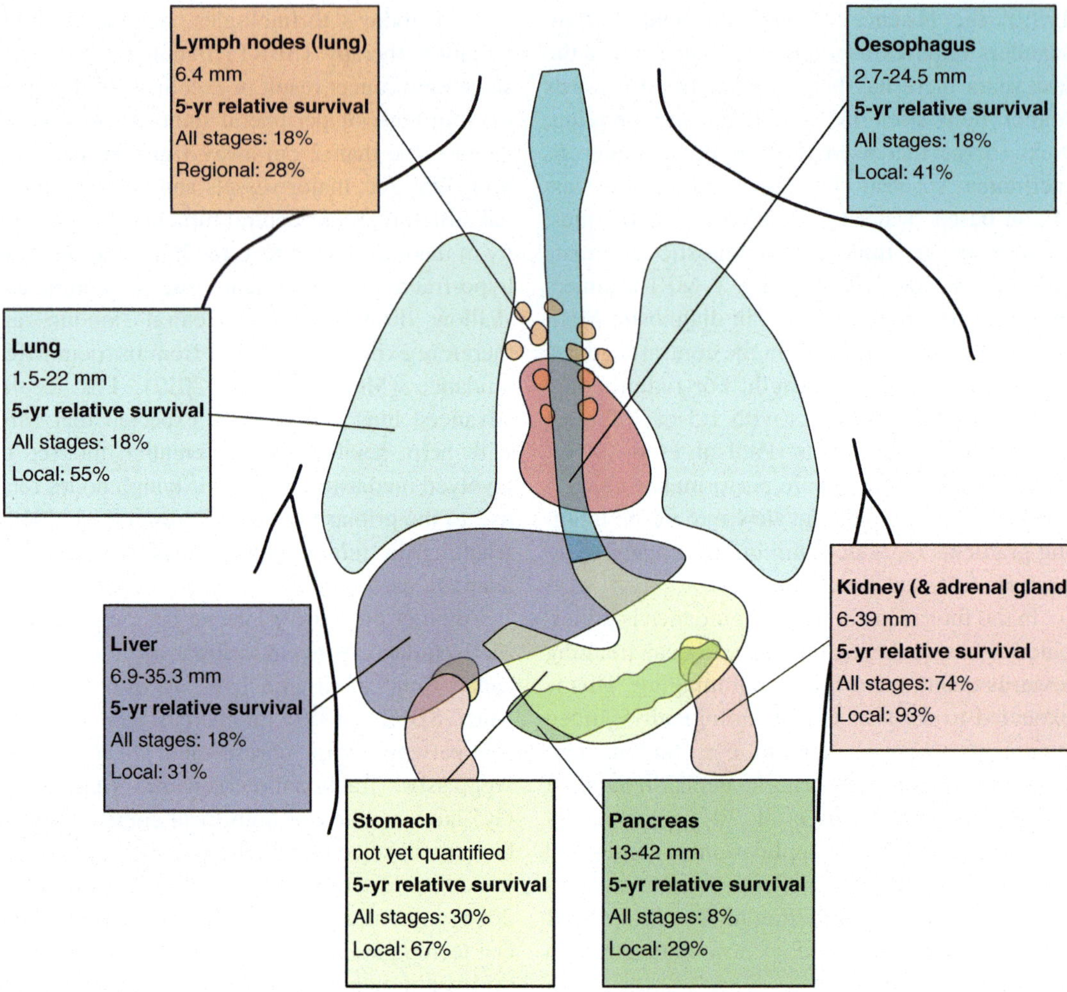

Fig. 3 Target sites for in-room MRI-guidance in the thorax and upper abdomen. Relative survival data was retrieved from Howlader et al. (2016). Cranial-caudal (CC) motion was quantified using cine MRI (Kirilova et al. 2008; Feng et al. 2009; Lever et al. 2014; Stam et al. 2013; Poulsen et al. 2016; Fast et al. 2017)

(5×6 Gy) increases the 1-year local control to 80% (from 40 to 60% for conventional fractionation) and is associated with less pancreatic pain and low gastrointestinal toxicity (Balaban et al. 2016). Substantial motion of the tumour (Feng et al. 2009) and surrounding OARs especially the duodenum and stomach makes it difficult to deliver the appropriate radiation dose.

Renal cell carcinoma (kidney cancer) is traditionally assumed to be radio-resistant, although this belief rests on experience gained with conventionally fractionated radiotherapy. In recent years, high radiation doses have been associated with an increased radio-sensitivity through activation of the ceramide pathway (De Meerleer et al. 2014). The required hypo-fractionation (e.g. 3×12 Gy) can only be delivered safely with high conformality (resulting in dose inhomogeneity in the target) achieved with SBRT. Although prospective trial data is missing, it is hypothesized that kidney SBRT could become a viable treatment option for medically inoperable patients.

Adrenal gland metastases commonly occur in about 20% of patients with malignant tumours. SBRT is emerging as a useful local ablation technique for some of these patients. Since the adrenal glands are adjacent to the kidney, motion characteristics are similar for those sites.

Besides tumour sites in thorax and upper abdomen, motion can also displace or deform organs in the pelvis such as rectum, prostate and cervix. Here, motion is usually not periodic and may occur on a time-scale of seconds to minutes. Typical causes are rectal activity, muscle clenching, bladder filling and leg motion (Nederveen et al. 2002). Depending on the source of motion, the tumour can be deformed momentarily or for a sustained period of time.

1.5 High-Field In-Room Guidance Systems

In-room guidance systems based on high-field MRI have recently entered routine clinical service. The most comprehensive integration of MRI and radiation treatment is achieved with hybrid MR-linac devices. Table 2 lists some of the technical characteristics that influence imaging and therapy. Note that the low-field Viewray MRIdian system (ViewRay Inc., Oakwood Village, OH, USA) is discussed in Chap. 9.

The first clinically available integrated high-field in-room guidance solution is the Elekta Unity MR-linac (Elekta AB, Stockholm, Sweden). Unity combines a 1.5 T MRI scanner based on the Philips Ingenia with a 7 MV Elekta linac. The system is set up in such a way that the beam generation resides outside the closed-bore magnet. Since both subsystems are sensitive to electromagnetic interference, the radio frequency (RF) coupling between the two sub-systems needs to be minimized. To prevent the strong magnetic field of the magnet to deflect accelerated electrons in the beam generation, active shielding coils are driven in such a way as to obtain a field-free zone in an annulus around the bore (Overweg et al. 2009). To protect the acquisition chain of the MRI scanner from the RF interference of the linac, the MRI scanner is isolated by an RF cage. Beam absorption is minimized by deploying a split gradient coil with a 20 cm gap between the two halves.

Another hybrid MRI/radiotherapy device is currently being developed in Australia (Keall et al. 2014). The Australian MR-linac combines a split magnet design with a 6 MV linac. The system is prepared to inject the photon beam either perpendicular to or parallel with the B_0 field directions in order to investigate the impact of the configuration on dose generation.

Siemens recently presented another more experimental MR-linac concept (Heid et al. 2015). Here, a Siemens Magnetom Espree magnet is combined with a compact linac assembly inside the MRI bore. The reduced bore width of 40 cm limits the applicability of this approach to head or extremity treatments. In the initial experiments, the magnet was ramped up to 0.5 T, less than its full capability of 1.5 T.

An alternative approach pioneered in Toronto but not widely available is a retractable ceiling mounted MRI scanner (Jaffray et al. 2014). This

Table 2 High-field MRI-guided radiotherapy system

System	Field strength (T)	Max. gradient amplitude (mT/m)	Patient gap (bore) (cm)	Magnet design	Beam orientation (w.r.t. B_0)	Treatment beam	Field inhomogeneity (ppm)
Australian	1.0	10	50 (62)	Split	In-line or perpendicular	4 and 6 MV, 120 leaves	0.47[a]
Elekta Unity	1.5	15	70	Closed	Perpendicular	7 MV, 160 leaves	0.59[b]
Philips Ingenia	1.5	30	70	Closed	n/a	n/a	0.46[b]
ViewRay MRIdian	0.35	18	70	Split	Perpendicular	6 MV, 138 leaves	<25[c]

Specifications for the Philips Ingenia MRI scanner and the Viewray MRIdian linac are shown for comparison
[a] Peak-to-peak inhomogeneity in a 20 cm diameter of spherical volume (DSV)
[b] Root-mean-squared field inhomogeneity in a 30 cm DSV
[c] 45 cm DSV

system design minimizes modifications of the therapy and imaging components as they are not used at the same time. Instead, the MRI scanner is retracted beyond the treatment room prior to commencement of treatment. After the patient is scanned, the patient support system has to be moved from the position of the MRI to the linear accelerator. By design, the system is not able to monitor intra-fractional motion.

2 MR Imaging Techniques for Radiotherapy Adaptations

In contrast to the on-board imaging techniques in Table 1, on-line MRI can extract internal volume of interests (VOIs) by means of volume excitation and *Fourier* encoding. Therefore, unlike backprojection-based techniques, it is not necessary to image the entire anatomy, when only small volumes are of interest. As the acquisition time in MRI scales overproportionally with the size of the field-of-view (FOV), proper FOV selection can translate directly into imaging speed-up, which is essential for on-line and especially real-time applications.

MR image formation is determined for one part by the invariant physical properties of tissue, such as relaxation parameters T1 and T2 and proton density ρ. To configure the contrast in tissue the excitation volume and the resolution of the images, pulse sequences are played out during the examinations, which define the shape, strength and duration of RF pulses, imaging gradients and acquisition intervals.

2.1 Anatomic Imaging

Depending on the anatomic site and contrast requirement, various pulse sequence types are used. In Fig. 4, a selection of imaging techniques for abdominal and thoracic sites available on

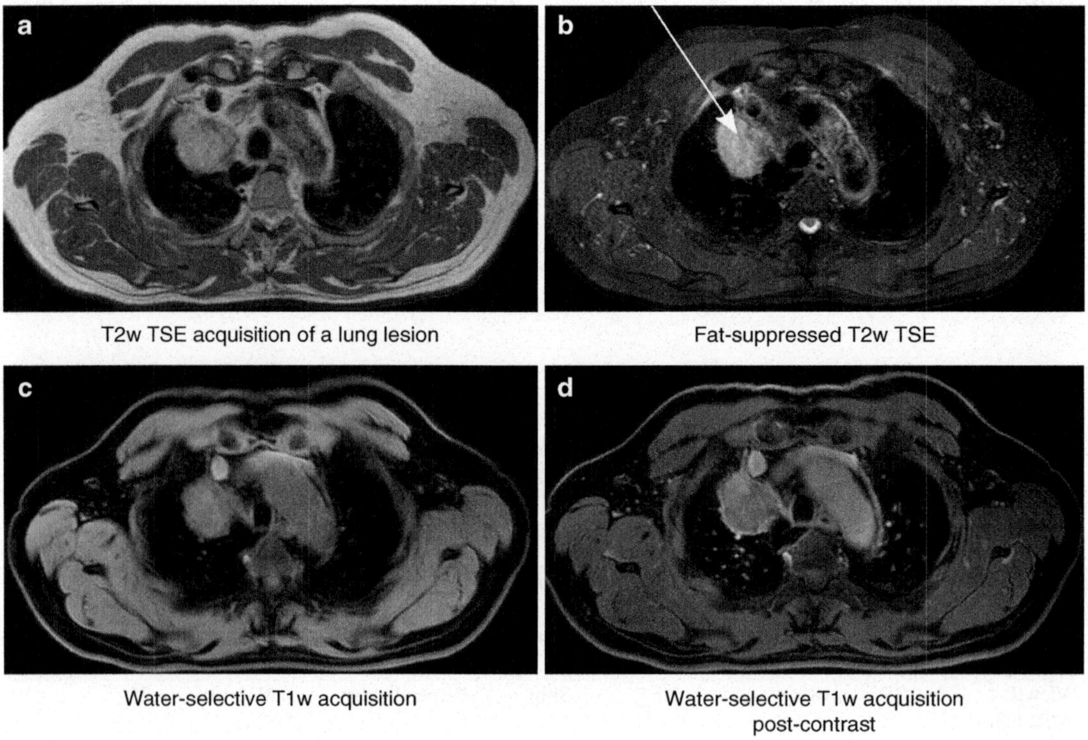

Fig. 4 Different MRI contrasts in abdominal sites at 1.5 T high-field MRI: In (**a**) and (**b**), selective spectral attenuated inversion recovery (SPAIR) fat-suppression highlights the tumour (white arrow). Similarly, comparison of pre-(**c**) and post-contrast image (**d**) is of value for target identification and localization. *Images courtesy of Rob Tijssen (UMC Utrecht)*

high-field MRI is presented. In addition to weightings to the relaxation parameters T1 and T2, spectrally selective pulses can be employed in order to improve tumour contrast as shown in Fig. 4a and b, where a spectrally selective fat suppression yields largely improved tumour contrast. Similarly, contrast injections offer increased significant sensitivity in the well perfused tumour volume (Fig. 4c, d) and allows the extraction of functional parameters such as k_{trans}.

In anatomic imaging for the definition and characterization of tissue, images are resolved in 3D. Volumetric encoding can be accomplished by either stacking multiple individually acquired 2D slices (as in CT) or by *Fourier* encoding the entire VOI in all three dimensions. The latter is generally accomplished by a significantly increased SNR, but suffers from increased sensitivity to intra-scan motion artefacts. Anatomic imaging in 3D is lengthy (in the order of minutes). Along with pulse sequence settings defining the contrast, such as repetition time, echo time and flip angle, imaging time is mainly dependent on the pixel density and volume size. As a rule of thumb, each line of voxels in the VOI requires one repetition time to be acquired. Hence, a 3D volume with $0.5 \times 0.5 \times 0.2$ m^3 and 2 mm^3 isotropic voxel size requires

$$T_{acq} = 250 \times 100 \times T_R \approx 1.7 \text{ min} \qquad (1)$$

with an exemplary repetition time of 4 ms. In this regime real-time imaging is neither intended nor possible.

Similar to CT, encoding moving anatomy over lengthy acquisition times merges data from different respiratory states which leads to blurring and ghosting as shown at the abdominal wall in Fig. 5a. To alleviate these adverse effects, motion compensation techniques such as *gating* or *triggering* are applied, which reduce the data acquisition of the stable inhale or exhale periods detected by either MRI or other surrogate signals such as respiratory bellows. Figure 5b shows a triggered acquisition, essentially eliminating the breathing-induced blur around the abdomen.

2.2 Dynamic 2D Cine MRI

In contrast to 3D image sequences, 2D MRI can sample the anatomy with high temporal resolution approaching the real-time imaging domain. For example, on the current Elekta Unity MR-linac system imaging rates of 4 Hz are feasible with T1-weighted or balanced steady-state free precession (bSSFP)-type contrasts and in-plane resolutions similar to anatomic imaging.

Fast imaging is generally performed using bSSFP sequences (Scheffler and Lehnhardt 2003). Depending on the manufacturer, these sequences are also known as TrueFisp (Siemens), balanced fast-field echo (b-FFE) (Philips) and FIESTA (GE). These sequences are based on gradient-echoes and maintain a steady transverse magnetization. bSSFP requires very short

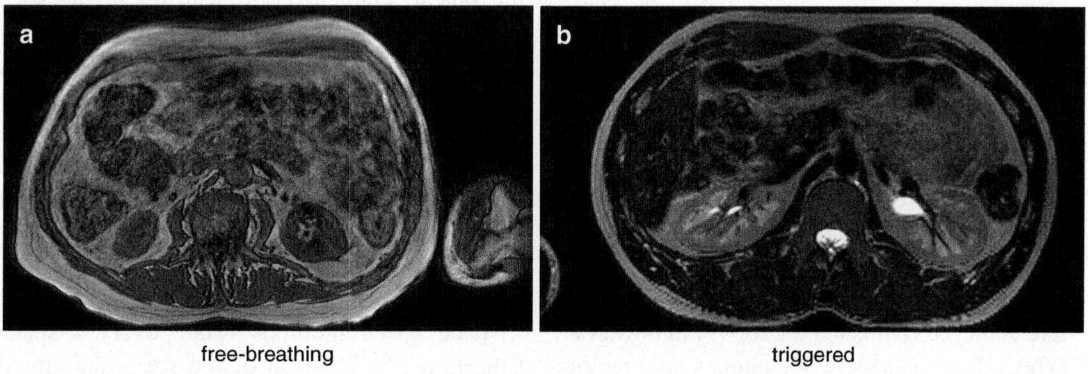

Fig. 5 Motion during the acquisition process: (**a**) and (**b**) shows the differences in body outline depending on motion compensation strategies during acquisition

repetition times (TR, 3–6 ms) which are only possible with fast-switching gradients. Its mixed T2/T1-weighted contrast is considered suitable for morphological imaging but does not usually have enough T2-weighting for diagnostic purposes at high-field strengths.

Another alternative for fast 2D cine acquisitions is the spoiled gradient-echo sequence (Plathow et al. 2005). Here, any residual transversal magnetization is destroyed at the end of each excitation cycle. The resulting images show more T1-weighting. Magnetization spoiling at low repetition times translates into a reduced SNR and could lead to a loss in contrast-to-noise ratio (CNR), especially compared to bSSFP-type sequences.

Besides the choice of sequence, the FOV, slice thickness and orientation of the cine slice are also crucial. The FOV needs to cover the relevant anatomy and be large enough to minimize fold-over artefacts in the phase-encoding direction. When this is not possible (e.g. large patients, involvement of arms), additional saturation bands outside the FOV can help mitigate the problem. For 2D cine acquisitions, slice thickness is usually in the 3–10 mm range and thus tends to be larger compared to 3D acquisitions. Thicker slices are needed to achieve sufficient SNR and better defined slice profiles. They also increase robustness against through-plane motion. This can be an issue if the predominant axes of motion do not coincide with the preselected slice orientation.

2.3 4D MRI

Due to the lengthy image encoding, real-time or *true* 3D MRI is currently only feasible when the spatio-temporal resolution is vastly reduced, resulting in compromised image quality. Combining parallel imaging with sparse sampling techniques, a spatial resolution of approximately 4 mm and a temporal resolution of 1 s were achieved (Dinkel et al. 2009; Plathow et al. 2009). However, these techniques are neither widely available nor proven to generate sufficient image quality for radiotherapy applications. 4D MRI describes the process of acquiring a respiratory-correlated volumetric image representation of an average respiratory cycle. Similar to sorting approaches in 4D (CB)CT, image data acquired over multiple respiratory cycles is retrospectively binned according to phase or amplitude. Sorting requires an external surrogate (e.g. a belt-mounted pressure sensor, or a tidal flow measurement) or an internal surrogate (e.g. a 1D navigator signal, or a self-navigation signal). Image acquisition schemes can be divided into 2D or 3D k-space methods.

Within the 2D k-space methods, interleaved multi-slice 2D acquisitions have proven very popular due to their wide-spread availability and simple reconstruction (von Siebenthal et al. 2007; Paganelli et al. 2015; van de Lindt et al. 2018a, b). Here, a respiratory phase is assigned to each image slice. The interleaved acquisition pattern minimizes cross talk between slices and ensures that the magnetization is recovered in between acquisitions of the same slice. Prominent image features such as the diaphragm motion captured in sagittal/coronal images or a navigator signal can be used as to extract internal surrogates, minimizing errors compared to an external motion surrogate. Image acquisition times are usually around 5 min, while image reconstruction takes seconds. A common issue of any 2D k-space based 4D MRI method is the lack of spatial resolution in the through-plane direction, although super-sampling approaches might be able to compensate for this (Reeth et al. 2015). 2D imaging techniques are also susceptible to slice warping due to gradient non-linearities in the slice selection gradient field. While slice warping can be corrected in multi-slice 2D sequences (Keesman et al. 2019), these distortions are only a real issue at the very edge of the FOV, outside of the VOI relevant for radiotherapy applications. Furthermore, incorrectly binned slices might degrade image quality in the individual respiratory phases.

Unlike the 2D k-space acquisitions, 3D k-space based methods relate every k-space sample to the position of the surrogate signal (Stemkens et al. 2015; Deng et al. 2016; Rank et al. 2017). By continuously looping over the

3D k-space, each respiratory phase is filled with enough k-space lines to reconstruct a 3D image. This effectively yields a full 4D stack in both k and image domain. Compared to sliced-bases acquisition, image volumes do not suffer from slice stacking artefacts due to ambiguous surrogate signals. Figure 6 illustrates the difference between Cartesian and radial filling of k-space. Furthermore, using radial acquisitions, intra-phase motion artefacts have less of an impact on image quality due to the relatively dense sampling of the k-space centre. The disadvantage compared to Cartesian acquisitions are mainly the loss of sampling efficiency and

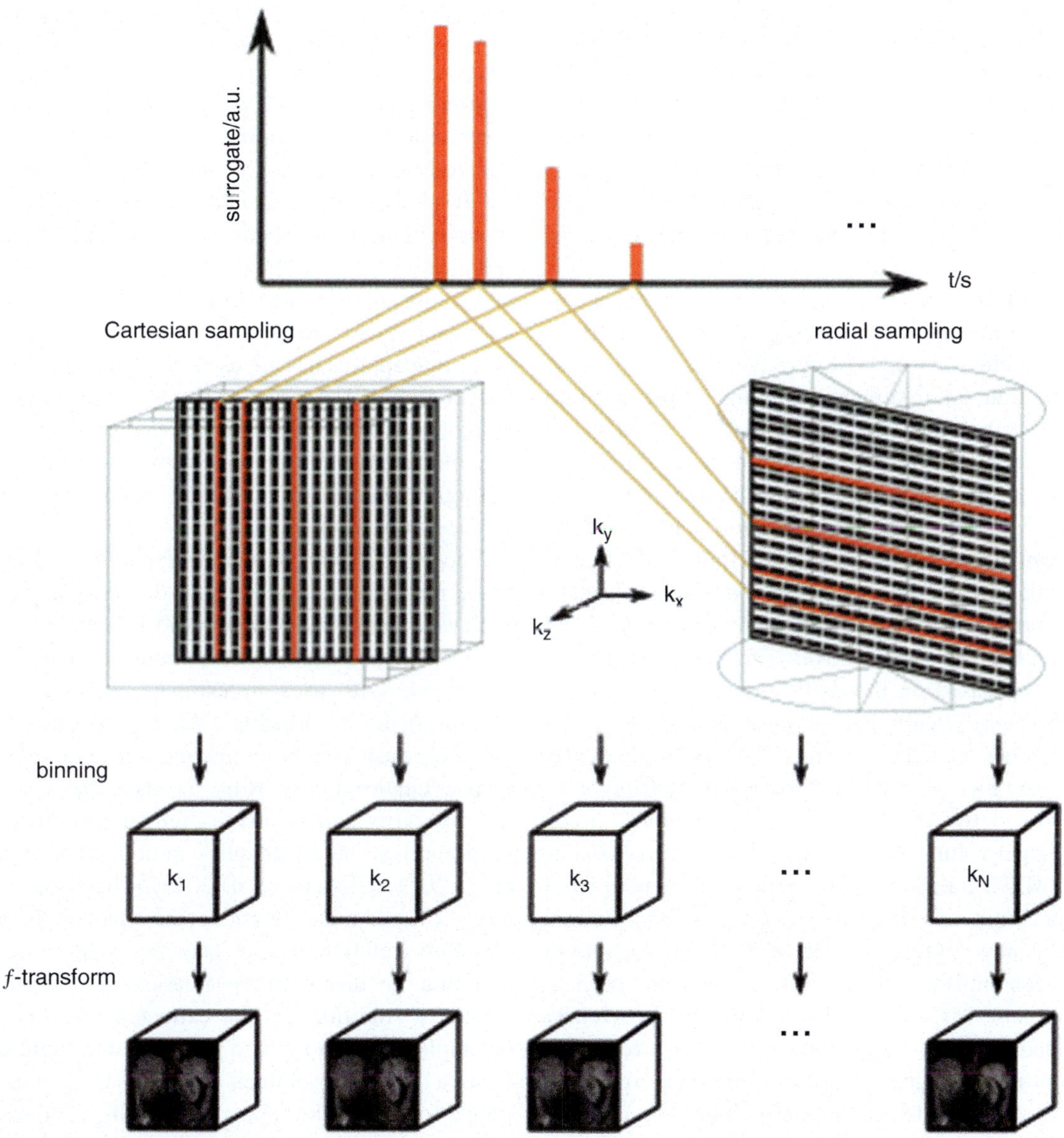

Fig. 6 Concept of k-space based retrospective binning for 4D MRI: each read-out line (dashed) is assigned to a respiratory phase. In the Cartesian example (left figure), each k-space plane is consecutively filled. In radial acquisitions, read-out lines are either collected per *blade* (right figure) or in a *stack-of-stars* fashion (not shown). The anatomy is sampled until enough data to fill all individual k-spaces k_i for each respiratory phase i has been acquired. Respiratory-correlated 3D images are then obtained by Fourier transformation of k_i

the necessary gridding (i.e. interpolating the radially acquired k-space to a Cartesian grid). Given the large FOV and fine spatial resolution required in radiotherapy applications, 4D image acquisition times are a big challenge and one way to accelerate this is under-sampling k-space. Using a gradient-echo sequence with a radial stack-of-stars sampling scheme may facilitate under-sampling factors of up to 16.8 (Rank et al. 2017). This results in acquisition times below 1 min but currently comes at the penalty of reconstruction times of a few hours. The radial stack-of-stars acquisition pattern has the additional advantage that the signal intensity at the centre of k-space can be used to derive a surrogate respiratory signal for retrospective binning.

4D MR images can be used in a variety of situations pre-, intra- and post-treatment. In the planning phase, 4D CT indicating the range of motion for treatment planning purposes could be substituted or augmented by MRI-based motion models. In addition to the non-ionizing imaging, a further advantage compared to CT is the superior soft-tissue contrast of the MRI which can aid delineations. High-field 4D MR images acquired using the on-board scanner immediately before treatment can replace 4D CBCT for patient positioning and plan alterations based on the daily anatomy and motion. During treatment, continuous anatomical images and the machine configuration of the linac can be combined to reconstruct the actually delivered dose and to continuously track target volumes using, e.g., multi-leaf collimator (MLC) tracking. Both applications benefit from a continuous stream of 3D images with minimal latency. As real-time 3D MRI is not feasible in such on-line applications, models are used to obtain 3D images based on the previously acquired 4D motion model and a fast, real-time surrogate signal. Next to simple interpolation models, the use of parametric models was investigated. Such models infer the 3D image from a parametric description of the retrospectively binned 4D dataset using a fast lower-dimension surrogate, such as sliced or low-resolution images (Stemkens et al. 2016; Li et al. 2017; Stemkens et al. 2018; Paganelli et al. 2018).

2.4 Motion Estimation and Contour Propagation for On-Line MRI

The increased dimensionality of on-line MRI compared to surrogate based observations requires new paradigms for tracking motion-induced changes in anatomy. The complex anatomical motion cannot be fully described by the translations, rotations and scaling used in rigid image transformations. Instead, methods accounting for the elasticity of tissue should be used to interpret motion in the continuous image stream of an MR-linac treatment. Mainly, two classes of image processing are being investigated. First, in order to automatically identify entire structures, auto-segmentation approaches are used (Sharp et al. 2014; Fast et al. 2017). Automated contouring is crucial in treatment paradigms, in which the machine has to automatically re-plan or change the machine settings (tracking/gating) based on the current position of structures.

Second, deformable image registration (DIR)-based methods are used to trace the trajectory of each voxel over time (Oliveira and Tavares 2014). Rather than segmenting the contour of anatomic structures, DIR tries to estimate a per-voxel motion field (deformable vector field (DVF)) matching each voxel of a moving image to a reference (static) image (Fig. 7). This per-voxel description is particularly useful for dose mapping applications of adaptive radiotherapy (Wu et al. 2011; Glitzner et al. 2015). There partial doses of treatment fractions are mapped to a common (reference) dose map for adaptive re-planning or dosimetric evaluation over many fractions. Additionally, the extracted DVF may be employed as an input to propagate the contour from a manually defined structure in a static image to the moving image. Generally, segmentation and registration methods benefit greatly from the adjustable and improved tissue contrast of MR-images compared to attenuation-based CT or CBCT.

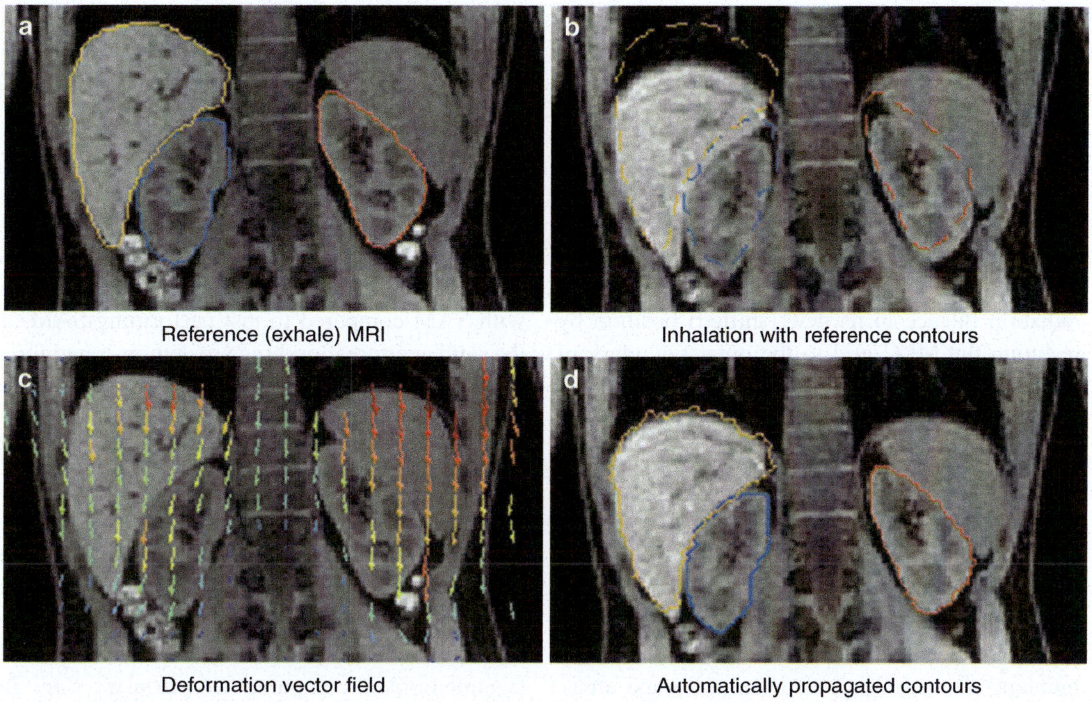

Fig. 7 Image registration and contour propagation: a reference image (**a**) is selected and contours added to the structures of interest. During treatment, the MRI captures changes in anatomy, for instance due to breathing (**b**). Using DIR, DVFs are estimated (**c**) which can be used to map the reference contours onto the current anatomy during treatment (**d**)

3 Inter-Fractional Treatment Adaptations

Hybrid MR-linac systems provide superior online imaging capabilities. This can be utilized to capture day-to-day variations in patient anatomy and daily patient set-up. In this section we will detail some of the adaptation options available on the Elekta Unity MR-linac. Due to the system design of the Unity MR-linac, the ability of the treatment operator to use the treatment couch to compensate for changes in relative beam-to-target position is limited to CC couch movement. Positioning the patient on the treatment couch outside of the treatment bore will likely result in larger initial beam-to-target misalignment compared to on the conventional linac, especially if no room laser system is available. Inter-fractional target shifts in anterior-posterior (AP) or left-right (LR) direction, or more complex deformable changes require an on-line adaptation of the treatment plan.

Any on-line change in the treatment plan needs to be validated on the anatomy of the day using a pre-treatment MRI scan. Since MRI does not provide the electron density information required for dose calculation purposes, this pre-treatment image can either be directly converted to a pseudo-CT image (although this is challenging outside the pelvis or brain (Edmund and Nyholm 2017)), or be registered to a planning CT image using DIR. Updated planning contours can be generated by warping initial planning contours to the pre-treatment MR image or by manually delineating while the patient is on the treatment couch. As manual delineations are time-consuming, a hybrid method, combining manual re-delineation where necessary with automatic contour propagations is often desirable.

3.1 Rigid Aperture Morphing

Instead of using the treatment couch to compensate for beam-to-target misalignment, the individual beam apertures can be realigned with the treatment target by shifting the beam aperture according to the offset in 3D target position projected into the beam's-eye-view (BEV). Beam aperture morphing attempts to recover the desired radiation fluence in its new (shifted) position by re-fitting the MLC grid to the outer boundary of the desired fluence area (Sawant et al. 2008; Tacke et al. 2010). This simple first order correction strategy ignores any relative motion between target and surrounding anatomy and resulting density changes in the beam path. Beam aperture morphing will work reasonably well for relatively small target shifts and treatment plans with a medium or low degree of modulation. For high degrees of modulation, the finite leaf width results in more unintended over-dosage and under-dosage areas. For target shifts in excess of 1 cm the flattening-filter free (FFF) beam profile introduces systematic changes in delivered dose (c.f. Fig. 8) which cannot be addressed without adjusting the number of monitor units or segment apertures.

3.2 Warm-Start Optimization

In patients where relatively simple aperture morphing is not sufficient to ensure that the plan objectives and constraints are met, more complex adaptations of beam weights and segment apertures are necessary. A pragmatic approach is to take the treatment plan generated prior to treatment and to use it for the daily adaptation (*warm-starting*). Using the initial plan as prior information dramatically reduces computational complexity and reduces re-planning times to a few minutes. Bol et al. (2013) presented an approach they termed virtual couch shift (VCS). The VCS is based on translating and rotating the pre-treatment dose distribution according to the pre-treatment MR image. A new plan is then generated that tries to mimic this goal dose distribution as closely as possible. Another approach is segment aperture morphing (SAM) (Ahunbay et al. 2008, 2010) in combination with segment weight optimization (SWO) or even segment shape optimization (SSO) (Winkel et al. 2019). The SAM algorithm is especially suitable for deformed anatomies as it preserves the distance of each leaf to the edge of the PTV. In addition, SWO rebalances the weights of all apertures and SSO modifies the shape of each aperture if necessary. The dosimetric advantages of warm-start optimization (WSO) in combination with SAM compared to just performing SAM or the rigid aperture morphing are demonstrated for a liver SBRT patient in Fig. 8.

3.3 Full Re-planning

From a theoretical point of view, starting a completely new optimization (*cold-starting*) based on the pre-treatment images with patient in treatment position is expected to yield a more optimal treatment plan compared to *warm-starting*. In practice, *cold-starting* treatment planning can be challenging as it is computationally expensive. Traditionally, treatment planning is a time-consuming task, often requiring several user interventions or inspections. In recent years, several automation methods for treatment planning were developed (Winkel et al. 2016). Once full re-planning is accelerated and will take no more than a few minutes, it is expected that *warm-starting* will be rendered obsolete. For the first-in-man Elekta Unity trial at UMC Utrecht (The Netherlands), full re-planning was performed for simple palliative treatments of bone metastasis in 5–11 min depending on plan complexity.

4 Intra-Fractional Treatment Adaptations

While inter-fractional variations in patient anatomy and patient set-up can be sufficiently addressed using rigid aperture morphing or warm-start optimization, intra-fractional anatomical variations require real-time treatment adaptations such as respiratory gating, dynamic tumour tracking or intra-fractional re-planning.

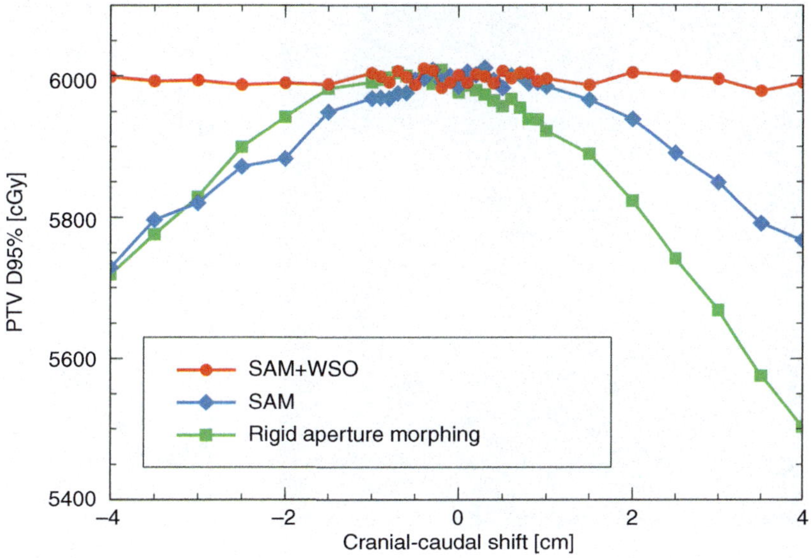

Fig. 8 Example WSO for a liver SBRT patient. Target dose is shown as function of CC positional shift. *Data courtesy of Wouter van den Wollenberg (The Netherlands Cancer Institute). Abbreviations: segment aperture morphing (SAM), warm-start optimization (WSO)*

4.1 Respiratory Gating

For moving targets in the abdomen and thorax, high-field MRI-guidance allows to continuously image the anatomic target (Fig. 9) rather than deducing the target position from indirect surrogate signals with questionable correlation. In those sites, respiratory gating can be used for motion compensation of both MRI and treatment delivery. Restricting the delivery to stable states of the respiratory cycle largely reduces the dose dispersion and image blurring due to respiratory motion. This effectively reduces geometric margins around the target and dose exposure to vicinal OARs and normal tissue. The gating efficiency (duty cycle) is for the most part dependent on the width of the gating window, i.e. the residual range of target motion during beam-on. Commonly, the efficiency ranges from 25 to 50 % (Jiang 2006), and the gating windows from 3 to 5 mm.

Depending on the treatment site, breath-holds can introduce dosimetric benefits by shifting OARs away from the target. However, gating free-breathing has been shown to obtain more reproducible expiration positions than repeated breath holds (Stam et al. 2013). Due to its technological simplicity, respiratory gating has been widely adopted on conventional linacs (Giraud and Houle 2013). High-field MRI-guided gating was shown to be fast enough (Glitzner et al. 2017) to perform gating in a clinical setting in accordance with recommendations by AAPM Task Group 76 (Keall et al. 2006).

4.2 Dynamic Tumour Tracking

The motion signal from the real-time cine MRI can also be used to dynamically steer the treatment beam according to the target motion using the MLC. Keall coined the term “breathing leaves” to describe how the MLC moves in synchrony with the tumour (Keall et al. 2001). MLC tracking is an emerging technique that is currently being tested in first clinical trials (Colvill et al. 2015). Treatment deliveries based on MLC tracking have two main advantages over conventional deliveries: the reduction in PTV/margin, and the ability to compensate for motion not anticipated during treatment planning or from the pre-beam imaging. The reduction of PTV is especially pronounced for more mobile or smaller tumours. Any reduction in PTV shrinks the amount of patient anatomy needlessly exposed to high dose, and consequently reduces dose-limiting toxicities. Compared to gating, the delivery efficiency is much higher as the beam is not paused.

The first proof-of-principle MLC tracking study on an earlier MR-linac prototype was

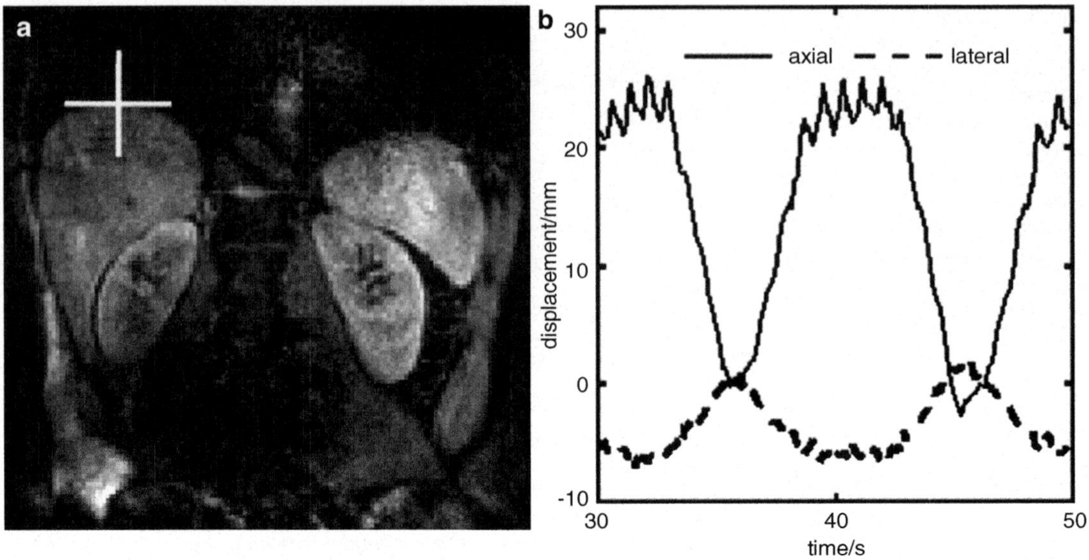

T1w EPI

Respiratory trace

Fig. 9 Mobility of the abdomen. (**a**) Continuous EPI acquisition (10 Hz) of a coronal plane through the abdomen. (**b**) After DIR, a point (white cross in (**a**)) in the DVF was traced over time. *Data courtesy of Baudouin Denis de Senneville (UMC Utrecht)*

conducted in 2012 (Crijns et al. 2012). Using a 1D pencil-beam MRI navigator, the translational motion of a simple phantom was fully compensated by MLC tracking. The total system latency was estimated at 200 ms for the prototype system. In research-mode, the commercial Unity system showed similar tracking latencies in a comparable experimental set-up, yet with full 2D image information (Glitzner et al. 2019). A simpler form of tracking, which requires a less strict synchronization between imaging and MLC adaptation, is tumour trailing (Fast et al. 2019). Here, only the baseline drift/shift motion component is compensated. Beyond tracking of the tumour centroid, it is also expected that the MR-linac will prove useful for deformation tracking. Tumour deformations can occur periodically for a single tumour during respiration, or as differential motion between tumour and involved lymph nodes (Ge et al. 2014). 2D cine MR images can be used to either directly observe the deformed tumour contour over time (Fast et al. 2017) or to derive a DVF for each image. Both inputs can be used to adapt the MLC apertures to the deformation.

For thoracic tumours there are concerns that the electron-return effect (ERE) in combination with the tissue-air interfaces prominent in lungs could affect the ability to perform MLC tracking safely. A treatment simulation study for lung SBRT vindicated this concern (Menten et al. 2016). With or without the influence of the magnetic field, the peak-to-peak tumour motion was the main predictor for the reduction in PTV achievable with MLC tracking. Limiting the high-dose volume to the tumour resulted in a clear sparing of healthy tissues.

4.3 Impact of Imaging in Real-Time Applications

Real-time MRI during therapy increases the sensitivity of target detection compared to other onboard techniques due to its superior image quality and higher image dimensionality. Using MR images for real-time feedback applications such as tracking or gating requires an analysis of image latencies and image quality, which both determine the performance of the feedback system.

The image quality of fast MRI is restricted by the physical and anatomical properties of the tissue, which translate into limited SNR in fast T1w acquisitions or artefacts in images with large blood vessels, pulsating in the same frequency range as the acquisition frequency of the MRI. Furthermore, technical limitations of imaging gradient or shim performance cause significant geometric distortions due to field inhomogeneities in EPI- or banding artefacts in bSSFP-type acquisitions.

The contribution of data acquisition to the overall delay feedback is complex, as data acquisition in MRI takes place in *Fourier*-domain. A phenomenological and intuitive description of imaging feedback has been established for MRI-guided high intensity focussed ultrasound (HIFU) (Ries et al. 2010), quantifying the imaging latency as the remaining imaging time after sampling the centre of k-space. Assuming fully linear k-space coverage, image sampling ($T_{sampling}$) adds a delay of half the acquisition time T_{acq} to the feedback system. Furthermore, due to the restricted imaging frequency, an average age of an image ($\langle T_{age}\rangle = T_{acq}/2$) adds to the system delay (Poulsen et al. 2010). Additionally, image and data transport, image processing and the eventual machine state change as a reaction to the observed anatomy must be considered in the latency calculations.

$$\begin{aligned}\Delta T_{feedback} &= \Delta T_{sampling} + \langle \Delta T_{age} \rangle \\ &\quad + \Delta T_{processing\ and\ transport} + \Delta T_{adaptation} \\ &= 250\ \text{ms} + \Delta T_{processing\ and\ transport} \\ &\quad + \Delta T_{adaptation}\ (\text{at 4 Hz})\end{aligned} \tag{2}$$

As shown in Eq. (2), real-time MRI with currently feasible frame rates of 4 Hz (equivalent to 250 ms delay) contributes the major share to the overall system latency, particularly compared to the gating and tracking adaptation times of the linac hardware (Fast et al. 2014; Glitzner et al. 2015, 2019). Therefore, improving image acquisition speed will have the highest impact on system latency for real-time high-field MRI. A more thorough analysis showed that the choice of image readout has a significant impact on the imaging latency (Borman et al. 2018). More specifically, imaging latency is highly dependent on the point in time, k_0 is sampled after the start of image acquisition (see Fig. 10).

In this light, image dimension reduction (navigator echoes), utilization of motion models and sparse sampling are viable starting points to reduce acquisition time and therefore improve the reaction time of the feedback system.

4.4 Real-Time Dose Accumulation and Intra-Fractional Re-planning

In their current form, both respiratory gating and dynamic tumour tracking are focused on allowing the safe delivery of dose to a comparatively small PTV, thus sparing surrounding healthy tissue from irradiation. These treatment techniques are especially suitable if the tumour motion is periodic and predictable. In some cases, however, anatomical motion is erratic and unpredictable. Coughing, peristalsis or other gastrointestinal motion events can cause systematic changes of the tumour position with respect to OARs. In such cases, the dosimetric trade-offs between target and OARs used for optimizing the initial treatment plan might not apply to the current anatomy, resulting in sub-optimal treatments. Intra-fractional re-planning creates a new treatment plan for the remainder of the treatment fraction based on the most recently observed anatomy and the already delivered dose (Kamerling et al. 2016a; Kontaxis et al. 2017). Accounting for the already delivered dose up to the time point of re-planning is crucial for ensuring that the desired target coverage and OAR dose constraints are met.

Accumulating dose on-line is challenging both from a computational and an imaging point of view (Glitzner et al. 2015; Fast et al. 2016; Kamerling et al. 2016b; Stemkens et al. 2017). For dose accumulation, each anatomical patient instance (a 3D image representation for each time point sampled) is paired with the full linac state for this time point. As volumetric MRI is currently too slow to sufficiently capture respiratory motion, a 3D anatomical patient instance must be estimated from 2D cine MRI. One option is to use the 2D cine MRI to deform a 3D/4D MR

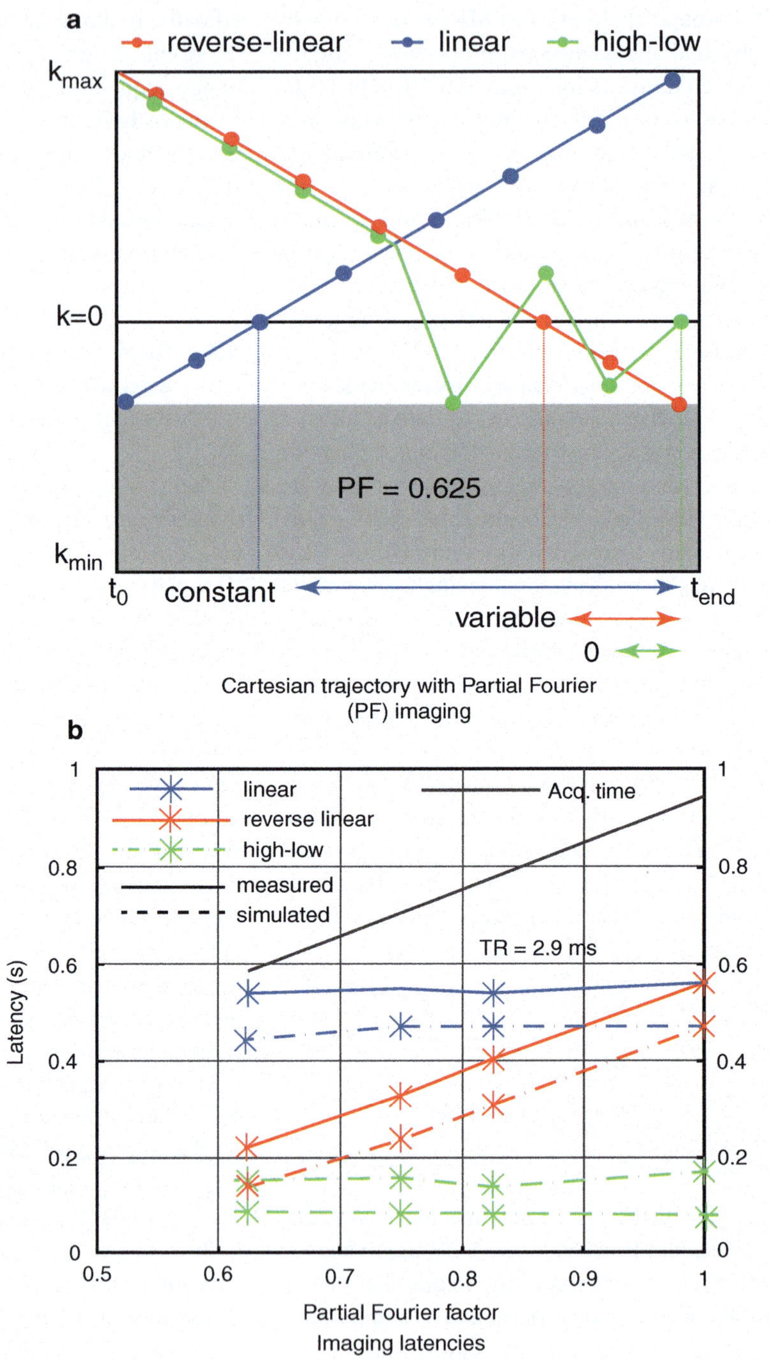

Fig. 10 MR imaging latency is dependent on the read-out scheme of the MRI sequence. In (**a**), the temporal sampling order of three sampling trajectories commonly available on MRI systems, i.e. reverse-linear, linear and high-low are depicted. According to the choice of readout, k_0 is sampled at different points in time after start of image acquisition (t_0). Accordingly, the apparent imaging latency differs greatly (**b**) (Courtesy Pim Borman, Copyright IOP (Borman et al. 2018))

image acquired prior to treatment. This immediately provides the contours required for treatment planning. The pre-treatment image can in turn be registered with a CT image from treatment planning, providing the necessary ED values for dose calculation.

Intra-fractional re-planning is a novel technique which needs to be developed further before it can be used clinically. Important unsolved research questions are related to the accuracy of automated (unsupervised) decision making, on-line quality assurance (QA) and the required frequency and accuracy of on-line dose accumulation and intra-fractional re-planning.

5 Conclusions and Outlook

High-field MRI in-room guidance is a game changing technology that facilitates on-line treatment adaptations in external beam radiotherapy. A new generation of hybrid MR-linac underwent sustained technological development over the last decade. Using a high-field strength for in-room imaging ensures that an image quality en par with diagnostic MRI scanners is achieved. The Elekta Unity MR-linac was successfully tested in a first-in-man clinical trial at UMC Utrecht (The Netherlands) in 2017, and has now entered routine clinical service.

Importantly, hybrid MR-linac systems go beyond simply setting up the patient based on soft-tissue contrast. In future, treatments should be truly personalized by creating a new treatment plan based on the on-line acquired MR images. Real time guidance using dynamic cine MRI could then be used to drive adaptation strategies such as MLC tracking and intra-fractional re-planning. Finding the optimal image acquisition and treatment adaptation strategy for each clinical target site is work in progress. Beyond adaptations driven by morphological imaging, the high-field strength might offer additional opportunities for on-line adaptations driven by quantitative functional MRI.

Acknowledgements The University Medical Center Utrecht (UMCU) is part of the Elekta MR-linac Consortium and we acknowledge financial and technical support from Elekta AB under research agreements. We are grateful to Uulke van der Heide, Tessa van de Lindt (both NKI) and Rob Tijssen (UMCU) for very useful discussions.

References

Ahunbay EE, Peng C, Chen GP, Narayanan S, Yu C, Lawton C, Li XA (2008) An on-line replanning scheme for interfractional variations. Med Phys 35(8):3607–3615

Ahunbay EE, Peng C, Holmes S, Godley A, Lawton C, Li XA (2010) Online adaptive replanning method for prostate radiotherapy. Int J Radiat Oncol Biol Phys 77(5):1561–1572

Balaban EP, Mangu PB, Khorana AA, Shah MA, Mukherjee S, Crane CH, Javle MM, Eads JR, Allen P, Ko AH, *et al* (2016) Locally advanced, unresectable pancreatic cancer: American Society of Clinical Oncology Clinical Practice guideline. J Clin Oncol 34(22):2654–2668

Bley TA, Wieben O, François CJ, Brittain JH, Reeder SB (2010) Fat and water magnetic resonance imaging. J Magn Reson Imaging 31(1):4–18

Bol G, Lagendijk J, Raaymakers B (2013) Virtual couch shift (VCS): accounting for patient translation and rotation by online IMRT re-optimization. Phys Med Biol 58(9):2989. https://doi.org/10.1088/0031-9155/58/9/2989

Borman PTS, Tijssen RHN, Bos C, Moonen CTW, Raaymakers BW, Glitzner M (2018) Characterization of imaging latency for real-time MRI-guided radiotherapy. Phys Med Biol 63(15):155023. https://doi.org/10.1088/1361-6560/aad2b7

Colvill E, Booth JT, O'Brien RT, Eade TN, Kneebone AB, Poulsen PR, Keall PJ (2015) Multileaf collimator tracking improves dose delivery for prostate cancer radiation therapy: results of the first clinical trial. Int J Radiat Oncol Biol Phys 92(5):1141–1147

Crijns S, Raaymakers B, Lagendijk J (2012) Proof of concept of MRI-guided tracked radiation delivery: tracking one-dimensional motion. Phys Med Biol 57(23):7863

De Meerleer G, Khoo V, Escudier B, Joniau S, Bossi A, Ost P, Briganti A, Fonteyne V, Van Vulpen M, Lumen N, *et al* (2014) Radiotherapy for renal-cell carcinoma. Lancet Oncol 15(4):e170–e177

Deng Z, Pang J, Yang W, Yue Y, Sharif B, Tuli R, Li D, Fraass B, Fan Z (2016) Four-dimensional MRI using three-dimensional radial sampling with respiratory self-gating to characterize temporal phase-resolved respiratory motion in the abdomen. Magn Reson Med 75(4):1574–1585

Dinkel J, Hintze C, Tetzlaff R, Huber PE, Herfarth K, Debus J, Kauczor HU, Thieke C (2009) 4D-MRI analysis of lung tumor motion in patients with hemidiaphragmatic paralysis. Radiother Oncol 91(3):449–454

Edmund JM, Nyholm T (2017) A review of substitute CT generation for MRI-only radiation therapy. Radiat Oncol 12(1):28

Fast MF, Nill S, Bedford JL, Oelfke U (2014) Dynamic tumor tracking using the Elekta Agility MLC. Med Phys 41(11):111719. https://doi.org/10.1118/1.4899175

Fast M, Kamerling C, Ziegenhein P, Menten M, Bedford J, Nill S, Oelfke U (2016) Assessment of MLC tracking performance during hypofractionated prostate radiotherapy using real-time dose reconstruction. Phys Med Biol 61(4):1546. https://doi.org/10.1088/0031-9155/61/4/1546

Fast MF, Eiben B, Menten MJ, Wetscherek A, Hawkes DJ, McClelland JR, Oelfke U (2017) Tumour auto-

contouring on 2d cine MRI for locally advanced lung cancer: a comparative study. Radiother Oncol 125(3):485–491. https://doi.org/10.1016/j.radonc.2017.09.013
Fast M, van de Schoot A, van de Lindt T, Carbaat C, van der Heide U, Sonke JJ (2019) Tumor trailing for liver SBRT on the MR-Linac. Int J Radiat Oncol Biol Phys 103(2):468–478. https://doi.org/10.1016/j.ijrobp.2018.09.011
Feng M, Balter JM, Normolle D, Adusumilli S, Cao Y, Chenevert TL, Ben-Josef E (2009) Characterization of pancreatic tumor motion using cine MRI: surrogates for tumor position should be used with caution. Int J Radiat Oncol Biol Phys 74(3):884–891
Ge Y, O'Brien RT, Shieh CC, Booth JT, Keall PJ (2014) Toward the development of intrafraction tumor deformation tracking using a dynamic multi-leaf collimator. Med Phys 41(6):061703. https://doi.org/10.1118/1.4873682
Gierga DP, Brewer J, Sharp GC, Betke M, Willett CG, Chen GT (2005) The correlation between internal and external markers for abdominal tumors: implications for respiratory gating. Int J Radiat Oncol Biol Phys 61(5):1551–1558. https://doi.org/10.1016/j.ijrobp.2004.12.013
Giraud P, Houle A (2013) Respiratory gating for radiotherapy: main technical aspects and clinical benefits. ISRN Pulmonol 2013: 1–13. http://dx.doi.org/10.1155/2013/519602
Glitzner M, Crijns S, De Senneville BD, Kontaxis C, Prins F, Lagendijk J, Raaymakers B (2015) On-line MR imaging for dose validation of abdominal radiotherapy. Phys Med Biol 60(22):8869
Glitzner M, Crijns S, De Senneville BD, Lagendijk J, Raaymakers B (2015) On the suitability of Elektas Agility 160 MLC for tracked radiation delivery: closed-loop machine performance. Phys Med Biol 60(5):2005–2017
Glitzner M, Woodhead PL, Lagendijk JJW, Raaymakers BW (2017) TU-FG-FS2-10: real-time performance of the Elekta MR-linac clinical prototype. Med Phys 44(6):3157
Glitzner M, Woodhead P, Borman P, Lagendijk J, Raaymakers B (2019) Technical Note: MLC-tracking performance on the Elekta unity MRI-linac. Phys Med Biol 64(15):15NT02
Heid O, Kleemann M, Heller J (2015) Integrated MRI-LINAC radiotherapy machine. In: Proceedings of the International Society for Magnetic Resonance in Medicine, vol 23
Howlader N, Noone A, Krapcho M, Miller D, Bishop K, Altekruse S, Kosary C, Yu M, Ruhl J, Tatalovich Z, *et al* (2016) Seer cancer statistics review, 1975–2013. National Cancer Institute, Bethesda
Jaffray DA, Langen KM, Mageras G, Dawson LA, Yan D, Mundt AJ, Fraass B (2013) Safety considerations for IGRT: executive summary. Pract Radiat Oncol 3(3):167–170
Jaffray DA, Carlone MC, Milosevic MF, Breen SL, Stanescu T, Rink A, Alasti H, Simeonov A, Sweitzer MC, Winter JD (2014) A facility for magnetic resonance-guided radiation therapy. Semin Radiat Oncol 24(3):193–195. https://doi.org/10.1016/j.semradonc.2014.02.012
Jiang SB (2006) Technical aspects of image-guided respiration-gated radiation therapy. Med Dosim 31(2):141–151. http://dx.doi.org/10.1016/j.meddos.2005.12.005. http://www.sciencedirect.com/science/article/pii/S0958394705001998. Image-Guided Radiation Therapy, Part 2: Cone-Beam Imaging and Respiratory Motion
Kamerling C, Fast M, Ziegenhein P, Nill S, Oelfke U (2016a) TH-CD-202-12: online inter-beam replanning based on real-time dose reconstruction. Med Phys 43(6):3879–3879. https://doi.org/10.1118/1.4958169
Kamerling CP, Fast MF, Ziegenhein P, Menten MJ, Nill S, Oelfke U (2016b) Real-time 4D dose reconstruction for tracked dynamic MLC deliveries for lung SBRT. Med Phys 43(11):6072–6081. https://doi.org/10.1118/1.4965045
Keall P, Kini V, Vedam S, Mohan R (2001) Motion adaptive X-ray therapy: a feasibility study. Phys Med Biol 46(1):1. https://doi.org/10.1088/0031-9155/46/1/301
Keall PJ, Mageras GS, Balter JM, Emery RS, Forster KM, Jiang SB, Kapatoes JM, Low DA, Murphy MJ, Murray BR, Ramsey CR, Van Herk MB, Vedam SS, Wong JW, Yorke E (2006) The management of respiratory motion in radiation oncology report of AAPM task group 76. Med Phys 33(10):3874–900. https://doi.org/10.1118/1.2349696
Keall PJ, Barton M, Crozier S, on behalf of the Australian MRI-Linac Program, including contributors from Ingham Institute Illawarra Cancer Care Centre Liverpool Hospital Stanford University Universities of Newcastle Queensland Sydney Western Sydney and Wollongong (2014) The Australian magnetic resonance imaging-linac program. Semin Radiat Oncol 24(3):203–206. https://doi.org/10.1016/j.semradonc.2014.02.015
Keesman R, van de Lindt TN, Juan-Cruz C, van den Wollenberg W, van der Bijl E, Nowee ME, Sonke JJ, van der Heide UA, Fast MF (2019) Correcting geometric image distortions in slice-based 4D-MRI on the MR-linac. Med Phys 46(7):3044–3054. https://doi.org/10.1002/mp.13602
Kirilova A, Lockwood G, Choi P, Bana N, Haider MA, Brock KK, Eccles C, Dawson LA (2008) Three-dimensional motion of liver tumors using cine-magnetic resonance imaging. Int J Radiat Oncol Biol Phys 71(4):1189–1195
Kontaxis C, Bol G, Stemkens B, Glitzner M, Prins F, Kerkmeijer L, Lagendijk J, Raaymakers B (2017) Towards fast online intrafraction replanning for free-breathing stereotactic body radiation therapy with the MR-linac. Phys Med Biol 62(18):7233
Kotte AN, Hofman P, Lagendijk JJ, van Vulpen M, van der Heide UA (2007) Intrafraction motion of the prostate during external-beam radiation therapy: analysis of 427 patients with implanted fiducial markers. Int J Radiat Oncol Biol Phys 69(2):419–425

Lever FM, Lips IM, Crijns SP, Reerink O, van Lier AL, Moerland MA, van Vulpen M, Meijer GJ (2014) Quantification of esophageal tumor motion on cine-magnetic resonance imaging. Int J Radiat Oncol Biol Phys 88(2):419–424

Li G, Wei J, Kadbi M, Moody J, Sun A, Zhang S, Markova S, Zakian K, Hunt M, Deasy JO (2017) Novel super-resolution approach to time-resolved volumetric 4-dimensional magnetic resonance imaging with high spatiotemporal resolution for multi-breathing cycle motion assessment. Int J Radiat Oncol Biol Phys 98(2):454–462. http://dx.doi.org/10.1016/j.ijrobp.2017.02.016. http://www.sciencedirect.com/science/article/pii/S0360301617303942

Maubon AJ, Ferru JM, Berger V, Soulage MC, DeGraef M, Aubas P, Coupeau P, Dumont E, Rouanet JP (1999) Effect of field strength on MR images: comparison of the same subject at 0.5, 1.0, and 1.5 T. Radiographics 19(4):1057–1067

Menten MJ, Fast MF, Nill S, Kamerling CP, McDonald F, Oelfke U (2016) Lung stereotactic body radiotherapy with an MR-linac – quantifying the impact of the magnetic field and real-time tumor tracking. Radiother Oncol 119(3):461–466. http://dx.doi.org/10.1016/j.radonc.2016.04.019

Menten MJ, Wetscherek A, Fast MF (2017) MRI-guided lung SBRT: present and future developments. Phys Med 44:139–149. https://doi.org/10.1016/j.ejmp.2017.02.003

Moran JM, Dempsey M, Eisbruch A, Fraass BA, Galvin JM, Ibbott GS, Marks LB (2011) Safety considerations for IMRT: executive summary. Med Phys 38(9):5067–5072

Nederveen AJ, van der Heide UA, Dehnad H, van Moorselaar RJA, Hofman P, Lagendijk JJ (2002) Measurements and clinical consequences of prostate motion during a radiotherapy fraction. Int J Radiat Oncol Biol Phys 53(1):206–214

Oliveira FP, Tavares JMR (2014) Medical image registration: a review. Comput Methods Biomech Biomed Eng 17(2):73–93

Overweg J, Raaymakers B, Lagendijk J, Brown K (2009) System for MRI guided radiotherapy. In: Proceedings of International Society on Magnetic Resonance in Medicine (ISMRM), Concord, 2009, p 593

Paganelli C, Summers P, Bellomi M, Baroni G, Riboldi M (2015) Liver 4DMRI: a retrospective image-based sorting method. Med Phys 42(8):4814–4821

Paganelli C, Kipritidis J, Lee D, Baroni G, Keall P, Riboldi M (2018) Image-based retrospective 4D MRI in external beam radiotherapy: a comparative study with a digital phantom. Med Phys 45(7):3161–3172. https://doi.org/10.1002/mp.12965

Paulson ES, Crijns SP, Keller BM, Wang J, Schmidt MA, Coutts G, van der Heide UA (2016) Consensus opinion on MRI simulation for external beam radiation treatment planning. Radiother Oncol 121(2):187–192

Plathow C, Klopp M, Fink C, Sandner A, Hof H, Puderbach M, Herth F, Schmähl A, Kauczor H (2005) Quantitative analysis of lung and tumour mobility: comparison of two time-resolved MRI sequences. Br J Radiol 78(933):836

Plathow C, Schoebinger M, Herth F, Tuengerthal S, Meinzer HP, Kauczor HU (2009) Estimation of pulmonary motion in healthy subjects and patients with intrathoracic tumors using 3D-dynamic MRI: initial results. Korean J Radiol 10(6):559–567

Poulsen PR, Cho B, Sawant A, Ruan D, Keall PJ (2010) Detailed analysis of latencies in image-based dynamic MLC tracking. Med Phys 37(9):4998–5005

Poulsen P, Knap M, Brix L, Sørensen T, Schmidt M, Pedersen E (2016) Real-time magnetic resonance imaging of simultaneous lung tumor motion and involved mediastinal lymph node motion. Int J Radiat Oncol Biol Phys 96(2):E686–E687

Rank CM, Heußer T, Buzan MT, Wetscherek A, Freitag MT, Dinkel J, Kachelrieß M (2017) 4d respiratory motion-compensated image reconstruction of free-breathing radial MR data with very high undersampling. Magn Reson Med 77(3):1170–1183

Reeth E, Tan CH, Tham IW, Poh CL (2015) Isotropic reconstruction of a 4-D MRI thoracic sequence using super-resolution. Magn Reson Med 73(2):784–793

Ries M, de Senneville BD, Roujol S, Berber Y, Quesson B, Moonen C (2010) Real-time 3D target tracking in mri guided focused ultrasound ablations in moving tissues. Magn Reson Med 64(6):1704–1712. https://doi.org/10.1002/mrm.22548

Rutt BK, Lee DH (1996) The impact of field strength on image quality in MRI. J Magn Reson Imaging 6(1):57–62. https://doi.org/10.1002/jmri.1880060111

Sawant A, Venkat R, Srivastava V, Carlson D, Povzner S, Cattell H, Keall P (2008) Management of three-dimensional intrafraction motion through real-time DMLC tracking. Med Phys 35(5):2050–2061

Scheffler K, Lehnhardt S (2003) Principles and applications of balanced SSFP techniques. Eur Radiol 13(11):2409–2418

Schlosser J, Salisbury K, Hristov D (2010) Telerobotic system concept for real-time soft-tissue imaging during radiotherapy beam delivery. Med Phys 37(12):6357–6367

Sharp G, Fritscher KD, Pekar V, Peroni M, Shusharina N, Veeraraghavan H, Yang J (2014) Vision 20/20: perspectives on automated image segmentation for radiotherapy. Med Phys 41(5):050902

Stam MK, Van Vulpen M, Barendrecht MM, Zonnenberg BA, Intven M, Crijns SP, Lagendijk JJ, Raaymakers BW (2013) Kidney motion during free breathing and breath hold for MR-guided radiotherapy. Phys Med Biol 58(7):2235

Stemkens B, Tijssen RH, de Senneville BD, Heerkens HD, van Vulpen M, Lagendijk JJ, van den Berg CA (2015) Optimizing 4-dimensional magnetic resonance imaging data sampling for respiratory motion analysis of pancreatic tumors. Int J Radiat Oncol Biol Phys 91(3):571–578. http://dx.doi.org/10.1016/j.ijrobp.2014.10.050. http://www.sciencedirect.com/science/article/pii/S0360301614043569

Stemkens B, Tijssen RH, de Senneville BD, Lagendijk JJ, van den Berg CA (2016) Image-driven, model-based 3D abdominal motion estimation for MR-guided radiotherapy. Phys Med Biol 61(14):5335

Stemkens B, Glitzner M, Kontaxis C, De Senneville BD, Prins FM, Crijns SP, Kerkmeijer LG, Lagendijk JJ, Van Den Berg CA, Tijssen RH (2017) Effect of intra-fraction motion on the accumulated dose for free-breathing MR-guided stereotactic body radiation therapy of renal-cell carcinoma. Phys Med Biol 62(18):7407

Stemkens B, Paulson ES, Tijssen RHN (2018) Nuts and bolts of 4D-MRI for radiotherapy. Phys Med Biol 63(21):21TR01. https://doi.org/10.1088/1361-6560/aae56d

Tacke MB, Nill S, Krauss A, Oelfke U (2010) Real-time tumor tracking: automatic compensation of target motion using the Siemens 160 MLC. Med Phys 37(2):753. https://doi.org/10.1118/1.3284543

van de Lindt T, Sonke JJ, Nowee M, Jansen E, van Pelt V, van der Heide U, Fast M (2018a) A self-sorting coronal 4D-MRI method for daily image guidance of liver lesions on an MR-Linac. Int J Radiat Oncol Biol Phys 102(4):875–884. https://doi.org/10.1016/j.ijrobp.2018.05.029

van de Lindt TN, Fast MF, van der Heide UA, Sonke JJ (2018b) Retrospective self-sorted 4D-MRI for the liver. Radiother Oncol 127(3):474–480. https://doi.org/10.1016/j.radonc.2018.05.006

van der Heide UA, Kotte AN, Dehnad H, Hofman P, Lagendijk JJ, van Vulpen M (2007) Analysis of fiducial marker-based position verification in the external beam radiotherapy of patients with prostate cancer. Radiother Oncol 82(1):38–45

van der Heide UA, Houweling AC, Groenendaal G, Beets-Tan RG, Lambin P (2012) Functional MRI for radiotherapy dose painting. Magn Reson Imaging 30(9):1216–1223

van Herk M, Remeijer P, Rasch C, Lebesque JV (2000) The probability of correct target dosage: dose-population histograms for deriving treatment margins in radiotherapy. Int J Radiat Oncol Biol Phys 47(4):1121–1135

von Siebenthal M, Szekely G, Gamper U, Boesiger P, Lomax A, Cattin P (2007) 4D MR imaging of respiratory organ motion and its variability. Phys Med Biol 52(6):1547

Welsh J, Settle SH, Amini A, Xiao L, Suzuki A, Hayashi Y, Hofstetter W, Komaki R, Liao Z, Ajani JA (2012) Failure patterns in patients with esophageal cancer treated with definitive chemoradiation. Cancer 118(10):2632–2640

Winkel D, Bol G, van Asselen B, Hes J, Scholten V, Kerkmeijer L, Raaymakers B (2016) Development and clinical introduction of automated radiotherapy treatment planning for prostate cancer. Phys Med Biol 61(24):8587

Winkel D, Bol GH, Kroon PS, van Asselen B, Hackett SS, Werensteijn-Honingh AM, Intven MP, Eppinga WS, Tijssen RH, Kerkmeijer LG, *et al* (2019) Adaptive radiotherapy: the Elekta Unity MR-linac concept. Clin Transl Radiat Oncol 18:54–59

Wu QJ, Li T, Wu Q, Yin FF (2011) Adaptive radiation therapy: technical components and clinical applications. Cancer J 17(3):182–189

Low Tesla MRI in-Room Gating during Radiotherapy

Davide Cusumano and Francesco Cellini

Contents

1 **Introduction** ... 129
2 **Rational for Hybrid Approach with Magnetic Resonance Imaging in Radiotherapy** ... 130
3 **The Low Tesla Hybrid Machines** ... 130
4 **Clinical Treatments Using Low Tesla Hybrid Machines** ... 131
5 **Clinical Perspective** ... 133
5.1 New Clinical Opportunities for RT Treatment Flow ... 133
5.2 New Clinical Opportunities for RT Delivery Approach ... 134
5.3 New Clinical Opportunities for Clinical Research ... 135
6 **Conclusions** ... 135
References ... 135

D. Cusumano
Dipartimento di Diagnostica per immagini, Radioterapia Oncologica ed Ematologia, UOC Fisica Sanitaria, Fondazione Policlinico Universitario "A. Gemelli" IRCCS, Rome, Italy
e-mail: davide.cusumano@policlinicogemelli.it

F. Cellini (✉)
Dipartimento di Diagnostica per immagini, Radioterapia Oncologica ed Ematologia, UOC Radioterapia Oncologica, Fondazione Policlinico Universitario "A. Gemelli" IRCCS, Rome, Italy
e-mail: francesco.cellini@policlinicogemelli.it

Abstract

Image-guided radiation therapy (IGRT) is commonly advocated as a key opportunity in the field of radio-oncological treatment approach. It allows more precise treatment delivery by combination of the rapid dose fall-off associated with intensity-modulated radiotherapy (IMRT) and daily imaging in regard to both tumour targeting and effective sparing of surrounding organs at risk (OARs) (Nguyen and Karlsson, 2015). One of the most innovative and promising opportunities in the context of the IGRT is represented by the use of magnetic resonance imaging (MRI) to support the delivery of radiotherapy (RT) treatment course.

1 Introduction

Image-guided radiation therapy (IGRT) is commonly advocated as a key opportunity in the field of radio-oncological treatment approach. It allows more precise treatment delivery by combination of the rapid dose fall-off associated with intensity-modulated radiotherapy (IMRT) and daily imaging in regard to both tumour targeting and effective sparing of surrounding organs at risk (OARs) (Nguyen and Karlsson, 2015). One of the most innovative and promising opportunities in the context of the IGRT is represented by the use of magnetic resonance imaging (MRI) to support the delivery of radiotherapy (RT) treatment course.

R. G. H. Beets-Tan et al. (eds.), *Imaging and Interventional Radiology for Radiation Oncology*, Medical Radiology, Diagnostic Imaging, https://doi.org/10.1007/978-3-030-38261-2_9

Hybrid machines combining MRI with RT delivery units provide the opportunity of in-room visualization of the region of interest (ROI) by MRI (both including target and organ at risk). Besides the visualization of ROIs, such systems support gated RT treatment delivery, improving the focus of delivered dose into the target while contemporary reducing the volume of irradiated normal tissues. Finally, some of these systems also provide the opportunity for on-board daily optimization of the treatment plan on the basis of the changes visualized by in-room daily MRI.

All these features open completely new opportunities to be exploited in both the clinical and research perspective. In this chapter, we will outline the background for introduction of in-room MRI systems in RT, the main issues and opportunities provided by such systems, the description of the clinically available ones and the new insights provided into the clinical practice.

2 Rational for Hybrid Approach with Magnetic Resonance Imaging in Radiotherapy

New hybrid machines have recently been designed to perform MRI in-room gating during RT. These machines combine an RT unit (constituted by either Linac- or cobalt-source-based device) with an MR scanner able to acquire volumetric image of patient before and after treatment and to perform planar acquisition in cine modality during the radiation treatment (Lagendijk et al. 2014).

Obtaining a daily MR acquisition of the ROIs offers the advantages provided by the excellent soft-tissue contrast of MR images, allowing a highly accurate verification of the patient's daily setup, also providing some additional information about the definition of target and organs at risk (OARs) in comparison with those obtainable by using the cone beam computed tomography (CBCT) for some treatment sites including the pelvis, upper abdomen and brain.

Moreover, the real-time continuous MR image acquisition enables the RT treatment delivery by using gating approach: it allows to treat the patients only when target and/or OARs are confirmed by the system to be in predefined conditions corresponding to the best planning option in terms of dose distribution.

Two basic features characterize the in-room gating by MRI during RT. First is the direct visualization of the target and OARs. Some gating approaches commonly refer to markers to be used as fiducials; some others follow the respiratory cycle of the patients by in-room cameras connected to breath detectors on the belly of the patients: the MRI in-room gating system directly tracks the target in itself instead of its surrogates. Second, the radiationless feature of MRI in-room gating system enhances the possibility to scan several times the patient without additional exposure.

Currently, only two hybrid machines designed for clinical purposes are available. The first model was the MRIdian system (ViewRay, Mountain View, California), introduced by the ViewRay company in 2014. This machine combined a 0.35 tesla (T) MR scanner with three cobalt-60 sources to deliver the radiation treatment (Mutic and Dempsey 2014). In 2017, the same company proposed MRIdian Linac, a second version of the machine where the Cobalt-60 sources of the radiant unit were replaced by a 6 MV flattening filter-free (FFF) linear accelerator (Linac).

In the same year, Elekta proposed Unity (Elekta, Stockholm, Sweden), a hybrid machine that combines a 1.5 tesla MR scanner with a 7 MV FFF Linac (Lagendijk et al. 2014).

More information about the low tesla models are provided in the following section; instead the high-field systems are described in Chap. 8.

3 The Low Tesla Hybrid Machines

The low tesla MRI-guided radiotherapy (MRgRT) machines mainly differ on the basis of the geometry system that determines the orientation of radiation beam with respect to the magnetic field.

Systems implementing longitudinal geometry are currently under development, where the central axis of the radiation source is oriented parallel to the magnetic field force lines, in order to avoid the perturbation of the magnetic field on the dose distribution. The Aurora RT™ Linac-MR system developed by the MagnetTx Oncology systems and the Australian MRI-Linac project of the Ingham Institute are two examples of this technology (Fallone 2014; Liney et al. 2018).

The MRIdian Linac system (ViewRay, Mountain View, California) uses instead a transverse geometry, and it has been licensed for clinical use since 2014. The last version of this machine joins a 0.35 tesla MR scanner equipped for parallel imaging with a 6 MV FFF Linac for radiation delivery.

The MR scanner is composed by an open split solenoid with a 28 cm-wide gap where the Linac is located. The two halves of the MR scanner are mechanically and thermally connected to guarantee the magnetic field stability.

The system is able to deliver fixed conformal RT or IMRT treatments in step and shoot modality, with a dose rate of 600 cGy/min. The Linac is equipped with a double-stack and double-focused multileaf collimator (MLC) with 138 leaves designed to project field sizes from 0.2×0.4 to 27.4×24.1 cm^2 at isocentre, capable of full overtravel and interdigitation.

It also provides a real-time imaging, acquiring four images per second on a sagittal plan using a true fast imaging with steady-state precession (TrueFISP) sequence. This type of sequence is determined by a mixture of T2$*$ and T1 properties of the tissues, and it is mostly depending on the relaxation time of the tissue protons (Hu et al. 2015).

MRIdian uses this sequence not only to perform real-time planar imaging but also to acquire volumetric images of the patient. The time of acquisition for a 3D scan ranges from 17 to 786 s, depending on the field of view and the spatial resolution. The short acquisitions (17 and 25 s) are mainly used for breath-hold treatments (abdomen and thorax sites), the longest ones (175 and 786 s) for free-breathing treatments (pelvic and head and neck districts).

The system provides also an intrafraction motion management, consisting in a gating system based on the real-time cine MR images, that makes this machine suitable for breath-hold treatments. Lamb et al. evaluated the latency of this motion management technique by using a dynamic phantom and film dosimetry, and they reported a maximum beam-off latency equal to 0.5 s (Lamb et al. 2017b).

The treatment planning system (TPS) uses a Monte Carlo algorithm integrated on a graphical power unit (GPU) architecture to calculate the dose distribution, and it is able to calculate IMRT complex plans in few minutes. This algorithm is based on PENELOPE, a computer code system developed in Fortran language in 1996 for research projects related to nuclear physics. The PENELOPE code was translated from Fortran to C++ language and then integrated on a GPU architecture to speed up the calculation time (Wang et al. 2016).

The importance of using a Monte Carlo algorithm lies in the need of taking into consideration the significant effects on the dose distribution due to the magnetic field presence. In fact, in the hybrid systems with transverse geometry, the electrons produced by the interaction of the radiation with the tissue of the patient are subjected to the Lorentz force due to the presence of magnetic field.

The magnetic field presence modifies the beam trajectory inside a homogeneous tissue, producing an asymmetrical penumbra and a reduced build-up region in the beam (Raaijmakers et al. 2008).

In presence of the interfaces between different medium densities, such as tissue-air interface, the magnetic field presence forces the electrons leaving the tissue to come back following an arc-shaped trajectory, with a curvature radius dependent by the magnetic field strength and electron energy.

This phenomenon, known as electron return effect (ERE), causes a dose increase at the tissue-air interface, whose entity is proportional to the magnetic field strength (Raaijmakers et al. 2008, 2007; Cusumano et al. 2018).

4 Clinical Treatments Using Low Tesla Hybrid Machines

One of the main advantages offered by the MRI-guided RT systems, independently by the magnetic field strength of the MR scanner, is represented by the possibility of adapting the treatment plan to the daily anatomy of the patient while the patient is positioned in treatment position.

All the low tesla MRgRT treatments start from a double treatment simulation: the patient is first positioned on the treatment couch of the hybrid device, using appropriated device immobilization and surface MR coils.

The MR simulation consists in acquiring volumetric MR images of the patient in different breathing conditions and evaluating its compliance in performing the treatment in breath-hold condition.

The MRIdian treatments of the abdomen and thorax districts are preferably administered in breath-hold technique, as it ensures more reproducible treatments and higher image quality with respect to free-breathing treatments, thanks to the elimination of the blurring effect and the motion artefact due to patient breathing. This allows a reduction of the margin expansion for the target and more precise contouring of all the therapy volumes (Bohoudi et al. 2017).

The patient is then moved to the CT simulation, where a CT scan is acquired in the same treatment conditions, to obtain the electron density map needed for the dose calculation.

The contouring and planning procedures are then carried out on the MR image that is co-registered to the CT image to obtain the electron density map. Different research groups are investigating the possibility to obtain the electron density information directly from the MR image, removing the CT simulation by the clinical workflow and paving the way towards the MRI-only radiotherapy. Although several approaches are currently under investigation, none of them has been already implemented in clinical practice (Edmund and Nyholm 2017).

The adaptive treatments differ from the conventional ones for the on-table procedure that is repeated every treatment fraction, and it consists in re-optimizing the original treatment plan on the basis of the daily situation of the patient therapy volumes.

Once the daily image is acquired, the radiation oncologist recontours the therapy volumes, and the medical physicist verifies the reliability of the electron density map. The treatment plan is then recalculated on the daily MRI and re-optimized if one or more dose constraints are not satisfied.

The time span represents a limiting factor in the adaptive workflow: Lamb et al. (2017a) have estimated on 80 cases a median execution time of 54 min before to start the beam delivery.

The online manual recontouring represents the more time-consuming activity, with a mean time of 22 min. Fu et al. (2018) have recently developed a convolutional neural network (CNN) deep-learning (DL) model to automatically segment the organs at risk typical of the pancreatic site (the liver, kidneys, stomach, bowel and duodenum), allowing a mean spare time equal to 75% with respect to the manual procedure.

As the deep-learning approaches are still not implemented in clinical practice, different manual strategies to speed up and standardize the adaptive procedure have been realized during the last years. In particular, for the application of the adaptive procedure on pancreatic cancer, it is common practice to contour only the therapy volumes that are located around the target volume (3 cm far to the target edges), in proximity of the high-dose region. Olberg et al. 2018 proposed a planning strategy that consists in grouping all the OARs surrounding the planning tumour volume (PTV) in a single structure and then cropping the PTV by 3 mm to this volume. The authors observed an average improvement of 3.87 ± 4.29% for the PTV coverage with respect to results of the conventional strategy, based on organ-specific constraint optimization.

On the other hand, Bohoudi et al. proposed an alternative approach defined as "stereotactic MR-guided adaptive radiotherapy" (SMART), consisting in the combination of all the surrounding OARs in optimization regions located at 1, 2 and 3 cm from the PTV edge.

In comparison with the approach proposed by Olberg et al., the SMART strategy requires a lower number of optimization steps (5 vs 18) to create optimal plans meeting the same dose constraints.

Once the treatment plan is adapted, the MRIdian TPS allows to execute a patient-specific quality assurance (QA), consisting in comparing, in terms of gamma analysis, the dose distribution calculated by the TPS with a secondary one obtained by using an independent algorithm (Li et al. 2015).

Alternative approaches of patient-specific QA (e.g. in vivo dosimetry with scintillators or electronic portal imaging device (EPID)) are currently under investigation for this type of machine.

Lastly, one of the unsolved questions related to the adaptive MRgRT treatments remains the summation of the dose distributions obtained from the different treatment fractions that is particularly challenging as the therapy volumes change position and volume every day. Although several approaches have been investigated, mainly based on dose warping or deformable image registration, a common methodology is not individuated yet (Simon et al. 2015).

5 Clinical Perspective

A low tesla MRI hybrid RT unit with in-room gating offers a wide spectrum of opportunities for clinicians to be investigated and exploited; such opportunities involve the treatment flow, the delivery approach, and some future research opportunity.

5.1 New Clinical Opportunities for RT Treatment Flow

A snapshot summarizing the innovations introduced in the conventional RT treatment flow by low tesla MRI in-room gating hybrid systems is depicted in Fig. 1 (Cellini 2017). As mentioned, the MR images provide a verification of the ROI based on high soft-tissue contrast, particularly useful in some areas of the body including the pelvis and upper abdomen. Thus, high-quality set-up verification is provided, potentially followed by conventional non-gated treatment course. One of the most interesting options is anyway presented by the real-time, radiationless, MR in-room imaging-guided and continuous (over the whole course of RT session), gating treatment by direct visualization of the specific ROI. As low tesla system, the MRIdian system in particular allows for a tuned definition of parameter for the personalization of the gating. The personalization of the gating includes the definition of the boundary around a certain structure that represents a limit to engage the gating of the dose delivery (e.g. setting a

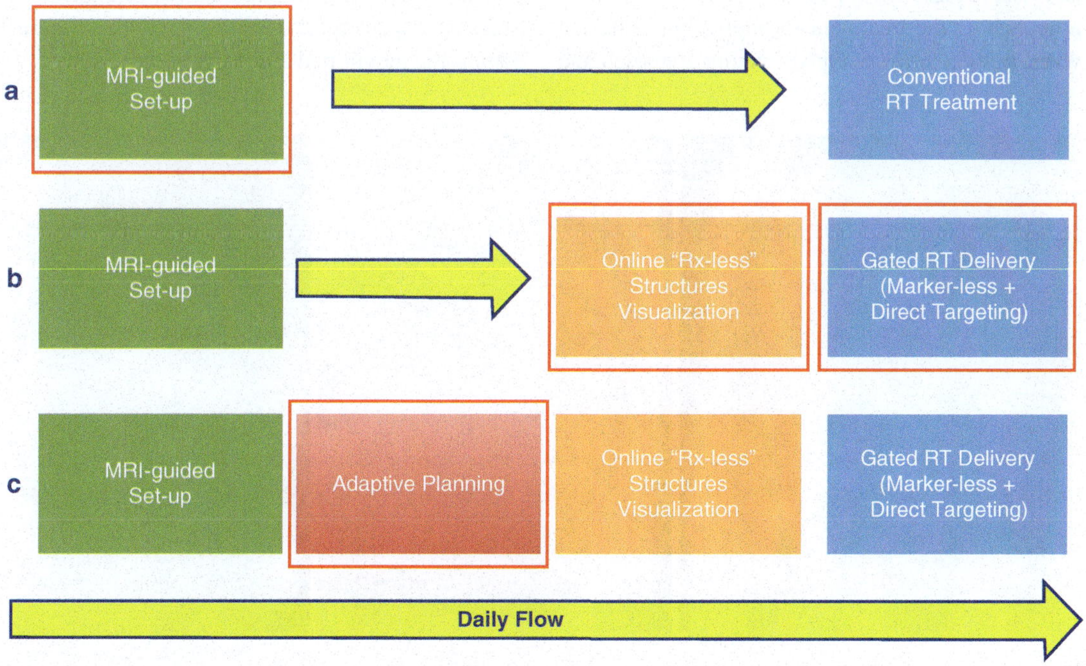

Fig. 1 Treatment procedure's flows. Red squares highlight the new clinical options provided by low Tesla MRI in-room systems

boundary of 3 mm around the GTV), the definition of the rate of the gated target surface enabling the gating of the treatment to temporary interrupt the RT delivery (e.g. "10% of the GTV" is the maximum percentage of such structure allowed to exceed the boundary) and the definition of a minimum delay before temporary interruption of the RT delivery when the defined rate of target structure actually exceeds the boundary (e.g. RT is gated if "10% of the GTV" exceeds the boundary of 3 mm around the GTV for at least 5 s). The potential to personalize the gating procedure day by day and/or patient by patient represents a challenging opportunity for clinicians. Finally, all the above-mentioned options can be associated to the adaptive daily optimization of the planned dose distribution, taking into account the modification due to target and organ displacement and different organ filling status, as mentioned in Sect. 4 (Mutic and Dempsey 2014).

5.2 New Clinical Opportunities for RT Delivery Approach

Low tesla MR in-room gating systems for RT allow approaching the treatment through some different ways, both in terms of type of gating approach and in terms of definition of kind of ROI to be gated. As for other gating systems, the patients can be asked to either freely breathe over the simulation procedure and each RT session or maintain a breath-hold (whether in mid or deep inspiration or mid or deep expiration): the choice is usually made accordingly to the best planning convenience and patient's compliance. The potentiality of the in-room low tesla gating device can be particularly exploited by personalizing the structure to be tracked through the RT session preforming the gating on. Since the visualization of the ROI is real time and direct moreover including all the structures within the field of view of the device, it can be applied not only to the target but also to any organ at risk needing a specific control in order to reduce the accumulated dose if the dose limits are close to the accepted tolerance. The former option is intuitively the most widely adopted with the aim of maximizing the dose delivered to the target while reducing the margins of normal tissues irradiated. The latter option can provide an added advantage in clinical settings requiring a different prioritization with less importance to gate a relatively stable target volume along the purpose to strictly reduce the irradiation of organs at risk presenting a narrow margin to the tolerance expected for the delivered doses. Figure 2 depicts the mentioned clinical approaches.

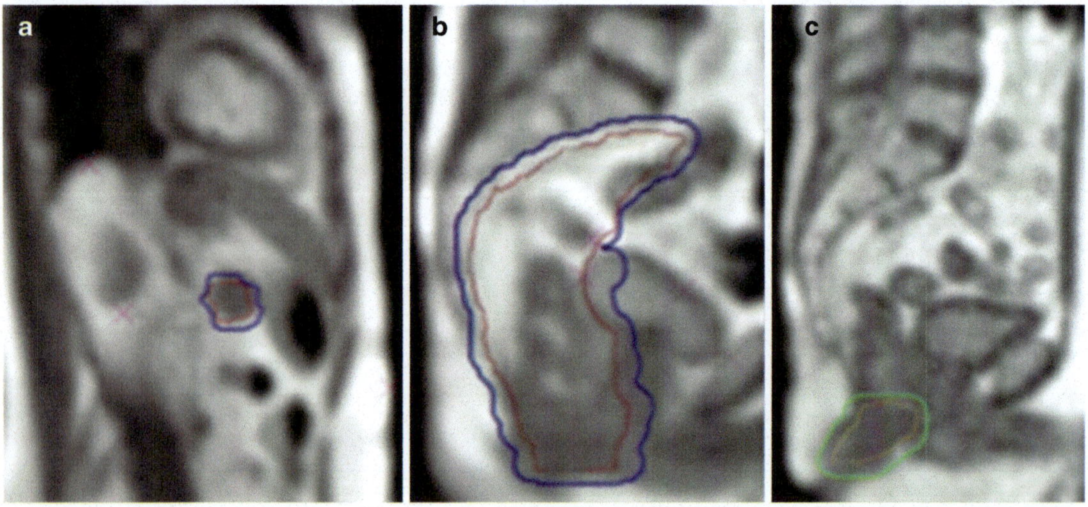

Fig. 2 Treatment approaches. (**a**) Target gating of a pancreatic lesion in breath-hold deep inspiration; (**b**) target gating of a rectal lesion in free breathing; (**c**) organ-at-risk gating for anal canal through a free-breathing treatment session for rectal cancer)

5.3 New Clinical Opportunities for Clinical Research

Since a low tesla in-room MRI-guided gating system allows a wide data collection in terms of imaging information through each treatment session and all over the whole RT course, the available applications of such an amount of data in the research field are of high importance. Currently, two main fields of research are ongoing. One is represented by the radiomic analysis: Radiomics refers to the comprehensive quantification of tumour phenotypes by applying a large number of quantitative image features (Lambin et al. 2012).

Radiogenomics analysis revealed that a prognostic radiomic signature, capturing intratumour heterogeneity, is associated with underlying gene expression patterns and thus can be adopted to personalize treatments. Also, MR imaging signatures allow prediction of survival and stratification of patients; moreover, the load of information retrievable by a daily and whole-treatment delivery opens a fully innovative and unexplored field of investigation. Boldrini et al. (2018) recently demonstrated on 16 patients that the variation of radiomic parameters extracted from low tesla MR images can predict clinical complete response in the case of locally advanced rectal cancer.

A second opportunity is represented by diffusion-weighted MR imaging (DWI) and apparent diffusion coefficient (ADC). DWI is a sequence that provides information on the degree of cellularity of lesions. ADC value provides information on the movement of water molecules outside the cells. Both the imaging data can be collected through the entire course of each RT session potentially providing new information to discriminate treatment and personalize patient's care. Very few and preliminary clinical experiences are available in this field, but those published are promising as much as interesting. Shaverdian et al. tested how ADC values obtained using a 0.35 T MRI RT system over the course of neoadjuvant chemoradiotherapy for rectal cancer correlate with pathological responses in three patients (Shaverdian et al. 2017).

6 Conclusions

In conclusion, the CBCT has assumed a key role in supporting the delivery of RT treatments, for IGRT integrating its potentialities with CT for planning; the low-field MR systems aim to provide a valid tool for evaluating the accurate delivery of high-precision RT treatment without using ionizing radiation, integrating their functionalities with those of the high tesla diagnostic MR.

References

Bohoudi O, Bruynzeel AME, Senan S, Cuijpers JP, Slotman BJ, Lagerwaard FJ, Palacios MA (2017) Fast and robust online adaptive planning in stereotactic MR-guided adaptive radiation therapy (SMART) for pancreatic cancer. Radiother Oncol 125:439–444

Boldrini L, Cusumano D, Chiloiro G, Casà C, Masciocchi C, Dinapoli N, Lenkowicz J, Cellini F, Gambacorta MA, Azario L, De Spirito M, Valentini V (2018) Delta Radiomics for rectal cancer response prediction with hybrid 0.35 T magnetic resonance guided radiotherapy (MRgRT) : a hypothesis generating study for an innovative personalized medicine approach. Radiol Med 124:145–153

Cusumano D, Teodoli S, Greco F, Fidanzio A, Boldrini L, Massaccesi M, Cellini F, Valentini V, Azario L, De Spirito M (2018) Experimental evaluation of the impact of low tesla transverse magnetic field on dose distribution in presence of tissue interfaces. Phys Med 53:80–85

Cellini F (2017) Oral presentation—International conference on advances in radiation oncology (ICARO2), Organized by the International Atomic Energy Agency, Vienna, Austria, 20–23 June 2017

Edmund JM, Nyholm T (2017) A review of substitute CT generation for MRI-only radiation therapy. Radiat Oncol 12:28

Fallone BG (2014) The rotating biplanar linac-magnetic resonance imaging system. Semin Radiat Oncol 24:200–202

Fu Y, Mazur TR, Wu X, Liu S, Chang X, Lu Y, Li HH, Kim H, Roach MC, Henke L, Yang D (2018) A novel MRI segmentation method using CNN-based correction network for MRI-guided adaptive radiotherapy. Med Phys 45:5129–5137

Hu Y, Rankine L, Green OL, Kashani R, Li HH, Li H, Nana R, Rodriguez V, Santanam L, Shvartsman S, Victoria J, Wooten HO, Dempsey JF, Mutic S (2015) Characterization of the onboard imaging unit for the first clinical magnetic resonance image guided radiation therapy system. Med Phys 42:5828–5837

Lagendijk JJW, Raaymakers BW, van Vulpen M (2014) The magnetic resonance imaging-linac system. Semin Radiat Oncol 24:207–209
Lamb J, Cao M, Kishan A, Agazaryan N, Thomas DH, Shaverdian N, Yang Y, Ray S, Low DA, Raldow A, Steinberg ML, Lee P (2017a) Online adaptive radiation therapy: implementation of a new process of care. Cureus 9:e1618
Lamb JM, Ginn JS, O'Connell DP, Agazaryan N, Cao M, Thomas DH, Yang Y, Lazea M, Lee P, Low DA (2017b) Dosimetric validation of a magnetic resonance image gated radiotherapy system using a motion phantom and radiochromic film. J Appl Clin Med Phys 18:163–169
Lambin P, Rios-Velazquez E, Leijenaar R, Carvalho S, van Stiphout RGPM, Granton P, Zegers CML, Gillies R, Boellard R, Dekker A, Aerts HJWL (2012) Radiomics: extracting more information from medical images using advanced feature analysis. Eur J Cancer 48:441–446
Li HH, Rodriguez VL, Green OL, Hu Y, Kashani R, Wooten HO, Yang D, Mutic S (2015) Patient-specific quality assurance for the delivery of (60)co intensity modulated radiation therapy subject to a 0.35-T lateral magnetic field *Int*. J Radiat Oncol Biol Phys 91:65–72
Liney GP, Whelan B, Oborn B, Barton M, Keall P (2018) MRI-linear accelerator radiotherapy systems. Clin Oncol (R Coll Radiol) 30:686–691
Mutic S, Dempsey JF (2014) The ViewRay system: magnetic resonance-guided and controlled radiotherapy. Semin Radiat Oncol 24:196–199
Nguyen NP, Karlsson UL (2015) Editorial: image-guided radiotherapy for effective radiotherapy delivery. Front Oncol 18(5):253. https://doi.org/10.3389/fonc.2015.0025
Olberg S, Green O, Cai B, Yang D, Rodriguez V, Zhang H, et al. (2018) Optimization of treatment planning workflow and tumor coverage during daily adaptive magnetic resonance image guided radiation therapy (MR-IGRT) of pancreatic cancer. Radiat Oncol 13:51
Raaijmakers AJE, Raaymakers BW, Lagendijk JJW (2007) Experimental verification of magnetic field dose effects for the MRI-accelerator. Phys Med Biol 52:4283–4291
Raaijmakers AJE, Raaymakers BW, Lagendijk JJW (2008) Magnetic-field-induced dose effects in MR-guided radiotherapy systems: dependence on the magnetic field strength. Phys Med Biol 53:909–923
Shaverdian N, Yang Y, Hu P, Hart S, Sheng K, Lamb J, Cao M, Agazaryan N, Thomas D, Steinberg M, Low DA, Lee P (2017) Feasibility evaluation of diffusion-weighted imaging using an integrated MRI-radiotherapy system for response assessment to neoadjuvant therapy in rectal cancer. Br J Radiol 90:20160739
Simon A, Nassef M, Rigaud B, Cazoulat G, Castelli J, Lafond C, Acosta O, Haigron P, de Crevoisier R (2015) Roles of deformable image registration in adaptive RT: from contour propagation to dose monitoring. Conf Proc IEEE Eng Med Biol Soc 2015:5215–5218
Wang Y, Mazur TR, Green O, Hu Y, Li H, Rodriguez V, Wooten HO, Yang D, Zhao T, Mutic S, Li HH (2016) A GPU-accelerated Monte Carlo dose calculation platform and its application toward validating an MRI-guided radiation therapy beam model. Med Phys 43:4040

Endoluminal Brachytherapy: Technicalities and Main Clinical Evidences

G. C. Mattiucci, L. Tagliaferri, R. Autorino, and G. Kovacs

Contents

1 **Introduction** 138

2 **Application Technique** 138
2.1 Biliary Duct Cancer 138
2.2 Oesophagus Cancer 139

3 **Clinical Indications** 140
3.1 Biliary Duct Cancer 140

4 **Conclusion** 144

References 146

Abstract

Intraluminal brachytherapy (BT) can be used in upper gastrointestinal cancers such as bile duct or esophageal tumor in curative or palliative setting. The application technique depends on the anatomical site to be treated. The endoluminal brachytherapy technique seems to provide good results in the treatment of cholangiocarcinoma or esophageal cancer. It is an important component in the multimodality approach of the bile duct. With a high local dose to the tumor, surrounding normal tissues, the brachytherapy may be applied as radical treatment alone or in combination with external beam radiotherapy or may prolong patency of biliary tract as palliative treatment.

Also in esophageal cancer, endoluminal brachytherapy can be used as a radical treatment in inoperable patients alone in early stage or in combination with external radiotherapy in advanced stages; in palliative cases, it is the treatment of choice to improve dysphagia and quality of life.

G. C. Mattiucci
U.O.C. Radioterapia Oncologica, Dipartimento di Diagnostica per immagini, Radioterapia Oncologica ed Ematologia, Fondazione Policlinico Universitario A. Gemelli IRCCS, Rome, Italy

Istituto di Radiologia, Università Cattolica del Sacro Cuore, Rome, Italy

L. Tagliaferri (✉) · R. Autorino
U.O.C. Radioterapia Oncologica, Dipartimento di Diagnostica per immagini, Radioterapia Oncologica ed Ematologia, Fondazione Policlinico Universitario A. Gemelli IRCCS, Rome, Italy
e-mail: luca.tagliaferri@policlinicogemelli.it

G. Kovacs
Gemelli-INTERACTS, Università Cattolica del Sacro Cuore, Rome, Italy

R. G. H. Beets-Tan et al. (eds.), *Imaging and Interventional Radiology for Radiation Oncology*, Medical Radiology, Diagnostic Imaging, https://doi.org/10.1007/978-3-030-38261-2_10

1 Introduction

Intraluminal brachytherapy (BT) can be used in upper gastrointestinal cancers such as bile duct or esophageal tumor in curative or palliative setting.

2 Application Technique

The application technique depends of the anatomical site to be treated. For catheter/applicator positioning a percutaneous or endoluminal approach, a radiography-/CT-/MRI-based approach or the endoscopy guidance or the combination of the listed methods can also be used.

2.1 Biliary Duct Cancer

Interventional radiotherapy in the biliary ducts can be performed using two different techniques: the transduodenal endoscopic technique and the transhepatic technique.

Transduodenal endoscopic technique: In this technique, an endoscopic retrograde cholangiography is used for defining the length of the involved biliary duct length and the effective extension of the disease. A flexible radiopaque guide wire is inserted under endoscopy and fluoroscopy guidance inside the biliary duct until lesion's cranial margin was passed. Then, a naso-biliary tube is pushed into the biliary tree following the guide wire. A flexible, usually 5–6, French interventional radiotherapy catheter including a radiopaque marker wire is positioned inside the naso-biliary tube under fluoroscopy control and fixed to the skin with the tip over the lesion. The entire tumor plus the safety margins needs to correspond the part of the applicator that has the possibility of containing active treatment source positions.

Transhepatic technique: For the second way of application technique, a cholangiography is used. The cholangiogram allows identifying the position and the length of the macroscopic disease in the biliary tree. A biliary drain will be positioned by a transhepatic approach, and an interventional radiotherapy catheter with radiopaque dummy sources will be fixed covering the target area. This technique allows the use of interventional radiotherapy also in lesions that can be reached and treated by an endoscopic approach. Using a noncovered metal stent and anchoring "handmade" flaps on the tip of the biliary catheters can be performed to avoid migration and dislodgement (Skowronek and Zwierzchowski 2017; Nori et al. 2001).

Treatment planning: A 2D planning using orthogonal radiography images could be used, but a 3D CT-based planning, defining tumor volume et OARs, is recommended. In case of 2D planning, the location and length of the stenotic bile duct tumor should be identified at PTC and/or ERCP or magnetic resonance cholangiopancreatography (MRCP). For the CTL, a 1 cm margin is taken proximally and distally of the visible stenosis. In case of 3D CT-based planning, CTV is obtained by adding 1–1.5 cm margin to the GTV, defined as any visible tumor at CE CT or MRI, especially along the bile duct. A PTL or PTV margin of 0.5–1 cm, in agreement to the approach, is added to CTL/CTV to encompass the uncertainties in catheter reconstruction. When possible, it is recommended to perform a breath-hold simulation CT scan or a 4D simulation CT scan to reduce errors in the catheter reconstruction caused by catheter deformation due to breathing (Skowronek 2002: The GEC-ESTRO Handbook of Brachytherapy second Edition) (Ash 2002, The GEC-ESTRO Handbook of Brachytherapy first Edition).

The reference dose is usually defined at 10 mm from the source axis, and in the 3D CT-based approach, the dose distribution is optimized to the target volumes and AORs, in particular to the liver, pancreas, duodenum, small bowel, stomach, and spinal cord based on dose distribution parameters calculated from the cumulative dose volume histogram (Skowronek and Zwierzchowski 2017).

Several dose schedules are reported in the literature, and HDR interventional radiotherapy is nowadays the most common in the clinical practice. In the boost setting with HDR, the recommended dose prescription is 15–20 Gy in 2–3 fractions. In the palliation setting with HDR, the dose prescription ranges from 15 to 25 Gy in 3–5 fractions (Mattiucci et al. 2015) or 16 Gy in two weekly fractions (Aggarwal et al. 2013).

2.2 Oesophagus Cancer

Pretreatment evaluation: To be able to perform esophagus interventional radiotherapy, the organ lumen cannot have a tight stenosis, or, at least, the grade of the stenosis should allow the applicator passage. In some situations, the stenosis can be dilated or opened by a laser intervention by an expert in endoscopic manipulations. In addition, before the interventional radiotherapy procedure, the tumor location—a pretreatment esophagoscopy—is mandatory.

Tumor localization: For localizing the tumor during the radiotherapy procedure, multiple methods can be used. These include the use of endoluminal radiopaque markers, skin radiopaque markers, or tumor margins measured from the dental arch (incisors). For the first method, some submucosal clips are fixed on the visible distal and/or proximal tumor margins, while with the second method, the markers are fixed on the patient's skin, and endoscopy combined with fluoroscopy is used in order to know the exact projection of the tumor margins on the skin. This last one is less accurate because the skin marker's position can vary with different thorax positions; for this reason, it is not advisable. However, the exact positioning of the patient in both marking and treatment sessions is mandatory to avoid inaccuracies.

Choice of applicator size: The applicator diameter should be as large as possible. The choice depends on the residual lumen in correspondence of the tumor. There are applicators with some balloons along the surface that can be inflated with water; this allows the optimal applicator adherence to the target mucosa and at the same time keeps it also in varying lumen diameters stable. The recommended external diameter of the applicator for esophageal brachytherapy is not less than 0.6 cm and not more than 1.0 cm. Narrower (<0.6 cm in diameter) catheters deliver a significantly larger dose to the mucosa. The use of larger caliber catheters (>1 cm diameter) may be associated with an increased risk of esophageal abrasions or perforations.

Applicator positioning: With or without endoscopic guidance, a flexible radiopaque guide wire is pushed through the esophagus lumen into the stomach. A fluoroscopy is mandatory in this time. The macroscopic tumor margins can be detected by the rapports between the wire and the intraluminal or skin markers. As the next step, the applicator with a radiopaque dummy source inside is introduced in the esophagus using the guide wire. The macroscopic tumor plus the safety margins needs to be in correspondence with the part of the applicator which has the possibility of active treatment source positions. The caudal part of the catheter should be positioned at least 3–4 cm distal from the caudal tumor margin in order to ensure the dose coverage also corresponding to the safety margins—these are usually 1–2 cm. If only control method is the measurement of the distance between the dental arch as a point of reference and the cranial/caudal macroscopic tumor boarders, the applicator needs to have distance indicators on its surface. The introduction of the applicator on the guide wire can be controlled easily by controlling the distance indicators at the dental line.

Some authors described different methods using 16-gauge nasogastric catheters. The HDR applicator is passed and fixed into it. The system is introduced inside the esophagus, and using the markers position or oral contrast, the tumor margins are detected by fluoroscopy and the catheter is fixed in the right position. However, 16-gauge nasogastric catheter does not always result in an appropriate surface contact over the full target length (Marinello et al. 1992; Flores 2001).

Treatment planning: A 2D planning using orthogonal radiography images could be used, but a 3D CT-based planning, defining tumor volume et OARs, is recommended. The target volume is defined taking in account the diagnostic findings from pretreatment barium swallow, esophagoscopy, and sectional imaging (Gaspar et al. 1997a, b, c; Rovirosa et al. 2015; Lettmaier and Strnad 2014; Potter and Van Limberger 2002, The GEC-

ESTRO Handbook of Brachytherapy first Edition). For better tumor delineation, fusion images with diagnostic CT or PET-CT may be useful (Rovirosa et al. 2015). In case of 2D planning for the clinical target length (CTL), a 2 cm margin is taken proximally and distally from the visible stenosis. In case of 3D CT-based planning, the clinical target volume is comprised of the gross tumour volume (GTV) plus a variable caudal and distal margin, usually of 2 cm, to take into account the microscopic spread (CTV). A planning target length or a planning target volume, in agreement to the approach, is added to encompass uncertainties in applicator placement and reconstruction. Margin size depends on the clinical and technical aspects of the procedure (Rovirosa et al. 2015; Lettmaier and Strnad 2014; Potter and Van Limberger 2002, The GEC-ESTRO Handbook of Brachytherapy first Edition).

The prescription dose is usually at 5 mm from the applicator or at 10 mm from MIDsource position, and in 3D CT-based approach, the dose distribution is optimized to target volumes and AORs basing on dose distribution parameters calculated from cumulative dose volume histogram (Gaspar et al. 1997a, b, c; Rovirosa et al. 2015).

Several dose schedules are reported in the literature. In the boost setting with HDR is recommended, 3–4 weeks after 50–60 Gy EBRT, a dose prescription of 10–12 Gy in two weekly fractions of 5–6 Gy. In the palliation setting with HDR, the dose prescription ranges from 7 to 28 Gy in fractions of 5–7 Gy (Gaspar et al. 1997a, b, c; Rovirosa et al. 2015).

3 Clinical Indications

The endoluminal brachytherapy technique seems to provide good results in the treatment of cholangiocarcinoma or esophageal cancer, when indicated.

3.1 Biliary Duct Cancer

Extrahepatic cholangiocarcinoma is an uncommon adenocarcinoma, which arises from the epithelial cells of bile ducts. It has an incidence of less than 1.5 cases per 100,000 inhabitants in Western countries (Parkin et al. 2002).

There is a marked geographic variability, largely due to variations in regional environmental risk factors. The majority of patients are older than 65, with the peak incidence occurring in the seventh decade of life (Curado et al. 2008).

Complete surgical resection is the gold standard for cure in extrahepatic bile duct cancers (Chao and Greager 1991; Lillemore 1994; Klempnauer et al. 1997).

Even in patients who undergo surgical resection for cure, 5-year survival rate can be as low as about 10% (Nakeeb et al. 1996).

While surgical resection provides the best chances of long-term survival and quality of life, the majority of patients are not candidates for curative resection due to locally advanced disease at diagnosis, poor physical conditions, and/or tumor location (Erickson and Nag 1998). In this setting, given the short life expectancy, palliation is often the therapeutic goal. In particular, palliative surgery, biliary drainage, chemotherapy, and radiotherapy with either external beam irradiation or intraluminal brachytherapy (ILBT) can be performed for the relief of obstructive jaundice and other symptoms.

In patients with unresectable biliary tract cancer, intraluminal brachytherapy can be used separately or in combination with external beam RT.

In order to minimize radiation exposure to the critical normal tissues and to administer higher doses to a well-defined and limited volume, intraluminal brachytherapy has been increasingly applied during the past two decades (Johnson et al. 1985; Vallis et al. 1996; Milella et al. 1998; Green et al. 1973). Small carcinomas that do not spread beyond the extrahepatic bile ducts can be treated effectively with this technique.

Intraluminal brachytherapy alone appears to have limited effectiveness for advanced inoperable carcinoma, partly because of the frequent recurrences within the nonirradiated portion of the bile ducts (Schnapauff et al. 2012; Fletcher et al. 1984; Molt et al. 1986; Montemaggi et al. 1996). For these reasons, several investigators have advocated a combination of EBRT and intraluminal brachytherapy (ILBT) (Lee et al. 1997; Conroy et al. 1982). However, most clinical experience for a combined approach has been confined to EBRT and low-dose-rate ILBT using radium needles, iridium seeds, or iridium wire. Only a few studies have taken high-dose-rate ILBT into consideration for these patients (Kamada et al. 1996; González González et al. 1999). Fritz et al. (1994) reported encouraging results for bile duct cancer patients treated with a combination of EBRT and high-dose rate intraluminal brachytherapy, but their responses were not compared with a control group.

Shin et al. (2003) retrospectively reviewed 31 patients in order to assess the feasibility and therapeutic benefits of a combination of EBRT and high-dose rate ILBT. Out of 31 patients, 17 patients only underwent EBRT (Group 1), and 14 patients were treated with EBRT in combination with high-dose-rate ILBT (Group 2). EBRT was delivered with a median dose of 50.4 Gy. ILBT was prescribed at 1.5 cm from the center of the source with a single daily dose of 5 Gy to a total of 15 Gy given in three fractions. With a median follow-up of 12 months, the overall actuarial 2-year survival rate for Group 2 patients was significantly better than that for Group 1 patients (0% for Group 1 vs. 21% for Group 2; $p = 0.015$) (Table 1).

Morganti et al. (2000) published a study demonstrating that chemo-RT plus ILBT was relatively well tolerated and resulted in reasonable local control and survival.

Twenty patients with unresectable (16 patients) or residual (4 patients), nonmetastatic extrahepatic bile tumors received external beam radiation. Twelve patients received a boost by intraluminal brachytherapy using (192) iridium wires. Four patients treated with external beam (39.6–50.4 Gy) plus intraluminal brachytherapy (30–50 Gy) had a clinical response (two partial, two complete) after treatment. For the total patient group, the median survival and time to local progression was 21.2 and 33.1 months, respectively (Table 1).

Recently, a retrospective analysis by Ghafoori et al. (2011) on a group of 37 patients who underwent EBRT with concurrent chemotherapy and/or brachytherapy for locally advanced extrahepatic cholangiocarcinoma found that long-term

Table 1 Biliary duct cancer: radiotherapy or chemoradiation and intraluminal brachytherapy

	Radiotherapy and intraluminal brachytherapy						
Author	Journal	Year	No. pts	Type and design of the study	Radiation therapy	Results	*P*
Fritz et al. (1994)	Int J Radiat Oncol Biol Phys	1994	30	*Retrospective study*		*Median survival (months)*	
				EBRT + ILBT	EBRT: 30–45 Gy and ILBT: 20–45 Gy	10	
Shin et al. (2003)	Int J Radiat Oncol Biol Phys	2003	31	*Retrospective study*		*2-ys OS*	0.015
				EBRT	MD EBRT: 50.4 Gy	0%	
				RT + ILBT	ILBT dose: 15 Gy	21%	
Morganti et al. (2000)	Int J Radiat Oncol Biol Phys	2000	20	*Retrospective study*		*Response rate*	<0.05
				RTCT + ILBT Vs	EBRT: 3960–5040 cgy	44.4%	
				RTCT	ILBT: 3000–5000 cGy	0%	
Ghafoori et al. (2011)	Int J Radiat Oncol Biol Phys	2011	37	*Retrospective study*		*1 year LC*	0.096
				EBRT± ILBT Vs	MD EBRT: 45 Gy	97%	
				ILT	ILBT: 40 Gy	56%	

EBRT external beam radiation therapy, *ILBT* intraluminal brachytherapy *MD EBRT* mean dose of external beam radiotherapy survival is rare, but the majority had local control at the time of death. Symptoms due to local tumor effect might thus be effectively controlled with RT. Multifield external beam techniques were used to treat gross disease to a median dose of 45 Gy (range, 30–62 Gy) using 1.8 to 3 Gy daily fractions. BT using iridium-192 (dose rate, 45–150 cGy/h) prescribed to a depth of 5 to 10 mm via percutaneous catheters was administered to six patients (median dose, 40 Gy; range, 25–50 Gy) without external beam treatment and as a boost to eight patients who received EBRT (median BT dose, 25 Gy, range, 20–35 Gy; median combined radiation dose, 70 Gy, range, 64–81 Gy).

Foo et al. (1997) confirmed that external beam irradiation combined with a transcatheter boost can result in long-term survival of patients with extrahepatic bile duct cancer. Both distant metastases and local recurrence develop in 25–30% of patients despite irradiation. Survival may be improved by using chemotherapy in combination with EBRT to impact disease relapse (local and distant). Because there may be a dose response with irradiation, survival may also be improved by increasing the dose of radiation delivered by transcatheter boost.

Alden and Mohiuddin (1994) published a study regarding the impact of radiation dose in combined external beam and intraluminal Ir-192 brachytherapy for bile duct cancer. They enrolled 48 patients and concluded that a dose response is shown with more than double the 2-year and median survival for doses >55 Gy. A brachytherapy dose of 25 Gy, plus 44–46 Gy external beam is well tolerated. High-dose-combined brachytherapy and external beam radiation (60–75 Gy) appears to be the most effective modality for extrahepatic bile duct cancer.

In brief, it can be assumed that the combined use of EBRT and high-dose-rate ILBT is a beneficial, relatively safe, and effective approach to improve the outcome in selected patients.

Due to the advanced stage of the disease at diagnosis or the presence of substantial comorbidities that preclude surgical therapy, more than half of the patients with cholangiocarcinoma are candidates for only palliative treatments (Tamada and Sugano 2000). Palliative surgery, biliary drainage (endoscopic or percutaneous), and RT with either external beam or ILBT can be performed for the treatment of obstructive jaundice and other symptoms. Endoscopic biliary drainage with a self-expandable metal endoprosthesis (metal stent) has become a favored palliative drainage procedure. However, it is often difficult to achieve long-term biliary patency by stenting alone, secondary to high rates of stent occlusion caused by tumor ingrowth or overgrowth (36). Some authors have reported that ILBT (mean dose: 25 Gy) is effective in preventing tumor ingrowth, prolongs biliary patency, and may be the treatment of choice for patients with poor performance status (Table 2) (28-37-38). Bowling et al. (1996) presented a retrospective study that showed a survival advantage in the RT group (Table 2) in the first 9 months after diagnosis. The patients received a combination of external beam radiotherapy (30 Gy in 10 fractions) followed by brachytherapy (60 Gy). Chen et al. (2004) came up with a study to evaluate the feasibility and safety of ILBT in the treatment of malignant obstructive jaundice. Mean stent patency was significantly longer in the ILBT Group (8.3 vs. 12.6 months, $p < 0.05$, Table 2), but there was no significant difference in mean survival (9.4 vs. 6.0 months). HDR 192-Ir was used in the therapy; fractional doses of 4–7 Gy were given every 3–6 days for 3–4 times. Kocak et al. (2005) published a study on eight patients with similar findings.

In conclusion, based on retrospective studies, HDR ILBT plus metallic stenting for inoperable patients with obstructive jaundice from biliary duct carcinoma appears to be feasible and may lead to an improved quality of life in terms of the control of symptoms.

Esophageal cancer brachytherapy can be used also in esophageal tumors as both definitive treatment in unresectable cancers and salvage or palliative therapy in patients with advanced or recurrent cancer. Radiation therapy oncology group (RTOG) 92-07 was a prospective single-arm phase I/II study investigating combination EBRT, 50 Gy in 25 fractions, followed by HDRBT (using an applicator with an external

Table 2 Biliary duct cancer: palliative treatment

	Radiotherapy and intraluminal brachytherapy						
Author	Journal	Year	No. pts	Type and design of the study	Radiation therapy	Results	*P*
Bruha et al. (2001)	Hepatogastroenterology	2001	32	*Retrospective study*		*Stent patency*	
				Stent implantation + ILBT	ILBT: 30 Gy	418 days	
Eschelman et al. (1996)	Radiology	1996	22	*Retrospective study*		*Stent patency*	
				Percutaneous biliary drainage + ILBT	MD ILBT: 25 Gy	19.5 months	
Bowling et al. (1996)	Gut	1996	56	*Retrospective study*		*Median survival (months)*	<0.05
				Endoscopic biliary stenting		7	
				Endoscopic biliary stenting + EBRT + ILBT	EBRT: 30 Gy ILBT: 60 Gy	11	
Chen et al. (2004)	World J Gastroenterol	2004	34	*Prospective study*		*Stent patency (months)*	<0.05
				Biliary stenting Vs		8.3	
				Biliary stenting + ILBT	ILBT dose: 1200–2800 cGy	12.6	

MD ILBT mean dose of intraluminal brachytherapy, *EBRT* external beam radiotherapy diameter of 4–6 mm), 15 Gy in three fractions. The protocol was amended to 10 Gy in two fractions after early toxicity reports, but initial publication revealed a 26% rate of life-threatening toxicity and a median overall survival less than 12 months (Gaspar et al. 1997a, b, c). RTOG 92-07 was criticized for its extreme dose escalation, concurrent chemotherapy (CT), and use of unsecured HDR sources allowing for poor prediction of dose falloff. Shortly after publication of RTOG 92-07, the American Brachytherapy Society (ABS) established treatment guidelines for definitive and palliative use of HDRBT in esophageal cancer (Gaspar et al. 1997a, b, c). Optimal candidates include patients with thoracic esophageal lesions ≤10 cm in length, confined to the esophageal wall. The ABS guidelines do not recommend using HDRBT in patients with a tumor >10 cm in length or in those with extraesophageal disease or lymph node involvement. Contraindications include involvement of the cervical esophagus, nontraversable esophageal stenosis, or tracheoesophageal fistula. A Japanese study of 21 patients with superficial esophageal squamous cell carcinoma (SCC) treated with either EBRT alone to a total dose of 60–69 Gy or a combination of EBRT to 50–56 Gy followed by an HDRBT boost of two to three fractions of 4 Gy revealed significantly higher local control and disease-specific survival in patients receiving combination treatment (Nishimura et al. 1999) Patients treated with EBRT alone had 3-year LC and disease-specific survival of 45% and 67%, respectively, compared to 85% and 100% in patients treated with EBRT + HDRBT. Treatment-related toxicity was mild and consisted of two patients in the combination treatment arm developing transient esophageal ulcers. There were no treatment-related fatalities. In a study of 26 patients with nonmetastatic esophageal SCC treated with definitive concurrent chemoradiation (CRT) to a median dose of 50.4 Gy followed by HDRBT of 8 Gy in two fractions, Sharan et al. (2014) also reported high LC of 61.5%. Tables 3 and 4 show the most relevant results in the literature on external beam and brachytherapy in early and advanced stages of esophageal cancer, respectively.

High-dose rate brachytherapy (HDRBT) is an established technique for palliation of pain, dysphagia, and obstruction in esophageal cancer, either alone or in combination with stenting and/or EBRT. In a Norwegian trial randomizing 41 patients to either self-expanding metal stent (SEMS) placement followed by HDRBT to a total prescribed dose of 24 Gy in three fractions or HDRBT alone, Amdal et al. (2013) reported faster improvement in dysphagia following combination treatment with both SEMS and HDRBT but no difference in total dysphagia relief with extended follow-up. The authors concluded that combination treatment with SEMS + HDRBT may be indicated for patients needing immediate dysphagia relief, while HDRBT alone may be preferable for less urgent cases due to the lower complication rate.

To date, there is no clear consensus on the optimal palliative approach for patients with incurable esophageal cancer.

HDRBT has been shown to be an efficacious treatment for the palliation of esophageal cancer-related dysphagia. A study by Sur et al. (2004) did not find an improvement in dysphagia-free survival (Dy-FS) or OS in 60 patients with inoperable advanced esophageal carcinoma randomized to treatment with either HDRBT alone or HDRBT + EBRT. Other studies have found HDRBT + EBRT to be superior to HDRBT alone in providing dysphagia relief. In a prospective study of 219 patients randomized to HDRBT of 8 Gy with or without EBRT of 30 Gy in fractions, Rosenblatt et al. (2010) reported an absolute benefit in dysphagia relief of 18% at 200 days in patients treated with combination HDRBT + EBRT compared to those treated with HDRBT alone. There were four treatment-related fatalities due to perforations or dehydration, with no significant difference in OS or toxicity between the two treatment arms.

4 Conclusion

Endoluminal brachytherapy is an important component in the multimodality approach of the bile duct. With a high local dose to the tumor, surrounding normal tissues, the brachytherapy

Table 3 Esophagus cancer early stage: external beam irradiation plus brachytherapy

	N	*T* (TNM)	EBI (Gy)	BT (Gy)	Chemotherapy	Complete response (%)	Local control	DFS (%)	Complications
Yorozu et al. (1999)	124	T1–T2	40–60	8–24 in 2–4 fractions	Yes (41%)	73	1 year 68% 2 years 58%		12 Gy: 17% 24 Gy 80%
Murakami et al. (2015)	32	T1–T2	50–66	10–12 in 2 fractions	Yes (32%)	100	1 year 85–93% 2 years 70–83%		Ulcers 8/32
Yamada et al. (2006)	63	T1	55–59.4	12 in 2–3 fractions	Yes	98		5 years 63.7%	3 ulcers or stenosis
Ishikawa et al. (2010)	36	T1	60	10–9 in 2–3 fractions	Yes	87		5 years 59%	6
Tamaki et al. (2012)	51	T1	56–60	LDR: 10 in 2 fractions HDR: 9 in 3 fractions	No	80	81%		2 deaths

Table 4 Esophagus cancer advanced stage: external beam irradiation plus brachytherapy

	N	Stage	EBI (Gy)	BT (Gy)	Chemotherapy	Complete response (%)	OS
Hujala et al. (2002)	40	III–IV	40	10 in 4 fractions	No	–	1 years 30% 2 years 17.5%
Vuong et al. (2005)	70	T1–T3 N0–N1	50	20 in 5 fractions	Yes	–	5 years 28%
López Carrizosa et al. (2007)	23	II–IV	44.2	21 in 5 fractions	No	23	5 years 10.1%
Calais et al. (1997)	53	IIB–III	60	10 in 5 fractions	Yes	1 years LC 74% 3 years LC 30%	3 years 27%
Someya et al. (2002)	–	IIIB–IV	60	–	–	2 years LC: 83.3% < 5 cm 25% ≥ 5 cm	Biliary duct

may be applied as radical treatment alone or in combination with external beam radiotherapy or may prolong patency of biliary tract as palliative treatment.

Also in esophageal cancer, endoluminal brachytherapy can be used as a radical treatment in inoperable patients alone in early stage or in combination with external radiotherapy in advanced stages; in palliative cases, it is the treatment of choice to improve dysphagia and quality of life.

References

Aggarwal R, Patel FD, Kapoor R, Kang M, Kumar P, Sharma SC (2013) Evaluation of high-dose-rate intraluminal brachytherapy by percutaneous transhepatic biliary drainage in the palliative management of malignant biliary obstruction a pilot study. Brachytherapy 12:162–170

Alden ME, Mohiuddin M (1994) The impact of radiation dose in combined external beam and intraluminal Ir-192 brachytherapy for bile duct cancer. Int J Radiat Oncol Biol Phys 28(4):945–951

Amdal CD et al (2013) Palliative brachytherapy with or without primary stent placement in patients with oesophageal cancer, a randomised phase III trial. Radiother Oncol 107(3):428–433

Ash D (2002) Bile duct tumours. Cap. 25 The GEC-ESTRO Handbook of Brachytherapy 1st Edition. 539–542

Bowling TE, Galbraith SM, Hatfield AR, Solano J, Spittle MF (1996) A retrospective comparison of endoscopic stenting alone with stenting and radiotherapy in non-resectable cholangiocarcinoma. Gut 39(6):852–855

Bruha R, Petrtyl J, Kubecova M, Marecek Z, Dufek V, Urbanek P et al (2001) Intraluminal brachytherapy and self-expandable stents in non-resectable biliary malignancies—the question of long-term palliation. Hepato-Gastroenterology 48:631–637

Calais G, Dorval E, Louisot P, Bourlier P, Klein V, Chapet S, Reynaud-Bougnoux A, Huten N, De Calan L, Aget H, Le Floch O (1997) Radiotherapy with high dose rate brachytherapy boost and concomitant chemotherapy for Stages IIB and III esophageal carcinoma: results of a pilot study. Int J Radiat Oncol Biol Phys 38(4):769–775

Chao TC, Greager JA (1991) Carcinoma of the extrahepatic bile ducts. J Surg Oncol 46:145–150

Chen Y, Wang XL, Yan ZP, Cheng JM, Wang JH, Gong GQ, Qian S, Luo JJ, Liu QX (2004) HDR-192Ir intraluminal brachytherapy in treatment of malignant obstructive jaundice. World J Gastroenterol 10(23):3506–3510

Conroy RM, Shahbazian AA, Edwards KC, Moran EM, Swingle KF, Lewis GJ et al (1982) A new method for treating carcinomatous biliary obstruction with intracatheter radium. Cancer 49:1321–1327

Curado MP, Edwards B, Shin HR, Storm H, Ferlay J, Heanue M et al (2008) Cancer incidence in five continents, vol. IX. IARC Scientific Publications, Lyon. [No. 160]

Erickson BA, Nag S (1998) Biliary tree malignancies. J Surg Oncol 67:203–210

Eschelman DJ, Shapiro MJ, Bonn J, Sullivan KL, Alden ME, Hovsepian DM et al (1996) Malignant biliary duct obstruction: long-term experience with Gianturco stents and combined modality radiation therapy. Radiology 200:717–724

Fletcher MS, Brinkley D, Dawson JL, Nunnerley H, Williams R (1984) Radiotherapy of high bile duct carcinoma using intracatheter iridium 192 wire. Cancer 54:2069–2073

Flores AD (2001) Brachytherapy in cancer of the oesophagus. In: Joslin CAF, Flynn A, Hall EJ (eds) Principles and practice of brachytherapy using afterloading systems, pp 243–256

Foo ML, Gunderson LL, Bender CE, Buskirk SJ (1997) External radiation therapy and transcatheter iridium in the treatment of extrahepatic bile duct carcinoma. Int J Radiat Oncol Biol Phys 39(4):929–935

Fritz P, Brambs HJ, Schraube P, Freund U, Berns C, Wannenmacher M (1994) Combined external beam radiotherapy and intraluminal high dose rate brachytherapy on bile duct carcinomas. Int J Radiat Oncol Biol Phys 29:855–861

Gaspar LE, Nag S, Herskovic A, Mantravadi O, Speiser B, The Clinical Research Committee (1997a) American Brachythefuypy Society: American Brachytherapy Society (ABS) consensus guidelines for brachytherapy of esophageal cancer. Int J Radiat Oncol Biol Phys 38(1):127–132

Gaspar LE et al (1997b) A phase I/II study of external beam radiation, brachytherapy and concurrent chemotherapy in localized cancer of the esophagus (RTOG 92-07): preliminary toxicity report. Int J Radiat Oncol Biol Phys 37(3):593–599

Gaspar LE et al (1997c) American brachytherapy society (ABS) consen- sus guidelines for brachytherapy of esophageal cancer. Clinical Research Committee, American Brachytherapy Society, Philadelphia, PA. Int J Radiat Oncol Biol Phys 38(1):127–132

Ghafoori AP, Nelson JW, Willett CG, Chino J, Tyler DS, Hurwitz HI et al (2011) Radiotherapy in the treatment of patients with unresectable extrahepatic cholangiocarcinoma. Int J Radiat Oncol Biol Phys 81:654–659

González González D, Gouma DJ, Rauws EA, van Gulik TM, Bosma A, Koedooder C (1999) Role of radiotherapy, in particular intraluminal brachytherapy in the treatment of proximal bile duct carcinomas. Ann Oncol 10(Suppl. 4):215–220

Green N, Mikkelsen WP, Kernen JA (1973) Cancer of the common hepatic bile ducts. Palliative radiotherapy. Radiology 109:687–689

Hujala K, Sipilä J, Minn H, Ruotsalainen P, Grenman R (2002) Combined external and intraluminal radiotherapy in the treatment of advanced oesophageal cancer. Radiother Oncol 64(1):41–45

Ishikawa H, Nonaka T, Sakurai H, Tamaki Y, Kitamoto Y, Ebara T, Shioya M, Noda SE, Shirai K, Suzuki Y, Takahashi T, Nakano T (2010) Usefulness of intraluminal brachytherapy combined with external beam radiation therapy for submucosal esophageal cancer: long-term follow-up results. Int J Radiat Oncol Biol Phys 76(2):452–459

Johnson DW, Safai C, Goffinet DR (1985) Malignant obstructive jaundice: treatment with external-beam and intracavitary radiotherapy. Int J Radiat Oncol Biol Phys 11:411–416

Kamada T, Saitou H, Takamura A, Nojima T, Okushiba SI (1996) The role of radiotherapy in the management of extrahepatic bile duct cancer: an analysis of 145 consecutive patients treated with intraluminal and/or external beam radiotherapy. Int J Radiat Oncol Biol Phys 34:767–744

Klempnauer J, Ridder GJ, Werner M, Weimann A, Pichlmayr R (1997) What constitutes long-term survival after surgery for hilar cholangiocarcinoma? Cancer 79:26–347

Kocak Z, Ozkan H, Adli M, Garipagaoglu M, Kurtman C, Cakmak A (2005) Intraluminal brachytherapy with metallic stenting in the palliative treatment of malignant obstruction of the bile duct. Radiat Med 23(3):200

Lee CK, Barrios BR, Bjarnson H (1997) Biliary tree malignancies: the University of Minnesota experience. J Surg Oncol 65:298–305

Lettmaier S, Strnad V (2014) Intraluminal brachytherapy in oesophageal cancer: defining its role and introducing the technique. J Contemp Brachytherapy 6(2):236–241

Lillemore KD (1994) Current status of surgery for Klatskin tumors. Curr Opin Gen Surg:161–167

López Carrizosa MC, Samper Ots PM, Rodríguez Pérez A et al (2007) High dose rate brachytherapy (HDR-BT) in locally advanced oesophageal cancer. Clinic response and survival related to biological equivalent dose (BED). Clin Transl Oncol 9:385–391. https://doi.org/10.1007/s12094-007-0071-y

Marinello G, Pierquin B, Grimard L et al (1992) Dosimetry of intraluminal brachytherapy. Radiother Oncol 23:213–216

Mattiucci GC, Autorino R, Tringali A, Perri V, Balducci M, Deodato F, Gambacorta MA, Mantini G, Tagliaferri L, Mutignani M, Morganti AG, Phase A (2015) I study of high-dose-rate intraluminal brachytherapy as palliative treatment in extrahepatic biliary tract cancer. Brachytherapy 14:401–404.12: 162–170

Milella M, Salvetti M, Cerrotta A, Cozzi G, Uslenghi E, Tavola A et al (1998) Interventional radiology and radiotherapy for inoperable cholangiocarcinoma of the extrahepatic bile ducts. Tumori 84:467–471

Molt P, Hopfan S, Watson RC, Botet JF, Brennan MF (1986) Intraluminal radiation therapy in the management of malignant biliary obstruction. Cancer 57:536–544

Montemaggi P, Morganti AG, Dobelbower RR Jr, Brizi G, Smaniotto D, Costamagna G et al (1996) Role of intraluminal brachytherapy in extraheptic bile duct and pancreatic cancers: is it just for palliation? Radiology 199:861–866

Morganti AG, Trodella L, Valentini V, Montemaggi P, Costamagna G, Smaniotto D et al (2000) Combined modality treatment in unresectable extrahepatic biliary carcinoma. Int J Radiat Oncol Biol Phys 46:913–919

Murakami Y, Takahashi I, Nishibuchi I, Doi Y, Okabe T, Kenjo M, Kimura T, Nagata Y (2015) Long-term results of definitive concurrent chemoradiotherapy for patients with esophageal submucosal cancer (T1bN0M0). Int J Clin Oncol 20(5):897–904

Nakeeb A, Pitt HA, Sohn TA, Coleman J, Abrams RA, Piantadosi S et al (1996) Cholangiocarcinoma. A spectrum of intrahepatic, perihilar and distal tumors. Ann Surg 224:463–473

Nishimura Y et al (1999) External beam radiation therapy with or without high-dose-rate intraluminal brachytherapy for patients with superficial esophageal carcinoma. Cancer 86(2):220–228

Nori D, Parikh S, Sundararaman S, Heernan M (2001) Brachytherapy in the treatment of pancreas and bile

duct cancer. In: Joslin CA, Flynn A, Hall EJ (eds) Principles and practice of brachytherapy using afterloading systems. Arnold, New York, pp 325–332
Parkin DM, Whelan SL, Ferlay J, Teppo L, Thomas DB (2002) Cancer incidence in five continents, vol VIII. IARC Press, Lyon. [IARC Scientific Publications No. 155]
Potter R, Van Limberger E. (2002) Oesophagel Cancer. Cap. 24 The GEC-ESTRO Handbook of Brachytherapy 1st Edition, 515–537
Rosenblatt E et al (2010) Adding external beam to intra-luminal brachy- therapy improves palliation in obstructive squamous cell oesophageal cancer: a prospective multi-centre randomized trial of the International Atomic Energy Agency. Radiother Oncol 97(3):488–494
Rovirosa A, Anchuelo J, Crispin V, Gutierrez C, Herreros A, Herruzo I, Menendez JC, Pino P, Polo A, Rodriguez S (2015) Recommendations of the Spanish brachytherapy group of SEOR for HDR endoluminal treatments. Part 1: Oesophagus. Clin Transl Oncol 17(8):581–589
Schnapauff D, Denecke T, Grieser C, Colletini F, Seehofer D, Sinn M et al (2012) Computed tomography-guided interstitial HDR brachytherapy (CT-HDRBT) of the liver in patients with irresectable intrahepatic cholangiocarcinoma. Cardiovasc Intervent Radiol 35:581–587
Sharan K et al (2014) Treatment outcomes after intraluminal brachytherapy following definitive chemoradiotherapy in patients with esophageal cancer. J Cancer Res Ther 10(2):337–341
Shin HS, Seong J, Kim WC, Lee HS, Moon SR, Lee IJ et al (2003) Combination of external beam irradiation and high-dose rate intraluminal brachytherapy for inoperable carcinoma of the extrahepatic bile ducts. Int J Radiat Oncol Biol Phys 57:105–112
Skowronek J (2002) Bile duct cancer. Cap. 28 The GEC-ESTRO Handbook of Brachytherapy 1st Edition
Skowronek J, Zwierzchowski G (2017) Brachytherapy in the treatment of bile duct cancer – a tough challenge. J Contemp Brachytherapy 9(2):187–195
Someya M, Sakata K, Saito A, Nagakura H, Oouchi A, Hareyama M (2002) Results of external irradiation and low-dose-rate intraluminal brachytherapy for esophageal cancer. Acta Oncol 41(1):63–68
Sur R et al (2004) Randomized prospective study comparing high-dose- rate intraluminal brachytherapy (HDRILBT) alone with HDRILBT and external beam radiotherapy in the palliation of advanced esophageal cancer. Brachytherapy 3(4):191–195
Tamada K, Sugano K (2000) Diagnosis and non-surgical treatment of bile duct carcinoma developments in the past decade. J Gastroenterol 35:319–325
Tamaki T, Ishikawa H, Takahashi T, Tamaki Y, Kitamoto Y, Okamoto M, Noda SE, Katoh H, Shirai K, Sakurai H, Nakano T (2012) Comparison of efficacy and safety of low-dose-rate vs. high-dose-rate intraluminal brachytherapy boost in patients with superficial esophageal cancer. Brachytherapy 11(2):130–136. https://doi.org/10.1016/j.brachy.2011.05.008. Epub 2011 Jun 22
Vallis KA, Benjamin IS, Munro AJ, Adam A, Foster CS, Williamson RC et al (1996) External beam and intraluminal radiotherapy for locally advanced bile duct cancer: role and tolerability. Radiother Oncol 41:61–66
Vuong T, Szego P, David M, Evans M, Parent J, Mayrand S, Corns R, Burtin P, Faria S, Devic S (2005) The safety and usefulness of high-dose-rate endoluminal brachytherapy as a boost in the treatment of patients with esophageal cancer with external beam radiation with or without chemotherapy. Int J Radiat Oncol Biol Phys 63(3):758–764
Yamada K, Murakami M, Okamoto Y, Okuno Y, Nakajima T, Kusumi F, Takakuwa H, Matsusue S (2006) Treatment results of chemoradiotherapy for clinical stage I (T1N0M0) esophageal carcinoma. Int J Radiat Oncol Biol Phys 64(4):1106–1111
Yorozu A, Dokiya T, Oki Y (1999) High-dose-rate brachytherapy boost following concurrent chemoradiotherapy for esophageal carcinoma. Int J Radiat Oncol Biol Phys 45(2):271–275

Part III

Imaging for Tumor Staging and Volume Definition (Wim J. G. Oyen, Monique Maas, Ursula Nestle)

Staging and Target Volume Definition by Imaging in CNS Tumors

Bas Jasperse and Gerben Borst

Contents

1 **Imaging Recommendations for Brain Tumor Imaging** ... 151
1.1 Basic MRI Protocol ... 151
1.2 Therapy-Related Changes That Mimic Tumor Progression ... 152

2 **Tumors Arising from Glial Cells** ... 154
2.1 Tumor Classification WHO Criteria ... 154
2.2 Low-Grade Astrocytoma (WHO II) and Anaplastic Astrocytoma (WHO III) ... 154
2.3 Low-Grade Glioma: Oligodendroglioma (WHO II) ... 155
2.4 High-Grade Glioma: Glioblastoma (WHO IV) ... 157

3 **Primary Central Nervous System Lymphoma** ... 158
3.1 MR Imaging ... 158
3.2 Radiotherapy ... 158

4 **Metastases** ... 162
4.1 MR Imaging ... 162
4.2 Radiotherapy ... 162

5 **Meningioma** ... 164
5.1 MR Imaging ... 164
5.2 Radiotherapy ... 165

References ... 166

B. Jasperse (✉) · G. Borst
Netherlands Cancer Institute/Antoni van Leeuwenhoek Ziekenhuis Amsterdam, Amsterdam, The Netherlands
e-mail: g.borst@nki.nl

Abstract

This chapter will comprise of staging, target volume definition, and radiotherapy planning for low-grade gliomas, oligodendrogliomas, glioblastomas, primary central nervous system lymphoma, and metastases. Ependymomas, pleomorphic xanthoastrocytomas, and pilocytic astrocytomas will not be included in this chapter due to their low prevalence in adults. Imaging will focus on MRI imaging, as this is the most important modality used in daily clinical practice.

1 Imaging Recommendations for Brain Tumor Imaging

1.1 Basic MRI Protocol

The standard brain MRI protocol should at least include a T1 pre- and postcontrast, T2, FLAIR, and DWI sequence. A slice thickness of 3 mm or less is preferred, with a maximum slice thickness of 5 mm. The inclusion of at least a postcontrast 1 mm 3D T1 sequence is highly recommended for optimal detail of enhancing brain tumors and the possibility of multiplanar reconstruction (ACR-ASNR guidelines 2013, https://www.acr.org/-/media/ACR/Files/Practice-Parameters/MR-Brain.pdf, Ellingson et al. 2015).

R. G. H. Beets-Tan et al. (eds.), *Imaging and Interventional Radiology for Radiation Oncology*, Medical Radiology, Diagnostic Imaging, https://doi.org/10.1007/978-3-030-38261-2_11

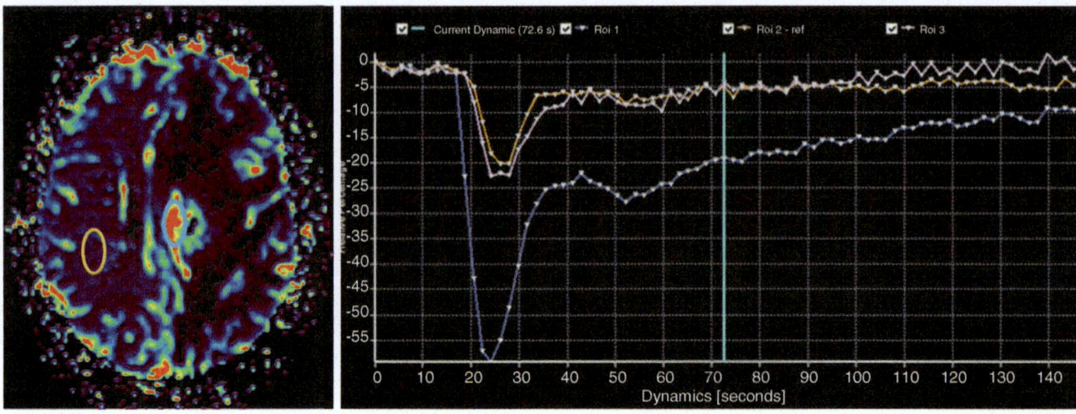

Fig. 1 DSC perfusion imaging. Regions of interest placed in normal appearing white matter (orange) and tumor (blue) on the CBV map. The signal intensity over time within the ROIs is plotted in the time intensity curve, from which different perfusion metrics can be calculated, as presented in the tables. The RCBV is calculated by dividing the CBV in the tumor by the CBV in the normal appearing white matter

To better distinguish radionecrosis/pseudoprogression from recurrent tumor, perfusion MRI should be performed at least after radiotherapy treatment for primary brain tumors (Abbasi et al. 2018; Patel et al. 2017; Chuang et al. 2016). The usefulness of perfusion MRI to make this distinction for brain metastasis is less established (Kerkhof et al. 2018), but may be helpful. Arterial spin labeling (ASL), dynamic contrast enhancement (DCE), and dynamic susceptibility contrast (DSC) are the MRI techniques used to measure tissue perfusion. DSC (Fig. 1) is easy to implement, measure, and interpret and is therefore regarded as the preferred MRI perfusion method in brain tumor imaging by most neuroradiologists. The relative cerebral blood volume (RCBV) of suspicious tissue versus normal appearing white matter is the variable of interest in DSC imaging. RCBV is calculated by dividing the cerebral blood volume (CBV) within a region of interest (ROI) placed in suspicious tissue by the CBV within an ROI placed in normal appearing white matter.

1.2 Therapy-Related Changes That Mimic Tumor Progression

Obviously, the expected finding after brain surgery is a skull defect with underlying effusion and/or thickening of the dura, a fluid-filled resection cavity with or without surrounding edema, intracranial air, and enhancement depending on the time since the surgical intervention. These findings are easily recognizable as postsurgical changes on MRI imaging. Distinguishing between surgery-related enhancement and residual tumor can be challenging and takes radiological expertise and experience for optimal interpretation. Thin linear contrast enhancement in the edge of the resection cavity is a common tissue reaction that usually starts to occur 24–48 h *after* surgery. Thick/nodular enhancement at in the surgical area present *within* 24–48 h of resection should raise the suspicion of residual tumor. A baseline MRI of the brain within 48 h after brain surgery is therefore recommended for the detection residual tumor and as a reference for follow-up studies (Albert et al. 1995; Ekinci et al. 2003). Comparison of tumor enhancement on the presurgical MRI and enhancement around the surgical cavity on the postsurgical MRI is helpful to further distinguish residual tumor from postsurgical enhancement.

Another source of contrast enhancement is (surgery induced) ischemia. Ischemia does not enhance immediately after onset, but may start enhancing in the following weeks to months (Fig. 2) and can be mistaken for tumor progression. Relating the area of contrast enhancement

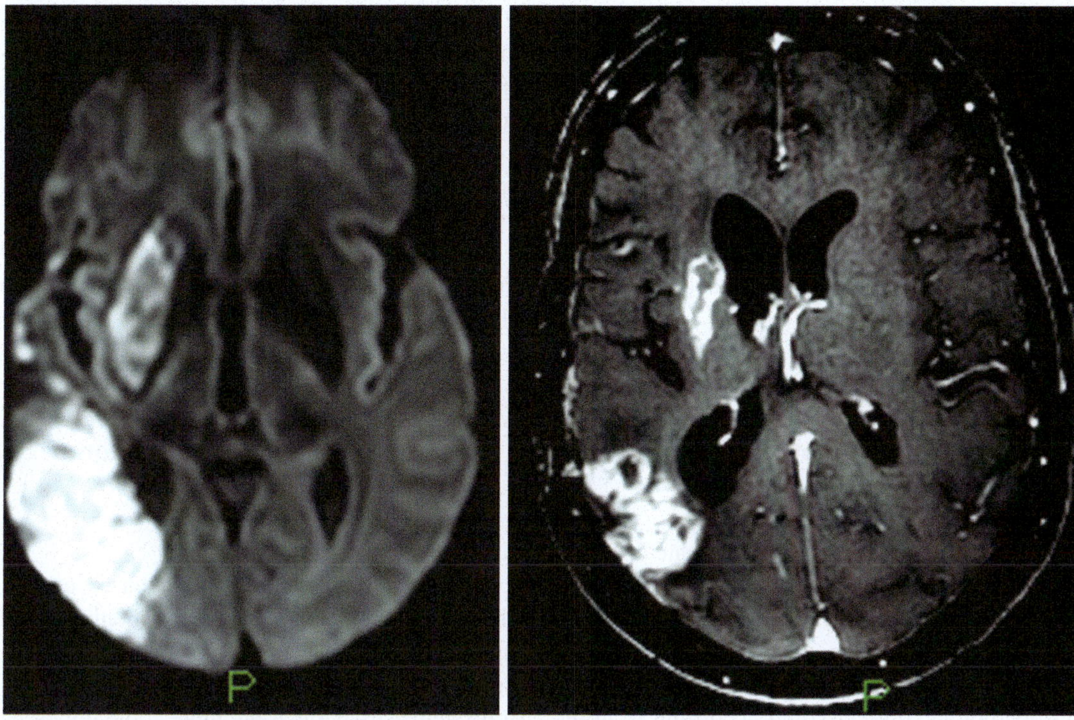

DWI at stroke   T1C after 3 months

Fig. 2 Imaging findings after ischemic stroke. The DWI shows acute infarction in right basal ganglia and right temporal/parietal region. Fulminant contrast enhancement developed within the areas of acute infarction as seen on the 3-month follow-up MRI

to a corresponding area of nonenhancing diffusion restriction on the MRI scan made within days after surgery can prove ischemia as the cause of contrast enhancement. Follow-up is another way to prove ischemia as the cause of contrast enhancement, showing a resolution of the enhancement with or without corresponding tissue loss and/or signal abnormalities as time progresses.

Increased size of previous contrast enhancement, or new enhancement of brain tissue can occur in response to, especially high dose, brain irradiation. The term pseudoprogression is used when this occurs within months after brain irradiation and radionecrosis when the increase occurs after 3–6 months after brain irradiation. Strictly speaking, these areas of increased enhancement are indistinguishable from tumor progression, although the pattern of enhancement may favor one over the other. Ring enhancement with a necrotic center or a diffuse fluffy enhancement pattern can be seen in radiation-induced enhancement and shows similarities to tumoral enhancement. RCBV perfusion measurements within the area of enhancement are extremely helpful to distinguish radiation-induced from tumor-induced enhancement. As a rule, low perfusion (i.e., similar or lower than normal appearing white matter) is seen in radiation-induced enhancement and high perfusion in high-grade glioma. Perfusion characteristics of brain metastases probably depend on the underlying primary tumor, making the perfusion harder to interpret. Perfusion of the brain metastases before radiation treatment may be useful as a reference.

Nonenhancing glioma tissue can be difficult to distinguish from signal abnormalities due to surgery or radiotherapy-induced brain tissue damage. Brain edema can be expected shortly after radiotherapy and brain surgery, presenting as an area of nonenhancing high T2 signal in white matter that respects the gray-white matter boundary, exhibits some mass effect, and occurs shortly after the therapeutic intervention. Late post-therapeutic brain tissue damage presents as nonenhancing T2 signal abnormalities with no mass effect or even mass-sparing effect. The main differential diagnosis of these late post-therapeutic signal abnormalities is diffusely growing glial tumor. Stability over time is the most certain sign of late post-therapeutic tissue damage.

2 Tumors Arising from Glial Cells

2.1 Tumor Classification WHO Criteria

The term "glial cells" is used to indicate different nonneuronal cell types that form the supportive tissue of brain parenchyma, including oligodendrocytes, astrocytes, microglia, and ependymal cells. Tumors that arise from these glial cells are histopathologically classified according to criteria defined by the World Health Organization (WHO) based on microscopic similarities with different types of glial cells (hence the names astrocytoma, oligoastrocytoma, and oligodendroglioma) and graded from I to IV according to their presumed growth rate, likelihood of further dedifferentiation, and extent of invasive growth (Louis et al. 2007).

In recent years, new evidence has emerged implicating the prognostic value of several genetic markers of brain tumors, resulting in a major update of the WHO criteria in 2016. These new criteria aim to combine both histopathological and genetic features in tumor classification, for which in some cases the genetics can overrule histopathologic features (Louis et al. 2016). With regard to astrocytomas, oligodendrogliomas, and glioblastomas, the major genotypes that are considered in this classification are presence of IDH mutation, 1p/19q codeletion, and H3K27M mutation. To do justice to this new classification, a new nomenclature has been developed in which the histopathological classification is named first, followed by details regarding the genetic tumor characteristics (for example: *Oligodendroglioma, IDH-mutant,* and *1p/19q-codeleted*). The 2016 WHO criteria update for brain tumors aims to improve tailoring of patient therapy, better classification for clinical trials, and more precise categorization for epidemiological purposes. Further updates are expected to come in the near future with the accumulation of knowledge on brain tumor genotype and its clinical implications.

At present, the 2016 WHO brain tumor criteria are the standard for tumor classification on which treatment decisions are based.

2.2 Low-Grade Astrocytoma (WHO II) and Anaplastic Astrocytoma (WHO III)

2.2.1 MR Imaging

Low-grade astrocytoma's (Fig. 3) can occur anywhere in the brain, but are most commonly located supratentorially adjacent or arising from the cortex, especially in the frontal or temporal lobes in adults. Brain stem astrocytomas are more commonly seen in children. *Low-grade astrocytomas* have homogeneous high signal intensity on T2 and FLAIR sequences with corresponding low T1 signal intensity. The margins of these tumors can vary from well-circumscribed to less-defined borders. As with all astrocytomas, the extent of signal abnormalities does not accurately reflect the true tumor extent. Normal underlying structures are usually distorted or destroyed. Low-grade tumors show no enhancement and have a low relative cerebral blood volume on perfusion MRI. In some cases, low-grade astrocytomas present as diffuse signal abnormalities in gray and white matter across multiple lobes and even across hemispheres through the corpus callosum, massa intermedia, and anterior commissure, referred to as *gliomatosis cerebri*. With this growth pattern, brain structures are typically slightly enlarged with preservation of underlying brain structures. Although the infiltration can go anywhere in the brain and even into the spinal cord, the most affected areas are the thalamus, basal ganglia, brainstem, corpus callosum, and cerebellum. Gliomatosis cerebri has been deleted from the latest WHO criteria, as this is regarded as a growth pattern that can occur in astrocytic as well as oligodendroglial tumors.

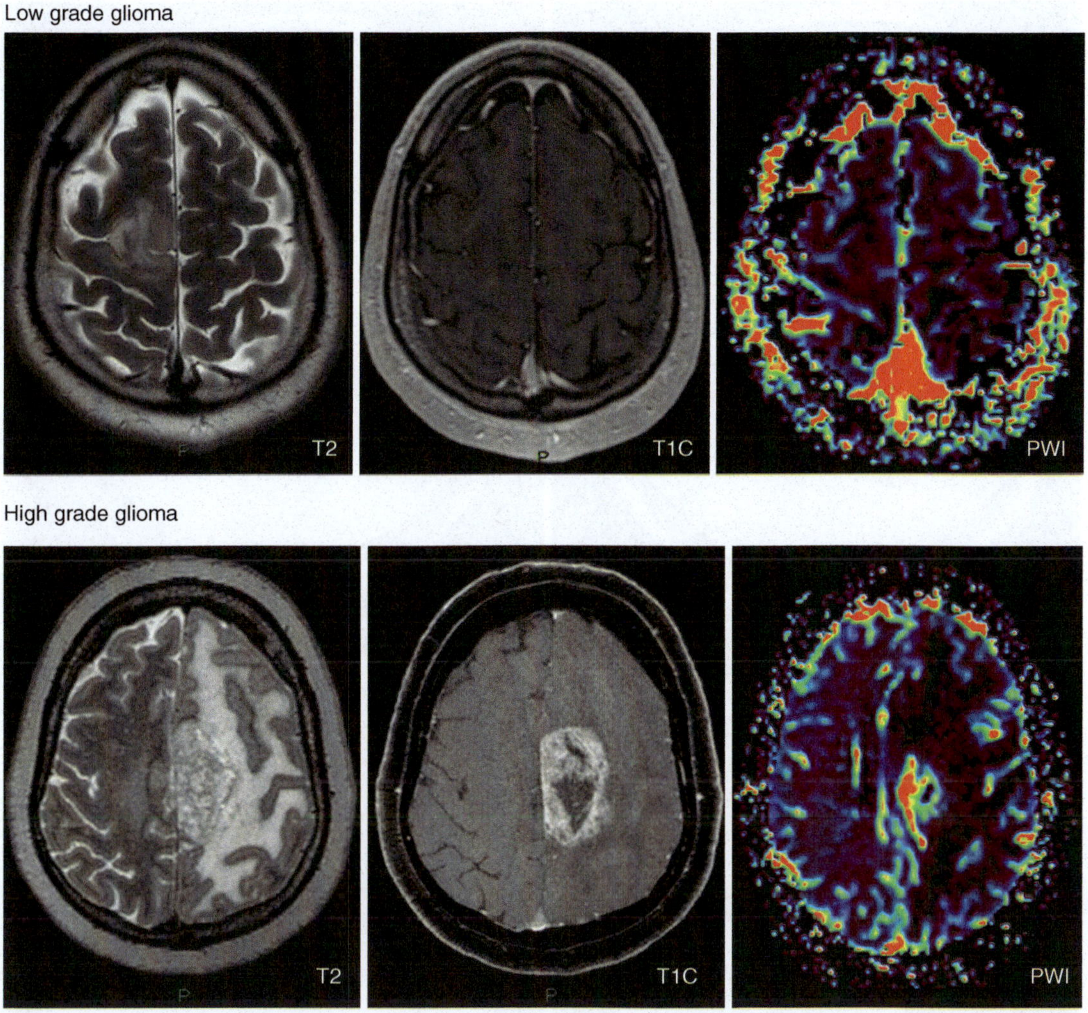

Fig. 3 Low-grade and high-grade glioma. Nonenhancing region of increased T2 signal intensity including both cortex and adjacent white matter in the right frontal lobe in a low-grade glioma (top). Perfusion was not increased. Heterogenous enhancing tumor with necrotic components, surrounding edema, and regions of increased perfusion in the left frontal lobe in a high-grade glioma/glioblastoma (bottom)

For all low-grade gliomas, enlargement at follow-up, enhancement, or increased RCBV within the tumor is suggestive of progression to a higher grade and is commonly referred to as *anaplastic astrocytoma (WHO III)*. Anaplastic astrocytomas may exhibit a more heterogeneous signal intensity on T1- and T2-weighted sequences and may show greater mass effect as compared to low-grade astrocytomas. Perfusion imaging usually shows an increased RCBV. Focal, patchy, or homogeneous contrast enhancement can occur. Evident enhancement with non-enhancing necrotic components is suspicious for further progression to glioblastoma (WHO IV).

2.3 Low-Grade Glioma: Oligodendroglioma (WHO II)

2.3.1 MR Imaging

Oligodendrogliomas (Fig. 4) are usually cortically or subcortically based and most commonly occur in the frontal lobes but may arise in other parts of the supratentorial brain. An infratentorial

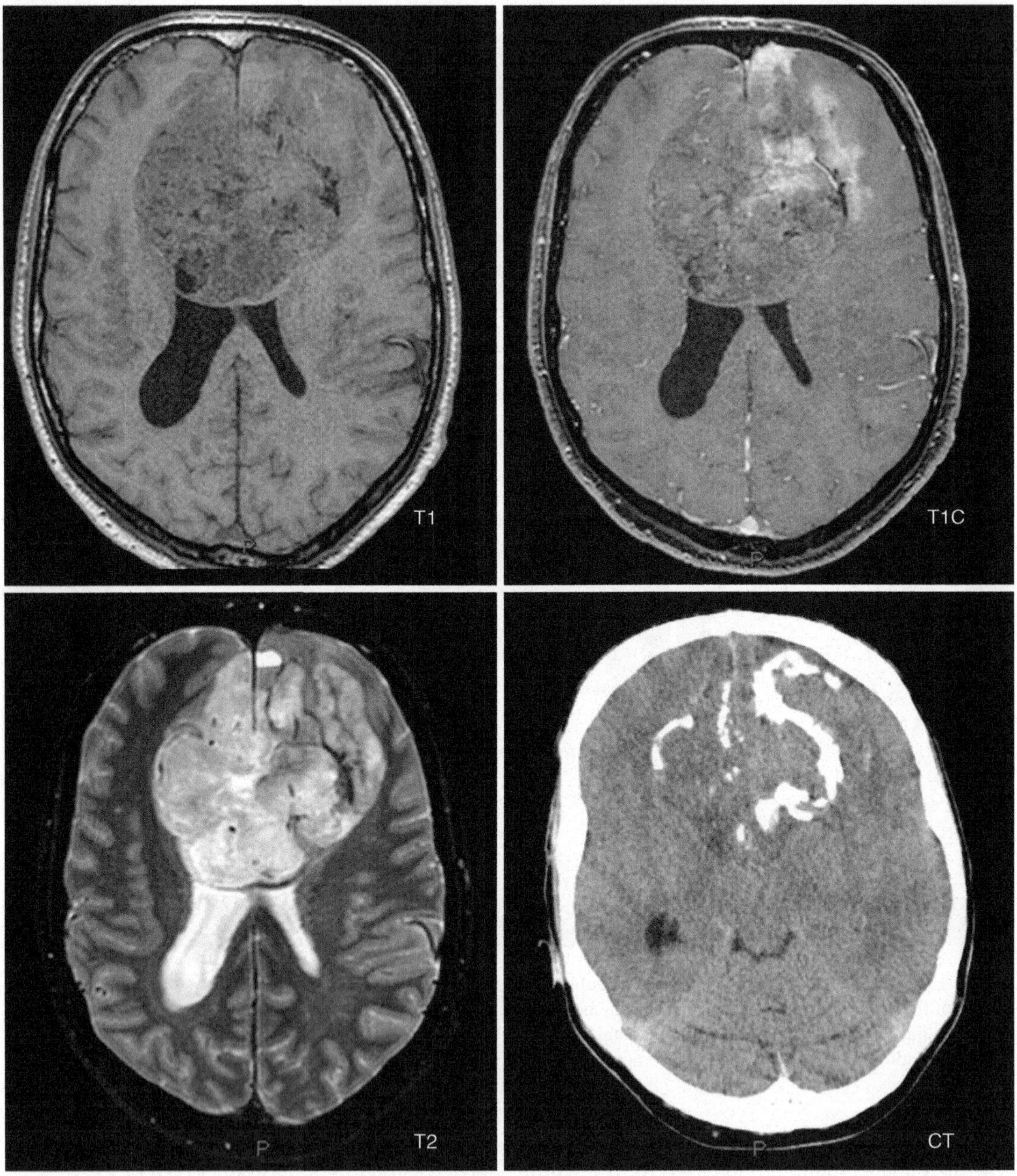

Fig. 4 Oligodendroglioma. Frontal tumor with heterogeneous signal intensity on T1 and T2, some enhancing components, and coarse calcifications. The calcifications are seen as low signal intensity on especially T2 sequences and as high-density components on CT

location is uncommon. Signal characteristics are heterogeneously low on T1 and heterogeneously high on T2-/FLAIR-weighted sequences. These tumors can have cystic components and a varying degree of perifocal edema. Calcifications are common and explain part of the heterogeneity. When in doubt, susceptibility-weighted MRI (SWI), T2 gradient echo, or, especially, CT can be used to better characterize these calcifications. Contrast enhancement is variable from no enhancement to heterogeneous patchy enhancement. Enhancement and increased RCBV on perfusion imaging are not sure signs of high-grade tumor components and should not be interpreted as such on initial imaging. Short-term follow-up can be considered in the setting of tumor enhancement, increased perfusion, and changes in tumor size or tumor characteristics (especially new enhancement and/or increased RCBV) on follow-up imaging.

2.3.2 Radiotherapy Planning

The diagnosis of diffuse low-grade astrocytoma needs to be confirmed by tissue examination after biopsy or surgery. Therapeutic options include radiation, chemotherapy, or careful observation.

Radiation therapy can be used to reduce the size of the tumor and may improve symptoms. The optimal timing and dose of radiation for this type of tumor is still being studied. There is a longstanding discussion on the advantages and disadvantage between immediate ("early") radiotherapy and delayed ("deferred") radiotherapy at the time of progression. A large randomized European trial (EORTC 22845 study) recently examined this question of early versus deferred radiation therapy. Although early radiation slightly delayed the average time until regrowth, the overall survival outcome of both the early and deferred groups was identical. Results from two clinical trials (EORTC 22844 and ECOG/RTOG) focusing on low-grade gliomas suggest that high-dose radiotherapy is not preferable to lower-dose radiotherapy, and patients should receive doses in the range of 50.4–54 Gy in 1.8 Gy fractions. A randomized phase II clinical trial is comparing proton beam versus photon-based intensity-modulated radiation in IDH mutant grade II or III glioma regarding side effects (NCT03180502).

MRI-based target definition for radiotherapy dose planning is the standard practice for neuro-oncology (Schmidt and Payne 2015). As most low-grade tumors usually do not have contrast-enhancing lesions, the target volume is determined by the surgical cavity and/or MRI FLAIR or T2 abnormalities (Fig. 3). Since the survival of patients treated for low-grade tumors is sufficient to experience long-term neurocognitive deficits (Douw et al. 2009; Klein 2012), the target definition with regard to normal tissue is very relevant. Unfortunately, previous randomized trials have never explored failure patterns and neurocognitive sequelae based on target definition and margins. The most commonly used target definition is the surgical cavity and/or MRI FLAIR or T2 abnormalities plus a margin of 2 cm (edited to anatomical borders) (Sarmiento et al. 2015). Intensity modulated radiation therapy (IMRT) modifies the dose distribution as conformal to the target volume as possible. Using a volumetric arc therapy (VMAT) technique, the normal tissue dose can be better spared than with IMRT and is now widely implemented (Briere et al. 2017). The normal tissue dose is especially important in low-grade glioma because of the long-term survival and the risks associated with radiation dose to the normal tissue. Whereas protons have physical properties that reduce the dose to the normal tissue, superior toxicity profiles of proton therapy compared with those of photon therapy have not been established (Combs 2017).

2.4 High-Grade Glioma: Glioblastoma (WHO IV)

2.4.1 MR Imaging

Microvascular proliferation and necrosis are the microscopic hallmarks of *glioblastoma* (Fig. 3). Similarly, the typical MRI characteristic of glioblastoma is jagged thick enhancement around a nonenhancing necrotic core. Solid, nodular, ring, or patchy enhancement is seen less often. The tumor is usually surrounded by a large area of high signal on T2/FLAIR sequences that can partly be due to infiltrating tumor in combination with perifocal edema. As with other astrocytomas, tumor tissue may extend far beyond the observed signal abnormalities. Perfusion imaging shows markedly increased RCBV within the enhancing tumor components, due to microvascular proliferation. Glioblastoma is relentlessly destructive and can invade through all brain structures, including cranial nerves, subependymal lining of the ventricles, and into the leptomeningeal space.

2.4.2 Radiotherapy Planning

For high-grade glioma, two radiation schemes are mostly applied, either 60Gy in 30 fraction combined with temozolomide (Hegi et al. 2005; Stupp 2006; Stupp et al. 2007) or a shortened scheme of 40 Gy in 15 fractions (Perry et al. 2017). Different guidelines exist for target delineation in high-grade gliomas. The ESTRO-ACROP guidelines recommend a target definition that is based on the postoperative T1/T2 FLAIR abnormalities (Niyazi et al. 2016). These guidelines propose a 1.5–2 cm volumetric expansion around the tumor to create a clinical target volume (CTV) to encompass microscopic disease as 80% of recurrences occurs within a 2 cm margin. In general, this expansion is adjusted to anatomical borders and to some extent by T2/FLAIR abnormalities (Fig. 5a, b). To accommodate for individual patient setup uncertainties and registration errors, a margin of 2–5 mm is recommended dependent on the experience within the institute where the patient is treated.

Although the tumor definition on both the preoperative as the postoperative MRI correlates with the recurrence pattern, most institutes define the target on the postoperative MRI scan because of superior target definition (Farace et al. 2011). A dedicated radiotherapy MRI scan is recommended for planning purposes since significant (and prognostic important) regrowth and changes can be observed in the time interval between the postoperative MRI and the start of the radiotherapy (Pirzkall et al. 2009; Villanueva-Meyer et al. 2017) (Fig. 6).

Other imaging modalities are currently not the standard for delineation purposes, although much research is being done to optimize the target volume of the individual patient. MRI diffusion tensor imaging (DTI) may be able to improve detection of microscopic spread of the tumor cells and improve target definition (Jensen et al. 2017; Price et al. 2007). Positron emission tomography (PET) modality has not been introduced as standard modality. Functional imaging might be especially helpful in the recurrent setting to differentiate between radiation necrosis and tumor recurrence (Hoijati et al. 2018).

3 Primary Central Nervous System Lymphoma

3.1 MR Imaging

High nuclear/cytoplasmic ratio is an important histologic feature of primary central nervous system lymphomas (Fig. 7). This feature is reflected in the typical finding of diffusion restriction (high signal on DWI and low signal on ADC) and relatively low T2 signal intensity on MRI and high density on CT images.

Lymphomas are classically periventricular in location and can involve the corpus callosum and deep gray matter structures. A more peripheral location in close relationship with the gray-white matter junction can also be observed. Strong and homogeneous tumor enhancement is typical. High T2 signal of surrounding tissue due to edema is a common feature. These tumors can be solitary or multiple.

The expected imaging and pathological features of lymphomas are drastically altered in immunocompromised patients. Although homogeneous imaging features can occur, heterogeneity is a typical feature of lymphomas in immunocompromised patients. The pattern of enhancement is heterogeneous and can include peripheral enhancement with central necrosis. T1 and T2 signal intensities can be heterogeneous depending on the degree of necrosis and hemorrhage. The appearance of lymphoma in immunocompromised patients frequently leads to differential diagnostic challenges, as the imaging features mimic that of glioblastoma, toxoplasmosis, metastasis, and brain abscess.

3.2 Radiotherapy

The role of radiotherapy is excellently discussed in the review of Kasenda et al. (2016). The technique is whole brain radiotherapy (WBRT) using a CT scan and mask-based approach of two lateral fields. SRS may be used in highly selected patients (e.g., relapse or refractory) (Shin et al. 2017) using contrast-enhanced MRI for target delineation.

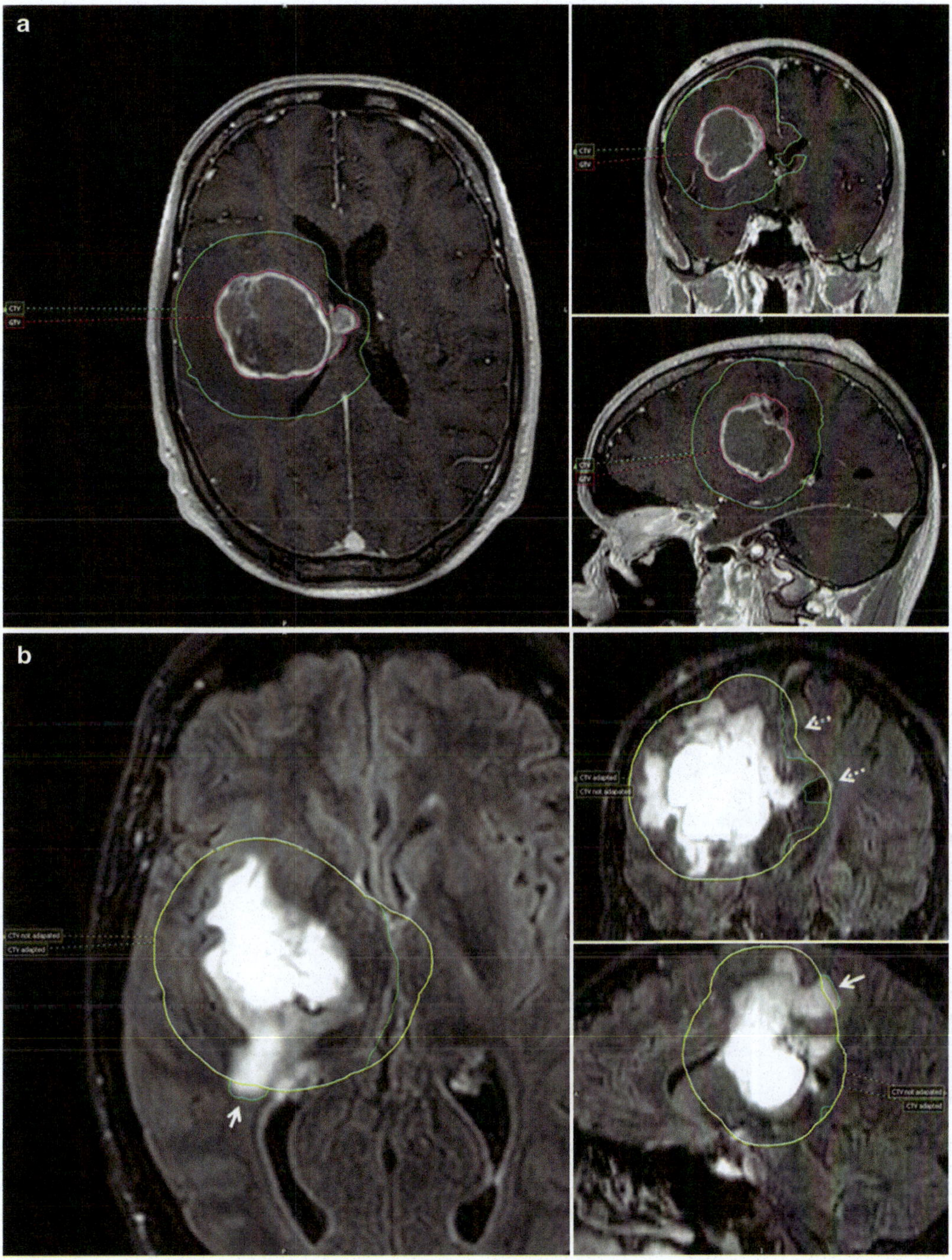

Fig. 5 (**a**) Anatomical borders; the gross total volume (GTV, purple line) is defined by the T1 contrast-enhancing lesion. This volume is expended with 1.5 cm to encompass the microscopic disease (clinical target volume (CTV, green line). Anatomical borders (in this case, the falx cerebri, white arrow) should be taken into account and will prevent unnecessary irradiation dose. (**b**) Beside the adaptation to anatomical border, also margin editing may be performed to include the areas that are at risk for microscopic spread. In this case, the 1.5 cm CTV margin did not include all the FLAIR intense region, and the CTV (green line) was manually adapted from the original CTV (yellow line) to include this region as well (solid arrows). As was already shown in Fig GB1A, the CTV (green line) was also edited according to the falx cerebri and ventricle (dashed arrows)

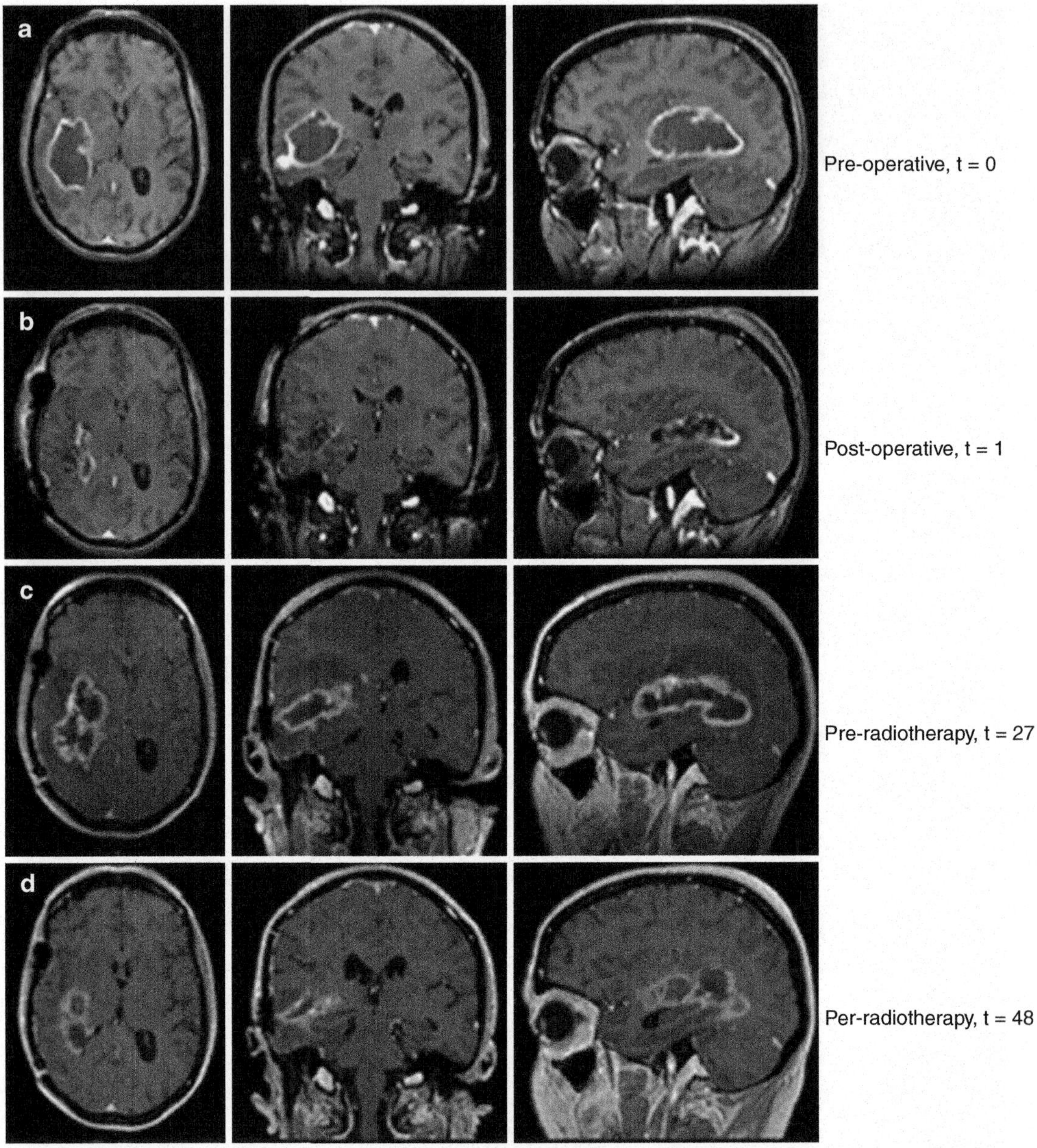

Fig. 6 This patient has a right temporal tumor as can be seen on the navigation MRI made for neurosurgery purposes (**a**, $t = 0$ days). After subtotal resection as defined on the postoperative MRI made within 48 h (**b**, $t = 1$ day), the patient was prepared for radiotherapy with a dedicated planning MRI on day 27 (**c**). Significant tumor regrowth occurred within this period of time. This tumor did respond to the radiotherapy as can be seen on the MRI in the third week of irradiation (**d**)

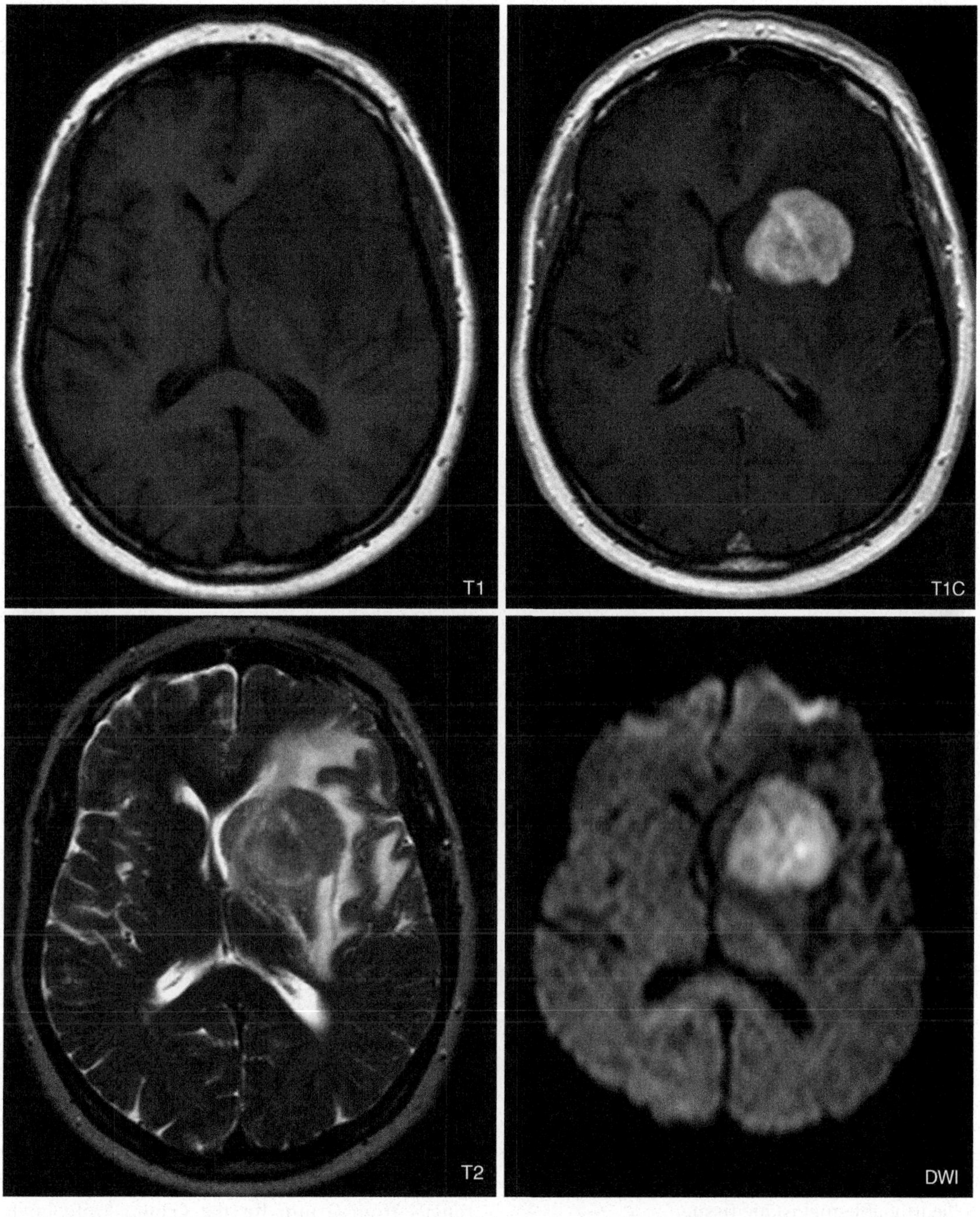

Fig. 7 Lymphoma. Solid-enhancing tumor in the left basal ganglia with surrounding edema in a 77-year-old woman with right-sided hemiparesis and aphasia. Low T2 signal intensity and high signal on DWI is caused by high cellularity of this tumor

4 Metastases

4.1 MR Imaging

Contrast enhancement within lesions is the conclusive feature to look for when assessing the brain for metastatic disease (Fig. 8). A simple and common solid parenchymal brain metastasis will have a low T1, high T2, and homogeneous enhancement. However, T1/T2 characteristics and pattern of enhancement can vary depending on the composition of the metastasis, depending on necrosis, hemorrhage, melanin content, calcifications, and cystic components. In some instances, the T1/T2 characteristics can provide a clue to the original primary tumor. Mucinous metastases tend to have a low T2 signal and is suggestive of metastasis from a primary gastrointestinal mucinous adenocarcinoma. Melanoma metastases can show a high T1 signal and low T2 signal due to melanin content. Hemorrhage is frequently encountered in metastases from melanoma, renal cell carcinoma, choriocarcinoma, thyroid cancer, lung cancer, and breast cancer. Special caution should be observed when distinguishing hemorrhagic components from viable metastatic tissue. In most cases, this distinction should not pose a problem when the enhancing metastasis is well defined with some small intratumoral hemorrhagic components. The extent of metastatic lesions is harder if not impossible to distinguish in larger hemorrhage that extend beyond the metastasis margins (Fig. 8), as hemorrhage can entirely obscure the enhancing component of the metastasis. Additionally, hemorrhage can show enhancement over time. Thin ring enhancement at the margins of hemorrhage is the most typical pattern, although a more diffuse enhancement can sometimes be observed. Nodular enhancing components in or at the margin of the hemorrhage give a clue to viable metastatic tissue.

Most brain metastases occur within brain parenchyma at any location, with a predilection for the interface between cortex and gray matter. Leptomeningeal enhancement presents as contrast enhancement on the surface of the brain, that is, within the sulci of the supratentorial brain, foliae of the cerebellum, the surface of the brain stem/cervical spinal cord, and cranial nerves (most easily observed on the vestibulocochlear and trigeminal nerves). The extent of leptomeningeal enhancement is probably not representative of the full extent of the leptomeningeal metastases. Absence of leptomeningeal enhancement does not rule out leptomeningeal metastasis and should prompt consideration of lumbar puncture depending on the degree of clinical suspicion. Hydrocephalus can occur due to changes in CSF flow dynamics and is highly suspicious of leptomeningeal in the appropriate clinical setting. Dural metastasis can arise from the dura or can occur as direct extension from skull metastasis. Dural metastases are most frequently observed in patients with breast carcinoma. The dural metastases can present as an enhancing mass lesions attached to the dura or a plaque similar to enhancing thickening of the dura. These tumors can be hard to distinguish from meningiomas on imaging alone.

4.2 Radiotherapy

Radiotherapy for brain metastasis is a dynamic field in which the indication and technique undergo rapid changes and development. Because of the toxicity (neurocognitive decline), WBRT is more and more abandoned for the sake of the quality of life. Stereotactic radiosurgery (SRS) is a technique in which high-dose radiotherapy is applied in a single or in several fractions. The T1 plus contrast is being used to delineate the tumor, and usually no CTV margin is taken into account since brain metastasis do not have an infiltrative character (Baumert et al. 2006). The PTV margin is dependent on the technique that is used and ranges from 0 mm for the Gammaknife up to 1–3 mm for Linac-based or Cyberknife based SRS. Seymour et al. (2015) showed that the interval between the imaging and the treatment delivery is of importance. Whereas it was assumed that target lesions within the brain were not subject to

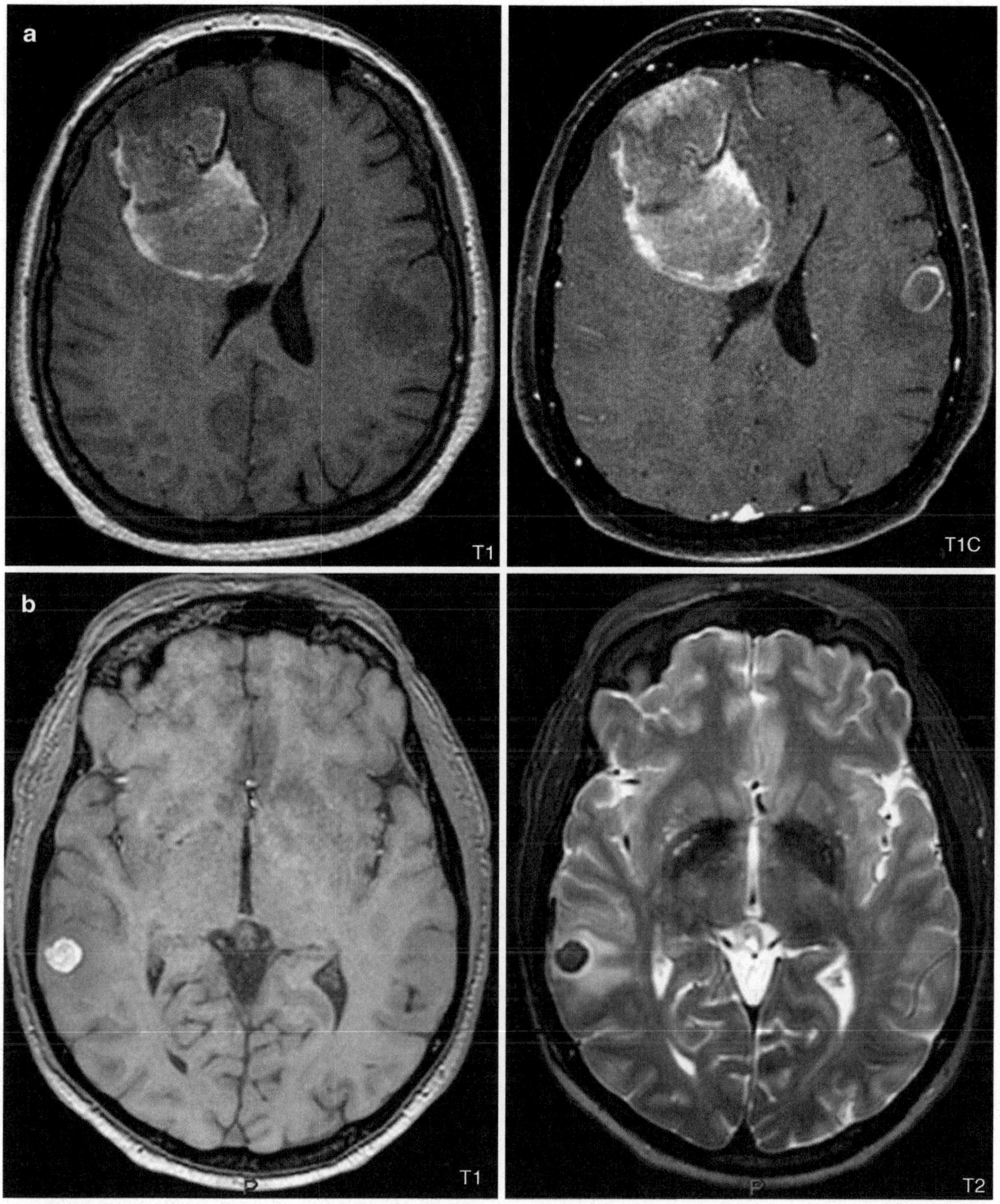

Fig. 8 (**a**) Brain metastases. Large hemorrhage in the right frontal lobe with heterogeneously high signal intensity on the T1 sequence without contrast. The T1 sequence with contrast shows enhancing tissue at the anterior side of the hemorrhage, making the diagnosis of hemorrhagic brain metastasis. A smaller ring-enhancing brain metastasis is seen in the left frontal lobe. (**b**) Metastasis in the right temporal lobe with high signal on the T1-weighted sequence without contrast and very low signal intensity on T2. The signal intensities are consistent with melanin within this melanoma metastasis

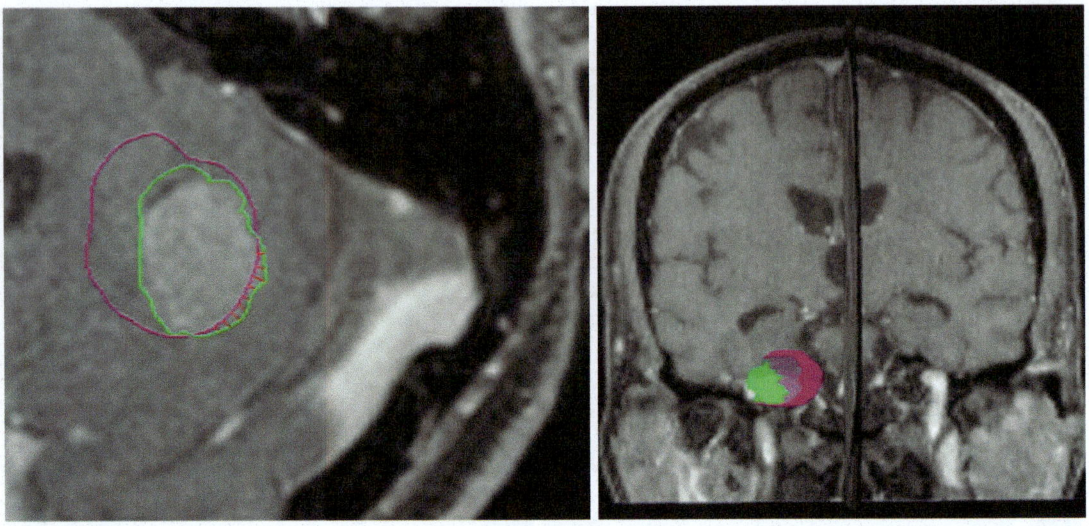

Fig. 9 Example of a patient who received one dose of dexamethasone the day before the MRD and continued dexamethasone intake hereafter (2dd4mg). The MRRT was made 8 days later, and the tumor contours overlaid on sagittal (left) and coronal (right) view of the MRRT T1w+c image. The pink contour is the reference contour from the MRD examination, whereas the green contour is delineated on the data from the MRRT examination. The red lines in the left image represent the positive distances between the two tumor surfaces. The right image shows a 3D depiction of these tumor contours. Here, the MRRT tumor volume is shifted outside the MRD tumor volume as indicated in green (Hessen et al. 2017)

movements, Hessen et al. (2017) showed that significant location shifts of brain metastases can occur (Fig. 9). For this reason, it is important to limit the time interval between the MRI and treatment delivery and to not change the steroid prescription within this interval. For fractionated SRS, tumor location shifts can have a major impact on the delivered radiotherapy dose, and for some patients, a repeated MRI during fractionated SRS is indicated (Hessen et al. 2019; Fig. 10).

For all target areas in radiotherapy planning and delivery, it is important to take MRI distortion and patient position into account (Schmidt and Payne 2015). This is especially important when safety margins around the GTV are small or not applied.

5 Meningioma

5.1 MR Imaging

Meningiomas (Fig. 11) arise from the meningothelial cells and are therefore typically extra-axial in location. The typical MRI pattern is that of a strongly enhancing mass attached to the meninges that, depending on the size, pushes away adjacent brain structures. Signs of extra-axial location are a cleft between the tumor and brain parenchyma, splaying of the cortex, and dural tail. Keep in mind that the dural tail is not only specific for meningioma but can also be seen with other pathologies such as dural metastases. The T1 signal of the parenchyma is similar to that of gray matter, whereas the T2 signal can be variable. Calcifications are commonly seen and are best observed using CT. A central feeding artery arising from the dura may be appreciated especially on T2-weighted images (flow voids) and is virtually pathognomonic for meningioma. Thickening of the adjacent bone is highly suggestive of meningioma. Edema and even cyst-like structures can be observed in adjacent brain parenchyma.

Meningiomas are mostly located supratentorially arising from the convexities or falx. Less common but classical locations are the olfactory groove, parasellar region, and sphenoid wing. When infratentorially located, meningiomas tend to occur at the cerebellopontine angle, with schwannoma as the most important differential diagnosis.

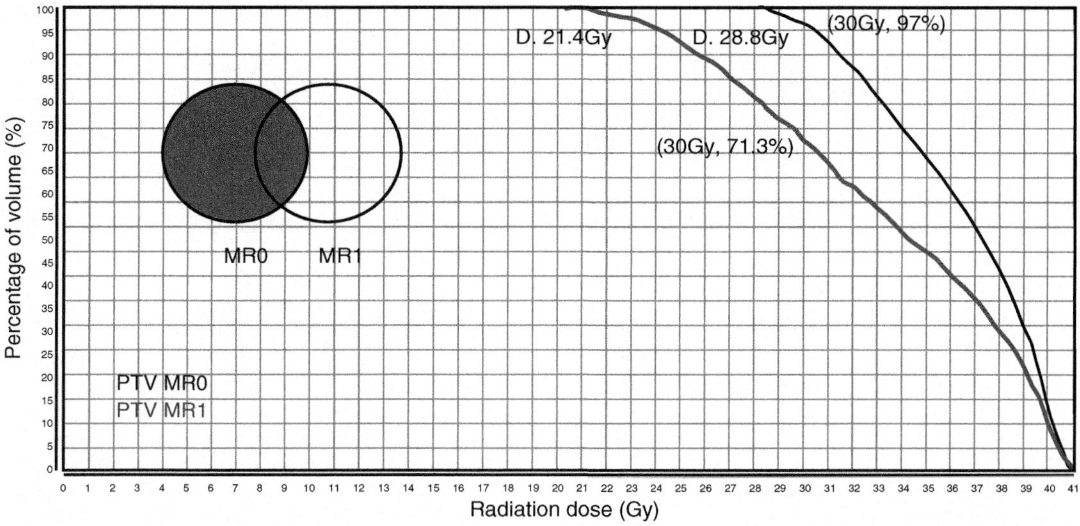

Fig. 10 Schematic view of the two target volumes with tumor shift. MR0 = planning MRI; MR1 = repeated MRI during fractionated SRS. As can be seen in a clinical example, the dose volume histogram of a radiotherapy plan for the target defined on MR0 has a minimum dose of 28.8Gy. However, the minimum dose half way the treatment as defined on MR1 is 21.4Gy. Also, the PTV coverage decreased by 25.7 percentage points within this time frame (time = 8 days). PTV = planning target volume; MR0 = planning MRI; MR1 = repeated MRI; fSRS = fractionated stereotactic radiosurgery (Hessen et al. 2019)

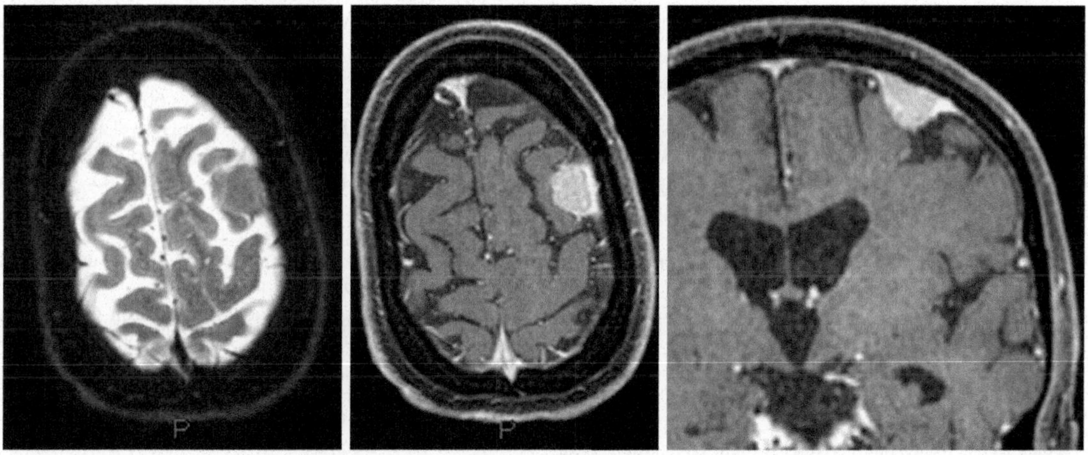

Fig. 11 Meningioma. Extra-axial solidly enhancing mass attached to the dura with intermediate T2 signal. The brain is pushed away by the tumor. A dural tail can be appreciated on the coronal image

Although a mass lesion is the most common presentation of meningioma, meningiomas may present as a more plaque-like thickening of the dura (meningioma en plaque) or can be entirely intraosseous. Meningioma can in some instance be found within the lateral ventricle, around the optic nerve, or the pineal region.

5.2 Radiotherapy

Treatment options for meningioma is dependent on many different factors such as WHO grade, size, growth rate, symptoms, location and patient performance, and preference. Whereas WHO I lesions can be treated with surgery or radiotherapy alone, WHO grade II and III lesions are often treated by the combination of surgery and radiotherapy. Whether radiotherapy is given in a single, several, or multiple fractions is dependent on the size and location. Gammaknife-based radiotherapy has the advantage of a no PTV margins and steeper dose gradient, resulting in less unwanted radiotherapy dose to the normal tissue (Ma et al. 2014) as compared with other radiotherapeutic modalities. Postoperative radiotherapy encompasses residual disease and/or the postoperative cavity determined on contrast-enhanced MRI. For some locations (e.g., the skull base), the additional value of functional imaging is under investigation to improve the target delineation (Stade et al. 2018).

In general, no margin is taken into account for microscopic spread even though meningiomas often show a dural tail sign (Fig. 11) which is a thickening of the dura adjacent to the tumor (Wilms et al. 1989). Although some studies show tumor cells in the dural tail, others described the dural tail as a vascular effect of the dura from proliferating connective tissue (Aoki et al. 1990, Rokni-Yazdi et al. 2009). Whether or not to include the dural tail in the target definition is an ongoing debate. Based on retrospective studies, it seemed safe to not include the whole dural tail and to consider only inclusion of the dural tail that is directly adjacent to the tumor (Dibiase et al. 2004, Bulthuis et al. 2014).

References

Abbasi AW, Westerlaan HE, Holtman GA, Aden KM, van Laar PJ, van der Hoorn A (2018) Incidence of tumour progression and pseudoprogression in high-grade Gliomas: a systematic review and meta-analysis. Clin Neuroradiol 28:401. https://doi.org/10.1007/s00062-017-0584-x

Albert FK, Forsting M, Sartor K, Adams HP, Kunze S (1995) Early postoperative magnetic resonance imaging after resection of malignant glioma: objective evaluation of residual tumor and its influence on regrowth and prognosis. Neurosurgery 36:873. https://doi.org/10.1227/00006123-199504000-00045

Aoki S, Sasaki Y, Machida T, Tanioka H (1990) Contrast-enhanced MR images in patients with meningioma: importance of enhancement of the dura adjacent to the tumor. AJNR Am J Neuroradiol 11(5):935–938

Baumert BG, Rutten I, Dehing-Oberije C, Twijnstra A, Dirx MJM, Debougnoux-Huppertz RMTL et al (2006) A pathology-based substrate for target definition in radiosurgery of brain metastases. Int J Radiat Oncol Biol Phys 66:187. https://doi.org/10.1016/j.ijrobp.2006.03.050

Briere TM, McAleer MF, Levy LB, Yang JN (2017) Sparing of normal tissues with volumetric arc radiation therapy for glioblastoma: single institution clinical experience. Radiat Oncol. 12(1):79. https://doi.org/10.1186/s13014-017-0810-3

Bulthuis VJ, Hanssens PE, Lie ST, van Overbeeke JJ (2014) Gamma Knife radiosurgery for intracranial meningiomas: Do we need to treat the dural tail? A single-center retrospective analysis and an overview of the literature. Surg Neurol Int. 5(Suppl 8):S391–S395. https://doi.org/10.4103/2152-7806.140192. eCollection 2014

Chuang MT, Liu YS, Tsai YS, Chen YC, Wang CK (2016) Differentiating radiation-induced necrosis from recurrent brain tumor using MR perfusion and spectroscopy: a meta-analysis. PLoS One 11:e0141438. https://doi.org/10.1371/journal.pone.0141438

Combs SE (2017) Does proton therapy have a future in CNS tumors? Curr Treat Options Neurol 19(3):12. https://doi.org/10.1007/s11940-017-0447-4

DiBiase SJ, Kwok Y, Yovino S, Arena C, Naqvi S, Temple R, Regine WF, Amin P, Guo C, Chin LS (2004) Factors predicting local tumor control after gamma knife stereotactic radiosurgery for benign intracranial meningiomas. Int J Radiat Oncol Biol Phys 60(5):1515–1519

Douw L, Klein M, Fagel SS, van den Heuvel J, Taphoorn MJ, Aaronson NK, Postma TJ, Vandertop WP, Mooij JJ, Boerman RH, Beute GN, Sluimer JD, Slotman BJ, Reijneveld JC, Heimans JJ (2009) Cognitive and radiological effects of radiotherapy in patients with low-grade glioma: long-term follow-up. Lancet Neurol 8(9):810–818

Ekinci G, Akpinar IN, Baltacioğlu F, Erzen C, Kiliç T, Elmaci I, Pamir N (2003) Early-postoperative magnetic resonance imaging in glial tumors: prediction of tumor regrowth and recurrence. Eur J Radiol 45:99. https://doi.org/10.1016/S0720-048X(02)00027-X

Ellingson BM, Bendszus M, Boxerman J, Barboriak D, Erickson BJ, Smits M et al (2015) Consensus recommendations for a standardized brain tumor imaging protocol in clinical trials. Neuro-Oncology. https://doi.org/10.1093/neuonc/nov095

Farace P, Giri MG, Meliadò G, Amelio D, Widesott L, Ricciardi GK et al (2011) Clinical target volume delineation in glioblastomas: pre-operative versus post-operative/pre-radiotherapy MRI. Br J Radiol 84:271. https://doi.org/10.1259/bjr/10315979

Hegi ME, Diserens A-C, Gorlia T, Hamou M-F, de Tribolet N, Weller M et al (2005) MGMT gene silencing and benefit from Temozolomide in Glioblastoma. N Engl J Med 352:997. https://doi.org/10.1056/nejmoa043331

Hessen ED, van Buuren LD, Nijkamp JA, de Vries KC, Kong Mok W, Dewit L, van Mourik AM, Berlin A, van der Heide UA, Borst GR (2017) Significant tumor shift in patients treated with stereotactic radiosurgery for brain metastasis. Clin Transl Radiat Oncol 2:23–28

Hessen E, Nijkamp J, Damen P, Hauptmann M, Jasperse B, Dewit L, Lutkenhaus L, Lamers E, van der Heide U, Damen E, Hanssens P, Borst G (2019) Predicting and implications of target volume changes of brain metastases during fractionated stereotactic radiosurgery. Radiother Oncol. pii: S0167-8140(19)33001-4

Jensen MB, Guldberg TL, Harbøll A, Lukacova S, Kallehauge JF (2017) Diffusion tensor magnetic resonance imaging driven growth modeling for radiotherapy target definition in glioblastoma. Acta Oncol 56:1639. https://doi.org/10.1080/0284186X.2017.1374559

Karim AB, Maat B, Hatlevoll R, Menten J, Rutten EH, Thomas DG, Mascarenhas F, Horiot JC, Parvinen LM, van Reijn M, Jager JJ, Fabrini MG, van Alphen AM, Hamers HP, Gaspar L, Noordman E, Pierart M, van Glabbeke M (1996) A randomized trial on dose-response in radiation therapy of low-grade cerebral glioma: European Organization for Research and Treatment of Cancer (EORTC) Study 22844. Int J Radiat Oncol Biol Phys 36(3):549–556. https://clinicaltrials.gov/ct2/show/NCT03180502

Kasenda B, Loeffler J, Illerhaus G, Ferreri AJM, Rubenstein J, Batchelor TT (2016) The role of whole brain radiation in primary CNS lymphoma. Blood 128:32. https://doi.org/10.1182/blood-2016-01-650101

Kerkhof M, Ganeff I, Wiggenraad RGJ, Lycklama à Nijeholt GJ, Hammer S, Taphoorn MJB et al (2018) Clinical applicability of and changes in perfusion MR imaging in brain metastases after stereotactic radiotherapy. J Neuro-Oncol 138:133. https://doi.org/10.1007/s11060-018-2779-7

Klein M (2012) Neurocognitive functioning in adult WHO grade II gliomas: impact of old and new treatment modalities. Neuro Oncol 14(Suppl 4):iv17–iv24

Louis DN, Ohgaki H, Wiestler OD, Cavenee WK, Burger PC, Jouvet A et al (2007) The 2007 WHO classification of tumours of the central nervous system. Acta Neuropathol 114:97. https://doi.org/10.1007/s00401-007-0243-4

Louis DN, Perry A, Reifenberger G, von Deimling A, Figarella-Branger D, Cavenee WK et al (2016) The 2016 World Health Organization classification of tumors of the central nervous system: a summary. Acta Neuropathol 131:803. https://doi.org/10.1007/s00401-016-1545-1

Ma L, Nichol A, Hossain S, Wang B, Petti P, Vellani R, Higby C, Ahmad S, Barani I, Shrieve DC, Larson DA, Sahgal A (2014) Variable dose interplay effects across radiosurgical apparatus in treating multiple brain metastases. Int J Comput Assist Radiol Surg 9(6):1079–1086. Published online 2014 Apr 20. https://doi.org/10.1007/s11548-014-1001-4

Niyazi M, Brada M, Chalmers AJ, Combs SE, Erridge SC, Fiorentino A et al (2016) ESTRO-ACROP guideline "target delineation of glioblastomas.". Radiother Oncol 118:35–42

Patel P, Baradaran H, Delgado D, Askin G, Christos P, Tsiouris AJ, Gupta A (2017) MR perfusion-weighted imaging in the evaluation of high-grade gliomas after treatment: a systematic review and meta-analysis. Neuro-Oncology 19:118. https://doi.org/10.1093/neuonc/now148

Perry JR, Laperriere N, O'Callaghan CJ, Brandes AA, Menten J, Phillips C et al (2017) Short-course radiation plus Temozolomide in elderly patients with Glioblastoma. N Engl J Med 376:1027. https://doi.org/10.1056/NEJMoa1611977

Pirzkall A, McGue C, Saraswathy S, Cha S, Liu R, Vandenberg S et al (2009) Tumor regrowth between surgery and initiation of adjuvant therapy in patients with newly diagnosed glioblastoma. Neuro-Oncology 11:842. https://doi.org/10.1215/15228517-2009-005

Price SJ, Jena R, Burnet NG, Carpenter TA, Pickard JD, Gillard JH (2007) Predicting patterns of glioma recurrence using diffusion tensor imaging. Eur Radiol 17:1675. https://doi.org/10.1007/s00330-006-0561-2

Rokni-Yazdi H, Azmoudeh Ardalan F, Asadzandi Z, Sotoudeh H, Shakiba M, Adibi A, Ayatollahi H, Rahmani M (2009) Pathologic significance of the "dural tail sign". Eur J Radiol 70(1):10–16

Sarmiento JM, Venteicher AS, Patil CG (2015) Early versus delayed postoperative radiotherapy for treatment of low-grade gliomas. Cochrane Database Syst Rev 6:CD009229. https://doi.org/10.1002/14651858.CD009229.pub2

Schmidt MA, Payne GS (2015) Radiotherapy planning using MRI. Phys Med Biol. Author manuscript; available in PMC 2016 Dec 5

Seymour ZA, Fogh SE, Westcott SK, Braunstein S, Larson DA, Barani IJ, Nakamura J, Sneed PK (2015) Interval from imaging to treatment delivery in the radiation surgery age: how long is too long? Int J Radiat Oncol Biol Phys 93(1):126–132. https://doi.org/10.1016/j.ijrobp.2015.05.001. Epub 2015 May 7

Shin SM, Silverman JS, Bowden G, Mathieu D, Yang HC, Lee CC, Tam M, Szelemej P, Kaufmann AM, Cohen-Inbar O, Sheehan J, Niranjan A, Lunsford LD, Kondziolka D (2017) Relapsed or refractory primary central nervous system lymphoma radiosurgery: report of the International Gamma Knife Research Foundation. J Radiosurg SBRT 4(4):247–253

Stade F, Dittmar J-O, Jäkel O, Kratochwil C, Haberkorn U, Debus J, Combs SE (2018) Influence of 68Ga-DOTATOC on sparing of normal tissue for radiation therapy of skull base meningioma: differential impact of photon and proton radiotherapy. Radiat Oncol 13(58). https://doi.org/10.1186/s13014-018-1008-z. Published online 2018 Apr

Stupp R (2006) Changing paradigms—an update on the multidisciplinary management of malignant

glioma. Oncologist 11:165. https://doi.org/10.1634/theoncologist.11-2-165
Stupp R, Hegi ME, Gilbert MR, Chakravarti A (2007) Chemoradiotherapy in malignant glioma: standard of care and future directions. J Clin Oncol 25:4127. https://doi.org/10.1200/JCO.2007.11.8554
van den Bent MJ, Afra D, de Witte O, Ben Hassel M, Schraub S, Hoang-Xuan K, Malmström PO, Collette L, Piérart M, Mirimanoff R, Karim AB, EORTC Radiotherapy and Brain Tumor Groups and the UK Medical Research Council (2005) Long-term efficacy of early versus delayed radiotherapy for low-grade astrocytoma and oligodendroglioma in adults: the EORTC 22845 randomised trial. Lancet 366(9490):985–990
Wilms G, Lammens M, Marchal G, Van Calenbergh F, Plets C, Van Fraeyenhoven L, Baert AL (1989) Thickening of dura surrounding meningiomas: MR features. J Comput Assist Tomogr 13(5):763–768

T-Staging and Target Volume Definition by Imaging in Head and Neck Tumors

Ivan Platzek, Linda Agolli, Bettina Beuthien-Baumann, and Esther G. C. Troost

Contents

1 **Introduction** 170

2 **T-Staging Using Computed Tomography** 170

2.1 Image Acquisition 170

3 **Magnetic Resonance Imaging** 172

4 **T-Staging Using Positron Emission Tomography** 175

5 **PET for HNSCC Characterization** 176

6 **Definition of the Radiation Target Volume** 177

References 178

Abstract

Anatomical and functional imaging by means of computed tomography, magnetic resonance imaging, and positron emission tomography are, besides a thorough physical examination, of utmost importance for accurate staging of primary tumors in the head and neck region. This chapter deals with the particular advantages and disadvantages of those imaging techniques and gives practical guidance on how to employ these in radiation treatment planning.

I. Platzek
Institute and Polyclinic for Diagnostic and Interventional Radiology, Faculty of Medicine and University Hospital Carl Gustav Carus, Technische Universität Dresden, Dresden, Germany

L. Agolli
Department of Radiotherapy and Radiation Oncology, Faculty of Medicine and University Hospital Carl Gustav Carus, Technische Universität Dresden, Dresden, Germany

OncoRay—National Center for Radiation Research in Oncology, Dresden, Germany

B. Beuthien-Baumann
Department of Radiology, German Cancer Research Center (DKFZ), Heidelberg, Germany

E. G. C. Troost (✉)
Department of Radiotherapy and Radiation Oncology, Faculty of Medicine and University Hospital Carl Gustav Carus, Technische Universität Dresden, Dresden, Germany

OncoRay—National Center for Radiation Research in Oncology, Dresden, Germany

Institute of Radiooncology — OncoRay, Helmholtz-Zentrum Dresden-Rossendorf, Dresden, Germany

Faculty of Medicine and University Hospital Carl Gustav Carus, Technische Universität Dresden, Dresden, Germany
e-mail: esther.troost@uniklinikum-dresden.de

R. G. H. Beets-Tan et al. (eds.), *Imaging and Interventional Radiology for Radiation Oncology*,
Medical Radiology, Diagnostic Imaging, https://doi.org/10.1007/978-3-030-38261-2_12

1 Introduction

Ultrasound imaging, computed tomography (CT), and magnetic resonance imaging (MRI) are the main imaging modalities used in the head and neck region. In staging of head and neck squamous cell carcinoma (HNSCC), the use of ultrasound is limited to the assessment of cervical lymph nodes due to artifacts caused by bones and air cavities. Both CT and MRI allow for a complete assessment of all anatomical structures of the head and neck including the primary tumor. The choice between CT and MR for staging of primary HNSCC is greatly influenced by the tumor location, the availability of the respective imaging modality, and the preferences of the referring physicians or the radiologists.

The clinical TNM classification is essential for both the choice of treatment and prognosis in head and neck cancer (Kademani et al. 2005). T-staging of head and neck cancer varies according to the tumor location taking into account the tumor size and the presence of invasion of adjacent anatomical structures (Table 1, Sobin et al. 2010).

2 T-Staging Using Computed Tomography

2.1 Image Acquisition

CT scans are routinely obtained in supine position, and modern multi-slice CT scanners allow for very short acquisition times of even less than 1 s. CT examinations of the head and neck region are routinely performed after injection of iodinated contrast media (typically 80 to 100 ml with an injection rate of 2–5 ml/s) in order to improve the inherently low soft tissue contrast of CT. Recommendations regarding the interval between initiation of contrast injection and of CT data acquisition vary between 35–40 s and 70 s (Baum et al. 2000).

In some cases, dynamic maneuvers may be helpful to evaluate anatomical structures of the head and neck. Such maneuvers are possible due to the short acquisition times of CT. Examples of these maneuvers are puffing the cheeks for improved visualization of the buccal plane and modified Valsalva maneuver for improved visualization of the pyriform sinuses (Weissman and Carrau 2001).

A complete examination of the head and neck region should cover the area between the sella turcica (upper border) and the sternoclavicular joints (lower border). Both soft tissue window images and bone window images are routinely calculated from CT examinations of the head and neck. Soft tissue images are used for assessment of tumor spread and of cervical lymph nodes, while bone window images are indispensable for reviewing bony structures, including possible destruction caused by a tumor. With current CT scanners, a slice thickness of 0.6 mm can be achieved. In general, a slice thickness of 3 mm is adequate for the evaluation of the head and neck. Besides the routinely obtained axial images, reconstructions with axial and coronal orientation are recommended and can be very helpful for assessment of tumor extent.

CT is widely used for T-staging of HNSCC for the primary tumors which usually show stronger contrast enhancement when compared to surrounding tissues, e.g., muscles. Smaller HNSCC may be visible as a focal mucosal thickening, while larger tumors tend to be enhancing masses disturbing the normal symmetry, and they may include necrotic areas. CT is of particular use for identifying clinical T4 disease, which is associated with invasion into surrounding tissues, such as bone, for several HNSCC subsites (Mukherji et al. 2001). CT is also the preferred imaging modality for evaluation of laryngeal cancer, for destruction of the cartilage can be detected, which also influences the clinical T-staging and thus the treatment choice. The soft tissue contrast of CT is usually insufficient to visualize perineural tumor spread encountered in, for example, adenoid cystic carcinoma. An indirect sign of perineural tumor spread may be bone destruction adjacent to neuroforamina, which, in turn, is well visible on CT.

Apart from the clinical indications of CT for T-staging, other advantages of CT include its wide availability, short scan times, and relatively

Table 1 Overview of clinical T-staging for the primary head and neck squamous cell carcinoma (according to eighth edition of AJCC TNM Staging Manual)

HNSCC subsite	cT0	cT1	cT2	cT3	cT4
Nasopharynx[a]	No primary tumor identified	Tumor confined to nasopharynx or extends to oropharynx and/or nasal cavity without parapharyngeal involvement	Tumor with parapharyngeal extension and/or adjacent soft tissue involvement (medial or lateral pterygoid, and/or prevertebral muscles)	Tumor invades bony structures of skull base cervical vertebra, pterygoid structures, and/or paranasal sinuses	Tumor with intracranial extension and/or involvement of cranial nerves, hypopharynx, orbit, parotid gland, and/or infiltration beyond the lateral surface of the lateral pterygoid muscle
Oropharynx, p16 positive[a]	No primary tumor identified	Tumor 2 cm or smaller in greatest dimension	Tumor more than 2 cm but not more than 4 cm	Tumor more than 4 cm or extension to lingual surface of epiglottis	Tumor invades any of the following: Larynx, deep/ extrinsic muscle of tongue, medial pterygoid, hard palate, mandible, or beyond
Oropharynx, p16 negative[a]	No primary tumor identified	Tumor 2 cm or smaller in greatest dimension	Tumor more than 2 cm but not more than 4 cm	Tumor more than 4 cm or extension to lingual surface of epiglottis	Tumor invades any of the following: Larynx, deep/ extrinsic muscle of tongue, medial pterygoid, hard palate, mandible, or beyond
Oral cavity	No primary tumor identified	Tumor 2 cm or smaller in greatest dimension	Tumor more than 2 cm but not more than 4 cm	Tumor more than 4 cm or extension	**cT4a** Tumor invades adjacent structures only (through cortical bone [mandible, maxilla], into deep [extrinsic] muscle of tongue, maxillary sinus, skin of face) **cT4b** Tumor invades masticator space, pterygoid plates, or skull base and/or encases internal carotid artery
Larynx, supraglottis	No primary tumor identified	Tumor limited to one subsite of supraglottis with normal vocal cord mobility	Tumor invades mucosa of more than one adjacent subsite of supraglottis or glottis or region outside supraglottis	Tumor limited to larynx with vocal cord fixation and/or invades any of the following: Postcricoid area, pre-epiglottic space, paraglottic space, and/or inner cortex of thyroid cartilage	**cT4a** Tumor invades through the outer cortex of the thyroid cartilage and/or invades tissues beyond the larynx **cT4b** Tumor invades prevertebral space, encases carotid artery, or invades mediastinal structures

(continued)

Table 1 (continued)

HNSCC subsite	cT0	cT1	cT2	cT3	cT4
Larynx glottis	No primary tumor identified	**cT1a** Tumor limited to one vocal cord **cT1b** Tumor involves both vocal cords	Tumor extends to supraglottis and/or subglottis, and/or impaired vocal cord mobility	Tumor limited to the larynx with vocal cord fixation and/or invasion of paraglottic space, and/or inner cortex of thyroid cartilage	**cT4a** Tumor invades through the outer cortex of the thyroid cartilage and/or invades tissues beyond the larynx **cT4b** Tumor invades prevertebral space, encases carotid artery, or invades mediastinal structures
Larynx subglottis	No primary tumor identified	Tumor limited to the subglottis	Tumor extends to vocal cord(s) with normal or impaired mobility	Tumor limited to larynx with vocal cord fixation and/or invasion of paraglottic space and/or inner cortex of the thyroid cartilage	**cT4a** Tumor invades cricoid or thyroid cartilage and/or invades tissues beyond the larynx **cT4b** Tumor invades prevertebral space, encases carotid artery, or invades mediastinal structures
Hypopharynx	No primary tumor identified	Tumor limited to hypopharynx and 2 cm or smaller in greatest dimension	Tumor extending to more than one part of the hypopharynx, or invades the nearby structures, or is larger than 2 cm but smaller than 4 cm in greatest dimension and has not affected the vocal cords	Tumor larger than 4 cm in greatest dimension, or tumor affecting the movement of the vocal cords, or invasion in the esophagus	**cT4a** Tumor invades the thyroid or cricoid cartilage, the hyoid bone, the thyroid gland, or nearby areas of muscle or fat **cT4b** Tumor invades prevertebral space, encases carotid artery, or invades mediastinal structures

[a]Major modification in eighth Edition of the AJCC TNM Cancer Staging Manual

low cost. Due to the short scan times, CT suffers less from motion artifacts than MR, and it holds the possibility to perform a complete staging examination (covering head and neck, thorax, abdomen, and pelvis) in a single scan.

Nowadays, the CT scans obtained in routine clinical practice are mainly obtained using a single x-ray source with only one energy. Stemming from the urge to characterize kidney stones, CT techniques have been further developed to (simultaneously or sequentially) acquire two images using two x-ray energies, thus enabling more in-depth tissue characterization. This so-called "dual energy CT" technique has the potential to improve tumor delineation due to better visibility of contrast media (Kuno et al. 2012).

3 Magnetic Resonance Imaging

Modern clinical MRI scanners typically have a magnetic field strength of 1.5 or 3 Tesla and are thus well suited for imaging of primary head and neck tumors. MR examinations are performed with the patient in a supine position using a head–neck coil. For radiation treatment planning purposes, the MR scan may be acquired with the patient in treatment position, i.e., wearing a head and neck mask. However, imaging equipment needs to be modified for this purpose (Paulus et al. 2014). Current MR scanner uses multielement coils capable of parallel acquisition, which help reduce acquisition times. However, acquisition times are substantially longer when compared to CT (approx. 20–30 min).

MR examinations typically consist of several MR measurements (sequences) for obtaining complementary anatomical and functional information. In HNSCC patients, one sequence (i.e., T1 weighted) acquires contrast-enhanced images after the administration of small quantities of gadolinium chelates, since contrast media improve tumor detection and delineation. Moreover, a typical MR protocol in HNSCC patients includes T1-weighted images in axial orientation, short tau inversion recovery (STIR) images in axial and coronal orientation, and T1-weighted contrast-enhanced images with fat suppression in axial and coronal orientation. For HNSCC staging, a slice thickness of $\leq$3 mm is recommended.

MRI has a high soft tissue contrast and is therefore the preferred imaging modality in patients suspected of having or proven to have a carcinoma of the oral cavity (i.e., the tongue, oropharynx, or floor of mouth) (Ong and Chong 2006). Moreover, MR is superior to CT for the detection and delineation of skull base infiltration in nasopharyngeal tumors, and it is more sensitive to the detection of perineural tumor spread (Ong and Chong 2006; Caldemeyer et al. 1998). In most cases, HNSCCs are hypointense on non-enhanced T1-weighted images and hyperintense on STIR images. Most HNSCCs show strong gadolinium enhancement on T1-weighted images with the exception of non-enhancing necrotic tumor areas.

Besides anatomical imaging, MRI can also be used for tissue characterization, e.g., to assess tumor perfusion or water molecule diffusion. In order to assess tissue perfusion, dynamic contrast-enhanced MR can be acquired. Analysis of MR perfusion data allows for several parameters to be quantified, i.e., blood plasma volume per unit tissue volume (V_p), volume transfer constant (K_{trans}), and volume per unit tissue volume (VE) (Gaddikeri et al. 2016). Perfusion parameters are possible biomarkers for tumor cell hypoxia, which in turn is an important adverse prognostic factor in HNSCC, and hold prognostic value with respect to both radiochemotherapy response and disease-free survival (Chawla et al. 2011; Kim et al. 2009; Nordsmark et al. 2005). Water molecule diffusion (i.e., Brownian motion) in tissues, which is linked to tissue cellularity, can be assessed by diffusion-weighted imaging (DWI). Most malignant tumors, including HNSCC, have a high cell density, which leads to diffusion restriction compared to healthy tissues. While the use of DWI of the HNSCC has been evaluated in numerous studies, it is currently not part of routine MRI protocols in patients with HNSCC. The most promising indications for DWI in HNSCC include nodal staging, evaluation of treatment response, and suspected tumor recurrence. Even though this is not the prime subject of this chapter, these applications are briefly highlighted here (Fig. 1).

Since all lymph nodes have a high cell density and thus less diffusion than the surrounding fat and muscles, visual evaluation of unprocessed DWI images is not appropriate for differentiating between benign and malignant lymph nodes. Instead, the so-called apparent diffusion coefficient (ADC), derived from DWI MRI, can be used to quantify diffusion in the lymph nodes. This approach is more time consuming than visual evaluation, as it is currently necessary to define regions of interest (ROIs) for the evaluated lymph nodes manually.

In a recently published meta-analysis, Suh et al. (2018) were able to show that in patients with HNSCC of the head and neck, ADC values derived from metastatic lymph nodes are significantly lower than those derived from benign lymph nodes. Suh et al. (2018) have calculated an optimal cutoff ADC value of 0.965 × 10^3mm^2/s and a sensitivity and specificity of 90% and 88%, respectively. It should be mentioned, however, that the number of studies (and patients) summarized in this meta-analysis was rather low (9 studies, 337 patients) and that the meta-analysis did not include a direct comparison with conventional MR sequences used in HNSCC imaging (i.e., turbo spin echo sequences). Noteworthy, a meta-analysis on the accuracy of conventional

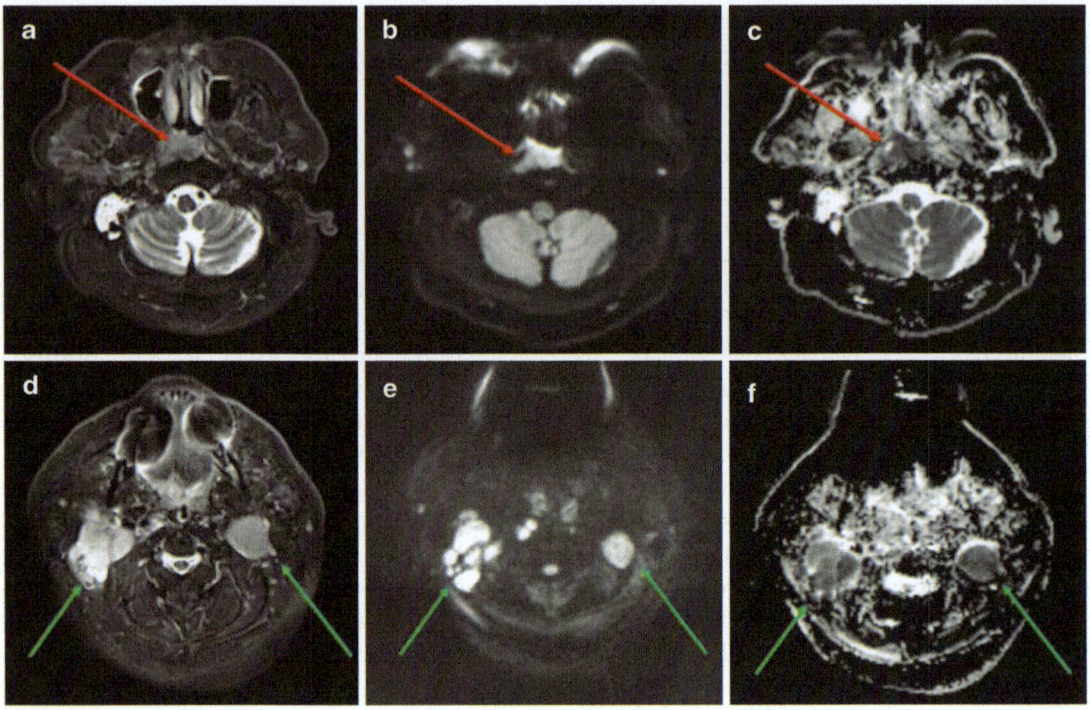

Fig. 1 Patient with a squamous cell carcinoma of the nasopharynx (red arrow) and bilateral lymph node metastases (green arrows). (**a**) and (**d**) are conventional short tau inversion recovery turbo spin echo images shown for comparison. The tumor and lymph node metastases present with high signal intensity on high *b*-value DWI images [$b = 1000$ s/mm^2, (**b**, **e**)] and low signal intensity on apparent diffusion coefficient (ADC) maps (**c**, **f**)

MRI has calculated a pooled sensitivity and specificity of 65% and 81% (Liao et al. 2012).

Another potential use of DWI in HNSCC is the prediction of treatment response. For this, the primary tumor needs to be delineated to calculate the ADC and potentially other quantitative diffusion parameters. The mode of evaluating treatment response, however, is not standardized. In a recent meta-analysis, Zhou et al. (2018) determined the pooled sensitivity and specificity of ADC for predicting locoregional failure after radiochemotherapy to be 82% and 70%, respectively. Also, ADC was found to correlate with disease-free survival and overall survival (Hatakenaka et al. 2014).

Finally, DWI may aid identifying persistent or recurrent HNSCC, which is difficult with conventional MRI sequences. Early studies were able to demonstrate that ADCs of persistent or recurrent HNSCC are significantly lower than those of benign tissues (Vandecaveye et al. 2007; Abdel Razek et al. 2006). The combination of DWI and conventional MRI is able to improve the detection of HNSCC recurrence in comparison with standalone conventional MRI (Tshering Vogel et al. 2013). In addition, Yu et al. (2017) have shown that the accuracy of DWI for persistent HNSCC after radiochemotherapy compares favorably with that of positron emission tomography using F18-fluoro-deoxy-glucose ([^{18}F]FDG-PET/CT; see next paragraph). At present, though, [^{18}F]FDG-PET/CT is the better-validated method for assessment of recurrent disease in HNSCC.

Overall, despite promising results, the adoption of DWI in head and neck imaging has been hampered by lack of standardization of acquisition parameters, by the time-consuming nature of quantitative evaluation, and also by partly conflicting results of early studies. Recent meta-analyses provide an argument for the use DWI in HNSCC, especially for lymph node staging. Larger, ideally multicenter studies are necessary to improve standardization of acquisition parameters and evaluation of DWI of the head and neck.

Overall, the main advantages of MRI over CT are its superior soft tissue contrast, and the variety of anatomical and functional sequences available for tumor characterization and possibly in the future personalized treatment. Important contraindications for MR include most types of cardiac pacemakers, nerve simulators, insulin or analgesic pumps, and metal implants. As for CT, MRI of the head and neck region suffers from dental implant artifacts.

4 T-Staging Using Positron Emission Tomography

If positron emission tomography (PET) is included into the staging procedure of HNSCC patients for the assessment of the local and regional disease extent as well as possible distant metastases, the radiopharmaceutical most frequently applied is the glucose analogue [^{18}F]FDG. In malignant processes, [^{18}F]FDG uptake reflects metabolic activity of tumors and thus can be seen as a surrogate of the total viable tumor cell density. Most primary HNSCC and their metastases exhibit an increased glucose metabolism, which is in general higher than the glucose uptake of the surrounding structures. Nevertheless, physiologic uptake in moderate hypermetabolic structures, such as the ring of Waldeyer or the salivary glands, may render the differentiation between tumor and benign lymphoid tissue difficult (Burrell and Van den Abbeele 2005). Furthermore, tracer uptake is found in inflammatory tissue and subsequent reactive lymph nodes, which may lead to false-positive readings in proximity of the tumor and/or on regional lymph nodes. Due to the inherent restriction of the spatial resolution of PET, very small (<<1 cm) and/or only superficially spreading tumors with intermediate glucose metabolism may be missed using [^{18}F]FDG-PET, although they may be readily detectable by clinical examination.

In general, exact T-staging is not considered the domain for PET, since exact size and/or infiltration of surrounding structures can only be judged by morphologic imaging modalities, i.e., CT or MRI. Since PET scans are most often being performed on hybrid scanners such as PET/CT or more recently PET/MR, T-staging can be gathered from the morphologic component, whereas the glucose uptake and its distribution pattern serve as one of the multiple possible characteristics of the primary HNSCC. Nonetheless, occasionally small tumors undetectable by morphologic imaging and lacking uptake of contrast agent may exhibit substantial glucose metabolism and can only be detected by [^{18}F]FDG-PET. This may also be true in HNSCC patients with substantial artifacts on CT or MRI imaging originating from, for example, dental fillings (Fig. 2) (O'Daniel et al. 2007; Platzek et al. 2014).

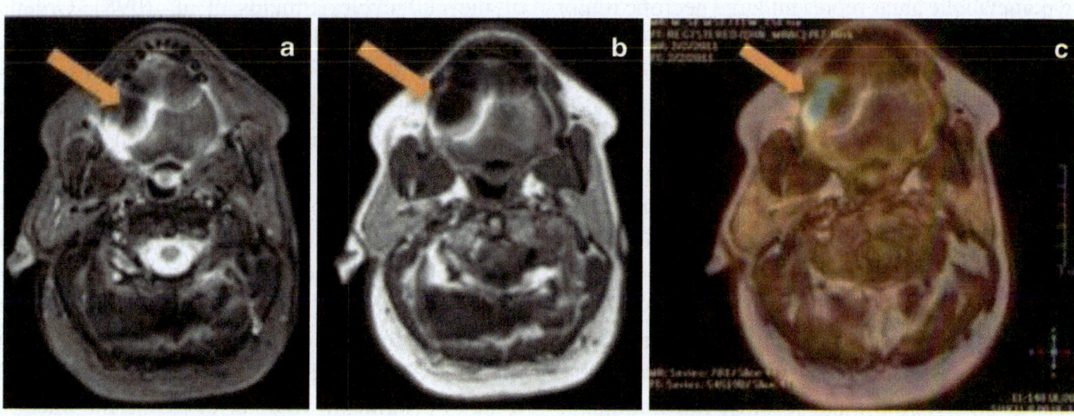

Fig. 2 (**a**) Turbo inversion recovery magnitude (TIRM), turbo spin echo (TSE) MRI, (**b**) T1-weighted TSE-MRI without contrast enhancement, and (**c**) fused [^{18}F]FDG-PET-MR of a patient with a cT2N0M0 squamous cell carcinoma of the right tongue. The tumor diagnosis and staging on MRI was heavily hampered by dental metal artefacts and relied on [^{18}F]FDG-PET instead (orange arrows)

In patients with cervical lymph node metastases of squamous cell origin, a primary tumor in the head and neck region is often anticipated. [^{18}F]FDG-PET (combined with CT or MRI) is a valuable tool for identification of the unknown primary tumor and is recommended in case the conventional work-up, i.e., panendoscopy under general anesthesia with tonsillectomy and blind biopsies and anatomical imaging has not revealed conclusive results. The detection rate of [^{18}F]FDG-PET was found to be between 30% and 50% in these circumstances (Johansen et al. 2011; Ruhlmann et al. 2016). Noteworthy, false-positive readings may occur, if [^{18}F]FDG-PET is performed after panendoscopy with multiple biopsies.

5 PET for HNSCC Characterization

Primary HNSCC display various, often heterogeneous tumor characteristics, e.g., tumor cell hypoxia and proliferation. These tumor characteristics adversely affect treatment outcome and can be incorporated in personalized treatment decisions (Corvo et al. 1993; Gray et al. 1953; Kim and Tannock 2005; Troost et al. 2010a). Tumor cell hypoxia stems from a chaotic and inferior vascular network hampering the supply of oxygen and nutrients thus leading to chronic hypoxia or from acutely blocked perfusion due to infarction or vessel breakdown resulting in acute hypoxia (Bussink et al. 2003). When using [^{18}F]FDG for PET imaging, hypometabolic areas represent large necrotic tumor subvolumes, whereas vital tumor shows enhanced glucose metabolism. Both hypoxia and proliferation may be underlying mechanisms for pronounced [^{18}F]FDG-uptake, but to what degree both characteristics contribute to the PET signal cannot be gathered from the [^{18}F]FDG-image alone.

A well-characterized hypoxia-related PET tracer that has been used in various (pre-)clinical studies is the nitroimidazole-derivative F18-fluoro-misonidazole (FMISO) (Löck et al. 2017; Thorwarth et al. 2005; Troost et al. 2006, 2008; Zips et al. 2012). Similar to other nitroimidazole derivatives (i.e., EF3, EF5, FAZA, HX4), FMISO is taken up by the cells and is trapped under hypoxic conditions, when the compound is reduced. FMISO will leave the normoxic cell unchanged and thus not lead to enhanced tracer accumulation under normoxic circumstances (Koch et al. 1995). Generally, the tumor-to-background ratio (TBR) for FMISO and the other nitroimidazole PET tracers is rather low (Peeters et al. 2015). Therefore, strategies leading to higher TBR have been pursued, such as static FMISO-PET imaging 3–4 h post injection or analysis of dynamic FMISO-PET uptake (Abolmaali et al. 2011; Welz et al. 2017). Several studies have investigated the prognostic value of FMISO-PET for outcome after radio(chemo)therapy in HNSCC. Data indicate that not only the baseline scan may hold prognostic information for the outcome after radio(chemo)therapy but also reoxygenation as detected by FMISO occurring early during the course of treatment was found to be of high prognostic value in recently published exploration and validation cohorts (Löck et al. 2017; Thorwarth et al. 2005; Troost et al. 2006, 2008; Zips et al. 2012). Also FAZA-PET has been used for the assessment of its prognostic value in HNSCC patients, and it is part of an ongoing EORTC study (Servagi-Vernat et al. 2014).

The proliferative activity of the primary tumor can be assessed in vivo using the thymidine-analogue 3'-deoxy-3'[^{18}F]fluorothymidine (FLT). FLT is transported into the cell via the human nucleoside transporter-1 and trapped after phosphorylation by the cytosolic thymidine kinase 1, which is upregulated during the S-phase of the cell cycle (Shields et al. 1998). Organs with physiologically high proliferative activity, such as bone marrow, exhibit an intense FLT-uptake. However, the FLT-uptake in HNSCC is generally lower compared with [^{18}F]FDG, most likely reflecting the situation that only a proportion of tumor cells are proliferating (Hoshikawa et al. 2015). Troost et al. (2007, 2010b) found FLT-PET to reflect proliferative activity of HNSCC tumors of the oral cavity, whereas the tracer is of no value for the diagnosis of lymph node metastases. Moreover, FLT-PET was found to be of prognostic value prior to and the tracer's decline in the second week of radio(chemo)therapy in a cohort of 48 HNSCC patients (Hoeben et al. 2013; Troost et al. 2010c).

6 Definition of the Radiation Target Volume

During the past two decades, innovative radiotherapy techniques such as intensity-modulated radiation therapy (IMRT) and volumetric-modulated arc therapy (VMAT) have been developed and widely introduced for the treatment of HNSCC patients. This modern technique allows for the highly precise delivery of high-radiation doses to the target volume, i.e., primary tumor and lymph nodes, while delivering a relatively low dose to the surrounding radiation-sensitive organs at risk (OAR) (Bortfeld 2006; Gregoire et al. 2015). Consequently, too large target volumes may lead to unnecessary damage to the OARs, whereas incorrectly too small target volumes may lead to a marginal miss.

Even though there are atlases for contouring the primary tumor volume, elective nodal area, and OARs in HNSCC, the definition of the gross tumor volume (GTV) is highly variable and interobserver dependent (Brouwer et al. 2015; Gregoire et al. 2003; Jager et al. 2016). In order to define the GTV, it is mandatory to carefully take the patient's medical history, to thoroughly examine the patient's head and neck region, depending on the center's experience to perform an ultrasound examination with fine needle aspiration, and to finally acquire the aforementioned imaging, i.e., CT and/or MRI, possibly combined with [^{18}F]FDG-PET. Besides, the process of defining the GTV is influenced by other factors, such as patient positioning, image characteristics (resolution, slice thickness), image registration accuracy, and the administration of contrast during the simulation CT (Leibfarth et al. 2013; Weiss and Hess 2003). Also, the definition of the margin required for coverage of the macroscopically invisible microscopic tumor extension, resulting in the so-called clinical target volume (CTV), depends on the guidelines of the treating institute and/or observer and may range from 5 mm to 2 cm in HNSCC (Campbell et al. 2012; Hong et al. 2012; Moeckli et al. 2009; Apolle et al. 2019).

In general, a treatment planning CT (with intravenous iodine-containing contrast agent) is obtained with the patient in supine position immobilized by a customized head-and-neck support and mask. The CT scan is thus far compulsory for it holds valuable information on electron density and Hounsfield units compulsory for high-energy photon treatment planning. This CT scan can be fused with diagnostic (e.g., preoperative) CT, MR, or ([^{18}F]FDG-)PET scans.

The prime question to be addressed before using imaging in target volume delineation is its geometric accuracy and correlation with the actual tumor volume as measured in the resection specimen. This measurement is ideally performed in tumors attached to or originating from a rather rigid environment, such as the larynx, in order to avoid deformations during the fixation process. Two studies have validated the tumor size depicted on anatomical (CT and MRI) and functional ([^{18}F]FDG-PET) imaging using laryngeal resection specimens. Daisne et al. (2004) assessed 29 patients with pharyngolaryngeal carcinomas, of whom nine underwent a total laryngectomy enabling correlation of the GTVs derived by imaging with that of the surgical resection specimen. Overall, no significant difference was observed between the average GTVs delineated on CT or MRI, whereas the PET GTVs were smaller. Interestingly, the GTVs gathered from the resection specimens were even significantly smaller, illustrating that all imaging modalities actually overestimate the tumor size. In those patients having undergone a total laryngectomy, none of the imaging modalities adequately depicted the superficial tumor extension. Moreover, false-positive delineations of the cartilage, the extra laryngeal space, and pre-epiglottic extensions were detected. Only recently, Ligtenberg et al. (2017) assessed CT, MRI, and [^{18}F]FDG-PET for GTV and CTV definition in 25 laryngeal/hypopharyngeal carcinoma patients scheduled to undergo a laryngectomy. The GTVs on CT and MRI were delineated in consensus, whereas the PET volumes were automatically segmented (using a Gaussian mixture model adapted for laryngeal and hypopharyngeal tumors) (Aristophanous et al. 2007). Modality-specific CTV margins were derived based on the resection specimen and added to the GTV to achieve adequate tumor coverage. These CTVs were compared to a standard CTV, resulting from the GTV on CT with an additional margin of 10 mm. The median GTVs contoured/segmented on CT, MRI, and PET were 17.5, 15.5, and 14.5 ml, respectively, so in accordance with Daisne et al. (2004), the PET-derived GTV was the smallest. Based on the pathological specimen, the CTV margins could be substantially reduced, being 4.3 mm for CT, 6.1 mm for MRI, and 5.2 mm for PET, leading to a target volume reduction of 48–52%.

For optimal visualization and delineation of the GTV, adequate window-width/window-level (WW/WL) settings need to be chosen for CT and the optimal sequence for MR imaging. No such evidence-based recommendation can be given for PET imaging. Schinagl et al. (2007) compared five PET segmentation tools in a cohort of 78 HNSCC and reported the fixed standardized uptake value (SUV) of 2.5 to be unsuccessful in 45% of the cases. Moreover, the threshold-based PET-GTVs were on average smaller than on CT. During the past 15 years, numerous (semi-) automatic segmentation tools have been developed and applied to HNSCC, resulting in the "YAPETISM" phenomenon (yet another PET image segmentation method) (Belhassen and Zaidi 2010; Geets et al. 2007; Lee 2010; van Dalen et al. 2007). Consequently, in clinical practice, the PET-based GTV definition is often based on manual contouring or the contour defined by 50% of the maximum SUV of the tumor. Clinicians employing these approaches should be aware of their shortcomings and refrain from defining a PET-based GTV, but instead contour the GTV on anatomical imaging.

The interobserver variability can be reduced if a second observer reviews the delineation. Geets et al. (2005) found the interobserver variability among five observers contouring 20 pharyngolaryngeal GTVs, the spinal cord, and parotid glands not to differ depending on the anatomical imaging modality used, i.e., CT or MRI. Conversely, Anderson et al. (2014) assessed GTVs of 14 patients contoured by three observers and found the largest interobserver agreement to be in PET-CT imaging (48%), followed by T1-weighted MRI and CT (47%); MRI combined with PET-CT provided the least agreement in generated GTVs. These recent data suggest that efforts needed for optimal patient positioning, choice of imaging techniques and sequences, the image registration as well as their geometric accuracy cannot be underestimated.

In advancing image-guided high-precision radiotherapy, radiologists, nuclear medicine physicians, and radiation oncologists, as well as their medical physicists and technologists, should join forces with the aim to increase the tumor control probability and decrease the normal tissue complication probability for patients with squamous cell carcinomas of the head and neck. In the future, the introduction of new (combined) imaging techniques, e.g., 7 Tesla MRI, and new radiotracers for PET imaging may augment these efforts.

References

Abdel Razek AA, Soliman NY, Elkhamary S, Alsharaway MK, Tawfik A (2006) Role of diffusion-weighted MR imaging in cervical lymphadenopathy. Eur Radiol 16(7):1468–1477

Abolmaali N, Haase R, Koch A, Zips D, Steinbach J, Baumann M et al (2011) Two or four hour [(1)(8)F] FMISO-PET in HNSCC. When is the contrast best? Nuklearmedizin 50(1):22–27

Anderson CM, Sun W, Buatti JM, Maley JE, Policeni B, Mott SL et al (2014) Interobserver and intermodality variability in GTV delineation on simulation CT, FDG-PET, and MR images of head and neck Cancer. Jacobs J Radiat Oncol 1(1):006

Apolle R, Appold S, Bijl HP, Blanchard P, Bussink J, Faivre-Finn C et al (2019) Inter-observer variability in target delineation increases during adaptive treatment of head-and-neck and lung cancer. Acta Oncol 58(10):1378–1385

Aristophanous M, Penney BC, Martel MK, Pelizzari CA (2007) A Gaussian mixture model for definition of lung tumor volumes in positron emission tomography. Med Phys 34(11):4223–4235

Baum U, Greess H, Lell M, Nomayr A, Lenz M (2000) Imaging of head and neck tumors--methods: CT, spiral-CT, multislice-spiral-CT. Eur J Radiol 33(3):153–160

Belhassen S, Zaidi H (2010) A novel fuzzy C-means algorithm for unsupervised heterogeneous tumor quantification in PET. Med Phys 37(3):1309–1324

Bortfeld T (2006) IMRT: a review and preview. Phys Med Biol 51(13):R363–R379
Brouwer CL, Steenbakkers RJ, Bourhis J, Budach W, Grau C, Gregoire V et al (2015) CT-based delineation of organs at risk in the head and neck region: DAHANCA, EORTC, GORTEC, HKNPCSG, NCIC CTG, NCRI, NRG oncology and TROG consensus guidelines. Radiother Oncol 117(1):83–90
Burrell SC, Van den Abbeele AD (2005) 2-Deoxy-2-[F-18]fluoro-D-glucose-positron emission tomography of the head and neck: an atlas of normal uptake and variants. Mol Imaging Biol 7(3):244–256
Bussink J, Kaanders JH, van der Kogel AJ (2003) Tumor hypoxia at the micro-regional level: clinical relevance and predictive value of exogenous and endogenous hypoxic cell markers. Radiother Oncol 67(1):3–15
Caldemeyer KS, Mathews VP, Righi PD, Smith RR (1998) Imaging features and clinical significance of perineural spread or extension of head and neck tumors. Radiographics 18(1):97–110. quiz 47
Campbell S, Poon I, Markel D, Vena D, Higgins K, Enepekides D et al (2012) Evaluation of microscopic disease in oral tongue cancer using whole-mount histopathologic techniques: implications for the management of head-and-neck cancers. Int J Radiat Oncol Biol Phys 82(2):574–581
Chawla S, Kim S, Loevner LA, Hwang WT, Weinstein G, Chalian A et al (2011) Prediction of disease-free survival in patients with squamous cell carcinomas of the head and neck using dynamic contrast-enhanced MR imaging. AJNR Am J Neuroradiol 32(4):778–784
Corvo R, Giaretti W, Sanguineti G, Geido E, Orecchia R, Barra S et al (1993) Potential doubling time in head and neck tumors treated by primary radiotherapy: preliminary evidence for a prognostic significance in local control. Int J Radiat Oncol Biol Phys 27(5):1165–1172
Daisne JF, Duprez T, Weynand B, Lonneux M, Hamoir M, Reychler H et al (2004) Tumor volume in pharyngolaryngeal squamous cell carcinoma: comparison at CT, MR imaging, and FDG PET and validation with surgical specimen. Radiology 233(1):93–100
Gaddikeri S, Gaddikeri RS, Tailor T, Anzai Y (2016) Dynamic contrast-enhanced MR imaging in head and neck Cancer: techniques and clinical applications. AJNR Am J Neuroradiol 37(4):588–595
Geets X, Daisne JF, Arcangeli S, Coche E, De Poel M, Duprez T et al (2005) Inter-observer variability in the delineation of pharyngo-laryngeal tumor, parotid glands and cervical spinal cord: comparison between CT-scan and MRI. Radiother Oncol 77(1):25–31
Geets X, Lee JA, Bol A, Lonneux M, Gregoire V (2007) A gradient-based method for segmenting FDG-PET images: methodology and validation. Eur J Nucl Med Mol Imaging 34(9):1427–1438
Gray LH, Conger AD, Ebert M, Hornsey S, Scott OC (1953) The concentration of oxygen dissolved in tissues at the time of irradiation as a factor in radiotherapy. Br J Radiol 26(312):638–648
Gregoire V, Daisne JF, Geets X, Levendag P (2003) Selection and delineation of target volumes in head and neck tumors: beyond ICRU definition. Rays 28(3):217–224
Gregoire V, Langendijk JA, Nuyts S (2015) Advances in radiotherapy for head and neck Cancer. J Clin Oncol 33(29):3277–3284
Hatakenaka M, Nakamura K, Yabuuchi H, Shioyama Y, Matsuo Y, Kamitani T et al (2014) Apparent diffusion coefficient is a prognostic factor of head and neck squamous cell carcinoma treated with radiotherapy. Jpn J Radiol 32(2):80–89
Hoeben BA, Troost EG, Span PN, van Herpen CM, Bussink J, Oyen WJ et al (2013) 18F-FLT PET during radiotherapy or chemoradiotherapy in head and neck squamous cell carcinoma is an early predictor of outcome. J Nucl Med 54(4):532–540
Hong TS, Tome WA, Harari PM (2012) Heterogeneity in head and neck IMRT target design and clinical practice. Radiother Oncol 103(1):92–98
Hoshikawa H, Mori T, Yamamoto Y, Kishino T, Fukumura T, Samukawa Y et al (2015) Prognostic value comparison between (18)F-FLT PET/CT and (18)F-FDG PET/CT volume-based metabolic parameters in patients with head and neck cancer. Clin Nucl Med 40(6):464–468
Jager EA, Ligtenberg H, Caldas-Magalhaes J, Schakel T, Philippens ME, Pameijer FA et al (2016) Validated guidelines for tumor delineation on magnetic resonance imaging for laryngeal and hypopharyngeal cancer. Acta Oncol 55(11):1305–1312
Johansen J, Petersen H, Godballe C, Loft A, Grau C (2011) FDG-PET/CT for detection of the unknown primary head and neck tumor. Q J Nucl Med Mol Imaging 55(5):500–508
Kademani D, Bell RB, Bagheri S, Holmgren E, Dierks E, Potter B et al (2005) Prognostic factors in intraoral squamous cell carcinoma: the influence of histologic grade. J Oral Maxillofac Surg 63(11):1599–1605
Kim JJ, Tannock IF (2005) Repopulation of cancer cells during therapy: an important cause of treatment failure. Nat Rev Cancer 5(7):516–525
Kim S, Loevner L, Quon H, Sherman E, Weinstein G, Kilger A et al (2009) Diffusion-weighted magnetic resonance imaging for predicting and detecting early response to chemoradiation therapy of squamous cell carcinomas of the head and neck. Clin Cancer Res 15(3):986–994
Koch CJ, Evans SM, Lord EM (1995) Oxygen dependence of cellular uptake of EF5 [2-(2-nitro-1H-imidazol-1-yl)-N-(2,2,3,3,3-pentafluoropropyl)acetamide]: analysis of drug adducts by fluorescent antibodies vs bound radioactivity. Br J Cancer 72(4):869–874
Kuno H, Onaya H, Iwata R, Kobayashi T, Fujii S, Hayashi R et al (2012) Evaluation of cartilage invasion by laryngeal and hypopharyngeal squamous cell carcinoma with dual-energy CT. Radiology 265(2):488–496
Lee JA (2010) Segmentation of positron emission tomography images: some recommendations for target

delineation in radiation oncology. Radiother Oncol 96(3):302–307
Leibfarth S, Monnich D, Welz S, Siegel C, Schwenzer N, Schmidt H et al (2013) A strategy for multimodal deformable image registration to integrate PET/MR into radiotherapy treatment planning. Acta Oncol 52(7):1353–1359
Liao LJ, Lo WC, Hsu WL, Wang CT, Lai MS (2012) Detection of cervical lymph node metastasis in head and neck cancer patients with clinically N0 neck-a meta-analysis comparing different imaging modalities. BMC Cancer 12:236
Ligtenberg H, Jager EA, Caldas-Magalhaes J, Schakel T, Pameijer FA, Kasperts N et al (2017) Modality-specific target definition for laryngeal and hypopharyngeal cancer on FDG-PET, CT and MRI. Radiother Oncol 123(1):63–70
Löck S, Perrin R, Seidlitz A, Bandurska-Luque A, Zschaeck S, Zöphel K et al (2017.:In press) Residual tumour hypoxia in head-and-neck cancer patients undergoing primary radiochemotherapy, final results of a prospective trial on repeat FMISO-PET imaging. Radiother Oncol 124:533
Moeckli R, Sozzi WJ, Mirimanoff RO, Ozsahin M, Zouhair A, Valley JF et al (2009) Physical considerations on discrepancies in target volume delineation. Z Med Phys 19(4):224–235
Mukherji SK, Isaacs DL, Creager A, Shockley W, Weissler M, Armao D (2001) CT detection of mandibular invasion by squamous cell carcinoma of the oral cavity. AJR Am J Roentgenol 177(1):237–243
Nordsmark M, Bentzen SM, Rudat V, Brizel D, Lartigau E, Stadler P et al (2005) Prognostic value of tumor oxygenation in 397 head and neck tumors after primary radiation therapy. An international multi-center study. Radiother Oncol 77(1):18–24
O'Daniel JC, Rosenthal DI, Garden AS, Barker JL, Ahamad A, Ang KK et al (2007) The effect of dental artifacts, contrast media, and experience on interobserver contouring variations in head and neck anatomy. Am J Clin Oncol 30(2):191–198
Ong CK, Chong VF (2006) Imaging of tongue carcinoma. Cancer Imaging 6:186–193
Paulus DH, Thorwath D, Schmidt H, Quick HH (2014) Towards integration of PET/MR hybrid imaging into radiation therapy treatment planning. Med Phys 41(7):072505
Peeters SG, Zegers CM, Lieuwes NG, van Elmpt W, Eriksson J, van Dongen GA et al (2015) A comparative study of the hypoxia PET tracers [(1)(8)F]HX4, [(1)(8)F]FAZA, and [(1)(8)F]FMISO in a preclinical tumor model. Int J Radiat Oncol Biol Phys 91(2):351–359
Platzek I, Beuthien-Baumann B, Schneider M, Gudziol V, Kitzler HH, Maus J et al (2014) FDG PET/MR for lymph node staging in head and neck cancer. Eur J Radiol 83(7):1163–1168
Ruhlmann V, Ruhlmann M, Bellendorf A, Grueneisen J, Sawicki LM, Grafe H et al (2016) Hybrid imaging for detection of carcinoma of unknown primary: a preliminary comparison trial of whole-body PET/MRI versus PET/CT. Eur J Radiol 85(11):1941–1947
Schinagl DA, Vogel WV, Hoffmann AL, van Dalen JA, Oyen WJ, Kaanders JH (2007) Comparison of five segmentation tools for 18F-fluoro-deoxy-glucose-positron emission tomography-based target volume definition in head and neck cancer. Int J Radiat Oncol Biol Phys 69(4):1282–1289
Servagi-Vernat S, Differding S, Hanin FX, Labar D, Bol A, Lee JA et al (2014) A prospective clinical study of (1)(8)F-FAZA PET-CT hypoxia imaging in head and neck squamous cell carcinoma before and during radiation therapy. Eur J Nucl Med Mol Imaging 41(8):1544–1552
Shields AF, Grierson JR, Dohmen BM, Machulla HJ, Stayanoff JC, Lawhorn-Crews JM et al (1998) Imaging proliferation in vivo with [F-18]FLT and positron emission tomography. Nat Med 4(11):1334–1336
Sobin LH, Gospodarowicz MK, Wittekind C, International Union against Cancer (2010) TNM classification of malignant tumours, 7th edn. Chichester, West Sussex, UK, xx. Wiley-Blackwell, Hoboken, NJ, p 309
Suh CH, Choi YJ, Baek JH, Lee JH (2018) The diagnostic value of diffusion-weighted imaging in differentiating metastatic lymph nodes of head and neck squamous cell carcinoma: a systematic review and meta-analysis. AJNR Am J Neuroradiol 39(10):1889–1895
Thorwarth D, Eschmann SM, Scheiderbauer J, Paulsen F, Alber M (2005) Kinetic analysis of dynamic 18F-fluoromisonidazole PET correlates with radiation treatment outcome in head-and-neck cancer. BMC Cancer 5:152
Troost EG, Bussink J, Hoffmann AL, Boerman OC, Oyen WJ, Kaanders JH (2010c) 18F-FLT PET/CT for early response monitoring and dose escalation in oropharyngeal tumors. J Nucl Med 51(6):866–874
Troost EG, Bussink J, Slootweg PJ, Peeters WJ, Merkx MA, van der Kogel AJ et al (2010b) Histopathologic validation of 3′-deoxy-3'-18F-fluorothymidine PET in squamous cell carcinoma of the oral cavity. J Nucl Med 51(5):713–719
Troost EG, Laverman P, Kaanders JH, Philippens M, Lok J, Oyen WJ et al (2006) Imaging hypoxia after oxygenation-modification: comparing [18F]FMISO autoradiography with pimonidazole immunohistochemistry in human xenograft tumors. Radiother Oncol 80(2):157–164
Troost EG, Laverman P, Philippens ME, Lok J, van der Kogel AJ, Oyen WJ et al (2008) Correlation of [(18)F]FMISO autoradiography and pimonodazole immunohistochemistry in human head and neck carcinoma xenografts. Eur J Nucl Med Mol Imaging 35(10):1803–1811
Troost EG, Schinagl DA, Bussink J, Boerman OC, van der Kogel AJ, Oyen WJ et al (2010a) Innovations in radiotherapy planning of head and neck cancers: role of PET. J Nucl Med 51(1):66–76
Troost EG, Vogel WV, Merkx MA, Slootweg PJ, Marres HA, Peeters WJ et al (2007) 18F-FLT PET does not discriminate between reactive and metastatic lymph nodes in primary head and neck cancer patients. J Nucl Med 48(5):726–735
Tshering Vogel DW, Zbaeren P, Geretschlaeger A, Vermathen P, De Keyzer F, Thoeny HC (2013) Diffusion-

weighted MR imaging including bi-exponential fitting for the detection of recurrent or residual tumour after (chemo)radiotherapy for laryngeal and hypopharyngeal cancers. Eur Radiol 23(2):562–569

van Dalen JA, Hoffmann AL, Dicken V, Vogel WV, Wiering B, Ruers TJ et al (2007) A novel iterative method for lesion delineation and volumetric quantification with FDG PET. Nucl Med Commun 28(6):485–493

Vandecaveye V, De Keyzer F, Nuyts S, Deraedt K, Dirix P, Hamaekers P et al (2007) Detection of head and neck squamous cell carcinoma with diffusion weighted MRI after (chemo)radiotherapy: correlation between radiologic and histopathologic findings. Int J Radiat Oncol Biol Phys 67(4):960–971

Weiss E, Hess CF (2003) The impact of gross tumor volume (GTV) and clinical target volume (CTV) definition on the total accuracy in radiotherapy theoretical aspects and practical experiences. Strahlenther Onkol 179(1):21–30

Weissman JL, Carrau RL (2001) "Puffed-cheek" CT improves evaluation of the oral cavity. AJNR Am J Neuroradiol 22(4):741–744

Welz S, Monnich D, Pfannenberg C, Nikolaou K, Reimold M, La Fougere C et al (2017) Prognostic value of dynamic hypoxia PET in head and neck cancer: results from a planned interim analysis of a randomized phase II hypoxia-image guided dose escalation trial. Radiother Oncol 124:526

Yu Y, Mabray M, Silveira W, Shen PY, Ryan WR, Uzelac A et al (2017) Earlier and more specific detection of persistent neck disease with diffusion-weighted MRI versus subsequent PET/CT after definitive chemoradiation for oropharyngeal squamous cell carcinoma. Head Neck 39(3):432–438

Zhou Q, Zeng F, Ding Y, Fuller CD, Wang J (2018) Meta-analysis of diffusion-weighted imaging for predicting locoregional failure of chemoradiotherapy in patients with head and neck squamous cell carcinoma. Mol Clin Oncol 8(1):197–203

Zips D, Zophel K, Abolmaali N, Perrin R, Abramyuk A, Haase R et al (2012) Exploratory prospective trial of hypoxia-specific PET imaging during radiochemotherapy in patients with locally advanced head-and-neck cancer. Radiother Oncol 105(1):21–28

T-Staging and Target Volume Definition by Imaging in Breast Tumours

Roberto C. Delgado Bolton, Adriana K. Calapaquí Terán, and Philip Poortmans

Contents

1	**Introduction**	184
1.1	T-Staging	184
2	**Imaging Techniques**	186
2.1	Mammography	186
2.2	MRI	188
2.3	PET	191
3	**Target Volume Delineation**	195
4	**Radiation Oncology Treatments**	197
4.1	Radiation Therapy in Conservative Surgery	197
4.2	Radiation Therapy after Mastectomy	199
5	**Conclusions**	200
References		200

R. C. Delgado Bolton (✉)
Department of Diagnostic Imaging (Radiology) and Nuclear Medicine, University Hospital San Pedro and Centre for Biomedical Research of La Rioja, Logroño, La Rioja, Spain
e-mail: rcdelgado@riojasalud.es

A. K. Calapaquí Terán
Department of Pathology, University Hospital "Marqués de Valdecilla,", Santander, Spain

Department of Radiation Oncology, Hospital Central de la Defensa "Gómez Ulla", Madrid, Spain
e-mail: adrianakatherine.calapaqui@scsalud.es

P. Poortmans
Department of Radiation Oncology, Institut Curie, Paris, France

Paris Sciences and Lettres, PSL University, Paris, France
e-mail: Philip.poortmans@curie.fr

Abstract

Breast cancer is the most frequent cancer in women in both developed and developing countries. Early detection of breast cancer is of great importance, as it allows carrying out less mutilating or aggressive treatments, thus achieving a better quality of life and higher survival rates. The standard of care in breast cancer therefore includes organized screening programs. Mammography and MRI play a key role in both staging of breast lesions and target volume definition. The treatment of breast cancer should be multidisciplinary, involving gynecologists, pathologists, radiologists, surgeons, medical oncologists, and radiation oncologists and nuclear medicine physicians, among others, in order to personalize the treatment of each patient. With the aim of offering the best radiation therapy to patients, but in turn to limit radiation to organs at risk, several imaging techniques are used, which help to define the volumes of treatment: clinical tumour volume (CTV) and planning tumour volume (PTV). Throughout the world, computed tomography (CT) is the most used imaging technique for treatment planning, but we can use the information provided by ultrasound, magnetic resonance, etc., to assist in correctly defining the primary tumour bed and the lymph node regions. Radiation therapy is adapted to the patients' risks and may include whole-breast, chest wall, regional nodes, or be

R. G. H. Beets-Tan et al. (eds.), *Imaging and Interventional Radiology for Radiation Oncology*, Medical Radiology, Diagnostic Imaging, https://doi.org/10.1007/978-3-030-38261-2_13

limited to (accelerated) partial breast irradiation ((A)PBI). Regarding [^{18}F]FDG PET/CT, it has a limited role in the diagnosis of breast cancer, but it can provide relevant information for detecting locoregional and distant disease, for helping to plan surgical and medical treatment, monitoring response, and locating recurrent disease. PET also has the potential to quickly assess new treatments by detecting their effects on specific receptors and has evidenced it improves the prediction of the clinical outcome in previously treated breast cancer patients.

1 Introduction

According to the WHO, breast cancer is the most frequent cancer in women in both developed and developing countries. It is estimated that one in eight women will develop breast cancer throughout her life. The majority of cases occur between 45 and 65 years.

Early detection of breast cancer is of great importance, as it allows carrying out less aggressive treatments combined with achievement of superior results, thus achieving a better quality of life and higher survival rates. In recent years, mortality from this tumor has decreased relatively between 25% and 35%. Five-year survival in initial stages exceeds 90%.

The standard of care in breast cancer includes screening programs. The screening program begins at the age of 50 (age of highest incidence) through mammograms performed every 2 years, but earlier in certain groups: (a) 25–30 years of age for carriers of the breast cancer 1 gene and untested relatives of carriers (Hendrick et al. 1997); (b) 25–30 years of age or 10 years earlier than the age of the affected relatives at diagnosis (whichever is later) for women with first-degree relatives with premenopausal breast cancer or for women with lifetime risk for breast cancer 20% on the basis of family history (Tabár et al. 2001; Brekelmans et al. 2001); (c) eight years after radiation therapy but not before 25 years of age for women who received radiation between the ages of 10 and 30 years (Lee et al. 2010); and (d) any age for women with biopsy-proven lobular neoplastic lesion, atypical ductal hyperplasia, ductal carcinoma in situ, or invasive breast cancer (Lee et al. 2010). The addition of ultrasound, magnetic resonance imaging, and breast examination to mammography would be necessary in high-risk cases.

To standardize the description of breast lesions in imaging techniques since 1992, the American College of Radiology (ACR) created the breast imaging reporting and data system (BI-RADS) to reduce the variability in radiological reports and facilitate communication between different specialists and enable monitoring results. The fifth update of the BI-RADS is currently in use (ACR BI-RADS Atlas® n.d.); see Table 1 (concordance between BI-RADS assessment categories and management recommendation). Concordance between BI-RADS assessment categories and management recommendations (ACR) allows us to know the radiological classification of lesions of the breast, to know the clinical attitude to be followed and the probability that the lesion is positive for cancer.

The histopathologic types of breast carcinoma are the following: in situ carcinomas (ductal carcinoma in situ; Paget disease); invasive carcinomas (not otherwise specified, NOS); ductal, inflammatory, medullary, NOS; medullary with lymphoid stroma; mucinous; papillary, predominantly micropapillary pattern; tubular, lobular; Paget disease and infiltrating; undifferentiated; squamous cell; adenoid cystic; secretory; cribriform (NCCN 2019).

1.1 T-Staging

The internationally accepted system for the staging of tumours including breast cancer is the tumour, node, and metastasis (TNM) of the American Joint Committee on Cancer (AJCC), the eighth edition of 2018 being currently in use. The TNM anatomic staging system for breast cancer classifies tumours on the basis of the primary tumour type (invasive or in situ) and size (T) (Table 2), the presence or absence of regional

Table 1 Concordance between BI-RADS assessment categories and management recommendations (ACR BI-RADS Atlas® n.d.)

Assessment	Management	Likelihood of cancer
Category 0: Incomplete—Need additional imaging evaluation and/or prior mammograms for comparison	Recall for additional imaging and/or comparison with prior examination(s)	N/A
Category 1: Negative	Routine mammography screening	Essentially 0% likelihood of malignancy
Category 2: Benign	Routine mammography screening	Essentially 0% likelihood of malignancy
Category 3: Probably benign	Short-interval (6-month) follow-up or continued surveillance mammography	>0% but ≤2% likelihood of malignancy
Category 4: Suspicious Category 4A: *Low suspicion* for malignancy Category 4B: *Moderate suspicion* for malignancy Category 4C: *High suspicion* for malignancy	Tissue diagnosis	>2% but <95% likelihood of malignancy >2% to ≤10% likelihood of malignancy >10% to ≤50% likelihood of malignancy >50% to <95% likelihood of malignancy
Category 5: Highly suggestive of malignancy	Tissue diagnosis	≥95% likelihood of malignancy
Category 6: Known biopsy-proven malignancy	Surgical excision when clinically appropriate	N/A

Table 2 American Joint Committee on Cancer (AJCC), Eighth Edition (2017). TNM staging for breast cancer (Definitions for the primary tumour (T) (NCCN 2019))

T-staging	Primary tumor	
TX	Primary tumour cannot be assessed	
T0	No evidence of primary tumour	
Tis (DCIS)	Ductal carcinoma in situ	
Tis (Paget)	Paget disease of the nipple NOT associated with invasive carcinoma and/or carcinoma in situ (DCIS) in the underlying breast parenchyma. Carcinomas in the breast parenchyma associated with Paget disease are categorized based on the size and characteristics of the parenchymal disease, although the presence of Paget disease should still be noted	
T1	Tumour ≤20 mm in greatest dimension	
	T1mi	Tumour ≤1 mm in greatest dimension
	T1a	Tumour >1 mm but ≤5 mm in greatest dimension (round any measurement >1.0–1.9 mm to 2 mm)
	T1b	Tumour >5 mm but ≤10 mm in greatest dimension
	T1c	Tumour >10 mm but ≤20 mm in greatest dimension
T2	Tumour >20 mm but ≤50 mm in greatest dimension	
T3	Tumour >50 mm in greatest dimension	
T4	Tumour of any size with direct extension to the chest wall and/or to the skin (ulceration or macroscopic nodules); invasion of the dermis alone does not qualify as T4	
	T4a	Extension to chest wall; invasion or adherence to pectoralis muscle in the absence of invasion of chest wall structures does not qualify as T4
	T4b	Ulceration and/or ipsilateral macroscopic satellite nodules and/or edema (including *peau d'orange*) of the skin, which do not meet the criteria for inflammatory carcinoma
	T4c	Both T4a and T4b are present
	T4d	Inflammatory carcinoma

Table 3 American Joint Committee on Cancer (AJCC), Eighth Edition (2017). TNM staging for breast cancer (TNM staging for breast cancer. Definitions for the regional lymph nodes. Clinical (cN) staging (NCCN 2019))

Clinical N (cN) staging	Regional lymph nodes (N)	
cNX	Regional lymph nodes cannot be assessed (e.g., previously removed)	
cN0	No regional lymph node metastases (by imaging or clinical examination)	
cN1	Metastases to movable ipsilateral level I, II axillary lymph node(s)	
	cN1mi	Micrometastases (approximately 200 cells, larger than 0.2 mm, but none larger than 2.0 mm)
cN2	Metastases in ipsilateral level I, II axillary lymph nodes that are clinically fixed or matted; *or* in ipsilateral internal mammary nodes in the absence of axillary lymph node metastases	
	cN2a	Metastases in ipsilateral level I, II axillary lymph nodes fixed to one another (matted) or to other structures
	cN2b	Metastases only in ipsilateral internal mammary nodes in the absence of axillary lymph node metastases
cN3	Metastases in ipsilateral infraclavicular (level III axillary) lymph node(s) with or without level I, II axillary lymph node involvement; *or* in ipsilateral internal mammary lymph node(s) with level I, II axillary lymph node metastases; *or* metastases in ipsilateral supraclavicular lymph node(s) with or without axillary or internal mammary lymph node involvement	
	cN3a	Metastases in ipsilateral infraclavicular lymph node(s)
	cN3b	Metastases in ipsilateral internal mammary lymph node(s) and axillary lymph node(s)
	cN3c	Metastases in ipsilateral supraclavicular lymph node(s)

American Joint Committee on Cancer (AJCC), Eighth Edition (2017)

lymph node involvement (N) (Tables 3 and 4), and the presence or absence of distant metastases (M) (Table 5). AJCC anatomic stage groups are presented in Table 6 (NCCN 2019).

- Primary tumour (T)—The stage is assessed by clinical examination and abnormal imaging findings in mammographic, breast ultrasound, and/or magnetic resonance imaging that permits assessing tumor size. See Table 2 (the eighth edition TNM staging system—focus on T-staging).
- Lymph nodes (N)—The status of the regional lymph nodes is one of the most important prognostic factors in early-stage breast cancer. N-staging can be clinical (cN) or pathological (pN). See Table 3 and Table 4 (the eighth edition TNM staging system—focus on N-staging).
- Metastasis (M)—Most patients with breast cancer have disease limited to the breast (stages I to II) without nodules or with limited nodules (i.e., less than three), and patients who have locally advanced disease (T3 or higher, N2 or N3, M0)) or inflammatory breast cancer should be studied to rule out disease at a distance. See Table 5 (the eighth edition TNM staging system—focus on M staging).

AJCC anatomic stage groups are presented in Table 6 (NCCN 2019).

2 Imaging Techniques

2.1 Mammography

Mammography is the recommended method for breast cancer screening of women in the general population and in patients diagnosed with breast cancer. The preoperative diagnostic mammography can help to define the extent of disease and may identify multifocal or multicentric cancer that could preclude breast conservation or signal a potential difficulty in achieving clear surgical margins.

Table 4 American Joint Committee on Cancer (AJCC), Eighth Edition (2017). TNM staging for breast cancer (TNM staging for breast cancer. Definitions for the regional lymph nodes. Pathologic (pN) staging (NCCN 2019))

Pathologic (pN) staging	Regional lymph nodes (N)	
pNX	Regional lymph nodes cannot be assessed (e.g., not removed for pathological study or previously removed)	
pN0	No regional lymph node metastases identified or ITCs only	
	pN0(i+)	ITCs only (malignant cell clusters no larger than 0.2 mm) in regional lymph node(s)
	pN0(Mol+)	Positive molecular findings by reverse transcriptase polymerase chain reaction (RT-PCR); no ITCs detected
pN1	Micrometastases; *or* metastases in 1–3 axillary lymph nodes; *and/or* clinically negative internal mammary nodes with micrometastases or macrometastases by sentinel lymph node biopsy	
	pN1mi	Micrometastases (approximately 200 cells, larger than 0.2 mm, but none larger than 2.0 mm)
	pN1a	Metastases in 1–3 axillary lymph nodes, at least one larger than 2.0 mm
	pN1b	Metastases in ipsilateral internal mammary sentinel nodes, excluding ITCs
	pN1c	pN1a and pN1b combined
pN2	Metastases in 4–9 axillary lymph nodes; *or* positive ipsilateral internal mammary lymph nodes by imaging in the absence of axillary lymph node metastases	
	pN2a	Metastases in 4–9 axillary lymph nodes, at least one larger than 2.0 mm
	pN2b	Metastases in clinically detected internal mammary lymph nodes with or without microscopic confirmation; with pathologically negative axillary nodes
pN3	Metastases in 10 or more axillary lymph nodes; *or* in infraclavicular (level III axillary) lymph nodes; *or* positive ipsilateral internal mammary lymph nodes by imaging in the presence of one or more positive level I, II axillary lymph nodes; *or* in more than three axillary lymph nodes and micrometastases or macrometastases by sentinel lymph node biopsy in clinically negative ipsilateral internal mammary lymph nodes; *or* in ipsilateral supraclavicular lymph nodes	
	pN3a	Metastases in 10 or more axillary lymph nodes (at least one larger than 2.0 mm); *or* metastases to the infraclavicular (level III axillary) lymph nodes
	pN3b	pN1a o pN2a in the presence of cN2b (positive internal mammary nodes by imaging); *or* pN2a in the presence of pN1b
	pN3c	Metastases in ipsilateral supraclavicular lymph nodes

American Joint Committee on Cancer (AJCC), Eighth Edition (2017)

Table 5 American Joint Committee on Cancer (AJCC), Eighth Edition (2017). TNM staging for breast cancer (TNM staging for breast cancer. Definitions for distant metastases (M). M staging (NCCN 2019))

M stage	Distant metastases (M)	
M0	No clinical or radiographic evidence of distant metastases	
	cM0(i+)	No clinical or radiographic evidence of distant metastases in the presence of tumor cells or deposits no larger than 0.2 mm detected microscopically or by molecular techniques in circulating blood, bone marrow, or other nonregional nodal tissue in a patient without symptoms or signs of metastases
cM1	Distant metastases detected by clinical or radiographic means	
pM1	Any histologically proven metastases in distant organs; or if in nonregional node, metastases greater than 0.2 mm	

American Joint Committee on Cancer (AJCC), Eighth Edition (2017)

Table 6 AJCC anatomic stage groups (NCCN 2019)

	TNM stage		
Stage group	T stage	N stage	M stage
Stage 0	Tis	N0	M0
Stage IA	T1	N0	M0
Stage IB	T0	N1mi	M0
	T1	N1mi	M0
Stage IIA	T0	N1	M0
	T1	N1	M0
	T2	N0	M0
Stage IIB	T2	N1	M0
	T3	N0	M0
Stage IIIA	T0	N2	M0
	T1	N2	M0
	T2	N2	M0
	T3	N1	M0
	T3	N2	M0
Stage IIIB	T4	N0	M0
	T4	N1	M0
	T4	N2	M0
Stage IIIC	Any T	N3	M0
Stage IV	Any T	Any N	M1

American Joint Committee on Cancer (AJCC), Eighth Edition (2017)

A significant limitation of mammographic assessment of disease extent is the obscuring of the borders or extent of the primary tumor by dense overlying tissue. Dense breasts can limit the sensitivity of mammography both for detection of breast cancers and for delineating disease extent. Mammographic sensitivity is 80% among women with predominantly fatty breasts but just 30% in women with extremely dense breasts (Mandelson et al. 2000).

Another limitation of mammography is invasive cancers that are contiguous to the chest wall and are not completely included in the mammographic projections, since they need other techniques such as MRI to evaluate the posterior tumor extension and the pectoral fascia or muscular involvement, if that determines a change in the therapeutic approach (extension of surgery and the use of primary systemic therapy) (Morris et al. 2000). Figures 1, 2, 3 and 4 present cases in which mammography studies were performed.

2.2 MRI

The use of breast MRI in the preoperative evaluation of patients recently diagnosed with breast cancer has increased significantly in recent years due to its well-documented high sensitivity to detect breast cancer hidden in affected and contralateral breasts (Lee et al. 2010).

MRI may be used for staging evaluation to define the extent of cancer or presence of multifocal or multicentric cancer in the ipsilateral breast or as screening of the contralateral breast cancer at time of initial diagnosis (Lee et al. 2010; Houssami et al. 2008). Two examples are presented in Figs. 2 and 4.

According the National Comprehensive Cancer Network (NCCN), MRI can be used for women with Paget's disease of the breast who have a negative physical examination and mammogram, as breast MRI can define the extent of disease and aid in treatment planning (Lee et al. 2010).

For women in whom extensive reconstructive surgery is being planned, breast MRI may be used to identify occult contralateral cancers. MRI staging causes more extensive breast surgery in an important proportion of women by identifying additional cancer lesions; however, false-positive findings on breast MRI are common. Therefore, surgical decisions should not be based solely on the MRI findings (Houssami et al. 2008). All suspicious findings on MRI require pathologic confirmation.

In patients with very high risk for contralateral disease (e.g., because of an inherited predisposing condition or prior chest wall irradiation) (Lee et al. 2010), MRI may be useful.

MRI may be helpful for breast cancer evaluation before and after preoperative systemic therapy to define extent of disease, response to treatment, and potential for breast-conserving therapy (NCCN 2019). However, MRI can overestimate residual invasive cancer and is not accurate for predicting pathologic response.

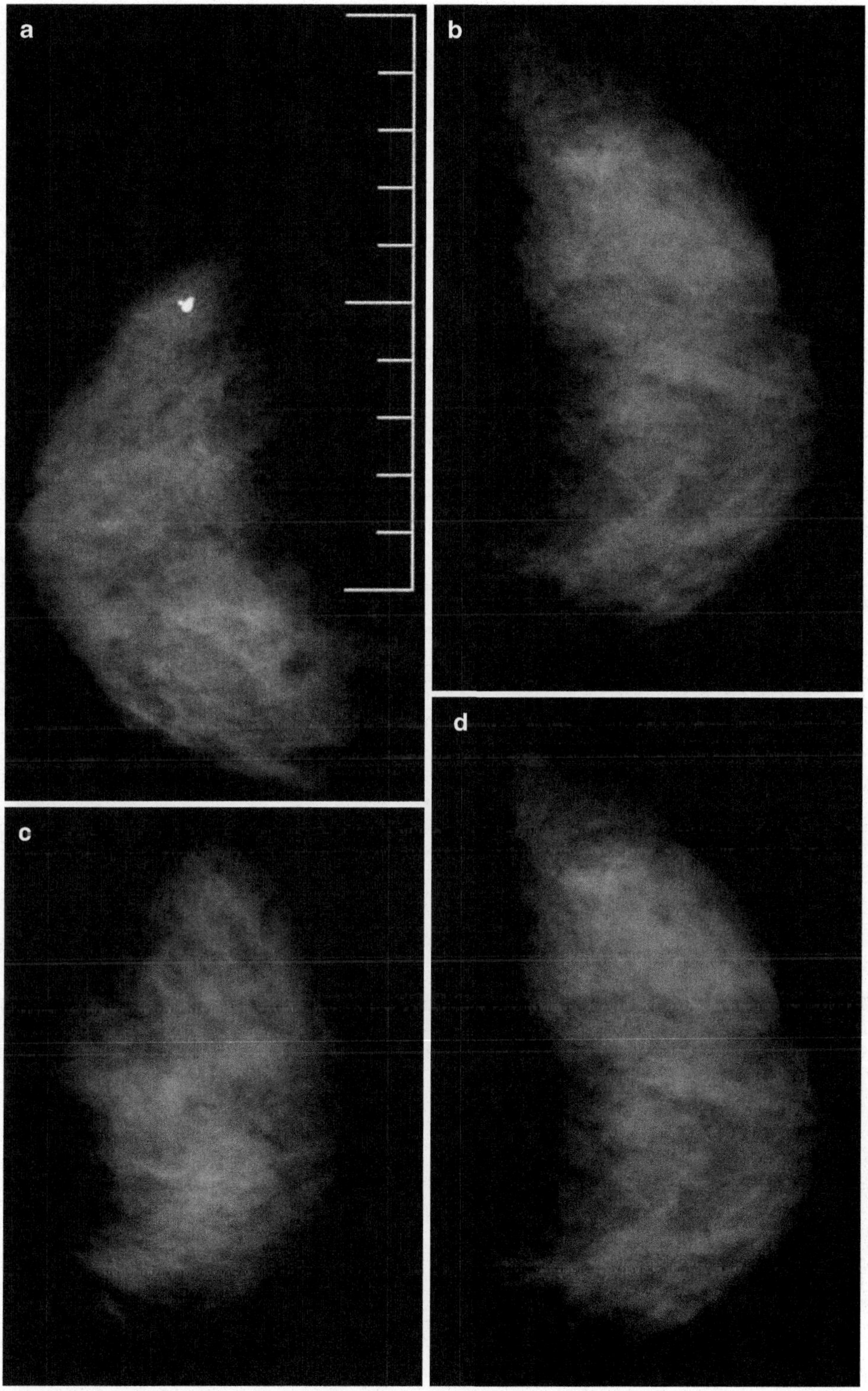

Fig. 1 A 61-year-old woman followed in the breast cancer screening program. The mammography (**a**–**d**) is reported as negative for malignancy, categorized as BI-RADS 2, to be followed 2 years later

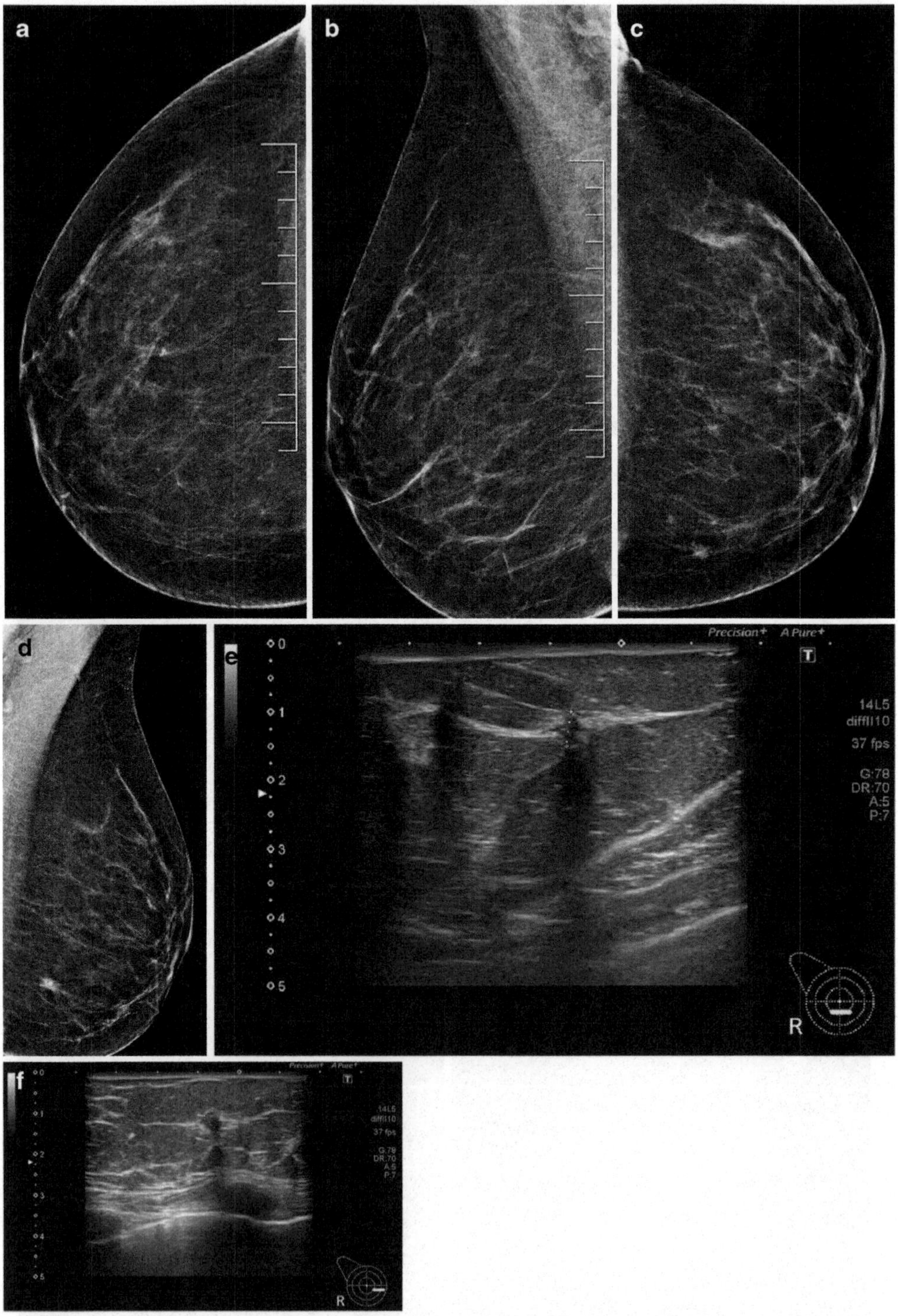

Fig. 2 A 53-year-old woman followed in the breast cancer screening program. The mammography (**a–d**) is reported as BI-RADS 4C due to two lesions in the right breast. The patient is referred to breast ultrasound and biopsy (punch, gross needle aspiration, and tru-cut). The ultrasound (**e**, **f**) evidences two lesions in the right breast, both in the inferior quadrants, both measuring 5 mm, one with microcalcifications in its interior. The left axilla is negative. The pathology study shows an intraductal micropapiloma in one of the lesions and an infiltrating micropapilar carcinoma in the other lesion. The breast MRI (**g–j**) reported the presence of two lesions in the right breast with a negative axilla, confirming the diagnosis of multicentric carcinoma in the right breast

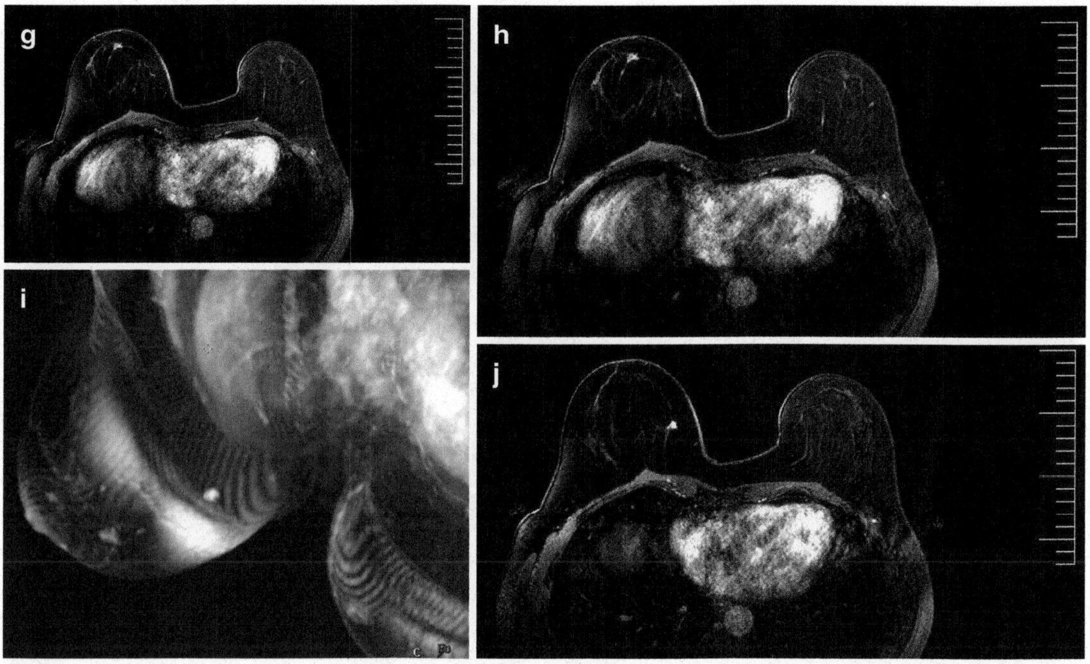

Fig. 2 (continued)

2.3 PET

The use of [^{18}F]FDG PET or PET/CT scanning is not indicated in the staging of clinical stage I, II, or operable III (T3 N1) breast cancer. The recommendation against the use of PET scanning is supported by (a) the high false-negative rate in the detection of lesions that are small (<1 cm) and/or low grade (Kumar et al. 2006), (b) the low sensitivity for detection of axillary nodal metastases, (c) the low prior probability of these patients having detectable metastatic disease, and (d) the high rate of false-positive scans (Wahl et al. 2004). [^{18}F]FDG PET/CT is most helpful in situations where standard staging studies are equivocal or suspicious, especially in the setting of locally advanced or metastatic disease (NCCN 2019).

A recent systematic review analyzing the role of [^{18}F]FDG PET/CT in restaging and treatment response assessment of malignant disease has described the appropriate use of PET/CT in several cancer types, including breast cancer (Jadvar et al. 2017). The goal of these recommendations is to guide the appropriate use of this technique. As mentioned above, PET/CT has a limited role in the diagnosis of breast cancer (Raylman et al. 2008), but it can provide relevant information for detecting locoregional (including nodal) as well as distant disease, for helping to plan surgical and medical treatment, for monitoring response to treatment, and for locating recurrent disease (Buscombe et al. 2004; Byrne et al. 2004; Esserman 2005; Isasi et al. 2005; Quon and Gambhir 2005; Rieber et al. 2002; Zangheri et al. 2004). PET also has the potential to quickly assess new treatment by detecting their effects on specific receptors (Jadvar et al. 2017; Esserman 2005; Flanagan et al. 1998) and has evidenced it improves the prediction of the clinical outcome in previously treated breast cancer patients (Bombardieri and Crippa 2001; Vranjesevic et al. 2002). A retrospective study that included 133 breast cancer patients showed that PET results provided information on 6-month outcome that was independent of the stage or past treatments, significantly influencing patient management (Santiago et al. 2006).

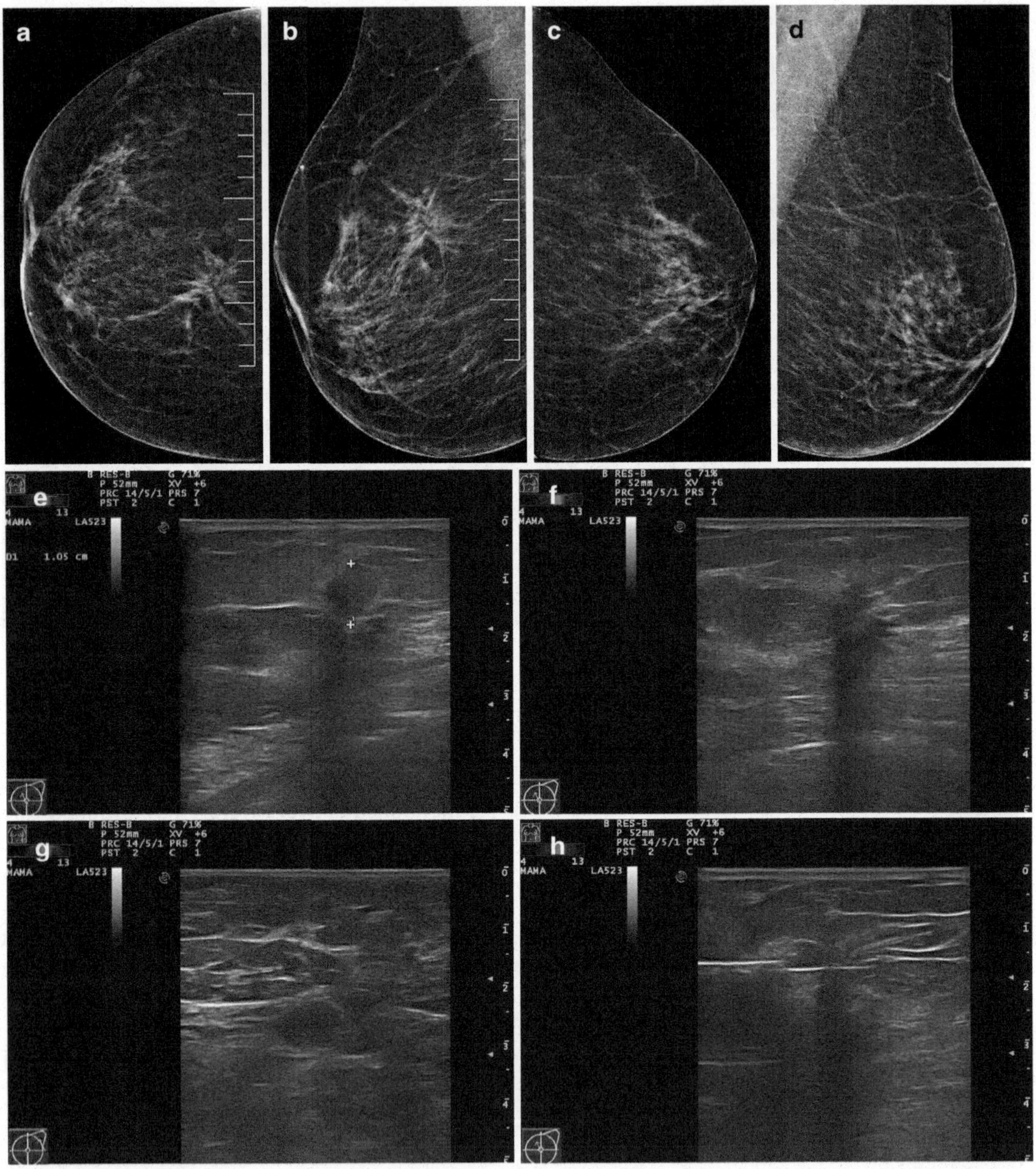

Fig. 3 An 81-year-old woman who refers a nodule in the upper external quadrant of the left breast. The mammography (**a**–**d**) is reported as BI-RADS 5 due to a lesion in the upper internal quadrant of the left breast measuring 15 mm in the ultrasound (**e**–**h**). The biopsy (punch, gross needle aspiration, and tru-cut) evidences infiltrant carcinoma in the breast lesion, whereas the fine needle aspiration of the axillary lymph node was suspicious of malignancy due to atypical epithelial cells

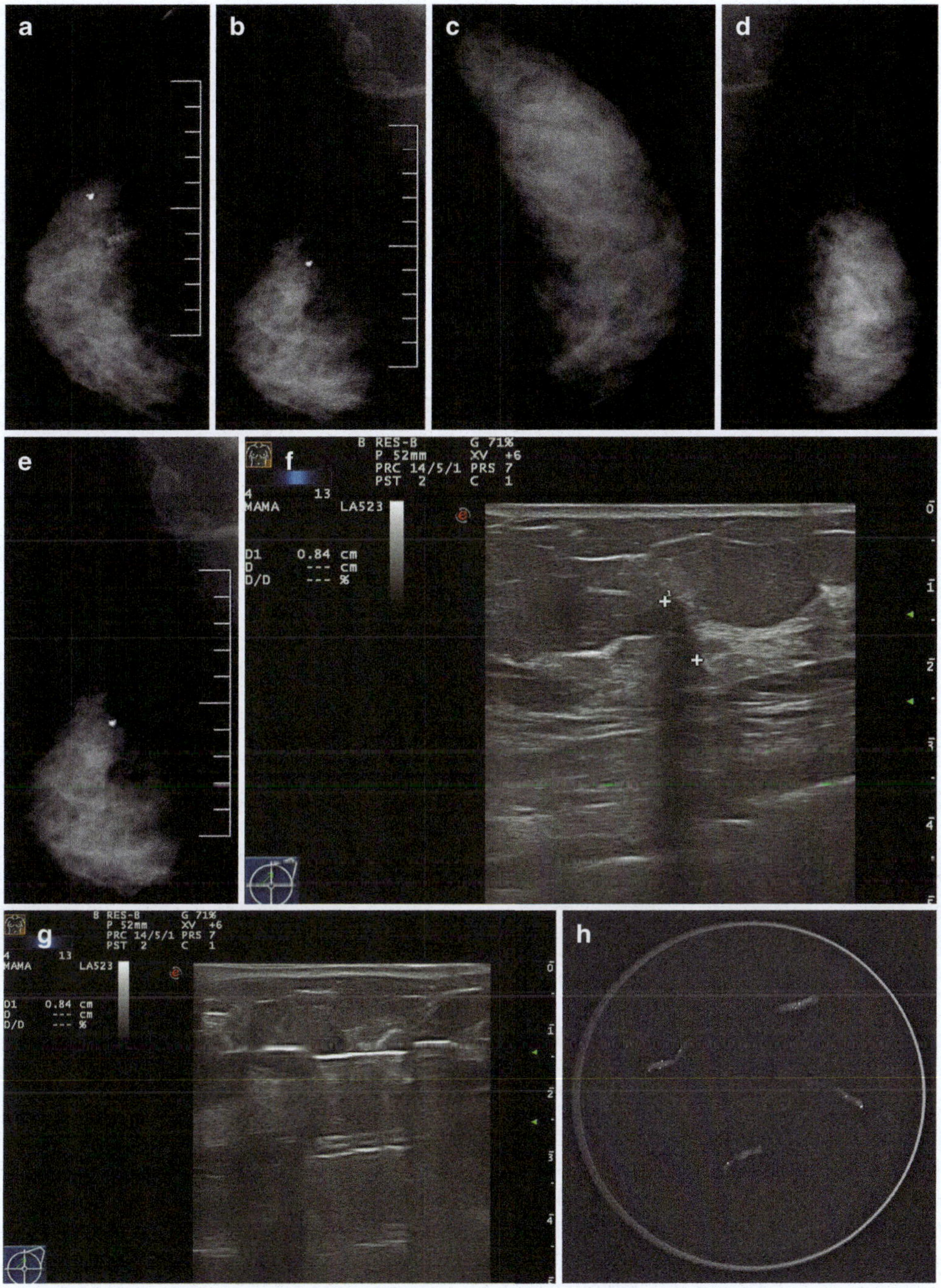

Fig. 4 A 63-year-old woman followed in the breast cancer screening program. The mammography (**a–e**) is reported as BI-RADS 5 due to a 20 mm area with microcalcifications in the left breast. The patient is referred to breast ultrasound and biopsy (punch, gross needle aspiration, and tru-cut). The ultrasound (**f, g**) evidences an 8 mm nodule in the upper quadrants of the left breast. The four cylinders (**h**) present microcalcifications with the diagnosis of pleomorphic high-grade in situ lobular carcinoma. MRI (**i, j**) confirms the presence of a 15 × 24 mm lesion suspicious of malignancy in the upper quadrants of the left breast where the biopsy had been performed. The right breast presents a nodule with benign characteristics. Presurgical location of the lesions (**k, l**) is done, confirming the correct excision in the surgical specimen

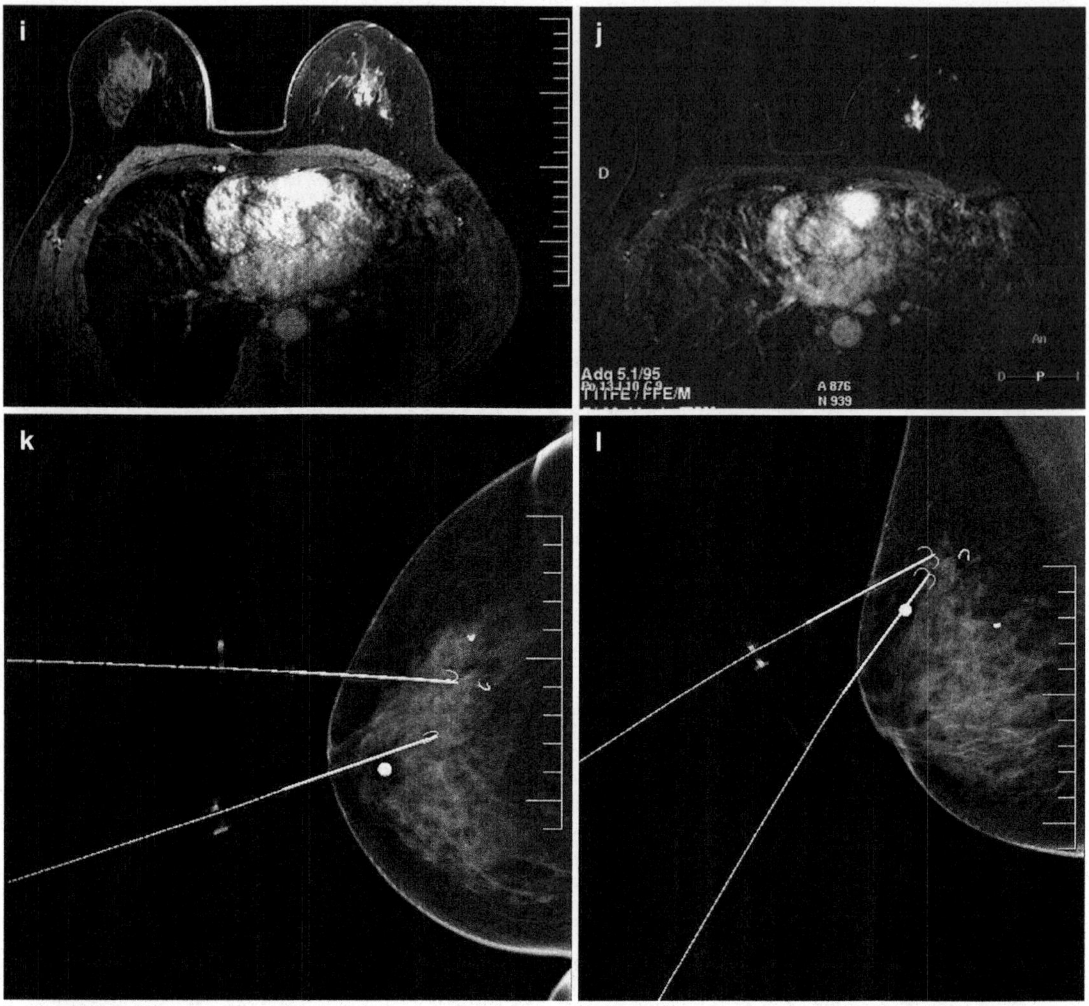

Fig. 4 (continued)

2.3.1 Restaging for Detection of Local Recurrence

This indication is considered appropriate with a score of 8 of 9 in the aforementioned systematic review (Jadvar et al. 2017). A meta-analysis by Pennant et al. (2010) evaluating PET/CT in the detection of recurrence in patients with a history of breast cancer evidenced that PET/CT had a significantly higher sensitivity compared with CT [95% (95% CI: 88–98%) vs. 80% (95% CI: 65–90%)], but the increase in specificity was not significant [89% (95% CI: 69–97%) vs. 77% (95% CI: 50–92%)]. The differences in the sensitivity or specificity of PET when compared with MRI were not significant. A study by Champions et al. reported sensitivity, specificity, positive predictive value, negative predictive value, and accuracy of PET/CT for detecting breast cancer recurrences were 93.6%, 85.4%, 96.7%, 74.5%, and 92.1%, respectively. The comparison with the standard workup was available in 67 patients; in these PET/CT had a higher sensitivity and accuracy (94.5% vs. 33% and 94% vs. 48%, respectively) (Champion et al. 2011). Another study indicated the sensitivity, specificity, negative predictive value, and positive predictive value for disease relapse or progression were 89% vs. 77%, 73% vs. 53%, 90% vs. 75%, and 72% vs. 55%, respectively, for PET/CT and CT (Evangelista et al. 2012).

2.3.2 Restaging for Detection of Metastases

This indication is considered appropriate with a score of 7 of 9 in the aforementioned systematic review (Jadvar et al. 2017). A study by Veit-Haibach et al. comparing the value of combined PET/CT, PET+CT (viewed side by side), CT alone, and PET alone in the restaging of patients with recurrent breast cancer showed that, overall, the TNM tumour stage was correctly determined in 40/44 patients with PET/CT, in 38/44 with PET+CT, in 36/44 with PET alone, and in 36/44 patients with CT alone. The authors conclude that combined PET/CT appeared to be more accurate in restaging and showed a moderate impact on therapy over PET and CT (Veit-Haibach et al. 2007). In another study, sensitivity, specificity, positive predictive value, and negative predictive value were 98.7%, 85.3%, 92.5%, and 97.2%, respectively, in the same clinical scenario of restaging patients with known breast cancer (Manohar et al. 2012). Moreover, another study reported that the sensitivity and specificity of recurrent lesion detection for PET, CT, and PET/CT were 84%, 66%, and 93% and 100%, 92%, and 100%, respectively (Dirisamer et al. 2010).

2.3.3 Treatment Response Evaluation

This indication is considered appropriate with a score of 7 of 9 in the abovementioned systematic review (Jadvar et al. 2017). The findings described below are mainly based on chemotherapy given in the neoadjuvant setting. Results can vary for immunotherapy, targeted therapy, and in more advanced disease settings (Jadvar et al. 2017).

A meta-analysis by Cheng et al. (2012) included 17 studies (with 781 subjects) that fulfilled the inclusion criteria with the aim of determining the diagnostic performance of PET/CT for the evaluation of response to neoadjuvant chemotherapy in patients with breast cancer. The results show a pooled sensitivity of 85% (95% CI: 79–89%) and a pooled specificity of 66% (95% CI: 60–72%). The pooled likelihood ratio (LR+), negative likelihood ratio (LR–), and diagnostic odds ratio (DOR) were 2.835 (95% CI: 1.640–4.900), 0.221 (95% CI: 0.160–0.305), and 17.628 (95% CI 7.431–41.818). The area under the curve (AUC) was 0.8934. However, a worse efficacy was reported by another study with 76 patients receiving neoadjuvant chemotherapy, evidencing PET after two cycles and PET after the final cycle of chemotherapy had a sensitivity, specificity, positive, and negative predictive value of PET of 52%, 45%, 50%, and 47%, and 33%, 84%, 67%, and 56%, respectively (García Vicente et al. 2014), for predicting lymph node histopathological response in patients with locally advanced breast cancer (Jadvar et al. 2017).

3 Target Volume Delineation

The treatment of breast cancer should be multidisciplinary, involving gynecologists, pathologists, radiologists, surgeons, medical oncologists, and radiation oncologists and nuclear medicine physicians, among others, in order to personalize the treatment of each patient and offer better results. Figure 5 presents the case of a patient in which the importance of a multidisciplinary approach is key to success.

Radiation therapy, which purpose is to eliminate possible tumour cells from the area at risk for bearing residual cancer cells, aims to avoid local and distant recurrences, while causing as little damage as possible to healthy organs (organs at risk, OAR). In general, in cases of conservative surgery, postoperative radiation therapy is always performed, and in cases of mastectomy, radiation therapy is indicated in the presence of risk factors for recurrence.

In order to offer the best radiation therapy to patients, while limiting radiation dose to risk organs, several imaging techniques are used, which help to define the volumes of treatment correctly (clinical tumor volume, CTV; planning tumor volume, PTV). Throughout the world, the most used imaging technique for treatment planning is computed tomography (CT), but we can use the information provided by ultrasound, magnetic resonance, etc., to correctly identify the primary tumor bed and the lymph node regions.

To properly contour all the volumes related to treatment preparation, the first step is to perform a correct positioning of the patient. Patients are most often treated in the supine position using an immobilization system adaptable to the patient's anatomy.

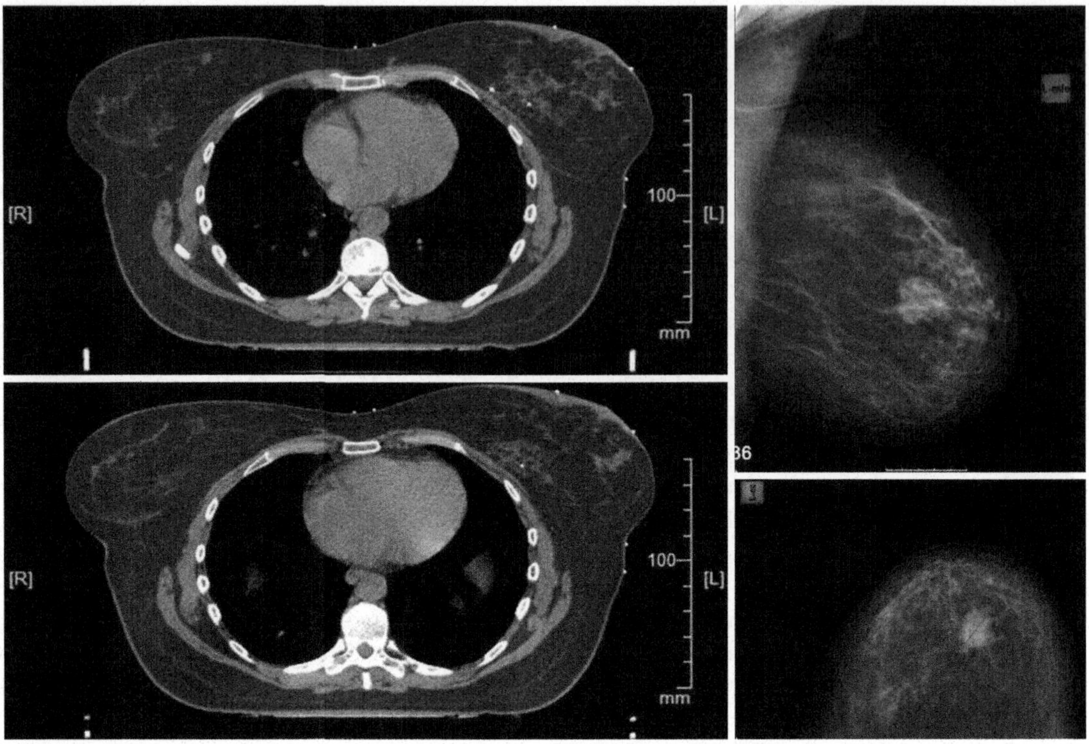

Fig. 5 Patient with a primary tumour in the left breast after oncoplastic surgery. The clips on the CT scan in radiation therapy position could easily misguide target volume contouring as they only indicate the deep site of the surgical bed but do not indicate the original position of the primary tumour to contour the primary tumour bed for boost or partial breast irradiation

- The immobilization is performed preferably with both arms abducted and rotated externally.
- All surgical scars should be marked with a radiopaque marker wire and the breast area with a circular wire.

Then, the volumes of treatment are defined according to the extent of the disease and the type of treatment received (conservative surgery, mastectomy, primary systemic chemotherapy) (Offersen et al. 2015; Strnad et al. 2015):

- Gross target volume (GTV): Primary tumour bed.
- Clinical target volume (CTV):
  - CTV breast (after conservative surgery): Includes the entire mammary gland.
  - CTV boost or APBI (after conservative surgery): Includes the primary tumour bed with a margin accounting for microscopic extension.
  - CTV chest wall (after mastectomy): Includes the subcutaneous tissue that covered the removed breast including the lymphatic drainage to the axilla.
  - CTV nodal for regional lymph node areas:
    - CTVn L1: Level 1.
    - CTVn L2: Level 2.
    - CTVn L3: Level 3.
    - CTVn L4: formerly called supraclavicular region.
    - CTVn IMN: the internal mammary nodes (IMN).
- Planning target volume (PTV): The CTV with a margin to accommodate for uncertainties related to treatment delivery including the variation in daily patients' positioning.

4 Radiation Oncology Treatments

4.1 Radiation Therapy in Conservative Surgery

Postoperative radiation therapy is indicated in all patients undergoing conservative surgery, unless there is a contraindication for its administration.

4.1.1 Whole-Breast Radiation

Radiation therapy of the entire breast reduces by ±3/4 the risk of recurrence of the disease versus surgery alone and reduces the risk of death, regardless of whether the armpit is affected or not (Early Breast Cancer Trialists' Collaborative Group (EBCTCG) et al. 2011).

Target and doses:

- The whole-breast should receive a dose of 40–42.5 Gy in 15–16 fractions moderately hypofractionated or 45–50.4 Gy in 25–28 fractions conventionally fractionated.
- A boost to the tumour bed is recommended in patients at higher risk for recurrence. Typical boost doses are 10–16 Gy in 4–8 fractions. It reduces the risk of local recurrence to a clinically significant level especially in high-grade young patients (under 50 years), reducing the need for mastectomy after lumpectomy, however affecting negatively the aesthetic result. It does not improve overall survival (Bartelink et al. 2001).

4.1.1.1 Volumes

CTV breast: The ESTRO consensus guideline on target volume delineation for elective radiation therapy of early-stage breast cancer defines the following limits for the CTV of the breast (Offersen et al. 2015): The dorsal border of the CTVp_breast is the ventral side of the major pectoral muscle and where that is not present the exterior side of the ribs and intercostal muscles. Nevertheless, at the caudal part of the breast, the dorsal border can be adjusted in ventro/ventrolateral direction—in particular in obese patients—since this rather represents subcutaneous fat extending from the abdominal wall which is not part of the CTV. This may decrease the dose to the heart in left-sided cases. The ventral border is 5 mm under the skin surface except in cases with T4b, T4c, and T4d cancer, where a full radiation dose up to the skin is advised, which can be obtained by using a bolus. The cranial border extends usually maximally up to the level of the caudal edge of the sternoclavicular joint, without this being a strict criterion (Offersen et al. 2015). The caudal border is the lowest CT slice with breast shape still visible. The medial border extends maximally to the ipsilateral edge of the sternal bone, without this being a strict criterion especially in the cases of ptotic breasts. Moreover, even in non-IV contrast-enhanced CT scans, it is usually possible to identify in some CT slices the medial mammary branches originating from the internal thoracic artery, and the breast glandular tissue is positioned lateral to these vessels—allowing for a reduction in the medial extension of the CTVp. At the lateral border, the breast tissue may produce a helpful—for delineation—fold, but in particular in obese patients, it may be very difficult to define this border clearly. Here again help is provided from the vessels, since it is usually possible to identify the lateral thoracic artery from which the lateral part of the breast is nourished, and the CTVp_breast should be delineated ventral/medial to this vessel. Irrespective of the position of the primary tumor bed in the breast, care should be taken that the CTVp_breast encompasses the primary tumour bed, including relevant margins around (Offersen et al. 2015).

GTV and CTV Boost: While the radiation dose can be delivered using several techniques, including external beam or intraoperative electrons, photons, or brachytherapy, the tumour bed remains always the same as described by Strnad et al. and by Boersma et al., most often on a CT scan in treatment position, although other imaging modalities, including ultrasound, can be used as well (Strnad et al. 2015; Boersma et al. 2012).

CTV Nodal Areas: Since 2000, after the results of the trial were published in the J. Clinical Oncology (Katz et al. 2000), and even more after the publication of the EBCTCG meta-analyses in 2005 (Clarke et al. 2005; Early Breast Cancer Trialists' Collaborative Group (EBCTCG) 2005; Chia et al. 2005), regional lymph node irradiation

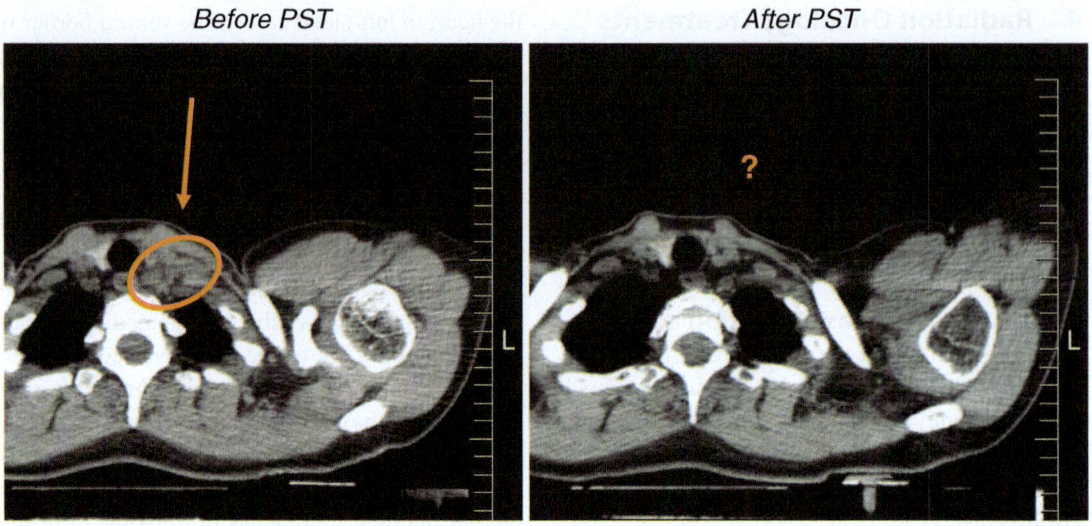

Fig. 6 Patient with locoregionally advanced left-sided breast cancer. The CT scan in radiation therapy (RT) position at the left shows the clinically enlarged lymph nodes in axilla level 4 (supraclavicular) before the primary systemic therapy (PST). The CT scan in RT position at the right shows complete remission of these nodes. Without the pre-PST scan, a geographical miss or, to avoid this, excessively large target volumes could have been caused

is at least to be considered for patients with 1–3 involved axillary nodes and recommended from four affected lymph nodes on, as it reduces recurrences and improves overall survival (Katz et al. 2000).

In recent years, research has focused on groups of patients with low nodal involvement N1. These patients represent a heterogeneous group that includes affectation of 1–3 lymph nodes and microscopic involvement of the sentinel lymph node. It is currently recommended to administer locoregional radiation therapy to patients with more than one lymph node involved, as it improves disease-free survival and metastasis-free survival by reducing the risk of recurrence and potentially improving overall survival (EBCTCG (Early Breast Cancer Trialists' Collaborative Group) et al. 2014).

The ESTRO consensus guideline on target volume delineation for elective radiation therapy of early-stage breast cancer also defines the limits for the CTV of the nodal areas (Offersen et al. 2015). The general principle is that the lymphatics follow the veins (axillary, subclavian, jugular, internal mammary). Because of this, the axilla is divided into five parts, using the pectoral muscles and the clavicle as anatomical borders. The ESTRO consensus guideline defines the boundaries of the following lymph node areas: axilla level 1 (CTVn_L1), axilla level 2 (CTVn_L2), axilla level 3 (CTVn_L3), lymph node level 4 (CTVn_L4), and the internal thoracic veins (CTVn_IMN) (Offersen et al. 2015). Figure 6 presents the case of a patient with clinically enlarged lymph nodes in axilla level 4 (supraclavicular) before the primary systemic therapy.

4.1.2 (Accelerated) Partial Breast Irradiation ((a)PBI)

For low-risk patients, a radiation therapy technique combined with conservative surgery is proposed as an alternative to whole-breast irradiation, delivering the doses to a limited volume of tissue surrounding the primary tumour bed. This can be done with 1–15 treatment fractions, varying between 1 day and 3 weeks, although most often a 1-week schedule is used.

Studies of APBI suggest that rates of local control in well-selected patients, using the ASTRO or the GEC_ESTRO criteria, with early-stage breast cancer are comparable to those treated with standard whole-breast RT for at least external beam and interstitial brachytherapy techniques (Offersen et al. 2015; Strnad et al. 2015, 2018; Montagne et al. 2019; Marta et al. 2019; Rahimy et al. 2019; Miranda et al. 2019; Schäfer et al. 2018). However, compared to standard whole-breast radiation, some but not all recent studies document an inferior cosmetic outcome with APBI.

The patients selected must generally meet the abovementioned criteria.

4.2 Radiation Therapy after Mastectomy

Postmastectomy radiation therapy has two important benefits for adequately selected patients: decreasing recurrence rates and increasing overall survival. Figure 7 presents the case of a patient after mastectomy.

The candidates for postmastectomy radiation therapy are those who are at greater risk of local recurrence of the disease:

- Tumour size (T3 or more).
- Lymph node involvement.
- Involved, especially deep, resection margins.
- Unfavorable histology including triple-negative and lobular types.

4.2.1 Chest Wall Irradiation (Including Breast Reconstruction)

Target and doses:

- The target volume consists of the draining lymphatics, mainly subcutaneously, and residual breast tissue. The CTV thereby includes the part of the chest wall that originally covered the removed breast, most or all of the mastectomy scar, and in high-risk patients the drain sites. The prescribed dose is identical to that for whole-breast irradiation.

4.2.1.1 Volumes

CTV Chest Wall: The ESTRO consensus guideline also defines the boundaries for the CTV of the thoracic wall (Offersen et al. 2015). In mastectomy patients, radiopaque wires should be positioned around the—imaginary—original site of the breast and also corresponding to the mastectomy scar. Whereas the position of the contralateral breast can be helpful for this if both arms are symmetrically elevated, generally the surface of the CTVp_thoracic wall is reduced by the surgical procedure following the pulling on adjacent skin and subcutaneous tissue to close the defect after removal of the breast (Offersen et al. 2015). Therefore, careful palpation of the thoracic wall

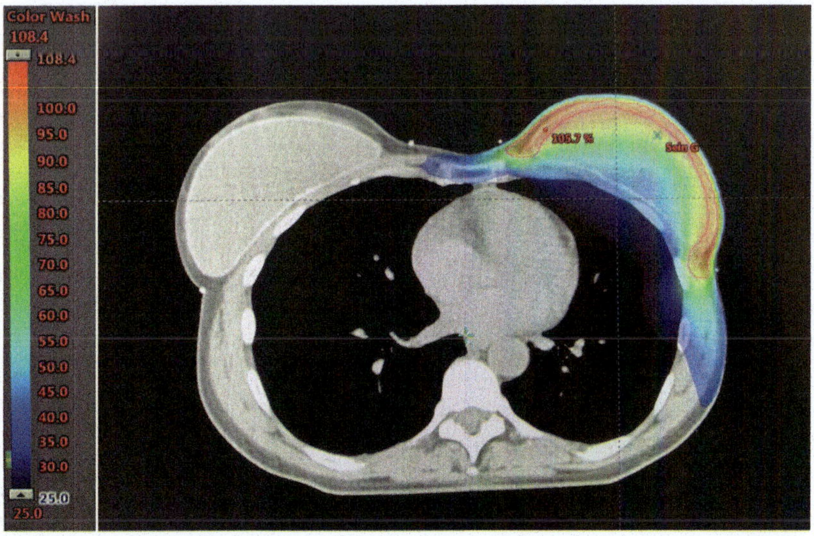

Fig. 7 Patient with bilateral breast augmentation after left-sided skin-sparing mastectomy. The target volume only includes the subcutaneous lymphatic plexus (red). With volumetric IMRT, a conformal dose distribution with sparing of nontarget tissues could be obtained

while positioning the radiopaque markers and the position of the mastectomy scar should be used as well. In some countries, e.g., Denmark, it is standard to apply a 3-mm bolus alongside the mastectomy scar extending a total of 6 cm in cranio-caudal direction (DBCG consensus). This is to achieve a full radiation dose in the skin to avoid skin recurrences. In general, the boundaries of the CTVp_thoracic wall are similar to those of the CTVp_breast as described above. In slim patients, the thoracic wall may be so thin that the CTV_thoracic wall disappears when cropping the volume 5 mm beneath the skin. In such cases, a 5-mm bolus may be applied, and the CTVp_thoracic wall should be extended up to the level of the skin. Unless invasion was demonstrated (tumor stage T4a and T4c), there is no reason for routinely including the major pectoral muscle and the ribs in the CTVp_thoracic wall (Offersen et al. 2015).

Chest Wall Scar Boost: This technique is mostly used in the USA. In Europe, its application is minimal. Different techniques using photons and/or electrons are appropriate, depending of the kind of surgery (mastectomy only or mastectomy plus reconstruction).

CTV Nodal: As mentioned above, with the aim of reducing recurrence and potentially improving overall survival, locoregional RT is indicated in patients undergoing mastectomy with one or more affected lymph nodes (EBCTCG (Early Breast Cancer Trialists' Collaborative Group) et al. 2014). The limits of CTV nodal for regional lymph node areas are the same as the CTV nodal in radiation therapy after conservative surgery (see previous section).

5 Conclusions

Breast cancer is the most frequent cancer in women. Early detection is of great importance, as it allows carrying out less aggressive treatments, maintaining identical or even better results, combined with a better quality of life, thereby the importance of including screening programs in the standard of care. Mammography, MRI, and ultrasound play a key role in staging and target volume definition, with additional benefits from PET scanning and other imaging modalities. The treatment of breast cancer requires a full multidisciplinary organization in order to personalize the treatment of each patient and to obtain better results adapted to each single patient. With the aim of offering the best radiation therapy treatment to patients, but in turn to limit radiation to organs at risk, several imaging techniques are used to delimit all volumes related to treatment correctly. Throughout the world, CT is the most frequently used imaging technique for treatment planning, but we can use the information provided by ultrasound, magnetic resonance, etc., to more precisely define the tumour bed and the lymphatic drainage pathways. Regarding [^{18}F] FDG PET/CT, it has a limited role in the diagnosis of breast cancer, but it can provide relevant information for detecting locoregional (including nodal) as well as distant disease, for helping to plan surgical and medical treatment, for monitoring response to treatment, and for locating recurrent disease. PET also has the potential to quickly assess new treatments by detecting their effects on specific receptors and has evidenced it improves the prediction of the clinical outcome in previously treated breast cancer patients.

References

ACR BI-RADS Atlas® (n.d.) 5th Edition. https://www.acr.org/Clinical-Resources/Reporting-and-Data-Systems/Bi-Rads

Bartelink H, Horiot JC, Poortmans P, Struikmans H, Van den Bogaert W, Barillot I, European Organization for Research and Treatment of Cancer Radiotherapy and Breast Cancer Groups et al (2001) Recurrence rates after treatment of breast cancer with standard radiotherapy with or without additional radiation. N Engl J Med 345:1378–1387

Boersma LJ, Janssen T, Elkhuizen PH, Poortmans P, van der Sangen M, Scholten AN et al (2012) Reducing interobserver variation of boost-CTV delineation in breast conserving radiation therapy using a preoperative CT and delineation guidelines. Radiother Oncol 103:178–182

Bombardieri E, Crippa F (2001) PET imaging in breast cancer. Q J Nucl Med 45:245–256

Brekelmans CT, Seynaeve C, Bartels CC, Tilanus-Linthorst MM, Meijers-Heijboer EJ, Rotterdam Committee for Medical and Genetic Counseling et al

(2001) Effectiveness of breast cancer surveillance in BRCA1/2 gene mutation carriers and women with high familial risk. J Clin Oncol 19:924–930
Buscombe JR, Holloway B, Roche N, Bombardieri E (2004) Position of nuclear medicine modalities in the diagnostic work-up of breast cancer. Q J Nucl Med Mol Imaging 48:109–118
Byrne AM, Hill AD, Skehan SJ, McDermott EW, O'Higgins NJ (2004) Positron emission tomography in the staging and management of breast cancer. Br J Surg 91:1398–1409
Champion L, Brain E, Giraudet AL, Le Stanc E, Wartski M, Edeline V et al (2011) Breast cancer recurrence diagnosis suspected on tumor marker rising: value of whole-body 18FDG-PET/CT imaging and impact on patient management. Cancer 117:1621–1629
Cheng X, Li Y, Liu B, Xu Z, Bao L, Wang J (2012) 18F-FDG PET/CT and PET for evaluation of pathological response to neoadjuvant chemotherapy in breast cancer: a meta-analysis. Acta Radiol 53:615–627
Chia S, Bryce C, Gelmon K (2005) The 2000 EBCTCG overview: a widening gap. Lancet 365:1665–1666
Clarke M, Collins R, Darby S, Davies C, Elphinstone P, Evans V, Early Breast Cancer Trialists' Collaborative Group (EBCTCG) et al (2005) Effects of radiotherapy and of differences in the extent of surgery for early breast cancer on local recurrence and 15-year survival: an overview of the randomised trials. Lancet 366:2087–2106
Dirisamer A, Halpern BS, Flöry D, Wolf F, Beheshti M, Mayerhoefer ME, Langsteger W (2010) Integrated contrast-enhanced diagnostic whole-body PET/CT as a first-line restaging modality in patients with suspected metastatic recurrence of breast cancer. Eur J Radiol 73:294–299
Early Breast Cancer Trialists' Collaborative Group (EBCTCG) (2005) Effects of chemotherapy and hormonal therapy for early breast cancer on recurrence and 15-year survival: an overview of the randomised trials. Lancet 365:1687–1717
Early Breast Cancer Trialists' Collaborative Group (EBCTCG), Darby S, McGale P, Correa C, Taylor C, Arriagada R, Clarke M et al (2011) Effect of radiotherapy after breast-conserving surgery on 10-year recurrence and 15-year breast cancer death: meta-analysis of individual patient data for 10,801 women in 17 randomised trials. Lancet 378:1707–1716
EBCTCG (Early Breast Cancer Trialists' Collaborative Group), McGale P, Taylor C, Correa C, Cutter D, Duane F, Ewertz M et al (2014) Effect of radiotherapy after mastectomy and axillary surgery on 10-year recurrence and 20-year breast cancer mortality: meta-analysis of individual patient data for 8135 women in 22 randomised trials. Lancet 383:2127–2135
Esserman L (2005) Integration of imaging in the management of breast cancer. J Clin Oncol 23:1601–1602
Evangelista L, Baretta Z, Vinante L, Bezzon E, De Carolis V, Cervino AR et al (2012) Comparison of 18F-FDG positron emission tomography/computed tomography and computed tomography in patients with already-treated breast cancer: diagnostic and prognostic implications. Q J Nucl Med Mol Imaging 56:375–384
Flanagan FL, Dehdashti F, Siegel BA (1998) PET in breast cancer. Semin Nucl Med 28:290–302
García Vicente AM, Soriano Castrejón Á, León Martín A, Relea Calatayud F, Muñoz Sánchez Mdel M, Cruz Mora MÁ et al (2014) Early and delayed prediction of axillary lymph node neoadjuvant response by (18)F-FDG PET/CT in patients with locally advanced breast cancer. Eur J Nucl Med Mol Imaging 41:1309–1318
Hendrick RE, Smith RA, Rutledge JH III, Smart CR (1997) Benefit of screening mammography in women aged 40–49: a new meta-analysis of randomized controlled trials. J Natl Cancer Inst Monogr 1997:87–92
Houssami N, Ciatto S, Macaskill P, Lord SJ, Warren RM, Dixon JM, Irwig L (2008) Accuracy and surgical impact of magnetic resonance imaging in breast cancer staging: systematic review and meta-analysis in detection of multifocal and multicentric cancer. J Clin Oncol 26:3248–3258
Isasi CR, Moadel RM, Blaufox MD (2005) A meta-analysis of FDG-PET for the evaluation of breast cancer recurrence and metastases. Breast Cancer Res Treat 90:105–112
Jadvar H, Colletti PM, Delgado-Bolton R, Esposito G, Krause BJ, Iagaru AH et al (2017) Appropriate use criteria for FDG PET/CT restaging and treatment response assessment of malignant disease. J Nucl Med 58:2026–2037
Katz A, Strom EA, Buchholz TA, Thames HD (2000) Locoregional recurrence patterns after mastectomy and doxorubicin-based chemotherapy: implications for postoperative irradiation. J Clin Oncol 18:2817–2827
Kumar R, Chauhan A, Zhuang H, Chandra P, Schnall M, Alavi A (2006) Clinicopathologic factors associated with false negative FDG-PET in primary breast cancer. Breast Cancer Res Treat 98:267–274
Lee CH, Dershaw DD, Kopans D, Evans P, Monsees B, Monticciolo D et al (2010) Breast cancer screening with imaging: recommendations from the Society of Breast Imaging and the ACR on the use of mammography, breast MRI, breast ultrasound, and other technologies for the detection of clinically occult breast cancer. J Am Coll Radiol 7:18–27
Mandelson MT, Oestreicher N, Porter PL, White D, Finder CA, Taplin SH, White E (2000) Breast density as a predictor of mammographic detection: comparison of interval- and screen-detected cancers. J Natl Cancer Inst 92:1081–1087
Manohar K, Mittal BR, Senthil R, Kashyap R, Bhattacharya A, Singh G (2012) Clinical utility of F-18 FDG PET/CT in recurrent breast carcinoma. Nucl Med Commun 33:591–596
Marta GN, Barrett J, Porfirio GJM, Martimbianco ALC, Bevilacqua JLB, Poortmans P, Riera R (2019) Effectiveness of different accelerated partial breast irradiation techniques for the treatment of breast cancer patients: systematic review using indirect comparisons of randomized clinical trials. Rep Pract Oncol Radiother 24:165–174

Miranda FA, Teixeira LAB, Heinzen RN, de Andrade FEM, Hijal T, Buchholz TA et al (2019) Accelerated partial breast irradiation: current status with a focus on clinical practice. Breast J 25:124–128

Montagne L, Gal J, Chand ME, Schiappa R, Falk AT, Kinj R et al (2019) GEC-ESTRO APBI classification as a decision-making tool for the management of 2nd ipsilateral breast tumor event. Breast Cancer Res Treat. https://doi.org/10.1007/s10549-019-05221-z. [Epub ahead of print]

Morris EA, Schwartz LH, Drotman MB, Kim SJ, Tan LK, Liberman L et al (2000) Evaluation of pectoralis major muscle in patients with posterior breast tumors on breast MR images: early experience. Radiology 214:67–72

NCCN Clinical practice guidelines in oncology (NCCN guidelines®) guidelines version 1.2019 — march 14, 2019. NCCN.org. Breast Cancer Accessed 31 March 2019. https://www.nccn.org/professionals/physician_gls/pdf/breast.pdf

Offersen BV, Boersma LJ, Kirkove C, Hol S, Aznar MC, Biete Sola A et al (2015) ESTRO consensus guideline on target volume delineation for elective radiation therapy of early stage breast cancer. Radiother Oncol 114:3–10

Pennant M, Takwoingi Y, Pennant L, Davenport C, Fry-Smith A, Eisinga A et al (2010) A systematic review of positron emission tomography (PET) and positron emission tomography/computed tomography (PET/CT) for the diagnosis of breast cancer recurrence. Health Technol Assess 14:1–103

Quon A, Gambhir SS (2005) FDG-PET and beyond: molecular breast cancer imaging. J Clin Oncol 23:1664–1673

Rahimy E, Weidhaas J, Wei W, Lannin D, Horowitz N, Higgins S et al (2019) Patient-reported outcomes and cosmesis in a feasibility study of 4-dimensional simulated image guided accelerated partial breast irradiation. Pract Radiat Oncol. https://doi.org/10.1016/j.prro.2019.01.013. pii: S1879–8500(19)30047–5. [Epub ahead of print]

Raylman RR, Majewski S, Smith MF, Proffitt J, Hammond W, Srinivasan A et al (2008) The positron emission mammography/tomography breast imaging and biopsy system (PEM/PET): design, construction and phantom-based measurements. Phys Med Biol 53:637–653

Rieber A, Schirrmeister H, Gabelmann A, Nuessle K, Reske S, Kreienberg R et al (2002) Pre-operative staging of invasive breast cancer with MR mammography and/or PET: boon or bunk? Br J Radiol 75:789–798

Santiago JF, Gonen M, Yeung H, Macapinlac H, Larson S (2006) A retrospective analysis of the impact of 18F-FDG PET scans on clinical management of 133 breast cancer patients. Q J Nucl Med Mol Imaging 50:61–67

Schäfer R, Strnad V, Polgár C, Uter W, Hildebrandt G, Ott OJ, Groupe Européen de Curiethérapie of European Society for Radiotherapy and Oncology (GEC-ESTRO) et al (2018) Quality-of-life results for accelerated partial breast irradiation with interstitial brachytherapy versus whole-breast irradiation in early breast cancer after breast-conserving surgery (GEC-ESTRO): 5-year results of a randomised, phase 3 trial. Lancet Oncol 19:834–844

Strnad V, Hannoun-Levi JM, Guinot JL, Lössl K, Kauer-Dorner D, Resch A, Working Group Breast Cancer of GEC-ESTRO et al (2015) Recommendations from GEC ESTRO Breast Cancer Working Group (I): target definition and target delineation for accelerated or boost partial breast irradiation using multicatheter interstitial brachytherapy after breast conserving closed cavity surgery. Radiother Oncol 115:342–348

Strnad V, Major T, Polgar C, Lotter M, Guinot JL, Gutierrez-Miguelez C et al (2018) ESTRO-ACROP guideline: interstitial multi-catheter breast brachytherapy as accelerated partial breast irradiation alone or as boost – GEC-ESTRO Breast Cancer Working Group practical recommendations. Radiother Oncol 128:411–420

Tabár L, Vitak B, Chen HH, Yen MF, Duffy SW, Smith RA (2001) Beyond randomized controlled trials: organized mammographic screening substantially reduces breast carcinoma mortality. Cancer 91:1724–1731

Veit-Haibach P, Antoch G, Beyer T, Stergar H, Schleucher R, Hauth EA, Bockisch A (2007) FDG-PET/CT in restaging of patients with recurrent breast cancer: possible impact on staging and therapy. Br J Radiol 80:508–515

Vranjesevic D, Filmont JE, Meta J, Silverman DH, Phelps ME, Rao J et al (2002) Whole-body (18)F-FDG PET and conventional imaging for predicting outcome in previously treated breast cancer patients. J Nucl Med 43:325–329

Wahl RL, Siegel BA, Coleman RE, Gatsonis CG (2004) Prospective multicenter study of axillary nodal staging by positron emission tomography in breast cancer: a report of the staging breast cancer with PET Study Group. J Clin Oncol 22:277–285

Zangheri B, Messa C, Picchio M, Gianolli L, Landoni C, Fazio F (2004) PET/CT and breast cancer. Eur J Nucl Med Mol Imaging 31(Suppl 1):S135–S142

T-Staging and Target Volume Definition by Imaging in GI Tumors

Maria Isabel Morales, Feyza Sen, Bülent Polat, Philip Kleine, and Andreas Buck

Contents

1 **Esophageal Cancer and Cancer of the Gastroesophageal Junction** 203
2 **Gastric Cancer** 208
3 **Colorectal Cancer** 209
4 **Pancreatic Cancer** 213
References 217

M. I. Morales
Department of Nuclear Medicine, University Hospital of Würzburg, Würzburg, Germany

Department of Nuclear Medicine, University of Navarra, Pamplona, Navarra, Spain

F. Sen
Department of Nuclear Medicine, University Hospital of Würzburg, Würzburg, Germany

Department of Nuclear Medicine, Uludag University Hospital, Bursa, Turkey

B. Polat · P. Kleine
Department of Radiation Oncology, University Hospital of Würzburg, Würzburg, Germany

A. Buck (✉)
Department of Nuclear Medicine, University Hospital of Würzburg, Würzburg, Germany
e-mail: buck_a@ukw.de

1 Esophageal Cancer and Cancer of the Gastroesophageal Junction

This chapter focuses on analyzing the ability of tomographic imaging techniques including PET/CT to detect the primary tumor of esophageal cancer and cancer of the gastroesophageal junction (GEJ) by means of T-staging and determining the added value of tomographic imaging including PET/CT for target volume delineation in radiotherapy planning procedures (Fig. 1). Gastric cancers are addressed separately because of the low sensitivity of [^{18}F]FDG-PET in frequent subtypes of these cancers, limiting its use in staging and in the delineation process.

In North America and Europe, a relevant change in incidence of esophageal and GEJ cancers in favor of adenocarcinoma has been observed in the last decades (Lagergren and Lagergren 2013; Zhang 2013). Worldwide, squamous cell carcinoma (SCC) still represents the most common histologic subtype. Both subtypes differ in a number of features including risk factors, tumor location, tumor biology, and outcomes. Smoking and alcohol consumption are the major risk factors for SCC, while acid reflux and Barrett's esophagus are the main underlying mechanisms in the development of esophageal adenocarcinoma. A diagnosis of esophageal and GEJ cancer, either SCC or adenocarcinoma subtype, generally implies a poor prognosis. At least half of the

R. G. H. Beets-Tan et al. (eds.), *Imaging and Interventional Radiology for Radiation Oncology*, Medical Radiology, Diagnostic Imaging, https://doi.org/10.1007/978-3-030-38261-2_14

patients are diagnosed at an advanced stage (Courrech Staal et al. 2009). This occurs because of early and rapid dissemination of tumor cells to regional lymph nodes and distant organs. This aggressive tumor biology underscores the need of early diagnosis and accurate selection of patients who might benefit from curatively intended therapy. After new refinements in endoscopic and imaging techniques and major recent advances such as new strategies of neoadjuvant treatment and molecular therapies, the diagnosis can be established also at earlier stages. Consequently, the morbidity rate has been lowered considerably, but recent prognostic trends have not yet found its way to a noteworthy improvement in patient outcome. In esophageal adenocarcinoma, the clinical feature of locally circumscribed tumors is silent with no tumor-related symptoms and rarely manifests with gastrointestinal bleeding in patients having ulcers (Behrens et al. 2011). The underlying reflux may present itself with heartburn and retrosternal pain and should prompt for endoscopy. Late in the course of the disease of both subtypes, dysphagia predominates clinically besides general, tumor-related symptoms.

Precise staging is a key component in the initial workup and subsequent patient management. The staging classification of esophageal and GEJ cancer has been recently refined with the newest eighth edition of the American Joint Committee on Cancer (AJCC) TNM system with incorporation of anatomic and nonanatomic categories (Rice et al. 2017). New to the eighth edition, the treatment strategy has taken into consideration not only the classification by clinical stage (cTNM) before any treatment and pathologic stage after surgery (pTNM) but also the pathologic stage after neoadjuvant treatment (ypTNM). Early esophageal carcinoma includes tumors which are restricted to the submucosa with no lymph nodes involved (T1a/b, N0) (NCCN guidelines esophageal and esophagogastric cancers; version 2020). The treatment options include endoscopic resection or esophagectomy in case of resectable disease. However, the use of surgery alone in curative intent results in suboptimal outcomes, especially in patients with locally advanced disease due to inadequate local or systemic tumor control. Therefore, the management of these cancers requires a multidisciplinary decision-making process for either staging or treatment, regardless of the histological subtype (Cools-Lartigue and Ferri 2019). Combined chemoradiotherapy, either as definitive therapy or in the neoadjuvant setting, is nowadays applied more frequently. Recent randomized controlled clinical trials have confirmed the efficacy of preoperative chemoradiation (CROSS study) and perioperative chemotherapy (MAGIC trial, including gastric cancers predominantly with lower esophageal and GEJ cancers) followed by surgery with improved survival rates, hence becoming accepted standards for therapeutic management (Van Hagen et al. 2012; Cunningham et al. 2006). Recently, targeted therapies have shown encouraging results as an alternative treatment of advanced GEJ adenocarcinoma which are refractory to first-line chemotherapy.

SCC tends to be more sensitive to radiation therapy and chemotherapy than adenocarcinoma. However, neoadjuvant CRT has also demonstrated a benefit in patients with esophageal adenocarcinoma, albeit the benefit is less pronounced compared to patients with SCC (Cools-Lartigue and Ferri 2019). Though the surgical pathology (pTNM) produces the most accurate staging, the advent of better imaging techniques with high resolution has improved clinical staging (Kim et al. 2009) and provides the baseline for subsequent treatment decisions. After diagnosis with endoscopic biopsy, patients usually undergo endoscopic ultrasonography (EUS), which has excellent sensitivity and specificity and accurately determines T stage and locoregional node involvement in esophageal and GEJ cancer (Walker et al. 2011). The depth of tumor invasion is one of the criteria used to select multimodality treatment protocols instead of primary surgery (Kim et al. 2009). Accuracy of EUS for T determination is around 80–89% with the best accuracy for T3–T4 tumors (Lu et al. 2016; Lightdale and Kulkarni 2005). Should EUS raise a suspicion for paraesophageal nodal involvement, this can further be clarified histologically by means of EUS-guided fine-needle aspiration.

Computed tomography (CT) plays an important role in the initial staging process to assess local invasion of adjacent mediastinal structures as well as regional nodal involvement and to rule out distant metastases. T-staging at CT depends on esophageal wall thickening (>5 mm); therefore, CT is less accurate to differentiate T1, T2, and T3 tumors (Lu et al. 2016) (Fig. 2). The ability of positron emission tomography (PET) to visualize metabolic characteristics of tumors has been a major advance in staging of gastrointestinal malignancies. PET imaging is primarily performed using [^{18}F]fluorodeoxyglucose ([^{18}F] FDG), a radiolabeled metabolite which accumulates in tissues with a high turnover of glucose, representing viability and proliferative activity of tumors. The standardized uptake value (SUV) is a semiquantitative measure of [^{18}F]FDG-uptake and metabolic activity of tumors. Incorporation of [^{18}F]FDG-PET to the anatomical CT dataset, referred to as integrated [^{18}F]FDG-PET/CT, has a proven value for tumor staging by precise depiction of the tumor extent and locoregional lymph node involvement, especially nonadjacent lymph nodes and distant metastasis. According to the current NCCN (2020) practice guideline, [^{18}F] FDG-PET/CT is being considered a routine component of initial staging workup for esophageal and GEJ cancers and recommended to be performed when there is no evidence of metastatic disease. [^{18}F]FDG-PET/CT provides more accurate staging and prognostic stratification than CT alone and can lead to a change of management in more than one third of patients. However, [^{18}F] FDG-PET/CT has some limitations in the assessment of the primary tumor and particularly in the detection of peritumoral nodal disease (Barber et al. 2012). Because such lymph nodes are likely to be resected with the primary tumor or included in the radiation field, the clinical significance of false negative lymph nodes is expected to be less relevant from a clinical point of view.

Several studies have assessed the detection rate of [^{18}F]FDG-PET in primary tumors. Increased uptake of [^{18}F]FDG was seen in 68–100% of esophageal tumors (Muijs et al. 2010). Early-stage disease, particularly T1, is less likely to be visualized on PET. Especially T1a tumors remaining within the muscularis mucosa are found difficult to be detected by [^{18}F]FDG-PET/CT (Muijs et al. 2010; Kato et al. 2005). In one study, only 43% of pT1 tumors demonstrated focal [^{18}F]FDG-uptake, whereas almost all pT2-T4 tumors were visualized by PET (Kato et al. 2005). [^{18}F]FDG accumulation was observed in 18% of patients with pT1a tumors and 61% of patients with pT1b tumors involving the submucosa. Detection rates in patients with pT2, pT3, and pT4 tumors were 83%, 97%, and 100%, respectively. It has been suggested that PET imaging detects primary esophageal tumors with an invasion status of T1b or greater, whereas T1a tumors cannot be adequately detected (Himeno et al. 2002). The relationship between the intensity of [^{18}F]FDG-uptake, expressed as SUV, and the depth of tumor invasion has been assessed in some studies, but there is no final agreement on a significant correlation (Kato et al. 2002; Flamen et al. 2000). T-staging of GEJ tumors is based on histologic depth of invasion rather than absolute size. Hence, the resolution of [^{18}F]FDG-PET/CT seems not sufficient enough to replace endoscopic ultrasonography (EUS) or CT (Wu and Goodman 2013).

In esophageal cancers, radiotherapy represents the treatment modality of choice. Accurate delineation and subsequent irradiation of the gross tumor volume (GTV) is a prerequisite for a successful radiotherapy in patients with esophageal or GEJ cancers (Muijs et al. 2010). The major aim of radiotherapy is the delivery of an optimal radiation dose to the tumor with minimum geographic misses and minimum of radiation injury to neighboring healthy tissues. Target volume definition is challenging as it is observer dependent. The terminology of target volumes include delineation of the gross tumor volume (GTV, i.e., primary tumor and locoregional lymph node metastases), the clinical target volume (CTV, i.e., GTV plus safety margin in all directions and elective nodal areas to cover potential microscopic disease), and planning target volume (PTV) to account for set-up inaccuracies and esophageal, gastric, and respiratory movements during radiation (Schreurs et al. 2010). Currently, target volume definition for treatment planning is based on intravenous contrast-enhanced CT. Despite some inherent limitations,

CT, in combination with endoscopic ultrasound, is considered as standard imaging modality for state-of-the-art radiotherapy. Definition of the cranio-caudal tumor extent is demanding on CT images. However, on CT, poor soft tissue discrimination of esophagus and adjacent lymph nodes and the difficulty in depiction of pathologic alteration in normal-sized structures remain as limiting factors which are responsible for a large interobserver variability in target volume delineation. As mentioned previously, EUS is useful in determining the depth of invasion, T stage, and peritumoral lymph node involvement. However, the translation of EUS findings into the treatment planning process is difficult (Konski et al. 2005).

[^{18}F]FDG-PET/CT has emerged as newest functional imaging modality in order to guide target delineation and to more precisely define the GTV (Fig. 1). The role of [^{18}F]FDG-PET/CT in radiotherapy planning of esophageal carcinoma is less developed, though changes in target volume with potential impact on treatment planning have been reported in preliminary studies (Muijs et al. 2010; Muijs et al. 2013; Muijs et al. 2014; le Grange et al. 2015). Muijs et al. have established two treatment plans for each of 21 patients: one based on CT data alone and the other incorporating also PET/CT images. The CT-based treatment plan inadequately covered PET-based target volume in 36% of patients (Muijs et al. 2010). Cranial and caudal adjustment of the primary tumor demarcation, as defined by CT planning alone versus PET/CT, resulted in discordancies of geographic misses (Leong et al. 2006; Schreurs et al. 2010). Leong et al. reported that CT-based GTV excluded PET-avid disease in 69% of patients, and a geographic miss of gross tumor appeared in 31% of patients, respectively. When compared with CT alone, PET/CT is assumed to more accurately represent true disease extent. In several studies, PET/CT has shown a significant impact on defining GTV, CTV, and PTV and may result in a reduction of radiation-induced toxicity and improvement of locoregional control of disease. Moureau-Zabotto et al. (2005) reported that PET/CT resulted in a decrease in GTV in 12 of 34 patients examined (35%). In 7 patients of the same group, PET/CT also appeared to increase the GTV, owing to an increased detection of primary tumor and occult lymph node metastases (Moureau-Zabotto et al. 2005). Small but suspicious lymph nodes at CT may be missed on [^{18}F]FDG-PET because of the limited spatial resolution (approx. 5 mm). The significance of [^{18}F]FDG-negative tumor margins remains to be determined since long-term outcome data are not available right now. Conversely, if target volume includes false-positive nodes, this may cause an increased radiation field with the possibility of late radiation toxicity such as radiation pneumonitis or even cardiac mortality. An important issue regarding the use of [^{18}F]FDG-PET for tumor volume delineation is the methodology employed to define the functional volume of interest. Different methods have been proposed including visual judgement (Schreurs et al. 2010; Moureau-Zabotto et al. 2005) and semiautomated contouring methods applying SUV thresholds on PET/CT images (Mamede et al. 2007; Zhong et al. 2009; Thomas et al. 2015). Visual discrimination of tumor boundaries is observer dependent and can lead to significant bias. None of the thresholding approaches have been standardized. Especially in small-sized tumors, image count levels are affected by partial volume effects. Also, heterogeneous tracer uptake may cause difficulties for image interpretation, introducing additional bias. Another challenge is the precise delineation of motion artefacts. It has been reported that the distal esophagus shows more mobility compared with the proximal region (Dieleman et al. 2007) and the lower third is affected in a stronger way by respiratory-induced motion (Yamashita et al. 2011). Motion artefacts can severely influence tumor volume estimation and require correction algorithms such as respiratory gating. Target definition in esophageal cancer based on PET-images may not provide clear tumor margins due to the presence of peritumoral inflammation, which frequently occurs. A standard [^{18}F]FDG-PET cannot reliably differentiate between inflammation and increased glucose uptake in a malignant lesion. However, there are other radiopharmaceuticals available which could potentially aid in differentiation, e.g., [^{18}F]fluorothymidine (FLT) (van Westreenen et al. 2005).

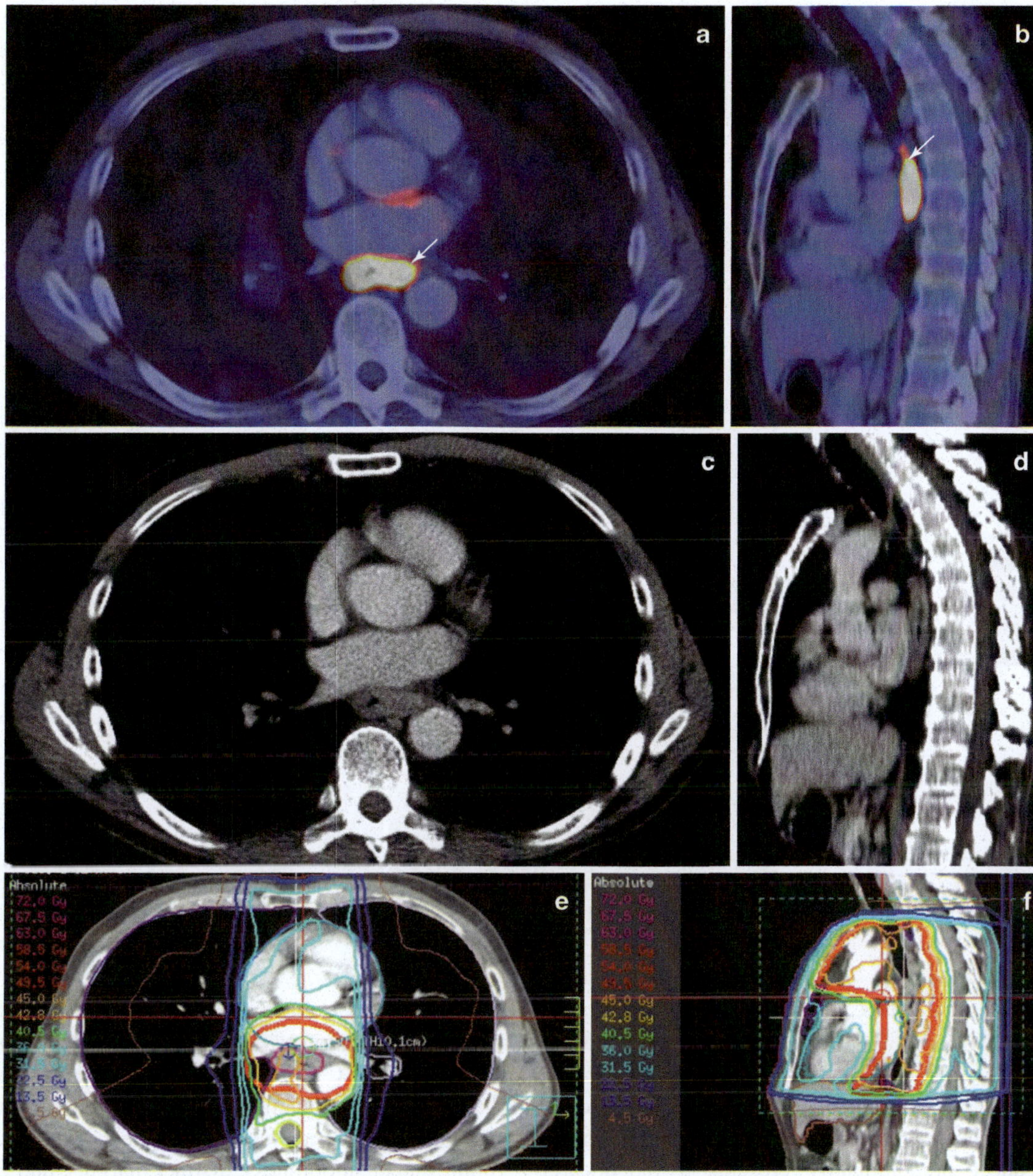

Fig. 1 [18F]FDG-PET/CT for radiotherapy planning. Transversal (**a**) and sagittal (**b**) section of PET/CT reveal intense uptake of the glucose analog [18F]FDG in the primary tumor (esophageal cancer, arrow). Corresponding sections of contrast-enhanced CT are shown in transversal (**c**) and sagittal view (**d**). Definition of the GTV based on [18F]FDG-PET/CT is shown in (**e**, transversal section) and (**f**, sagittal view)

In summary, the addition of PET to CT-based radiation treatment planning has improved target volume definition by more accurate localization of the primary tumor and involved locoregional lymph nodes, which in turn improves local disease control and reduces radiation-induced risks and complications (Muijs et al. 2013). There is currently no uniformly accepted method for incorporating the PET information into target delineation, and there is an obvious lack of prospectively validated data. Incorporation of [18F]FDG-PET imaging into CT-assisted volume definition seems to have great impact on target volume definition with the potential to avoid geographical misses (Fig. 2).

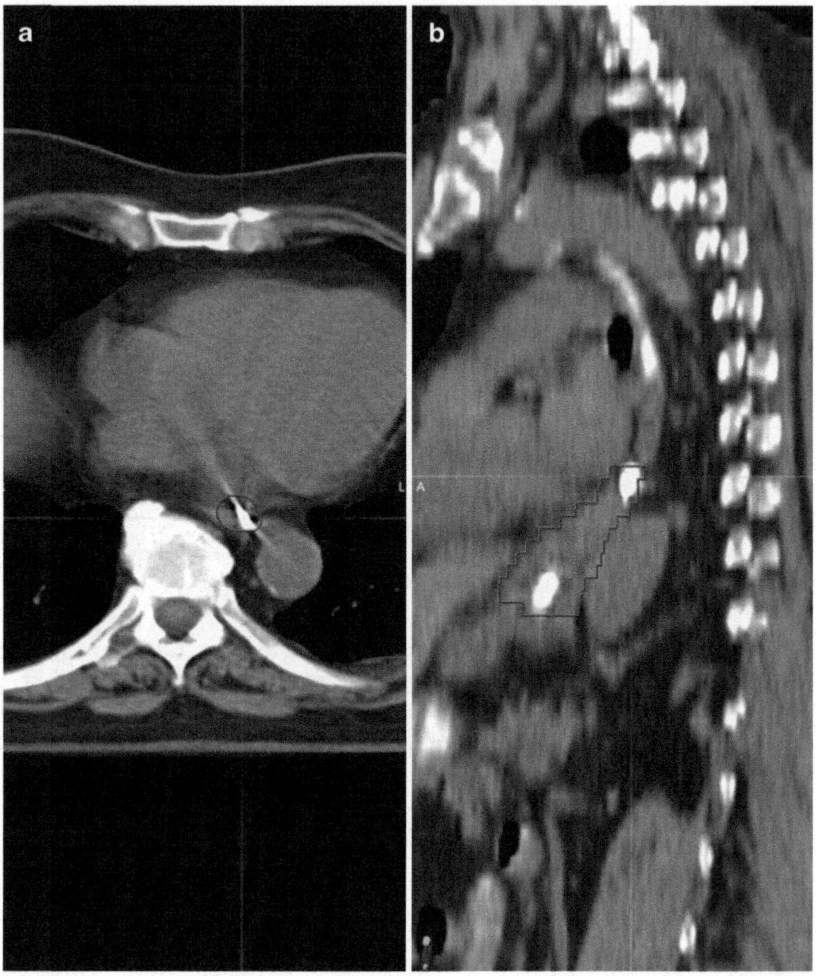

Fig. 2 Enhanced definition of the GTV based on CT-visible clips. With this approach, precise delineation of the GTV based on pretherapeutic PET/CT can be ensured (Thomas et al. Radiother Oncol 2015; with permission)

2 Gastric Cancer

Despite significant advances in diagnosis and treatment, gastric cancer remains a leading cause of cancer death worldwide. In general, gastric cancer predominantly presents as adenocarcinoma. The individual prognosis depends mainly on tumor stage and histology, surgical curability, and response to adjuvant or neoadjuvant therapies. Early gastric cancer is defined as limited to mucosa or submucosa, and endoscopic resection is considered with or without lymphadenectomy for T1a and T1b tumors, respectively. Until a distant metastasis has been identified, the patient is a candidate for respective surgery. Adjuvant and neoadjuvant therapies are necessary options before and/or after surgery. Whereas EUS is used routinely to determine the T- and N-stage, it is less useful in distal tumors (Smhty et al. 2016). When compared with CT, EUS is more accurate for the diagnosis of lymphatic involvement based on malignancy criteria such as hypoechogenicity, round shape, smoothness, distinct margins, and a size >1 cm (Bhutani et al. 1997). Other than considered as routine component of initial staging workup for esophageal and GEJ cancers NCCN 2020, [^{18}F]FDG-PET is less sensitive for identifying primary gastric cancers. Nearly 20–30% of gastric cancers cannot be detected by [^{18}F]FDG-PET (Dassen et al. 2009). This is related to a highly variable [^{18}F]FDG-avidity in different histological subtypes. In diffuse and mucinous tumor types or signet ring cell carcinoma, detection rate is low (Dębiec et al. 2017).

Distal gastric tumors tend not to take up [^{18}F]FDG when compared with proximal gastric and GEJ cancers as they are more likely to be of a non-intestinal subtype (Mukai et al. 2006; Stahl et al. 2003). The role of PET/CT is limited in T-staging due to its low spatial resolution (Yun et al. 2014). An improvement by means of sensitivity may be achieved using alternative PET radiotracers such as [^{18}F]fluorothymidine (FLT) rather than [^{18}F]FDG (Ott et al. 2011).

Technical and histopathological factors affect the visibility of primary gastric tumors at [^{18}F]FDG-PET/CT. Inflammatory conditions (e.g., gastritis) can lead to false-positive PET findings, and physiological [^{18}F]FDG-uptake adds to potential confusion. Distension of the stomach with water is a simple approach to overcome physiological [^{18}F]FDG-uptake and improve diagnostic performance of PET/CT for detecting primary tumors. The role of [^{18}F]FDG-PET/CT in the tumor delineation process remains unclear with very few studies existing in literature (Dębiec et al. 2017). This may be related to the low tracer accumulation and low sensitivity frequently seen in gastric cancer subtypes. Thus, no definite conclusions can be drawn on the use of [^{18}F]FDG-PET/CT for this purpose.

3 Colorectal Cancer

Worldwide, colorectal cancer is the third most common cancer with over 1.8 million new cases in 2018 according to the American Institute for Cancer Research (AICR) and World Cancer Research Foundation (WCRF). Its overall survival at 5 years varies from 50% to 60%, with high dependency on disease stage (Chouwhury et al. 2010; National Institute for Health and Clinical Excellence 2004). In contrast, cancer of the anal canal is an uncommon disease that accounts for up to 4% of all anorectal malignancies, with a higher incidence reported in people with HIV infection (Crum-Cianflone et al. 2010; D'Souza et al. 2008; Bedimo et al. 2004; Piketty et al. 2008). According to the American College of Radiology (ACR) Appropriateness Criteria guidelines (Fowler et al. 2017), colon cancer diagnosis is based on its clinical presentation (blood in stools, anemia, obstruction) or on its incidental diagnosis in asymptomatic stages during a routine colonoscopy surveillance. The last version of the TNM classification, suggested by the American Joint Committee on Cancer (AJCC), is the eighth edition, with other historical staging systems no longer in use (Dukes or Astler-Coller) (Amin et al. 2016). Nevertheless, it must be taken into account that the final diagnosis is established after tumor excision based on histopathology. Current treatment strategies are divided into two branches, the primary tumor management and distant/metastatic disease management. The primary tumor management in colon and rectal cancer usually consists of surgery together with selective chemotherapy or multimodal treatment in case of high-risk tumors, including systemic options (adjuvant/neoadjuvant chemotherapy), novel drugs (e.g., bevacizumab, cetuximab), and local radiation, with demonstrated prognostic impact in rectal cancer (Nappi et al. 2018). Concerning cancer of the anal canal, standard chemotherapy is considered as first-line therapeutic option due to an attempt of sphincter preservation and avoidance of colostomy.

Unlike the widely accepted use of imaging techniques in locally advanced stages (cT3–4 or cN1) or metastatic colorectal cancer (cM1), their use remains controversial when used for locoregional staging. ACR discourages the use of imaging for the T/N evaluation, but, on the contrary, the European Society of Medical Oncology (ESMO) considers the use of abdominal/pelvic CT scan or MRI as appropriate (Labianca et al. 2013). Conversely, in rectal cancer, transrectal ultrasound and pelvic MRI are considered appropriate as well. In fact, pelvic MRI not only predicts the risk of local recurrence according to extramural vascular invasion and distance to the circumferential resection margin but also detects synchronous or metachronous metastases. An exception is the eligible use of abdominal and pelvic CT for the evaluation of complications or disease spread. The clinical benefit of routine chest CT in colorectal cancer remains controversial and is therefore not generally recommended.

The most common indication for [^{18}F]FDG-PET/CT is the screening for extrahepatic distant metastases and nodal evaluation (Figs. 3 and 4). Hybrid imaging has higher sensitivity compared with CT alone. Regarding the evaluation of liver metastases, [^{18}F]FDG-PET/CT has been historically considered a less sensitive tool due to enzymatic reasons such as overexpression of glucose-6-phosphatase that allows the exit of [^{18}F]FDG from the cell. However, new strategies including multiphase studies, contrast bolus administration, or optimization of timing and technical parameters can overcome this limitation. Contrary to metastatic colorectal assessment, [^{18}F]FDG-PET/CT is not routinely considered for tumor staging, despite some evidence in the literature. Current NCCN guidelines (NCCN 2020) discourage the routine application of [^{18}F]FDG-PET/CT for colorectal cancer staging, follow-up, response evaluation after chemotherapy, or in case of non-resectable or clear evidence of metastatic disease. However, both NCCN and ESMO guidelines accept that [^{18}F]FDG-PET/CT has a leading role in those patients in which intravenous contrast administration is not possible, when there are equivocal or suspicious findings at standard imaging techniques (contrast-enhanced CT or MRI) or when there are prior anatomic images available indicating potentially curable M1 disease. In case of relapse, e.g., suspected by elevated tumor marker levels (carcinoembryonic antigen), [^{18}F]FDG-PET/CT can be useful in detecting tumor lesions with high sensitivity and specificity (94.1% and 77.2%, respectively) and with a recommendation for using PET/CT in that scenario, as suggested by the most current version of the NCCN practice guideline.

Recently, new hybrid techniques such as PET/MRI with multiplanar high-resolution fused images have emerged, providing important information about cell density and metabolic activity. Some preliminary studies (Paspulati et al. 2015) have compared PET/MRI with PET/CT regarding T-staging of rectal cancer, obtaining higher diagnostic accuracy and, at least, similar accuracy regarding N- and M-staging as well as restaging. On the other hand, increased examination time was observed when PET/MRI was performed (median 97 min vs. 38 min, respectively), needing significant improvement. Regarding lymph node assessment, standard imaging techniques have limited value because size itself is not an adequate criterion. [^{18}F]FDG-PET/CT is not routinely recommended but could support correct N-classification according to lymph node uptake and size (Lu et al. 2012). With reference to anal cancer, [^{18}F]FDG PET/CT is recommended for local staging of T2–T4, N0, or N+ primary tumors (Benson et al. 2016), because it usually determines the primary extension of the tumor, lymph node involvement, and distant metastases with higher sensitivity (92.9–100%) compared with CT (67–99%, respectively). Despite the fact that most anal cancers are [^{18}F]FDG-avid according to the NCCN guideline and a recent meta-analysis (Mahmud et al. 2017), the NCCN expert panel does not consider [^{18}F]FDG-PET/CT as a replacement for a diagnostic CT study. In summary, [^{18}F]FDG-PET/CT is considered as a second-line technique for locoregional staging in colorectal cancer. Further analysis is needed in order to recommend its routine use. Given the additional information in inconclusive, potentially surgically curable metastases, some guidelines consider the use of [^{18}F]FDG-PET/CT in rectal cancer in conjunction to CT and MRI. In particular, this applies to those high-risk patients presenting with increased CEA levels or high likelihood for the presence of metastases.

Once the indications and contraindications for imaging in colorectal and anal cancer are established, it is now time to evaluate the role of [^{18}F]FDG-PET/CT for radiation therapy planning. Chemoradiation is considered as a treatment of choice in case of carcinoma of the anal canal and advanced stages of colorectal cancer due to an organ-preserving strategy. For this purpose, CT has traditionally been used to guide the delineation process or to perform 3D dose planning. In recent years, the emergence of more conservative, efficient radiation techniques (i.e., less high-dose radiation in healthy tissues and less long-term side effects) makes it necessary to consider more precise parameters, mainly the gross tumor volume (GTV) and the clinical target volume (CTV). To address these requirements, functional imaging with [^{18}F]FDG-PET/CT has been considered as suitable tool which is superior to CT alone

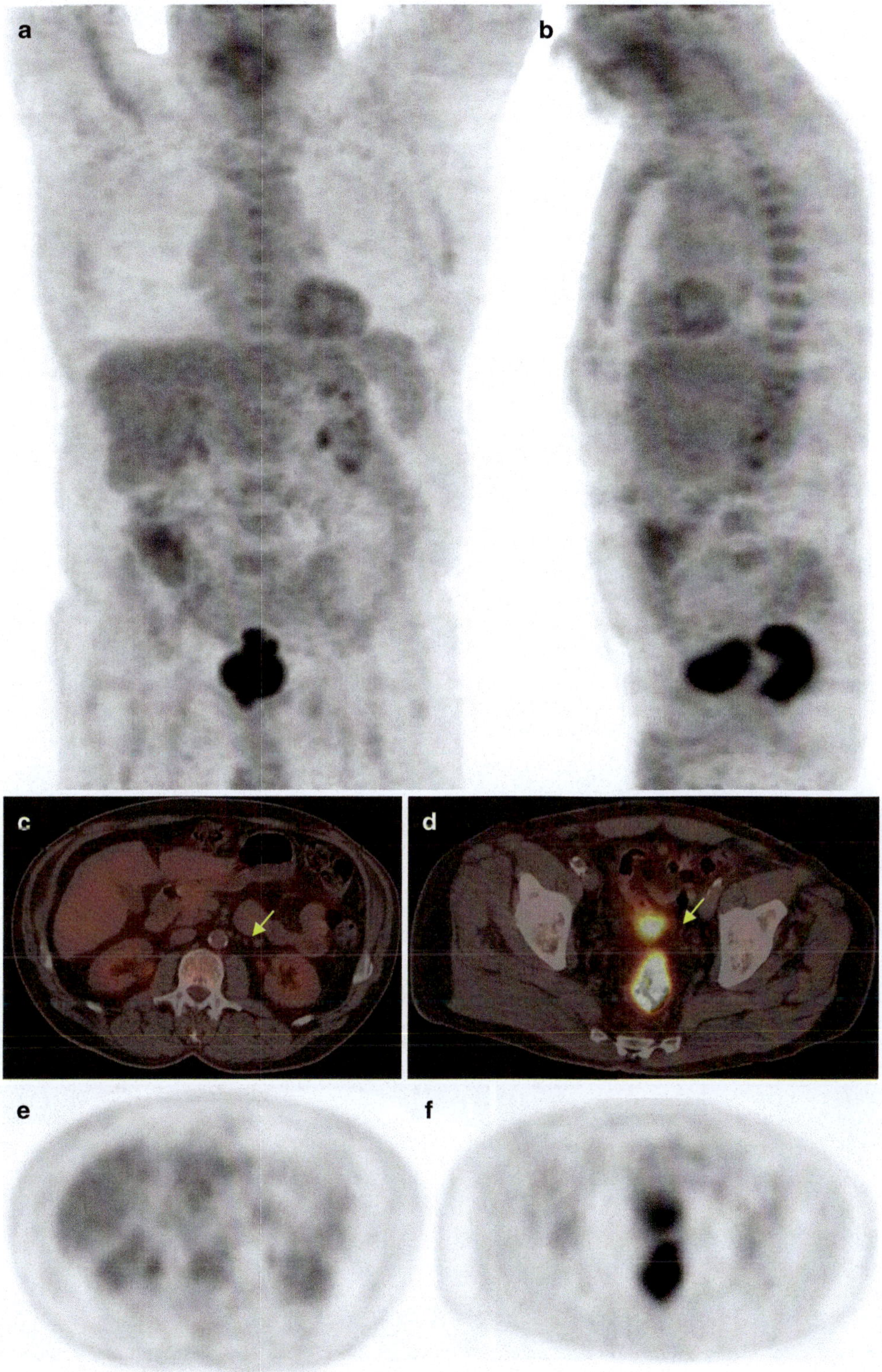

Fig. 3 A 68-year-old patient with locally advanced rectal cancer and suspicious lymph node enlargement in the pelvis, as identified by MRI. [^{18}F]FDG-PET/CT showed focal tracer uptake only in the rectum without other pathological lesions. Surgical biopsy confirmed rectal cancer without lymphatic invasion

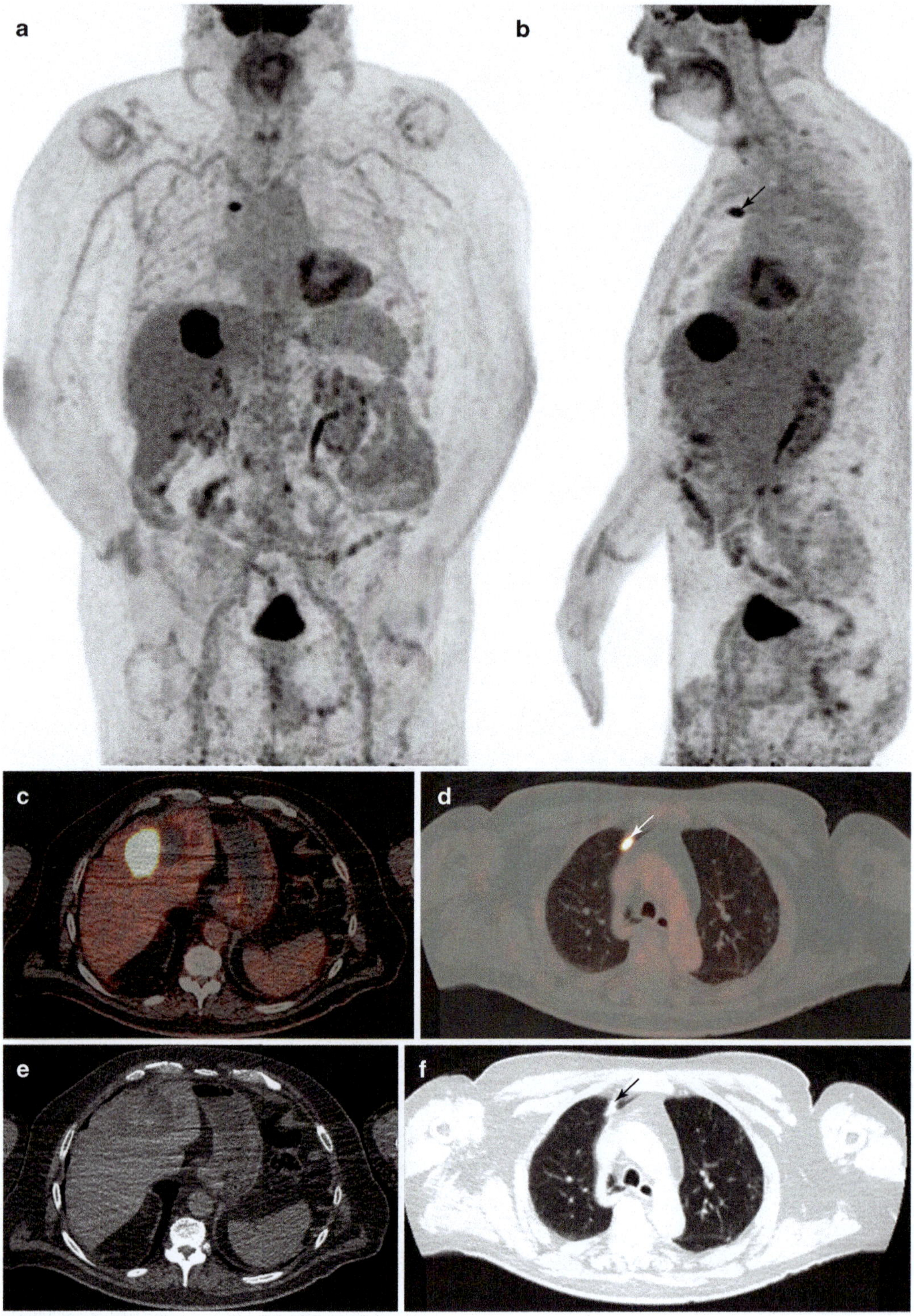

Fig. 4 A 74-year-old patient with colorectal cancer and metachronous liver metastases and subsequent resection and percutaneous ablation. [^{18}F]FDG-PET/CT showed residual hepatic metastases and an unexpected solitary pulmonary metastasis (right lung, arrow)

(Jones et al. 2015), providing also prognostic information (Gauthé et al. 2017). In addition, in a systematic review and a meta-analysis including 10 cross-sectional studies (Albertsson et al. 2018), [^{18}F]FDG-PET/CT results changed the definition of the target volume in one out of four patients. According to these results, the NCCN practice guideline suggests that [^{18}F]FDG-PET/CT should be considered for therapy planning, although there were no data available on the effect of PET/CT on progression-free or overall survival. Other publications compare the role of [^{18}F]FDG-PET/CT, MRI, and colonoscopy after preoperative hyperthermic chemoradiotherapy in rectal cancer. Parameters of PET quantification (SUVmax) emerged as most reliable and as independent predictor of complete pathological response (Murata et al. 2018). [^{18}F]FDG-PET/CT is not only relevant for therapy planning, but also plays a role for evaluating tumor heterogeneity, an important factor regarding resistance to treatment. Furthermore, it is strongly related to prognosis and prediction of response to neoadjuvant chemoradiotherapy. In some studies of adenocarcinoma and mucinous variants of colorectal cancer (Lovinfosse et al. 2017), the prognostic value of baseline texture analysis as part of a radiomics approach in locally advanced rectal cancer was assessed. These studies allowed the identification of different tumor phenotypes, classifying patients at high-risk/poor survival according to the characteristics of tumor heterogeneity, which could lead to a change of the therapeutic management and consideration of a more aggressive chemotherapy and/or radiotherapy, as well as a closer monitoring in those cases with poor prognostic profile. Another added value of [^{18}F]FDG-PET/CT is the evaluation of metabolic tumor volume (MTV), defined as sum of the estimated volumes of all lesions with increased uptake, a known prognostic marker associated with poor prognosis of solid tumors, including also anal cancer (Mahmud et al. 2017). On the other hand, a high variability of physiological distribution of [^{18}F]FDG is frequently observed in the GI tract and is also present in inflammatory lesions and after administration of some drugs (e.g., metformin), which could complicate the detection of colorectal cancer and adequately define the tumor size. Similar to diffuse [^{18}F]FDG-uptake, focal uptake could be correlated with other nonspecific features or even premalignant conditions, including dysplastic adenomas (28–67%) (Kitajima et al. 2017). In summary, there is increasing evidence that [^{18}F]FDG-PET/CT is beneficial not only in anal cancer but also in colorectal cancer due to its prognostic impact, detection rate, and clinical impact after radiotherapy. In addition, its role in the evaluation of tumor heterogeneity has been demonstrated. This aspect needs additional research because it is part of complex algorithms necessary to achieve a comprehensive management of the patient.

4 Pancreatic Cancer

With 5-year survival rates of 1–5%, pancreatic cancer represents one of the most lethal cancers and ranks as the fourth leading cause of cancer-related death in the United States. Approximately 54.000 patients are diagnosed in the USA every year (NCCN 2020). Surgery is the only curative treatment option but can be offered to only a very limited number of patients. At initial diagnosis, most patients present with an advanced stage, and only 20% are potential candidates for surgery. Despite complete resection of the primary tumor, the 5-year survival rate can be as low as 32% (NCCN 2020) proof of lymph node metastases (Lemke AJ et al. 2004). Most of pancreatic cancers arise from ductal or acinar cells and related stem cells. Risk factors of pancreatic adenocarcinoma include cigarette smoking, heavy alcohol consumption, and exposure to chemicals including beta-naphthylamine and benzidine. Chronic pancreatitis is also an established risk factor being associated with a 7-fold increased risk. A genetic predisposition can be assigned to a small number of patients (≤10%). Mutations were described in the CDKN2A gene or the BRCA2, PALB2, HER2, BRAFm KRAS and MSH2 genes. Neuroendocrine cancers or islet cell tumors represent rare-type cancers of the pancreas, accounting for less than 5% of all pancreatic tumors (Nakamoto et al. 2000).

The prognosis of patients with adenocarcinoma of the pancreas can be improved by adjuvant or neoadjuvant chemo- or chemoradiotherapy. Today, there is no accepted consensus regarding the most effective adjuvant treatment, and guidelines in the USA and European countries vary considerably. Therefore, it has been generally suggested that adjuvant or neoadjuvant therapy should be provided within clinical trials, whenever feasible. Outside of controlled clinical studies, the NCCN practice guideline suggests the use of 5-fluorouracil or gemcitabine-based protocols as adjuvant therapy, with or without the addition of radiotherapy (NCCN 2020). Recently, a German multicenter-controlled phase 3 trial (CONCO) reported a significant delay of disease recurrence when patients had adjuvant treatment with gemcitabine, as compared with a control group receiving no further treatment after resective surgery (DFS at 3 years, 23.5% vs. 7.5%, respectively) (Oettle et al. 2007). However, overall survival was not significantly different (22.1 and 20.2 months, respectively). Regarding chemo- and/or chemoradiotherapy prior to surgery (i.e., applied in a neo-adjuvant setting), no randomized trials are available comparing both approaches. In principle, additional treatment prior to surgery may result in higher patient numbers achieving margin-negative resections and delivers treatment also to micrometastatic disease. Since no controlled trials are available, implementation of neoadjuvant treatment is suggested only within ongoing clinical trials.

Sensitive detection of early cancers and lymph node metastases, differential diagnosis of pancreatic cancer and chronic, mass-forming pancreatitis, or the assessment of tumor resectability using noninvasive imaging modalities remain challenging. Usually, clinical symptoms including epigastric pain, weight loss, or jaundice raise a clinical suspicion on pancreatic cancer. For the diagnostic workup, imaging techniques including abdominal ultrasound (US), endoscopic ultrasound (EUS), contrast-enhanced computed tomography (CT), and magnetic resonance imaging (MRI) represent the mainstay diagnostic tests. In patients with newly diagnosed pancreatic tumors, the sensitivity of spiral CT for detecting pancreatic cancer is 65–90% and the specificity 46–85%, respectively. The positive (PPV) and negative predictive values (NPV) were reported to be as high as 79–87% and 31–61%, respectively (Bipat et al. 2005). For prediction of resectability, heterogeneous results have been reported for CT with a PPV of 89% and an NPV of 28% (Megibow et al. 1995). Tumors are considered resectable in case of no distant metastases and no radiographic evidence of encasement of the superior mesenteric artery more than 180 degrees and no aortic invasion. Also, lymph node metastases beyond the area of resection are considered to be non-resectable. In a recent meta-analysis, Bipat and colleagues reported sensitivity and specificity values from pooled data of 81% or 82%, respectively (Bipat et al. 2005). With the availability of modern multi-slice CT scanners using more advanced imaging protocols such as dynamic multiphase CT, the accuracy of CT imaging is steadily increasing. Using a triple-phase spiral CT technique, sensitivity for pancreatic cancer has been reported to be as high as 97% (Fletcher et al. 2003).

Abdominal ultrasound (US) is widely used and less costly but insufficient for assessment of resectability. US has a high sensitivity to detect tumors of the pancreas; however, sensitivity is reduced in tumors <3 cm. Endoscopic ultrasound (EUS) has been shown to be significantly more sensitive. Detection rates of pancreatic cancer are reported between 93% and 98%, respectively (Borbath et al. 2005; DeWitt et al. 2004; Mertz et al. 2000). The resectability can be predicted correctly in 88% of patients. T-staging at EUS was reported to be correct in 67% and nodal staging in 44%, respectively. Today, EUS is regarded as a complementary imaging modality to CT or MRI. EUS is particularly relevant to assess tumor invasion of vascular structures, e.g., the portal vein. MRI offers superior soft tissue contrast compared with CT and other imaging modalities. Regarding detection of pancreatic cancer, MRI has a sensitivity of 84–88% and a specificity of 78%, respectively (Bipat et al. 2005; Borbath et al. 2005). In multicenter trials, an overall accuracy of 70% and a PPV of 88% have been reported for differentiating resectable and non-resectable pancreatic cancer. However, the corresponding NPV was as low as 23% (Megibow et al. 1995). Novel, diffusion-weighted imaging protocols have the potential to increase the accuracy of MRI. Recently, dedicated pancreatic MRI has been suggested by the NCCN practice guideline as an equivalent alternative to CT imaging at initial workup.

Endoscopic retrograde cholangiopancreatography (ERCP) is regarded as a therapeutic rather than a diagnostic tool. ERCP is especially important in case of significant biliary obstruction needing decompression by stent placement. Patients who cannot undergo ERCP may have a magnetic resonance-based examination (MRCP). To establish the diagnosis of pancreatic cancer, histologic confirmation is not necessary. A percutaneous biopsy results in sensitivity and specificity values ranging between 80–90% and 98–100%, respectively. The risk for disseminating tumor cells is considered to be low; however, as recommended by the NCCN practice guideline, EUS-guided fine-needle aspiration biopsy is preferred to CT-guided biopsy due to better diagnostic yield and safety issues.

For [^{18}F]FDG-PET without coregistration of CT data, meta-analyses including more than 1.000 patients report a median sensitivity and specificity value of 91% and 78%, respectively. However, there is a wide range of sensitivity and specificity values reported in individual studies (sensitivity, 64–96%; specificity, 64–94%) (Bares et al. 1994; Delbeke et al. 1999, Diederichs et al. 1998; Friess et al. 1995; Heinrich et al. 2005, Inokuma et al. 1995; Lemke et al. 2004; Nakamoto et al. 2000). More recent clinical trials including also contrast-enhanced CE as part of PET/CT protocols report high sensitivity of 96% but also reduced specificity (67%) (Buchs et al. 2011). The performance of [^{18}F]FDG-PET for differentiating pancreatic tumors is somewhat lower compared to other solid tumors. This observation is presumably related to increased blood sugar values which can be frequently observed in patients with pancreatic tumors (20–30%). In a series from Zimny and colleagues, 25% of the study collective suffered from diabetes (Zimny et al. 1997). Whereas in patients with normal blood sugar values PET sensitivity was appropriate (98%, 46/47), the sensitivity dropped to 68% (17/27) in patients with hyperglycemia. Tumoral [^{18}F]FDG-uptake, as measured by calculation of the SUV, was significantly higher in patients with normal blood glucose values (6.9 ± 3.7) as compared to patients with hyperglycemia (5.5 ± 3.4). Therefore, it has been suggested that medication with insulin should be performed in hyperglycemic patients to increase the sensitivity. Delbeke and colleagues applied insulin i.v. (2–10 I.E.) every 15 min to achieve blood sugar values below 150 mg/dl (Delbeke et al. 1999). This approach resulted in a sensitivity value of 80% in diabetic patients. A recent guideline of the Society of Nuclear Medicine (SNM) admits the use of insulin for this purpose (Delbeke 2006). However, it is recommended that the time point for injecting [^{18}F]FDG should be delayed to reduce unspecific tracer uptake in muscle tissue. The second drawback of [^{18}F]FDG-PET in pancreatic cancer is a frequently observed coexistence of malignant tumors and inflammatory processes such as acute or chronic pancreatitis. Diederichs et al. showed that the specificity of [^{18}F]FDG-PET significantly drops if C-reactive protein is elevated or leucocyte count is increased (Diederichs et al. 2000). The specificity was as low as 40% compared to 87% in patients with normal CRP values or normal white blood cell count. Due to these drawbacks, [^{18}F]FDG-PET or [^{18}F]FDG-PET/CT should not be routinely used for differential diagnosis of pancreatic tumors but can serve as a problem-solving tool in patients with inconclusive findings at CT or MRI.

In patients with pancreatic cancer, detection of regional lymph node and distant metastases is of paramount importance to select patients who will benefit from resective surgery. Many studies have shown that the performance of [^{18}F]FDG-PET for lymph node staging is poor with sensitivity values between 17% and 33%, respectively (Delbeke et al. 1999; Lemke et al. 2004; Heinrich et al. 2005). Also, integrated PET/CT imaging does not lead to a significant increase of sensitivity, as recently reported by Heinrich and Asagi (Heinrich et al. 2005; Asagi et al. 2013). Better sensitivity values of PET and PET/CT have been reported for the detection of liver, peritoneal, or extra-abdominal metastases. In the study of Heinrich, the sensitivity of PET regarding detection of liver metastases was 81% (13/16) and significantly higher to that of contrast-enhanced CT (56%, 9/16). The specificity of CT regarding detection of liver metastases was 95% compared to 100% of PET/CT. Due to the sensitive detection of distant metastases, two publications reported a significant impact of PET and PET/CT regarding patient management. In the series of Delbeke et al., the therapeutic regimen was changed in 8/56 (13%) patients due to detection of previously unknown metastases (Delbeke et al. 1999). Heinrich reported an impact of PET/CT on therapeutic decision making in 16%, predominantly due to prevention of surgery in patients with distant metastases detected exclusively at [^{18}F] FDG-PET or PET/CT (Heinrich et al. 2005). Superiority of PET/CT including contrast-enhanced CT over CE-CT has been described also in a retrospective trial of Asagi and coworkers including 108 patients with pancreatic cancer (Asagi et al. 2013).

Recently, the following chemotherapeutic regimens have shown improvement of the time to progression and overall survival: FOLFIRINOX (5-FU/leucovorin, oxaliplatin, irinotecan), gemcitabine + erlotinib, gemcitabine + cisplatin, or gemcitabine + NAB-pacletaxel. Most recent guidelines on the management of pancreatic cancer do not suggest a specific imaging modality for response monitoring. In clinical trials, endoscopic techniques including EUS, CT, and MRI are currently most widely used for this purpose, and response is described according to response criteria in solid tumors (RECIST 1.1) (Eisenhauer et al. 2009). The most recent version of the NCCN guideline does not report on the suitability

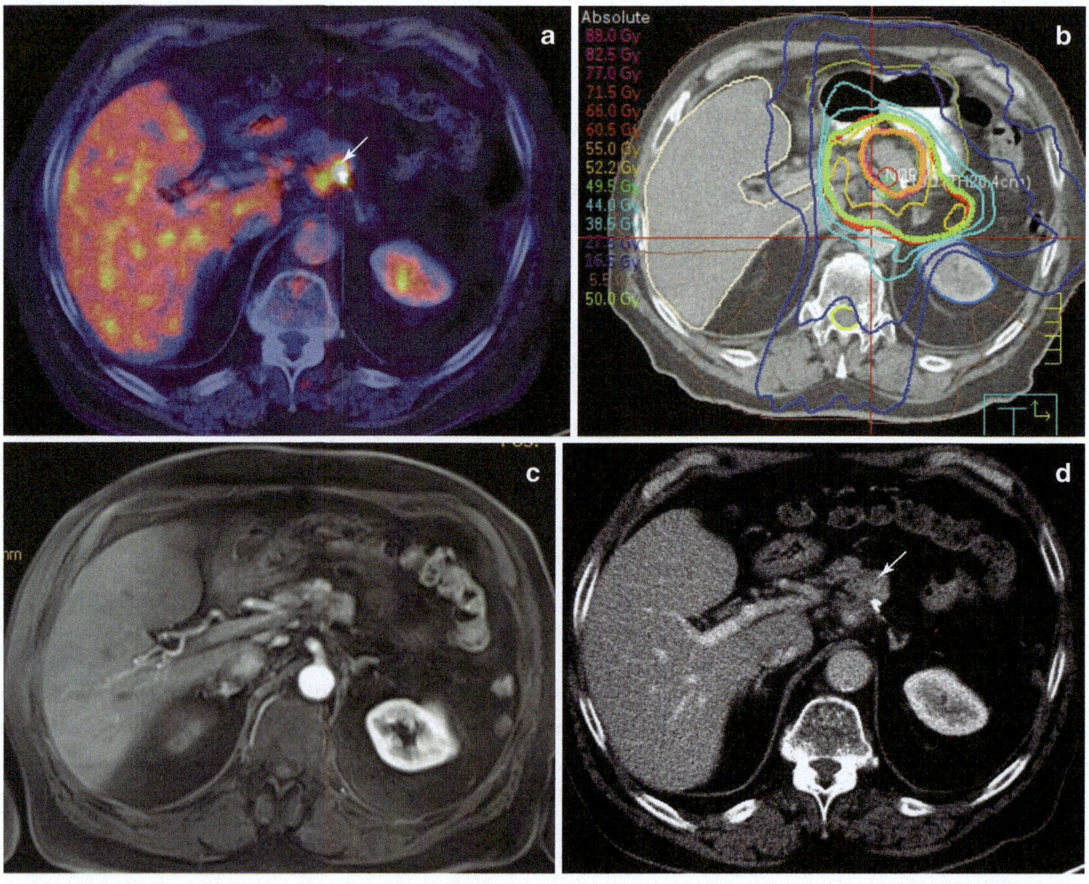

Fig. 5 Local recurrence of pancreatic cancer, as identified by [^{18}F]FDG-PET/CT (**a**, arrow). The tumor shows intense [^{18}F]FDG-uptake. (**b**) indicates the GTV based on tumor extension as defined by [^{18}F]FDG-PET/CT. (**c**) Visualization of the tumor at contrast-enhanced MRI (T2). (**d**) Corresponding section of contrast-enhanced spiral CT. Local recurrence appears as soft tissue mass (indicated by an arrow)

of PET or PET/CT for this purpose (Diederichs et al. 2000).

Currently, nuclear imaging plays only a minor role for management of pancreatic cancer, including radiotherapy planning (Fig. 5). With the increasing availability of novel cancer biomarkers, pilot trials on the diagnostic utility of surrogate markers for tumor hypoxia, proliferation, integrin expression, or chemokine receptor expression will provide interesting insights into the biology of pancreatic cancer. Imidazole derivatives such as [^{18}F]misonidazole (FMISO) can be used for specific imaging of hypoxic tumor tissue potentially leading to more efficient radiotherapy by increasing the radiation dose to the hypoxic fraction of tumors. However, the future role of these PET tracers for imaging pancreatic cancer remains to be determined. It is also expected that MR/PET-scanners will enhance the diagnostic accuracy of tomographic imaging. The superior soft tissue contrast offered by MRI will complement molecular information provided by PET. However, given the aggressive nature of the disease with disseminated cancer cells present in the majority of patients, the appropriateness of imaging, especially regarding T- and N-staging, will remain challenging. M-staging appears more promising, but it will be challenging to demonstrate superiority of MR/PET over the available PET/CT-technology.

References

Albertsson P, Alverbratt C, Liljegren A et al (2018) Positron emission tomography and computed tomographic (PET/CT) imaging for radiation therapy planning in anal cancer: a systematic review and meta-analysis. Crit Rev Oncol Hematol 126:6–12

Amin MB, Edge S, Greene F, Byrd DR, Brookland RK, American Joint Committee on Cancer, Colon and Rectum et al (2016) AJCC cancer staging manual, 8th edn. Springer, New York, NY

Asagi A et al (2013) Utility of contrast-enhanced FDG-PET/CT in the clinical Management of Pancreatic Cancer: impact on diagnosis, staging, evaluation of treatment response, and detection of recurrence. Pancreas 42(1):11–19

Barber TW et al (2012) 18F-FDG PET/CT has a high impact on patient management and provides powerful prognostic stratification in the primary staging of esophagealcancer: a prospective study with mature survival data. J Nucl Med 53(6):864–871

Bares R et al (1994) F-18 fluorodeoxyglucose PET in vivo evaluation of pancreatic glucose metabolism for detection of pancreatic cancer. Radiology 192(1):79–86

Bedimo R, Chen RY, Accortt NA, Raper JL, Linn C, Allison JJ et al (2004) Trends in AIDS-defining and non-AIDS-defining malignancies among HIV-infected patients: 1989–2002. Clin Infect Dis 39:1380

Behrens A (2011) Barret's adenocarcinoma of the esophagus-better outcomes through new methods of diagnosis and treatment. Dtsch Arztebl Int 108:313–319

Benson AB, Venook AP, Bekaii-Saab T, Chan E, Chen YJ, Cooper HS (2016) Anal carcinoma. In: NCCN clinical practice guidelines in oncology. National Comprehensive Cancer Network

Bhutani MS, Hawes RH, Hoffman BJ (1997) A comparison of the accuracy of echo features during endoscopic ultrasound (EUS) and EUS-guided fine-needle aspiration for diagnosis of malignant lymph node invasion. Gastrointest Endosc 45(6):474–9

Bipat S et al (2005) Ultrasonography, computed tomography and magnetic resonance imaging for diagnosis and determining resectability of pancreatic adenocarcinoma: a meta-analysis. J Comput Assist Tomogr 29(4):438–445

Borbath I et al (2005) Preoperative assessment of pancreatic tumors using magnetic resonance imaging, endoscopic ultrasonography, positron emission tomography and laparoscopy. Pancreatology 5(6):553–561

Buchs NC et al (2011) Value of contrast-enhanced 18F-fluorodeoxyglucose positron emission tomography/computed tomography in detection and presurgical assessment of pancreatic cancer: a prospective study. J Gastroenterol Hepatol 26(4):657–662

Chouwhury FU, Shah N, Scarsbrook AF, Bradley KM (2010) [18F]FDG PET/CT imaging of colorectal cancer: a pictorial review. Postgrad Med J 86: 174–182

Cools-Lartigue J, Ferri L (2019) Should Multidisciplinary Treatment Differ for Esophageal Adenocarcinoma versus Esophageal Squamous Cell Cancer? Ann Surg Oncol 26:1014–1027

Courrech Staal EF et al (2009) Outcome of low-volume surgery for esophageal cancer in a high-volume referral center. Ann Surg Oncol 16:3219–3226

Crosby T, Hurt CN, Falk S et al (2013) Chemoradiotherapy with or without cetuximab in patients with oesophageal cancer (SCOPE1): a multicenter phase 2/3 randomised trial. Lancet Oncol 14(7):627–637

Crum-Cianflone NF, Hullsiek KH, Marconi VC, Ganesan A, Weintrob A, Barthel RV et al (2010) Anal cancers among HIV-infected persons: HAART is not slowing rising incidence. AIDS 24:535

Cunningham D et al (2006) MAGIC Trial Participants Perioperative chemotherapy versus surgery alone for resectable gastroesophageal cancer. N Engl J Med 355(1):11–20

Dassen AE et al (2009) FDG-PET has no definite role in preoperative imaging in gastric cancer. Eur J Surg Oncol 35(5):449–55

Dębiec K et al (2017) 18-Fluorodeoxy-Glucose Positron Emission Tomography- Computed Tomography (18-FDG-PET/CT) for Gross Tumor Volume (GTV) Delineation in Gastric Cancer Radiotherapy. Asian Pac J Cancer Prev 18(11):2989–2998

Delbeke D et al (1999) Optimal interpretation of FDG PET in the diagnosis, staging and management of pancreatic carcinoma. J Nucl Med 40(11): 1784–1791

Delbeke D et al (2006) Procedure guideline for tumor imaging with 18F-FDG PET/CT 1.0. J Nucl Med 47(5):885–895

DeWitt J et al (2004) Comparison of endoscopic ultrasonography and multidetector computed tomography for detecting and staging pancreatic cancer. Ann Intern Med 141(10):753–763

Diederichs CG et al (1998) FDG PET: elevated plasma glucose reduces both uptake and detection rate of pancreatic malignancies. J Nucl Med 39(6):1030–1033

Diederichs CG et al (2000) Values and limitations of 18F-fluorodeoxyglucose-positron-emission tomography with preoperative evaluation of patients with pancreatic masses. Pancreas 20(2):109–116

Dieleman EM et al (2007) Four-dimensional computed tomographic analysis of esophageal mobility during normal respiration. Int J Radiat Oncol Biol Phys 67:775–780

D'Souza G, Wiley DJ, Li X, Chmiel JS, Margolick JB, Cranston RD et al (2008) Incidence and epidemiology of anal cancer in the multicenter AIDS cohort study. J Acquir Immune Defic Syndr 48:491–499

Eisenhauer EA et al (2009) New response evaluation criteria in solid tumours: revised RECIST guideline (version 1.1). Eur J Cancer 45(2):228–247

Flamen P et al (2000) Utility of positron emission tomography for the staging of patients with potentially operable esophageal carcinoma. J Clin Oncol 18:3202–3210

Fletcher JG et al (2003) Pancreatic malignancy: value of arterial, pancreatic, and hepatic phase imaging with multi-detector row CT. Radiology 229(1):81–90

Friess H et al (1995) Diagnosis of pancreatic cancer by 2[18F]-fluoro-2-deoxy-D-glucose positron emission tomography. Gut 36(5):771–777

Fowler KJ, Kaur H, Cash BD, Feig BW, Gage KL, Garcia EM, Hara AK, Herman JM, Kim DH, Lambert DL, Levy AD, Peterson CM, Scheirey CD, Small W Jr, Smith MP, Lalani T, Carucci LR (2017) ACR Appropriateness Criteria Pretreatment Staging of Colorectal Cancer. Expert Panel on Gastrointestinal Imaging. J Am Coll Radiol 14(5S): S234–S244

Gauthé M, Richard-Molard M, Fayard J, Alberini JL, Cacheux W, Lievre A (2017) Prognostic impact of tumor burden assessed by metabolic tumor volume on FDG PET/CT in anal canal cancer. Eur J Nucl Med Mol Imaging 44:63–70

Heinrich S et al (2005) Positron emission tomography/computed tomography influences on the management of resectable pancreatic cancer and its cost-effectiveness. Ann Surg 242(2):235–243

Himeno S et al (2002) Evaluation of esophageal cancer by positron emission tomography. Jpn J Clin Oncol 32: 340–346

Inokuma T et al (1995) Evaluation of pancreatic tumors with positron emission tomography and F-18 fluorodeoxyglucose: comparison with CT and US. Radiology 195(2):345–352

Jones M, Hruby G, Solomon M, Rutherford N, Martin J (2015) The role of FDG PET/CT in the initial staging and response assessment of anal cancer: a systematic review and meta-analysis. Ann Surg Oncol 22(11):3574–3581

Kato H et al (2002) Comparison between positron emission tomography and computed tomography in the use of the assessment of esophageal carcinoma. Cancer 94:921–928

Kato H et al (2005) The incremental effect of positron emission tomography on diagnostic accuracy in the initial staging of esophageal carcinoma. Cancer 103:148–156

Kim TJ et al (2009) Multimodality assessment of esophageal cancer: preoperative staging and monitoring of response to therapy. Radiographics 29(2): 403–421

Kitajima K, Nakajo M, Kaida H, Minamimoto R, Hirata K, Tsurusaki M, Doi H et al (2017) Present and future roles of FDG PET/CT imaging in the management of gastrointestinal cancer: an update. Nagoya J Med Sci 79(4):527–543

Konski A et al (2005) The integration of 18-fluoro-deoxy-glucose positron emission tomography and endoscopic ultrasound in the treatment-planning process for esophageal carcinoma. Int J Radiat Oncol Biol Phys 61(4):1123–8

Labianca R, Nordlinger B, Beretta GD, Mosconi S, Mandalà M, Cervantes A, Arnold D (2013) Early colon cancer: ESMO clinical practice guidelines. Ann Oncol 24(Suppl 6):vi64–vi72

Lagergren J, Lagergren P (2013) Recent developments in esophageal adenocarcinoma. CA Cancer J Clin 63:232–248

le Grange et al (2015) Defining the target in Cancer of the Oesophagus: direct radiotherapy planning with Fluorodeoxyglucose positron emission tomography-computed tomography. Clin Oncol 27:160–167

Lemke AJ et al (2004) Retrospective digital image fusion of multidetector CT and 18F-FDG PET: clinical value in pancreatic lesions--a prospective study with 104 patients. J Nucl Med 45(8):1279–1286

Lightdale CJ, Kulkarni KG (2005) Role of endoscopic ultrasonography in the staging and follow-up of esophageal cancer. J Clin Oncol 23:4483–4489

Leong T et al (2006) A prospective study to evaluate the impact of FDG-PET on CT-based radiotherapy treatment planning for oesophageal cancer. Radiother Oncol 78(3):254–61

Lorchel F et al (2006) Esophageal cancer determination of internal target volume for conformal radiotherapy. Radiother Oncol 80:327–332

Lovinfosse P, Polus M, Van Daele D, Martinive P, Daenen F, Hatt M et al (2017) FDG PET/CT radiomics for predicting the outcome of locally advanced rectal cancer. Eur J Nucl Med Mol Imaging 45:365

Lu J et al (2016) Impact of PET/CT on radiation treatment in patients with esophageal cancer: A systematic review. Crit Rev Oncol Hematol 107:128–137

Lu YY, Chen JH, Ding HJ, Chien CR, Lin WY, Kao CH (2012) A systematic review and meta-analysis of pretherapeutic lymph node staging of colorectal cancer by 18F-FDG PET or PET/CT. Nucl Med Commun 33:1127–1133

Mahmud A, Poon R, Jonker D (2017) PET imaging in anal canal cancer: a systematic review and meta-analysis. Br J Radiol 90:20170370

Mamede M et al (2007) Pre-operative estimation of esophageal tumor metabolic length in FDG-PET images with surgical pathology confirmation. Ann Nucl Med 21:553–562

Megibow AJ et al (1995) Pancreatic adenocarcinoma: CT versus MR imaging in the evaluation of resectability--report of the radiology diagnostic oncology group. Radiology 195(2):327–332

Mertz HR et al (2000) EUS, PET, and CT scanning for evaluation of pancreatic adenocarcinoma. Gastrointest Endosc 52(3):367–371

Moureau Zabotto L et al (2005) Impact of CT and 18F-deoxyglucose positron emission tomography image fusion for conformal radiotherapy in esophageal carcinoma. Int J Radiat Oncol Biol Phys 63(2):340–5

Muijs CT et al (2010) A systematic review of the role of FDG-PET/CT in tumour delineation and radiotherapy planning in patients with esophageal cancer. Radiother Oncol 97(2):165–171

Muijs CT et al (2013) Oesophageal tumour progression between the diagnostic 18-F-FDG-PET and the 18-F-FDG-PET for radiotherapy treatment planning. Radiother Oncol 106:283–287

Muijs CT et al (2014) Clinical validation of FDG-PET/CT in the radiation treatment planning for patients with oesophageal cancer. Radiother Oncol. 113:188–192

Mukai K et al (2006) Usefulness of preoperative FDG-PET for detection of gastric cancer. Gastric Cancer 9(3):192–6

Murata H, Okamoto M, Takayashi T, Motegi M et al (2018) SUVmax-based parameters of FDG-PET/CT reliably predict pathologic complete response after preoperative hyperthermo-chemoradiotherapy in rectal cancer. Anticancer Res 38:5909–5916

Nakamoto Y et al (2000) Delayed (18)F-fluoro-2-deoxy-D-glucose positron emission tomography scan for differentiation between malignant and benign lesions in the pancreas. Cancer 89(12):2547–2554

Nappi A, Berretta M, Romano C, Tafuto S, Cassata A, Casaretti R, Silvestro L, De Divitiis C, Alessandrini L, Fiorica F, Ottaiano A, Nasti G (2018) Metastatic colorectal cancer: role of target therapies and future perspectives. Curr Cancer Drug Targets 18: 421–429

National Institute for Health and Clinical Excellence (2004) Improving outcomes in colorectal cancer. Manual update. National Institute for Health and Clinical Excellence, London

NCCN practice guideline. Colon cancer. Version 1.2020; www.nccn.org; accessed 03/2020

NCCN practice guideline Colorectal cancer, Version 1.2020; www.nccn.org; accessed 03/2020

NCCN practice guideline. Esophageal and esophagogastric junction cancers. Version 1.2020; www.nccn.org; accessed 03/2020

NCCN practice guideline. Gastric cancer. Version 1.2020; www.nccn.org; accessed 03/2020

NCCN practice guideline. Pancreatic cancer. Version 1.2020; www.nccn.org; accessed 03/2020

NCCN practice guideline. Rectal cancer. Version 1.2020; www.nccn.org; accessed 03/2020

Oettle H et al (2007) Adjuvant chemotherapy with gemcitabine vs observation in patients undergoing curative-intent resection of pancreatic cancer: a randomized controlled trial. JAMA 297(3):267–277

Ott K et al (2011) Molecular imaging of proliferation and glucose utilization: utility for monitoring response and prognosis after neoadjuvant therapy in locally advanced gastric cancer. Ann Surg Oncol 18(12):3316–23

Paspulati R, Partovi S, Herrmann K, Krishnamurthi S, Delancy C, Nguyen N (2015) Comparison of hybrid FDG PET/MRI compared with PET/CT in colorectal cancer staging and restaging: a pilot study. Abdom Imaging 40:1415–1425

Piketty C, Selinger-Leneman H, Grabar S, Duvivier C, Bonmarchand M, Abramowitz L et al (2008) Marked increase in the incidence of invasive anal cancer among HIV-infected patients despite treatment with combination antiretroviral therapy. AIDS 22:1203–1211

Rice TW et al (2017) Cancer of the esophagus and esophagogastric junction: an eight edition staging primer. J Thorac Oncol 12:36–42

Schreurs LM et al (2010) Impact of 18-fluorodeoxyglucose positron emission tomography on computed tomography defined target volumes in radiation treatment planning of esophageal cancer: reduction in geographic misses with equal inter-observer variability: PET/CT improves esophageal target definition. Dis Esophagus 23(6):493–501

Smhty EC et al (2016) Gastric cancer: ESMO Clinical Practice Guidelines for diagnosis, treatment and follow-up. Annals of Oncology 27, Supll5:38–49

Stahl A et al (2003) FDG PET imaging of locally advanced gastric carcinomas: correlation with endoscopic and histopathological findings. Eur J Nucl Med Mol Imaging 30(2):288–95

Strobel K et al (2008) Contrast-enhanced 18F-FDG PET/CT: 1-stop-shop imaging for assessing the resectability of pancreatic cancer. J Nucl Med 49(9):1408–1413

Thomas L et al (2015) Tumour delineation in oesophageal cancer – A prospective study of delineation in PET and CT with and without endoscopically placed clip markers. Radiother Oncol 116(2):269–75

van Westreenen HL, Cobben DC, Jager PL, van Dullemen HM, Wesseling J, Elsinga PH, Plukker JT (2005) Comparison of 18F-FLT PET and 18F-FDG PET in esophageal cancer. J Nucl Med 46(3):400–4

Walker AJ et al (2011) Integrated PET/CT fusion imaging and endoscopic ultrasound in the pre-operative staging and evaluation of esophageal cancer. Mol Imaging Biol 13:166–171

Wu AJ, Goodman KA (2013) Positron emission tomography imaging for gastroesophageal junction tumors. Semin Radiat Oncol 23(1):10–15

Yamashita H et al (2011) Four-dimensional measurement of the displacement of internal fiducial markers during 320-multislice computed tomography scanning of thoracic esophageal cancer. Int J Radiat Oncol Biol Phys 79:588–595

Yun M (2014) Imaging of Gastric Cancer Metabolism Using 18 F-FDG PET/CT. J Gastric Cancer 14(1):1–6

Zhang Y (2013) Epidemiology of esophageal cancer. World J Gastroenterol 19(34):5598–5606

Zhong X et al (2009) Using 18F-fluorodeoxyglucose positron emission tomography to estimate the length of gross tumor in patients with squamous cell carcinoma of the esophagus. Int J Radiat Oncol Biol Phys 73(1):136–141

Zimny M et al (1997) Fluorine-18 fluorodeoxyglucose positron emission tomography in the differential diagnosis of pancreatic carcinoma: a report of 106 cases. Eur J Nucl Med 24(6):678–682

T Staging and Target Volume Definition by Imaging in GU Tumors

Paolo Castelluci, Stefano Fanti, Stefano Bracci, Valeria Panebianco, Alessio Giuseppe Morganti, and Rezarta Frakulli

Contents

1 **Male Genital Tract Malignancies** 221
1.1 Prostate Cancer 221
1.2 Cancers of the Testis and the Penis 229

2 **Female Genital tract Malignancies** 232
2.1 Cervical Cancer 232
2.2 Endometrial Cancer 237
2.3 Vulvar and Vaginal Cancer 241

3 **Urological Malignancies** 243
3.1 Bladder Cancer 243

References 247

P. Castelluci (✉) · S. Fanti
Nuclear Medicine Unit, S. Orsola-Malpighi University Hospital, University of Bologna, Bologna, Italy
e-mail: paolo.castellucci@aosp.bo.it; s.fanti@unibo.it

S. Bracci · V. Panebianco
Department of Radiological Sciences, Oncology and Pathology, Sapienza University of Rome, Rome, Italy
e-mail: valeria.panebianco@uniroma1.it

A. G. Morganti · R. Frakulli
Radiation Oncology Center, Department of Experimental, Diagnostic and Specialty, Medicine—DIMES University of Bologna, S. Orsola-Malpighi Hospital, Bologna, Italy

1 Male Genital Tract Malignancies

1.1 Prostate Cancer

Abstract

The diagnosis of prostate cancer is usually performed with random transrectal ultrasonography-guided biopsies in patients that are found with elevated serum PSA or positive digital rectal examination. PSMA *positron emission tomography/computed tomography* (PET/CT) imaging showed good accuracy to stage prostate cancer, but the sensitivity of this method remains suboptimal, particularly in the detection of small lymph nodal metastasis.

Magnetic resonance imaging (MRI) currently plays a main role in the different phases of prostate cancer management such as the detection, local staging, active surveillance, and follow-up. Instead CT is limited to the assessment of distant metastases as it shows low sensitivity in the identification of both localized lesions and lymph-node metastases. The use of multiparametric MRI has been demonstrated to improve the accuracy of tumor localization, making MRI the modality of choice for local staging of prostate tumor.

Radiotherapy (RT) for prostate cancer can be modulated in terms of dose, target volumes, and integration with androgen deprivation therapy. This modulation is performed by defining different risk groups based on PSA value, Gleason score, and tumor/nodal stage. According to the

R. G. H. Beets-Tan et al. (eds.), *Imaging and Interventional Radiology for Radiation Oncology*, Medical Radiology, Diagnostic Imaging, https://doi.org/10.1007/978-3-030-38261-2_15

different risk groups, the clinical target volume includes only the prostatic gland in low-risk prostate cancer, and prostate, seminal vesicles, and pelvic lymph nodes (LNs) in high-risk prostate cancer. Using external beam radiotherapy (EBRT), MRI allows reduction of delineated target volumes while improving extracapsular extension and seminal vesicle invasion detection with potential impact on clinical outcome. Also, in brachytherapy treatments, MRI can accurately identify prostate gland, extra-prostatic tissues, and normal structures.

1.1.1 PET Tracers for Imaging Prostate Cancer

- **[^{18}F]FDG (FDG)**
  [^{18}F]FDG is the most used radiopharmaceutical in oncology. However, in some cancers (tumors showing low glycolytic activity such as prostate cancer), [^{18}F]FDG-PET/CT is of limited use. As for many other cancers, [^{18}F]FDG uptake in prostate cancer depends on tumor differentiation. [^{18}F]FDG-PET/CT may be useful in the evaluation of extent and treatment response in metastatic disease and in prediction of patient outcome (Jadvar 2013). However, nowadays [^{18}F]FDG is not routinely used in clinical practice for prostate cancer.
- **[^{18}F]FACBC**
  [^{18}F]FACBC (anti-1-amino-3–[^{18}F]fluorocyclobutane-1-carboxylic acid) is a L-leucine analogue that has recently been applied to the study of prostate cancer. In some preliminary reports, it has been shown that FACBC might have a small superiority over choline (Schuster et al. 2016) in terms of accuracy. However, the literature is still limited to few centers and limited patients' populations.
- **^{11}C- [^{18}F]** Choline
  Choline is a precursor of phosphatidylcholine, a membrane phospholipid. Choline can be labeled with either ^{11}C- or [^{18}F]. The two tracers gave similar results in literature in terms of specificity and sensitivity, but no direct comparison is ever been performed.
  Choline is currently used in all the steps of the natural history of the disease: intraprostatic detection of prostate cancer before biopsy, staging, and restaging in case of biochemical recurrence and evaluation of the extent of the disease and therapy response in metastatic castrate-resistant patients (Castellucci et al. 2017).
- **PSMA**
  The molecule PSMA (prostate-specific membrane antigen) corresponds to the enzyme glutamate carboxypeptidase II. The enzyme is overexpressed in many cancer cells including prostate cancer. It has been used for the first time to image human prostate cancer in 2013 (Afshar-Oromieh et al. 2013). PSMA is very versatile since it can be labeled to a large number of radiotracers either for imaging (^{68}Ga- [^{18}F]- ^{111}In- ^{99}Tc) or therapy (^{177}Lu- ^{131}I- ^{225}Ac).

Nowadays, Gallium 68 (Ga) is the most widely used isotope to label PSMA for imaging since it can be produced by a Ge–Ga (Germanium–Gallium) generator, allowing even centers not equipped with a cyclotron to produce it. In the last few years, Ga PSMA has gained a key role in prostate molecular imaging, and probably this molecule will represent the next standard to image prostate cancer mostly to stage, restage the disease, and select patients who may benefit from radio receptor therapy (RRT).

1.1.2 Prostate Cancer Staging with PET/CT

- **Intraprostatic Diagnosis and Nodal Staging**
  The use of choline for intraprostatic diagnosis or for nodal and distant staging of prostate cancer is not recommended by any of the main international guidelines (Mottet et al. 2017). This is mainly due to a suboptimal accuracy that has been shown in the past decades by choline PET/CT either in the detection of intraprostatic foci of disease or in the detection of nodal lesions (Evangelista et al. 2013). More recently, interesting results have been obtained by the use of other radiopharmaceuticals such as ^{68}Ga-PSMA PET/CT and by the clinical applications of the novel hybrid tomograph PET/MRI.

Fendler et al. (Fendler et al. 2016) studied 21 patients with an initial diagnosis of PCa using PET/CT with ^{68}Ga-PSMA to localize cancer in the prostate and surrounding tissue. Authors showed a suboptimal sensitivity of 67%, but remarkable specificity and accuracy of 92% and 72%, respectively, a PPV of 97%, and an NPV of 42%. Zamboglou et al. (2017) studied seven patient candidates and scheduled for a subsequent radical prostatectomy with ^{68}Ga-PSMA PET/MR: interestingly, the information provided by both ^{68}Ga-PSMA PET and by MRI alone resulted to be complementary. Using both information to delineate the extent of intraprostatic PCa foci, the authors reached a sensitivity of 82% and a specificity of 89%. Eiber et al. confirmed these results (Eiber et al. 2016), showing in 53 patients that simultaneous PET/MRI scan statistically outperformed mpMRI and PET imaging alone for a precise localization of intraprostatic prostate cancer foci.

In conclusion, the application of PSMA PET/CT or PSMA PET/MRI could be very useful in clinical practice mainly in the following applications: (1) in patients at high risk of prostate cancer, but with negative or inconclusive biopsy, PSMA PET could guide, together with MRI, subsequent re-biopsies and (2) in patients at high risk for nodal involvement at presentation, to guide the primary treatment (either surgical or using EBRT) in case of detection of extraprostatic disease.

- **Lymph Nodal Staging**

Preoperative nomograms are able to graduate with good accuracy the individual risk of lymph-node metastasis (Briganti et al. 2012). However, the main limitation of preoperative nomograms is the lack of information about the site of disease. That is why, when the risk of nodal metastases is greater than 5%, there is an indication to perform an extended nodal dissection (ePLND) (Mottet et al. 2017). An accurate staging using different imaging methods may have a role in guiding clinicians (surgeons or radiation oncologists) in performing image-guided GTV or extended PLND or to exclude from primary aggressive treatments those patients already showing distant metastatic spread of the disease.

Some recent reports showed very good results in the application of ^{68}Ga-PSMA PET/CT in order to stage prostate cancer. Maurer et al. (2016) studied 130 patients with a presurgical ^{68}Ga-PSMA PET/CT in order to assess the presence of lymph nodal metastasis. In the intermediate and high-risk selected population, 117/734 (15.9%) lymph-node templates showed metastases. On a patient basis, authors showed a sensitivity of 65.9%, a specificity of 98.9%, and an accuracy of 88.5%. On a per-side-based analysis, the sensitivity, specificity, and accuracy of ^{68}Ga-PSMA PET/CT were 68.3%, 99.1%, and 95.2%, respectively.

Similar results were later on published by van Leeuwen et al. (2017). Authors enrolled 30 intermediate and high-risk PCa patients scheduled for radical prostatectomy. In this population, about 37% of patients resulted to be positive at final diagnosis after lymph-node dissection. On a patient basis, ^{68}Ga-PSMA PET/CT showed a sensitivity of 64%, a specificity of 95%, a PPV of 88%, and an NPV of 82%. On a lymph-node region-based analysis, the sensitivity dropped down to 56%, the specificity was 98%, the PPV was 90%, and the NPV was 94%. Interestingly in this study, authors reported the mean size of the missed lymph nodes at ^{68}Ga-PSMA PET/CT that resulted to be equal to 2.7 mm.

In conclusion, PSMA PET/CT imaging showed good accuracy to stage PCa prior to curative treatment, but the sensitivity of this method remains suboptimal, particularly in the detection of small lymph-nodal metastasis. In order to minimize this limitation, an optimal patient population selection should be performed before a PSMA PET/CT. Probably only patients showing high or very high risk for the presence of LNs or distant lesions could benefit from PSMA PET/CT. In this way, it could be possible to reduce the presence of false-negative results, increase the percentage of patients who have uncommon location of the disease that could be detected by PSMA PET/CT (e.g., retroperitoneal lymph nodes), and finally exclude from aggressive treatments patients showing multiple distant lesions at presentation.

1.1.3 Staging with CT or MRI

The diagnosis of prostate cancer is usually performed with random transrectal ultrasonography (US)-guided biopsies in patients that are found with elevated serum PSA or positive digital rectal examination (Kitzing et al. 2016). The high soft-tissue contrast resolution of MRI combined with its capability to provide anatomic, biologic, metabolic, and functional information (i.e., multiparametric MRI), however, has dramatically changed the current approach to prostate cancer. In fact, MRI currently plays a main role in the different phases of prostate cancer management such as the detection, local staging, active surveillance, and follow-up (Kitzing et al. 2016).Moreover, mpMRI is a useful tool to guide prostate biopsy as it showed a higher detection rate of significant prostate cancer as compared to TRUS-guided biopsy (Schoots et al. 2015).Differently from MRI, the use of CT is limited to the assessment of distant metastases as it shows low sensitivity in the identification of both localized lesions and lymph-node metastases (Panebianco et al. 2012).The use of multiparametric MRI has been demonstrated to improve the accuracy of tumor localization, making MRI the modality of choice for local staging of prostate tumor (Boonsirikamchai et al. 2013; Delongchamps et al. 2011; Fütterer et al. 2006a). The addition of MRI to the conventional approaches (i.e., serum PSA, digital rectal examination, transrectal US) brought to an improvement of staging accuracy, in particular in the assessment of extraprostatic disease (Kayat Bittencourt et al. 2015). The distinction between organ-confined and extraprostatic disease has several practical consequences in terms of risk of recurrence and risk of locoregional and distant metastases (Kayat Bittencourt et al. 2015; Boccon-Gibod et al. 2003; Yamada et al. 1994). Furthermore, its use has several therapeutical implications as it is a useful tool in the planning of surgery and radiotherapy (RT), both representing the main treatment modality used to treat prostate cancer (Beyersdorff et al. 2005). In case of potential surgical candidates, MRI is essential to differentiate between intraprostatic (i.e., T2) and extraprostatic (i.e., T3) disease; moreover, it is able to assess the infiltration of the prostate capsule, seminal vesicles, and adjacent organs (Murphy et al. 2013). It can improve the planning of nerve-sparing radical prostatectomy in case of localized tumor as it can predict the absence of tumor in the areas of the neurovascular bundles (Labanaris et al. 2009; Panebianco et al. 2009). Additionally, it helps RT planning, allowing for an accurate delineation of the prostate as well as of the surrounding organs that must be spared with the aim to reduce the risk of radiation-induced complications. Finally, mpMRI is a valid tool to evaluate the prostatic bed after radical prostatectomy when a recurrence is suspected based on elevated serum PSA helping the treatment planning of salvage RT (Panebianco et al. 2012; Boonsirikamchai et al. 2013).A routine mpMRI study includes T2wi for anatomical details obtained in three orthogonal planes (i.e., axial, sagittal, and coronal) and functional imaging as DWI that gives information about cellular density, membrane permeability, and space between cells and DCE that are obtained during and after intravenous bolus contrast material injection reflecting tumor neoangiogenesis (Kitzing et al. 2016; Panebianco et al. 2012). Overall, the normal prostate is divided in several anatomic zones: the transitional zone, the central zone, the peripheral zone that contains around the 80% of the glandular tissue, and the anterior fibromuscular stroma. On T2wi, the peripheral zone is hyperintense while the central and the transitional zone (i.e., the central gland) are often inseparable on MRI due to the presence of benign prostatic hypertrophy and shows a variegated signal because of the association of glandular and fibrotic tissue. The prostate has a fibrous capsule that must be assessed in case of extraprostatic extension of a tumor. Adjacent to the capsule, posterolaterally and bilaterally, pass the neurovascular bundle, and infiltration is a sign of extraprostatic extension (Boonsirikamchai et al. 2013; Kayat Bittencourt et al. 2015). The seminal vesicles are located posterosuperiorly with respect to the prostate and appears hyperintense on T2wi as they are filled with seminal fluid.Prostate cancer has a hypointense signal on T2wi compared to the hyperintense signal of the peripheral zone. However, there are several benign conditions that are hypointense on T2wi such post-biopsy changes, prostatitis, or posttreatment changes. Even if the majority of cancer are localized in the peripheral zone, about 30% of cancer develops in the central zone, making its assessment difficult because of the variable signal intensity in the central gland as previously reported. Tumors arising in the central gland often shows a homogenously hypointense signal with lenticular shape and well-defined margins (erased charcoal sign) (Kitzing et al. 2016; Panebianco et al. 2015a). On T2wi, findings that suggests extraprostatic disease with a sensitivity of about 90% and specificity of up 100% are the presence of asymmetry of the neurovascular bundle, tumor encasement of the neurovascular bundle, a bulging prostatic contour, a spiculated margin, obliteration of the recto-prostatic angle, capsular retraction, and a tumor-capsule interface of greater than 1 cm (Boonsirikamchai et al. 2013; Kayat Bittencourt et al. 2015; Hricak et al. 2007; Fütterer et al. 2006b). Infiltration of seminal vesicles is suggested with high specificity by a tumor that directly extends to the seminal vesicles itself and the presence of hypointense and enlarged ejaculatory ducts and/or seminal vesicles (Boonsirikamchai et al. 2013; Sala et al. 2006). However, there are several potential pitfalls in the local staging of prostate cancer that makes the differentiation between T3 and T2 stage disease challenging: at the apex, the presence of peripheral zone prostatic tissue due to an anatomical variation involved by a tumor can simulate a pseudo T3a disease; at the base, a bulging benign prostatic hyperplasia nodule near the root of the seminal vesical can mimic its infiltration (i.e., T3b stage); the neurovascular bundles can sometimes be considered a lesion of the peripheral zone; finally, granulomatous prostatitis can infiltrate the periprostatic fat simulating a T3a disease (Panebianco et al. 2015a).The association of functional imaging such as DWI and DCE to anatomical imaging has improved the specificity of tumor diagnosis and localization (Panebianco et al. 2015a; Tan et al. 2012; Caivano et al. 2012).DWI reflects the diffusion of free water molecules at the cellular level. In case of prostate tumor, because of the cellular density, there is a restriction of water motion that is displayed with bright pixels on DWI and dark pixels on ADC, the quantitative parameters of DWI. Several studies showed that DWI improved tumor detection when associated with T2wi with respect to T2wi alone. In meta-analyses, Wu et al. found that the sensitivity and specificity of T2wi + DWI in the detection of prostate cancer were 0.72 and 0.81, respectively, with respect to T2wi that showed a sensitivity and specificity of 0.62 and 0.77, respectively (Wu et al. 2012). Moreover, Delongchamps et al. found that only T2W + DWI performed better than T2W alone ($P = 0.02$) for tumor detection in the transition zone (Vargas et al. 2012). DWI is also useful to differentiate between benign and malignant lesion. In study performed on 29 patients, Sato et al. found a mean ADC value of 1.11 mm^2/s for malignant lesion versus 1.68 mm^2/s for benign lesion (Sato et al. 2005). Finally, several authors demonstrate that the median ADC value in the tumors has a negative relationship with Gleason score and that there is a statistically significant difference among low-, intermediate-, and high-grade tumors (Hambrock et al. 2011; Panebianco et al. 2015b).DCE-MRI, a technique based on contrast media administration, can detect and quantify the vascularity and angiogenesis of the tumor. Prostate cancer typically shows an early and rapid enhancement with early wash-out in the delayed phases as compared to prostate normal tissue (Boonsirikamchai et al. 2013). The reported sensitivity and specificity vary among different studies, but there is general consensus that it improves the performance of T2wi alone (Murphy et al. 2013). In a study that compared DWI, DCE, and DWI + DCE for the detection of prostate cancer, the authors found that DWI and DWI + DCE were more accurate and sensitive than DCE alone in the detection of prostate cancer (Iwazawa et al. 2011). In another study, Kim et al. investigated the combination of DWI and DCE-MRI in predicting the local stage with respect to pathologic results obtained at RP as the reference standard. The combination of DWI and DCE-MRI displayed 82.4% sensitivity, 87.2% specificity, 70% PPV, and 93.2% NPV in detecting extraprostatic extension (Kim et al. 2010). However, benign prostate tissue such as BPH nodules and prostatitis can show high vascularity that reduces the accuracy of DCE in tumor detection. Thus, DCE should be used in association with T2wi and DWI to improve sensitivity and specificity of mpMRI (Purysko et al. 2016). Overall, MRI has a high specificity but low sensitivity in the diagnostic accuracy for local staging. A recent metanalysis showed that the sensitivity and specificity for detection of ECE (i.e., T3a), SVI (i.e., T3b), and overall stage T3 disease (i.e., T3a + T3b) were 0.57 (95% CI 0.49–0.64) and 0.91 (95% CI 0.88–0.93), 0.58 (95% CI 0.47–0.68) and 0.96 (95% CI 0.95–0.97), and 0.61 (95% CI 0.54–0.67) and 0.88 (95% CI 0.85–0.91), respectively (De Rooij et al. 2016). Moreover, MRI showed a limited accuracy for detection of microscopic ECE, a disease category with favorable prognosis compared to extensive ECE (De Rooij et al. 2016).Finally, it has been demonstrated that the use of a higher field strength (i.e., 3.0 T) improves the detection sensitivity for ECE. However, when higher field strength is not available or in the absence of mpMRI, endorectal coil should be used, while its use exhibited no additional benefit for ECE detection in case of lower field strength even if it can slightly improve sensitivity for SVI detection (De Rooij et al. 2016).Lymph-node metasteses are poorly detected with either MRI or CT as the main criteria used is based on nodal size. Overall, CT and MRI show a sensitivity of around 30% in revealing lymph-node metastases (Hövels et al. 2008).

1.1.4 Target Volume Definition by Imaging

1.1.4.1 External Beam Radiotherapy

Target Definition

The prescription of radiotherapy for prostate cancer (PCa) can be modulated in terms of dose, target volumes, and integration with androgen deprivation therapy. This modulation is performed by defining different risk groups based on PSA value, Gleason score, and tumor/nodal stage.

According to the different risk groups, the clinical target volume (CTV) includes only the prostatic gland in low-risk PCa and prostate, seminal vesicles, and pelvic lymph nodes in high-risk PCa (https://www.nccn.org/professionals/physician_gls/f_guidelines.asp).

Computed Tomography

Computed tomography (CT) is the standard imaging modality for external beam radiotherapy (EBRT) planning by providing tissues electron density needed for dose calculation algorithms.

However, several studies showed significant interobserver variability in CTV delineation based on CT scan (Villeirs et al. 2005; Rasch et al. 1999), and the same results were reported about seminal vesicles delineation (Valicenti et al. 1999).

Therefore, coregistration and fusion of CT with other imaging modalities is considered to be useful in PCa irradiation.

Magnetic Resonance Imaging

Magnetic resonance imaging (MRI) is superior to CT scan in prostate gland delineation. In a multi-observer study on 18 patients, comparing CT to conventional MRI for prostate borders definition, using CT the authors found a 1.4 times larger volume compared to conventional MRI. The CT-defined prostatic volume was 8 mm larger at the base of the seminal vesicles and 6 mm larger at the prostatic apex compared to axial MRI. No significant differences in terms of interobserver variability were found in MRI-based prostate definition (Valicenti et al. 1999). Debois and coworkers reported a larger interobserver variation of the prostatic apex location on CT compared to conventional MRI (CT: 0.54–1.07 cm vs. MRI: 0.17–0.25 cm) (Debois et al. 1999). Hentschel and colleagues confirmed these results in a series of 294 patients. The mean prostate volume defined by MRI (44.3 cm^3, range: 8.8–182.8 cm^3) was 35% smaller compared to the one defined by CT (68.5 cm^3, range: 15.2–241.3 cm^3) (Hentschel et al. 2011).

The reduction of CTV achievable by MRI might have a potential impact on toxicity reduction. In fact, Steenbakkers et al., in a study on 18 patients, reported a dose reduction of 2.0–7.0 Gy to rectal wall and penile bulb by using MRI-based delineation (Steenbakkers et al. 2003).

Recently, six observer teams delineated intraprostatic tumor lesions by multiparametric-MRI in 20 PCa patients before radical prostatectomy. A total of 89 neoplastic lesions were found at pathological evaluation. About 18 of 89 lesions were identified by all teams, and all were dominant lesions. The median pathological volume of these lesions was 2.4 cm^3. The median interobserver standard deviation of the delineations was 0.23 cm^3. The kappa indices for the agreement between the delineations of teams were 0.61 ± 0.19. The kappa indices for the agreement between delineations of teams and pathologist were 0.45 ± 0.16. The authors concluded that identification of most dominant lesions is possible, and therefore dose escalation to the dominant lesion is feasible (Steenbergen et al. 2015).

Few clinical trials are available in literature on the use of intraprostatic boost, and most of them are feasibility studies (Schild et al. 2014; Aluwini et al. 2013). Aluwini and coworkers reported the results of 50 hormone-naïve patients with low- and intermediate-risk prostate cancer treated with stereotactic body radiotherapy (SBRT) to a total dose of 38 Gy delivered in 4 daily fractions of 9.5 Gy. An integrated boost to 11 Gy per fraction was applied to the dominant lesion visible on MRI. Median follow-up was 23 months. The two-year actuarial biochemical control rate was 100%. Median International Prostate Symptoms Score (IPSS) was 9/35 before treatment, with a median increase of 4 points at 3 months and remaining stable at 13/35 thereafter. No late Grade 3 toxicity was reported (Aluwini et al. 2013). Schild and coworkers reported the data of a feasibility study incorporating an MRI-directed boost to the intraprostatic lesion. A total of 78 men received EBRT for localized prostate cancer. The whole prostate received 77.4 Gy in 43 fractions, and simultaneous intraprostatic boost up to 83 Gy was delivered to the MRI identified lesion. In 16 (21%) patients, the MRI did not detect a neoplasm, and these patients received a simultaneous boost of 81 Gy to the posterior prostate. Three-year biochemical control, local control, distant control, and survival were 92%, 98%, 95%, and 95%, respectively. Only two patients reported Grade 3 toxicity (Schild et al. 2014).

Positron Emission Tomography/Computed Tomography (PET/CT)

[^{18}F]FDG or choline PET/CT are the most used tracers in prostate cancer. However, the sensitivity reported for the detection of primary prostate cancer shows a large variation (66–79%) (Aluwini et al. 2013; Farsad et al. 2005; Giovacchini et al. 2008), and specificity has shown in several studies to be low due to the limited ability in differentiating benign prostatic lesions from prostate cancer (Martorana et al. 2006). There are also limitations in delineation of prostate cancer using choline PET/CT due to choline uptake in benign lesions, and even the use of absolute and relative SUV thresholds for prostate cancer delineation must be viewed critically.

In patients with local recurrence, choline PET/CT might be useful to detect and delineate the recurrence within the prostatic bed, allowing a boost to metabolic tumor volume (MTV) (PET positive sites) (Farsad et al. 2012). Casamassima et al. evaluated SBRT in the treatment of nodal recurrence of prostate cancer detected by ^{11}C-choline PET/CT in 71 patients with biochemical recurrence. Of these patients, 32 (45%) with negative PET results were referred for systemic treatment (androgen ablation). Again, PSA velocity was significantly higher in ^{11}C-choline PET/CT-positive compared to ^{11}C-choline PET/CT-negative patients ($p < 0.05$). Sixty-four percent of ^{11}C-choline PET/CT-positive patients had locally confined lymph-node lesions and underwent curative SBRT to pathological nodes using ^{11}C-choline PET/CT images (SBRT to the recurrence site only or whole pelvis irradiation plus a boost to MTV lymph nodes). Three-year OS, disease-free survival, and local control were 92%, 17%, and 90%, respectively. The authors concluded that high SBRT doses are effective in the treatment of limited nodal recurrence and that

^{11}C-choline PET/CT might improve gross tumor delineation and SBRT response monitoring (Castellucci et al. 2014).

A recent review evaluated the role of ^{11}C- or [^{18}F]choline PET/CT in biochemical recurrence of prostate cancer. The authors reported a low accuracy in detecting local recurrence. The correlation of PSA levels and PSA kinetics with the rate of detection by choline PET/CT should be considered to achieve a better patient selection (Casamassima et al. 2011).

^{68}Ga-prostate-specific membrane antigen (^{68}Ga-PSMA) is a new promising tracer still under investigation. Some preliminary data about the impact on radiotherapy planning have been reported (Mapelli et al. 2016). Bluemel et al. evaluated the impact of ^{68}Ga-PSMA PET/CT on radiotherapy planning in 45 patients with recurrent prostate cancer. The median PSA level was 0.67 ng/ml. Suspected lesions were detected in 53.3% of patients. In 62.5% of patients, lesions were only detected by ^{68}Ga-PSMA PET. Treatment was changed in 42.2% of patients, extending salvage radiotherapy to metastases (9/19), administering dose escalation in patients with macroscopic local recurrence (6/19) or replacing radiotherapy by systemic therapy (2/19). All but one showed biochemical response (mean PSA decline 78 ± 19%) within a mean follow-up of 8.1 ± 5.2 months (Bluemel et al. 2016). Table 1 shows a summary of studies reporting the impact of PET/CT on radiotherapy planning.

1.1.4.2 Brachytherapy (BT)

The current standard of care for PCa brachytherapy (BT) simulation and treatment planning is based on transrectal ultrasound imaging of the prostate. However, MRI-based simulation and treatment planning are under investigation (Vigneault et al. 2016; D'Amico et al. 1998).

Vigneault and colleagues reported the long-term outcomes of image-guided high-dose- BT boost to the dominant intraprostatic lesion using multiparametric MRI. Twenty patients with intermediate-risk prostate cancer were included. All patients were treated with an EBRT dose of 40 Gy, combined with a high-dose-rate BT boost of 15 Gy. Concurrently, the dominant intraprostatic lesion received a boost of 18 Gy. The 5-year biochemical failure-free survival rate was 94.7%. The mean IPSS rose from 7 (baseline) to 10.4 (1 month after treatment) and rapidly decreased to 6.9 (after 3 months). Acute genitourinary Grade 3 toxicities were reported in 5% of patients. No Grade 3 late genitourinary toxicities were reported. Only Grade 1 acute and late gastrointestinal toxicities were reported (Vigneault et al. 2016).

D'Amico and coworker evaluated the dose-localization capability and acute toxicity of a real-time intraoperative MRI-guided approach to prostate BT. Nine patients with clinical stage T1cNxM0 prostate cancer, PSA <10 ng/mL, Gleason score ≤3 + 4, and endo-rectal coil MRI-based stage T2 disease were included. The prescribed minimum peripheral dose was 160 Gy to the clinical target volume, which was the MRI-defined peripheral zone of the prostate. Each catheter containing the ^{125}Iodine sources was placed under real-time MR guidance. For the 9 study patients, 89–99% (median 94%) of the clinical target volume received a minimum peripheral dose of 160 Gy, and ≥95% of the volume of the prostatic urethra and 70% (median) of the volume of the anterior rectal wall received doses below the constraints. The authors concluded that real-time MRI-guided interstitial BT

Table 1 Summary of studies reporting the impact of PET/CT in radiotherapy planning

Authors (publication year)	Study design	Treatment aim	Tracer	No. of patients	Stage changes (%)	Target definition changes (%)
Casamassima et al. (2011)	Retrospective	Salvage	Choline	71	55	35
Castellucci et al. (2014)	Retrospective	Salvage	Choline	605	29	14.8
Souvatzoglou et al. (2011)	Retrospective	Salvage	Choline	37	30	13
Bluemel et al. (2016)	Retrospective	Salvage	PSMA	45	53	42.2
Dewes et al. (2016)	Retrospective	Definitive	PSMA	15	53	33.3

is able to achieve the planned dose–volume histogram results for CTV and healthy juxtaposed structures with minimal acute morbidity (D'Amico et al. 1998).

1.1.4.3 Conclusions

Using EBRT, MRI allows the reduction of delineated target volumes while improving extracapsular extension and seminal vesicle invasion detection with potential impact on clinical outcome. Even in BT treatments, MRI can accurately identify prostate gland, extra-prostatic tissues, and normal structures (rectal wall, urethra, and bladder).

^{11}C- or [^{18}F]choline PET/CT has a limited role in primary prostate cancer due to large variation in reported sensitivity and specificity. In recurrent prostate cancer ^{11}C- or [^{18}F]choline PET/CT, accuracy is higher in the presence of fast PSA kinetics or increasing PSA levels despite ongoing androgen deprivation. New promising tracers are under investigation.

1.2 Cancers of the Testis and the Penis

Abstract

Testicular cancer is the most frequent malignancy in men between the ages of 20 and 34 years. Germ cell tumors represent 95% of histological types, divided in seminoma and non-seminoma tumors.

The typical lymphatic spread is in the retroperitoneum, while the hematogenous spread is mostly to the lungs. Ultrasonography represents often the only imaging modalities used to diagnose and evaluate a testicle tumor. PET/CT using [^{18}F]FDG has shown good results in order to stage the disease.

MRI has a higher tissue contrast resolution that helps in differentiating benign from malignant lesion and also identifying the lesion as intra- or extratesticular. Radical inguinal orchiectomy is the standard treatment for Stage I seminoma being adjuvant EBRT considered optional while EBRT is recommended in stages IIA–IIB after orchiectomy. The role of MRI in radiotherapy planning is limited because the RT target is outside the surgical bed. [^{18}F]FDG-PET/CT could theoretically improve delineation of positive lymph nodes.

Squamous cell carcinoma of the penis is an uncommon neoplasm. The role of imaging in the staging of the primary tumor is mostly based on US and MRI. Conversely, the role of CT is mostly confined in the evaluation of lymph-node and distant metastases. MRI provides excellent soft-tissue contrast, permitting the assessment of the normal penile anatomy as well as the tumor extent. In early-stage and low-grade cancers, an organ-sparing approach with surgical excision is possible. In high-grade or more advanced stage, a partial or total penectomy with or without lymph-node dissection is recommended. However, even in this group of patients, an organ-sparing strategy is still feasible. MRI is the imaging modality of choice in identification of patients with penile cancer recommended for brachytherapy due to high accuracy in depth of infiltration definition.

1.2.1 Staging with PET/CT

Testicular cancer is the most frequent malignancy in men between the ages of 20 and 34 years. The most frequent histological type is the germ cell tumors (GCT) (Manecksha and Fitzpatrick 2009). The diagnosis is, in most cases, performed by physical examination and US. The typical lymphatic spread is in the retroperitoneum, while the hematogenous spread is mostly to the lungs (Albers et al. 2012).

Testicular cancers have high response rates to therapies (Albers et al. 2012), but an accurate staging, an adequate early systemic treatment (with or without radiotherapy and surgery), and a very strict follow-up are mandatory in order to obtain the best chance of cure for the patients.

Imaging plays an important role in the clinical management of testicular cancer. PET/CT using [^{18}F]FDG has shown good results in order to stage the disease (Hain et al. 2000).

1.2.1.1 [^{18}F]FDG PET/CT

To rule out the presence of metastatic spread to the retro peritoneum is the goal of any imaging method in the staging of testicular cancer. CT is the most available imaging technique for this purpose; however, [^{18}F]FDG PET/CT may provide complementary information to the ones provided by CT and may play a role in the initial staging of patients with testicular cancer (Richie 2015).

In a retrospective study, Ambrosini et al. (Ambrosini et al. 2014) applied [^{18}F]FDG PET/CT in 51 seminoma patients. PET/CT showed a sensitivity of 92% and a specificity of 84%. In the same study, in 70 patients with non-seminoma testicular cancers, the sensitivity and specificity for [^{18}F]FDG PET/CT were 77% and 95%, respectively. In the whole population, the clinical management has been changed according to the information provided by [^{18}F]FDG PET/CT in 92% (47/51) of seminomas patients and in 84% (59/70) of non-seminoma patients. Sharma et al. (Sharma et al. 2014) confirmed the high accuracy of [^{18}F]FDG PET/CT in this condition, showing a sensitivity, specificity, PPV, NPV, and accuracy of 94.2%, 75.0%, 83.0%, 90.9%, and 85.8%, respectively.

1.2.2 Staging with CT or MRI

US represents often the only imaging modalities used to diagnose and evaluate a testicle tumor, even if MRI can provide some useful information in case of inconclusive findings in US. MRI has a higher tissue contrast resolution and shows the ability to better characterize certain lesions based on their features, such the presence of fat-containing lesions or the presence of hemoglobin degradation products, helping in differentiating benign from malignant lesion. MRI is also useful to localize the lesion as intra- or extratesticular (Huges Cassidy et al. 2010).

At MRI, the normal adult testis appears has an oval structure with homogeneous hyperintense signal on T2wi, while it has a hypo-isointense signal on T1wi. The testis is surrounded by the tunica albuginea that is hypointense in both the T1wi and T2wi. The epididymis, which lies above the testis, appears isointense to the testis on T1wi and more hypointense with respect to the testis on T2wi. Both the testicles and the epididymis enhance after the administration of contrast agents. The tunica vaginalis envelopes both the testis and the epididymis with his visceral layer, while the parietal layer forms the internal portion of the scrotal sac. These two layers form a virtual space that became a real space in case of fluid collections. The scrotal sac has a hypointense signal on both T1wi and T2wi (Parker III et al. 2015).

Tumors that arise in the scrotum can be subdivided in extratesticular tumors that are in the majority of cases of benign nature and in intratesticular tumors that conversely are generally malignant. The most common testicular malignant tumors are germ cells tumors (Huges Cassidy et al. 2010).

Moreover, some overlaps exist between testicular tumor and nonneoplastic conditions in terms of imaging appearance, and in some recent article, MRI showed a sensitivity up to 100% in differentiating benign from malignant lesions (Moreno et al. 2015).

MRI has a high accuracy in the local staging of testicle cancer of more than 90%. In fact, it can show the interruption of the hypointense signal of the tunica albuginea in case of T2 lesion or the infiltration of the spermatic cord or scrotal skin in case of T3 and T4 lesion, respectively (Tsili et al. 2010).

However, the role of imaging in staging testicular cancer is limited to the evaluation of lymph-node and distant metastases because the T-staging is generally determined on the basis of pathologic analysis after orchiectomy (Moreno et al. 2015; Winter and Albers 2011).

Physical examination, consisting in the palpation of penis and inguinal region, is essential for a correct evaluation and staging of penile tumor and lymph-node involvement. The role of imaging in the staging of the primary tumor is mostly based on US and MRI. Conversely, the role of CT is mostly confined in the evaluation of lymph-node and distant metastases.

MRI provides excellent soft-tissue contrast, permitting the assessment of the normal penile anatomy as well as the tumor extent.

At MRI, the normal corpus spongiosum and the corpora cavernosa are hyperintense on T2wi and are of intermediate intensity on T1wi. The corpus spongiosum surrounds the musculature of urethra that has a hypointense signal in T2wi. The tunica albuginea, which is the fascial sheath that envelopes both the corpora cavernosa and the corpus spongiosum, appears hypointense on both T1wi and T2wi. Both the corpus spongiosum and the corpora cavernosa enhance after the administration of contrast media (Lont et al. 2003a).

Squamous cell carcinoma is the most frequent type of penile cancer and in general arises in the glans or prepuce. It usually appears as an infiltrative hypointense mass on T1wi and T2wi, which enhances after intravenous contrast media infusion. Urethral carcinomas, another type of penile cancer, are generally squamous cell carcinomas, even if transitional cell carcinoma or adenocarcinoma can also occur. They are commonly localized in the bulbo-membranous portion of the urethra and appear as hypointense mass with respect to corpora cavernosa (Lont et al. 2003a).

In a study that compared physical examination, MRI, and US in the evaluation of the extension of penile cancer, physical examination had the better positive predictive value for estimating tumor size and infiltration into the corpora cavernosa. However, MRI showed the higher sensitivity for the evaluation of deep infiltration and therefore is the imaging method of choice in determining infiltration depth, especially when it cannot be determined accurately by physical examination only (Hakenberg et al. 2015). Moreover, a concurrent phimosis could hide an underlying penile cancer, which conversely is easily diagnosed with imaging (Kayes et al. 2007).

Intracavernosal prostaglandin injection with artificial erection can emphasize the boundary between the tunica albuginea and the corpora cavernosa on T2-weighted images, allowing for a more accurate local staging. Kayes et al. showed that the use of MRI with intracavernosal prostaglandin injection has a high accuracy in predicting the involvement of corpora cavernosa (Moreno et al. 2015). However, intracavernosal prostaglandin is not indicated in case of penile implants or conditions that may cause priapism such as sickle cell anemia (Lont et al. 2003a).

1.2.3 Target Volume Definition by Imaging

1.2.3.1 External Beam Radiotherapy (EBRT)

Testicular cancer is the most common solid tumor in men aged 20–34 years. Germ cell tumors represent 95% of histological types, divided in seminoma and non-seminoma tumors (Manecksha and Fitzpatrick 2009). Radiotherapy is a therapeutic option in seminoma. Radical inguinal orchiectomy is the standard treatment for Stage I seminoma being adjuvant EBRT considered optional while EBRT is recommended in stages IIA–IIB after orchiectomy.

The CTV in Stage I include para-caval, precaval, and inter-aorto-caval lymph nodes for right-sided testicular seminomas and at least the para-aortic and pre-aortic lymph nodes for left-sided testicular seminomas. In Stage IIA–IIB, the CTV includes ipsilateral common, external, and proximal internal iliac lymph nodes down to the top of the acetabulum (https://www.nccn.org/professionals/physician_gls/f_guidelines.asp). In Stage IIA–IIB, a boost to positive lymph nodes is recommended.

Magnetic Resonance Imaging (MRI)

MRI can accurately differentiate intratesticular from extra-testicular lesions. Furthermore, MRI can accurately estimate the local extent of testicular carcinomas in patients for whom testis-sparing surgery is planned (Tsili et al. 2014). The role of MRI in radiotherapy planning is limited because the RT target is outside the surgical bed.

Positron Emission Tomography/Computed Tomography (PET/CT)

PET/CT using [^{18}F]FDG has shown a high accuracy in assessment of lymph nodes (Ambrosini et al. 2014). Although no study directly evaluated the impact of [^{18}F]FDG-PET/CT in RT planning, [^{18}F]FDG-PET/CT could theoretically improve delineation of positive lymph nodes.

1.2.4 Penile Cancer

1.2.4.1 External Beam Radiotherapy

Squamous cell carcinoma of the penis is an uncommon neoplasm representing 0.4% to 0.6% of all tumors in men (Ambrosini et al. 2014). Surgery is the standard treatment. In early-stage (Tis, T1a) and low-grade (G1–G2) cancers, an organ sparing approach with surgical excision is possible. In high-grade (G3) or more advanced stage, a partial or total penectomy with or without lymph node dissection is recommended. However, even in this group of patients, an organ sparing strategy is still feasible. In fact, circumcision followed by radiotherapy (EBRT with or without chemotherapy or BT) may achieve an organ sparing (https://www.nccn.org/professionals/physician_gls/f_guidelines.asp; Crook et al. 2013).

In EBRT a bolus to primary penile lesions is required for a better target coverage. Even in lesions less than 4 cm, a prophylactic inguinal irradiation is recommended, and in larger tumors, the target includes also to pelvic lymph nodes (https://www.nccn.org/professionals/physician_gls/f_guidelines.asp).

The presence and extent of lymph-node metastases from penile cancer have a negative impact on outcomes. In case of patients unfit for lymphadenectomy, imaging tools may allow the delivery of a boost to the positive lymph nodes. In their review, Mueller-Lisse and colleagues evaluated the impact of different imaging modalities in penile cancer staging. Sensitivity and specificity of [^{18}F]FDG PET/CT for lymph-node metastasis were 80% and 100%, respectively, and MRI sensitivity and specificity were 100% and 97%, respectively (Mueller-Lisse et al. 2008).

1.2.4.2 Brachytherapy

Circumcision and BT are recommended in selected patients being 87% the 5-year organ sparing rate. Inclusion criteria of patients candidate to BT are T1b or T2 and maximum diameter less than 4 cm. Only T3 tumors with extension into the penile urethra without mucosal disruption might be considered to BT with an increased risk of meatal stenosis (Crook et al. 2013). MRI is the imaging modality of choice in identification of patients with penile cancer recommended for BT due to high accuracy in depth of infiltration definition (Lont et al. 2003b).

2 Female Genital tract Malignancies

2.1 Cervical Cancer

Abstract
Cervical cancer is the third most common cancer in young women. Squamous cell carcinoma is the most frequent histotype, while about 20% of cases are adenocarcinoma and adenosquamous carcinoma. The main role of [^{18}F]FDG-PET/CT in cervical cancer at presentation is assessing lymph-node status particularly in patients with advanced stages, in which extra pelvic spread could be potentially present.

CT scan has a limited role in the local staging of cervical carcinoma as it shows a low soft-tissue contrast resolution. Conversely, MRI represents the best imaging method for an accurate assessment of tumor location, tumor size, and local staging as it can best evaluate local invasion into the parametria, pelvic sidewall, or adjacent organs.

The standard primary treatment of very early-stage disease is surgery, and, for more advanced disease, pelvic external beam radiotherapy combined with concurrent chemotherapy plus brachytherapy boost are recommended. MRI is the most important imaging tool in radiotherapy. In fact, the contouring guidelines for external beam planning of cervical cancer (Gynecologic IMRT Consortium and the Japanese Radiation Oncology Group) recommend delineation of both target and organs at risk on T2-weighted MRI. Also, in the brachytherapy planning, MRI is the recommended imaging. Several studies reported a significant impact of [^{18}F]FDG-PET/CT performed before radiotherapy in terms of radiotherapy fields change. However, in the only randomized trial, no impact in overall survival has been recorded.

2.1.1 Staging with PET/CT

Cervical cancer is the third most common cancer in young women (Jemal et al. 2008), but the incidence of cervical cancer varies significantly among different countries ranging from 1 to more than 50 cases per 100,000 (Arbyn et al. 2011). Squamous cell carcinoma is the most frequent histotype, while about 20% of cases are adenocarcinoma and adenosquamous carcinoma. As for many other gynecological malignancies, the standard staging system is FIGO classification; however, this method, although easy and simple to apply, has some limitations since it does not consider some prognostic factors such as tumor size, histologic grade, and local or retroperitoneal lymph node status. Initial staging of cervical cancer is usually performed with CT, or MRI and [^{18}F]FDG PET/CT (Grigsby 2008). Recently, the application of the hybrid PET/MRI has shown some promising results (Grueneisen et al. 2015). The combination of radio- and chemotherapy, EBRT, and brachytherapy is the treatment of choice in locally advanced disease.

2.1.1.1 [^{18}F]FDG PET/CT

In almost all primary cervical cancers, there is an increased [^{18}F]FDG activity that depends on the histological type and differentiation. As in many other tumors, also in cervical cancer, squamous tumors and poorly differentiated tumors showed a higher SUV_{max} if compared with the other types of cervical cancers (Kidd et al. 2009). The intensity of [^{18}F]FDG uptake is strictly correlated with tumor proliferation and aggressiveness: higher SUV_{max} values are associated with an increased risk of lymph-node involvement. Kidd et al. (2009) enrolled 240 patients with cervical cancer at presentation: tumor mean SUV_{max} higher than 11.62 was associated with poorly differentiated tumor types. Interestingly, SUV_{max} was found to be a stronger predictive factor of risk of lymph-node involvement if compared with stage, histology, and differentiation. In another well-conducted study, Lee et al. (Lee et al. 2009) confirmed these results in 44 patients with FIGO Stage IB–IIA invasive cervical carcinoma. The mean SUV_{max} was significantly higher in patients with deep stromal invasion and pathologically confirmed large tumors if compared with the patients without these characteristics.

The main limitation of [^{18}F]FDG PET/CT in staging cervical cancer is the limited spatial resolution so that small lesions (theoretically lower than 5mm in diameter) and micro metastasis cannot be detected by [^{18}F]FDG PET/CT. However, the information provided by [^{18}F]FDG PET may give complementary information to MRI in the evaluation of local extent of disease. Gruniesen et al. (Grueneisen et al. 2015) showed that PET/MRI enabled the detection of all 27 primary tumor lesions of the uterine cervix and allowed for the correct determination of the T-stage in 23 out of the 27 patients.

The main goal of [^{18}F]FDG PET/CT in cervical cancer at presentation is assessing lymph-node status particularly in patients with advanced stages (≥IB2), in which extra pelvic spread (mainly retroperitoneal lymph node involvement) could be potentially present (Gouy et al. 2012). The assessment of lymph-node status with [^{18}F]FDG PET/CT may lead to a significant change in treatment planning (Magné et al. 2008). Moreover, lymph-node status assessed by [^{18}F]FDG PET has been found to be the most significant independent pretreatment predictor factor of progression-free and overall survival in patients with cervical cancer (Grigsby 2008). [^{18}F]FDG PET/CT may show unexpected extrapelvic spread such as retroperitoneum or supraclavicular nodal metastasis which is a dramatic impact on disease management. Havrilesky et al. (Havrilesky et al. 2005) published a meta-analysis showing a pooled sensitivity of 84% and a pooled specificity of 95% in the detection of retroperitoneal lymph nodes, while the sensitivity and specificity was 79% and 99%, respectively, in the detection of pelvic lesions.

Chao et al. (2008) reported the results of a prospective trial that included 47 cervical cancer patients with paraaortic, inguinal, or supraclavicular nodal involvement found at CT or MRI. Additional [^{18}F]FDG PET/CT had a major impact in 21/47 patients showing the presence of other sites of disease, downstaging the disease, enabling metabolic biopsy of involved sites, and changing the treatment strategy to palliation. Overall, [^{18}F]FDG PET/CT altered management either by extension of the radiation field to include the para-aortic area or by a change in the total administered dose to the involved nodes in the pelvic area. Finally, the use of hybrid PET/MRI tomograph (Grueneisen et al. 2015) in 27 patients at presentation showed a sensitivity, specificity, and diagnostic accuracy for the detection of nodal positive patients of 91%, 94%, and 93%, respectively. PET/MRI correctly identified regional metastatic disease in 80% of the patients and nonregional lymph-node metastases in 100% of the patients.

2.1.2 Staging with CT or MRI

In the assessment of cervical cancer, it is recommended to perform CT scan or MRI to correctly stage the tumor. CT scan has a limited role in the local staging of cervical carcinoma as it shows a low soft-tissue contrast resolution even if it can demonstrate the spread to the bladder and rectum, the presence of enlarged lymph-node, or distant metastases (Freeman et al. 2012a).

Conversely, MRI has the best soft-tissue contrast resolution and has a paramount role in the local staging of cervical cancer. MRI, in fact, represents the best imaging method for an accurate assessment of tumor location, tumor size, and local staging as it can best evaluate local invasion into the parametria, pelvic sidewall, or adjacent organs (Okamoto et al. 2003; Sala et al. 2013a). Actually, clinical assessment of tumor size and parametrial or pelvic sidewall invasion shows an accuracy of 60% or less, carrying to an overall underestimation of tumor staging (Okamoto et al. 2003; Zand et al. 2007). Moreover, MRI has a negative predictive value of up the 100% for exclusion of bladder and rectal invasion and around the 95% for exclusion of parametrial invasion, revesting a main role for selecting patients who are candidates for surgery (Sala et al. 2013a; Sahdev et al. 2007; Sheu et al. 2001; Rockall et al. 2006).

MRI has then a main role in the correct risk stratification of patients affected by cervical cancer with the aim to determine the most appropriate therapeutic approach (Freeman et al. 2012a).

On the basis of these characteristics, MRI is currently used in the monitoring of treatment response, the detection of recurrence, the assessment of complications due to the disease or treatment, and the planning of radiation therapy in case of advanced disease (Sala et al. 2013a; Addley et al. 2010; Beddy et al. 2011).

T2wi represents the key sequence of cervical carcinoma staging showing an accuracy rate of more than 85% in the correct evaluation of tumor size and of more than 80% in the assessment of parametrial invasion (Sheu et al. 2001; Balleyguier et al. 2011). To better evaluate cervical cancer, T2wi is commonly obtained on the axial oblique plane (i.e., orthogonal to the longitudinal axis) and sagittal plane, allowing the correct assessment of cervical stroma and the relationship of the tumor with the parametria, bladder, rectosigmoid, and pelvic sidewall (Sala et al. 2013a).

DCE sequences have a marginal role in the evaluation of cervical cancer as it could be useful in the depiction of small tumors; conversely, it has no value in the assessment of parametrial invasion. Similarly to DCE, DWI is useful in association with T2wi to localize small cervical tumors or poorly circumscribed lesions (Sala et al. 2013a).

The assessment of cervical anatomy is best performed on high-resolution T2wi that shows an optimal soft-tissue contrast resolution. Typically, the cervix is characterized by several layers that present different signal intensity at MRI: the inner layer has a high signal intensity and represents the endocervical canal; the inner layer is surrounded by the epithelium of the cervix that is a line showing a high signal intensity lower than that of the endocervical canal; surrounding the endocervical line there is the cervical stroma that shows a low signal intensity; and the outer layer is a rim of intermediate signal intensity represented by myometrial cervical extension.

Cervical cancer appears at T2wi as a lesion of intermediate to high signal intensity that substitutes the low signal intensity of cervical stroma (Freeman et al. 2012a; Noël et al. 2014).

On DCE, cervical cancer shows early enhancement, similar to that of cervical mucosa. On delayed phase, most lesions are isointense or hypointense relative to the stroma (Noël et al. 2014; Seki et al. 1997).

Usually, cervical cancer demonstrates high signal intensity on DWI and low signal intensity on corresponding ADC maps with the ADC value lower than that of the normal cervical tissue (Freeman et al. 2012a).

FIGO Stage I disease represents a disease that is confined to the cervix and is subdivided into two categories: Stage IA that represents by definition a microinvasive disease and then is not seen on MRI and Stage IB that is further classified into Stages IB1 and IB2 whether it measures less (IB1) or more than 4 cm (IB2). MRI is then not indicated in the case of Stage IA1 while it is recommended in clinical Stage IB or higher, given the needs of an accurate assessment of tumor size, the involvement of parametrial or lower vaginal, and to assess the presence of lymph node or distant metastases as the identification of such adverse prognostic factors precludes surgery (Freeman et al. 2012a; Scheidler and Heuck 2002; Cheng et al. 2004).

Stage II disease is a tumor that grows beyond the cervix but does not spread to the pelvic sidewall or the lower one-third of the vagina (Freeman et al. 2012a). Stage IIA represents lesions that invades the upper two-thirds of vagina without parametrial invasion and is recognized on T2wi as the presence of an interruption of the hypointense vaginal wall. Stage IIA is further subdivided into Stages IIA1 and IIA2 if the greatest dimension of the tumor is less (IIA1) or more than 4 cm (IIA2).

Stage IIB disease is the presence of parametrial invasion without extension to the pelvic sidewall and is seen on T2wi as a tumor that disrupts the low signal intensity cervical stromal ring and invades the parametrium (Freeman et al. 2012a; Nicolet et al. 2000). The correct assessment of parametrial invasion is of paramount importance as it represents a poor prognostic factor; on T2wi it can be excluded with a specificity of up to 99% and a negative predictive value of up to 100% if the low signal intensity cervical stroma is wider for more than 3 mm (Sala et al. 2007, 2013a; Zand et al. 2007). A potential pitfall is the correct evaluation of parametrial invasion in larger lesion. In large tumors, the compression of the cervical stroma may cause stromal edema that can lead to an overestimation of parametrial invasion that reduces the accuracy of MRI to 70%, while in smaller lesion, it reaches 96% (Freeman et al. 2012a; Zand et al. 2007).

According to the revised FIGO staging system, Stage III is a disease that extends into the lower three-thirds of the vagina without extension to the pelvic sidewall (IIIA) or that extends to the pelvic sidewall or cause hydronephrosis (IIIB). A lesion that is depicted within 3 mm of the internal obturator, levator ani, and piriformis muscles or the iliac vessels should be considered a Stage IIIB disease (Freeman et al. 2012a; Sala et al. 2013a; Zand et al. 2007).

Stage IV disease is the invasion of the surrounding organs by the tumor or the presence of distant metastases. In particular, Stage IVA is the invasion of rectal or bladder mucosa and is best showed on T2wi as the interruption of the low signal intensity bladder or rectal wall by the tumor that infiltrates into the mucosa. Usually, the infiltration of the bladder is more common than that of the rectum. Overall, MRI shows a negative predictive value of around 100% in the assessment of bladder or rectal invasion (Sala et al. 2013a; Rockall et al. 2006).

Stage IVB is the presence of distant metastases including paraaortic and inguinal lymph nodes.

2.1.3 Target Volume Definition by Imaging

2.1.3.1 External Beam Radiotherapy (EBRT)

Target Volume

Cervical cancer is the second most common gynecological cancer. Squamous cell carcinoma is the most frequent histological type (80%). The standard primary treatment of very early stage disease is surgery, and, for more advanced disease, pelvic EBRT combined with concurrent chemotherapy plus brachytherapy boost are recommended (https://www.nccn.org/professionals/physician_gls/f_guidelines.asp). In the CTV are included the entire GTV (intermediate/high signal seen on T2-weighted MR images), entire cervix (if not already included within GTV contour), uterus, parametria including ovaries, and entire mesorectum if uterosacral ligament involved. Furthermore, the upper half of the vagina (if minimal or no vaginal extension) or upper two-thirds of the vagina (if upper vaginal involvement) or entire vagina (if extensive vaginal involvement) are included (Fütterer et al. 2006b).

Magnetic Resonance Imaging (MRI)

MRI is considered the best imaging tools to define soft tissue and parametrial involvement. In fact, both contouring guidelines for external beam planning of cervical cancer (Gynecologic IMRT Consortium and the Japanese Radiation Oncology Group) recommend delineation of both target and organs at risk on T2-weighted MRI (Lim et al. 2011; Toita et al. 2011).

Recently, Song et al. analyzed the GTV delineation according to different imaging tools. A total of 23 patients with locally advanced cervical cancer were studied using a 3-Tesla MRI and CT. For each patient, the GTVs were delineated manually on CT (GTV-CT) and 4 MRI sequences, including T1, T2, T1 with fat suppression and contrast, and apparent diffusion coefficient–diffusion-weighted imaging (ADC-DWI) (GTV-T1, GTV-T2, GTV-T1F+, and GTV-ADC). The average GTV volumes for T1, T2, ADC, and T1F+ were (in cm^3) 62.8 ± 62.1, 58.4 ± 61.2, 50.9 ± 59.8, 66.4 ± 64.9, respectively. The differences between T2 and other MRI sequences were significant ($p < 0.05$). There was no significant difference between GTV-T1 and GTV-T1F+. GTV-T1 was larger than GTVT2 mainly due to the lower soft-tissue contrast at the tumor boundary in T1 compared to T2 sequences. GTV-ADC was smaller than GTV-T2 being the uncovered volume accounting for up to 16% of the GTV-T2. The authors concluded that MRI-based GTV (fusion of the GTV-T2 and GTV-ADC) may be more appropriate than individual GTV-T2 and GTV-ADC. There was a significant difference between GTV-MRI and GTV-CT in terms of volumes. On average, GTV-MRI was smaller (18.4%) than GTV-CT for the cases studied (Song et al. 2016).

Positron Emission Tomography/Computed Tomography (PET/CT)

Pathological uptake of [^{18}F]FDG-PET/CT may modify treatment strategy, either by extending the radiation volumes to the para-aortic area or by detecting affected lymph nodes (Chao et al. 2008; Yildirim et al. 2008; Tsai et al. 2010; Lazzari et al. 2014). Table 2 reported a summary of these studies (Chao et al. 2008; Yildirim et al. 2008; Tsai et al. 2010; Lazzari et al. 2014). Tsai and colleagues evaluated in a prospective randomized study the impact of [^{18}F]FDG-PET/CT on extra-pelvic metastases detection, radiation field design, and survival outcome in cervical cancer patients with enlarged pelvic nodes on MRI imaging. Whole pelvis was the standard irradiation field for the control group and for patients without extra-pelvic findings in the PET group. From January 2002 to April 2006, 129 patients were included, and 66 of them were randomized to receive [^{18}F]FDG-PET/CT. The authors confirmed the impact on treatment changes in patients undergoing [^{18}F]FDG-PET/CT. [^{18}F]FDG-PET/CT detected para-aortic lymph-node metastases in 6 patients and omental node metastases in 1 patient. Four patients remained disease-free after treatment modification. No difference between [^{18}F]FDG-PET/CT group and [^{18}F]FDG-PET/CT group was observed in 4-year overall survival (79% vs. 85%, $p = 0.65$), disease-free survival (75% vs. 77%, $p = 0.64$), and distant metastasis-free survival (82% vs. 78%, $p = 0.83$) (Tsai et al. 2010).

2.1.3.2 Brachytherapy

Target Volume

The GEC ESTRO guidelines recommend T2-weighted MRI images for target and OAR delineation (Haie-Meder et al. 2005). According to these guidelines, the CTV includes a high-risk (HR) and intermediate-risk (IR) area. HR CTV includes the area with a higher risk of local recurrence because of residual macroscopic disease after EBRT. The intent is to deliver a total dose as high as possible and appropriate to eradicate all residual macroscopic tumor. IR CTV includes the initial macroscopic extent of disease with significant risk of residual microscopic disease at time of BT. Therefore, this area should receive a total radiation dose appropriate to cure significant microscopic disease (Haie-Meder et al. 2005).

Pötter and coworkers reported the results of a study based on EBRT with 45–50.4 Gy ± concomitant cisplatin chemotherapy plus 4 × 7 Gy high dose rate (HDR) BT. BT was delivered according GEC ESTRO recommendations. A total of 156 consecutive patients (median age 58 years) with cervical cancer FIGO stages IB–IVA were treated. The 3-year local control was 95–100% in limited/favorable (IB/IIB) and

Table 2 Summary of studies reporting the impact of [18F]FDG-PET/CT in radiotherapy planning

Authors (publication years)	Study type	No of patients	Stage changes (%)	Target definition changes (%)	Other results
Chao et al. (2008), Briganti et al. (2012)	Prospective	47	45	17	75% of the patients with modified radiotherapy field remained disease free (at 2-year follow-up)
Yildirim et al. (2008), Panebianco et al. (2012)	Prospective	16	12.5 25	25	NR
Tsai et al. (2010), Boonsirikamchai et al. (2013)	Prospective randomized trial	66	11	11	57% of patients with modified radiotherapy field remained disease free with 53 months median follow-up
Lazzari et al. (2014), Delongchamps et al. (2011)	Prospective	66	18	18	NR

NR not reported

85–90% in large/poor responding (IIB/III/IV) cervical cancer patients. Compared to a historical series, there was relative reduction in pelvic recurrence by 65–70% and reduction in major morbidity. The 3-year overall survival was 68%: 72% for larger tumors (2–5 cm diameter), 65% for larger tumors (>5 cm diameter), 74% for IB, 78% for IIB, and 45% for IIIB stage, respectively (Pötter et al. 2011).

In another larger series from Aarhus, 140 patients underwent MRI-guided brachytherapy according to GEC ESTRO recommendations. The 3-year local control was 91%. Comparisons with historical controls from the same institution showed that the improved local control translated into a significant improvement in overall survival by 16% (from 63 to 79%) (Lindegaard et al. 2013).

Positron Emission Tomography/Computed Tomography (PET/CT)

Few studies assessed the role of [18F]FDG-PET/CT-guided brachytherapy (Malyapa et al. 2002; Lin et al. 2007). Malyapa and colleagues compared two-dimensional (2D) treatment planning brachytherapy with three-dimensional (3D) treatment planning based on [18F]FDG-PET/CT in 11 patients with cervical cancer. Patients underwent two [18F]FDG-PET/CTs: a first one to visualize the tumor and a second one with [18F]FDG placed inside the tandem and ovoid applicators to visualize the treatment source positions for 3D treatment planning. The tumor volumes were delineated using a binary threshold technique in which the threshold [18F]FDG-PET/CT image intensity was 40% of the peak tumor intensity. [18F]FDG-PET/CT provided a reliable estimate of the cervical cancer volume and 3D spatial relationship of the tumor to tandem and ovoid applicators. The authors concluded that this technique was feasible and more accurate compared to 2D treatment planning (Malyapa et al. 2002).

2.1.3.3 Conclusions

MRI is considered the standard imaging tool to define soft tissue and parametrial involvement. Further improvements of MRI technique might increase the accuracy of target definition. [18F]FDG-PET/CT is more effective in detecting positive lymph nodes. Several studies reported a significant impact of [18F]FDG-PET/CT performed before RT in terms of RT fields change. However, in the only randomized trial, no impact in OS has recorded. MRI is the recommended imaging in BT planning. Data regarding [18F]FDG-PET/CT are limited being mostly a series of feasibility studies.

2.2 Endometrial Cancer

Abstract
Endometrial cancer is the most common gynecologic malignancy in the developed countries. Histopathologic cervical invasion, depth of

myometrial invasion, lymph node status, and distant metastases are the most relevant prognostic factors.

The main aim of [^{18}F]FDG PET/CT in the endometrial cancer is the assessment of nodal status with highly specific and suboptimal sensitivity and could not replace lymphadenectomy.

However, because of the higher tissue contrast resolution, the role of MRI in the preoperative setting as a useful tool for a correct staging as well as a guide for an accurate surgery treatment has been established. As a result, MRI has been recently incorporated in the preoperative assessment of endometrial cancer in the majority cancer imaging guidelines.

The primary treatment in patients affected by endometrial cancer is usually surgery. According to risk factors and stage, adjuvant radiotherapy with or without chemotherapy may represent an option of adjuvant therapy. Radiotherapy can also be used as primary treatment in patients with unresectable disease or in patients with medical contraindications to surgery.

2.2.1 Staging with PET/CT

Endometrial cancer is the most common gynecologic malignancy in the developed countries (Amant et al. 2005). Histopathologic cervical invasion, depth of myometrial invasion, lymph-node status, and distant metastases are the most relevant prognostic factors (Amant et al. 2005). An accurate preoperative staging is crucial since it may provide clinical and prognostic information. In fact, the overall 5-year overall survival rate is 80%, but it dramatically drops down to 50% in patients showing lymph-node metastases (Lewin et al. 2010).

Imaging is usually performed with transvaginal ultrasound, MRI, and CT who provide detailed anatomic information, while functional/metabolic characteristics may be assessed with [^{18}F]FDG PET/CT (Faria et al. 2015).

As well as in cervical cancer, the intensity of [^{18}F]FDG uptake in the primary lesion may provide useful prognostic information (Kitajima et al. 2012). However, the main aim of [^{18}F]FDG PET/CT in this pathologic condition is the assessment of nodal status. Many evidences have showed that preoperative [^{18}F]FDG PET/CT may assess the status of pelvic and abdominal lymph nodes with high accuracy.

Chang et al. (2012) published a meta-analysis including 243 patients from seven studies. The overall pooled sensitivity and specificity of [^{18}F]FDG PET/CT scans in the detection of pelvic and/or paraaortic metastasis were 63.0% and 94.7%, respectively. These results have been recently confirmed by a prospective multicenter clinical trial (Atri et al. 2017). The study has been designed to evaluate the accuracy of [^{18}F]FDG PET/CT in the evaluation of nodal metastasis in women with high-risk endometrial cancer. The trial enrolled 215 women with high-risk endometrial cancer at presentation. In the abdomen, authors found a sensitivity for [^{18}F]FDG PET/CT that ranged from 0.52 to 0.74 and a specificity that ranged from 0.85 to 0.92. Results in the pelvis were sensitivity 0.65 and specificity 0.93. Authors concluded that [^{18}F]FDG PET/CT can improve detection of *LN* metastasis in the abdomen compared with the current standard of contrast-enhanced diagnostic CT.

Finally in a recent meta-analysis, Bollineni et al. (2016) evaluated 13 studies and 861 patients with endometrial cancer at presentation. For the detection of nodal involvement, authors found a pooled sensitivity and specificity of 0.72 and 0.94, respectively. Authors also assessed the accuracy of [^{18}F]FDG PET/CT in the detection of cancer relapse in 8 studies and 378 patients. The pooled sensitivity was 0.95 (95% CI, 0.91–0.98), and the pooled specificity was 0.91 (95% CI, 0.86–0.94).

In conclusion, the evidences in literature showed that although highly specific [^{18}F]FDG PET/CT showed suboptimal sensitivity and could not replace lymphadenectomy. However, it could show the presence of nodal lesions in sites not generally removed with a standard lymph-node dissection.

2.2.2 Staging with CT or RM

The primary treatment in patients affected by endometrial cancer is usually surgery. As the majority of prognostic factors and information for the correct management and risk stratification of endometrial cancer are generally obtained based on preoperative and postoperative histologic specimen (i.e., depth of myometrial invasion, cervical stroma invasion, tumor grading, lympho-vascular space invasion), the preoperative assessment is mostly performed with ultrasound in patients found with early stage disease, while in advanced disease, CT and/or PET-CT are routinely performed for the assessment of lymph-node and distant metastases (Meissnitzer and Forstner 2016).

However, because of the higher tissue contrast resolution, the role of MRI in the preoperative setting as a useful tool for a correct staging as well as a guide for an accurate surgery treatment has been established. As a result, MRI has been recently incorporated in the preoperative assessment of endometrial cancer in the majority of cancer imaging guidelines (Kinkel et al. 2009; Querleu et al. 2011; Remedios and McCoubrie 2007).

The added role of MRI with respect to US or CT in the local assessment and staging of endometrial cancer is based on its high-contrast resolution, providing an accurate evaluation of the depth of myometrial invasion and of cervical stromal invasion (Meissnitzer and Forstner 2016; Rockall et al. 2007). Moreover, it provides some additional information such as the tumor dimension or the presence of adnexal or peritoneal disease that may contraindicate or change the surgical approach (Amant et al. 2007).

MRI has also a role in the correct staging of young patients. The exclusion of myometrial invasion at MRI is an indication for a conservative surgery with the aim to preserve fertility in such young patients. Finally, it is a useful tool for the radiation therapy planning when a neoadjuvant RT is indicated instead of surgery (Meissnitzer and Forstner 2016).

At MRI, the normal uterine anatomy is best depicted on T2wi. The normal endometrium shows high signal intensity surrounded by the lower signal intensity of the junctional zone and the intermediate signal intensity of the myometrium (Freeman et al. 2012b; Sala et al. 2013b).

Endometrial carcinoma commonly demonstrates a hypointense signal with respect to the endometrium on T2-weighted images. After contrast material administration, the tumor shows a mild and slow enhancement demonstrating lower signal intensity with respect to the myometrium that shows the maximal enhancement after 1–2 min (Freeman et al. 2012b). On DWI, which is mainly used to depict small lesion and small pelvic metastases in the case of extrauterine spread, endometrial carcinoma shows high signal intensity corresponding to the low signal intensity in the ADC maps which indicates a restricted diffusion (Freeman et al. 2012b; Beddy et al. 2012; Rechichi et al. 2010).

The FIGO Stage I tumor was revised in 2009 and includes Stage IA tumor corresponding to lesion that infiltrates the endometrium and the myometrium for less than 50% and Stage IB cancer that includes lesion that invades the myometrium for more than 50%. The use of DCE sequences can help to identify the deep myometrium infiltration based on the signal intensity difference after contrast media administration, as previously reported. Potential pitfalls in the estimation of myometrium depth infiltration is the presence of leiomyomas, adenomyosis, loss of junctional zone definition, or peritumoral inflammation. These pitfalls may potentially be reduced using DCE and DWI along with T2wi, reaching a sensitivity and specificity for the evaluation of depth of myometrial invasion of almost 95% in several studies (Rockall et al. 2007; Sala et al. 2009, 2013b; Beddy et al. 2012).

Stage II endometrial cancer denotes a carcinoma that directly invades cervical stroma. On T2wi, cervical stroma invasion is represented by the interruption of the hypointense cervical stroma ring. To better evaluate stromal interruption, T2wi should be evaluated in an axial plane orthogonal to the cervix (axial oblique plane) (Meissnitzer and Forstner 2016; Sala et al. 2013b). On delayed phase images after contrast media administration (i.e., 2–3 min after gadolinium media injection), the preservation of the normal enhancement of the cervical mucosa excludes stromal invasion (Freeman et al. 2012b). Overall, accuracy of MRI imaging in the assessment of cervical stroma invasion is around 92% (Sala et al. 2009; Manfredi et al. 2004).

Stage III disease represents the locoregional invasion spread of the tumor which is a carcinoma that goes beyond the uterus but that remains in the true pelvis. Stage IIIa represents a tumor invading the uterine serosa or infiltrates the adnexa. T2wi depicts the interruption of the outer hypointense contour of the uterine representing the serosa. DWI is useful to improve the identification of metastatic deposits to the adnexa (Sala et al. 2013b). Stage IIIb is a tumor that infiltrates the parametrium and the vagina, directly or by metastatic spread. On T2wi is depicted by the interruption of the hypointense vaginal wall (Freeman et al. 2012b). Stage IIIc is the presence of metastatic lymph node to the pelvis (IIIC1) or to the para-aortic nodes with or without pelvic nodal involvement (IIIC2).

Stage IV disease is the direct invasion of the bladder or rectal mucosa (Stage IVA) or the occurrence of distant metastases (Stage IVB) (Freeman et al. 2012b). The presence of a lesion of the same intensity of the tumor that disrupts the normal hyperintense signal of the bladder or rectal mucosa on T2wi represents the direct invasion of bladder and rectum. The sagittal plane is mostly used to best evaluate the rectum and bladder wall invasion. The preservation of the fat plane between the tumor and these two organs excludes the Stage IVA (Meissnitzer and Forstner 2016).

Stage IVB disease is the observation of distant metastases including nodal metastases different from Stages IIIC1 and IIIC2, malignant ascites, or peritoneal deposits (Freeman et al. 2012b).

2.2.3 Target Volume Definition by Imaging

2.2.3.1 External Beam Radiotherapy

Target Volume

Endometrial cancer is the most frequent gynecological cancer in developed countries (Siegel et al. 2017). Hysterectomy and bilateral salpingo-oophorectomy are the first steps in treatment of potentially resectable endometrial cancer patients. Surgery includes resection of the pelvic and para-aortic nodes to assess nodal stage. According to risk factors and stage, adjuvant RT with or without chemotherapy may represent an option of adjuvant therapy (https://www.nccn.org/professionals/physician_gls/f_guidelines.asp). RT can also be used as primary treatment in patients with unresectable disease or in patients with medical contraindications to surgery (Podzielinski et al. 2012; Fishman et al. 1996). Adjuvant RT is generally based on brachytherapy (BT) alone or in combination with EBRT.

The clinical target volume (CTV) includes gross tumor volume (GTV) (where present), lower common iliacs, external–internal iliacs and presacral nodes, parametria, and upper vaginal/paravaginal tissues. Extended filed RT includes para-aortic lymph nodes (https://www.nccn.org/professionals/physician_gls/f_guidelines.asp).

Magnetic Resonance Imaging

MRI is the imaging modality of choice to localize and assess tumor extension (myometrial invasion, cervical invasion) and adjacent organ involvement due to its superior spatial and contrast resolution (Fennell et al. 2016). This is particularly important in patients unfit for surgery and therefore undergoing definitive RT.

Positron Emission Tomography/Computed Tomography (PET/CT)

As previously reported above in the section of staging with PET/CT, [^{18}F]FDG-PET/CT has an important role in the detection of pelvic and para-aortic lymph nodes. This information is important especially in the case of definitive RT because of the possibility to boost the dose to positive nodes. However, Simcock et al. reported interesting results even in resected patients who are candidates to adjuvant RT while showing that [^{18}F]FDG-PET/CT can change treatment decision also in this setting. A total of 73 patients with either high-risk disease after hysterectomy or with recurrent disease were included. [^{18}F]FDG-PET/CT found residual disease in 35% of post-operative patients, changing the planned treatment in 31% of them. In the group with known recurrence, additional disease compared to standard imaging was found in 72% of cases, changing therapeutic management in 36% (Simcock et al. 2015).

2.2.3.2 Brachytherapy

Recently, a consensus from the American Brachytherapy Society recommended MRI to define the GTV, CTV, and the organs at risk for the treatment of medically inoperable endometrial cancer (Schwarz et al. 2015).

However, most of the published studies included patients who underwent CT- or MRI-based planning for BT treatment (Gill et al. 2014; Weitmann et al. 2005). Gill and coworkers reported the results of one of largest series including 38 patients with medically inoperable clinical Stage I endometrial adenocarcinoma who received definitive high-dose rate BT with or without EBRT. BT planning was based on MRI or CT. Dose was prescribed to the clinical target volume (CTV: entire uterus, cervix, and upper 1–2 cm of vagina). Median dose of BT alone was 37.5 Gy in 5–6 fractions. For combined therapy, median EBRT and BT doses were 45 and 25 Gy (in 4–5 fractions), respectively. Two-year actuarial local control and overall survival were 90.6% and 94.4%. No Grade 2–5 late toxicities were recorded (Gill et al. 2014).

2.3 Vulvar and Vaginal Cancer

Abstract

Vulvar cancer represents only 3–5% of gynecological cancers. The dissemination is mainly lymphatic, with prevalent involvement of inguinal nodes, while hematogenous spread is rare.

[18F]FDG PET/CT gives promising results in the assessment of nodal status.

The role of CT in the local staging of vulvar tumor is marginal and is confined in locally advanced lesion. Instead of MRI, it permits an accurate local staging of vulvar cancer. Radiotherapy has a major role in curative treatment of vulvar cancer patients in both postoperative and radical setting.

MRI imaging has a higher soft-tissue contrast as compared to CT and has a paramount role in the local staging of vaginal tumors because it demonstrates the size and the location of the lesion, its extension to the parametria, and the involvement of the pelvic sidewall; moreover, it shows the involvement of other surrounding organs as the bladder or urethra, rectum, and lymph nodes. Organ-sparing surgery usually is difficult due to the proximity of rectum, bladder, and urethra. External beam radiotherapy and brachytherapy with or without chemotherapy are the most used primary treatments.

2.3.1 Staging with PET/CT

Vulvar cancer is relatively rare since it represents only 3–5% of gynecological cancers and less than 1% of all cancers in women (Siegel et al. 2013). The dissemination is mainly lymphatic, with prevalent involvement of inguinal nodes, while hematogenous spread is rare (Van der Steen et al. 2010).

Lymph-node status, the size of the primary tumor, and stromal invasion of the primary tumor are the main risk factors in this pathological condition (Van der Steen et al. 2010). As well as in other gynecological malignancies, the knowledge of nodal status may provide useful prognostic and clinical information to clinicians: overall survival rate at five years in early stages is 90%, while in patients with nodal involvement, it drops down to 50% (Howlader et al. n.d.).

For this purpose, sentinel node biopsy it is suggested, and it has been extensively used in this condition with excellent results (Oonk et al. 2017). Considering the low incidence of vulvar cancer, there are few data on the utility of imaging such as CT, MR, or PET in the staging of these patients.

[18F]FDG PET/CT gave promising results in the assessment of nodal status. Collarino et al. (2017) studied with [18F]FDG PET/CT 33 patients with vulvar cancer at presentation and 56 inguinal regions. [18F]FDG PET/CT showed on a groin-by-groin basis a sensitivity of 95.2% and a specificity of 75%, NPV of 96.4%, PPV of 69%, and accuracy of 82.5%.

Robertson et al. (2016) studied the clinical impact of [18F]FDG PET/CT in a population of 54 patients with vulvar cancer and 29 patients with vaginal cancer. [18F]FDG-PET/CT detected nodes suspicious for metastases on 29/83 (35%) patients. Distant metastases were identified in 10 patients. All suspicious lesions seen on CT were positively identified on PET/CT. According to [^{18}F]FDG-PET/CT, prognosis changed in 51% of cases, and a major change in the clinical management has been performed in 36% of the patients. Authors concluded that [^{18}F]FDG-PET/CT may play a significant role in the management of vaginal and vulvar cancer.

2.3.2 Staging with CT or MRI

MR imaging has a higher soft-tissue contrast as compared to CT and has a paramount role in the local staging of vaginal tumors because it demonstrates the size and the location of the lesion, its extension to the parametria, and the involvement of the pelvic sidewall; moreover, it shows the involvement of other surrounding organs as the bladder or urethra, rectum, and lymph nodes. Finally, MR imaging is useful for the evaluation of pelvic anatomy for surgical and RT planning (Chang 2002).

At MRI, primary vaginal squamous cell carcinoma may appear in the majority of cases as an irregular, diffuse mass. However, it may appear also as a well-defined lobulated mass or as a circumferential vaginal thickening. At T1wi, squamous cell carcinoma appears as isointense to muscle and can be evaluated only in case of large lesions. T1wi sequences are mostly used for the assessment of tissue enhancement after contrast media administration since the vagina shows a uniform intermediate signal intensity on T1wi, making the anatomic definition inadequate with these sequences (Walker et al. 2011).

High-resolution T2wi is used to accurately assess the location and the extension of the lesion as squamous cell tumor shows a homogeneous intermediate signal intensity well separated from the low signal intensity of the vaginal wall (Parikh et al. 2008). The presence of high signal intensity foci within the tumor may be due to tumoral necrosis and then demonstrating the presence of a poorly differentiated squamous cell carcinoma (Randall et al. 1986). In this situation should be considered an adeno-squamous carcinoma, mucinous adenocarcinoma, or metastases originating from the cervix or uterus (Fetissof et al. 1990).

On T2wi, Stage I tumors appear as plaque of tissue of intermediate signal intensity that expands and fills the vagina without any sign of involvement of the vaginal wall that has a normal low intensity signal as descripted above. On the contrary, in Stage II lesions, the low intensity signal of the outer vaginal muscularis layer is lost, indicating the extension to the paravaginal tissues (Parikh et al. 2008).

In Stage III, the tumor extends laterally to the pelvic sidewall, which is best seen on T2wi. The intermediate signal intensity of the tumor invades through the low signal intensity of the sidewall muscle and pelvic floor (Hricak et al. 1991).

Stage IVA is better evaluated on T2wi with the tumor that invades through the low signal intensity of the bladder or rectal wall. Moreover, the loss of the vesicovaginal fat plane or the rectovaginal septum is seen (Tsuda et al. 1999).

The assessment of distant and nodal metastases is well evaluated with either MRI or CT (Parikh et al. 2008). The role of CT in the local staging of vulvar tumor is marginal and is confined in locally advanced lesion in the assessment of the invasion of organ such as the bladder and rectum or in the assessment of groin, pelvic, and extrapelvic lymph-node metastases in case of tumors >2 cm (Fuh and Berek 2012). In case of small primary lesion, the tumor may appear on CT as an area of vulvar thickening or vulvar mass (Viswanathan et al. 2013). Differently from CT, MRI permits an accurate local staging of vulvar cancer.

To better evaluate the vaginal wall and its involvement from vulvar tumors, the vagina may be distended using ultrasound gel. The distension of the vagina also permits the visualization of small vulvar lesions and their local extension (Viswanathan et al. 2013). Vulvar tumors are generally isointense to muscle on T1wi, show intermediate to high signal intensity on T2wi, and have an early enhancement after contrast administration. The use of T2wi with fat suppression permits a better evaluation of the tumor because of its signal intensity characteristics (Griffin et al. 2008). Gross tumor with internal necrosis can demonstrate high signal intensity on T2wi. The involvement of surrounding organs, such as the vagina, anus, and rectum, may appear as an intermediate signal soft-tissue mass and will show intense enhancement on dynamic sequences (Viswanathan et al. 2013).

2.3.3 Target Volume Definition by Imaging

2.3.3.1 Vulvar Cancer

Vulvar cancer is a relatively uncommon neoplasm, responsible for 5% of gynecologic malignancies (Howlader et al. n.d.). RT has a major role in curative treatment of vulvar cancer patients in both postoperative and radical setting (https://www.nccn.org/professionals/physician_gls/f_guidelines.asp).

Recently, a consensus guideline on vulvar cancer target contouring has been published (Gaffney et al. 2016). According to the involvement of surrounding organs, the CTV includes the GTV plus a 2–3 cm margin or whole organ and pelvic nodes. More in details, the consensus guidelines recommended that if the primary vulvar lesion involves the vagina, then the GTV plus 3 cm margin should be included in the CTV. If there is any uncertainty as to the proximal extent of the vaginal extension, the entire vaginal length should be included in the CTV. If the primary vulvar lesion involves the anus, anal canal, or bladder, the GTV plus at least 2 cm of anorectum or bladder is included in the CTV. If the primary vulvar lesion is in periurethral position, the GTV plus at least 2 cm of urethra is included in the CTV. If the disease extends into the mid- or proximal urethra, the entire urethra and bladder neck should be included in the CTV. For clitoral lesions, GTV plus at least 2 cm is included in the CTV, and in many cases, the CTV should cover the suspensory ligament of the clitoris which extends to the pubic bone (Walker et al. 2011). The lymph nodes included are inguinal-femoral nodes, bilateral external iliac nodes, obturator, and internal iliac nodes.

Due to rarity of this disease, evidences on the impact of MRI in radiotherapy planning are lacking. However, MRI is the optimal imaging tool to evaluate local extent of disease which has an obvious impact in target definition. As previously reported in the staging section about [^{18}F]FDG-PET/CT, this imaging modality shows high sensitivity in positive node detection, with potential impact in modifying treatment strategy and radiation fields.

2.3.3.2 Vaginal Cancer

Vaginal cancer is very uncommon. Organ-sparing surgery usually is difficult due to proximity of the rectum, bladder, and urethra. EBRT and BT with or without chemotherapy are the most used primary treatments. Due to rarity of this tumor, no randomized trial is available, and therefore current guidelines are extrapolated from retrospective studies (Chyle et al. 1996; Frank et al. 2005).

The EBRT CTV includes the GTV with 1–2 cm expansion, the entire vagina, paravaginal area up to the pelvic sidewalls, and bilateral pelvic lymph nodes. The included nodes are common iliac, external iliac, internal iliac, obturator, and presacral lymph nodes. In case of involvement of the distal one-third of the vagina, the inguinal lymph nodes should also be included (Beriwal et al. 2012).

Being [^{18}F]FDG-PET/CT more sensitive in positive nodes detection, compared to CT, in all gynecological cancers (Lee et al. 2015), also in patients with vaginal cancer [^{18}F]FDG-PET/CT might change the radiation fields by extending them to adjacent areas or by delivering a boost to positive lymph nodes.

MRI is more sensitive compared to CT scan in defining tumor site and local extensions (Parikh et al. 2008). Particularly, MRI play an important role in selecting patients with vaginal cancer candidate for BT. According to the American Brachytherapy Society guidelines for vaginal cancer, superficial lesions ($\leq$0.5 cm thick at the time of BT) may be treated with intracavitary BT. Deeper lesion should be treated with or also with interstitial BT (Beriwal et al. 2012).

3 Urological Malignancies

3.1 Bladder Cancer

Abstract

Bladder cancer is the most frequent neoplasm in the urinary tract. The role of PET/CT in tumor or nodal staging of bladder cancer probably deserves further investigations to better understand if there is a real added value of this method over standard cross-sectional imaging. CT scan is the most common imaging technique used to detect bladder lesion and to stage bladder tumor once the initial diagnosis is performed. CT urography, that is useful to assess both the upper urinary tract and the bladder, shows a sensitivity and specificity of 90% or more for the diagnosis of bladder cancer in patients with hematuria. The role of CT in terms of local staging is confined to the assessment of tumors that macroscopically infiltrate the perivisceral fat or that invade the surrounding organs. MRI shows a high soft-tissue contrast resolution that permits to differentiate the bladder wall layers, which potentially allow for a more accurate local tumor staging and the differentiation between muscle-invasive and non-muscle-invasive disease.

Organ preservation therapy based on radiotherapy or radiochemotherapy represents an alternative treatment in patients unfit for surgery. Recently, organ preservation with trimodality strategy including maximal transurethral resection of the tumor and chemoradiation can be offered also to patients fit for surgery with outcomes similar to those of radical surgery. MRI is the most appropriate imaging tool to define tumor extension and to better delineate the target for boost irradiation.

3.1.1 Staging with PET/CT

Bladder carcinoma (BC) is the most frequent type of cancer of the urinary tract. Leading symptom is the painless hematuria (Witjes et al. 2014). Urothelial (transitional cell) carcinoma is the most frequent type of bladder cancer representing more than 90%. Much less frequent are squamous cell carcinomas and adenocarcinoma (Kaufman et al. 2009). Unfortunately, about 30% of patients have muscle invasion at presentation, and this condition has a high rate of early systemic dissemination. Main sites of dissemination are the liver, lung, bone, and adrenal glands (Witjes et al. 2014). First diagnosis is based on cystoscopy and subsequent biopsy. If no metastatic spread is detected by imaging, muscle-invasive bladder-confined cancer is treated with radical cystectomy with pelvic lymph node dissection (PLND). Systemic therapy is based on cisplatin-based combination chemotherapy (Witjes et al. 2014). Cross-sectional imaging (CT and MRI) are widely used for imaging primary BC. The role of [^{18}F]FDG PET/CT in the detection of localized BC is limited because the bladder is usually filled with radioactive urine, masking the presence of primary tumor. Early or late images, catheterization or bladder irrigation, are some of the methods that have been used to overcome this problem (Bouchelouche et al. 2012). Finally, other tracers showing low or absent urinary excretion have been proposed such as ^{11}C-choline (Ceci et al. 2015).

3.1.1.1 [^{18}F]FDG-PET/CT

In a meta-analysis (Wang et al. 2014) that evaluated six studies, the pooled sensitivity and specificity for [^{18}F]FDG PET/CT in the detection of primary tumor was 80.0% and 84.0%. Apolo et al. (Apolo et al. 2010) showed a better accuracy of [^{18}F]FDG PET/CT in comparison with CT/MRI for the assessment of lymph node (LN). In this population, [^{18}F]FDG PET/CT changed the clinical management in up to 68% of the patients. Jensen et al. (2011) compared [^{18}F]FDG PET CT versus CT and MRI for lymph-node staging in 48 patients studied before surgery. Authors did not find any advantage for combined [^{18}F]FDG PET/CT over CT alone for LN staging. Whereas, [^{18}F]FDG PET/CT showed an advantage over MRI. Finally, Ceci et al. (2015) studied with ^{11}C-choline 39 patients for preoperative lymph-node evaluation before radical cystectomy and extended pelvic LN dissection. ^{11}C-choline PET/CT showed a sensitivity, specificity, positive predictive value, negative predictive value, and accuracy of 59%, 90%, 71%, 84%, and 81%, respectively. In conclusion, the clinical role of PET/CT in T- or N-staging of bladder cancer probably deserves further investigations to better understand if there is a real added value of this method over standard cross-sectional imaging.

3.1.2 Staging with CT or MRI

CT scan is the most common imaging technique used to detect bladder lesion (e.g., in case of hematuria) and to stage bladder tumor once the initial diagnosis is performed (Lee et al. 2017). CT urography, that is useful to assess both the upper urinary tract and the bladder, shows a sensitivity and specificity of 90% or more for the diagnosis of bladder cancer in patients with hematuria (Caterino et al. 2001).

In the staging of bladder cancer is of paramount importance the assessment of the upper urinary tract since 2% of these patients have a synchronous upper tract tumor, but the incidence increases to 7.5% in tumors located in the trigone (Brown et al. 2005; Palou et al. 2005; Babjuk et al. 2017). Moreover, during follow-up, metachronous tumor in the upper tract is detected in 3.9% of such patients, and the risk of developing metachronous lesions tend to increase in patients with multiple and high-risk tumors (Lee et al. 2017; Babjuk et al. 2017; Yousem et al. 1988; Millán-Rodríguez et al. 2000). Furthermore, it is essential the assessment of the presence of potential hydronephrosis since it may have an influence on the treatment strategies and is also considered a poor prognostic factor (Bartsch et al. 2007; Bostrom et al. 2010).

CT urography is generally performed with images acquired before and after the administration of intravenous iodinated contrast material, sometimes using a split bolus technique that allows the acquisition of the urothelial (nephrographic) and pyelographic (excretory) phases together. However, the urothelial and pyelographic phases may be obtained also separately with sequential acquisition for a better evaluation of early enhancing lesions in the urothelial phase and assess the presence of filling defects within the ureters or the bladder filled with contrast material in the pyelographic phase (Lee et al. 2017; Kim et al. 2004).

The role of CT in terms of local staging is confined to the assessment of tumors that macroscopically infiltrates the perivisceral fat or that invades the surrounding organs (i.e., T3b or T4). In fact, T3a tumors that indicate lesions that microscopically infiltrates perivisceral fat cannot be evaluated with CT (Verma et al. 2012; Alfred Witjes et al. 2017; Vikram et al. 2009; Panebianco et al. 2010; Tsampoulas et al. 2008; Tekes et al. 2005; Liedberg et al. 2013; Malayeri et al. 2015). Moreover, the assessment of local invasion of adjacent organs may be difficult because the correct evaluation of anatomic planes is not always possible, as well as for the presence of tissue reactions after TURB makes challenging the evaluation for any possible residual cancer (Bostrom et al. 2010; Malayeri et al. 2015).

The intravesical instillation of negative contrast agents such as air or carbon dioxide has been used to perform virtual cystoscopy. In small series virtual cystoscopy showed a sensitivity higher than 90% in the detection of bladder cancer, permitting a more accurate evaluation of local staging also in T1 tumors (Caterino et al. 2001; Panebianco et al. 2010; Tsampoulas et al. 2008). However, this procedure is not routinely performed because of the invasiveness of the procedure and the fact that conventional cystoscopy is still required to discover small lesions and to obtain tissue specimen (Verma et al. 2012).

Otherwise from CT, MRI shows a high soft-tissue contrast resolution that permits to differentiate the bladder wall layers, that potentially allows for a more accurate local tumor staging and the differentiation between muscle-invasive and non-muscle-invasive disease (Lee et al. 2017; Tekes et al. 2005).

The use of multiparametric MRI, that uses both conventional and functional sequences is currently the most useful approach to assess the local staging of bladder cancer. On T1wi, the urine shows low signal intensity, while the bladder wall and the perivesical fat show intermediate signal intensity and high signal intensity, respectively. On T2wi, the bladder wall shows low signal intensity, while the urine is hyperintense. The detrusor muscle appears on T2wi as a hypointense linear structure; its interruption indicates a muscle invasive tumor while it is not interrupted in case of superficial or papillary tumors (Liedberg et al. 2013; Malayeri et al. 2015). The acquisition of images on three orthogonal planes permit a better evaluation of deep invasion based on the localization of the tumor; in fact, the use of coronal plane is useful when the lesion is located on the lateral bladder wall or the dome while the sagittal plane is better for tumor localized on the anteroposterior bladder wall or the dome (Verma et al. 2012; Tekes et al. 2005).

The presence of a nodule of intermediate signal intensity similar to that of tumor on T2wi into the hyperintense perivisceral fat is a sign of extravesical extension, while an enlargement of the surrounding organ showing the same intensity of the tumor is a sign of an invading lesion. However, the assessment of microscopic extravesical disease (T3a) is mostly not possible with MRI and CT (Lee et al. 2017; Malayeri et al. 2015). Nevertheless, similar to CT, potential pitfalls of extravesical evaluation with MRI are the post-TURB alteration and the inflammatory reaction due to the tumor itself mimicking an extension of the tumor to the perivesical fat (Tekes et al. 2005).

The main question in the local staging of bladder cancer is whether it is possible to distinguish non-muscle-invasive cancer from muscle-invasive cancer (stage T2 or more) as this issue has an implication in the treatment approach.

The use of conventional MRI sequences however shows an accuracy for staging bladder cancer of around 15% in T1 and T2 lesions (El-Assmy et al. 2009). The rationale of using DCE and DWI MRI sequences is to increase the accuracy of local staging of bladder lesion, mainly to assess T1 and T2 lesions (Lee et al. 2017). T1wi sequences are acquired before and after gadolinium-based contrast material administration. In the early phase (20 s after injection), the tumor, the mucosa, and submucosa enhance more than the bladder muscle layer that remains hypointense, and this may help to differentiate T1 from T2 lesion. On the delayed phase (after 5 min), the contrast within the bladder may help to delineate the intraluminal contour of the lesion. The reported accuracy of DCE imaging in differentiating muscle-invasive from non-muscle-invasive lesion ranged from 84 to 87% in several studies (Lee et al. 2017; El-Assmy et al. 2009; Watanabe et al. 2009).

Differently from DCE, DWI is obtained without exogenous contrast material injection and reflects the facilitation or the restrictions of water movements within a tissue (i.e., water diffusivity), a characteristic that is influenced by interactions of water with cell structures and molecules.

It has been reported that DWI may improve MRI accuracy in staging bladder tumor. In fact, the use of DWI is useful in the identification of small lesion not visible with other MRI sequences, and it is also helpful in case of suspicion of muscle invasion or extravesical extension on T2wi (Lee et al. 2017). In particular, DWI can improve the differentiation between the tumor and the different bladder wall layers including the detrusor layer and the submucosa that show different intensities at DWI (Verma et al. 2012).

The combination of T2wi, DCE, and DWI could achieve an accuracy of more than 90% in differentiating T1 and T2 or higher-stage disease (Verma et al. 2012; Takeuchi et al. 2009). Recently, Panebianco et al. used diffusion tensor imaging (DTI), an MRI technique based on water diffusivity, in case of inconclusive DWI in the assessment of invasion of the muscle layer, reaching an overall accuracy of 94% in differentiating NMIBC from MIBC (Panebianco et al. 2017).

3.1.3 Target Volume Definition by Imaging

3.1.3.1 External Beam Radiotherapy

Target Volume

Bladder cancer is the most frequent neoplasm in the urinary tract. In early-stage Ta, Tis and T1 RT are not recommended. However, organ preservation therapy based on RT or radiochemotherapy represents an alternative treatment in patients unfit for surgery with results comparable to the ones of surgery (Booth et al. 2014). Recently, organ preservation with trimodality strategy including maximal transurethral resection of the tumor and chemoradiation can be offered also to patients fit for surgery with outcomes similar to those of radical surgery (https://www.nccn.org/professionals/physician_gls/f_guidelines.asp).

The recommended dose to the whole bladder (with or without prophylactic nodal irradiation) is 39.6–50.4 Gy. The delivery of prophylactic nodal RT (presacral nodes, bilateral distal common iliac, external iliac, internal iliac, and obturator nodes) should be based on patient comorbidities and risk of toxicities (Baumann et al. 2016). A boost to the primary tumor or to the whole bladder up to 60–66 Gy and to positive pelvic lymph nodes up to 54–66 Gy is recommended (Lee et al. 2017).

Magnetic Resonance Imaging (MRI)

MRI is the most promising imaging modality to define tumor site, extension, and adjacent organ involvement due to its superior spatial and contrast resolution. Whalley and coworkers evaluated the feasibility of image-guided IMRT with accelerated hypofractionation based on simultaneously integrated boost. A total of 20 patients with Stage II or III disease and 8 patients with Stage IV were included. The volumes of interest delineation were performed using MRI with the aid of a radiologist. GTV was defined as the anatomical area of the bladder at highest risk of gross residual disease. The intermediate risk CTV was defined as the whole bladder (expanded by 10 mm to define the intermediate risk PTV), and the GTV was expanded by 0.5 cm to define the high-risk PTV. If treated, the uninvolved obturator and internal and external iliac nodes were contoured as a separate low-risk CTV and then expanded by a 1 cm margin to define the low-risk PTV. Macroscopic disease received 66 Gy in 30 fractions in 11 patients or 55 Gy in 20 fractions in patients with worse performance status or treated with palliative intent. Ten patients received concurrent chemotherapy. Grade ≥2 acute toxicity rate was 21% in genitourinary (GU) and gastrointestinal (GI) toxicity. Five patients (18%) developed late GU toxicity, and no patient showed ≥2 late GI toxicity. Nineteen patients underwent cystoscopy 6 weeks after RT, with complete response in 86% of patients including all patients treated with chemoradiation. In patients treated with curative aim, local–regional control and overall survival were 90 and 100% in the chemoradiation group versus 86 and 69% in the RT alone group (Whalley et al. 2015).

Positron Emission Tomography/Computed Tomography (PET/CT)

As reported in the [^{18}F]FDG-PET/CT section, the clinical role of this imaging modality in T- and N-staging of bladder cancer needs further investigations to detect an added value over standard cross-sectional imaging. To our knowledge, no studies directly investigated the impact of [^{18}F]FDG-PET/CT in RT planning in patients with bladder cancer. However, in case of positive lymph nodes at [^{18}F]FDG-PET/CT, this information could improve target definition.

3.1.3.2 Conclusions

MRI is the most appropriate imaging tool to define tumor extension and to better delineate the target for boost irradiation. The role of [^{18}F]FDG-PET/CT in radiotherapy planning needs to be investigated.

References

Addley HC, Vargas HA, Moyle PL, Crawford R, Sala E (2010) Pelvic imaging following chemotherapy and radiation therapy for gynecologic malignancies. Radiographics 30:1843–1856

Afshar-Oromieh A, Malcher A, Eder M, Eisenhut M, Linhart HG, Hadaschik BA et al (2013) PET imaging with a [68Ga]gallium-labelled PSMA ligand for the diagnosis of prostate cancer: biodistribution in humans and first evaluation of tumour lesions. Eur J Nucl Med Mol Imaging 40:486–495. https://doi.org/10.1007/s00259-012-2298-2

Albers P, Albrecht W, Algaba F, Bokemeyer C, Cohn-Cedermark G, Fizazi K et al (2012) EAU Guidelines on testicular cancer. Update 2011. European Association of Urology. Actas Urol Esp 36:127–145

Alfred Witjes J, Lebret T, Compérat EM, Cowan NC, De Santis M, Bruins HM et al (2017) Updated 2016 EAU guidelines on muscle-invasive and metastatic bladder cancer. Eur Urol 71:462–475

Aluwini S, van Rooij P, Hoogeman M, Kirkels W, Kolkman-Deurloo IK, Bangma C (2013) Stereotactic body radiotherapy with a focal boost to the MRI—visible tumor as monotherapy for low- and intermediate-risk prostate cancer: early results. Radiat Oncol. https://doi.org/10.1186/1748-717X-8-84

Amant F, Moerman P, Neven P, Timmerman D, Van Limbergen E, Vergote I (2005) Endometrial cancer. Lancet 366:491–505

Amant F, Moerman P, Neven P, Timmerman D, Van Limbergen E, Vergote I (2007) Treatment modalities in endometrial cancer. Curr Opin Oncol 19:479–485

Ambrosini V, Zucchini G, Nicolini S, Berselli A, Nanni C, Allegri V et al (2014) 18F-FDG PET/CT impact on testicular tumours clinical management. Eur J Nucl Med Mol Imaging 41:668

Apolo AB, Riches J, Schoder H, Akin O, Trout A, Milowsky MI et al (2010) Clinical value of fluorine-18

2-fluoro-2-deoxy-D-glucose positron emission tomography/computed tomography in bladder cancer. J Clin Oncol 28:3973–3978

Arbyn M, Castellsagué X, de Sanjosé S, Bruni L, Saraiya M, Bray F et al (2011) Worldwide burden of cervical cancer in 2008. Ann Oncol 22:2675–2686

Atri M, Zhang Z, Dehdashti F, Lee SI, Marques H, Ali S et al (2017) Utility of PET/CT to evaluate retroperitoneal lymph node metastasis in high-risk endometrial cancer: results of ACRIN 6671/GOG 0233 trial. Radiology 283(2):450–459. https://doi.org/10.1148/radiol.2016160200

Babjuk M, Böhle A, Burger M, Capoun O, Cohen D, Compérat EM et al (2017) EAU Guidelines on non–muscle-invasive urothelial carcinoma of the bladder: update 2016. Eur Urol 71:447–461

Balleyguier C, Sala E, Da Cunha T, Bergman A, Brkljacic B, Danza F et al (2011) Staging of uterine cervical cancer with MRI: guidelines of the European Society of Urogenital Radiology. Eur Radiol 21:1102–1110

Bartsch GC, Kuefer R, Gschwend JE, de Petriconi R, Hautmann RE, Volkmer BG (2007) Hydronephrosis as a prognostic marker in bladder cancer in a cystectomy-only series. Eur Urol 51:690–698

Baumann BC, Bosch WR, Bahl A, Birtle AJ, Breau RH, Challapalli A et al (2016) Development and validation of consensus contouring guidelines for adjuvant radiation therapy for bladder cancer after radical cystectomy. Int J Radiat Oncol Biol Phys 96:78–86

Beddy P, Rangarajan RD, Sala E (2011) Role of MRI in intracavitary brachytherapy for cervical cancer: what the radiologist needs to know. AJR Am J Roentgenol 196:341–347

Beddy P, Moyle P, Kataoka M, Yamamoto AK, Joubert I, Lomas D et al (2012) Evaluation of depth of myometrial invasion and overall staging in endometrial cancer: comparison of diffusion-weighted and dynamic contrast-enhanced MR imaging. Radiology 262:530–537

Beriwal S, Demanes DJ, Erickson B, Jones E, De Los Santos JF, Cormack RA et al (2012) American Brachytherapy Society consensus guidelines for interstitial brachytherapy for vaginal cancer. Brachytherapy 11:68–75

Beyersdorff D, Taymoonan K, Knösel T, Schnorr D, Felix R, Hamm B et al (2005) MRI of prostate cancer at 1.5 and 3.0 T: comparison of image quality in tumor detection and staging. AJR 185:1214–1220

Bluemel C, Linke F, Herrmann K, Simunovic I, Eiber M, Kestler C et al (2016) Impact of 68Ga-PSMA PET/CT on salvage radiotherapy planning in patients with prostate cancer and persisting PSA values or biochemical relapse after prostatectomy. EJNMMI Res 6(1):78–85

Boccon-Gibod L, Bertaccini A, Bono AV, Dev Sarmah B, Höltl W, Mottet N et al (2003) Management of locally advanced prostate cancer: a European consensus. Int J Clin Pract 57:187–194

Bollineni VR, Ytre-Hauge S, Bollineni-Balabay O, Salvesen HB, Haldorsen IS (2016) high diagnostic value of 18f-fdg pet/ct in endometrial cancer: systematic review and meta-analysis of the literature. J Nucl Med 57(6):879–885. https://doi.org/10.2967/jnumed.115.170597

Boonsirikamchai P, Choi S, Frank SJ, Ma J, Elsayes KM, Kaur H et al (2013) MR imaging of prostate cancer in radiation oncology: what radiologists need to know. Radiographics 33:741–761

Booth CM, Siemens DR, Li G, Peng Y, Kong W, Berman DM et al (2014) Curative therapy for bladder cancer in routine clinical practice: a population-based outcomes study. Clin Oncol 26(8):506–514

Bostrom PJ, Van Rhijn BWG, Fleshner N, Fleshner N, Finelli A, Jewett M et al (2010) Staging and staging errors in bladder cancer. European Urology Supplements 9:2–9

Bouchelouche K, Turkbey B, Choyke PL (2012) PET/CT and MRI in bladder cancer. J Cancer Sci Ther Suppl 14:1–18. https://doi.org/10.4172/1948-5956.S14-001

Briganti A, Larcher A, Abdollah F, Capitanio U, Gallina A, Suardi N et al (2012) Updated nomogram predicting lymph node invasion in patients with prostate cancer undergoing extended pelvic lymph node dissection: the essential importance of percentage of positive cores. Eur Urol 61:480–487

Brown RF, Meehan CP, Colville J, Power R, Torreggiani WC (2005) Transitional cell carcinoma of the upper urinary tract: spectrum of imaging findings. Radiographics 25:1609–1627

Caivano R, Cirillo P, Balestra A, Lotumolo A, Fortunato G, Macarini L et al (2012) Prostate cancer in magnetic resonance imaging: diagnostic utilities of spectroscopic sequences. J Med Imaging Radiat Oncol 56:606–616

Casamassima F, Masi L, Menichelli C, Bonucci I, Casamassima E, Lazzeri M et al (2011) Efficacy of eradicative radiotherapy for limited nodal metastases detected with choline PET scan in prostate cancer patients. Tumori 97:49–55

Castellucci P, Ceci F, Graziani T, Schiavina R, Brunocilla E, Mazzarotto R et al (2014) Early biochemical relapse after radical prostatectomy: which prostate cancer patients may benefit from a restaging 11C-choline PET/CT scan before salvage radiation therapy? J Nucl Med 55:1424–1429

Castellucci P, Ceci F, Fanti S (2017) Imaging of prostate cancer using ^{11}C-choline PET/computed tomography. PET Clin 12:137–143. https://doi.org/10.1016/j.cpet.2016.11.002

Caterino M, Giunta S, Finocchi V, Giglio L, Mainiero G, Carpanese L et al (2001) Primary cancer of the urinary bladder: CT evaluation of the T parameter with different techniques. Abdom Imaging 26:433–438

Ceci F, Bianchi L, Graziani T, Castellucci P, Pultrone C, Eugenio B et al (2015) 11C-choline PET/CT and bladder cancer: lymph node metastasis assessment with pathological specimens as reference standard. Clin Nucl Med 40(2):124–128. https://doi.org/10.1097/RLU.0000000000000604

Chang SD (2002) Imaging of the vagina. Radiol Clin North Am 40:637–658

Chang MC, Chen JH, Liang JA, Yang KT, Cheng KY, Kao CH (2012) 18F-FDG PET or PET/CT for detection of metastatic lymph nodes in patients with endometrial cancer: a systematic review and meta-analysis. Eur J Radiol 81(11):3511–3517. https://doi.org/10.1016/j.ejrad.2012.01.024.

Chao A, Ho K, Wang CC, Cheng HH, Lin G, Yen TC et al (2008) Positron emission tomography in evaluating the feasibility of curative intent in cervical cancer patients with limited distant lymph node metastases. Gynecol Oncol 110:172–178

Cheng X, Cai S, Li Z, Tang M, Xue M, Zang R (2004) The prognosis of women with stage IB1-IIB node-positive cervical carcinoma after radical surgery. World J Surg Oncol 2:47

Chyle V, Zagars GK, Wheeler JA, Wharton JT, Delclos L (1996) Definite radiotherapy for carcinoma of the vagina: Outcome and prognostic factors. Int J Radiat Oncol Biol Phys 35:891–895

Collarino A, Garganese G, Valdés Olmos RA, Stefanelli A, Perotti G et al (2017) Evaluation of dual time point imaging ^{18}F-FDG PET/CT for lymph node staging in vulvar cancer. J Nucl Med. https://doi.org/10.2967/jnumed.117.194332

Crook JM, Haie-Meder C, Demanes DJ, Mazeron JJ, Martinez AA, Rivard MJ (2013) American Brachytherapy Society-Groupe Européen de Curiethérapie-European Society of Therapeutic Radiation Oncology (ABS-GEC-ESTRO) consensus statement for penile brachytherapy. Brachytherapy 12(3):191–198. https://doi.org/10.1016/j.brachy.2013.01.167

D'Amico AV, Cormack R, Tempany CM, Kumar S, Topulos G, Kooy HM et al (1998) Real-time magnetic resonance image-guided interstitial brachytherapy in the treatment of select patients with clinically localized prostate cancer. Int J Radiat Oncol Biol Phys 42(3):507–515

De Rooij M, Hamoen EH, Witjes JA, Barentsz JO, Rovers MM (2016) Accuracy of magnetic resonance imaging for local staging of prostate cancer: a diagnostic meta-analysis. Eur Urol 70:233–245

Debois M, Oyen R, Maes F, Verswijvel G, Gatti G, Bosmans H et al (1999) The contribution of magnetic resonance imaging to the three-dimensional treatment planning of localized prostate cancer. Int J Radiat Oncol Biol Phys 45:857–865

Delongchamps NB, Rouanne M, Flam T, Beuvon F, Liberatore M, Zerbib M et al (2011) Multiparametric magnetic resonance imaging for the detection and localization of prostate cancer: combination of T2-weighted, dynamic contrast-enhanced and diffusion-weighted imaging. BJU Int 107:1411–1418

Dewes S, Schiller K, Sauter K, Eiber M, Maurer T, Schwaiger M et al (2016) Integration of (68) Ga-PSMA-PET imaging in planning of primary definitive radiotherapy in prostate cancer: a retrospective study. Radiat Oncol 11:73–80

Eiber M, Weirich G, Holzapfel K, Souvatzoglou M, Haller B, Rauscher I et al (2016) Simultaneous (68) Ga-PSMA HBED-CC PET/MRI improves the localization of primary prostate cancer. EurUrol 70:829–836. https://doi.org/10.1016/j.eururo.2015.12.053

El-Assmy A, Abou-El-Ghar ME, Mosbah A, El-Nahas AR, Refaie HF, Hekal IA et al (2009) Bladder tumor staging: comparison of diffusion- and T2-weighted MR imaging. Eur Radiol 19:1575–1581

Evangelista L, Guttilla A, Zattoni F, Muzzio PC, Zattoni F (2013) Utility of choline positron emission tomography/computed tomography for lymph node involvement identification in intermediate- to high-risk prostate cancer: a systematic literature review and meta-analysis. Eur Urol 63:1040–1048

Faria SC, Sagebiel T, Devine C, Lal C, Balachandran A, Bhosale P (2015) Imaging in endometrial carcinoma. Indian J Radiol Imaging 25:137–147

Farsad M, Schiavina R, Castellucci P, Nanni C, Corti B, Martorana G et al (2005) Detection and localization of prostate cancer: correlation of (11)C-choline PET/CT with histopathologic step-section analysis. J Nucl Med 46:1642–1649

Farsad M, Schwarzenbock S, Krause BJPET (2012) CT and choline: diagnosis and staging. Q J Nucl Med Mol Imaging 56(4):343–353

Fendler WP, Schmidt DF, Wenter V, Thierfelder KM, Zach C, Stief C et al (2016) 68Ga-PSMA PET/CT detects the location and extent of primary prostate cancer. J Nucl Med 57:1720–1725

Fennell J, Scholb r J, Grosu AL, Volegova-Neher N, Henne K, Langer M et al (2016) MRI and FDG-PET/CT imaging in gynecological malignancies: the radiation oncology perspective. Q J Nucl Med Mol Imaging 60(2):117–123

Fetissof F, Haillot O, Lanson Y, Arbeille B, Lansac J (1990) Papillary tumour of the vagina resembling transitional cell carcinoma. Pathol Res Pract 186:358–364

Fishman DA, Roberts KB, Chambers JT, Kohorn EI, Schwartz PE, Chambers SK (1996) Radiation therapy as exclusive treatment for medically inoperable patients with stage I and II endometrioid carcinoma with endometrium. Gynecol Oncol 61:189–196

Frank SJ, Jhingran A, Levenback C, Eifel PJ (2005) Definitive radiation therapy for squamous cell carcinoma of the vagina. Int J Radiat Oncol Biol Phys 62:138–147

Freeman SJ, Aly AM, Kataoka MY et al (2012a) The revised FIGO staging system for uterine malignancies: implications for MR imaging. Radiographics 32:1805–1827

Freeman SJ, Aly AM, Kataoka MY, Addley HC, Reinhold C, Sala E (2012b) The revised FIGO staging system for uterine malignancies: implications for MR imaging. Radiographics 32:1805–1827

Fuh KC, Berek JS (2012) Current management of vulvar cancer. Hematol Oncol Clin North Am 26:45–62

Fütterer JJ, Heijmink SW, Scheenen TW, Veltman J, Huisman HJ, Vos P et al (2006a) Prostate cancer localization with dynamic contrast-enhanced MR imaging and proton MR spectroscopic imaging. Radiology 241:449–458

Fütterer JJ, Heijmink SW, Scheenen TW, Jager GJ, Hulsbergen-Van de Kaa CA, Witjes JA et al (2006b) Prostate cancer: local staging at 3-T endorectal MR imaging—early experience. Radiology 238:184–191

Gaffney DK, King B, Viswanathan AN, Barkati M, Beriwal S, Eifel P et al (2016) Consensus recommendations for radiation therapy contouring and treatment of vulvar carcinoma. Int J Radiat Oncol Biol Phys 95(4):1191–1100. https://doi.org/10.1016/j.ijrobp.2016.02.043

Gill BS, Kim H, Houser C, Olsen A, Kelley J, Edwards RP et al (2014) Image-based three-dimensional conformal brachytherapy for medically inoperable endometrial carcinoma. Brachytherapy 13:542–547

Giovacchini G, Picchio M, Coradeschi E, Scattoni V, Bettinardi V, Cozzarini C et al (2008) [(11)C]choline uptake with PET/CT for the initial diagnosis of prostate cancer: relation to PSA levels, tumour stage and anti-androgenic therapy. Eur J Nucl Med Mol Imaging 35:1065–1073

Gouy S, Morice P, Narducci F, Uzan C, Gilmore J, Kolesnikov-Gauthier H et al (2012) Nodal-staging surgery for locally advanced cervical cancer in the era of PET. Lancet Oncol 13:212–220

Griffin N, Grant LA, Sala E (2008) Magnetic resonance imaging of vaginal and vulval pathology. Eur Radiol 18:1269–1280

Grigsby PW (2008) The prognostic value of PET and PET/CT in cervical cancer. Cancer Imaging 8:146–155

Grueneisen J, Schaarschmidt BM, Heubner M, Aktas B, Kinner S, Forsting M et al (2015) Integrated PET/MRI for whole-body staging of patients with primary cervical cancer: preliminary results. Eur J Nucl Med Mol Imaging 42(12):1814–1824. https://doi.org/10.1007/s00259-015-3131-5

Haie-Meder C, Pötter R, Van Limbergen E, Briot E, De Brabandere M, Dimopoulos J et al (2005) Gynaecological (GYN) GEC-ESTRO Working Group. Recommendations from Gynaecological (GYN) GEC-ESTRO Working Group (I): concepts and terms in 3D image based 3D treatment planning in cervix cancer brachytherapy with emphasis on MRI assessment of GTV and CTV. Radiother Oncol 74(3):235–245

Hain SF, O'Doherty MJ, Timothy AR, Leslie MD, Partridge SE, Huddart RA (2000) Fluorodeoxyglucose PET in the initial staging of germ cell tumours. Eur J Nucl Med 27:590–594

Hakenberg OW, Compérat EM, Minhas S, Necchi A, Protzel C, Watkin N et al (2015) EAU guidelines on penile cancer: 2014 update. Eur Urol 67:142–150

Hambrock T, Somford DM, Huisman HJ, van Oort IM, Witjes JA, Hulsbergen-van de Kaa CA et al (2011) Relationship between apparent diffusion coefficients at 3.0-T MR imaging and Gleason grade in peripheral zone prostate cancer. Radiology 259:453–461

Havrilesky LJ, Kulasingam SL, Matchar DB, Myers ER (2005) FDG-PET for management of cervical and ovarian cancer. Gynecol Oncol 97:183–191

Hentschel B, Oehler W, Strauss D, Ulrich A, Malich A (2011) Definition of the CTV prostate in CT and MRI by using CT-MRI image fusion in IMRT planning for prostate cancer. Strahlenther Onkol 1187:183–190

Hövels AM, Heesakkers RA, Adang EM, Jager GJ, Strum S, Hoogeveen YL et al (2008) The diagnostic accuracy of CT and MRI in the staging of pelvic lymph nodes in patients with prostate cancer: a meta-analysis. Clin Radiol 63:387–395

Howlader N, Noone AM, Krapcho M et al (eds) (n.d.) SEER cancer statistics review, 1975–2011. National Cancer Institute, Bethesda, MD, http://seer.cancer.gov/statfacts/html/vulva.html, based on November 2013 SEER data submission, posted to the SEER web site, April 2014.

Hricak H, Secaf E, Buckley DW, Brown JJ, Tanagho EA, McAninch JW (1991) Female urethra: MR imaging. Radiology 178:527–535

Hricak H, Choyke PL, Eberhardt SC, Leibel SA, Scardino PT (2007) Imaging prostate cancer: a multidisciplinary perspective. Radiology 243:28–53

Huges Cassidy F, Ishioka KM, McMahon CJ, Chu P, Sakamoto K, Lee KS et al (2010) MR imaging of scrotal tumors and pseudotumors. Radiographics 30:665–683

Iwazawa J, Mitani T, Sassa S, Ohue S (2011) Prostate cancer detection with MRI: is dynamic contrast-enhanced imaging necessary in addition to diffusion-weighted imaging? Diagn Interv Radiol 17:243–248

Jadvar H (2013) Imaging evaluation of prostate cancer with 18F-fluorodeoxyglucose PET/CT: utility and limitations. Eur J Nucl Med Mol Imaging 40(Suppl 1):5–10

Jemal A, Siegel R, Ward E, Hao Y, Xu J, Murray T et al (2008) Cancer statistics, 2008. CA Cancer J Clin 58:71–96

Jensen TK, Holt P, Gerke O, Riehmann M, Svolgaard B, Marcussen N et al (2011) Preoperative lymph-node staging of invasive urothelial bladder cancer with 18F-fluorodeoxyglucose positron emission tomography/computed axial tomography and magnetic resonance imaging: correlation with histopathology. Scand J Urol Nephrol 45:122–128

Kaufman DS, Shipley WU, Feldman AS (2009) Bladder cancer. Lancet 374:239–249

Kayat Bittencourt L, Litjens G, Hulsbergen-van de Kaa CA, Turkbey B, Gasparetto EL, Barentsz JO (2015) Prostate cancer: The European Society of Urogenital Radiology Prostate Imaging Reporting and Data System criteria for predicting extraprostatic extension by using 3-T multiparametric MR. Radiology 276:479–489

Kayes O, Minhas S, Allen C, Hare C, Freeman A, Ralph D (2007) The role of magnetic resonance imaging in the local staging of penile cancer. Eur Urol 51:1313–1319

Kidd EA, Spencer CR, Huettner PC, Siegel BA, Dehdashti F, Rader JS et al (2009) Cervical cancer histology and tumor differentiation affect ^{18}F-fluorodeoxyglucose uptake. Cancer 115:3548–3554

Kim JK, Park SY, Ahn HJ, Kim CS, Cho KS (2004) Bladder cancer: analysis of multidetector row helical CT enhancement pattern and accuracy in tumor detection and perivesical staging. Radiology 231:725–731

Kim B, Breau RH, Papadatos D, Fergusson D, Doucette S, Cagiannos I et al (2010) Diagnostic accuracy of surface coil magnetic resonance imaging at 1.5 T for local staging of elevated risk prostate cancer. Can Urol Assoc J 4:257–262

Kinkel K, Forstner R, Danza FM, Oleaga L, Cunha TM, Bergman A et al (2009) Staging of endometrial cancer with MRI: guidelines of the European Society of Urogenital Imaging. Eur Radiol 19:1565–1574

Kitajima K, Kita M, Suzuki K, Senda M, Nakamoto Y, Sugimura K (2012) Prognostic significance of SUVmax (maximum standardized uptake value) measured by [18F]FDG PET/CT in endometrial cancer. Eur J Nucl Med Mol Imaging 39:840–845

Kitzing YX, Prando A, Varol C, Karczmar GS, Maclean F, Oto A (2016) Benign conditions that mimic prostate carcinoma: MR imaging features with histopathologic correlation. Radiographics 36:162–175

Labanaris AP, Zugor V, Takriti S, Smiszek R, Engelhard K, Nutzel R et al (2009) The role of conventional and functional endorectal magnetic resonance imaging in the decision of whether to preserve or resect the neurovascular bundles during radical retropubic prostatectomy. Scand J Urol Nephrol 43:25–31

Lazzari R, Cecconi A, Jereczek-Fossa BA, Travaini LL, Dell' Acqua V, Cattani F et al (2014) The role of [(18) F]FDG-PET/CT in staging and treatment planning for volumetric modulated Rapidarc radiotherapy in cervical cancer: experience of the European Institute of Oncology, Milan, Italy. Ecancermedicalscience 8. https://doi.org/10.3332/ecancer.2014.409

Lee YY, Choi CH, Kim CJ, Kang H, Kim TJ, Lee JW et al (2009) The prognostic significance of the SUVmax (maximum standardized uptake value for F-18 fluorodeoxyglucose) of the cervical tumor in PET imaging for early cervical cancer: preliminary results. Gynecol Oncol 115:65–68

Lee S, Catalano OA, Dehdashti F (2015) Evaluation of gynecologic cancer with MR imaging,^{18}F-FDG PET/CT, and PET/MR imaging. J Nucl Med 56:436–443

Lee CH, Tan CH, De Castro Faria S, Kundra V (2017) Role of imaging in the local staging of urothelial carcinoma of the bladder. AJR 208:1–13

van Leeuwen PJ, Emmett L, Ho B, Delprado W, Ting F, Nguyen Q et al (2017) BJU Int 119:209–215

Lewin SN, Herzog TJ, Barrena Medel NI, Deutsch I, Burke WM, Sun X et al (2010) Comparative performance of the 2009 international federation of gynecology and obstetrics' staging system for uterine corpus cancer. Obstet Gynecol 116:1141–1149

Liedberg F, Bendahl PO, Davidsson T, Gudjonsson S, Holmer M, Månsson W et al (2013) Preoperative staging of locally advanced bladder cancer before radical cystectomy using 3 tesla magnetic resonance imaging with a standardized protocol. Scand J Urol 47:108–112

Lim K, Small W Jr, Portelance L, Creutzberg C, Jürgenliemk-Schulz IM, Mundt A et al (2011) Consensus guidelines for delineation of clinical target volume for intensity modulated pelvic radiotherapy for the definitive treatment of cervix cancer. Int J Radiat Oncol Biol Phys 79(2):348–355. https://doi.org/10.1016/j.ijrobp.2009.10.075

Lin LL, Mutic S, Low DA, LaForest R, Vicic M, Zoberi I et al (2007) Adaptive brachytherapy treatment planning for cervical cancer using FDG-PET. Int J Radiat Oncol Biol Phys 67(1):91–96

Lindegaard JC, Fokdal LU, Nielsen SK, Juul-Christensen J, Tanderup K (2013) MRI-guided adaptive radiotherapy in locally advanced cervical cancer from a Nordic perspective. Acta Oncol 52(7):1510–1519

Lont AP, Besnard APE, Gallee MPW, van Tinteren H, Horenblas S (2003a) A comparison of physical examination and imaging in determining the extent of primary penile carcinoma. BJUi 91:493–495

Lont AP, Besnard AP, Gallee MP, van Tinteren H, Horenblas S (2003b) A comparison of physical examination and imaging in determining the extent of primary penile carcinoma. BJU Int 91(6):493–495

Magné N, Chargari C, Vicenzi L, Gillion N, Messai T, Magné J et al (2008) New trends in the evaluation and treatment of cervix cancer: the role of FDG-PET. Cancer rreat Rev 34:671–681

Malayeri AA, Pattanayak P, Apolo AB (2015) Imaging muscle-invasive and metastatic urothelial carcinoma. Curr Opin Urol 25:441–448

Malyapa RS, Mutic S, Low DA, Zoberi I, Bosch WR, Laforest R et al (2002) Physiologic FDG-PET three-dimensional brachytherapy treatment planning for cervical cancer. Int J Radiat Oncol Biol Phys 54(4):1140 1146

Manecksha RP, Fitzpatrick JM (2009) Epidemiology of testicular cancer. BJU Int 104:1329–1333

Manfredi R, Mirk P, Maresca G, Margariti PA, Testa A, Zannoni GF et al (2004) Local-regional staging of endometrial carcinoma: role of MR imaging in surgical planning. Radiology 231(2):372–378

Mapelli P, Incerti E, Ceci F, Castellucci P, Fanti S, Picchio M (2016) 11C- or 18F-choline PET/CT for imaging evaluation of biochemical recurrence of prostate cancer. J Nucl Med 57(Suppl 3):43–48

Martorana G, Schiavina R, Corti B, Farsad M, Salizzoni E, Brunocilla E et al (2006) 11C-choline positron emission tomography/computerized tomography for tumor localization of primary prostate cancer in comparison with 12-core biopsy. J Urol 176:954–960

Maurer T, Gschwend JE, Rauscher I, Souvatzoglou M, Haller B, Weirich G et al (2016) Diagnostic efficacy of (68)gallium-PSMA positron emission tomography compared to conventional imaging for lymph node staging of 130 consecutive patients with intermediate to high risk prostate cancer. J Urol 195: 1436–1443

Meissnitzer M, Forstner R (2016) MRI of endometrium cancer—how we do it. Cancer Imaging. https://doi.org/10.1186/s40644-016-0069-1

Millán-Rodríguez F, Chéchile-Toniolo G, Salvador-Bayarri J, Huguet-Pérez J, Vicente-Rodríguez J (2000) Upper urinary tract tumors after primary superficial bladder tumors: prognostic factors and risk groups. J Urol 164:1183–1187

Moreno CC, Small WC, Camacho JC, Master V, Kokabi N, Lewis M et al (2015) Testicular tumors: what radiologists need to know—differential diagnosis, staging, and management. Radiographics 35:400–415

Mottet N, Bellmunt J, Bolla M, Briers E, Cumberbatch MG, De Santis M et al (2017) EAU-ESTRO-SIOG Guidelines on Prostate Cancer. Part 1: screening, diagnosis, and local treatment with curative intent. Eur Urol 71:618–629

Mueller-Lisse UG, Scher B, Scherr MK, Seitz M (2008) Functional imaging in penile cancer: PET/computed tomography, MRI, and sentinel lymph node biopsy. Curr Opin Urol 18(1):105–110

Murphy G, Haider M, Ghai S, Sreeharsha B (2013) The expanding role of MRI in prostate cancer. AJR Am J Roentgenol 201:1229–1238

Nicolet V, Carignan L, Bourdon F, Prosmanne O (2000) MR imaging of cervical carcinoma: a practical staging approach. Radiographics 20:1539–1549

Noël P, Dubé M, Plante M, St-Laurent G (2014) Early cervical carcinoma and fertility-sparing treatment options: MR imaging as a tool in patient selection and a follow- up modality. Radiographics 34:1099–1019

Okamoto Y, Tanaka YO, Nishida M, Tsunoda H, Yoshikawa H, Itai Y (2003) MR imaging of the uterine cervix: imaging-pathologic correlation. Radiographics 23:425–445

Oonk MHM, Planchamp F, Baldwin P, Bidzinski M, Brännström M, Landoni F et al (2017) European Society of Gynaecological Oncology Guidelines for the management of patients with vulvar cancer. Int J Gynecol Cancer 27(4):832–837

Palou J, Rodriguez-Rubio F, Huguet J, Segarra J, Ribal MJ, Alcaraz A et al (2005) Multivariate analysis of clinical parameters of synchronous primary superficial bladder cancer and upper urinary tract tumor. J Urol 174:859–861

Panebianco V, Sciarra A, Osimani M, Lisi D, Ciccariello M, Salciccia S et al (2009) 2D and 3D T2-weighted MR sequences for the assessment of neurovascular bundle changes after nerve-sparing radical retropubic prostatectomy with erectile function correlation. Eur Radiol 19:220–229

Panebianco V, Sciarra A, Di Martino M, Bernardo S, Vergari V, Gentilucci A et al (2010) Bladder carcinoma: MDCT cystography and virtual cystoscopy. Abdom Imaging 35:257–264

Panebianco V, Sciarra A, Marcantonio A, Forte V, Biondi T, Laghi A et al (2012) Conventional imaging and multiparametric magnetic resonance (MRI, MRS, DWI, MRP) in the diagnosis of prostate cancer. Q J Nucl Med Mol Imaging 56:331–342

Panebianco V, Barchetti F, Barentsz J, Ciardi A, Cornud F, Futterer J et al (2015a) Pitfalls in interpreting mp-MRI of the prostate: a pictorial review with pathologic correlation. Insights Imaging 6:611–630

Panebianco V, Barchetti F, Sciarra A, Ciardi A, Indino EL, Papalia R et al (2015b) Multiparametric magnetic resonance imaging vs. standard care in men being evaluated for prostate cancer: a randomized study. Urol Oncol 33:17.e1–17.e7. https://doi.org/10.1016/j.urolonc.2014.09.013

Panebianco V, De Berardinis E, Barchetti G, Simone G, Leonardo C, Grompone MD et al (2017) An evaluation of morphological and functional multi-parametric MRI sequences in classifying non-muscle and muscle invasive bladder cancer. Eur Radiol 27(9):3759–3766. https://doi.org/10.1007/s00330-017-4758-3

Parikh JH, Barton DPJ, Ind TEJ, Sohaib SA (2008) MR imaging features of vaginal malignancies. Radiographics 28:49–63

Parker RA III, Menias CO, Quazi R, Hara AK, Verma S, Shaaban A et al (2015) MR imaging of the penis and scrotum. Radiographics 35:1033–1050

Podzielinski I, Randall ME, Breheny PJ, Escobar PF, Cohn DE, Quick AM et al (2012) Primary radiation therapy for medically inoperable patients with clinical stage I and II endometrial carcinoma. Gynecol Oncol 124:36–41

Pötter R, Georg P, Dimopoulos JC, Grimm M, Berger D, Nesvacil N et al (2011) Clinical outcome of protocol based image (MRI) guided adaptive brachytherapy combined with 3D conformal radiotherapy with or without chemotherapy in patients with locally advanced cervical cancer. Radiother Oncol 100(1):116–123

Purysko AS, Rosenkrantz AB, Barentsz JO, Weinreb JC, Macura KJ (2016) PI-RADS Version 2: a pictorial update. Radiographics 36:1354–1372

Querleu D, Planchamp F, Narducci F, Morice P, Joly F, Genestie C et al (2011) Clinical practice guidelines for the management of patients with endometrial cancer in France: recommendations of the Institut National du Cancer and the Société Française d'Oncologie Gynécologique. Int J Gynecol Cancer 21:945–950

Randall ME, Andersen WA, Mills SE, Kim JA (1986) Papillary squamous cell carcinoma of the uterine cervix: a clinicopathologic study of nine cases. Int J Gynecol Pathol 5:1–10

Rasch C, Barillot I, Remeijer P, Touw A, van Herk M, Lebesque JV (1999) Definition of the prostate in CT and MRI: a multiobserver study. Int J Radiat Oncol Biol Phys 43:57–66

Rechichi G, Galimberti S, Signorelli M, Perego P, Valsecchi MG, Sironi S (2010) Myometrial invasion in endometrial cancer: diagnostic performance of diffusion-weighted MR imaging at 1.5-T. Eur Radiol 20:754–762

Remedios D, McCoubrie P (2007) The Royal College of Radiologists. Making the best use of clinical radiology services: referral guidelines. Clin Radiol 62(10):919–920

Richie JP (2015) 18F-FDG PET/CT impact on testicular tumours clinical management. J Urol 194(4):991. https://doi.org/10.1016/j.juro.2015.07.003.

Robertson NL, Hricak H, Sonoda Y, Sosa RE, Benz M, Lyons G et al (2016) The impact of FDG-PET/CT in the management of patients with vulvar and vaginal cancer. Gynecol Oncol 140(3):420–424. https://doi.org/10.1016/j.ygyno.2016.01.011

Rockall AG, Ghosh S, Alexander-Sefre F, Babar S, Younis MT, Naz S et al (2006) Can MRI rule out bladder and rectal in- vasion in cervical cancer to help select patients for limited EUA? Gynecol Oncol 101:244–249

Rockall AG, Meroni R, Sohaib SA, Reynolds K, Alexander-Sefre F, Shepherd JH et al (2007) Evaluation of endometrial carcinoma on magnetic resonance imaging. Int J Gynecol Cancer 17:188–196

Sahdev A, Sohaib SA, Wenaden AE, S hepherd JH, Reznek RH (2007) The performance of magnetic resonance imaging in early cervical carcinoma: a long-term experience. Int J Gynecol Cancer 17:629–636

Sala E, Akin O, Moskowitz CS, Eisenberg HF, Kuroiwa K, Ishill NM et al (2006) Endorectal MR imaging in the evaluation of seminal vesicle invasion: diagnostic accuracy and multivariate feature analysis. Radiology 238:929–937

Sala E, Wakely S, Senior E, Lomas D (2007) MRI of malignant neoplasms of the uterine corpus and cervix. AJR Am J Roentgenol 188:1577–1587

Sala E, Crawford R, Senior E, Shaw A, Simcock B, Vrotsou K et al (2009) Added value of dynamic contrast-enhanced magnetic resonance imaging in predicting advanced stage disease in patients with endometrial carcinoma. Int J Gynecol Cancer 19:141–146

Sala E, Rockall AG, Freeman SJ, Mitchell DG, Reinhold C (2013a) The added role of MR imaging in treatment stratification of patients with gynecologic malignancies: what the radiologist needs to know. Radiology 266:717–740

Sala E, Rockall AG, Freeman SJ, Mitchell DG, Reinhold C (2013b) The added role of mR imaging in treatment strati cation of patients with gynecologic malignancies: what the radiologist needs to know. Radiology 266:717–740

Sato C, Naganawa S, Nakamura T, Kumada H, Miura S, Takizawa O et al (2005) Differentiation of noncancerous tissue and cancer lesions by apparent diffusion coefficient values in transition and peripheral zones of the prostate. J Magn Reson Imaging 21:258–629

Scheidler J, Heuck AF (2002) Imaging of cancer of the cervix. Radiol Clin North Am 40:577–590

Schild MH, Schild SE, Wong WW, Vora SA, Silva AC, Silva AM et al (2014) Early outcome of prostate Intensity Modulated Radiation Therapy (IMRT) incorporating a simultaneous intra-prostatic MRI directed boost. OMICS J Radiol. https://doi.org/10.4172/2167-7964.1000170

Schoots IG, Roobol MJ, Nieboer D, Bangma CH, Steyerberg EW, Hunink MG (2015) Magnetic resonance imaging-targeted biopsy may enhance the diagnostic accuracy of significant prostate cancer detection compared to standard transrectal ultrasound-guided biopsy: a systematic review and meta-analysis. Eur Urol 68:438–450

Schuster DM, Nanni C, Fanti S (2016) Evaluation of prostate cancer with radiolabeled amino acid analogs. J Nucl Med 57(Suppl 3):61–66

Schwarz JK, Beriwal S, Esthappan J, Erickson B, Feltmate C, Fyles A et al (2015) Consensus statement for brachytherapy for the treatment of medically inoperable endometrial cancer. Brachytherapy *14*(5):587–599

Seki H, Azumi R, Kimura M et al (1997) Stromal invasion by carcinoma of the cervix: assessment with dynamic MR imaging. AJR Am J Roentgenol 168:1579–1585

Sharma P, Jain TK, Parida GK, Karunanithi S, Patel C, Sharma A et al (2014) Diagnostic accuracy of integrated (18)F-FDG PET/CT for restaging patients with malignant germ cell tumours. Br J Radiol 87:20140263

Sheu MH, Chang CY, Wang JH, Yen M (2001) Preoperative staging of cervical carcinoma with MR imaging: a reappraisal of diagnostic accuracy and pitfalls. Eur Radiol 11:1828–1833

Siegel R, Naishadham D, Jemal A (2013) Cancer statistics, 2013. CA Cancer J Clin 63:11–30

Siegel RL, Miller KD, Jemal A (2017) Cancer Statistics, 2017. CA Cancer J Clin 67:7–30

Simcock B, Narayan K, Drummond E, Bernshaw D, Wells E, Hicks RJ (2015) The role of positron emission tomography/computed tomography in planning radiotherapy in endometrial cancer. Int J Gynecol Cancer 25(4):645–649

Song Y, Chen X, Erickson BA, Li A (2016) Improving delineation of gross tumor volume using magnetic resonance imaging for external beam radiation therapy of locally advanced cervical cancer. Int J Radiat Oncol Biol Phys 96(2):E303–E304

Souvatzoglou M, Krause BJ, Purschel A, Thamm R, Schuster T, Buck AK et al (2011) Influence of (11) C-choline PET/CT on the treatment planning for salvage radiation therapy in patients with biochemical recurrence of prostate cancer. Radiother Oncol 99(2):193–200

Steenbakkers RJ, Deurloo KE, Nowak PJ, Lebesque JV, van Herk M, Rasch CR (2003) Reduction of dose delivered to the rectum and bulb of the penis using MRI delineation for radiotherapy of the prostate. Int J Radiat Oncol Biol Phys 57:1269–1279

Steenbergen P, Haustermans K, Lerut E, Oyen R, De Wever L, Van den Bergh L et al (2015) Prostate tumor delineation using multiparametric magnetic resonance imaging: inter-observer variability and pathology validation. Radiother Oncol 115:186–190

Takeuchi M, Sasaki S, Ito M, Okada S, Takahashi S, Kawai T et al (2009) Urinary bladder cancer: diffusion-weighted MR imaging—accuracy for diagnosing T stage and estimating histologic grade. Radiology 251:112–121

Tan CH, Wei W, Johnson V, Kundra V (2012) Diffusion-weighted MRI in the detection of prostate cancer: meta-analysis. Am J Roentgenol 199:822–829

Tekes A, Kamel I, Imam K, Szarf G, Schoenberg M, Nasir K et al (2005) Dynamic MRI of bladder cancer: evaluation of staging accuracy. AJR Am J Roentgenol 184:121–127

Toita T, Ohno T, Kaneyasu Y, Kato T, Uno T, Hatano K et al (2011) A consensus-based guideline defining clinical target volume for primary disease in external beam radiotherapy for intact uterine cervical cancer. Jpn J Clin Oncol 41(9):1119–1126. https://doi.org/10.1093/jjco/hyr096

Tsai CS, Lai CH, Chang TC, Yen TC, Ng KK, Hsueh S et al (2010) A prospective randomized trial to study the impact of pretreatment FDG-PET for cervical cancer patients with MRI-detected positive pelvic but negative para-aortic lymphadenopathy. Int J Radiat Oncol Biol Phys 76(2):477–484

Tsampoulas C, Tsili AC, Giannakis D, Alamanos Y, So kitis N, Efremidis SC (2008) 16-MDCT cystoscopy in the evaluation of neoplasms of the urinary bladder. AJR 190:729–735

Tsili AC, Argyropoulou MI, Giannakis D, Sofikitis N, Tsampoulas K (2010) MRI in the characterization and local staging of testicular neoplasms. AJR 194:682–689

Tsili AC, Giannakis D, Sylakos A, Ntorkou A, Sofikitis N, Argyropoulou MI (2014) MR imaging of scrotum. Magn Reson Imaging Clin N Am 22(2):217–238

Tsuda K, Murakami T, Kurachi H, Narumi Y, Kim T, Takahashi S et al (1999) MR imaging of non-squamous vaginal tumors. Eur Radiol 9:1214–1218

Valicenti RK, Sweet JW, Hauck WW, Hudes RS, Lee T, Dicker AP et al (1999) Variation of clinical target volume definition in three-dimensional conformal radiation therapy for prostate cancer. Int J Radiat Oncol Biol Phys 44:931–935

Van der Steen S, de Nieuwenhof HP, Massuger L, Bulten J, de Hullu JA (2010) New FIGO staging system of vulvar cancer indeed provides a better reflection of prognosis. Gynecol Oncol 119:520–525

Vargas HA, Akin O, Franiel T, Goldman DA, Udo K, Touijer KA et al (2012) Normal central zone of the prostate and central zone involvement by prostate cancer: clinical and MR imaging implications. Radiology 262:894–802

Verma S, Rajesh A, Prasad SR, Gaitonde K, Lall CG, Mouraviev V et al (2012) Urinary bladder cancer: role of MR imaging. Radiographics 32:371–387

Vigneault E, Mbodji K, Racine LG, Chevrette E, Lavallée MC, Martin AG et al (2016) Image-guided high-dose-rate brachytherapy boost to the dominant intraprostatic lesion using multiparametric magnetic resonance imaging including spectroscopy: results of a prospective study. Brachytherapy 15(6):746–751

Vikram R, Sandler C, Ng C (2009) Imaging and staging of transitional cell carcinoma: part 1, lower urinary tract. AJR Am J Roentgenol 192:1481–1487

Villeirs GM, Van Vaerenbergh K, Vakaet L, Bral S, Claus F, De Neve WJ et al (2005) Interobserver delineation variation using CT versus combined CT+MRI in intensity-modulated radiotherapy for prostate cancer. Strahlenther Onkol 181:424–430

Viswanathan C, Kirschner K, Truong M, Balachandran A, Devine C, Bhosale P (2013) Multimodality imaging of vulvar cancer: staging, therapeutic response, and complications. AJR 200:1387–1400

Walker DK, Salibian RA, Salibian AD, Belen KM, Palmer SL (2011) Overlooked diseases of the vagina: a directed anatomic-pathologic approach for imaging assessment. Radiographics 31:1583–1598

Wang N, Jiang P, Lu Y (2014) Is fluorine-18 fluorodeoxyglucose positron emission tomography useful for detecting bladder lesions? A meta-analysis of the literature. Urol Int 92:143–149

Watanabe H, Kanematsu M, Kondo H, Goshima S, Tsuge Y, Onozuka M et al (2009) Pre- operative T staging of urinary bladder cancer: does diffusion-weighted MRI have supplementary value? AJR 192:1361–1366

Weitmann HD, Potter R, Waldhausl C, Nechvile E, Kirisits C, Knocke TH (2005) Pilot study in the treatment of endometrial carcinoma with 3D image-based high-dose-rate brachytherapy using modified Heyman packing: clinical experience and dose-volume histogram analysis. *Int J Radiat Oncol Biol Phys* 62:468–478

Whalley D, Caine H, McCloud P, Guo L, Kneebone A, Eade T (2015) Promising results with image guided intensity modulated radiotherapy for muscle invasive bladder cancer. Radiat Oncol 10:205. https://doi.org/10.1186/s13014-015-0499-0

Winter C, Albers P (2011) Testicular germ cell tumors: pathogenesis, diagnosis and treatment. Nat Rev Endocrinol 7(1):43–53

Witjes JA, Comperat E, Cowan NC, De SM, Gakis G, Lebret T et al (2014) EAU guidelines on muscle-invasive and metastatic bladder cancer: summary of the 2013 guidelines. Eur Urol 65:778–792

Wu LM, Xu JR, Ye YQ, Lu Q, Hu JN (2012) The clinical value of diffusion- weighted imaging in com- bination with T2-weighted imaging in diagnosing prostate carcinoma: a systematic review and meta-analysis. AJR 199:103–110

Yamada AH, Lieskovsky G, Petrovich Z, Chen SC, Groshen S, Skinner DG (1994) Results of radical prostatectomy and adjuvant therapy in the management of locally advanced, clinical stage TC, prostate cancer. Am J Clin Oncol 17:277–285

Yildirim Y, Sehirali S, Avci ME, Yilmaz C, Ertopcu K, Tinar S et al (2008) Integrated PET/CT for the evaluation of para-aortic nodal metastasis in locally advanced cervical cancer patients with negative conventional CT findings. Gynecol Oncol 108(1):154–159

Yousem DM, Gatewood OM, Goldman SM, Marshall FF (1988) Synchronous and metachronous transitional cell carcinoma of the urinary tract: prevalence, incidence, and radiographic detection. Radiology 167: 613–618

Zamboglou C, Drendel V, Jilg CA, Rischke HC, Beck TI, Schultze-Seemann W et al (2017) Comparison of (68) Ga-HBED-CC PSMA-PET/CT and multiparametric MRI for gross tumour volume detection in patients with primary prostate cancer based on slice by slice comparison with histopathology. Theranostics 7:228–237. https://doi.org/10.7150/thno.16638

Zand KR, Reinhold C, Abe H, Maheshwari S, Mohamed A, Upegui D (2007) Magnetic resonance imaging of the cervix. Cancer Imaging 7:69–66

T-Staging and Target Volume Definition by Imaging in GYN Tumors

A. Alessi, B. Pappalardi, A. Cerrotta, G. Calareso, and F. Crippa

Contents

1 **Cervical Cancer** 255
1.1 Imaging Modalities in Staging 256
1.2 Target Volume Definition 258

2 **Endometrial Cancer** 262
2.1 Imaging Modalities in Staging 263
2.2 Target Volume Definition 264

3 **Ovarian Cancer** 265
3.1 Imaging Modalities in Staging 266
3.2 Target Volume Definition 266

4 **Vaginal Cancer** 267
4.1 Imaging Modalities in Staging 267
4.2 Target Volume Definition 267

5 **Vulvar Cancer** 268
5.1 Imaging Modalities in Staging 269
5.2 Target Volume Definition 269

References 270

A. Alessi (✉) · F. Crippa
Division of Nuclear Medicine, Fondazione IRCCS Istituto Nazionale dei Tumori, Milan, Italy
e-mail: alessandra.alessi@istitutotumori.mi.it; flavio.crippa@istitutotumori.mi.it

B. Pappalardi · A. Cerrotta
Division of Radiation Oncology II, Fondazione IRCCS Istituto Nazionale dei Tumori, Milan, Italy

G. Calareso
Department of Radiology, Fondazione IRCCS Istituto Nazionale dei Tumori, Milan, Italy

Gynecological malignancies comprise a wide range of different tumors with various etiologies, risk factors, and treatment approaches/principles. Prevention, diagnosis, primary treatment, and management of recurrence are complex issues. A complete staging, which includes the evaluation of local tumor spread, lymph node involvement and distant metastases, is essential to choose the optimal treatment strategy. The impact of imaging has changed treatment approaches over the past 10 years with the development of Intensity Modulated Radiation Therapy (IMRT) and Image-Guided Brachytherapy (IGBT), allowing increasingly accurate and effective radiation dose delivery. Computer tomography (CT) and positron emission tomography (PET/CT) are widely used for IMRT. Magnetic resonance imaging (MRI) represents the gold standard for target definition in IMRT and IGBT.

In this chapter, we will discuss the role and the usefulness of imaging for primary tumor staging and target volume definition for gynecological malignancies.

1 Cervical Cancer

Cervical cancer (CC) is one of the most common female cancers and the leading cause of female cancer-related death worldwide (Ferlay et al. 2015). The major risk factor for development of cervical malignancy is infection with human papilloma virus (HPV). This cancer is clinically

R. G. H. Beets-Tan et al. (eds.), *Imaging and Interventional Radiology for Radiation Oncology*, Medical Radiology, Diagnostic Imaging, https://doi.org/10.1007/978-3-030-38261-2_16

Table 1 The International Federation of Gynecology and Obstetric (FIGO) stage in Cervical Cancer (CC)

Stage	Description
0	Carcinoma in situ
Ia1	Invasion of stroma <3 mm in depth and ≤7 mm in width
Ia2	Invasion of stroma >3 mm and ≤5 mm in depth and ≤7 mm in width
Ib1	Clinical lesions greater than stage Ia but no greater than 4 cm
Ib2	Clinical lesions confined to the cervix and >4 cm
IIa	Involvement of the upper 2/3 vagina
IIb	Involvement of the parametria without sidewall involvement
IIIa	Extension to lower 1/3 vagina
IIIb	Extension to pelvic sidewall or hydronephrosis or non- functional kidney
IVa	Extension to bladder or rectum
IVb	Distant metastases or disease beyond the pelvis

staged by the International Federation of Gynecology and Obstetrics (FIGO) system (Table 1) (FIGO Committed on Gynecologic Oncology (FCoG) 2014). The last revision of FIGO staging criteria encourages the use of cross-sectional imaging modalities to assess diagnostic and prognostic information such as tumor size, parametrial spread, and nodal involvement (Pecorelli 2009).

MRI is the modality of choice to determine local-regional tumor spread while contrast-enhanced CT (ce-CT) and 2-[fluorine 18]-fluoro-2-deoxy-D-glucose ([^{18}F]FDG) PET/CT are well suited to provide information on lymph node and distant metastases. Any available imaging modalities are useful to reliably stage disease in early cervical cancer (stage < IB) due to microscopic extension of disease. Patients with CC stage < IB are currently treated with surgery, while the standard treatment for locally advanced cervical cancer (LACC) is definitive chemo-radiation consisting of IMRT, IGBT, and concomitant chemotherapy (CHT) with Cisplatin. Radio-chemotherapy plays also a pivotal role as adjuvant treatment after surgery (Koh et al. 2016; Colombo et al. 2012) in patients with high-risk factors including positive surgical margins and/or positive parametria and/or positive lymph nodes.

1.1 Imaging Modalities in Staging

1.1.1 Magnetic Resonance Imaging

MRI is the best imaging modality to define the local extent of primary tumor because of its excellent soft-tissue contrast resolution (Nicolet et al. 2000; Okamoto et al. 2003). MRI is generally superior to CT in the evaluation of invasion of pelvic structures such as the parametria, vagina, bladder, and rectum. According to the European Section of Urological Research guidelines (ESUR), the essential MRI protocol includes a combination of at least two T2-weighted sequences (sagittal and oblique planes, perpendicular to the long axis of the cervical canal) and one axial T1-weighted sequence of the pelvis. Cervical malignancies are best visualized on T2-weighted images. High-resolution, small field of view axial oblique T2-weighted images perpendicular to the long axis of the cervix are routine when assessing for parametrial invasion (Figs. 1 and 2). The features indicating parametrial invasion include spiculated tumor–parametrium interface, soft-tissue extension into the parametria along the cardinal or uterosacral ligaments, encasement of the peri-uterine vessels and hydro-ureteronephrosis (Kaur et al. 2003). In large tumors, parametrial invasion may be overestimated on T2-weighted images, in

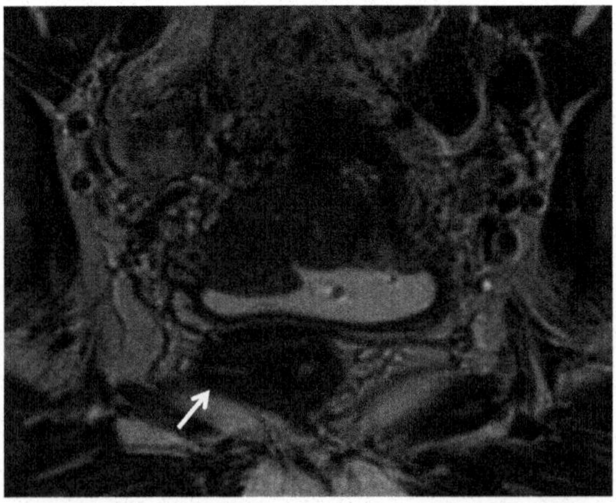

Fig. 1 Cervical carcinoma (FIGO IIB). Para-coronal T2-weighted MRI image shows solid signal tumor expanding out of cervix into adjacent right parametrial (arrowhead)

presence of stromal edema or peristromal stranding, caused respectively by tumor compression or postbiopsy hemorrhagic peristromal stranding. In these cases, a diffusion-weighted imaging (DWI) sequence may help to determine the true extent of the lesion.

The use of contrast-enhanced T1-weighted sequences is debated (Balleyguier et al. 2011); however, it may provide useful information to accurately delineate small cervical tumors (Akita et al. 2011) and differentiate residual or recurrent tumor from radiation fibrosis in the post-treatment setting.

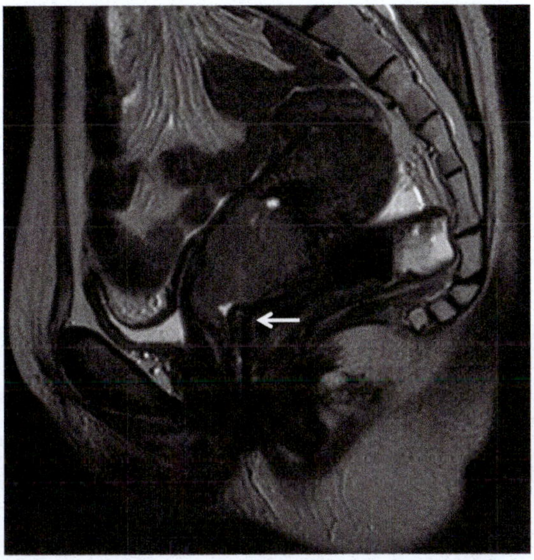

Fig. 2 Cervical carcinoma (FIGO stage III). Sagittal T2 weighted MRI image demonstrates a large signal mass in cervical cancer expanding on lower third of vagina (arrowhead)

Staging of lymph nodes, based on the size criterion (10 mm in short axis) still gives a low accuracy to MRI in the assessment of nodal status reported ranges of sensitivity and specificity of 38–89% and 78–99%, respectively (Hawighorst 1999; Scheidler et al. 1997). The presence of intranodal necrosis may be an adjunctive feature suggesting nodal metastasis.

1.1.2 [^{18}F]FDG PET-CT

PET-CT can detect primary and metastatic cervical cancer due to the intense [^{18}F]FDG uptake displayed by the majority of these tumors (Fig. 3). Poorly differentiated and squamous cell tumors have usually the highest [^{18}F]FDG uptake. Kidd et al. reported higher uptake in squamous tumors versus nonsquamous tumors (average SUVmax 11.9 vs. 8, respectively) and in poorly differentiate tumors versus well-differentiated tumors (average SUVmax 12.2 vs. 8.6, respectively) (Kidd et al. 2009). Tumors with high value of SUVmax have been demonstrated to be associated with increased risk of lymph node metastases (Yagi et al. 2016). However, PET/CT has some limitations for initial staging, due to poor spatial resolution of PET images and the potential interference of nonspecific uptake in normal pelvic organs (i.e., bladder and rectum) that can prevent tumor spreading detection in structures and organs close to the cervix. In early stages (stage IB and lower), PET/CT can give false negative results in small tumors and nodal micro-

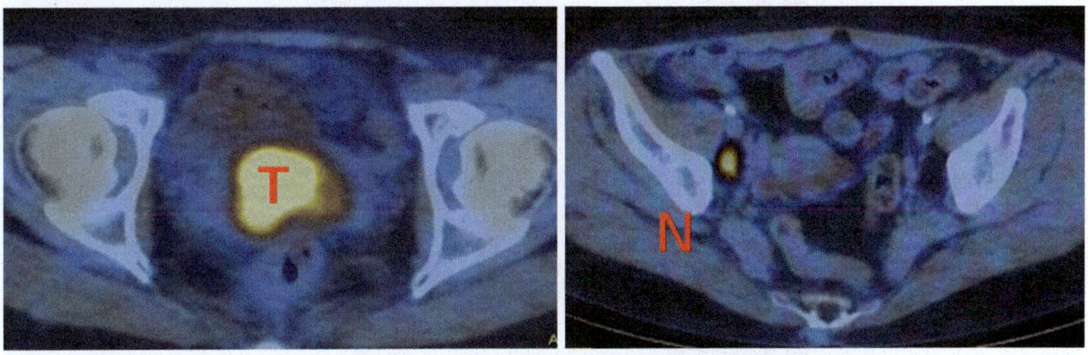

Fig. 3 Cervical carcinoma. Fused axial images PET-CT images show intense [^{18}F]FDG uptake by cervical tumor (*T*) and iliac right lymph node involvement (*N*)

metastases (Signorelli et al. 2011; Chung et al. 2010; Wright et al. 2005; Bentivegna et al. 2010). In locally advanced disease, PET/CT has higher sensitivity than CT and MRI in the detection of lymph node involvement with a reported sensitivity of 82% and specificity of 95% (Choi et al. 2010). The ability of PET-CT to assess nodal status can be useful in guiding therapies (Fig. 4); patients who have evidence of disease in the para-aortic lymph node at the time of initial diagnosis may benefit from extended radiation fields (Vargo et al. 2014). PET/MRI is an emerging potential noninvasive imaging tool for improved management of cervical carcinoma (Ohliger et al. 2017). Hybrid PET/MRI technology might become the preferred method to assess loco-regional extent of pelvic tumor, providing high-quality complimentary morphological and multiparametric functional information in one sitting. PET/MRI revealed with a significantly higher overall accuracy (83.3%) for T-staging of primary cervical cancers than PET/CT (53.3%) and a high diagnostic confidence in the evaluation of tumor metastasis, especially for tumor invasion into adjacent anatomical structure. Preliminary experience is encouraging but sufficient data are still lacking (Nie et al. 2017).

1.2 Target Volume Definition

Gynecological examination, diagnostic T2-weighted MRI, and treatment planning CT, with immobilization devices in supine position are important for target delineation and treatment planning. With the growing technical possibilities and availability of imaging, the field of intensity modulated image-guided external beam radiation therapy (EBRT) is rapidly evolving. [^{18}F]FDG PET/CT is strongly recommended to identify target loco-regional disease in IMRT/IGRT of CC (Grigsby 2009). Ideally, both PET/CT and MRI

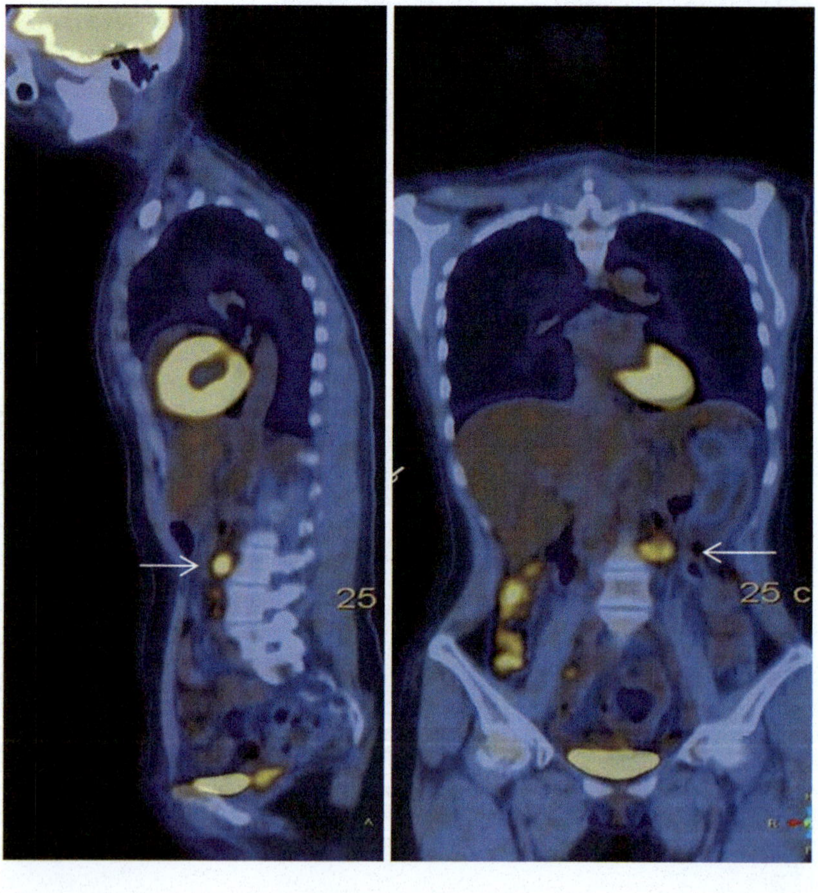

Fig. 4 Cervical carcinoma. Fused sagittal and coronal PET-CT images show [^{18}F]FDG-avid right iliac and retroperitoneal para-aortic lymph nodes (white arrow) consisting with nodal metastases

should be performed in treatment position, in order to enable optimal image fusion based on bony anatomy. The volumes of interest are in principle defined according to *ICRU 50/62/83*:

- GTV-T and GTV-N (Gross Tumor Volume at diagnosis) are defined and contoured based on imaging (MRI and PET-CT) and clinical characteristics (Fig. 5).
- CTV-T and CTV-N (Clinical Target Volume) are defined and contoured based on the extension of the GTV and the assumed microscopic spread for each specific tumor extension and its biological characteristics taking into account anatomical regions (e.g., vagina), compartments (e.g., parametrium), and borders (e.g., outer rectal wall).
- *CTV-T* is subdivided into:
  - CTV-T HR: GTV-T and any remaining cervix not infiltrated by tumor;
  - CTV-T LR: Initial CTV-T HR + complete parametria bilaterally + entire uterus + uninvolved vagina with a 20 mm margin measured from the most inferior position of the initial HR CTV-T, along the vaginal axis (not starting in the fornix), plus a margin of about 5 mm anterior and posterior toward bladder and rectum (excluding the noninvolved walls). In case of involvement of pelvic wall, sacro-uterine ligaments, mesorectum, or other involved structures at 20 mm, margin around the initial CTV-T HR will be extended into these structures and any pathological lymph nodes in the parametrium may be included.
- ITV (Internal Target Volume) is based on a standard or individualized margin; it accounts for uncertainties in size, shape, and position of the CTV-T within the patient, which include both inter- and intra-fraction motion.
- PTV (Planning Target Volume) is derived from the ITV or the CTV using an isotropic margin. The total CTV-T to PTV-T margin needs to accommodate random and systematic geometrical errors (i.e., positioning of patient during the course of EBRT, set-up errors).

In order to tailor the nodal target according to the assumed risk of microscopic nodal involvement, three risk groups are introduced with three different elective nodal target volumes:

- Small pelvis EBRT in low risk patients (LR LN)
- Large pelvis EBRT in intermediate risk patients (IR LN)
- Large pelvis + para-aortic EBRT in high risk patients (HR LN)

Risk allocation is based on primary tumor characteristics and nodal pathology at time of diagnosis and takes into account the probability

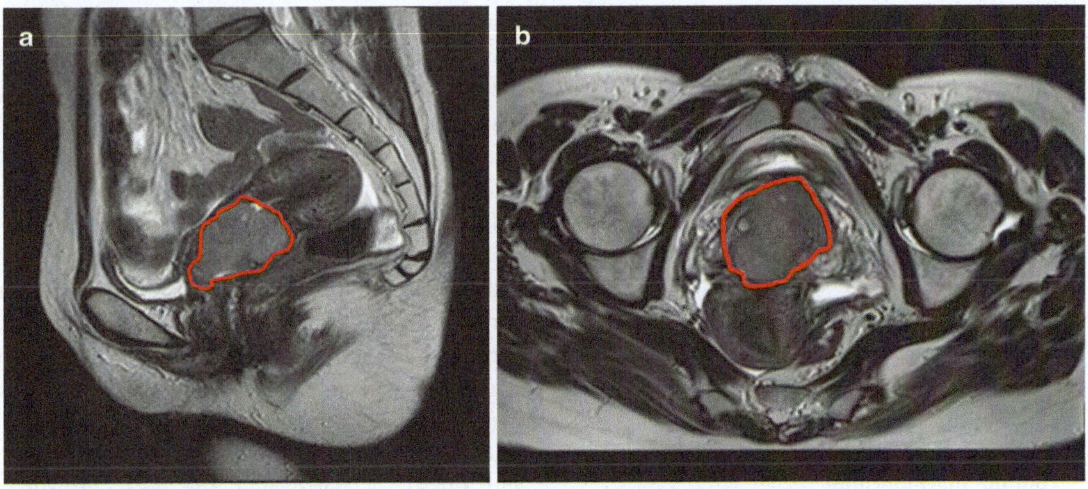

Fig. 5 Cervical cancer GTV (red) on sagittal and axial T2-weighted MRI images

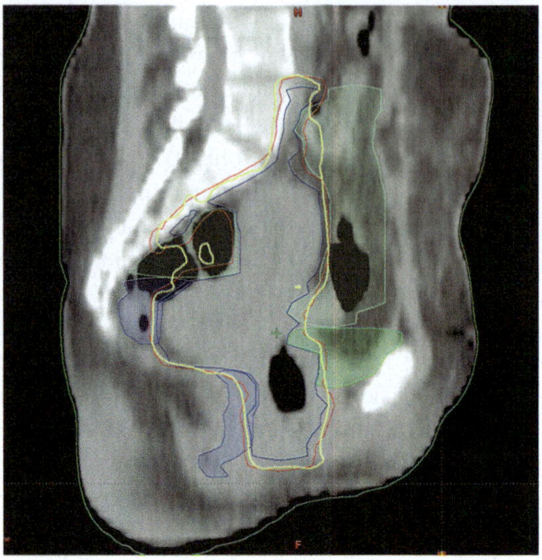

Fig. 6 Cervical cancer CTV-E (primary tumor and lymph nodes, blue), ITV (red), PTV (yellow) and OARs

of developing lymph node metastases in pelvic and para-aortic areas. PET-CT also may be useful for determining which patients benefit from the use of extended radiation fields. The pattern of lymph node recurrence has three predominant areas: within the radiation field in the obturator region (in-field), at the cranial field border (marginal), and in the para-aortic region (outside radiation field) (Verma et al. 2014). The elective nodal CTV (Fig. 6) of the combined draining nodal regions (CTV-E) is selected according to risk of nodal spread. No ITV is defined for the elective nodal target (CTV-E) as internal organ motion seems to play no important role for the CTV-E. In addition to IMRT radiation dose, simultaneous integrated boost (SIB) to [^{18}F]FDG-avid lymph nodes is currently recommended (Fig. 7) (Esthappan et al. 2008). The following organs at risk (OARs) should be delineated:

- Bladder: whole organ including the bladder neck;
- Rectum: from the ano-rectal sphincter to the recto-sigmoid junction;
- Sigmoid: from the recto-sigmoid junction to the left iliac fossa;
- Bowel: outer contour of bowel loops including the mesenterium;
- Femoral heads: both femoral head and neck to the level of the trochanter minor.

For para-aortic irradiation in addition:

- Kidneys: outer contour excluding renal pelvis;
- Spinal cord: outer contour.

In case of ovarian transposition:

- Ovary: Outer contour.

It is recommended to start contouring on MRI, exploiting the superior soft tissue resolution when delineating GTV-T and CTV-T; the next step of contouring normally proceeds on PET-CT to delineate nodal targets (GTV-Ns and CTV-E) and then on the treatment planning CT for OARs.

Standard treatment for locally advanced cervical cancer includes image-guided brachytherapy (IGBT) after EBRT. Even if CT planning brachytherapy (BT) is commonly used, MRI planning BT should be preferable as it allows a boost to be individually tailored, according to the residual tumor volume after typically 45–50 Gy of EBRT. For a small and/or well-responding tumor, IGBT may be initiated already during EBRT to shorten the overall treatment to 5–6 weeks. In any case, every effort should be made to keep the overall treatment time to <50 days. Before placement of the brachytherapy applicator, a clinical assessment of the tumor extension is performed describing tumor dimensions (width, height, and thickness) as well as the possible involvement of parametria, vagina, bladder, and rectum. MRI compatible applicator is chosen depending on the anatomical topography of tumor, uterus, cervix, and vagina. Additional implantation of MRI compatible needles in the peri-cervical tissues has to be used for appropriate target coverage. Sequences taken parallel to the applicator, i.e., paratransversal, paracoronal, and parasagittal, are superior to straight transversal, coronal, and sagittal images with regard to both target contouring and applicator reconstruction. Contouring for both tumor and OARs is performed for each insertion/

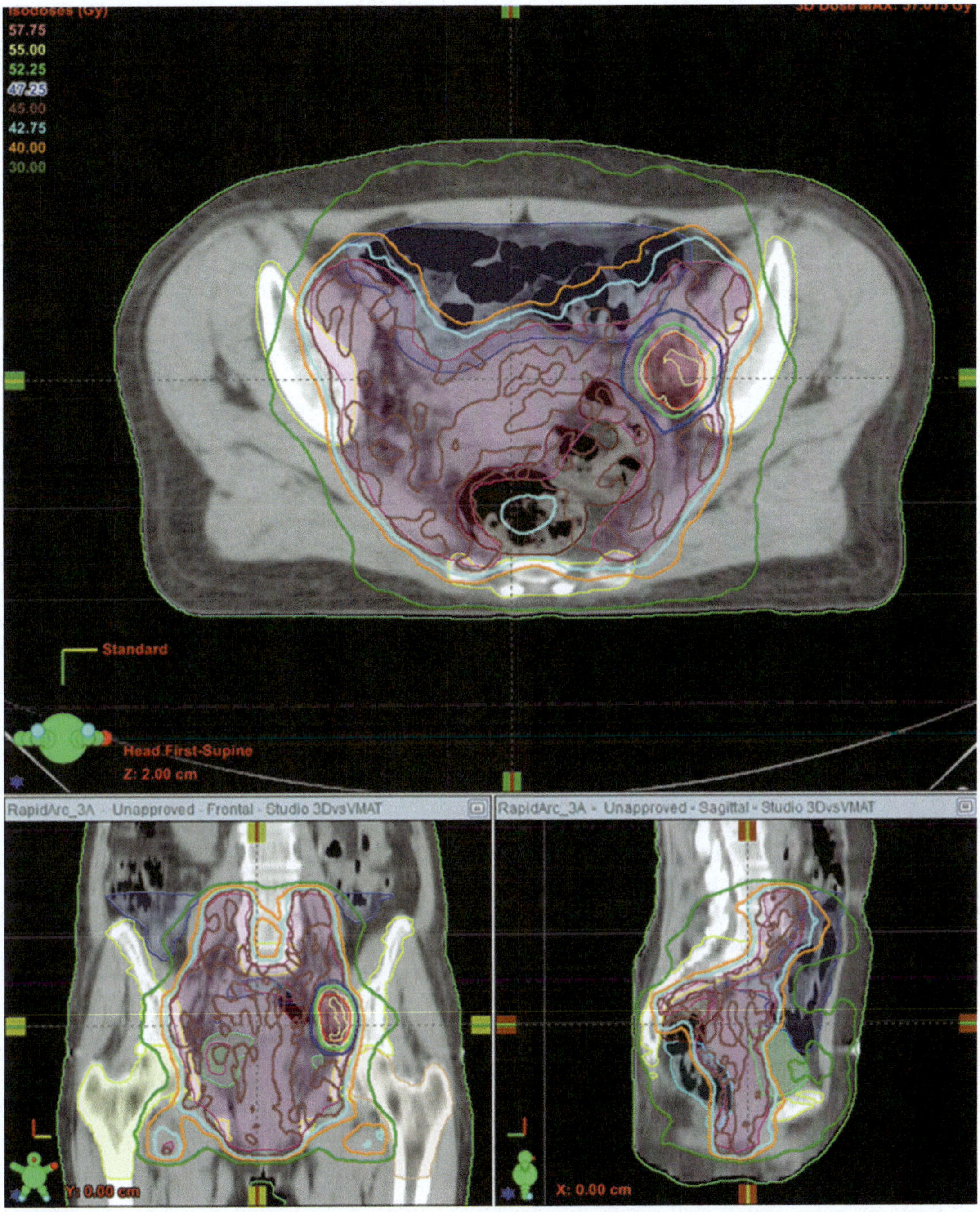

Fig. 7 Dose distribution with IMRT/VMAT in Cervical Cancer; this technique allows Simultaneous Integrated Boost (SIB) on PET-positives lymph nodes (left iliac internal)

implant of brachytherapy applicators by contouring on T2-weighted (para)-transversal MRI sequences in a dedicated 3D brachytherapy dose-planning system according to the *GEC ESTRO Recommendations and the ICRU/GEC ESTRO report 88* (ICRU report 88 2015; Dimopoulos et al. 2012; Pötter et al. 2006; Hellebust et al. 2010).

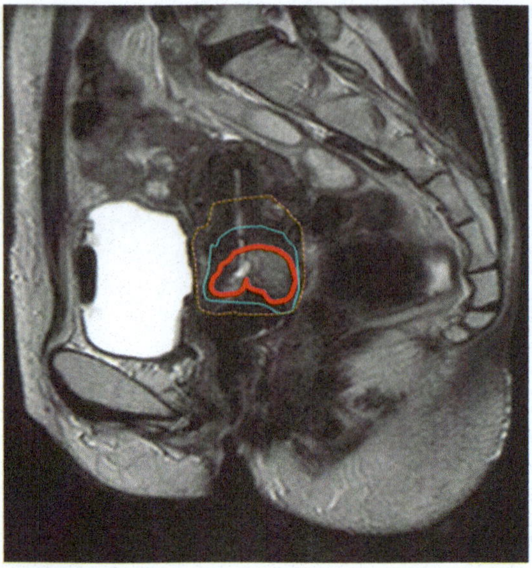

Fig. 8 Residual GTV (red), HR CTV (blue) and IR CTV (orange) at time of BT

Accurate tumor target contouring requires that information including clinical drawings from gynecological assessment and MRI at diagnosis have to be available at the contouring station.

The following targets should be contoured for IGBT (Fig. 8):

- GTV res: residual (high signal) Gross Tumor Volume of the primary tumor.
- HR-CTV: adaptive High Risk Clinical Target Volume of the primary tumor.
- IR-CTV: intermediate Risk Clinical Target Volume of the primary tumor.

The following organs are contoured (from at least 2 cm below the IR-CTV to 2 cm above the uterus):

- Bladder: outer bladder wall including the bladder neck.
- Rectum: outer rectal wall from the anal sphincter to the transition into the sigmoid.
- Sigmoid: outer sigmoid wall from the recto-sigmoid flexure to at least 2 cm above the parametria and the uterus.
- Bowel loops: outer contours of loops positioned within 3–4 cm to the uterus and applicator.

For cases with significant vaginal involvement, it is advised also to contour the urethra separately to be able to assess the dose to this structure. There is no specific DVH constraint known so far for urethra and vagina.

2 Endometrial Cancer

Endometrial cancer is the most common gynecologic malignancy and the fourth cancer in women. The majority of endometrial cancer cases occur in postmenopausal patients. Patients are staged according to FIGO staging system (Pecorelli 2009) (Table 2). The standard management of endometrial cancer is surgery, which includes hysterectomy, bilateral salpingo-oophorectomy, and pelvic and/or para-aortic lymph node dissection (Morice et al. 2016). There is no consensus about the necessity of performing extensive lymphadenectomy, because lymphadenectomy is associated with high morbidity. A combination of pre-operative imaging and intra-operative evaluation is

Table 2 Staging of endometrial cancer based on FIGO system

Stage	Description
I	Tumor confined to the corpus uteri
Ia	No or <half myometrial invasion
Ib	Invasion ≥half of the myometrium
II	Tumour invades cervical stroma, but does not extend beyond the uterus
III	Local and/or regional spread of the tumour
IIIa	Tumour invades the serosa of the corpus uteri and/or adnexa
IIIb	Vaginal and/or parametrial involvement
IIIc	Metastases to pelvic and/or para-aortic lymph nodes
IIIc1	Positive pelvic nodes
IIIc2	Positive para-aortic lymph nodes with or without positive pelvic lymph nodes
IV	Tumour invades bladder e/o bowel mucosa, and/or distant metastases
IVa	Tumour invades bladder e/o bowel mucosa
IVb	Distant metastases, including intra-abdominal metastasis and/or inguinal lymph nodes.

Table 3 Risk group classification of endometrial cancer based on ESMO-ESGO-ESTRO Consensus Conference

Risk group	Description
Low	Stage I endometrioid, grade 1–2, <50% MI, LVSI
Intermediate	Stage I endometrioid, grade 1–2, ≥50% MI, LVSI
High-intermediate	– Stage I endometrioid, grade 3, <50% MI, regardless of LVSI status; – Stage I endometrioid, grade 1-2, LVSI unequivocally+, regardless of MI;
High	– Stage I endometrioid, grade 3, ≥50% MI, regardless of LVSI status; – Stage II; – Stage III endometrioid, no residual disease; – Non endometrioid

therefore helpful in determining the optimal surgical strategy (Bell and Pannu 2011) (Table 3). Stratification of patient according to risk factors may guide the surgeon in avoiding unnecessary lymphoadenectomies in low-risk patients. Primary radiotherapy—oftentimes a combination of EBRT and brachytherapy—is reserved for medically inoperable patients (Schwarz et al. 2015).

2.1 Imaging Modalities in Staging

Pre-operative imaging is an essential part of diagnostic work-up in endometrial cancer, and it is important to define adjuvant treatment. MRI and [^{18}F]FDG PET/CT are complementary imaging modality in the initial staging of endometrial cancer.

MRI is the best imaging modalities in staging of endometrial cancer to accurately delineate the local extent of disease. MRI is significantly better than ultrasound or CT in the evaluation of both endocervical tumor extension and myometrial invasion (Kinkel et al. 2009). The MRI protocol includes T2-weighted sequences in the sagittal, axial oblique plane (perpendicular), and coronal oblique plane (parallel) to the uterine cavity and the high-resolution contrast-enhanced T1-weighted sequence. Endometrial carcinoma is usually isointense relative to the normal endometrium on T1-weighted images and hypointense relative to the endometrium on T2-weighted images. The staging accuracy of endometrial carcinoma by MR has been reported to be between 85 and 93% (Manfredi et al. 2004). Contrast-enhanced imaging is suggested for evaluation of deep myometrial invasion and it is especially recommended in presence of atrophic uteri, adenomyosis or fibroids, or in suspected advanced tumors (bladder or rectal wall invasion) (Sala et al. 2007).

A diffusion-weighted imaging is a tool in the assessment of endometrial malignancies, which may potentially aid in the differentiation of benign and malignant conditions of the uterus (Takeuchi et al. 2009). DWI may be used to depict drop metastases in the cervix and vagina and unexpected extra-uterine spread of disease within the adnexa and peritoneum. DWI may also depict endometrial cancer when endometrial biopsy is technically impossible because of cervical stenosis or when histopathologic results are inconclusive.

PET/CT has a limited diagnostic role in local staging of endometrial carcinoma. Physiological uptake of [^{18}F]FDG in the normal endometrium is most likely the cause of suboptimal sensitivity such as the ovulatory and menstrual phases or use of oral contraceptives. Due to limitations of spatial resolution, PET-CT is unlikely to assess the depth of myometrial and cervical stromal invasion and usually performed in patients where surgery is not indicated as the initial treatment choice (high-grade tumor histology, stage IVA and higher) (Fig. 9). For detection of lymph node metastases, PET-CT represents an important preoperative imaging method to differentiate patients that may benefit from lymphoadenectomy. The sensitivity of [^{18}F]FDG PET in detection of lymph node metastases is 63–95% (Chang et al. 2012). Nevertheless, the ability to identify lymph node involvement is affected by lymph node size: Kitajima et al. reported a sensitivity of 66.7% for lymph node between 5 and 9 mm and 16.7% for lymph node smaller than 5 mm (Kitajima et al. 2009). Similarly, in a study performed by Park et al. PET-CT was unable to detect lymph node <1 cm in diameter (Park et al. 2017). The

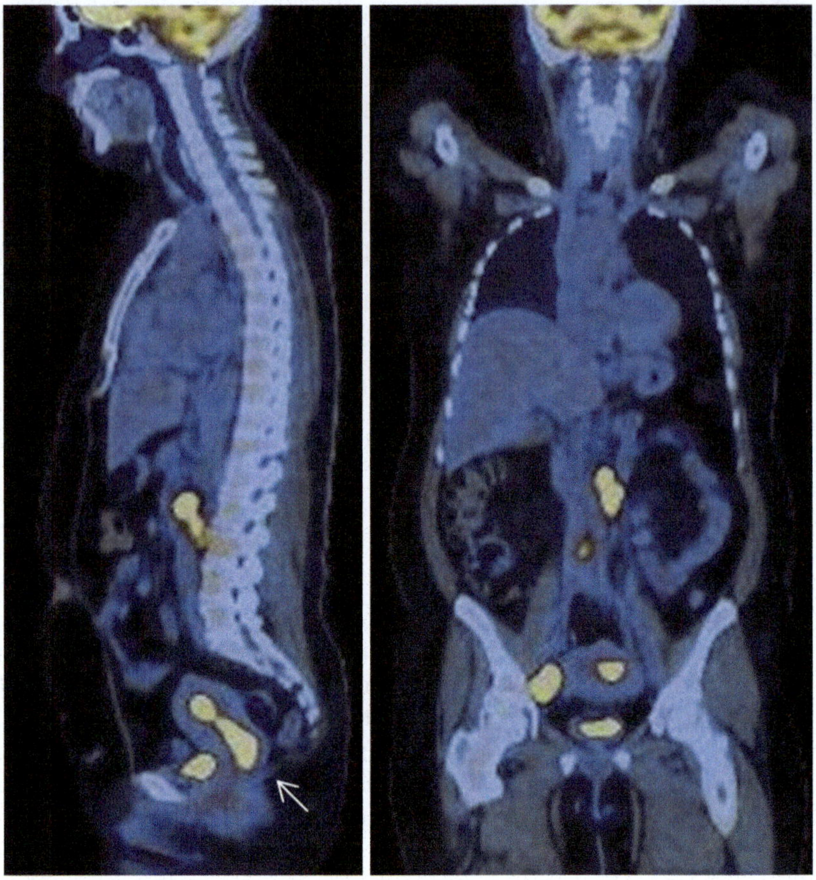

Fig. 9 Endometrial cancer (FIGO IV). Sagittal and coronal fused PET-CT images show intense [^{18}F]FDG uptake in endometrial cancer (white arrow) and [^{18}F]FDG-avid iliac and para-aortic lymph nodes

potential role of metabolic tumor parameters for predicting clinical outcome in endometrial cancer has been investigated. Several studies reported that high tumor SUVmax, SUVmean, metabolic tumor volume (MTV), and total lesion glycolysis (TLG) are prognostic factors of myometrial and cervical stromal invasion, lymph nodes metastases, and poor prognosis in endometrial cancer (Kitajima et al. 2015; Ghooshkhanei et al. 2014). Integrated PET/MRI has a potentially role in the planning of radiation therapy due high-resolution delineation of tumor obtained by the combination of both modalities into a single scan.

2.2 Target Volume Definition

Surgery is the therapeutic approach of choice in endometrial cancer; however, in patients who do not fit for surgery due to general medical conditions, such as obesity, high blood pressure, diabetes mellitus, and/or advanced age, radiation therapy is a good option in both early and advanced stages. It is recommended that an evaluation of the lymph nodes with CT or PET/CT as well as the use of MRI, whenever possible, will accurately determine the degree of myometrial infiltration.

Patients with stage I disease, grade I, can be treated with intracavitary BT alone. Patients with stage II, III, and IV (confined to the pelvis) should receive EBRT and intracavitary BT.

It was demonstrated that for patients with nonoperable endometrial cancer, the combined overall survival (OS) at 5 years is 53.2% and, even more important, the local control rate of the disease by using radiotherapy alone achieves 79.9% at 5 years (van der Steen-Banasik et al. 2016).

However, radiation therapy is more commonly employed as adjuvant setting (EBRT and/or BT, ±CHT). It is widely used dependent upon the individual risk factors, which include histological subtype, grading, lymphovascular space invasion (LVSI), myometrial invasion (MI), cervical invasion (CI), tumor size, and lymph node metastases (Pecorelli 2009).

To guide the choice of adjuvant therapy, patients should be stratified into risk groups (Table 3) based on European Society of Medical Oncology (ESMO) clinical practice guidelines (Koh et al. 2016). The first joint ESMO, European Society for Radiotherapy & Oncology (ESTRO), and European Society of Gynecological Oncology (ESGO) consensus conference on endometrial cancer addresses clinically relevant questions regarding adjuvant therapy and management of advanced/recurrent endometrial cancer. Currently, radiation oncologists employ several atlases for the definition, on treatment planning CT, of target volume for pelvic radiation in postoperative gynecologic malignancies (Small Jr et al. 2008). In general, CTV should include the common, external, and internal iliac lymph node regions, as well as the upper 3.0 cm of the vagina and paravaginal soft tissue lateral to the vagina. For patients with endometrial cancer with cervical stromal invasion, the presacral lymph node region should be included (Table 4). The CTV was defined by adding a 7 mm margin around the vasculature, based on research by Taylor et al. (2005) and extending it to include lymphoceles or surgical clips. The CTV was modified to exclude vertebral bodies and muscle and to limit the dose to the bowel. The major potential advantage of IGRT/IMRT, in the treatment of postoperative endometrial carcinomas, is not only the ability to more adequately cover the target volume but also the capability to shape a dose distribution that delivers a lower dose to intraperitoneal organs (i.e., small and large bowel), close to pelvic lymph nodes and other areas at risk (Mundt et al. 2002). Furthermore, IMRT has been shown to reduce normal tissue dose and is associated with decreased acute and chronic toxicity compared with conventional treatment (Mundt et al. 2003). Referring to adjuvant vaginal BT, in 2012, the American Brachytherapy Society (ABS) published recommendations for the treatment after surgical management of endometrial cancer: HDR is the most common delivery method; usual prescription for VBT alone is 7 Gy × 3 fractions generally at 0.5 cm depth; when combined with EBRT, the most common prescription is 5–5.5 Gy × 3 fractions generally at 0.5 cm depth (Harkenrider et al. 2014).

Table 4 CTV for adjuvant radiotherapy for endometrial cancer

Target site (CTV)	Definition
Common iliac lymph nodes	From 7 mm below L4–L5 interspace to level of bifurcation of common iliac arteries into external and internal iliac arteries
External iliac lymph nodes	From level of bifurcation of common iliac artery into external artery to level of superior aspect of femoral head where it becomes femoral artery
Internal iliac lymph nodes	From level of bifurcation of common iliac artery into internal artery, along its branches (obturator, hypogastric) terminating in paravaginal tissues at level of vaginal cuff
Upper vagina	Vaginal cuff and 3 cm of vagina inferior to cuff
Parametrial/ paravaginal tissue	From vaginal cuff to medial edge of internal obturator muscle/ischial ramus on each side
Presacral lymph nodes (If patient has endometrial cancer with cervical stromal invasion)	Lymph node region anterior to S1and S2 region

3 Ovarian Cancer

Ovarian cancer is the second most common gynecologic malignancy but it has the highest mortality mostly because it is usually diagnosed at a late stage. Primary cytoreductive surgery followed by chemotherapy is the treatment of choice for advanced ovarian cancer (du Bois et al. 2004).

Survival depends primarily on the success of the initial surgical procedure and residual disease after intervention is the most important prognostic factor in these patients (Elattar et al. 2011). In this setting, the evaluation of disease spread is essential to optimize surgery and to identify patients who may benefit from neo-adjuvant treatment (Rizzo et al. 2013).

3.1 Imaging Modalities in Staging

The ovarian cancer usually presents as unilateral or bilateral adnexal complex cystic masses; advanced stages are associated with pelvic organic invasion ascites and peritoneal carcinomatosis.

Ultrasound is usually the initial imaging modality for detection and characterization of adnexal masses and pelvic ascite. Ultrasound relies on morphologic features to distinguish between benign and malignant lesions; features such as thick irregular walls, papillary projections, and solid echogenic locules are considered signs of malignancy (Sassone et al. 1991; Ferrazzi et al. 1997).

MRI remains a problem-solving imaging modality after inconclusive ultrasound findings (Javadi et al. 2016; Forstner 2007). The addition of DWI sequences to gadolinium-enhanced MRI may improve the accuracy of tumor detection, especially for the assessment of mesentery, serosa of the small bowel and colon, and pelvis (surface of the uterus and bladder) and may also help to detect very small malignant deposits (Hricak et al. 2000).

CT provides clinically relevant information including size of the primary tumor, size and location of any peritoneal implants, lymph nodes, and it is essential to detect the presence of difficult-to-reach sites such as extra-abdominal lesions, porta hepatis, or mesenteric root lymph nodes, According to the ESUR guidelines (Forstner et al. 2010), CT should be extended from the distal thorax to the inguinal region. Inclusion of the lung bases in the field of view is recommended because this enables assessment of cardiophrenic lymph nodes and pleural effusion (Holloway et al. 1997). The most important limitation of CT is its inability to reliably depict implants with a maximal diameter of less than 5 mm on the bowel serosa, mesentery, or peritoneum, especially in the absence of ascites.

PET/CT has a low diagnostic value to characterize annessial masses because [^{18}F]FDG uptake may occur in ovaries of premenopausal women, endometriosis, pelvic inflammation, and benign cystic lesions. In addition, false negative results on PET/CT may occur in low grade or early tumors. Furthermore, some histological subtypes, in particular mucinous tumors and germ cell carcinoma, generally show low [^{18}F]FDG avidity (Tanizaki et al. 2014). However, PET/CT may play an important contribution in nodal staging also for evaluation of normal-sized lymph nodes involvement including those in the para-aortic, mediastinal, and supraclavicular regions. A meta-analysis by Yuan et al. reported that PET/CT is more accurate in detecting lymph node metastasis (sensitivity 64.1%, specificity 94.5%) than CT (sensitivity 42.6%, specificity of 95.0%) or MRI (sensitivity 54.7%, specificity 88.3%) (Yuan et al. 2012). PET/CT shows a higher detection rate of mesenteric tumor spread and subdiaphragmatic peritoneal disease compared to CT; false negative results may occur in case of peritoneal small tumor dissemination, with nodules smaller than 5 mm (De Iaco et al. 2011). [^{18}F]FDG PET-CT is essential for detecting recurrent disease, particularly in the setting of negative imaging findings but increasing tumor markers (Yoshida et al. 2004; Funicelli et al. 2010).

3.2 Target Volume Definition

Radiation therapy in ovarian cancers has been considered an outdated concept for many years, mainly due to its toxicity and failure to show benefit in terms of survival. Although there is no worldwide consensus, EBRT could be taken into consideration for nonserous variants (clear cell, endometrioid, and mucinous), intermediate risk patients (stage I, II, and stage III disease with grades 1, 2, and 3, but no residual disease postsurgery), stage II and stage III disease (with residuum less than 2 cm in diameter and confined to the pelvis), and recurrent disease (less than 2 cm in diameter and confined to the pelvis). Furthermore, EBRT (also as stereotactic modality) may be used in palliation of symptoms that cannot be treated by CHT alone (Rai et al. 2014).

4 Vaginal Cancer

Vaginal cancer is rare, representing only 2–3% of female genital tract malignancies (Hacker et al. 2015). The majority of primary vaginal cancers are squamous cell carcinoma (SCC) and the peak incidence occurs in the sixth and seventh decades of life. Adenocarcinomas and other histologists are more common in younger patients. Risk factors include older age and human papilloma virus infection. Vaginal cancer is most often diagnosed clinically. Staging is performed clinically according to the FIGO stage system (Table 5).

Table 5 Stage-based management of vaginal cancer

Stage	Description	Treatment
I	Tumor is confined to the vaginal wall	Surgical management ± adjuvant EBRT *or* primary EBRT with BT
II	Tumor involves sub-vaginal tissue but does not extend to the pelvic sidewall	EBRT ± BT ± CHT *or* Surgical management ± adjuvant EBRT
III	Tumor extends to the pelvic sidewall	EBRT ± BT ± CHT
IV		
IVa IVb	Tumor invades bladder or rectal mucosa or there is direct extension beyond the true pelvis Spread to distant organs	EBRT ± BT ± CHT *or* Pelvic exenteration ± EBRT ± chemotherapy Supportive care ± palliative CHT or EBRT

4.1 Imaging Modalities in Staging

Besides the standard procedures, such as gynecological examinations and biopsy, imaging modalities are not routinely recommended. The use of advanced imaging modalities such as CT, MRI, and PET-CT may be used to guide therapy, but it cannot reassign the stage. MRI can be useful in delineating tumor size and extent. At MRI imaging, vaginal tumors, and mostly squamous cell carcinomas, are best seen with T2-weighted sequences where they appear as a mass of homogeneous intermediate signal unlike the low signal intensity of the vaginal wall (Fig. 10). The presence of high-signal-intensity foci represents tumoral necrosis. At T1-weighted imaging, squamous cell carcinoma appears as an isointense to muscle lesion, and its presence can be appreciated only when the lesion is large enough to alter the vaginal contour. On DWI sequences, tumors show restricted diffusion. Fat saturades T2-weighted images and contrast-enhanced sequences are used for assessment of local invasion.

Limited data are available on the utility of [^{18}F]FDG PET/CT in vaginal cancer, but the modality appears to be of value in staging disease to detecting nodal and distant metastases. CT may be used to delineate the disease extent and evaluate nodal and distant metastatic spread although its sensitivity is lower compared to MRI and PET/CT. CT is primarily used for three-dimensional (3D) conformal treatment planning for radiotherapy delivery (Lee et al. 2013).

4.2 Target Volume Definition

Unlike cervical and endometrial cancer, no consensus guidelines currently exist regarding target delineation or treatment planning in vaginal cancer patients undergoing EBRT. Given the rarity of this disease, it is unlikely that such guidelines will ever be produced. In general, it is useful to delineate GTV and two CTV (Table 6). OARs include bowel, bladder, and rectum. In patients with involvement of the lower one-third of the vagina undergoing pelvic-inguinal IMRT, the

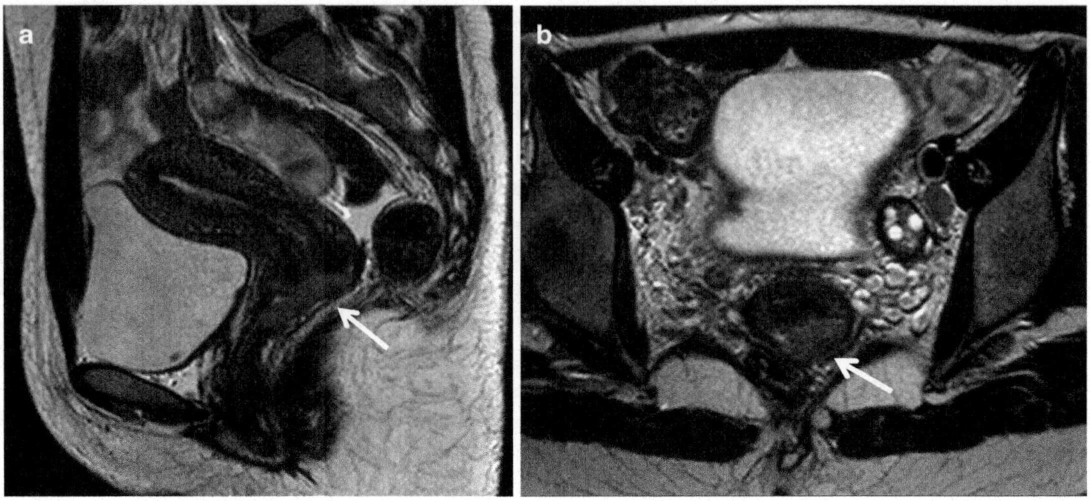

Fig. 10 Vaginal cancer. Sagittal and axial T2-weighted MRI images demonstrate tumor confined to the higher third of vagina

Table 6 Suggested target volumes for vaginal cancer

Target volumes	Description
GTV	Primary tumor de fined on CT/MRI and clinical examination
CTV_1	GTV plus a minimum of 3 cm of vagina superiorly and inferiorly
CTV_2	Paravaginal/parametrial tissues adjacent to CTV_1 and full vagina length PLUS pelvic lymph nodes (common iliac, external and internal iliac and presacral) if the cancer is limited to the upper two-thirds of the vagina: AND/OR bilateral inguinofemoral lymph nodes if the cancer involved the lower one-third of the vagina:
BT boost	
HR-CTV	For MRI-based planning: GTV, as well as the gray zones on MRI and the adjacent vaginal circumference at the level of the residual tumor (Dimopoulos et al. 2012) For CT-based planning: GTV demarcated by the placement of fiducial markers
IR-CTV	Initial GTV + the full vaginal length (given the risk of submucosal spread through the vaginal lymphatics) (Dimopoulos et al. 2012)

bilateral femoral heads and anus should also be included. All patients with locally advanced disease should receive a combination of EBRT and BT. The type of BT is dependent on disease extent, with intracavitary BT used for superficially invasive disease (<0.5 cm invasion) and interstitial BT for all other tumors. Chemotherapy is administered concomitantly at many centers in an attempt to augment patient outcomes (Frank et al. 2005).

5 Vulvar Cancer

Vulvar carcinoma is rare, accounting for 5–8% of gynecological malignancies (Stehman and Look 2006). Risk factors include age, lichen sclerosus, human papilloma virus infection, and vulvar intraepithelial neoplasia. Approximately 85% of cases of vulvar cancer are squamous cell carcinoma. Other histologic types include melanoma, Bartholin gland cancer, basal cell carcinoma, Paget disease, and adenocarcinoma. Vulvar carcinoma is diagnosed clinically according to FIGO classification system (Pecorelli 2009). In the early stage of disease (FIGO stage I), the role of imaging is limited. For locally advanced vulvar

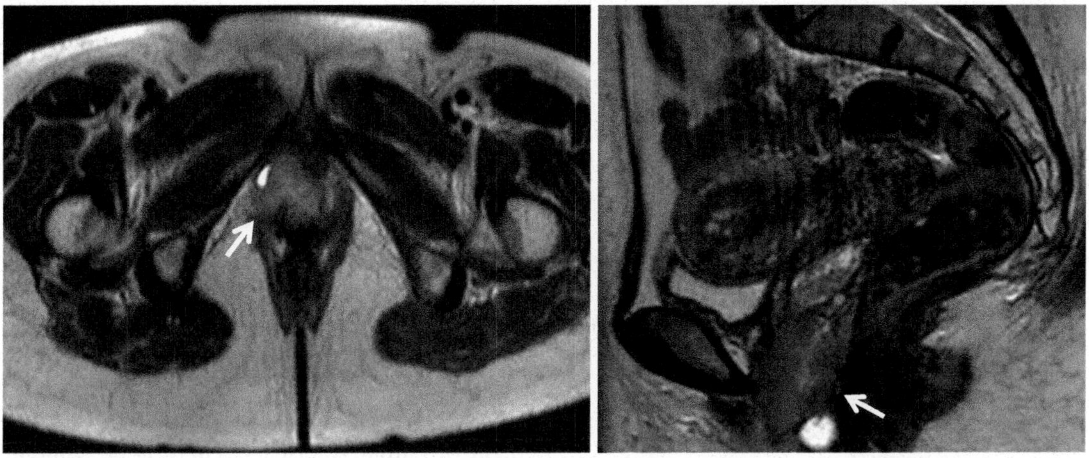

Fig. 11 Vulva cancer. Axial and sagittal T2 MRI images show vulvar tumor (white arrow) invading right para-vaginal tissues without pelvic wall extension

carcinomas (FIGO stages II and IVA), pretreatment imaging may be useful to evaluate the extent of local disease and distant metastases.

5.1 Imaging Modalities in Staging

MRI in locally advanced vulvar carcinomas is the main imaging modality to determine the involvement of adjacent structures (anal sphincter, urethra, or vaginal wall) and hence assisting surgical or radiotherapy planning. The MRI sequences generally used for vulvar lesions are T1-weighted, T2-weighted, fat- suppressed T1-weighted, and contrast-enhanced fat-suppressed T1-weighted imaging. On MRI, vulvar cancers appear as a solid mass with nonspecific low signal intensity on T1-weighted images and moderate-to-high signal intensity on T2-weighted images. Thin-section high-resolution T2-weighted sagittal and oblique axial images provide anatomic detail and tumor definition (Fig. 11). Fat-saturated T2-weighted images DWI and contrast-enhanced sequences are useful for assessment of local invasion.

CT of the abdomen and pelvis is routinely performed to evaluate for lymph node involvement and distant metastasis when tumor is larger than 2 cm. As regards PET/CT, vulvar carcinoma is usually an [^{18}F]FDG-avid cancer but the intense physiologic radiotracer activity within a urine-filled bladder may obscure and/or overestimate the degree of vulvar involvement. PET/CT may be performed for detection of lymph node involvement with sensitivity and specificity of 80% and 90%, respectively (Cohn et al. 2002).

5.2 Target Volume Definition

The standard treatment for vulvar squamous cell carcinoma (SCC) is surgery. External beam radiotherapy (EBRT), brachytherapy (BT), and chemotherapy are either adjuvant or definitive treatment options. Over the last two decades, the use of primary radiotherapy for patients at stage III-IVA vulvar cancer increased by 10–20% in women with early-stage disease, and 50–70% in advanced stages may return within 2 years after the primary treatment, and most of the recurrences are local. Loco-regional failure is an important risk factor for distant metastatic disease (Kellas-Ślęczka et al. 2016; Micheletti and Preti 2014). In regard to EBRT, in order to assist in delineation of the tumor, radiopaque wire is used to identify areas of gross disease or the postoperative tumor bed and a tailored bolus of 0.5–1 cm thickness is usually created for the

Table 7 Suggested target volumes and dose schemes for vulvar cancer

Target volume	Description	Dose schemes
GTV	Macroscopic disease, pathological nodes	**Adjuvant:** 50.4–59.4 (1.8 daily) **Radical**: 59.4–70.2 (1.8 daily)
CTV	GTV + 1 cm (including entire vulvar region, excluding anal sphincter) – The mons pubis could be excluded if it is not involved and/or the lesion is posterior – For posterior vulvar lesions: CTV includes perineum and if it is involved: • Anal verge: anal verge + 1–2 cm margin • Anal canal: entire mesorectum – For anterior periurethral lesion or to the bladder: 2 cm of urethra proximal to primary GTV **AND** Inguinal-femoral and pelvic lymph nodes (bilateral obturator and external and internal iliac) to the bifurcation of the external and internal iliac vessel **PLUS** Entire common iliac chain to the aortic bifurcation if pelvic node positive	**Adjuvant**: 45–50.4 (1.8 daily) **Radical**: 45–50.4 (1.8 daily)

vulvar region (at the time of treatment planning and is used for daily treatments) to remove the skin-sparing *effect* of a megavoltage X-ray beam. In Table 7, we summarize the target volumes and the suggested dose fractionation schemes used for vulvar cancer (Table 7). For organs at risk (OARs), we advocate contouring the anorectum (from the anal verge to rectosigmoid junction) the entire bladder, small bowel (from the rectosigmoid junction to 1–2 cm above the final CTV) femoral heads (to level of the lesser trochanter). Literature data suggested, in case of concurrent chemotherapy, to contour also the pelvic bone marrow including the lower lumbar spine, iliac, sacrum, and femoral heads. BT is an optimal treatment option for primary and recurrent carcinomas of the vulva: It allows the delivery of a very high radiation dose to the tumor while sparing OARs, and it is especially important for cases where the tumor is located close to dose-limiting organs. Interstitial BT in primary advanced disease allowed the achievement of palliative effects. There is no standard treatment schedule in BT and it is difficult to compare doses between the published studies because of the insufficient homogeneity of the groups, but in the available literature, doses range between 30 and 42 Gy as exclusive treatment.

References

Akita A, Shinmoto H, Hayashi S (2011) Comparison of T2-weighted and contrast enhanced T1-weighted MR imaging at 1.5 T for assessing the local extent of cervical carcinoma. Eur Radiol 21:1850–1857

Balleyguier C, Sala E, Da Cunha T et al (2011) Staging of uterine cervical cancer with MRI: guidelines of the European Society of Urogenital Radiology. Eur Radiol 21:1102–1110

Bell DJ, Pannu HK (2011) Radiological assessment of gynecologic malignancies. Obstet Gynecol Clin N Am 38(1):45–68

Bentivegna E, Uzan C, Gouy S, Leboulleux S, Duvillard P, Lumbroso J et al (2010) Correlation between [18f] fluorodeoxyglucose positron-emission tomography scan and histology of pelvic nodes in early-stage cervical cancer. Anticancer Res 30(3):1029–1032

Chang MC, Chen JH, Liang JA et al (2012) 18F FDG PET or PET-CT for detection metastatic lymph nodes in patients with endometrial cancer: a systematic review and meta-analysis. Eur J Radiol 81:3511–3517

Choi HJ, Ju W, Myung SK, Kim Y (2010) Diagnostic performance of computer tomography, magnetic resonance imaging, and positron emission tomography or positron emission tomography/computer tomography for detection of metastatic lymph nodes in patients with cervical cancer: Meta-analysis. Cancer Sci 101(6):1471–1479

Chung HH, Kang KW, Cho JY, Kim JW, Park NH, Song YS, Kim SH, Chung JK, Kang SB (2010) Role of magnetic resonance imaging and positron emission tomography/computed tomography in preoperative lymph node detection of uterine cervical cancer. Am J Obstet Gynecol 203(2):156

Cohn DE, Dehdashti F, Gibb RK, Mutch DG, Rader JS, Siegel BA, Herzog TJ (2002) Prospective evaluation of positron emission tomography for the detection of groin node metastases from vulvar cancer. Gynecol Oncol 85(1):179 84

Colombo N, Carinelli S, Colombo A, Marini C, Rollo D, Sessa C (2012) Cervical cancer: ESMO Clinical Practice Guidelines for diagnosis treatment and follow-up. Ann Oncol 23(Suppl 7):vii27–vii32

De Iaco P, Musto A, Orazi L, Zamagni C, Rosati M, Allegri V et al (2011) FDG-PET/CT in advanced ovarian cancer staging: value and pitfalls in detecting lesions in different abdominal and pelvic quadrants compared with laparoscopy. Eur J Radiol 80:e98–e103

Dimopoulos JC, Petrow P, Tanderup K, Petric P, Berger D, Kirisits C, Pedersen EM, van Limbergen E, Haie-Meder C, Pötter R (2012) Recommendations from Gynaecological (GYN) GEC-ESTRO Working Group (IV): basic principles and parameters for MR imaging within the frame of image based adaptive cervix cancer brachytherapy. Radiother Oncol 103(1):113–122

du Bois A, Quinn M, Thigpen T et al (2005) 2004 consensus statements on the management of ovarian cancer: final document of the 3rd International Gynecologic Cancer Intergroup Ovarian Cancer Consensus Conference (GCIG OCCC 2004). Ann Oncol 16(Suppl 8):viii7–viii12

Elattar A, Bryant A, Winter-Roach BA, Hatem M, Naik R (2011) Optimal primary surgical treatment for advanced epithelial ovarian cancer. Cochrane Database Syst Rev 10(8):CD007565

Esthappan J, Chaudhari S, Santanam L, Mutic S, Olsen J, Macdonald DM, Low DA, Singh AK, Grigsby PW (2008) Prospective clinical trial of positron emission tomography/computed tomography image-guided intensity-modulated radiation therapy for cervical carcinoma with positive para-aortic lymph nodes. Int J Radiat Oncol Biol Phys 72(4):1134–1139

Ferlay J, Soerjomataram I, Dikshit R, Eser S, Mathers C, Rebelo M, Parkin DM, Forman D, Bray F (2015) Cancer incidence and mortality worldwide: sources, methods and major patterns in GLOBOCAN 2012. Int J Cancer 136(5):E359–E386

Ferrazzi E, Zanetta G, Dordoni D, Berlanda N, Mezzopane R, Lissoni AA (1997) Transvaginal ultrasonographic characterization of ovarian masses: comparison of five scoring systems in a multicenter study. Ultrasound Obstet Gynecol 10(3):192–197

FIGO Committed on Gynecologic Oncology (FCoG) (2014) FIGO staging for carcinoma of the vulva, cervix, and corpus uteri. Int J Gynaecol Obstet 125(2):97–98

Forstner R (2007) Radiological staging of ovarian cancer: imaging findings and contribution of CT and MRI. Eur Radiol 17:3223–3235

Forstner R, Sala E, Kinkel K, Spencer JA (2010) European Society of Urogenital Radiology. ESUR guidelines: ovarian cancer staging and follow-up. Eur Radiol 20:2773–2780

Frank SJ, Jhingran A, Levenback C, Eifel PJ (2005) Definitive radiation therapy for squamous cell carcinoma of the vagina. Int J Radiat Oncol Biol Phys 62(1):138–147

Funicelli L, Travaini LL, Landoni F, Trifiro G, Bonello L, Bellomi M (2010) Peritoneal carcinomatosis from ovarian cancer: the role of CT and [(18) F] FDG-PET/CT. Abdom Imaging 35:701–707

Ghooshkhanei H, Treglia G, Sabouri G, Davoodi R, Sadeghi R (2014 Mar) Risk stratification and prognosis determination using (18)F-FDG PET imaging in endometrial cancer patients: a systematic review and meta-analysis. Gynecol Oncol 132(3):669–676

Grigsby PW (2009) PET/CT imaging to guide cervical cancer therapy. Future Oncol 5(7):953–958

Hacker NF, Eifel PJ, van der Velden J (2015) Cancer of the vagina. Int J Gynaecol Obstet 131(Suppl 2): S84–S87

Harkenrider M, Erickson B, Viswanathan A, Grover S, Small W (2014) Preliminary results of the American Brachytherapy Society survey of practice patterns for vaginal brachytherapy for postoperative endometrial cancer. Int J Radiat Oncol Biol Phys 90:S110

Hawighorst H (1999) Dynamic MR imaging in cervical carcinoma. Radiology 213:617–618

Hellebust TP, Kirisits C, Berger D, Pérez-Calatayud J, De Brabandere M, De Leeuw A, Dumas I, Hudej R, Lowe G, Wills R, Tanderup K, Gynaecologica(GYN)GEC-ESTRO Working Group (2010) Recommendations from Gynaecological (GYN) GEC-ESTRO Working Group: considerations and pitfalls in commissioning and applicator reconstruction in 3D image-based treatment planning of cervix cancer brachytherapy. Radiother Oncol 96(2):153–160

Hofmann W, Arvela HS, Harley NH, Marsh JW, McLaughlin J, Röttger A, Tokonami S (2012) J Int Comm Radiat Units Measurement Rep 88 12(2). (published December 2015)

Holloway BJ, Gore ME, A_Hern RP, Parsons C (1997) The significante of paracardiac lymph node enlargement in ovarian cancer. Clin Radiol 52:692–697

Hricak H, Chen M, Coakley FV, Kinkel K, Yu KK, Sica G, Bacchetti P, Powell CB (2000) Complex adnexal masses: detection and characterization with MR imaging—multivariate analysis. Radiology 214(1):39–46

Javadi S, Ganeshan DM, Qayyum A, Iyer RB, Bhosale P (2016) Ovarian Cancer, the revised FIGO staging system, and the role of imaging. AJR 206:1351–1360

Kaur H, Silverman PM, Iyer RB, Verschraegen CF, Eifel PJ, Charnsangavej C (2003) Diagnosis, staging, and surveillance of cervical carcinoma. AJR Am J Roentgenol 180:1621–1631

Kellas-Ślęczka S, Białas B, Fijałkowski M, Wojcieszek P, Szlag M, Cholewka A, Ślęczka M, Kołosza Z (2016) Interstitial high-dose-rate brachytherapy in locally advanced and recurrent vulvar cancer. J Contemp Brachyther 8(1):32–40

Kidd EA, Spencer CR, Huettner PC, Siegel BA, Dehdashti F, Rader JS, Grigsby PW (2009 Aug 1) Cervical cancer histology and tumor differentiation affect 18F-fluorodeoxyglucose uptake. Cancer 115(15):3548–3554

Kinkel K, Forstner R, Danza FM et al (2009) Staging of endometrial cancer with MRI: guidelines of the European Society of Urogenital Imaging. Eur Radiol 19:1565–1574

Kitajima K, Murakami K, Yamasaki E, Kaji Y, Sugimura K (2009) Accuracy of integrated FDG-PET/contrast-enhanced CT in detecting pelvic and para-aortic lymph node metastasis in patients with uterine cancer. Eur Radiol 19(6):1529–1536

Kitajima K, Suenaga Y, Ueno Y, Maeda T, Ebina Y, Yamada H, Okunaga T, Kubo K, Sofue K, Kanda T, Tamaki Y, Sugimura K (2015 Jul) Preoperative risk stratification using metabolic parameters of (18) F-FDG PET/CT in patients with endometrial cancer. Eur J Nucl Med Mol Imaging 42(8):1268–1275

Koh WJ, Greer BE, Abu-Rustum NR, Apte SM, Campos SM, Cho KR, Chu C, Cohn D, Crispens MA, Dorigo O, Eifel PJ, Fisher CM, Frederick P, Gaffney DK, Han E, Huh WK, Lurain JR 3rd, Mutch D, Fader AN, Remmenga SW, Reynolds RK, Teng N, Tillmanns T, Valea FA, Yashar CM, NR MM, Scavone JL (2016) Cervical cancer, Vers 1.2017. J Natl Compr Canc Netw 13(4):395–404; quiz 404

Lee LJ, Jhingran A, Kidd E, Cardenes HR, Elshaikh MA, Erickson B, Mayr NA, Moore D, Puthawala AA, Rao GG, Small W Jr, Varia MA, Wahl AO, Wolfson AH, Yashar CM, Yuh W, Gaffney DK (2013) Acr appropriateness criteria management of vaginal cancer. Oncology (Williston Park) 27(11):1166–1173

Manfredi R, Mirk P, Maresca G, Margariti PA, Testa A, Zannoni GF, Giordano D, Scambia G, Marano P (2004) Local-regional staging of endometrial carcinoma: role of MR imaging in surgical planning. Radiology 231(2):372–378

Micheletti L, Preti M (2014) Surgery of the vulva in vulvar cancer. Best Pract Res Clin Obstet Gynaecol 28:1074–1087

Morice P, Leary A, Creutzberg C, Abu-Rustum N, Darai E (2016) Endometrial cancer. Lancet 387(10023):1094–1108

Mundt AJ, Lujan AE, Rotmensch J et al (2002) Intensity-modulated whole pelvic radiotherapy in women with gynecologic malignancies. Int J Radiat Oncol Biol Phys 52:1330–1337

Mundt AJ, Mell LK, Roeske JC (2003) Analysis of chronic gastrointestinal toxicity in gynaecologic patients treated with intensity-modulated whole pelvic radiation therapy. Int J Radiat Oncol Biol Phys 56:1354–1360

Nicolet V, Carignan L, Bourdon F, Prosmanne O (2000) MR imaging of cervical carcinoma: a practical staging approach. Radiographics 20(6):1539–1549

Nie J, Zhang J, Gao J, Guo L, Zhou H, Hu Y, Zhu C, Li Q, Ma X (2017) Diagnostic role of 18F-FDG PET/MRI in patients with gynecological malignancies of the pelvis: a systematic review and meta-analysis. PLoS One 12(5):e0175401

Ohliger MA, Hope TA, Chapman JS, Chen LM, Behr SC, Poder L (2017) PET/MR imaging in gynecologic oncology. Magn Reson Imaging Clin N Am 25(3):667–684

Okamoto Y, Tanaka YO, Nishida M, Tsunoda H, Yoshikawa H, Itai Y (2003) MR imaging of the uterine cervix: imaging-pathologic correlation. Radiographics 23(2):425–445

Park JY, Lee JJ, Choi HJ, Song IH, Sung CO, Kim HO, Chae SY, Kim YT, Nam JH (2017) The value of preoperative positron emission tomography/computed tomography in node-negative endometrial cancer on magnetic resonance imaging. Ann Surg Oncol 24(8):2303–2310

Pecorelli S (2009) Revised FIGO staging for carcinoma of the vulva, cervix, and endometrium. Int J Gynaecol Obstet 105(2):103–104

Pötter R, Haie-Meder C, Van Limbergen E, Barillot I, De Brabandere M, Dimopoulos J, Dumas I, Erickson B, Lang S, Nulens A, Petrow P, Rownd J, Kirisits C, GEC ESTRO Working Group (2006) Recommendations from gynaecological (GYN) GEC ESTRO working group (II): concepts and terms in 3D image-based treatment planning in cervix cancer brachytherapy-3D dose volume parameters and aspects of 3D image-based anatomy, radiation physics, radiobiology. Radiother Oncol 78(1):67–77

Rai B, Bansal A, Patel FD, Sharma SC (2014) Radiotherapy for ovarian cancers—redefining the role. Asian Pac J Cancer Prev 15(12):4759–4763

Rizzo S, Calareso G, De Maria F, Zanagnolo V, Lazzari R, Cecconi A, Bellomi M (2013) Gynecologic tumors: how to communicate imaging results to the surgeon. Cancer Imaging 13(4):611–625

Sala E, Wakely S, Senior E, Lomas D (2007) MRI of malignant neoplasms of the uterine corpus and cervix. AJR Am J Roentgenol 188(6):1577–1587

Sassone AM, Timor-Tritsch IE, Artner A, Westhoff C, Warren WB (1991) Transvaginal sonographic characterization of ovarian disease: evaluation of a new scoring system to predict ovarian malignancy. Obstet Gynecol 78:70–76

Scheidler J, Hricak H, Yu KK, Subak L, Segal MR (1997) Radiological evaluation of lymph node metastases in patients with cervical cancer. A meta-analysis. JAMA 278:1096–1101

Schwarz JK, Beriwal S, Esthappan J, Erickson B, Feltmate C, Fyles A, Gaffney D, Jones E, Klopp A, Small W Jr, Thomadsen B, Yashar C, Viswanathan A (2015) Consensus statement for brachytherapy for the treatment of medically inoperable endometrial cancer. Brachytherapy 14(5):587

Signorelli M, Guerra L, Montanelli L, Crivellaro C, Buda A, Dell'Anna T et al (2011) Preoperative staging of cervical cancer: is 18-FDG-PET/CT really effective in patients with early stage disease? Gynecol Oncol 123(2):236–240

Small W Jr, Mell LK, Anderson P et al (2008) Consensus guidelines for delineation of clinical target volume for intensity-modulated pelvic radiotherapy in postoperative treatment of endometrial and cervical cancer. Int J Radiat Oncol Biol Phys 71:428–3453

Stehman FB, Look KY (2006) Carcinoma of the vulva. Obstet Gynecol 107(3):719–733

Takeuchi M, Matsuzaki K, Nishitani H (2009) Diffusion-weighted magnetic resonance imaging of endometrial cancer: differentiation from benign endometrial lesions and preoperative assessment of myometrial invasion. Acta Radiol 50:947–953

Tanizaki Y, Kobayashi A, Shiro M, Ota N, Takano R, Mabuchi Y et al (2014) Diagnostic value of preoperative SUVmax on FDG-PET/CT for the detection of ovarian cancer. Int J Gynecol Cancer 24:454–460

Taylor A, Rockall AG, Reznek RH et al (2005) Mapping pelvic lymph nodes: guidelines for delineation in intensity-modulated radiotherapy. Int J Radiat Oncol Biol Phys 63:1604–1612

van der Steen-Banasik E et al (2016) On behalf of the European Organisation for Research and Treatment of Cancer, Gynaecological Cancer Group (EORTC-GCG) systemic review: radiation therapy alone in medical non-operable endometrial carcinoma. Eur J Cancer 65:172. 181

Vargo JA, Kim H, Choi S, Sukumvanich P, Olawaiye AB, Kelley JL, Edwards RP, Comerci JT, Beriwal S (2014 Dec 1) Extended field intensity modulated radiation therapy with concomitant boost for lymph node-positive cervical cancer: analysis of regional control and recurrence patterns in the positron emission tomography/computed tomography era. Int J Radiat Oncol Biol Phys 90(5):1091–1098

Verma J, Sulman EP, Jhingran A, Tucker SL, Rauch GM, Eifel PJ, Klopp AH (2014) Dosimetric predictors of duodenal toxicity after intensity modulated radiation therapy for treatment of the para-aortic nodes in gynecologic cancer. Int J Radiat Oncol Biol Phys 88(2):357–362

Wright JD, Dehdashti F, Herzog TJ, Mutch DG, Huettner PC, Rader JS, Gibb RK, Powell MA, Gao F, Siegel BA, Grigsby PW (2005) Preoperative lymph node staging of early-stage cervical carcinoma by [18F]-fluoro-2-deoxy-D-glucose-positron emission tomography. Cancer 104(11):2484–2491

Yagi S, Yahata T, Mabuchi Y, Tanizaki Y, Kobayashi A, Shiro M, Ota N, Minami S, Terada M, Ino K (2016) Primary tumor SUV (max) on preoperative FDG-PET/CT is a prognostic indicator in stage IA2-IIB cervical cancer patients treated with radical hysterectomy. Mol Clin Oncol 5(3):216–222

Yoshida Y, Kurokawa T, Kawahara K et al (2004) Incremental benefits of FDG positron emission tomography over CT alone for the preoperative staging of ovarian cancer. AJR 182:227–233

Yuan Y, Gu ZX, Tao XF, Liu SY (2012) Computer tomography, magnetic resonance imaging, and positron emission tomography or positron emission tomography/computer tomography for detection of metastatic lymph nodes in patients with ovarian cancer: a meta-analysis. Eur J Radiol 81:1002–1006

N-stage Challenges

Jasenko Krdzalic, Michelle Versleijen, and Monique Maas

Contents

1 **Introduction** 275

2 **Imaging-Based Nodal Staging in Oncology** 276

2.1 Cross-Sectional Imaging 276

2.2 Functional Imaging: Positron Emission Tomography (PET-CT) 279

2.3 Ultrasound 279

3 **Nodal Evaluation with Imaging in Common Cancers** 281

3.1 Head and Neck Cancer 281

3.2 Lung Carcinoma 283

3.3 Cervical Cancer 285

3.4 Colorectal Carcinoma 286

3.5 Prostate Carcinoma 287

4 **Post-treatment Imaging of Nodes** 289

5 **Conclusion** 290

References 290

Abstract

Nodal involvement is an important determinant of treatment and prognosis in oncology. Nodal staging is performed with imaging, which comprises of cross-sectional imaging (CT, MRI), ultrasound and functional imaging (PET/CT). In this chapter, nodal staging criteria and pitfalls in nodal imaging for several tumour types are discussed.

1 Introduction

One of the main determinants of treatment and prognosis in cancer is the presence of nodal metastasis. Different imaging modalities play a fundamental role in determining the extent of lymph node involvement. Lymphatic dissemination indicates that the tumour has spread and thus reflects a higher risk for metastases. A higher number of involved nodes and a larger distance of the involved nodes to the primary tumour are both associated with a poorer prognosis (Kim et al. 2011; Detterbeck et al. 2016). Besides the involvement of nodes, it has also been proposed that the number of lymph nodes is predictive of survival (Aan de Stegge et al. 2016). So, assessment of nodes is of utmost importance in oncology.

J. Krdzalic
Department of Radiology, Zuyderland Medical Center, Heerlen, The Netherlands

M. Versleijen
Department of Nuclear Medicine, The Netherlands Cancer Institute—Antoni van Leeuwenhoek, Amsterdam, The Netherlands
e-mail: m.versleijen@nki.nl

M. Maas (✉)
Department of Radiology, The Netherlands Cancer Institute—Antoni van Leeuwenhoek, Amsterdam, The Netherlands
e-mail: m.maas@nki.nl

R. G. H. Beets-Tan et al. (eds.), *Imaging and Interventional Radiology for Radiation Oncology*, Medical Radiology, Diagnostic Imaging, https://doi.org/10.1007/978-3-030-38261-2_17

Traditionally, nodes have been imaged by cross-sectional techniques, and diagnosticians have mainly relied on size criteria. However, from many cancers, we know that size is not a reliable measure for determination of nodal involvement, e.g. in rectal, cervical and prostate cancer (Kim et al. 2011; Harisinghani et al. 2003; Liu et al. 2017). Small-sized nodes can harbour small metastases, while large nodes may be reactive (possibly as part of an immune response) (Wang et al. 2005). When measuring the size, the short axis diameter is most important, as the long axis diameter is variable and often large in healthy lymph nodes (e.g. in inguinal and obturator nodes), which will lead to extensive overstaging if size cut-offs are applied to the long axis diameter. Over time, morphological criteria have been added to the size criteria, which have improved results for nodal staging. Additionally, functional imaging techniques have been implemented in several cancers as a part of standard staging (e.g. PET/CT in lung cancer, head and neck cancer, prostate cancer and cervical cancer among others), improving the nodal staging accuracy even further.

Another important aspect of nodal staging in oncology is the assessment of nodes after treatment. This can be challenging due to the general size decrease of nodes after chemotherapy and/or radiotherapy, which makes the size cut-offs less reliable, but also hampers visual evaluation of nodal morphology due to the small size of nodes.

In this chapter, we will address the imaging modalities used in primary nodal staging and will shortly discuss evaluation of nodes after treatment. Subsequently, cancer types in which nodal staging with imaging is most important will be addressed, including head and neck cancer, lung cancer, colorectal cancer, cervical cancer and prostate cancer.

2 Imaging-Based Nodal Staging in Oncology

Currently, cross-sectional imaging (CT and MRI) and ultrasound are the mostly used modalities for nodal staging. Furthermore, in many cancers, the use of PET/CT is a standard care in the staging process and has proven to be a valuable adjunct for nodal staging. All of the mentioned modalities have their advantages and pitfalls. In this section, the value of the modalities for nodal staging will be discussed, and pitfalls in interpretation will be pointed out.

2.1 Cross-Sectional Imaging

2.1.1 Computed Tomography (CT)

Computed tomography is the mainstay of cancer staging, and almost every patient will undergo a CT with intravenous contrast in order to assess the primary tumour, nodes and metastases. Nodes are very easy to recognize on CT, as the node enhances and is hyperdense and is surrounded by the much more hypodense fat. Nodes normally have an oval shape, but can be very elongated. Specifically in larger nodes (e.g. in the inguinal, but also para-aortic nodes), it is possible to appreciate a fatty centre, consisting of the lymph node hilum (Fig. 1).

The presence of such a fatty hilum is indicative of a benign node. For nodal staging on CT, radiologists can mainly rely on size criteria (short axis diameter). The generally applied size cut-off is a

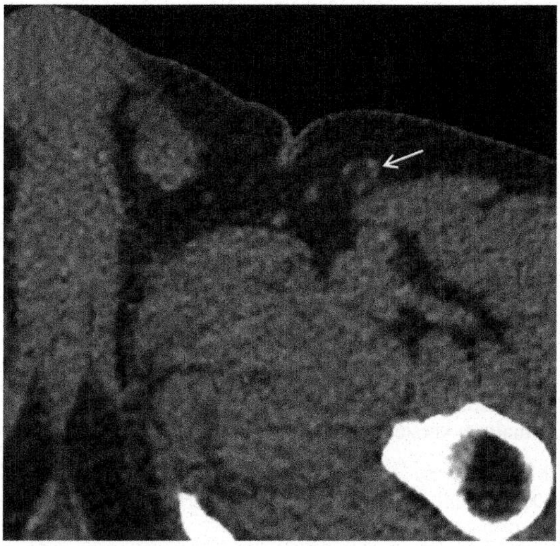

Fig. 1 CT image of an inguinal node (arrow) with a benign aspect. Short axis diameter is less than 10 mm; it has a central fatty hilum and is oval shaped

short-axis diameter of >1 cm to define a malignant node. However, this can differ between tumour types and nodal location. Besides size criteria, morphological criteria can be assessed with CT, but this can be difficult in nodes <1 cm. A clear indication of a malignant node on CT is the presence of necrosis, which makes a node appear heterogeneous with a hypodense centre (not consisting of hypodense fat). Additionally, a round shape, absence of a fatty hilum and irregular border are signs of malignancy in a node (Fig. 2). Also, asymmetrical thickening of the nodal cortex can be a sign of malignancy. These size and morphology criteria generally also apply to the appearance of malignant lymph nodes on MRI.

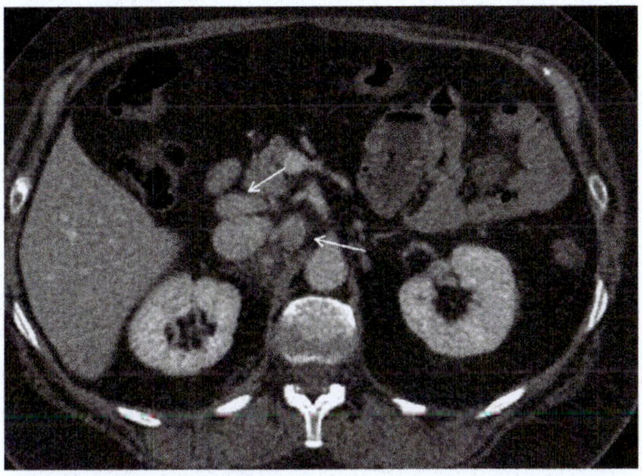

Fig. 2 CT image of enlarged lymph nodes in the upper abdomen (arrows). The short axis diameter is more than 10 mm, there is no fatty hilum and the node between the aorta and caval vein shows an irregular border

Sometimes normal structures and other pathologic processes can mimic abnormal lymph nodes. Normal ovaries can simulate external iliac nodal enlargement (Fig. 3). Also, (aberrant) blood vessels can be mistaken for lymph nodes, especially on non-contrast-enhanced CT. A prominent cisterna chyli can simulate retrocrural nodal enlargement. Peritoneal nodules are sometimes difficult to distinguish from mesenteric or pelvic lymph nodes, and after surgery, lymphoceles can mimic a low attenuation (necrotic) lymph node.

2.1.2 Magnetic Resonance Imaging (MRI)

Many tumour types will be additionally staged by other modalities than CT. MRI is often used for local staging of the regional primary tumour and nodes (e.g. rectal cancer, prostate cancer and head and neck cancer). On MRI, it is important to depict the distribution pattern of lymphatic metastases, in order to be able to evaluate all the regional lymph node areas.

Lymph nodes are best seen on T1-weighted images (T1WI). Normal lymph nodes are typically isointense to muscle and isointense or mildly hyperintense on T2 weighted imaging (T2WI). Both on T2WI and T1WI, there is a large contrast between the isointense node and

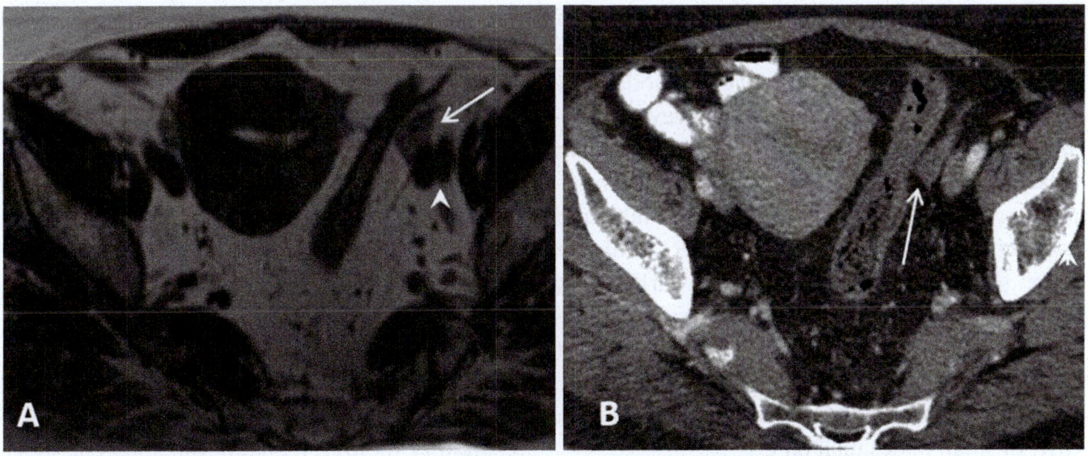

Fig. 3 Left ovary (arrow) adjacent to the external iliac vessels (arrow head) on T2-weighted MRI (**a**) and on CT (**b**). Due to its location near the vessels and ovoid shape, it can resemble an (enlarged) lymph node

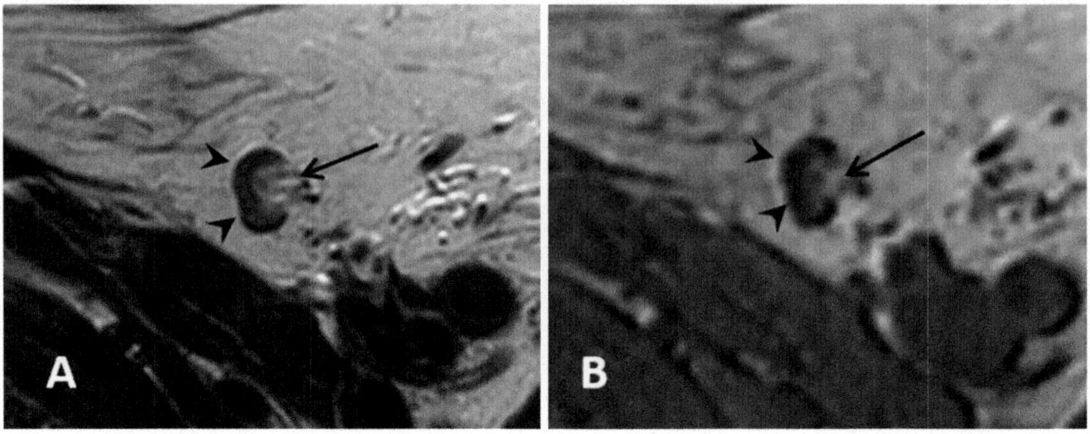

Fig. 4 T2-weighted image (**a**) and T1-weighted image (**b**) of an inguinal node with a typical benign aspect: normal short axis diameter of 5 mm, fatty hilum (arrow), symmetrical cortex (arrowheads) and elongated (not round) shape

the surrounding hyperintense fat (Fig. 4), making it easy to discriminate nodes from their surroundings.

Specifically in head and neck cancer, a fat-suppressed sequence (short tau inversion recovery, or STIR sequence) can be useful to identify nodes as the nodes can be of high signal intensity on T2WI, and by suppressing the fat, the nodes are easier to appreciate. Signal intensity of a node on MRI per se is not a discriminative factor to identify malignant nodes, except for necrotic nodes, which will be very hyperintense on T2W1 due to the fluid contents in necrosis. Heterogeneity of a node (as in CT) is a sign of malignancy. Also, nodal shape is a feature that can be used to differentiate benign from malignant nodes, where a round shape (without a fatty hilum) is indicative of a malignant node. Irregularity of the nodal border is also a malignant feature. However, over- and understaging occur regularly when using these morphological criteria. Besides these morphology criteria, size is also a feature to take into account when staging nodes with MRI, with the same limitations as mentioned earlier for CT. Generally, combining size and morphology leads to the highest accuracy to detect malignant nodes. Due to the higher resolution of MRI, the morphology of a node is easier to appreciate on MRI in small nodes than on CT.

Relatively new techniques have been introduced in MR imaging, with the most commonly evaluated technique being diffusion-weighted imaging (DWI). With this technique, the cell density of a tissue is evaluated by measuring the water movement between cells. Tumour tissue has a high cellular density (or high cellularity) and will therefore show restricted water movement and thus restricted diffusion of water molecules. This results in a high signal on DWI. Lymph nodes also have a high cellularity and therefore will also show restricted diffusion, whether they are malignant or not (Lambregts et al. 2011a). Therefore, DWI is not helpful to stage nodes. Figure 5 shows examples of nodes on T2WI and DWI. Due to the good visibility of nodes on DWI, it can be helpful to identify nodes that can consequently be correlated with T1WI and T2WI to assess size and morphology. Quantification of diffusion in a tissue by measuring the apparent diffusion coefficient (ADC) does not help in discriminating benign from malignant nodes, as there is a substantial overlap in ADC values between benign and malignant nodes. Contrast-enhanced imaging has been evaluated for nodal staging and has shown promising results in several tumour types, however, currently contrast-enhanced MRI is not part of routine nodal staging in nodal oncology (Lambregts et al. 2011b).

Different artefacts and pitfalls can sometimes simulate, or more often, obscure disease in MR imaging. The most common artefact is due to respiratory motion, reducing the apparent signal intensity of lesions. This applies mostly to thoracic organs and lymph nodes and structures adjacent to the diaphragm. Another common cause of artefacts is distortion of the magnetic

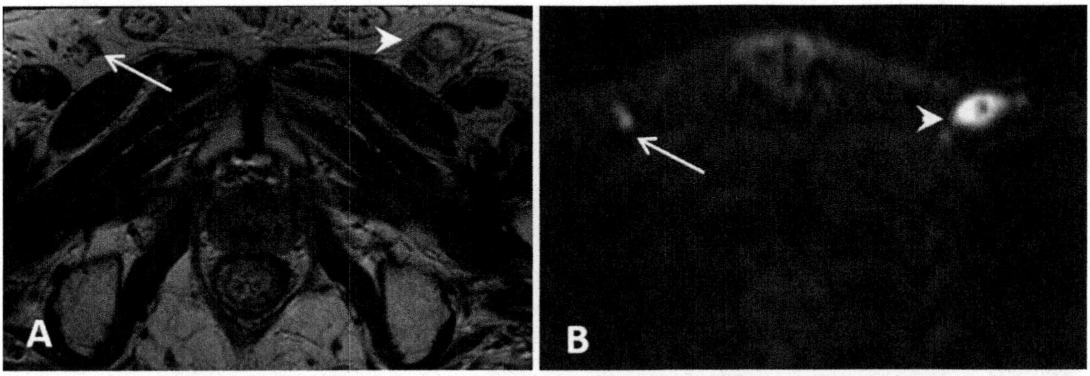

Fig. 5 T2-weighted MRI (**a**) and diffusion-weighted image (**b**) of a benign lymph node (right inguinal region, arrow) and a malignant node (arrow head in the left inguinal region). Notice that both the benign and malignant nodes have a high signal intensity on diffusion-weighted imaging. The central part of the malignant node in **b** is necrotic and only the rim of the node shows high cellularity, correlating with high signal on DWI

field from metallic objects (e.g. hip prosthesis) or air (susceptibility artefacts). This artefact can completely obscure the pelvic structures.

2.2 Functional Imaging: Positron Emission Tomography (PET-CT)

Currently, the PET working horse in oncology is [^{18}F]fluordeoxyglucose ([^{18}F]FDG). A characteristic of many tumour types is that glucose metabolism in tumour cells is increased. This results in an upregulation of membrane glucose transporters leading to an increased intracellular accumulation of [^{18}F]FDG in malignant lesions (Fig. 6).

However, some tumour types, amongst which (well-differentiated) prostate carcinoma, are non-hypermetabolic and other PET-tracers than [^{18}F]FDG are used for tumour detection.

Lesions with high uptake of the radiolabelled tracer are often highly suspicious for metastases. However, for several tracers, uptake may also be increased in physiological tissues or other processes, most importantly inflammation when using [^{18}F]FDG. Therefore, when assessing lymph nodes and predicting metastases, locoregional inflammatory processes, recent local interventions, surgery or other treatments such as radiotherapy should always be taken into account. The spatial resolution of PET is limited, and this progressively decreases sensitivity for detection of metastases in smaller lymph nodes. However, if the tracer uptake is high enough, even very small lymph nodes can become visible on PET. The intensity of uptake of the radiopharmaceutical in metastases is usually related to the uptake in the primary tumour. Thus, if the primary tumour has low uptake, the sensitivity for detection of nodal and distant metastases usually decreases as well. Furthermore, metastatic lymph nodes can show a false negative result on PET in case of necrosis, in which the necrotic tissue does not accumulate the PET tracer. In these cases, sometimes a hypermetabolic rim can be appreciated which in combination with the morphology of necrotic degeneration on CT or MRI makes a node highly suspicious for metastasis.

2.3 Ultrasound

Superficial lymph nodes, such as in the head and neck and inguinal regions, are easily accessible with ultrasound. Deeper located nodes (e.g. para-aortic and pelvic lymph nodes) are difficult to visualize with ultrasound and are not routinely evaluated with ultrasound. A normal lymph node on ultrasound is ovoid in shape, hypoechoic to the adjacent muscle and has an echogenic fatty hilum, while a malignant node will show a round shape, irregular border and absence of a fatty hilum. Also, internal structure of a malignant node on ultrasound is often heterogeneous (Fig. 7). Size thresholds vary with anatomic site and different cancers. Normal nodes have central

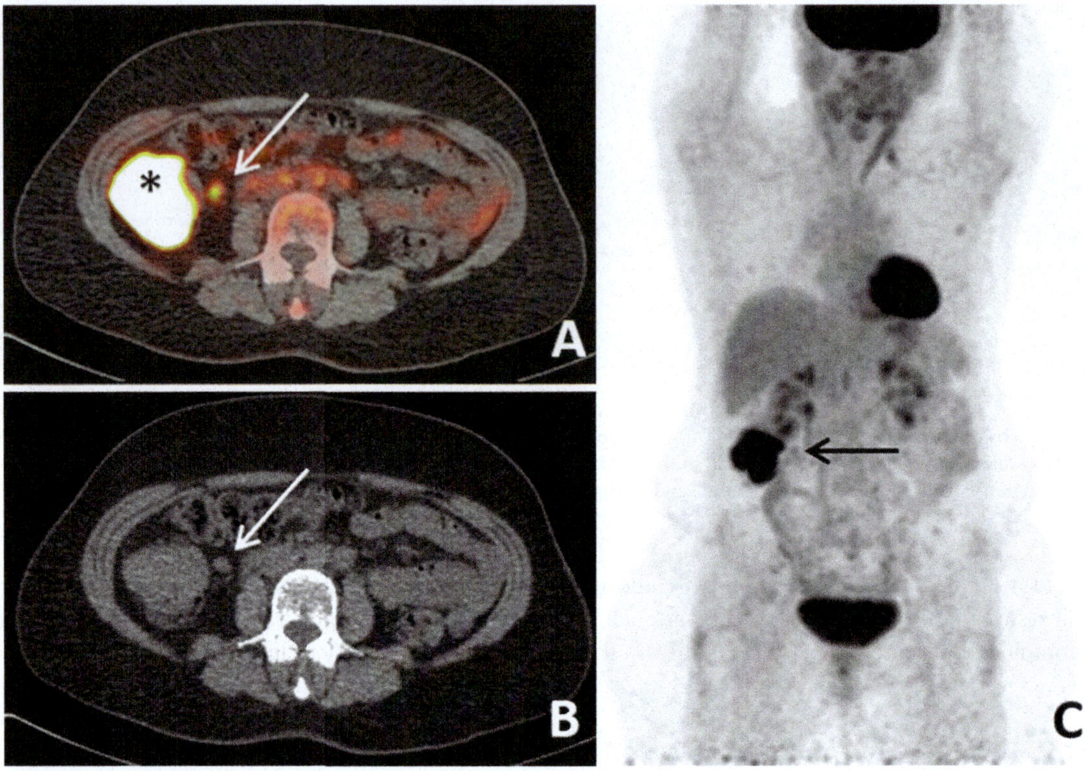

Fig. 6 [^{18}F]FDG PET/CT with intensely increased glucose metabolism in a primary colon ascendens carcinoma (asterisk) and a lymph node (<1 cm) medial to the tumour, suspicious of metastasis (arrows). Axial PET/CT (**a**), axial low dose CT (**b**) and maximal intensity projection (MIP) (**c**) are shown

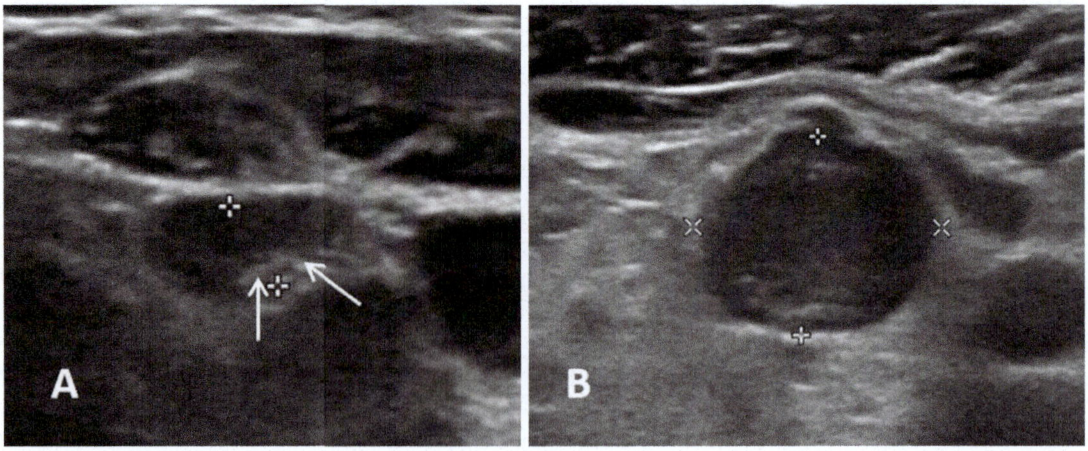

Fig. 7 (**a**) shows a normal node on ultrasound with 5 mm short axis diameter with a fatty hyper echogenic hilum (white arrows). In (**b**), a round enlarged (short axis 12 mm) node is shown with internal heterogeneity. This node is typically malignant

hilar and symmetric vascularity on power doppler imaging (Ganeshalingam and Koh 2009).

Ultrasound provides the opportunity to perform fine needle aspiration (FNA) or biopsy immediately during the examination. The drawback of ultrasound is the relatively high intra- and interoperator variability and its inability to evaluate deep (metastatic) lymph nodes.

3 Nodal Evaluation with Imaging in Common Cancers

3.1 Head and Neck Cancer

In head and neck cancer, nodal staging is a multimodal approach. Besides routine imaging with ultrasound and FNA for histopathological evaluation of suspicious nodes, this is usually a combination of MRI, CT and/or PET/CT. Depending on the primary tumour location, either CT or MRI is usually available for nodal evaluation. [^{18}F]FDG PET/CT outperforms MRI and CT in nodal staging with accuracies from 91 to 98%, while for MRI and CT accuracies between 60 and 84% have been reported (Al-Ibraheem et al. 2009). However, imaging with [^{18}F]FDG PET/CT introduces additional costs, radiation burden and potential delay, and is therefore usually reserved for patients with a relatively high risk of nodal metastases. When either CT, MRI, or PET suggests the presence of nodal involvement, ultrasound may be repeated with targeted FNA. Thus, nodal staging with imaging is tailored to specific patients and usually involves multiple modalities (Fig. 8).

The location of the primary tumour (nasal cavity, nasopharynx, oropharynx, oral cavity, hypopharynx, larynx, salivary gland and thyroid) determines the most likely location of nodal metastases. The neck is divided in seven levels of lymph node areas, as proposed by Som et al. (2000) Additional to these seven levels, nodal metastasis can also be found in the retropharyngeal space, occipital region, parotid gland and nasolabial area, depending on the primary tumour location. Normal nodes in the neck are largest in level 2, where a short axis up to 1.5 cm has been reported to be acceptable as a normal size (in absence of other signs of metastasis). For nodes in the other levels, a short axis size cut-off of >10 mm has been advised to identify malignant nodes (Yoon et al. 2009). Based on these criteria, however, understaging occurs in up to 31% of patients (Norling et al. 2014). Morphologic features that are indicative of malignancy include necrotic nodes (Fig. 9), round shape with absence of fatty hilum and border irregularity, which can be a sign of extracapsular extension (which is associated with poor prognosis) (Figs. 9 and 10).

Norling et al. reported that on sonography, an irregular nodal border, spherical shape and peripheral nodal blood flow and absence of a nodal hilum are the most important predictors of occult metastases in nodes 5 for the prediction of malignancy (Norling et al. 2014). The location of the malignant nodes is very important in head and neck staging as the more distant a node is from the primary tumour, the poorer the prognosis. Therefore, it is very relevant to describe the location of nodes per level and whether nodes are ipsilateral, bilateral, or contralateral. Midline nodes are considered to be ipsilaterally located for all head and neck cancers, except for thyroid cancer (Roland et al. 2016). The location of nodes is one of the determinants of the N-stage in the TNM staging system in head and neck cancer, besides size. To stage a node according to the TNM system, the largest dimension of a malignant node is used (contrary to the cut-off to differentiate malignant from benign nodes which is done by using the short axis). An important subgroup of patients in head and neck cancer are patients with human papilloma virus (HPV) positive tumours. These HPV+ tumours more often show cystic (not necrotic) nodes than HPV− tumours (Goldenberg et al. 2008). Patients with HPV+ tumours have a better prognosis than patients with HPV− tumours (Ang et al. 2010).

[^{18}F]FDG PET/CT is a very helpful tool in nodal staging of head and neck tumours as it can overcome the size criterion issues due to the detection of nodes <1 cm that are metabolically active and thus suspicious for metastasis (Abouzied et al.

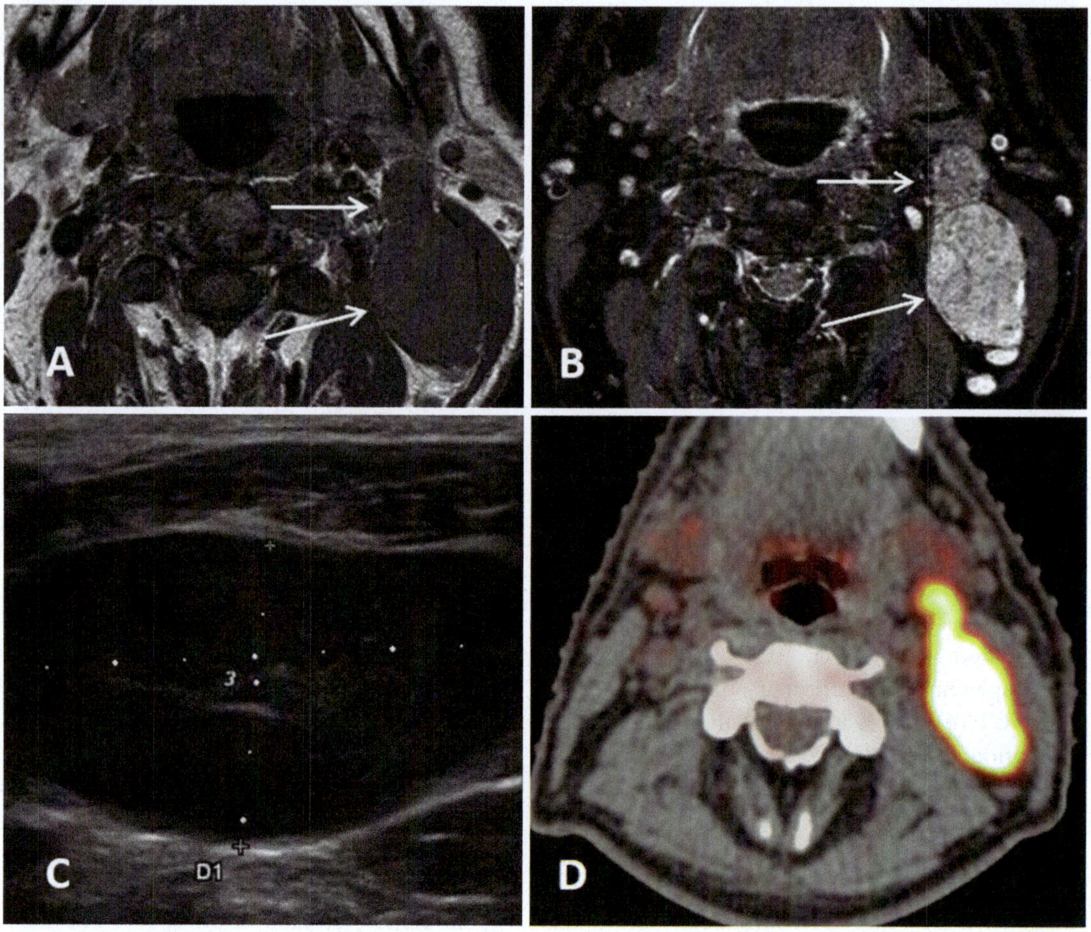

Fig. 8 Two malignant nodes (white arrows) in level II on the left side on T1-weighted MRI (**a**) and STIR (fat-suppressed T2-weighted MRI) (**b**). Corresponding ultrasound image (**c**) with a short axis diameter of 2.4 cm. Avid uptake of [^{18}F]FDG on PET-CT in (**d**)

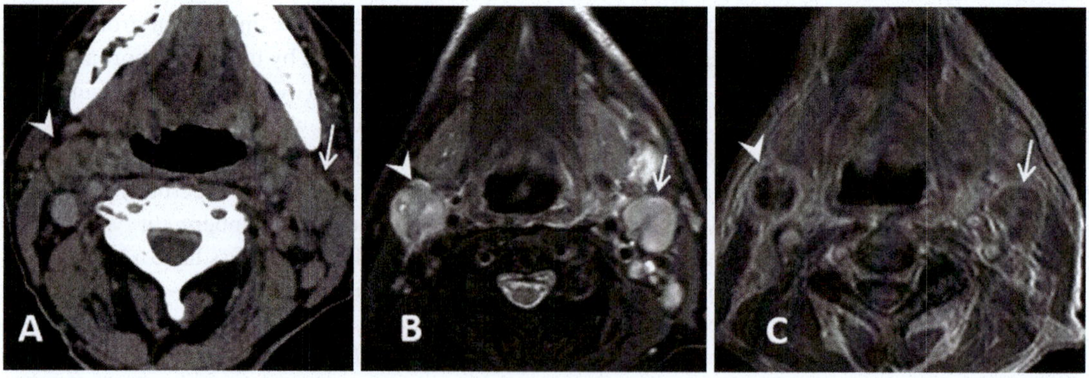

Fig. 9 Bilateral malignant nodes in level II on CT (**a**), STIR (**b**) and contrast-enhanced T1-weighted MRI (**c**). The node on the left side (white arrow) is clearly enlarged but shows a homogeneous internal structure. Conversely, the node on the right side (arrowhead) shows an irregular internal structure with hypo-enhancement centrally, indicating necrosis

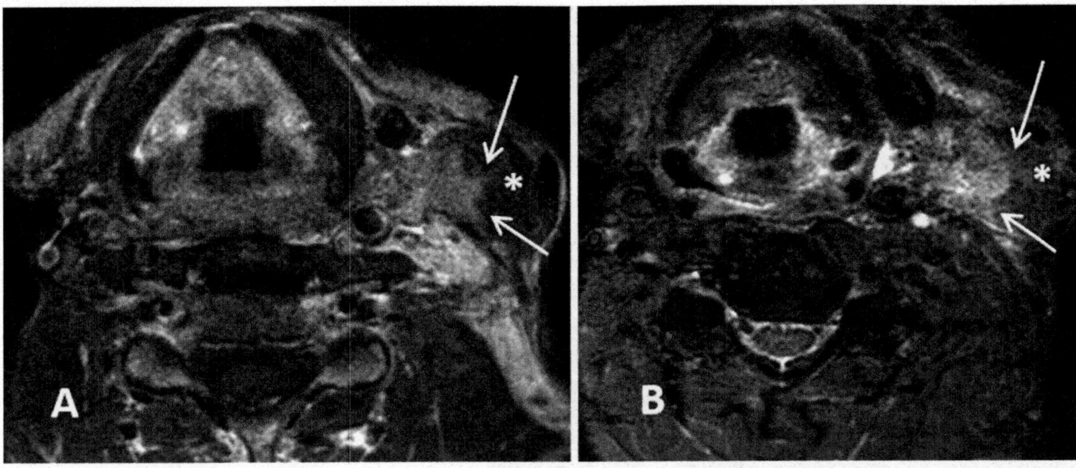

Fig. 10 Nodal metastasis in level II on the left side with extranodal extension and invasion of the sternocleidomastoid muscle (white arrows indicating extension beyond the nodal capsule; the muscle is indicated with asterisk). (**a**) Shows T1-weighted MRI and (**b**) STIR

2017). [^{18}F]FDG PET/CT is mainly used in staging of squamous cell head and neck carcinomas, which usually are intensely hypermetabolic (high [^{18}F]FDG uptake). To improve sensitivity for nodal metastases detection in the head and neck region, PET protocols with the arms down, longer acquisition times and high-resolution image reconstruction may be used to optimize image quality and sensitivity (Vogel et al. 2005). PET/CT has a high sensitivity of detecting (occult) metastases in non-enlarged lymph nodes (Ng et al. 2006; Kim et al. 2007). Hence, [^{18}F]FDG PET/CT is increasingly used in treatment planning, especially in radiotherapy planning in patients who are not undergoing neck dissection (Mazzola et al. 2017). For radiotherapy planning, scanning in radiotherapy position (flat table and personalized mask) is strongly advised (Thorwarth et al. 2012). An additional advantage of the use of [^{18}F]FDG PET/CT is its ability to detect distant metastases and second primary tumours. In patients with head and neck tumours, alcohol and tobacco use is frequently increased resulting in a higher risk for second primary tumours of the aerodigestive tract. Furthermore, [^{18}F]FDG PET/CT can identify approximately 30% of unknown primary tumours in patients presenting with cervical lymph node metastases, in whom the primary tumour was not detected by the comprehensive diagnostic work-up including endoscopy and conventional imaging methods (CT or MRI) (Cacicedo et al. 2016). [^{18}F]FDG false positive lesions (due to inflammation which may be related to recent biopsies) or false negative findings (due to small metastasis size, necrotic or cystic lymph nodes or (lymph node) metastases of non-[^{18}F]FDG avid primary tumours) can occur and should be kept in mind while evaluating [^{18}F]FDG PET/CT.

3.2 Lung Carcinoma

Lung cancer consists of different types of malignancies, with non-small cell lung cancer (NSCLC) being the most common. In patients with NSCLC, the intrathoracic lymph node stage is a major prognostic factor and determines the therapeutic approach. Early stage NSCLC can be treated with surgery. Contrast-enhanced CT is the most commonly used modality for the evaluation of the primary tumour and additionally for imaging of the lymph nodes. Several studies have evaluated the accuracy of CT for mediastinal nodal metastases, and a short axis diameter larger than 1 cm is considered enlarged, raising suspicion for metastasis (Kernstine et al. 1999). As in all other cancers, CT has the limitation that only shape and size of mediastinal lymph nodes can be evaluated, which are relatively unreliable criteria for discrimination between benign and malignant nodes. Overall, the pooled sensitivity and specificity of CT for identifying mediastinal metastases are 51% (95% CI

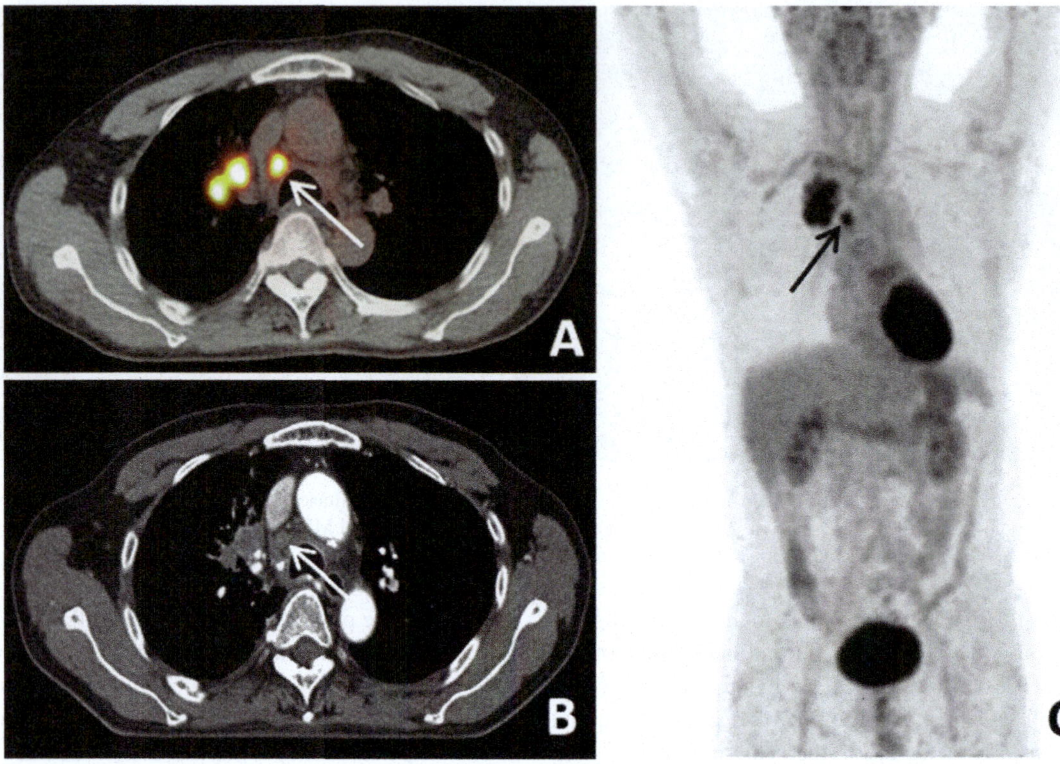

Fig. 11 [18F]FDG PET/CT with intense [18F]FDG uptake in a primary NSCLC in the right upper lobe, in the right hilar lymph nodes and in a non-enlarged pre-carinal lymph node of only 7 mm, highly suspicious of metastasis (arrows). Axial PET/CT (**a**), axial contrast enhanced CT (**b**) and maximal intensity projection (MIP) (**c**) are shown

47–54%) and 85% (95% CI 84–88%), respectively (Silvestri et al. 2007). Currently, MRI does not play a role in lung cancer staging outside research settings. This is mainly caused by the difficulty with cardiac and respiratory motion artefacts in MRI of the thorax. By the introduction of cardiac—and/or respiratory—triggered MRI sequences, MRI-based mediastinal lymph node assessment has become a feasible option, and it is expected that MRI will play a role in mediastinal evaluation in the future (Wielputz and Kauczor 2012).

[18F]FDG PET/CT has an important role in staging of mediastinal and hilar lymph nodes as it has a higher accuracy than contrast-enhanced CT (CECT), with a reported pooled sensitivity and specificity of 74% (95% CI 69–79%) and 85% (95% CI 82–88%), respectively (Silvestri et al. 2007; Murgu 2015). However, highest accuracy is achieved when [18F]FDG PET/CT and CECT are combined (Fig. 11).

Nodes in which [18F]FDG uptake is higher than the surrounding mediastinal tissue/blood pool are regarded positive. Risk for metastases increases with both lymph node size and intensity of metabolic activity ([18F]FDG uptake). False positive nodes on imaging can occur due to current or previous infections (such as tuberculosis) or inflammatory processes (e.g., related to emphysema, sarcoidosis, recent interventions, or radiotherapy-induced pneumonitis). False negative imaging results can be found in the case of small metastases (<6–8 mm), in which the tumour load is not high enough to cause increased [18F]FDG uptake or a size increase, or in necrotic nodes. In case the lymph nodes show increased accumulation of [18F]FDG and/or are enlarged on CECT, (histo)pathologic examination with lymph node sampling (transbronchial needle aspiration, and if negative, biopsy with endobronchial ultrasound or invasive mediastinoscopy) is performed selectively. Not every node needs to be biopsied, but only if biopsy outcome effects the choice of treatment, such as determining N3 metastasis. However, based on the very high negative predictive value for combined

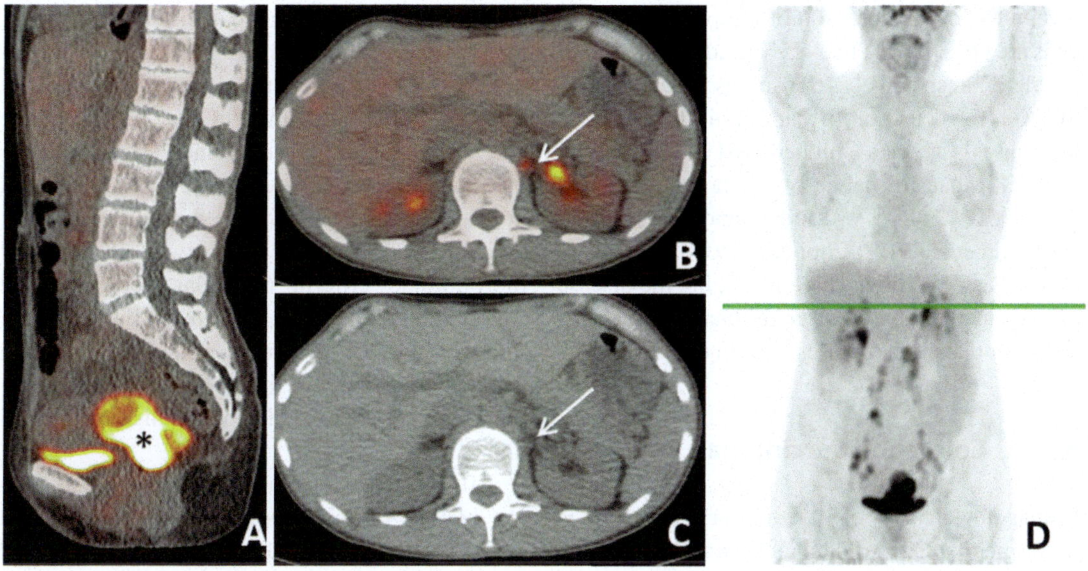

Fig. 12 [18F]FDG PET/CT with intense metabolic activity in a primary cervical cancer (asterisk) and in multiple bilateral pelvic and para-aortal lymph nodes suspicious for metastases. Sagittal (**a**) and axial PET/CT (**b**), axial low dose CT (**c**) and maximal intensity projection (MIP) (**d**) are shown. The green bar in the MIP indicates the level of the highest retroperitoneal suspicious lymph node, which is indicated with the white arrow on the axial planes

[18F]FDG PET/CT with CECT of around 90%, mediastinal lymph node sampling can generally be omitted in patients without enlarged or [18F]FDG-avid hilar and mediastinal lymph nodes. Exceptions are non-[18F]FDG-avid primary lung tumours or tumours that are in close contact with the mediastinum. The guidelines from the European Society of Thoracic Surgeons also recommend invasive nodal staging in patients with a primary tumour size >3 cm, based on higher probability of N2 disease, even when the CT and PET scans are negative for mediastinal lymph node involvement (De Leyn et al. 2014).

3.3 Cervical Cancer

The International Federation of Gynecology and Obstetrics (FIGO) staging system is mostly used for staging of patients with cervical cancer. Although not included in the FIGO clinical staging system, the lymph node status is an important prognostic factor, as patients with metastases have lower survival rates (Chung et al. 2009). Most diagnostic studies on nodal staging in cervical cancer concentrate on the pelvic and para-aortic lymph node regions.

For the locoregional evaluation of cervical cancer, imaging by MRI is the mostly used modality. Normal lymph nodes are ovoid and homogeneous, with intermediate signal intensity on T2WI, low signal intensity on T1WI and high signal intensity on DWI. They enhance homogeneously after intravenous injection of contrast, and a short axis of more than 1 cm is considered abnormal. Features suggestive of a nodal metastasis are similar to that of the other cancers that have been described in this chapter so far and include a round shape, irregular margins, or extracapsular mass/extension and central necrosis (Patel et al. 2010; Sala et al. 2007). As earlier mentioned, micrometastases or small lymph nodes with minimal nodal involvement are poorly detected (Bourgioti et al. 2016). This results in moderate sensitivity and specificity values for both CT (57% [95% CI 44–69%], 91% [95% CI 88–94%]) and MRI (54% [95% CI 46–61%], 93% [95% CI 91–95%]) (Liu et al. 2017). The addition of DWI only helps to identify more nodes, as explained before, but does not aid in discriminating benign from malignant nodes.

[18F]FDG PET/CT is a complementary modality in detecting lymph node and distant metastases in cervical cancer (Fig. 12). Sensitivity and specificity for the detection of lymph node metastases are 66% (95% CI 56–75%) and 97% (95% CI 95–98%), respectively. Sensitivity of [^{18}F]FDG PET/CT for detection of para-aortic lymph node metastases appears higher (81% [95% CI 52–95%]) than for pelvic lymph node metastases (55% [95% CI 42–67%]) and is superior to CT and MRI (Liu et al. 2017; Choi et al. 2010). [^{18}F]FDG PET/CT is of additive value in staging the disease extent, since it may detect additional pelvic, para-aortic, or distant metastases (Marth et al. 2017).

3.4 Colorectal Carcinoma

Primary evaluation of the tumour and nodes is performed by CT (colon cancer) and MRI (rectal cancer). Nodal staging in rectal cancer is one of the main challenges in imaging. Nodal staging in rectal cancer is performed by use of T2-weighted imaging, nodes are evaluated in the mesorectum and outside the mesorectum (obturator areas and para-iliac nodes, sometimes inguinal in distal rectal cancer). In earlier eras, size was mainly used for nodal staging, which led to substantial under- and overstaging (Wang et al. 2005). Addition of morphological criteria increased diagnostic performance, when compared to the lymph node size alone (Brown et al. 2003; Kim et al. 2004). Morphological criteria consist of assessment of border, shape and signal heterogeneity. For primary staging of rectal cancer, in the Dutch national guidelines, criteria based on size and morphology are recommended for the assessment of mesorectal nodes. In these guidelines, all nodes >8 mm short axis are deemed malignant, while nodes <5 mm should show three additional morphologic criteria (irregular border, round shape and heterogeneous signal) (Fig. 13). All nodes with short-axis diameters from 5–8 mm should (from two of the abovementioned morphological criteria) be deemed malignant (Beets-Tan et al. 2017).

Efforts have been made to improve nodal staging by use of diffusion-weighted imaging and contrast-enhanced MRI. Diffusion-weighted MRI mostly contributes to the identification of nodes, as earlier in this chapter, but is not helpful in distinguishing benign from malignant nodes. This is caused by the fact that all nodes have a dense tissue structure which leads to a high signal on DWI (Lambregts et al. 2011a). The addition of contrast-enhanced MRI (with USPIO or gadofosveset trisodium) significantly improved nodal staging with accuracies up to 84–96% (Lambregts et al. 2011b; Lahaye et al. 2008). Unfortunately, these contrast agents currently are not available for commercial use.

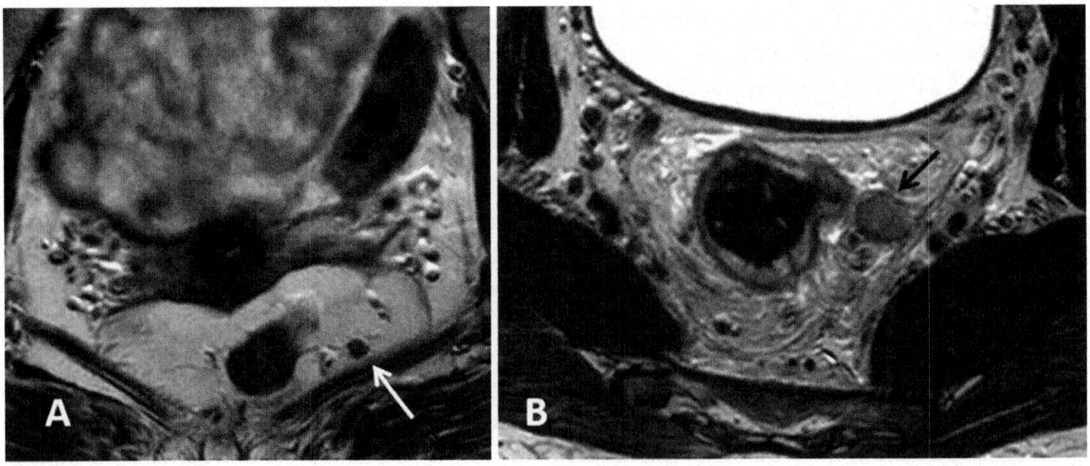

Fig. 13 On the left (**a**) a normal mesorectal node with a short axis of 4 mm, oval shape and regular border. On the right (**b**) a malignant node (black arrow) with a short axis diameter of 10 mm with a round shape and irregular border in the mesorectum

For colon cancer, CT is used to assess nodes. No reliable criteria exist for nodal staging in colon cancer. It is important to assess the presence of regional lymph node in the mesocolon and to distinguish them from para-aortic nodes, as the latter are considered distant metastases. Size is the main criterion, but has the same limitations as in rectal cancer. Mostly a size cut-off of 1 cm has been proposed, but this harbours a high risk for understaging. Alternatively, the presence of clusters of nodes neighbouring the tumour has been proposed to be a sign of nodal disease, but strong evidence to support this approach is lacking. So far, sensitivities for CT have been moderate around 71–83%. In research settings, MRI has been explored for the staging of colon cancer, but MRI does not aid in nodal staging with reported sensitivities between 43 and 71% (Nerad et al. 2017; Rollven et al. 2013). In a recent study by Rollven et al., the internal heterogeneity of at least one lymph node as a criterion yielded the best diagnostic performance for nodal staging in colon cancer with a sensitivity of 79%. Addition of the presence of outer border irregularity improved sensitivity to 85% (Rollven et al. 2017).

There is no routine role for [^{18}F]FDG PET/CT in primary lymph node staging of colorectal cancer. However, in case of inconclusive findings on CT or MRI, to exclude extrahepatic disease in case of liver-directed curative local therapies, unexplained CEA rise during follow-up or in restaging of resectable recurrence, additional [^{18}F]FDG PET/CT is recommended. Again, false positive lymph nodes (due to inflammation) or false negative findings (due to small metastasis size, necrotic, or mucinous lymph nodes) should be taken in to account.

3.5 Prostate Carcinoma

Imaging for the detection of lymph node metastases in prostate cancer is not performed routinely, as current management strategies mainly rely upon digital rectal examination, prostate-specific antigen (PSA) values and prostate biopsy (Gleason score) (Moghanaki et al. 2017). Role of MRI is to assess local tumour stage and nodal involvement in patients with already biopsy proven prostate cancer or for tumour detection in high-risk patients with previous negative prostate biopsies. MRI can direct (additional) biopsy for more accurate grading of the tumour (Barentsz et al. 2012). Nodal spread occurs to the obturator areas and can spread up to the para-aortic area. Lobulated or spiculated nodal borders, extracapsular growth and abnormal internal architecture (such as central necrosis) are suspicious (Vallini et al. 2016). Lymph nodes are considered abnormal if the short axis diameter exceeds 1 cm or if the lymph node is rounded and larger than 0.8 cm (Harisinghani et al. 2003). However, both CT and MRI have a low diagnostic performance in the detection of lymph node metastases from prostate cancer. For CT, sensitivity is 43% (95% CI 26–56) and specificity is 82% (95% CI 80–83); for MRI, the sensitivity is 39% (95% CI 22–56) and specificity is 82% (95% CI 79–83) (Hovels et al. 2008).

The most commonly used radiotracers in (re) staging of prostate carcinoma with PET/CT are choline or ligands against prostate-specific membrane antigen (PSMA). [^{18}F]- or ^{11}C-choline were commonly used until recently, mainly for restaging of prostate cancer in biochemical recurrence, but also for initial staging in high-risk prostate cancer. In prostate cancer cells, the uptake of choline, which is used to produce phosphatidylcholine, is frequently upregulated. In initial lymph node staging of intermediate and high-risk prostate carcinoma, choline PET/CT has a pooled sensitivity of 49% (95% CI 40–58) and pooled specificity of 95% (95% CI 92–97) (Evangelista et al. 2013). After prostatectomy, sensitivity of choline PET/CT increases with higher prostate-specific antigen (PSA) levels and shorter PSA doubling times (Schillaci et al. 2012). Besides choline, other PET tracers such as ^{11}C-acetate, [^{18}F] fluorocyclobutanecarboxylic acid (FACBC) and [^{18}F] and ^{68}Ga labelled PSMA ligands have been developed more recently. Of these, the PSMA-directed tracers appear to be the most valuable in prostate cancer imaging, and their use has increased progressively over the last few years (Incerti et al. 2017; Fendler et al. 2017). PSMA is a transmembrane protein that is overexpressed

(100–1000 fold) in up to 95% of prostate carcinomas. The level of PSMA expression increases with higher tumour stage and grade and in hormone-refractory disease (Schwarzenboeck et al. 2017). Due to the higher sensitivity and specificity in primary staging and recurrence detection of PSMA PET/CT, even at very low PSA levels, choline PET/CT has been replaced with PSMA PET/CT in many centres. In primary lymph node staging of patients with high or intermediate risk disease, PSMA PET/CT has been proven superior over morphological imaging (Maurer et al. 2016). PSMA expression often is very high, resulting in detection of otherwise occult metastases as small as 2–3 mm, despite the limited spatial resolution of PET (Fig. 14).

High dose (contrast-enhanced) CT or MRI, however, are superior to low dose CT to confirm the presence of small nodes at localization of increased PSMA ligand uptake. PSMA PET/CT has been proven valuable in treatment planning. It frequently results in alternation of N- or M-stage, requiring adjustment of radiotherapy planning (radiation field or dose) or modification of the treatment plan such as replacement of salvage surgery or radiotherapy by systemic treatment (Schwarzenboeck et al. 2017). Although PSMA ligand has a very high specificity for prostate cancer cells, various other malignancies (like renal cell carcinoma, hepatocellular carcinoma, breast cancer and others) have been shown to have increased uptake on PSMA PET/CT. In these tumours, neoexpression of PSMA in endothelial cells of capillary beds during tumour neovascularization occurs. Also, high uptake can be appreciated in benign diseases (such as Paget's disease, adrenal or thyroid adenoma, (rib) fractures, etc.) and organs (lacrimal glands, salivary glands, liver, spleen, small intestine, colon and kidneys). Furthermore, an important false positive pitfall is the uptake of PSMA ligand in ganglia of the autonomic nervous system, mainly in

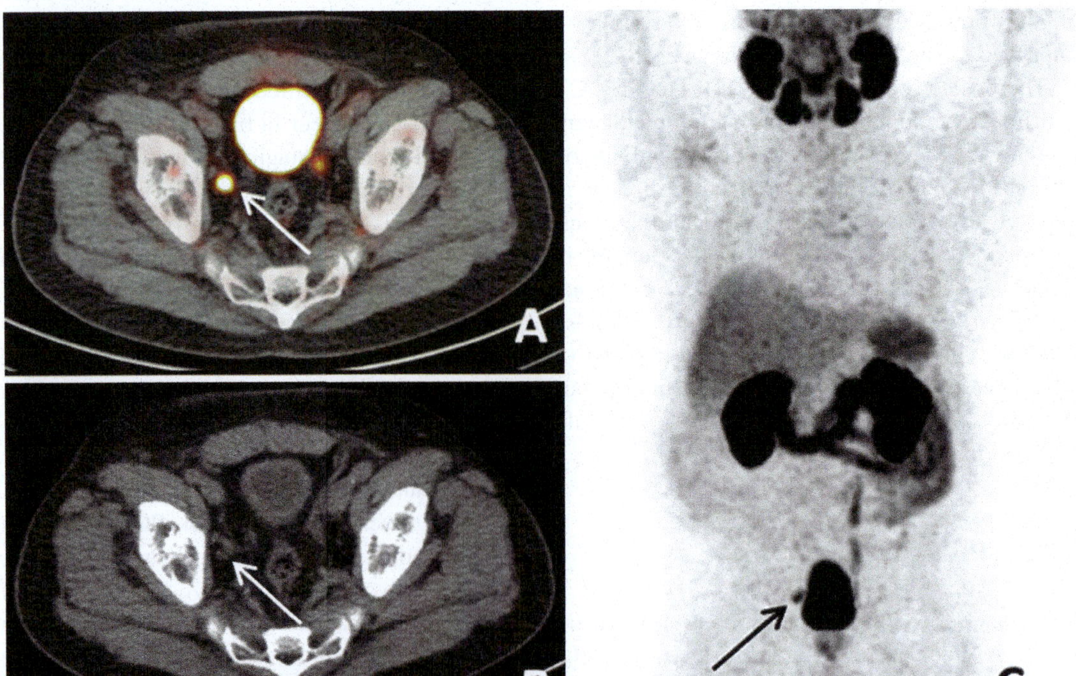

Fig. 14 ^{68}Ga-PSMA PET/CT showing a small lymph node of 6 mm (arrows) in the right obturator area which according to the very high PSMA expression is likely to harbour a metastasis of prostate carcinoma. Axial PET/CT (**a**), axial low dose CT (**b**) and maximal intensity projection (MIP) (**c**) are shown

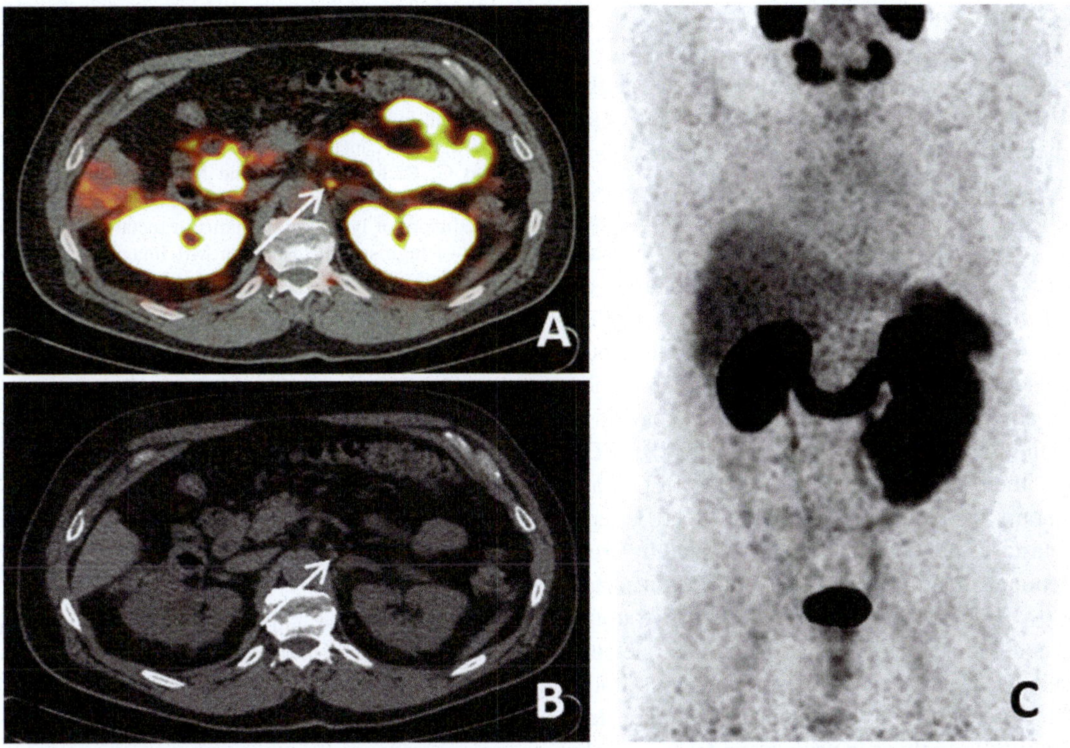

Fig. 15 ^{68}Ga-PSMA PET/CT with intense PSMA ligand binding (non pathologic) in a left-sided superior mesenteric ganglion (arrows). Axial PET/CT (**a**), axial low dose CT (**b**) and maximal intensity projection (MIP) (**c**) are shown

the sacral and coeliac region, which can be misinterpreted as lymph nodes (Fig. 15) (Silver et al. 1997; Kanthan et al. 2017).

4 Post-treatment Imaging of Nodes

The main aim of post-treatment (after chemotherapy, radiotherapy, or both) imaging of nodes is to identify residual metastatic nodes that will lead to the necessity to perform surgery or add another treatment. Generally, nodes (both benign and malignant) will decrease in size and some will disappear as a result of (chemo)radiation. Malignant nodes tend to be very responsive to radiotherapy, and nodal sterilization is often encountered. However, incomplete responses may occur and may involve clinically relevant discrepancies between nodal size on CT or MRI and the presence of tumour. PET/CT is often useful in these cases. For example, [^{18}F]FDG PET/CT has a high accuracy for excluding vital tumour in remaining enlarged residual nodes after (chemo)radiotherapy for node-positive squamous cell carcinoma in the head and neck area, preventing unneeded neck lymph node dissection (Mehanna et al. 2017). However, due to the general size decrease of benign and malignant nodes after (chemo)radiation, PET/CT can be more challenging.

In general, the same criteria and pitfalls as discussed in primary nodal staging are applicable to post-treatment imaging of nodes. However, pitfalls can occur more often in post-treatment imaging due to treatment-induced reactive changes which can lead to enlargement of nodes, increase in the number of nodes or changes in density or signal intensity. [^{18}F]FDG uptake can also increase due to inflammation, leading to false positive findings which can last for several months after therapy. Therefore, timing and follow-up imaging is of key importance to discriminate residual tumour activity from therapy-related inflammatory changes.

5 Conclusion

Imaging plays an important role in nodal staging. MRI and CT are commonly used and rely on size criteria and morphological criteria (shape, border and signal intensity or density). These criteria unfortunately are only moderately accurate, leading to under- and overstaging of N-stage. Furthermore, normal anatomic structures can sometimes be mistaken for nodes (e.g. ovary, cisterna chyli, or [small] lymphoceles). Ultrasound is often used for superficial nodes and provides the advantage to perform FNA to confirm or exclude nodal disease. PET/CT with [^{18}F]FDG, or other radiotracers in non [^{18}F]FDG-avid tumours, is a valuable adjunct to identify occult metastases in nodes that are undetected by cross-sectional imaging and ultrasound. Main pitfalls in ([^{18}F]FDG) PET/CT are false positive uptake in nodes due to inflammation or false negative findings in small, necrotic, or mucinous nodes. After (neoadjuvant) treatment, the same criteria and pitfalls apply as in primary nodal staging, but due to treatment-induced changes, pitfalls can occur more often than in a primary setting.

References

Aan de Stegge WB, van Leeuwen BL, Elferink MA, de Bock GH (2016) The evaluation of more lymph nodes in colon cancer is associated with improved survival in patients of all ages. PLoS One 11(5):e0155608

Abouzied MM, Fathala A, Alsugair A, Muhaideb AIA, Qahtani MHA (2017) Role of fluorodeoxyglucose-positron emission tomography/computed tomography in the evaluation of head and neck carcinoma. World J Nucl Med 16(4):257–265

Al-Ibraheem A, Buck A, Krause BJ, Scheidhauer K, Schwaiger M (2009) Clinical applications of FDG PET and PET/CT in head and neck cancer. J Oncol 2009:208725

Ang KK, Harris J, Wheeler R, Weber R, Rosenthal DI, Nguyen-Tan PF et al (2010) Human papillomavirus and survival of patients with oropharyngeal cancer. N Engl J Med 363(1):24–35

Barentsz JO, Richenberg J, Clements R, Choyke P, Verma S, Villeirs G et al (2012) ESUR prostate MR guidelines 2012. Eur Radiol 22(4):746–757

Beets-Tan RGH, Lambregts DMJ, Maas M, Bipat S, Barbaro B, Curvo-Semedo L et al (2017) Magnetic resonance imaging for clinical management of rectal cancer: updated recommendations from the 2016 European Society of Gastrointestinal and Abdominal Radiology (ESGAR) consensus meeting. Eur Radiol 28(4):1465–1475

Bourgioti C, Chatoupis K, Moulopoulos LA (2016) Current imaging strategies for the evaluation of uterine cervical cancer. World J Radiol 8(4):342–354

Brown G, Richards CJ, Bourne MW, Newcombe RG, Radcliffe AG, Dallimore NS et al (2003) Morphologic predictors of lymph node status in rectal cancer with use of high-spatial-resolution MR imaging with histopathologic comparison. Radiology 227(2):371–377

Cacicedo J, Navarro A, Del Hoyo O, Gomez-Iturriaga A, Alongi F, Medina JA et al (2016) Role of fluorine-18 fluorodeoxyglucose PET/CT in head and neck oncology: the point of view of the radiation oncologist. Br J Radiol 89(1067):20160217

Choi HJ, Ju W, Myung SK, Kim Y (2010) Diagnostic performance of computer tomography, magnetic resonance imaging, and positron emission tomography or positron emission tomography/computer tomography for detection of metastatic lymph nodes in patients with cervical cancer: meta-analysis. Cancer Sci 101(6):1471–1479

Chung HH, Park NH, Kim JW, Song YS, Chung JK, Kang SB (2009) Role of integrated PET-CT in pelvic lymph node staging of cervical cancer before radical hysterectomy. Gynecol Obstet Investig 67(1):61–66

De Leyn P, Dooms C, Kuzdzal J, Lardinois D, Passlick B, Rami-Porta R et al (2014) Revised ESTS guidelines for preoperative mediastinal lymph node staging for non-small-cell lung cancer. Eur J Cardio-thorac Surg 45(5):787–798

Detterbeck FC, Chansky K, Groome P, Bolejack V, Crowley J, Shemanski L et al (2016) The IASLC Lung Cancer Staging Project: methodology and validation used in the development of proposals for revision of the stage classification of NSCLC in the forthcoming (eighth) edition of the TNM classification of lung cancer. J Thorac Oncol 11(9):1433–1446

Evangelista L, Guttilla A, Zattoni F, Muzzio PC, Zattoni F (2013) Utility of choline positron emission tomography/computed tomography for lymph node involvement identification in intermediate- to high-risk prostate cancer: a systematic literature review and meta-analysis. Eur Urol 63(6):1040–1048

Fendler WP, Eiber M, Beheshti M, Bomanji J, Ceci F, Cho S et al (2017) (68)Ga-PSMA PET/CT: joint EANM and SNMMI procedure guideline for prostate cancer imaging: version 1.0. Eur J Nucl Med Mol Imaging 44(6):1014–1024

Ganeshalingam S, Koh DM (2009) Nodal staging. Cancer Imaging 9:104–111

Goldenberg D, Begum S, Westra WH, Khan Z, Sciubba J, Pai SI et al (2008) Cystic lymph node metastasis in patients with head and neck cancer: an HPV-associated phenomenon. Head Neck 30(7):898–903

Harisinghani MG, Barentsz J, Hahn PF, Deserno WM, Tabatabaei S, van de Kaa CH et al (2003) Noninvasive detection of clinically occult lymph-node metastases in prostate cancer. N Engl J Med 348(25):2491–2499

Hovels AM, Heesakkers RA, Adang EM, Jager GJ, Strum S, Hoogeveen YL et al (2008) The diagnostic accuracy of CT and MRI in the staging of pelvic lymph nodes in patients with prostate cancer: a meta-analysis. Clin Radiol 63(4):387–395

Incerti E, Mapelli P, Gianolli L, Picchio M (2017) PET imaging for lymph node dissection in prostate cancer. World J Urol 35(4):507–515

Kanthan GL, Hsiao E, Vu D, Schembri GP (2017) Uptake in sympathetic ganglia on (68) Ga-PSMA-HBED PET/CT: a potential pitfall in scan interpretation. J Med Imaging Radiat Oncol 61(6):732–738

Kernstine KH, Stanford W, Mullan BF, Rossi NP, Thompson BH, Bushnell DL et al (1999) PET, CT, and MRI with Combidex for mediastinal staging in non-small cell lung carcinoma. Ann Thorac Surg 68(3):1022–1028

Kim JH, Beets GL, Kim MJ, Kessels AG, Beets-Tan RG (2004) High-resolution MR imaging for nodal staging in rectal cancer: are there any criteria in addition to the size? Eur J Radiol 52(1):78–83

Kim MR, Roh JL, Kim JS, Lee JH, Cho KJ, Choi SH et al (2007) Utility of 18F-fluorodeoxyglucose positron emission tomography in the preoperative staging of squamous cell carcinoma of the oropharynx. Eur J Surg Oncol 33(5):633–638

Kim JS, Sohn DK, Park JW, Kim DY, Chang HJ, Choi HS et al (2011) Prognostic significance of distribution of lymph node metastasis in advanced mid or low rectal cancer. J Surg Oncol 104(5):486–492

Lahaye MJ, Engelen SM, Kessels AG, de Bruine AP, von Meyenfeldt MF, van Engelshoven JM et al (2008) USPIO-enhanced MR imaging for nodal staging in patients with primary rectal cancer: predictive criteria. Radiology 246(3):804–811

Lambregts DM, Maas M, Cappendijk VC, Prompers LM, Mottaghy FM, Beets GL et al (2011a) Whole-body diffusion-weighted magnetic resonance imaging: current evidence in oncology and potential role in colorectal cancer staging. Eur J Cancer (Oxford England: 1990) 47(14):2107–2116

Lambregts DM, Beets GL, Maas M, Kessels AG, Bakers FC, Cappendijk VC et al (2011b) Accuracy of gadofosveset-enhanced MRI for nodal staging and restaging in rectal cancer. Ann Surg 253(3):539–545

Liu B, Gao S, Li S (2017) A comprehensive comparison of CT, MRI, positron emission tomography or positron emission tomography/CT, and diffusion weighted imaging-MRI for detecting the lymph nodes metastases in patients with cervical cancer: a meta-analysis based on 67 studies. Gynecol Obstet Investig 82(3):209–222

Marth C, Landoni F, Mahner S, McCormack M, Gonzalez-Martin A, Colombo N (2017) Cervical cancer: ESMO Clinical Practice Guidelines for diagnosis, treatment and follow-up. Ann Oncol 28(Suppl 4):iv72–iv83

Maurer T, Gschwend JE, Rauscher I, Souvatzoglou M, Haller B, Weirich G et al (2016) Diagnostic efficacy of (68)gallium-PSMA positron emission tomography compared to conventional imaging for lymph node staging of 130 consecutive patients with intermediate to high risk prostate cancer. J Urol 195(5):1436–1443

Mazzola R, Alongi P, Ricchetti F, Fiorentino A, Fersino S, Giaj-Levra N et al (2017) 18F-Fluorodeoxyglucose-PET/CT in locally advanced head and neck cancer can influence the stage migration and nodal radiation treatment volumes. Radiol Med 122(12):952–959

Mehanna H, McConkey CC, Rahman JK, Wong WL, Smith AF, Nutting C et al (2017) PET-NECK: a multicentre randomised phase III non-inferiority trial comparing a positron emission tomography-computerised tomography-guided watch-and-wait policy with planned neck dissection in the management of locally advanced (N2/N3) nodal metastases in patients with squamous cell head and neck cancer. Health Technol Assess (Winchester, England) 21(17):1–122

Moghanaki D, Turkbey B, Vapiwala N, Ehdaie B, Frank SJ, McLaughlin PW et al (2017) Advances in prostate cancer magnetic resonance imaging and positron emission tomography-computed tomography for staging and radiotherapy treatment planning. Semin Radiat Oncol 27(1):21–33

Murgu SD (2015) Diagnosing and staging lung cancer involving the mediastinum. Chest 147(5):1401–1412

Nerad E, Lambregts DM, Kersten EL, Maas M, Bakers FC, van den Bosch HC et al (2017) MRI for local staging of colon cancer: can MRI become the optimal staging modality for patients with colon cancer? Dis Colon Rectum 60(4):385–392

Ng SH, Yen TC, Chang JT, Chan SC, Ko SF, Wang HM et al (2006) Prospective study of [18F]fluorodeoxyglucose positron emission tomography and computed tomography and magnetic resonance imaging in oral cavity squamous cell carcinoma with palpably negative neck. J Clin Oncol 24(27):4371–4376

Norling R, Buron BM, Therkildsen MH, Henriksen BM, von Buchwald C, Nielsen MB (2014) Staging of cervical lymph nodes in oral squamous cell carcinoma: adding ultrasound in clinically lymph node negative patients may improve diagnostic work-up. PLoS One 9(3):e90360

Patel S, Liyanage SH, Sahdev A, Rockall AG, Reznek RH (2010) Imaging of endometrial and cervical cancer. Insights Imaging 1(5–6):309–328

Roland N, Porter G, Fish B, Makura Z (2016) Tumour assessment and staging: United Kingdom national multidisciplinary guidelines. J Laryngol Otol 130(S2):S53–Ss8

Rollven E, Holm T, Glimelius B, Lorinc E, Blomqvist L (2013) Potentials of high resolution magnetic resonance imaging versus computed tomography for preoperative local staging of colon cancer. Acta Radiol (Stockholm Sweden: 1987) 54(7):722–730

Rollven E, Abraham-Nordling M, Holm T, Blomqvist L (2017) Assessment and diagnostic accuracy of lymph node status to predict stage III colon cancer using computed tomography. Cancer Imaging 17(1):3

Sala E, Wakely S, Senior E, Lomas D (2007) MRI of malignant neoplasms of the uterine corpus and cervix. AJR Am J Roentgenol 188(6):1577–1587

Schillaci O, Calabria F, Tavolozza M, Caracciolo CR, Finazzi Agro E, Miano R et al (2012) Influence of PSA, PSA velocity and PSA doubling time on contrast-enhanced 18F-choline PET/CT detection rate in patients with rising PSA after radical prostatectomy. Eur J Nucl Med Mol Imaging 39(4):589–596

Schwarzenboeck SM, Rauscher I, Bluemel C, Fendler WP, Rowe SP, Pomper MG et al (2017) PSMA ligands for PET imaging of prostate cancer. J Nucl Med 58(10):1545–1552

Silver DA, Pellicer I, Fair WR, Heston WD, Cordon-Cardo C (1997) Prostate-specific membrane antigen expression in normal and malignant human tissues. Clin Cancer Res 3(1):81–85

Silvestri GA, Gould MK, Margolis ML, Tanoue LT, McCrory D, Toloza E et al (2007) Noninvasive staging of non-small cell lung cancer: ACCP evidenced-based clinical practice guidelines (2nd edition). Chest 132(3 Suppl):178s–201s

Som PM, Curtin HD, Mancuso AA (2000) Imaging-based nodal classification for evaluation of neck metastatic adenopathy. AJR Am J Roentgenol 174(3):837–844

Thorwarth D, Beyer T, Boellaard R, de Ruysscher D, Grgic A, Lee JA et al (2012) Integration of FDG-PET/CT into external beam radiation therapy planning: technical aspects and recommendations on methodological approaches. Nucl Med 51(4):140–153

Vallini V, Ortori S, Boraschi P, Manassero F, Gabelloni M, Faggioni L et al (2016) Staging of pelvic lymph nodes in patients with prostate cancer: usefulness of multiple b value SE-EPI diffusion-weighted imaging on a 3.0 T MR system. Eur J Radiol Open 3:16–21

Vogel WV, Wensing BM, van Dalen JA, Krabbe PF, van den Hoogen FJ, Oyen WJ (2005) Optimised PET reconstruction of the head and neck area: improved diagnostic accuracy. Eur J Nucl Med Mol Imaging 32(11):1276–1282

Wang C, Zhou ZG, Wang Z, Chen DY, Zheng YC, Zhao GP (2005) Nodal spread and micrometastasis within mesorectum. World J Gastroenterol 11(23):3586–3590

Wielputz M, Kauczor HU (2012) MRI of the lung: state of the art. Diagn Interven Radiol (Ankara, Turkey) 18(4):344–353

Yoon DY, Hwang HS, Chang SK, Rho YS, Ahn HY, Kim JH et al (2009) CT, MR, US,18F-FDG PET/CT, and their combined use for the assessment of cervical lymph node metastases in squamous cell carcinoma of the head and neck. Eur Radiol 19(3):634–642

Tumor Biology Characterization by Imaging in Laboratory

Alberto Conficoni, Antonio Poerio, Eleonora Farina, and Alessio G. Morganti

Contents

1 **Introduction** ... 294
2 **Overview of Small-Animal Tumor Models** ... 295
2.1 Subcutaneous Engraftment Models ... 296
2.2 Orthotopic Patient-Derived Xenografts (PDX) Models ... 297
2.3 Genetically Engineered Mouse Models (GEMMs) ... 297
3 **Positron Emission Tomography (PET) in Tumor Biology Characterization** ... 298
4 **Micro-computed Tomography (μ-CT)** ... 301
5 **Micro-magnetic Resonance Imaging (μ-MRI)** ... 303
5.1 Diffusion-Weighted Magnetic Resonance Imaging ... 305
5.2 Perfusion Magnetic Resonance Imaging ... 307
5.3 Magnetic Resonance Spectroscopy ... 310
6 **Optical Imaging** ... 312
6.1 Bioluminescence Imaging (BLI) ... 313
6.2 Fluorescence Imaging (FLI) ... 313
6.3 Diffuse Optical Tomography (DOT) ... 314
References ... 314

Abstract

The practice of modern medicine in cancer treatment is moving toward an increasingly tailored approach. Current therapeutic strategies require careful pretreatment stratification and timely and effective monitoring during and after therapy, in order to maximize patient benefit. Accordingly, there is an increasing need to non-invasively delineate individual patient characteristics, with particular attention to the tumor biology underlying cellular and extracellular mechanisms involved in the development and progression of the disease, as well as in treatment response. For this purpose, one of the major priorities in oncological research has been identified in developing increasingly sensitive and specific imaging biomarkers for non-invasive characterization of cancer-related features. Different imaging methods are currently being developed in experimental murine models of human diseases in order to identify and implement innovative biomarkers with the perspective of clinical translation.

Alberto Conficoni and Antonio Poerio contributed equally to this work.

A. Conficoni · A. Poerio
Radiology Unit, Department of Experimental, Diagnostic and Specialty Medicine—DIMES, University of Bologna, S. Orsola-Malpighi Hospital, Bologna, Italy

E. Farina (✉) · A. G. Morganti
Radiation Oncology Center, Department of Experimental, Diagnostic and Specialty Medicine—DIMES, University of Bologna, S. Orsola-Malpighi Hospital, Bologna, Italy

R. G. H. Beets-Tan et al. (eds.), *Imaging and Interventional Radiology for Radiation Oncology*, Medical Radiology, Diagnostic Imaging, https://doi.org/10.1007/978-3-030-38261-2_18

After a brief review of the currently available tumor models of cancer, this chapter summarizes the current status of preclinical in vivo imaging techniques and the future perspectives of emerging imaging biomarkers for the characterization of tumor biology and behavior.

1 Introduction

The practice of modern medicine in cancer treatment is moving towards an increasingly tailored approach. Current therapeutic strategies require careful pretreatment stratification and timely and effective monitoring during and after therapy, in order to maximize patient benefit. According to this trend, there is an increasing need to non-invasively delineate individual patient characteristics, with particular attention to the tumor biology underlying cellular and extra-cellular mechanisms involved in the development and progression of the disease, as well as in treatment response. For this purpose, one of the major priorities in oncological research has been identified in developing increasingly sensitive and specific imaging biomarkers for non-invasive characterization of cancer-related features (Bernsen et al. 2015; O'Connor et al. 2016; Cyran et al. 2014).

Imaging plays a crucial role at all stages of a cancer's patient journey and, since it is non-invasive and readily amenable to longitudinal measurements, imaging is often the choice tool to evaluate the efficacy of treatments (Cunha et al. 2014; Wang et al. 2015). In addition, the growing knowledge on cancer pathophysiology, along with the development of modern imaging technologies, are moving preclinical and clinical imaging from exclusively assessing tumor size and morphology toward the visualization and quantification of cancer pathophysiological processes on a functional and molecular level (Cyran et al. 2014; Cunha et al. 2014).

Different imaging methods are currently being developed in experimental murine models of human diseases in order to identify and implement innovative biomarkers with the perspective of clinical translation. With the introduction and development of new miniaturized instrumentation specifically engineered for small animals, the ability to longitudinally study various experimental models of human cancer has exponentially grown in recent years, often with the main purpose of testing new pharmaceutical agents prior to translation into clinical practice (Cunha et al. 2014; Wang et al. 2015; Kagadis et al. 2016). In parallel, the escalating demand for preclinical imaging has been one of the factors behind the increasing use of advanced preclinical tumor models that could better represent human tumor biology, such as orthotopic and genetically engineered mouse models (GEMMs) (Wang et al. 2015).

Achievements in the field of small-animal in vivo imaging have led biomedical research to a higher level with inherent extraordinary advantages over traditional ex vivo techniques. Major strengths are real-time monitoring and the opportunity to capture an impressive amount of data in a nondestructive fashion, with substantial reduction in the number of animals required for studies, in full compliance with 3Rs (Replacement, Reduction, and Refinement) policies (Cunha et al. 2014; Kagadis et al. 2016). The most suitable methods for small-animal in vivo imaging are based on positron emission tomography (PET), optical imaging (OI), computerized tomography (CT) and magnetic resonance imaging (MRI). Each imaging technique has its strengths along with significant intrinsic limitations which restrict their application to specific research questions, but recent introduction of multimodality devices has proven to be capable of overcoming part of these limitations by exploiting the complementarity relationship between different imaging modalities: the combination of high-resolution modalities, like micro-CT or micro-MRI, with highly sensitive functional techniques, such as micro-PET, provides added value to the pursuit of new imaging biomarkers for cancer characterization (Cunha et al. 2014) (Table 1).

After a brief review of the currently available tumor models of cancer, in this chapter, we will

Table 1 Summary of the common in vivo small-animal imaging modalities

Imaging technique	Spatial resolution (mm)	Depth	Radiation exposure (Gy)	Relative costs	Type of probe	Advantages	Disadvantages
PET	1–2	No limit	0.1–1.0	$$$	Molecules labelled with positron emitters	High sensitivity; quantification; diversity of biological probes; physiological and molecular data	Short-lived radionuclides; impracticability of distribution of some of them; radiation exposure; expensive
CT	0.05	No limit	0.1–0.6	$$	Radiopaque contrast agents	Spatial resolution (especially for bone and lung imaging); quantification; morphological and physiological data	Poor soft tissue contrast; radiation exposure
MRI	0.1	No limit	None	$$$	Paramagnetic/ Superparamagnetic metal chelates, hyperpolarized contrast agents	Spatial resolution; high soft tissue contrast; quantifications; morphological, physiological, and molecular data	Low sensitivity and long acquisition times
OI	1–2	mm	None	$	Fluorophores or β-emitters	High sensitivity; high throughput; low cost; physiological and molecular data	Limited depth of penetration; poor translational power

PET positron emission tomography, *CT* computed tomography, *MRI* magnetic resonance imaging, *OI* optical imaging, mm millimetres, *Gy* gray

Adapted from Cunha, L.; Horvath, I.; Ferreira, S.; Lemos, J., Costa, P., Vieira, D., Veres, D.S.; Szigeti, K.; Summavielle, T.; Mathe, D.; et al. *Preclinical imaging: An essential ally in modern biosciences*. Mol. Diagn. Ther. 2014; 18: 153–173 (Cunha et al. 2014)

summarize the current status of preclinical in vivo imaging techniques and the future perspectives of the emerging imaging biomarkers for the characterization of tumor biology and behavior.

2 Overview of Small-Animal Tumor Models

In discussion of preclinical imaging, recent developments in the field of small-animal tumor models have to be mentioned. In fact, the choice of an accurate experimental model represents a cornerstone of translational research in the view to bridge the gap between promising in vitro concepts and their clinical applications (de Jong et al. 2014). In vivo murine models have become a mainstay in oncologic research as they are the most accessible animal models; technical progress in qualitative and, moreover, in quantitative imaging technologies have strongly promoted their use, in order to acquire new data on cancer biology and to also develop new effective anticancer drugs (de Jong et al. 2014; Cook et al. 2012). Our increasing knowledge of human cancer biology combined with technical improvements have contributed to the development of modern tumor models that are able to better reflect human disease (de Jong et al. 2014; Cook et al. 2012; Tentler et al. 2012; De Souza et al. 2015), as we will discuss in this section.

We have to keep in mind that, despite the progress in these experimental fields, the value of

Table 2 Overview of different in vivo animal models

Type of model	Cell type	Host	Site of tumor	Advantages	Disadvantages
Syngeneic or allograft	Mouse	Immunocompetent	Subcutaneous	Low cost Immunocompetent host Reproducible and easy Large numbers of animals Wide variety of tumor types	Poor representation of human disease Unsuitable for testing humanized antibodies Non-natural site of tumor
Xenograft	Human	Immune deficient	Subcutaneous	Low cost Reproducible and easy Homogenous Large numbers of animals	Immunosuppression Different representation of human disease Non-natural site of tumor Rodent tumor microenvironment
Orthotopic	Human	Immune deficient	Organ of interest	Lower cost than GEMMs Hosts readily available Tumors at natural sites Reliable metastatic pattern	Immunosuppressed Requires surgical skill Rodent tumor microenvironment Difficult to follow tumor kinetics
GEMMs	Mouse	Immunocompetent	Organ of interest	Good representation of human cancer Heterogeneous Immunocompetent Investigates the tumor cells and the microenvironment	Expensive Complicated breeding schemes Variable penetrance and tumor latency Difficult to follow tumor kinetics

GEMMs genetically engineered mouse models
Adapted from Cook, N., Jodrell, D. I. & Tuveson, D. A. *Predictive* in vivo *animal models and translation to clinical trials*. Drug Discov. Today 2012; 17: 253–260 (Cook et al. 2012).

many animal studies remains still controversial because preclinical data do not always translate into clinical application, often showing lack of predictive value in human disease (De Souza et al. 2015; Martic-Kehl et al. 2012; Perel et al. 2007). Clearly, despite the diversity of sophisticated models currently available, none of these models will reproduce all aspects of human cancer in a comprehensive manner and so it is crucial to select the right model for the right research topic. In the search for a more personalized approach to cancer therapy, selection of well-defined model systems and appropriate study designs (including the adequate imaging approach for the trial endpoint) is crucial to improve translational power (de Jong et al. 2014).

To date, multiple approaches are available for modelling human cancer in mice, and the power to predict clinical performance vary widely between each approach (de Jong et al. 2014; Cook et al. 2012; De Souza et al. 2015) (Table 2).

2.1 Subcutaneous Engraftment Models

The most common model currently used in laboratory remains the engraftment technique, in which cultured human (xenografts) or mouse (allograft) cells or tumor tissue explants are grafted into recipient immunodeficient or immune-competent mice (Cook et al. 2012).

The discovery of the athymic nude mouse (Rygaard and Povlsen 1969) opened a new era in cancer research providing an immunocompromised murine cancer model that could enable engraftment, preventing rejection of the same (de Jong et al. 2014; Cook et al. 2012). New syngeneic models, where murine cell lines are injected subcutaneously in immune-competent murine hosts, are those models that avoid the immunodeficiencies found in xenografts, allowing for the assessment of the immune system involvement in cancer progression and response to therapeutics and thus reflecting tumor–host interactions in a more reliable way (Cook et al. 2012; De Souza et al. 2015). These subcutaneous implantable models are relatively inexpensive, easy to handle, and also offer the advantage to rapidly examine large cohorts of relatively uniform tumors, and so they are still popular in many specific applications of preclinical research (Cook et al. 2012). Nevertheless, none of these models accurately reconstruct the complex interactions between tumor and host, often behaving differently than the corresponding human cancer (Cook et al. 2012; De Souza et al. 2015).

2.2 Orthotopic Patient-Derived Xenografts (PDX) Models

Although subcutaneous models are still popular in preclinical research, a specialized version of xenograft model has been elaborated by transplanting patient-derived tumor tissue or cancer cells into the tumor tissue of origin in the nude mouse (de Jong et al. 2014; Cook et al. 2012). Despite these patient-derived xenograft (PDX) models are more expensive and technically challenging to realize (Cook et al. 2012), they are considered to more accurately imitate the heterogeneity of the original tumor (Hoffman 1999) and other features of human tumors that are not evident in cell-line-based xenografts, such as a spontaneous metastatic spread that is more comparable to that seen in humans (De Souza et al. 2015; Hoffman 1999; Fidler 1990; Pettaway et al. 1996; Jin et al. 2010).

Such orthotopic PDX models have been established for several tumor types, including pancreas and colon tumors (Fu et al. 1992; Fu et al. 1991; Metildi et al. 2014). For other tumor types, such as prostate and breast tumors, they remain technically challenging, especially considering the hormone-receptor status of the engrafted outgrowth in relation to the original tumor (de Jong et al. 2014). Another advantage of a permanent PDX model lies in the opportunity to study human tumor responses to treatments in a longitudinal way (de Jong et al. 2014) although they have the drawback of developing a higher mutation rate away from the parent tumor over time (Cook et al. 2012).

Moreover, these engraftment models have a variable transplantation failure rate across different tumor types (de Jong et al. 2014; Cook et al. 2012; De Souza et al. 2015). To overcome this issue, recent developments have led to the generation of mice with more specifically compromised immune systems: these novel "triple-negative" mice combine T-cell and B-cell deficiency with a lack of functional natural killer cells, enabling significantly enhanced tumor take rate (de Jong et al. 2014; De Souza et al. 2015; Ito et al. 2012; Garcia and Freitas 2012; Shultz et al. 2007). However, the absence of a functional immune system in such models remains a major criticism to study the metastatic behavior of cancer (de Jong et al. 2014; De Souza et al. 2015). Therefore, in order to reconstitute the human immune system, chimeric "triple-negative" immunodeficient mice have been engrafted with human hematopoietic stem cells (Ito et al. 2008; Ji et al. 2012), generating a new humanized phenotype that has been further improved by introducing human cytokine genes (Ito et al. 2012).

2.3 Genetically Engineered Mouse Models (GEMMs)

Genetically engineered mouse models (GEMMs) are the most advanced animal models of human cancer, and many models now exist which closely recapitulate the human disease (Cook et al. 2012). Thanks to the use of transgenic and conditional knock-out and/or knock-in techniques, transgenic mice express oncogenes or dominant negative tumor suppressor genes in a nonphysiological manner in order to establish organ-specific autochthonous tumors similar to human disease (de Jong et al. 2014; Cook et al. 2012). In fact, besides providing similar genetic alterations compared to the analogous human cancer, GEMMs are able to reproduce in a comprehensive manner other crucial factors that drive cancer development and progression, constituting an intact mouse microenvironment, as well as an intact immune system, both of which are important advantages over most xenograft models (de Jong et al. 2014; Cook et al. 2012; Walrath et al. 2010). In addition, the progression of the cancer in GEMMs should recapitulate the histopathology and molecular abnormalities of the analogous human disease (Olive and Tuveson 2006).

Nonetheless, there are several shortcomings regarding the use of GEMMs that must be considered. First, GEMMs have variable penetrance and latency before tumor development and often require sophisticated imaging techniques to detect and monitor tumor growth (Cook et al. 2012). Second, GEMMs are more expensive than other models because they require complicated breeding schemes. We have also to consider that their usefulness is dependent on several further issues including fidelity of the genetic lesions and the kinetics of tumor progression (Cook et al. 2012) (controlling gene expression patterns is not always possible, often leading to unpredictable phenotypes (De Souza et al. 2015)), as well as the ability to detect disease and perform specific interventions (Cook et al. 2012). Finally, there are some research fields in which GEMMs cannot be used to evaluate drugs activity, particularly for highly specific monoclonal antibodies, which might only react with human epitopes (Ocana et al. 2010). However, such model systems are able to reproduce specific clinical aspects that are crucial to investigate tumor-related processes and the clinical applicability of probes and vectors for imaging and drugs studies. To date, more complex PDX models and GEMMs may be particularly relevant for imaging approaches that are clinically applicable, such as PET, SPECT, CT, and MRI (de Jong et al. 2014).

3 Positron Emission Tomography (PET) in Tumor Biology Characterization

PET is a functional imaging technique used to observe cellular metabolic processes. It is used in research to evaluate the in vivo biodistribution of radiotracers and consequently define biological processes (Tatsumi et al. 2003). The biochemical and metabolic informations obtained with this molecular imaging technique depend on the radiotracer used (Margolis et al. 2007). Recently, in literature, several studies focused on the searching of new radiotracers used in PET as biomarkers to understand different cellular mechanisms and consequently the tumor behaviors. Data from several biomarkers could help in different steps of the clinical process: from tumor diagnosis to be a guide in therapy choice, to predict, and to monitor therapy response and eventually disease progression (Stephen and Gillies 2007; Na et al. 2008; Tunariu et al. 2012; Avril and Weber 2005). In fact, PET is able to detect metabolic tumor evolution and to monitor therapy response also before clear anatomic changes. This result depends on its superior ability to detect vital cancer tissue in comparison to other instrumental tests as CT and MRI. Therefore, its use in a multimodal imaging approach may lead to a better tumor characterization, and it is potentially useful to develop new therapeutic strategies in preclinical area. Due to the complexity of tumor behavior, several probes about new radiotracers and also their ability to reveal different cellular mechanisms are investigated in laboratory. In the near future, their roles will be of major importance to understand the mechanism of anticancer therapy (Wang et al. 2009). There is an emerging need to develop, in laboratory, in vivo tests that can analyze the induced biological effect of new therapies in a neoplastic lesion. This could increase the feasibility and efficacy of therapies in selected patients with the result of a personalized cancer therapy, with a reduction of cost and side effects (Clark et al. 2017).

The emerging and the development of new therapeutic strategies as target therapy has strengthened the study of well-known and new biomarkers to better understand their interaction with in vivo cell lines, thanks to their integration as radiotracers in PET analysis.

Currently, [^{18}F]fluorodeoxyglucose (^{18}F]FDG) is the most widely used radiotracer in the oncology field. Its wide use in clinical practice is the result of numerous preclinical studies which continue to be published in literature. [^{18}F]FDG is able to measure the glucose metabolism, important to suggest a differential diagnosis between vital and necrotic areas within the same lesion. It has also the ability to detect changes in tumor glucose metabolism before changes in tumor morphology and size (Figs. 1 and 2). Rapid [^{18}F]FDG changes, in particular within 24–48 h after a therapy administration, provide data regarding treatment response reflecting drug effects at cellular levels (Wang et al. 2009; Avril and Propper 2007; Stroobants et al. 2003; Gayed et al. 2004). This characteristic is an optimal base to understand and develop new target therapies (Clark et al. 2017).

Another radiotracer is 3'-deoxy-3'-[^{18}F]-fluorothymidine ([^{18}F]FLT), whose metabolism in tumor cellular process of xenograft-bearing mice has been analyzed in several studies published in the last decade (McKinley et al. 2013). It is a pyrimidine analog phosphorylated by an enzyme within the salvage DNA synthesis pathway (thymidine kinase 1). The activity of thymidine kinase 1 and consequently the uptake of [^{18}F]FLT reflect cellular proliferation.

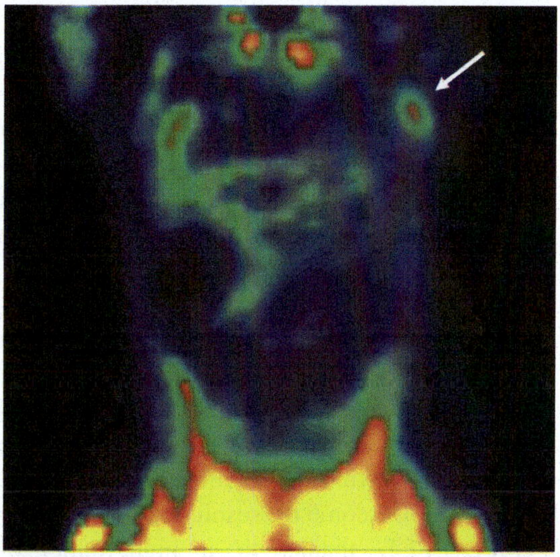

Fig. 1 Coronal small animal [^{18}F]FDG PET images of a mouse lung adenocarcinoma xenograft showing early detection of tumor engraftment (white arrow). The early confirmation of successful tumor engraftment, often before caliper detection, allows to test novel drugs when the tumor is still small and well vascularized (and therefore potentially more responsive to treatment)

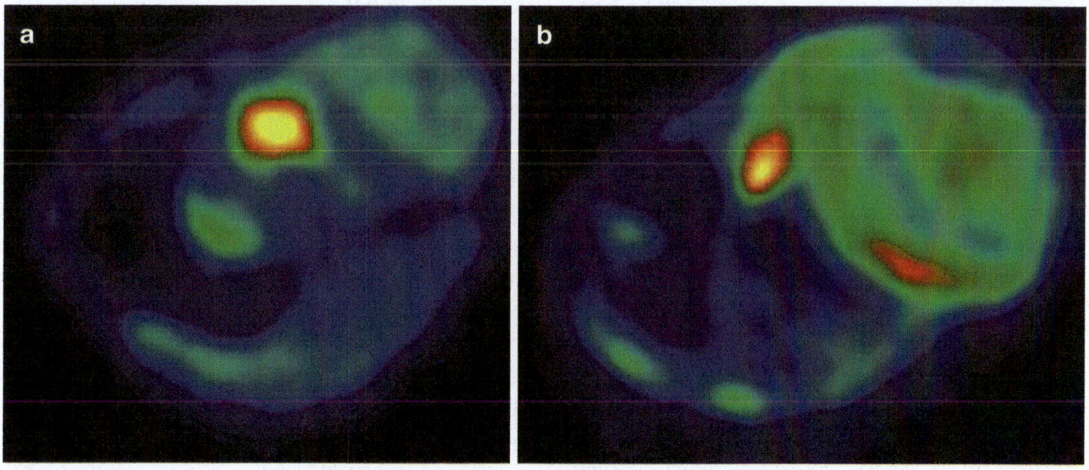

Fig. 2 Tansaxial small-animal [^{18}F]FDG PET images of a mouse lung adenocarcinoma xenograft showing tumor lesion increase in size and [^{18}F]FDG uptake over time. The possibility to re-scan small animals allows to monitor tumor growth over time and the metabolic response to novel drugs. Noninvasive small-animal imaging also allows to reduce the number of animals used for testing (avoiding the need to sacrifice the animals at fixed time points)

Modifications in [^{18}F]FLT level are usually indication of changes in cancer proliferation and also predict tumor shrinkage after therapy (Schelhaas et al. 2017; Perumal et al. 2012; Iommelli et al. 2014), although recently some reports showed doubts on this concept and consequently its use remains not clear in determined cases (Shields 2012; Schelhaas et al. 2014; Chalkidou et al. 2012). [^{18}F]FLT is also considered specific for differentiating cancer from inflammation (Lin et al. 2015). It is known for its correlation to cellular proliferation in several malignancies as in colorectal, esophageal, and breast cancer (Wang et al. 2009; Lin et al. 2015; Woolf et al. 2014).

Since last decade, O-(2-[^{18}F]fluoroethyl)-L-tyrosine ([^{18}F]FET) has also been largely used in neuro-oncology. [^{18}F]FET is capable of depicting cerebral gliomas, and for some authors it also has the capacity to differentiate low and high grade tissue using kinetic analysis (Pöpperl et al. 2006). It is able to overcome the resolution limitation of [^{18}F]FDG-PET, thanks to a high tumor-to-background contrast due to the relatively low uptake in normal brain tissue (Jansen et al. 2014). These important features lead to an intensive study of this biomarker in laboratory to improve preclinical in vivo imaging and monitoring tumor cells behavior that have undergone new therapies (Holzgreve et al. 2016).

Another of the most studied in laboratory radiotracer is 4-[^{18}F]-(2S,4R)-fluoroglutamine ([^{18}F]FGln). It is a glutamine analog involved in amino acid metabolism. Glucose and glutamine are the most abundant nutrients for producing energy in health and tumor cells. In fact, glutamine contributes to tumorigenesis (Zhu et al. 2017). [^{18}F]FGln-PET is used in monitoring therapeutic efficacy, assessing pharmacodynamic process. In fact, the biomarker can target the cellular glutamine metabolism that is altered in several kinds of cancer as in breast tumor (Son et al. 2013; Kim and Kim 2013; Zhou et al. 2017). Currently, several glutamine-based radiotracers are investigated with PET in preclinical area, but future studies are necessary to better understand their possible roles in therapeutic outcome assessment and in new drug development.

From previous data, numerous biomarkers are under investigation. The main biologic processes described concern glucose and amino acid metabolism, and also acetate and nucleotide metabolism, but currently preclinical research also pays attention on a wide range of different molecules that could be considered useful in PET analysis, for example, also in immunologic and hormonal fields. In particular, several immuno-PET are under preclinical investigation to identify predictive response biomarkers after the administration of anticancer immunotherapies (Tavaré et al. 2016; Rylova et al. 2016; Bhattacharyya et al. 2013).

Moreover, the recent clinical use of ^{68}Ga-labelled-prostate-specific membrane antigen-PET (^{68}Ga-PSMA-PET) is constantly increasing. Often in clinical practice, it is used in combination with multiparametric MRI providing important data about cancer sites and molecular information (Maurer et al. 2016). Its capacities are deeply analyzed in preclinical setting. In fact, PSMA is regulated by androgen receptor that is altered in a large sample of prostate cancer. A high level of PSMA is directly related to androgen receptor reduction. Therefore, PSMA-PET has the potential to obtain information about hormonal therapies (Miyamoto et al. 2012; Ahmad and Kumar 2011; Kumar 2016; Noss et al. 2002).

In laboratory, it can be useful also to test several radiotracers that could be involved in different features of a unique tumor biologic behavior as in the case of [^{18}F]FDG and [^{18}F]FLT in colorectal cancer. It is of interest also to understand the possible correlations and mechanisms between the tracers in PET (Wang et al. 2009). Another dual tracer used in research field is [^{18}F]FDG and ^{11}C choline: they are both tested in subcutaneous prostate cancer in mouse models resulting in better comprehension of the mechanisms of the tumor, especially of its typical grading heterogeneity (Belloli et al. 2009).

The use of PET in laboratory is not limited to the evaluation of the interactions in vivo of systemic therapies, but in literature, a considerable number of studies focuses on preclinical evaluation of radiation treatment. The main mechanism analyzed in laboratory is the biological repopulation that has a strong impact on the irradiated tissues also during therapy (Zhang et al. 2017; Yue et al. 2014; Yang et al. 2014). In specific, it is involved in the mechanism of radiation resistance and consequently in the use of higher doses in clinical practice, as in a dose-escalation setting, to overcome this problem and to reach a high disease control rate (Zhang et al. 2017; Yue et al. 2014; Yang et al. 2014; Wang and Li 2005; Røe et al. 2010). In these cases, a PET with [^{18}F]FLT can monitor tumor changes in growth, thanks to its characteristic to be related to Ki-67 as proliferation expression (Zhang et al. 2017; Yue et al. 2014; Wang et al. 2013). Moreover, results obtained by a [^{18}F]FLT PET have been compared with [^{18}F]FDG PET for colorectal cancer showing better results in early response monitory in xenograft-bearing mice with the former (Wang et al. 2010).

One important limitation in preclinical area is the tiny dimension of tumors in murine models, sometimes only few cubic millimeters, which is a challenge in terms of precision and require high technology imaging tools (Holzgreve et al. 2016). Another issue is the lack of a sufficient determination of intratumoral heterogeneity in radiotracer uptake, particularly in case of small size cancer[3]. If the tumor size is more than 1 cm, it is considered sufficient to obtain an adequate resolution without quantitative errors due to the partial volume effect, also if some authors have succeeded in characterizing even tumors of few millimeters in size (DiFilippo et al. 2012; Aubry et al. 2009). In fact, high spatial resolution is important to show volumes of interest and to reach a good accuracy. For this reason, an optimal solution may be the use of a dedicated PET for small animals that could lead to good results due to the use of a super-spatial resolution, but the high cost of this instrument makes impractical for easy accessibility. In the majority of cases, a clinical PET/CT scanner is used as an alternative in preclinical studies even if it leads to a lower image quality (DiFilippo et al. 2012; Chatziioannou 2002; Wolf and Abolmaali 2009). Some authors focused their studies on the use of a clinical PET to assess its feasibility in comparison with micro-PET obtained with dedicated tools. To evaluate the accuracy and analyze the results achieved after the radiotracer injection and after the PET scan, the mice were sacrificed and organs of interest, including the tumor, were measured in a ϒ-counter to compare the radioactivity (Tatsumi et al. 2003; Wang et al. 2017). The results showed a not optimal but acceptable resolution of images, in particular using small-animal-specific protocols with the help of thin-slice scans, and consequently at the moment clinical PET, in particular if hybrid with a CT, is the tool most used also in laboratory research. This is due also to their wide diffusion in contrast to the unavailability of dedicated small-animal PET/CT (Tatsumi et al. 2003; DiFilippo et al. 2012).

In conclusion, PET is currently an optimal instrument to analyze in preclinical area tumor biological processes with particular focus on molecular targets. The emerging studies on several radiolabeled probes will contribute to a better development and validation of new therapies.

4 Micro-computed Tomography (μ-CT)

Micro-computed Tomography (μCT) is a predominantly morphological imaging modality, which measures and compares differences in tissue density through the acquisition of hundreds of planar projections from multiple angles around the animal (usually, a micro-CT system is equipped with an X-ray tube and 2D X-ray detectors mounted in the opposite direction within the rotating gantry); in this way, it is possible to obtain volumetric 3D image dataset of bone structures and soft tissues with microscopic spatial resolution (50–100 μm) and subsecond temporal resolution (50 ms) (Cunha et al. 2014; Kagadis et al. 2010, 2016; Cavanaugh et al. 2004; de Kemp et al. 2010).

Initially introduced for the study of macroscopic and microscopic structures of bone tissue, in the last decades, this imaging technique has significantly improved, showing a great potential in many preclinical application, especially in cancer research (Cyran et al. 2014; Feldkamp et al. 1989).

In particular, μ-CT has proven to be an effective tool for the evaluation of tumor growth at a microscopic level, both for primitive lesions and metastases (e.g., Winkelmann and colleagues used μ-TC to evaluate bone metastases in murine prostate cancer models, detecting lesions as small as 0.3 mm in diameter) (Winkelmann et al. 2012).

Being based on the X-ray attenuation by tissues, the main limitation of this technique is the difficulty in differentiating tissues with similar attenuation characteristics, but it is possible to use contrast agents to improve tissue characterization through the enhancement of specific structures or regions. Among the contrast media normally used for in-vivo imaging, it is possible to distinguish two main categories, based on circulation time: conventional water-soluble nonionic iodine-based contrast agents (rapidly filtered from the blood by the kidneys) and blood-pool contrast agents (with higher blood half-life). Because of the relative slowness of the first μ-TC scanners (with acquisition time of up to a few hours), for a long time, it was not possible to use conventional iodinated contrast agents with the small living animals, because, as mentioned above, these agents are quickly eliminated from the blood immediately after intravenous injection (Schambach et al. 2010; Iacobellis et al. 2016). In humans, it is possible to acquire CT images in the first pass of the contrast medium, thanks to a sufficiently long circulation time, using a relative low contrast dose compared to total blood volume (Ritman 2004; Abruzzo et al. 2008; Dorr et al. 2007); in mice, this is not possible because the much faster circulation causes the contrast elimination just a few seconds after the injection, so it would be necessary to inject the contrast agent during the entire acquisition time, exceeding the renal filtration rate. (Previous studies on mice and rats showed that it is possible to obtain a sufficient anatomical definition of extra- and intracerebral compartments of the vascular system with the injection of 350 μL/30 g mouse of iodinated contrast, which was tolerated by all animals.)

Recent technological developments, especially in the field of X-rays detectors, currently allow acquisition time less than a minute, with superior quality images, thanks also to a higher SNR. This has made it possible not only the use of conventional contrast agents (similar to those used in CT-angiography) but also a significant reduction of the radiation dose, of the duration of anesthesia (and of the relative incidents), and of the motion artifacts (Schambach et al. 2009; Vogel 1997; Kiessling et al. 2004).

Blood-pool contrast agents allow very long acquisition time (hours) after a single injection, with a much smaller volume than that needed using conventional contrast media; in this way, it is possible to perform multiple measurements on the same animal with only one administration (thus without the problems linked to an excessive amount of contrast). Newer liposome-based blood-pool contrast agents, with longer blood half-life and with higher iodine concentration (>100 mg/mL), allow a much better anatomical definition, especially of the small structures (Barrett et al. 2006; Mukundan Jr et al. 2006).

Furthermore, over the years, new tumor-specific contrast media have been developed in order to improve the noninvasive characterization of neoplasms and the serial monitoring of disease before and during radio- or chemotherapy treatment in the preclinical setting: for example, Boll et al. studied liver lesions in a colon cancer metastasis murine model using a dedicated alkaline earth metal-based nano-particulate contrast agent, and they found that lesions as small as 300 μm were detectable after a single injection. Another example of liver-specific contrast agent is represented by the iodinated contrast agent DHOG (1,3-bis-[7-(3-amino-2,4,6-triiodophenyl)-heptanoyl]-2-oleoyl glycerol; *Fenestra LC; Art Technologies, San Diego, CA*), which is internalized by hepatocytes leading to a significant enhancement of the liver contrast after 2 hours from injection; this agent provides noninvasive quantification of liver metastases through the differentiation of normal hepatocytes and nonenhancing neoplastic cells (Boll et al. 2011; Gossl et al. 2006; Choukèr et al. 2008; Graham et al. 2008; Henning et al. 2008).

The use of contrast media has also allowed the development of more sophisticated CT-imaging techniques that can provide functional information, especially with regard to tissue perfusion (Cyran et al. 2012a). Using dynamic contrast-enhanced (DCE) imaging techniques, like CT-Perfusion, it is possible to quantify noninvasively functional parameters of tissue circulation like the regional blood flow (BF), the blood volume (BV), and the vessel permeability; these parameters allow a precise evaluation of tissue neoangiogenesis, which is a fundamental feature of neoplastic tissues.

The perfusion parameters related to the tumor microcirculation can be used to predict individual patient responses to radiotherapy and chemotherapy in various type of cancers (neck, lung, bowel, etc.), and are particularly useful in case of antiangiogenic tumor therapy, allowing the distinction between responder and nonresponder patients, through the quantification of therapeutic effect on tumor vascularization (Lind et al. 2010; Hermans et al. 2003).

Another very promising technique in CT imaging is the Dual Energy CT (DECT), in which the same anatomical structures (animals, organs, or tissue) are simultaneously scanned using two different energy spectra (usually 80 kV and 140 kV) to generate a set of matched images from which it is possible to obtain both anatomical, structural, and functional information (like tissue perfusion). In particular, DECT provides a clear distinction between iodine contrast and bone and soft tissues, and allows the reconstruction of iodine maps that show iodine distribution in a specific organ or tissue and that correlate very well with results obtained using Perfusion CT despite a much lower radiant exposure; also this technique is very useful in the serial monitoring of tumor angiogenesis, especially in case of radiation treatment associated with antiangiogenic factors (Zhang et al. 2009, 2012; Ashton et al. 2014; ; Clark et al. 2013).

5 Micro-magnetic Resonance Imaging (μ-MRI)

The Magnetic Resonance Imaging (MRI) is a noninvasive and nonionizing 3D imaging technique based on the physical phenomenon of nuclear magnetic resonance, through the study of nuclear magnetic behavior of different atoms of a specific organ or tissue positioned within a magnetic field.

It is beyond the scope of this review to explain the physics of MR, but we give a short description of the very basic principles: when a sample is placed into a magnetic field, its protons are aligned with (or against) the direction of the magnetic field; by applying a Radio-Frequency (RF) impulse, protons acquire energy that causes a misalignment in the magnetic field, but after a certain period of time, called "relaxation time", they return to the initial position generating another RF signal that is detected by the coils and processed to create digital images. The quality and the appearance of the images depend on the differences in the micro-environment of the protons within different tissues (and the signal intensity depends on the density of protons in tissues and on the relaxation properties of their spins).

By setting the resonance frequency of the coils at the proper value, it is possible to generate images encoding the signal emitted by a large variety of atomic nuclei (e.g., Sodium, Phosphorus, Carbon, Hydrogen), but the most used atom in MRI imaging is Hydrogen nucleo (proton—1H), because of its abundance in the body (water and fat) and thanks to its magnetic properties. (Hydrogen has a proton and an electron and it works as a little magnetic dipole.)

In recent years, we have witnessed rapid advances in MRI technique also in the preclinical research, thanks in particular to technological development and to the use of new scanners suitable for the study of small living animals (Cyran et al. 2014; Cunha et al. 2014; Albanese et al. 2013; Kauppinen and Peet 2011; Lewis et al. 2002; Pomper and Lee 2005; Koo et al. 2006).

Compared to normal MRI scanners routinely used in clinical practice, preclinical MRI scanners need a significant increase in spatial resolution that leads to a very marked signal reduction: for this reason, stronger magnets, stronger gradient sets, and specific receiver coils have been developed (Jakob 2011; Artemov 2016; Tremoleda et al. 2011).

Regarding the strength of the magnetic field, preclinical MRI systems work with magnetic fields strengths ranging from 4.7 to 11 T (as the

SNR increases with the strength of the magnetic field, small-animal MRI scanners should be at least 4.7 T), with corresponding proton resonance frequencies of 200–500 MHz, respectively. These scanners usually have horizontal superconducting magnets that allow an easier handling of the live animal during the examination. Actually, the most popular high-field magnets are cryomagnets, based on liquid cooling systems that provide low temperatures necessary for superconductivity.

Regarding the RF coils, these can be distinguished in two large categories: one for whole body and head imaging (of cylindrical shape and which generates uniform RF field) and one for the study of small, specific regions (surface coils). Multiple RF coil types have been developed by both main MR system manufacturers and independent producers (Jakob 2011; Brockmann 2007; Doty et al. 2007; Leroy-Willig and Geldwerth-Feniger 2007).

Among the various imaging modalities, MRI offers high spatial resolution (10–100 μm), an excellent soft tissue contrast (even without the administration of contrast media) and a very detailed anatomical definition; furthermore, MRI is a noninvasive and radiation-free technique. For these reasons, MRI is actually the most used technique for morphological study of tissues and organs, especially in the oncologic field, where it is widely used as a tool for cancer screening, lesion detection and characterization, for the visualization of changes that occur during neoplastic progression and to evaluate the response to therapy (Cyran et al. 2014; Lewis et al. 2002; Gore et al. 2011; Comley 2011).

In addition to its morphological skills, MRI is currently used for the study of many biological processes: as we will see next, a great variety of MRI techniques have been developed for functional and molecular imaging methods, like MR spectroscopy or perfusion- and diffusion-weighted imaging (Benz et al. 2016; Li and Padhani 2012).

In oncology, the application of these functional magnetic resonance pulse sequences allowed a more accurate assessment of the biology of many type of neoplasms (e.g., brain, lung, liver, breast) in various animal models, with important information on disease progression and therapy response (Cyran et al. 2014; Albanese et al. 2013; Kauppinen and Peet 2011; Li and Padhani 2012).

Perfusion MRI is used to quantify specific parameters of tissue microcirculation, such as regional blood volume or the rate of regional blood flow, which are indirect markers of angiogenesis and proliferation and can be used as markers of tumor viability and to predict the progression of disease and the response to therapy. Perfusion measurements can be obtained through different techniques, of which the most common is represented by the dynamic contrast-enhanced (DCE) imaging (with intravenous bolus injection of a contrast agent); however, it is possible to obtain quantitative information about perfusion also, without the administration of contrast media (for example, with the arterial spin labeling, or ASL, technique, in which the arterial blood water magnetization works as an endogenous contrast agent) (Barrett et al. 2007; Matsuo et al. 2014; Cyran et al. 2012b).

Diffusion-weighted imaging (DWI) is a functional MR technique based on the Brownian motion of free water within tissues. As specified below, this issue is particularly important in the study of neoplasms in which the increase in cellular density causes a reduction in water diffusion, which can be noninvasively detected through DWI sequences and quantified using the apparent diffusion coefficient (ADC) (Padhani and Khan 2010; Moffat et al. 2004).

Nuclear magnetic resonance spectroscopy (MRS) is a noninvasive and nonionizing technique based on the detection of the signal from specific compounds of low molecular weight (e.g., lactate, lipids, alanine, glutamine/glutamate, choline, N-acetylaspartate, creatine, etc.), the intensity of which depends on their concentration in the examined tissues. The most commonly used nuclei are 1H (proton), 31P (phosphorus), 23Na (sodium), and 13C (carbon). This technique is largely used to assess neoplastic tissue metabolism and can be used to serially monitor tumor biochemical changes; it has also been proved to be a valid tool for the evaluation of treatment response and the choice of the most appropriate therapy (Cunha et al. 2014; van der Graaf 2010; He et al. 2003).

5.1 Diffusion-Weighted Magnetic Resonance Imaging

Diffusion-weighted imaging (DWI) is a functional MRI technique used to evaluate structural tissue organization at a cellular level (Benz et al. 2016; Koh and Collins 2007).

Since the mid-1990s, diffusion imaging has been successfully applied to the evaluation of acute ischemic stroke as well as other intracranial diseases, and today its use is recommended in most brain MR studies (Schaefer et al. 2006; Schaefer et al. 2000). In the last two decades, new technological achievements on hardware and software, sequence design, and postprocessing methods have made DWI feasible also in body MRI (Koh and Collins 2007; Dietrich et al. 2010; Taouli et al. 2016) with applications in many extracranial sites such as liver (Taouli and Koh 2010), pancreas (Barral et al. 2015), kidneys (Taouli et al. 2009; Thoeny and De Keyzer 2011), prostate (Park et al. 2014; Gibbs et al. 2009), breast (Partridge et al. 2009), head and neck (Thoeny et al. 2012), and musculoskeletal system (Lecouvet 2016; Padhani and Gogbashian 2011). Despite its multiple fields of possible application, the growing interest in this technique is mainly due to its potential in detection and characterization of cancer both before and after therapy [126; 130] to such an extent that DWI is being actively supported by the National Cancer Institute as a noninvasive technique for imaging cancer biomarkers (Padhani et al. 2009). Furthermore, the innovative concept of diffusion-weighted whole body imaging with background body signal suppression (i.e., DWIBS) has proven to provide complementary information to CT and PET/CT, and it might even be able to replace tests using ionizing radiation in staging/restaging certain extra-cranial malignancies (Benz et al. 2016; Takahara et al. 2004; Kwee et al. 2008).

DWI exploits the incoherent three-dimensional thermally induced motion of water molecules in vivo (Brownian motion): the distance that water molecules can cover in a given time interval affects both signal intensity and contrast between tissues (Benz et al. 2016; Kwee et al. 2009; Winfield et al. 2015). In biological tissues, the free displacement of water molecules is constrained by the presence of restricting barriers (such as cell membranes, fibers, and macromolecules), and the signal intensity obtained with a diffusion-weighted sequence depends on the separation and permeability of these restricting boundaries (Kwee et al. 2009). In specific, water diffusion in biological tissues is composed of moving molecules within different compartments (i.e., intracellular, extracellular, intravascular, and transmembrane) (Kwee et al. 2009; Messiou and Kaiser 2015): every pathophysiological process which alters the volume ratio between these compartments or the physical nature of the impeding barriers (e.g. cell membrane) will thereby affect the diffusivity of the water molecules (Kwee et al. 2009).

Without going into technical details, diffusion-based contrast mainly depends on the choice of b value, which is a composite variable reflecting the strength and duration of application of two diffusion sensitized gradients applied on either side of the 180° refocusing pulse of a T2-weighted spin-echo sequence (Dietrich et al. 2010). Imaging with more than one *b*-value allows automated pixel-by-pixel calculation of the "apparent diffusion coefficient" (ADC), a mathematical parameter that represents a measure of the magnitude of water molecules displacement expressed in mm^2/s (Dietrich et al. 2010; Messiou and Kaiser 2015; Abramson et al. 2016). In general, since most malignant tumors are characterized by an increased cellular density with a higher intracellular/extracellular space volume ratio, they exhibit a relatively impeded diffusion, leading to a high signal intensity on high *b*-value DWI images and low ADC values when compared to healthy tissues (Benz et al. 2016; Kwee et al. 2009). Indeed, an impeded diffusion reflected by low ADC values has been reported for several malignant tumors with high cell density (Padhani et al. 2011; Thoeny and De Keyzer 2007). On the other hand, loss of cell membrane integrity in necrotic tumors and decrease in tumor cellularity, due to necrosis and/or apoptotic processes after successful treatment, may result in increased water diffusion in the extracellular space, leading to a decreased signal intensity on high b-value DWI images and corresponding increase in ADC values (Benz et al. 2016; Kwee et al. 2009; Padhani et al. 2011). This paradigm provides the basic model for DWI as a technique for tumor response assessment (Abramson et al. 2016).

Several correlations between ADC and histologic properties (such as proliferation index, tumor grade, and presence of necrosis) have shown that DWI could provide a potential imaging biomarker to characterize tumors in vivo; in several studies, lower ADC values have also been correlated with histologic features indicative of poor prognosis and with more aggressive tumors (Benz et al. 2016; Padhani et al. 2011; Hompland et al. 2014). Furthermore, it has been demonstrated both in preclinical and clinical settings that higher ADC values before treatment could predict an unfavorable response to therapies (Padhani et al. 2011; Roth et al. 2004; Koh et al. 2007; Cui et al. 2008), probably because a high ADC reflects the presence of tumor necrosis and low oxygen tensions, suggesting that ADC can be used as a predictor of the likelihood of a tumor responding to treatment (Padhani et al. 2011).

DWI shines also in assessing post-therapeutic changes, in preclinical tumor models as well as in clinical applications. Indeed, increases in ADC after successful chemotherapy and radiation therapy have been noted in several histological types of cancer, with strong negative correlations between ADC and tumor size (Padhani et al. 2011; Dudeck et al. 2008). Early changes in ADC values after treatment has been shown to be predictive of therapeutic response in several types of cancer (Winfield et al. 2015; Padhani et al. 2011), and failure to increase tumor ADC in response to therapy has predicted a poorer response to therapy (Hamstra et al. 2008; Eccles et al. 2009; Galbán et al. 2009; Giles et al. 2014), outlining the possible prognostic implications of this technique.

Studies on animal tumors and some human cancers have shown that a major advantage of DWI over traditional imaging modalities is that it is sensitive to changes occurring at a cellular level prior to changes in tumor size, after both chemotherapy and radiation treatment (Moffat et al. 2004; Abramson et al. 2016; Padhani et al. 2011). For preclinical drug studies, the ability of DWI to detect a small therapeutic effect is quite valuable because it provides the ability to quantify effects of varying the drug dosage and timings while reducing the number of animals by using the same animal as its own control. Another important aspect of DWI is that it is easily translatable from the animal model into clinical applications, thus providing a quantitative and sensitive surrogate marker for new drugs monitoring also in clinical trials (Moffat et al. 2004).

One of the major advantages of DWI includes the fact that it provides tumor characterization at baseline and after treatment without using ionizing radiation or any type of contrast media, relying only on endogenous contrast mechanisms, in reasonably short acquisition times (Koh and Collins 2007; Abramson et al. 2016; Padhani et al. 2011). However, we have to consider that this functional technique is burdened by technical limitations depending on its sensitivity to field inhomogeneities, especially in the proximity of interfaces of tissues with different susceptibilities and chemical shift artifacts due to the utilization of echoplanar imaging (EPI), which is necessary to reduce artifact movements (Dietrich et al. 2010; Winfield et al. 2015; Koh et al. 2012). EPI on higher field animal MRI scanners can be even more complicated due to the shortened tissue transverse relaxation and also due to the requirement for higher resolution (Moffat et al. 2004). The sequence needs also to be optimized in order to reduce eddy current effects, related to the diffusion sensitized gradients applied, and to achieve the best signal-to-noise ratio (Winfield et al. 2015; Koh et al. 2012).

To date, the major drawback in the validation of ADC as an imaging biomarker is the lack of standardization for data acquisition and analysis. There is currently no consensus on measurements or analysis methods, considering also that imaging protocols and analytic approaches vary significantly between different companies. This issue obviously limits the comparison between the results of different studies and also the feasibility of multicentre projects (Padhani et al. 2009; Winfield et al. 2015; Abramson et al. 2016). However, there is great potential for diffusion-weighted MRI to become an important surrogate biomarker for cancer in vivo evaluation, and future work includes optimization and standardization of the technique with validation of results on a large scale.

5.2 Perfusion Magnetic Resonance Imaging

Since angiogenesis is a critical process involved in tumor survival, growth, and metastatic spread, every method for assessing this phenomenon would potentially be quite useful in clinical oncology, especially after the introduction of novel antiangiogenic drugs in the current clinical practice (Gore et al. 2011; Barrett et al. 2007). By now, imaging represents the most powerful non-invasive method in order to visualize and quantify angiogenesis within the whole tumor, while giving functional data at baseline and also in the assessment of therapeutic response from the early stages, even before a noticeable change could be achieved with traditional imaging methods (Barrett et al. 2007). In recent years, in addition to clinical applications, there has been an increasing use of perfusion imaging techniques also in preclinical settings with studies regarding the efficacy of novel antiangiogenic treatment strategies and also drug delivery within tumor tissues (Bernsen et al. 2015; Barrett et al. 2007).

Among various imaging modalities, perfusion MRI techniques offer the greatest potential for imaging angiogenesis. Unlike nuclear medicine techniques, which evaluate tumor angiogenesis in a direct way through specific probes, perfusion MRI provides an indirect but very informative method for assessing vascular changes in tumors, mostly without radiation exposure and using relatively safe gadolinium-based contrast media. Through in vivo assessment and quantification of several microcirculatory parameters, we can exploit the differences between normal blood vessels and the immature and leaky vascular network of cancer in order to indirectly characterize the tumor itself (Cyran et al. 2014; Gore et al. 2011; Barrett et al. 2007).

In this section, perfusion MRI techniques will be briefly reviewed, focusing mainly on dynamic contrast-enhanced magnetic resonance imaging (DCE-MRI), because it is the most widely employed, especially in preclinical context.

5.2.1 Dynamic Contrast-Enhanced Magnetic Resonance Imaging

Dynamic contrast-enhanced magnetic resonance imaging (DCE-MRI) has emerged as a promising imaging technique that provides a noninvasive in vivo assessment of cancer- and treatment-related vascular alterations and, to date, it has settled as the most popular MRI method to evaluate angiogenesis (Sung et al. 2016).

Microscopic imaging studies and histologic evidences support the fact that angiogenesis increases the blood volume through the tumor tissue along with an enhanced transvascular leakage through the defective endothelial barrier of newly developed tumor vessels (Weidner 1995; McDonald and Baluk 2002). The assumption behind DCE-MRI relies on the hypothesis that a set of descriptive parameters used to characterize the vascular network of a given tissue (i.e., blood flow, vessel permeability, and intravascular/extravascular volume fractions) would eventually be different when considering healthy vessels in normal tissues and pathologic vessels in cancer tissues (Gore et al. 2011).

In simple terms, DCE-MRI is based on the measurements of how a paramagnetic tracer perfuses through such vessels, by evaluating the variation of MR signal intensity over time according to the dynamic changes in tracer's concentration in the tissue of interest (e.g., tumor). Such time-dependent signal changes will primarily depend on the flux of the paramagnetic tracer from the intravascular to the interstitial space, which is determined by the blood volume and transvascular permeability within each voxel (Gore et al. 2011; Sung et al. 2016).

In order to trace these changes, DCE-MRI involves serial acquisitions by using T1-weighted fast sequences heavily (usually three-dimensional spoiled gradient echo) before, during, and after intravenous injection of a low-molecular-weight gadolinium (Gd)-chelate, leading to an increase in signal intensity on T1-weighted images displaying a time-intensity curve that reflects the delivery and retention of the paramagnetic tracer within the tissue (Barrett et al. 2007; Abramson et al. 2016; Sung et al. 2016).

Such perfusion data could then be analyzed by a qualitative, semi-quantitative, or quantitative approach. The first two approaches examine the shape of the curve and other values such as the initial area under the gadolinium curve (IAUGC), time to peak, and wash-in/wash-out slopes, since most neoplasms are usually characterized by specific time-intensity curves. The quantitative approach fits the time-intensity curve to pharmacokinetic models in order to extract several parameters that directly measure tumor vessel perfusion and permeability (Abramson et al. 2016; Sung et al. 2016; Yankeelov and Gore 2007). The "extended Tofts and Kermode model" considers the contrast tracers distributed between the plasma space and the tissue space and, to date, is the most widely used. Standardized notation of this model considers *K*(trans) as the transvascular permeability, *V*(p)/*V*(e) as the volume fractions of plasma, and tissue space, respectively, and *K*(ep) as the redistribution rate constant between these two spaces (Yankeelov and Gore 2007; Walker-Samuel et al. 2006; Leach et al. 2003). Recent consensus recommendations drawn up by Leach and colleagues (2005) (Leach et al. 2005) regarding the use of DCE-MRI in early-stage clinical trials of antiangiogenic therapies state that IAUGC and K(trans) should be considered as the primary endpoints of such studies.

Evidences in literature showed that both healthy and tumor tissues exhibit characteristic pharmacokinetic parameter values, and that these parameters may be used to differentiate malignant from benign tumors, as in brain tumors (Kauppinen and Peet 2011; Gore et al. 2011).

As a vascular-specific biomarker, in the last decade, DCE-MRI has soon gained a primary role since the early stages of various novel antiangiogenic drugs development. Moreover, extended application of DCE-MRI parameters both in preclinical and clinical fields raises its advantages for supporting translational trials (Sung et al. 2016). Since its first applications in tumor xenografts, DCE-MRI has proven to be effective in monitoring treatment-related effects. Indeed, significant changes of some quantitative parameters, such as *K*(trans) or semi-quantitative IAUGC, were observed following several antiangiogenic chemotherapies, even much earlier than tumor size changes, both in small-animal tumor models (Rudin et al. 2005; Li et al. 2005; Ellingsen et al. 2009; Dafni et al. 2008; Moasser et al. 2007; Muruganandham et al. 2006; Marzola et al. 2005) and in early-phase clinical trials (Wedam et al. 2006; Lee et al. 2006; Mross et al. 2005; Liu et al. 2005; Medved et al. 2004; Morgan et al. 2003; Batchelor et al. 2007). This could be advantageous in the early selection of nonresponders or even in selecting candidates for a specific treatment (Barrett et al. 2007). Despite these encouraging premises, there is still a large variability on the values of DCE-MRI parameters as surrogate endpoint of monitoring treatment effect because of the controversy regarding baseline values and threshold validation to plan a treatment strategy (Sung et al. 2016).

Many studies also reported the ability of the DCE-MRI parameter *K*(trans) to predict treatment outcomes, both at baseline and early in the course of therapy (Zweifel and Padhani 2010; Bernstein et al. 2014; Flaherty et al. 2008; Ah-See et al. 2008; Johansen et al. 2009; Padhani et al. 2006). However, the right timing for the assessment of treatment response is still unclear and varies among different studies.

In conclusion, as one of the inherited drawbacks of every newly invented method such as DCE-MRI, there is still lacking on standardization of acquisition protocols, postprocessing elaborations, and also analytic approaches (Barrett et al. 2007; Abramson et al. 2016; Sung et al. 2016). Accuracy of the measured quantitative parameters can be influenced by the arterial input function, spatial and temporal resolutions, and by the pharmacokinetic models used in analyzing time-intensity curves (Abramson et al.

2016). Also, the optimal timing to ensure a reliable evaluation of treatment is still unknown (Winfield et al. 2015) and further reproducibility studies are needed in order to distinguish treatment-related effects from physiological fluctuation of parameters values (Abramson et al. 2016; Sung et al. 2016). However, DCE-MRI has become one the main imaging techniques used in antiangiogenic drugs trials, and it has the potential to become an important surrogate biomarker for cancer in vivo evaluation.

5.2.2 Other MRI Methods for Imaging Angiogenesis

Another available method to noninvasively interrogate the hemodynamic features of tumor vascular network is dynamic susceptibility contrast MRI (DSC-MRI). Like DCE-MRI, this technique relies upon serial acquisitions of dynamic MRI images before and after the intravenous injection of a gadolinium-chelate tracer in order to measure alterations in the native relaxation times of tissue water, T2 and T2∗. The magnitude of these alterations is related to the concentration of the contrast agent and the underlying geometry of its distribution in the tissue. Obtained data are then fitted to an appropriate pharmacokinetic model in order to estimate blood volume, blood flow, and mean transit time (Gore et al. 2011; Abramson et al. 2016).

DSC-MRI-derived maps of relative tumor blood flow and blood volume found their main applications in assessing the vascular microenvironment of brain tumors, showing a correlation with tumor grade (Aronen et al. 1994; Law et al. 2003; Weber et al. 2006) and treatment response (Fuss et al. 2001; Weber et al. 2004). It has been also hypnotized that DCS-MRI parameters could have a prognostic value in predicting clinical response in patients affected by low-grade glioma (Law et al. 2006) and also in patients with recurrent glioblastoma multiforme (Schmainda et al. 2015), respectively, before and after therapy. DSC-MRI has been also applied to evaluate the spatial and temporal development of the vascular network in brain metastases mouse models, underlining the role of the blood-to-tumor barrier in addition to the blood–brain barrier (Zhou et al. 2013).

Unlike other MRI techniques listed above, arterial spin labeling (ASL) is a noninvasive technique that gives a quantitative measure of tissue perfusion without any exogenous contrast agent. Indeed, ASL exploits radiofrequency pulses to invert the nuclear spin of the arterial blood protons flowing in the organ of interest. This magnetically labelled blood then exchanges with water in the tissue of interest, decreasing MRI signal intensity of the area proportionally to perfusion (Kauppinen and Peet 2011; Barrett et al. 2007). This technique was initially used to generate regional maps of cerebral blood flow in functional studies (van Laar et al. 2008), but it soon showed its potential also in assessing and monitoring tumor angiogenesis indirectly by measuring blood flow in brain tumors (Silva et al. 2000; Kimura et al. 2006), with interesting implications also in tumor grading (Wolf et al. 2005). Outside the brain, ASL has been successfully applied in quantifying blood flow in renal cell carcinoma (RCC) (De Bazelaire et al. 2005) and also in monitoring RCC recurrence after radiofrequency ablation therapy (Boss et al. 2006). These results are very promising in order to assess tumor perfusion, giving a potential tool also to monitor response to treatment, especially in the case of antiangiogenic drugs (Kauppinen and Peet 2011).

Finally, blood oxygenation level-dependent (BOLD) imaging is another functional MRI technique recently "lent" to oncology applications in order to demonstrate changes in tumor blood flow and oxygenation. BOLD imaging relies on the different magnetic properties of different hemoglobin state. Since deoxyhemoglobin has a paramagnetic activity, unlike oxyhemoglobin, its presence shortens the T2∗ of blood and surrounding tissues, while reducing MR signal intensity in T2∗-weighted gradient-echo sequences. Thus, oxyhemoglobin will act like an endogenous contrast agent and deoxyhemoglobin/oxyhemoglobin ratio will reflect the oxygenation state of a tissue (Kauppinen and Peet 2011; Barrett et al. 2007). Also in this case, most studies are concerned with brain tumor, and BOLD is able to demonstrate a signal heterogeneity within gliomas and meningiomas related to the patchy nature of perfusion and vascular reactivity in these tumors (Rijpkema et al. 2004; Rauscher et al. 2005; Müller et al. 2010). BOLD imaging could represent a noninvasive tool for mapping tumor hypoxia also in prostatic cancer (Jiang et al. 2004; Hoskin et al. 2007), providing a suitable method in order to monitor antivascular treatments and evaluate tumor oxygenation prior to radiotherapy (Kauppinen and Peet 2011; Matsuo et al. 2014).

The technique is affected by many inherited limitations, such as susceptibility artifacts, poor spatial resolution, and its sensitivity to other confounding factors like body temperature and use of medications. Its poor reproducibility and technical complexity are major drawbacks for translation into clinic, but BOLD imaging is a promising tool in radiation oncology in order to delineate areas of different oxygenation within tumors (Barrett et al. 2007).

5.3 Magnetic Resonance Spectroscopy

Since the 1980s, magnetic resonance spectroscopy (MRS) has been applied as an alternative noninvasive method to interrogate tissues composition, particularly neoplasms. Indeed, MRS permits tissue characterization from a biochemical and therefore metabolic point of view, allowing to detect spatial deviations from normal biochemistry in cancer (Pinker et al. 2012).

Employing almost the same hardware as conventional MRI, MRS is able to acquire signals from tissue metabolites present in very low concentration (i.e., a few millimoles) interrogating either a single specified voxel, as well as a 2D/3D array of voxels, without the need on any exogenous contrast agent (Winfield et al. 2015; Tee and Keshari 2015). The signal produced by a macroscopic sample after a radiofrequency pulse is composed of a set of single components generated by multiple spins precessing with different frequencies, each of them strictly dependent on the relationships with the surrounding molecular microenvironment (i.e., the chemical shift). Without going deep into technical details, the recorded free-induction decay (FID) is amplified with a phase detector and then fitted to the Fourier transformation in order to extract single spectral components, thus discriminating the different tissue compounds on the basis of chemical shift. Since water and fat protons are present in high concentrations, their signal would be confusing to the scopes, and so many approaches are applied in order to exclude their influence from the analysis (Cyran et al. 2014; Kagadis et al. 2016; Gore et al. 2011). The results of MRS could be displayed as a spectrum, where the concentration of a chemical specimen is proportional to its peak and also through specific maps on spectroscopic images. This method is able to detect specific biochemical and metabolic changes in neoplasms, which may be even pathognomonic for certain types of cancer, representing also a potential tool in evaluating treatment response and recurrence of the disease (Cyran et al. 2014; Cunha et al. 2014; Winfield et al. 2015).

To date, given their high representation in tissues, most clinical studies use signals from ^{1}H nuclei (i.e., proton) of tissue metabolites with high sensitivity performances and without the need for any hardware modification (Winfield et al. 2015; Tee and Keshari 2015). ^{1}H-MRS already represents a well-established tool in oncologic MRI for brain, breast, and prostate cancer, allowing tumor detection and characterization at diagnosis and also after treatment (Benz et al. 2016; Winfield et al. 2015; Pinker et al. 2012). Most brain tumors are characterized by low level of N-acetyl aspartate (normal neuronal marker) in conjunction with high total choline and other mobile lipids, due to an enhanced metabolic activity with high cell membrane turnover; due to their inherent high glycolytic activity, several tumor types are also characterized by high lactate concentration. Higher choline signals can also be found in prostate cancer, associated with reduced citrate signal, and breast cancer (Kauppinen and Peet 2011; Winfield et al. 2015). In addition, the application of ^{1}H-MRS is now expanding to the investigation of neoplasms in other body sites, such as soft tissue tumors (Sostman et al. 1994) and cervical and ovarian cancer (Stanwell et al. 2008; Mahon et al. 2004a, b).

Other accessible nuclei for MRS are ^{31}P, ^{13}C, ^{19}F, and ^{23}Na with different detectability related to variation in signal susceptibility, percentage isotope concentration, and tissue concentration (Benz et al. 2016).

^{31}P was one of the earliest nuclei employed to perform MRS studies. It gives a lower signal intensity than ^{1}H, due to its relatively low percentage concentration in tissues, but it has the advantage over ^{1}H-MRS of detecting separately choline metabolites, namely phosphomonoesters (i.e., phosphocholine) and phosphodiesters (i.e., glycerophosphocholine) (Winfield et al. 2015; Tee and Keshari 2015). High signals from choline metabolites tend to be related to aggressiveness of several neoplasms, whereas low levels are found in healthy tissues, and could also be employed in the assessment of treatment response (Kauppinen and Peet 2011; Pinker et al. 2012; Glaholm et al. 1989; Negendank 1992). In preclinical tumor models of cancer, some studies demonstrated significant changes in phospholipid precursors and catabolites detected by ^{31}P-MRS after chemotherapy, radiation therapy, and combined radio-chemotherapy, reflecting cell death or growth inhibition after successful treatment (Mahmood et al. 1994, 1995). ^{31}P-MRS provides also a panoramic view of tissue bioenergetics, extracting signals from nucleotide phosphates, phosphocreatine, and NADH. This application allows to noninvasively assess tumor activity and also measure pH in neoplastic environment (Kauppinen and Peet 2011; Winfield et al. 2015). Despite its potential, the low sensitivity of ^{31}P-MRS restricts its applications in cancer imaging, often requiring high field strength scanners (Kauppinen and Peet 2011; Pinker et al. 2012).

^{19}F gives a signal only slightly inferior to ^{1}H, and so ^{19}F-MRS is almost as sensitive as ^{1}H-MRS (Kauppinen and Peet 2011). Furthermore, because no background fluorine MR signal exists under physiological conditions (Gore et al. 2011), ^{19}F-MRS has been used to detect exogenous fluorine drugs (e.g., 5-fluorouracil) (McSheehy and Griffiths 1989; Stevens et al. 1984; Kamm et al. 2004) and to quantify tumor hypoxia using perfluorocarbons (Mason et al. 1996).

^{23}Na-MRS is already applied in studies regarding functional cardiac MRI, providing information on cellular metabolism in myocardial ischemic disease (Kim et al. 1997, 1999). Sodium imaging could represent a sensitive indicator of cell metabolism, since its intracellular levels rise under conditions of ATP deficiency when Na^+/K^+ ATPase pump is compromised (Pinker et al. 2012). Through the calculation of the parameter "tissue sodium concentration" (TSC), which relates extracellular and intracellular sodium content, ^{23}Na-MRS is able to evaluate a metabolic impairment also in cancer tissues. Studies demonstrated increased TSC in human brain tumors and also in breast cancer, providing a useful tool to improve the specificity of conventional breast MRI (Ouwerkerk et al. 2003, 2007). In a rat 9 L glioma model evaluated both with sodium imaging and proton diffusion imaging, changes in ^{23}Na signal and ADC were observed early after tumor treatment, even before reduction in tumor size (Schepkin et al. 2005).

The alternative nonproton MRS listed above are still under active investigation and further studies, as well as additional technical improvement, are needed in order to evaluate their added value in cancer biology characterization when compared to already well-established functional and molecular imaging techniques.

5.3.1 Hyperpolarized MRS with ^{13}C-labeled Molecules

As mentioned above, ^{1}H-MRS detection of cellular compounds has been shown to provide a sensitive tool for tumor diagnosis and post-therapeutic assessment in a variety of cancer. However, these measurements give only a static picture of cellular metabolism (Brindle et al. 2011). Last two decades have witnessed a growing interest in imaging molecules that can be administered even from the outside with spectroscopy. To date, ^{13}C-labeled molecules are the most widely used because of their capability to provide dynamic information on a variety of cellular pathways involved in tissue metabolism (Kauppinen and Peet 2011; Abramson et al.

2016; Brindle et al. 2011). However, of the total carbon naturally occurring, only 1.1% is present in the MR-active form of ^{13}C with a gyromagnetic ratio of about a quarter of that of ^{1}H (Tee and Keshari 2015) and, as a result, the sensitivity of ^{13}C-MRS is extremely poor when compared to ^{1}H-MRS (i.e., 0.02% considering 100% of ^{1}H-MRS) (Cyran et al. 2014; Tee and Keshari 2015; Brindle et al. 2011). In order to overcome this limitation, recent developments of several hyperpolarization methods have resulted in dramatic sensitivity gains in signal detection by over 10.000 fold. The term "hyperpolarization" encloses different techniques, achieved out of the body, that have been used to drive a given nucleus (e.g., ^{13}C) into a significant redistribution of energy levels to achieve, consequently, a larger magnetization for a given time (Gore et al. 2011; Benz et al. 2016; Tee and Keshari 2015). Unlike tracers used in nuclear medicine, hyperpolarized contrast agents are nonradioactive and have the advantage to report not only on their distribution in the tissue of interest but also on the distribution of their multiple metabolites, using only small concentrations (Gore et al. 2011; Abramson et al. 2016).

Since each of these tracers is characterized by a decay function of its T1-relaxation time, the main goal of hyperpolarization is to produce a nontoxic contrast agent with a sufficiently long T1 in conjunction with both rapid distribution and metabolism in the body (Abramson et al. 2016; Brindle et al. 2011). Among the different substrate that have been hyperpolarized, with varies lifetimes and uses, [1-^{13}C]pyruvate fulfils all the criteria above mentioned and, to date, it has been the most widely applied in MRS studies on animal cancer models (Abramson et al. 2016; Tee and Keshari 2015; Brindle et al. 2011).

Intravenous administration of hyperpolarized [1-^{13}C]pyruvate results in its rapid cellular conversion into labelled metabolites, namely lactate (through lactate dehydrogenase, i.e., LDH), alanine (through alanine transaminase), and carbon dioxide (through pyruvate dehydrogenase) (Tee and Keshari 2015; Brindle et al. 2011). Several preclinical studies demonstrated high levels of [1-^{13}C]lactate as a cancer biomarker that is able to distinguish tumor from healthy tissues (Golman et al. 2006; Park et al. 2010; Day et al. 2007a). This can be related to high levels of LDH activity in several types of neoplasms (Tee and Keshari 2015). A study conducted in transgenic adenocarcinoma of mouse prostate enlightened also that pyruvate-lactate exchange can be used to identify tumor grade (Albers et al. 2008). Early reduction in pyruvate-lactate conversion after chemotherapy and radiation therapy in a variety of cancer models (Day et al. 2007b; Day et al. 2011; Witney et al. 2010) showed also great potential for hyperpolarized [1-^{13}C]pyruvate-MRS in the evaluation of the response after conventional therapy. This technique has been also used in response assessment of targeted therapies administered in small-animal tumor models (Ward et al. 2010; Chaumeil et al. 2012). The first clinical trial conducted in 31 patients with untreated prostate cancer (Nelson et al. 2013) confirmed the safety of hyperpolarized [1-^{13}C] pyruvate in humans and showed high signal from labelled lactate in tumor regions.

Hyperpolarized MRS is a novel technology with great potential in the oncology field, but it is still in its primordial state. To date, the technique is affected by two major translational barriers represented by expensive hyperpolarization processes and technical limitations related to the need of multinuclear MRI scanner capability, which is not widely available on current MRI scanners. However, preliminary studies in preclinical research seem very promising in the view of providing new imaging biomarkers for cancer evaluation (Gore et al. 2011; Abramson et al. 2016; Tee and Keshari 2015).

6 Optical Imaging

Optical imaging (OI) includes a set of techniques that use light to assess tissue composition and molecular functions in the living body; images are obtained using light in the wavelength range from ultraviolet to near infrared. Various techniques are classified according to different types of light sources and photon detectors and on the presence of an external excitation source.

Thanks to the significant advantages offered by these techniques in temporal resolution, imaging contrast and, above all, cost-effectiveness, OI has quickly developed as a small-animal molecular imaging technology, and it has also been rapidly adapted to cancer research, with significant advances in the development of specific targeted probes which allow the quantification of the activity of specific molecular targets (Chen et al. 2016; Optical Imaging Fact Sheet 2012).

For the acquisition of images, the animal is placed in a light-tight imaging chamber, and the emitted light is detected using a charge-coupled device (CCD) detector; in the past decade, extremely sensitive detectors have been developed, capable of detecting visible to near infrared light emitted from the body (CCD cameras can convert light photons at wavelengths between 400 and 1000 nm). Actually, the most used OI techniques are "Bioluminescence, or BLI" (that uses a natural light produced by cells expressing emitting protein, like Luciferase species), "Fluorescence imaging, or FLI", and "near-infrared (NIR) Fluorescence imaging" (in which the optical probes can emit light only with the use of an external excitation source, like a laser), and "Diffuse optical tomography, or DOT" (based on diffuse light that penetrates tissue simultaneously at multiple projections) (Cunha et al. 2014; Massoud and Gambhir 2003; Bremer et al. 2003).

6.1 Bioluminescence Imaging (BLI)

This technique is based on the emission of visible photons at specific wavelengths produced by the oxidation of the molecule luciferin, a reaction catalyzed by the enzyme luciferase. Using BLI, it is possible to determine the location of specific chemical reaction or to identify the position and to follow the movement of specific cells within the body. Thanks to the development of specific DNA vectors including luciferase genes, actually with BLI, it is also possible to quantify small numbers of cells expressing the enzyme: target cells genetically modified to express the luciferase enzyme are inoculated (the most used is the firefly luciferase), then the luciferase substrate (e.g., luciferin) is systemically administered to obtain the emission of photons when it is captured and oxidized by the target cells. The photons generated are then captured by CCD cameras to create the image.

The possibility to modify almost any cell type for BLI led to a great development of this technique in the oncologic field, which can be used to detect very low levels of signal (thanks also to the absence of background light) and therefore a very small number of specific cells, resulting in an outstanding sensitivity that is particularly useful in the study of neoplasms and in the evaluation of therapy response (Cyran et al. 2014; Chen et al. 2016; Optical Imaging Fact Sheet 2012; Luker and Luker 2008; Wilson and Hastings 1988).

6.2 Fluorescence Imaging (FLI)

Unlike what happens in BLI, *Fluorescence Imaging (FLI)* requires the use of molecules (endogenous or exogenous) or materials that emit photons when activated by an external excitation source: a light of precise wavelength (in the visible range of 395–600 nm) is used to excite a target molecule, which responds emitting light characterized by lower energy and longer wavelength.

This technique involves the use of genetically modified cells that express fluorescent proteins, such as green-fluorescent protein (GFP) or the systemic administration of a fluorophore-based probe like a fluorescence-labeled antibody (Cunha et al. 2014; Chen et al. 2016; Optical Imaging Fact Sheet 2012; Massoud and Gambhir 2003).

NIR fluorescence imaging is performed using imaging photons in the 600–900 nm range, in order to optimize tissue penetration and to reduce the effect of auto-fluorescence from nontarget regions.

With FLI, it is possible to quantify specific gene expression and to monitor many physio-pathological process (at a cellular level), to identify specific cell types involved in the neoplastic process and to distinguish cancer cells from normal ones (Ntziachristos et al. 2003).

6.3 Diffuse Optical Tomography (DOT)

Diffuse Optical Tomography (DOT) is a computed tomography technique that generates three-dimensional images of a specific object (or of a region within the body) using diffuse light transmitted and scattered through the object at multiple projections. DOT imaging integrates the capabilities of computed tomography to those of OI; it has a good sensitivity and a very high spatial resolution (even 1–2 mm), and provides at the same time important quantitative information, as the signal intensity is an expression of the local concentration of fluorophore (with the possibility to visualize and to quantify the intensity of the fluorescent probe in a specific region of the small living animal) (Cunha et al. 2014; Chen et al. 2016; Optical Imaging Fact Sheet 2012; Gibson and Dehghani 2009; Culver et al. 2008).

Acknowledgments The authors would like to thank Professor Valentina Ambrosini for her contribution in figures collection.

Conflict of Interest Statement: All authors disclose any financial and personal relationships with other people or organizations that could inappropriately influence (bias) their work.

References

Abramson RG et al (2016) MR imaging biomarkers in oncology clinical trials. Magn Reson Imaging Clin N Am 24:11–29

Abruzzo T, Tumialan L, Chaalala C, Kim S, Guldberg RE, Lin A, Leach J, Khoury JC, Morgan AE, Cawley CM 3rd (2008) Microscopic computed tomography imaging of the cerebral circulation in mice: feasibility and pitfalls. Synapse 62(8):557–565

Ahmad N, Kumar R (2011) Steroid hormone receptors in cancer development: a target for cancer therapeutics. Cancer Lett 300:1–9

Ah-See ML, Makris A, Taylor NJ et al (2008) Early changes in functional dynamic magnetic resonance imaging predict for pathologic response to neoadjuvant chemotherapy in primary breast cancer. Clin Cancer Res 14:6580–6589

Albanese C, Rodriguez OC, VanMeter J, Fricke ST, Rood BR, Lee Y, Wang SS, Madhavan S, Gusev Y, Petricoin EF 3rd, Wang Y (2013) Preclinical magnetic resonance imaging and systems biology in cancer research. Am J Pathol 182(2):312–318

Albers MJ, Bok R, Chen AP, Cunningham CH, Zierhut ML, Zhang VY, Kohler SJ, Tropp J, Hurd RE, Yen YF, Nelson SJ, Vigneron DB, Kurhanewicz J (2008) Hyperpolarized 13C lactate, pyruvate, and alanine: noninvasive biomarkers for prostate cancer detection and grading. Cancer Res 68:8607–8615

Aronen HJ, Gazit IE, Louis DN et al (1994) Cerebral blood volume maps of gliomas: comparison with tumor grade and histologic findings. Radiology 191(1):41–51

Artemov D (2016) MRI imaging. In: Kagadis GC, Ford NL, Karnabatidis DN, Loudos GK (eds) Handbook of small animal imaging—preclinical imaging, therapy, and applications. CRC Press, Boca Raton, pp 121–137

Ashton JR, Clark DP, Moding EJ, Ghaghada K, Kirsch DG, West JL, Badea CT (2014) Dual-energy micro-CT functional imaging of primary lung cancer in mice using gold and iodine nanoparticle contrast agents: a validation study. PLoS One 9(2):e88129

Aubry K, Shao Z, Monteil J, Paraf F, Bessède JP, Rigaud M (2009) FDG-PET/CT of head and neck squamous cell carcinoma in a rat model. Mol Imaging Biol 11:88–93

Avril N, Propper D (2007) Functional PET imaging in cancer drug development. Future Oncol 3:215–228

Avril NE, Weber WA (2005) Monitoring response to treatment in patients utilizing PET. Radiol Clin North Am 43:189–204

Barral M, Taouli B, Guiu B et al (2015) Diffusion-weighted MR imaging of the pancreas: current status and recommendations. Radiology 274:45–63

Barrett T, Kobayashi H, Brechbiel M, Choyke PL (2006) Macromolecular MRI contrast agents for imaging tumor angiogenesis. Eur J Radiol 60(3):353–366

Barrett T, Brechbiel M, Bernardo M, Choyke PL (2007) MRI of tumor angiogenesis. J Magn Reson Imaging 26(2):235–249

Batchelor TT, Sorensen AG, di Tomaso E et al (2007) AZD2171, a pan-VEGF receptor tyrosine kinase inhibitor, normalizes tumor vasculature and alleviates edema in glioblastoma patients. Cancer Cell 11:83–95

Belloli S, Jachetti E, Moresco RM, Picchio M, Lecchi M, Valtorta S, Freschi M, Hess Michelini R, Bellone M, Fazio F (2009) Characterization of preclinical models of prostate cancer using PET-based molecular imaging. Eur J Nucl Med Mol Imaging 36:1245–1255

Benz MR, Vargas HA, Sala E (2016) Functional MR imaging techniques in oncology in the era of personalized medicine. Magn Reson Imaging Clin N Am 24(1):1–10

Bernsen MR, Kooiman K, Segbers M, van Leeuwen FW, de Jong M (2015) Biomarkers in preclinical cancer imaging. Eur J Nucl Med Mol Imaging 42(4):579–596

Bernstein JM, Homer JJ, West CM (2014) Dynamic contrast-enhanced magnetic resonance imaging biomarkers in head and neck cancer: potential to guide treatment? A systematic review. Oral Oncol 50:963–970

Bhattacharyya S, Kurdziel K, Wei L, Riffle L, Kaur G, Hill GC, Jacobs PM, Tatum JL, Doroshow JH, Kalen

JD (2013) Zirconium-89 labeled panitumumab: a potential immuno-PET probe for HER1-expressing carcinomas. Nucl Med Biol 40:451–457

Boll H, Nittka S, Doyon F, Neumaier M, Marx A, Kramer M, Groden C, Brockmann MA (2011) Micro-CT based experimental liver imaging using a nanoparticulate contrast agent: a longitudinal study in mice. PLoS One 6:e25692

Boss A, Martirosian P, Schraml C et al (2006) Morphological, contrastenhanced and spin labeling perfusion imaging for monitoring of relapse after RF ablation of renal cell carcinomas. Eur Radiol 27:1–11

Bremer C, Ntziachristos V, Weissleder R (2003) Optical-based molecular imaging: contrast agents and potential medical applications. Eur Radiol 13(2):231–243

Brindle KM, Bohndiek SE, Gallagher FA, Kettunen MI (2011) Tumor imaging using hyperpolarized 13C magnetic resonance spectroscopy. Magn Reson Med 66:505–519

Brockmann MA (2007) Use of clinical MR scanners for small rodent imaging. Methods 43(1):1

Cavanaugh D, Johnson E, Price RE, Kurie J, Travis EL, Cody DD (2004) In vivo respiratory-gated micro-CT imaging in small-animal oncology models. Mol Imaging 3(1):55–62

Chalkidou A, Landau DB, Odell EW, Cornelius VR, O'Doherty MJ, Marsden PK (2012) Correlation between Ki-67 immunohistochemistry and 18F-fluorothymidine uptake in patients with cancer: a systematic review and meta-analysis. Eur J Cancer 48:3499–3513

Chatziioannou AF (2002) Molecular imaging of small animals with dedicated PET tomographs. Eur J Nucl Med Mol Imaging 29:98–114

Chaumeil MM, Ozawa T, Park I, Scott K, James CD, Nelson SJ, Ronen SM (2012) Hyperpolarized 13C MR spectroscopic imaging can be used to monitor Everolimus treatment in vivo in an orthotopic rodent model of glioblastoma. Neuroimage 59:193–201

Chen X, Dongmei D, Liu FL, Cong W, Wang G, Liang J (2016) Optical-CT imaging. In: Kagadis GC, Ford NL, Karnabatidis DN, Loudos GK (eds) Handbook of small animal imaging—preclinical imaging, therapy, and applications. CRC Press, Boca Raton, pp 167–181

Choukèr A, Lizak M, Schimel D, Helmberger T, Ward JM, Despres D, Kaufmann I, Bruns C, Löhe F, Ohta A, Sitkovsky MV, Klaunberg B, Thiel M (2008) Comparison of Fenestra VC Contrast-enhanced computed tomography imaging with gadopentetate dimeglumine and ferucarbotran magnetic resonance imaging for the in vivo evaluation of murine liver damage after ischemia and reperfusion. Invest Radiol 43(2):77–91

Clark DP, Ghaghada K, Moding EJ, Kirsch DG, Badea CT (2013) In vivo characterization of tumor vasculature using iodine and gold nanoparticles and dualenergy micro-CT. Phys Med Biol 58(6):1683–1704

Clark PM, Ebiana VA, Gosa L, Cloughesy TF, Nathanson DA (2017) Harnessing preclinical molecular imaging to inform advances in personalized cancer medicine. J Nucl Med 58:689–696

Comley J (2011) In vivo preclinical imaging: an essential tool in translational research. Drug Discovery World 2011:58–71

Cook N, Jodrell DI, Tuveson DA (2012) Predictive in vivo animal models and translation to clinical trials. Drug Discov Today 17:253–260

Cui Y, Zhang XP, Sun YS, Tang L, Shen L (2008) Apparent diffusion coefficient: potential imaging biomarker for prediction and early detection of response to chemotherapy in hepatic metastases. Radiology 248(3):894–900

Culver J, Akers W, Achilefu S (2008) Multimodality molecular imaging with combined optical and SPECT/PET modalities. J Nucl Med 49(2):169–172

Cunha L, Horvath I, Ferreira S, Lemos J, Costa P, Vieira D, Veres DS, Szigeti K, Summavielle T, Mathe D et al (2014) Preclinical imaging: an essential ally in modern biosciences. Mol Diagn Ther 18:153–173

Cyran CC, von Einem JC, Paprottka PM, Schwarz B, Ingrisch M, Dietrich O, Hinkel R, Bruns CJ, Clevert DA, Eschbach R et al (2012a) Dynamic contrast-enhanced computed tomography imaging biomarkers correlated with immunohistochemistry for monitoring the effects of sorafenib on experimental prostate carcinomas. Invest Radiol 47:49–57

Cyran CC, Paprottka PM, Schwarz B, Sourbron S, Ingrisch M, von Einem J, Pietsch H, Dietrich O, Hinkel R, Bruns CJ et al (2012b) Perfusion MRI for monitoring the effect of sorafenib on experimental prostate carcinoma:a validation study. AJR Am J Roentgenol 198:384–391

Cyran CC, Paprottka PM, Eisenblatter M, Clevert DA, Rist C, Nikolaou K et al (2014) Visualization, imaging and new preclinical diagnostics in radiation oncology. Radiat Oncol 9:3

Dafni H, Kim SJ, Bankson JA, Sankaranarayanapillai M, Ronen SM (2008) Macromolecular dynamic contrast enhanced (DCE)-MRI detects reduced vascular permeability in a prostate cancer bone metastasis model following anti-platelet-derived growth factor receptor (PDGFR) therapy, indicating a drop in vascular endothelial growth factor receptor (VEGFR) activation. Magn Reson Med 60:822–833

Day SE et al (2007a) Detecting tumor response to treatment using hyperpolarized 13C magnetic resonance imaging and spectroscopy. Nat Med 13:1382–1387

Day SE, Kettunen MI, Gallagher FA, Hu DE, Lerche M, Wolber J, Golman K, Ardenkjaer-Larsen JH, Brindle KM (2007b) Detecting tumor response to treatment using hyperpolarized 13C magnetic resonance imaging and spectroscopy. Nat Med 13:1382–1387

Day SE, Kettunen MI, Krishna MC, Mitchell JB, Lizak MJ, Morris HD, Matsumoto S, Koretsky AP, Brindle KM (2011) Detecting response of rat C6 glioma tumors to radiotherapy using hyperpolarized [1-13C] pyruvate and 13C magnetic resonance spectroscopic imaging. Magn Reson Med 65:557–563

De Bazelaire C, Rofsky NM, Duhamel G et al (2005) Arterial spin labeling blood flow magnetic resonance imaging for the characterization of metastatic renal cell carcinoma. Acad Radiol 12:347–357

De Souza R et al (2015) Preclinical imaging and translational animal models of cancer for accelerated clinical implementation of nanotechnologies and macromolecular agents. J Control Release 10(219):313–330

Dietrich O, Biffar A, Baur-Melnyk A, Reiser MF (2010) Technical aspects of MR diffusion imaging of the body. Eur J Radiol 76:314–322

DiFilippo FP, Patel S, Asosingh K, Erzurum SC (2012) Small-animal imaging using clinical positron emission tomography/computed tomography and super-resolution. Mol Imaging 11:210–219

Dorr A, Sled JG, Kabani N (2007) Three-dimensional cerebral vasculature of the CBA mouse brain: a magnetic resonance imagingand micro computed tomography study. Neuroimage 35(4):1409–1423

Doty FD, Entzminger G, Kulkarni J, Pamarthy K, Staab JP (2007) Radio frequency coil technology for small-animal MRI. NMR Biomed 20(3):304–325

Dudeck O, Zeile M, Pink D et al (2008) Diffusion weighted magnetic resonance imaging allows monitoring of anticancer treatment effects in patients with soft-tissue sarcomas. J Magn Reson Imaging 27(5):1109–1113

Eccles CL, Haider EA, Haider MA, Fung S, Lockwood G, Dawson LA (2009) Change in diffusion weighted MRI during liver cancer radiotherapy: preliminary observations. Acta Oncol 48(7):1034–1043

Ellingsen C, Egeland TA, Gulliksrud K, Gaustad JV, Mathiesen B, Rofstad EK (2009) Assessment of hypoxia in human cervical carcinoma xenografts by dynamic contrast-enhanced magnetic resonance imaging. Int J Radiat Oncol Biol Phys 73:838–845

Feldkamp LA, Goldstein SA, Parfitt AM, Jesion G, Kleerekoper M (1989) The direct examination of three-dimensional bone architecture in vitro by computed tomography. J Bone Miner Res 4(1):3–11

Fidler IJ (1990) Host and tumour factors in cancer metastasis. Eur J Clin Invest 20:481–486

Flaherty KT, Rosen MA, Heitjan DF et al (2008) Pilot study of DCE-MRI to predict progression-free survival with sorafenib therapy in renal cell carcinoma. Cancer Biol Ther 7:496–501

Fu XY, Besterman JM, Monosov A, Hoffman RM (1991) Models of human metastatic colon cancer in nude mice orthotopically constructed by using histologically intact patient specimens. Proc Natl Acad Sci U S A 88:9345–9349

Fu X, Guadagni F, Hoffman RM (1992) A metastatic nude-mouse model of human pancreatic cancer constructed orthotopically with histologically intact patient specimens. Proc Natl Acad Sci U S A 89:5645–5649

Fuss M, Wenz F, Essig M, Muenter M, Debus J, Herman TS et al (2001) Tumor angiogenesis of low-grade astrocytomas measured by dynamic susceptibility contrast-enhanced MRI (DSC-MRI) is predictive of local tumor control after radiation therapy. Int J Radiat Oncol Biol Phys 51(2):478–482

Galbán CJ, Mukherji SK, Chenevert TL et al (2009) A feasibility study of parametric response map analysis of diffusion-weighted magnetic resonance imaging scans of head and neck cancer patients for providing early detection of therapeutic efficacy. Transl Oncol 2(3):184–190

Garcia S, Freitas AA (2012) Humanized mice: current states and perspectives. Immunol Lett 146:1–7

Gayed I, Vu T, Iyer R, Johnson M, Macapinlac H, Swanston N, Podoloff D (2004) The role of 18F-FDG PET in staging and early prediction of response to therapy of recurrent gastrointestinal stromal tumors. J Nucl Med 45:17–21

Gibbs P, Liney GP, Pickles MD, Zelhof B, Rodrigues G, Turnbull LW (2009) Correlation of ADC and T2 measurements with cell density in prostate cancer at 3.0 Tesla. Invest Radiol 44:572–576

Gibson A, Dehghani H (2009) Diffuse optical imaging. Philos Trans A Math Phys Eng Sci 367(1900):3055–3072

Giles SL, Messiou C, Collins DJ et al (2014) Whole-body diffusion-weighted MR imaging for assessment of treatment response in myeloma. Radiology 271:785–794

Glaholm J, Leach MO, Collins DJ, Mansi J, Sharp JC, Madden A et al (1989) In-vivo 31P magnetic resonance spectroscopy for monitoring treatment response in breast cancer. Lancet 1(8650):1326–1327

Golman K, Zandt RI, Lerche M, Pehrson R, Ardenkjaer-Larsen JH (2006) Metabolic imaging by hyperpolarized 13C magnetic resonance imaging for in vivo tumor diagnosis. Cancer Res 66:10855–10860

Gore JC, Manning HC, Quarles CC, Waddell KW, Yankeelov TE (2011) Magnetic resonance in the era of molecular imaging of cancer. Magn Reson Imaging 29(5):587–600

Gossl M, Bentley MD, Lerman LO (2006) Review--3D micro CT imaging of renal micro-structural changes. Nephron Clin Pract 103(2):c66–c70

van der Graaf M (2010) In vivo magnetic resonance spectroscopy:basic methodology and clinical applications. Eur Biophys J 39(4):527–540

Graham KC, Ford NL, MacKenzie LT, Postenka CO, Groom AC, MacDonald IC, Holdsworth DW, Drangova M, Chambers AF (2008) Noninvasive quantification of tumor volume in preclinical liver metastasis models using contrast-enhanced X-ray computed tomography. Invest Radiol 43(2):92–99

Hamstra DA, Galbán CJ, Meyer CR et al (2008) Functional diffusion map as an early imaging biomarker for high grade glioma: correlation with conventional radiologic response and overall survival. J Clin Oncol 26(20):3387–3394

He Q, Xu RZ, Shkarin P, Pizzorno G, Lee-French CH, Rothman DL et al (2003) Magnetic resonance spectroscopic imaging of tumor metabolic markers for cancer diagnosis, metabolic phenotyping. and characterization of tumor microenvironment Dis Markers 19(2–3):69–94

Henning T, Weber AW, Bauer JS, Meier R, Carlsen JM, Sutton EJ, Prevrhal S, Ziegler SI, Feussner H, Daldrup-Link HE, Rummeny EJ (2008) Imaging characteristics of DHOG, a hepatobiliary contrast agent for preclinical microCT in mice. Acad Radiol 15(3):342–349

Hermans R, Meijerink M, Van den Bogaert W, Rijnders A, Weltens C, Lambin P (2003) Tumor perfusion rate determined noninvasively by dynamic computed tomography predicts outcome in head-and-neck cancer after radiotherapy. Int J Radiat Oncol Biol Phys 57:1351–1356

Hoffman RM (1999) Orthotopic metastatic mouse models for anticancer drug discovery and evaluation: a bridge to the clinic. Invest New Drugs 17:343–359

Holzgreve A, Brendel M, Gu S, Carlsen J, Mille E, Böning G, Mastrella G, Unterrainer M, Gildehaus FJ, Rominger A, Bartenstein P, Kälin RE, Glass R, Albert NL (2016) Monitoring of tumor growth with [18F]-FET PET in a mouse model of glioblastoma: SUV measurements and volumetric approaches. Front Neurosci 10:260

Hompland T, Ellingsen C, Galappathi K, Rofstad EK (2014) DW-MRI in assessment of the hypoxic fraction, interstitial fluid pressure, and metastatic propensity of melanoma xenografts. BMC Cancer 15:14–92

Hoskin PJ, Carnell DM, Taylor NJ (2007) Hypoxia in prostate cancer: correlation of BOLD-MRI with pimonidazole immunohistochemistry-initial observations. Int J Radiat Oncol Biol Phys 68:1065–1071

Iacobellis F, Grassi R, Berritto D, Mansi L, et al. (2016) Preclinical techniques in animals. In: Sacerdoti F, Giordano A, Cavaliere C (eds) Advanced imaging techniques in clinical pathology. Springer, pp 113–121

Iommelli F, De Rosa V, Gargiulo S, Panico M, Monti M, Greco A, Gramanzini M, Ortosecco G, Fonti R, Brunetti A, Del Vecchio S (2014) Monitoring reversal of MET-mediated resistance to EGFR tyrosine kinase inhibitors in non-small cell lung cancer using 3'-deoxy-3'-[18F]-fluorothymidine positron emission tomography. Clin Cancer Res 20:4806–4815

Ito R et al (2008) Antigen-specific antibody production of human B cells in NOG mice reconstituted with the human immune system. Curr Top Microbiol Immunol 324:95–107

Ito R, Takahashi T, Katano I, Ito M (2012) Current advances in humanized mouse models. Cell Mol Immunol 9:208–214

Jakob P (2011) Small animal magnetic resonance imaging: basic principles, instrumentation and practical issues. In: Kiessling F, Pichler BJ (eds) Small animal imaging—basics and practical guide. Springer, Heidelberg, pp 151–164

Jansen NL, Suchorska B, Wenter V, Eigenbrod S, Schmid-Tannwald C, Zwergal A, Niyazi M, Drexler M, Bartenstein P, Schnell O, Tonn JC, Thon N, Kreth FW, la Fougère C (2014) Dynamic 18F-FET PET in newly diagnosed astrocytic low-grade glioma identifies high-risk patients. J Nucl Med 55:198–203

Ji M, Jin X, Phillips P, Yi S (2012) A humanized mouse model to study human immune response in xenotransplantation. Hepatobiliary Pancreat Dis Int 11:494–498

Jiang L, Zhao D, Constantinescu A, Mason RP (2004) Comparison of BOLD contrast and Gd-DTPA dynamic contrast-enhanced imaging in rat prostate tumor. Magn Reson Med 51:953–960

Jin K et al (2010) Patient-derived human tumour tissue xenografts in immunodeficient mice: a systematic review. Clin Transl Oncol 12:473–480

Johansen R, Jensen LR, Rydland J et al (2009) Predicting survival and early clinical response to primary chemotherapy for patients with locally advanced breast cancer using DCE-MRI. J Magn Reson Imaging JMRI 29:1300–1307

de Jong M, Essers J, van Weerden WM (2014) Imaging preclinical tumour models: Improving translational power. Nat Rev Cancer 14:481–493

Kagadis GC, Loudos G, Katsanos K, Langer SG, Nikiforidis GC (2010) In vivo small animal imaging: current status and future prospects. Med Phys 37(12):6421–6442

Kagadis GC, Ford NL, Karnabatidis DN, Loudos GK (2016) Handbook of small animal imaging: preclinical imaging, therapy, and applications. CRC Press, Boca Raton

Kamm YJ, Heerschap A, van den Bergh EJ, Wagener DJ (2004) 19F-magnetic resonance spectroscopy in patients with liver metastases of colorectal cancer treated with 5-fluorouracil. Anticancer Drugs 15:229–233

Kauppinen RA, Peet AC (2011) Using magnetic resonance imaging and spectroscopy in cancer diagnostics and monitoring: preclinical and clinical approaches. Cancer Biol Ther 12(8):665–679

de Kemp RA, Epstein FH, Catana C, Tsui BM, Ritman EL (2010) Small-animal molecular imaging methods. J Nucl Med 51(Suppl 1):18S–32S

Kiessling F, Greschus S, Lichy MP, Bock M, Fink C, Vosseler S, Moll J, Mueller MM, Fusenig NE, Traupe H, Semmler W (2004) Volumetric computed tomography (VCT): a new technology for noninvasive, high-resolution monitoring of tumor angiogenesis. Nat Med 10(10):1133–1138

Kim MH, Kim H (2013) Oncogenes and tumor suppressors regulate glutamine metabolism in cancer cells. J Cancer Prev 18:221–226

Kim RJ, Lima JA, Chen EL et al (1997) Fast 23Na magnetic resonance imaging of acute reperfused myocardial infarction. Potential to assess myocardial viability. Circulation 95(7):1877–1885

Kim RJ, Judd RM, Chen EL, Fieno DS, Parrish TB, Lima JA (1999) Relationship of elevated 23Na magnetic resonance image intensity to infarct size after acute reperfused myocardial infarction. Circulation 100(2):185–192

Kimura H, Takeuchi H, Koshimoto Y et al (2006) Perfusion imaging of meningioma by using continuous arterial spin-labeling: comparison with dynamic susceptibility-weighted contrast-enhanced MR images

and histopathologic features. AJNR Am J Neuroradiol 27:85–93
Koh DM, Collins DJ (2007) Diffusion-weighted MRI in the body: applications and challenges in oncology. AJR Am J Roentgenol 188:1622–1635
Koh DM, Scurr E, Collins D et al (2007) Predicting response of colorectal hepatic metastasis: value of pretreatment apparent diffusion coefficients. AJR Am J Roentgenol 188(4):1001–1008
Koh DM, Blackledge M, Padhani AR, Takahara T, Kwee TC, Leach MO, Collins DJ (2012) Whole-body diffusion-weighted MRI: tips, tricks, and pitfalls. AJR Am J Roentgenol 199(2):252–262
Koo V, Hamilton PW, Williamson K (2006) Non-invasive in vivo imaging in small animal research. Cell Oncol 28:127–139
Kumar R (2016) Steroid hormone receptors and prostate cancer: role of structural dynamics in therapeutic targeting. Asian J Androl 18:682–686
Kwee TC, Takahara T, Ochiai R, Nievelstein RA, Luijten PR (2008) Diffusion-weighted whole-body imaging with background body signal suppression (DWIBS): features and potential applications in oncology. Eur Radiol 18:1937–1952
Kwee TC, Takahara T, Ochiai R, Katahira K, Van Cauteren M, Imai Y, Nievelstein RA, Luijten PR (2009) Whole-body diffusion-weighted magnetic resonance imaging. Eur J Radiol 70:409–417
van Laar PJ, van der Grond J, Hendrikse J (2008) Brain perfusion territory imaging: methods and clinical applications of selective arterial spin-labeling MR imaging. Radiology 246:354–364
Law M, Yang S, Wang H, Babb JS, Johnson G, Cha S, Knopp EA, Zagzag D (2003) Glioma grading: sensitivity, specificity, and predictive values of perfusion MR imaging and proton MR spectroscopic imaging compared with conventional MR imaging. AJNR Am J Neuroradiol 24(10):1989–1998
Law M, Oh S, Babb JS et al (2006) Low-grade gliomas: dynamic susceptibility-weighted contrast-enhanced perfusion MR imaging—prediction of patient clinical response. Radiology 238(2):658–667
Leach MO, Brindle KM, Evelhoch JL, et al (2003) Assessment of antiangiogenic and antivascular therapeutics using MRI: recommendations for appropriate methodology for clinical trials. Br J Radiol 76(Spec No 1):S87–S91
Leach MO, Brindle KM, Evelhoch JL, Griffiths JR, Horsman MR, Jackson A et al (2005) The assessment of antiangiogenic and antivascular therapies in early-stage clinical trials using magnetic resonance imaging: issues and recommendations. Br J Cancer 92:1599–1610
Lecouvet FE (2016) Whole-body MR imaging: musculoskeletal applications. Radiology 279(2):345–365
Lee L, Sharma S, Morgan B et al (2006) Biomarkers for assessment of pharmacologic activity for a vascular endothelial growth factor (VEGF) receptor inhibitor, PTK787/ZK 222584 (PTK/ZK): translation of biological activity in a mouse melanoma metastasis model to phase I studies in patients with advanced colorectal cancer with liver metastases. Cancer Chemother Pharmacol 57:761–771
Leroy-Willig A, Geldwerth-Feniger G (2007) Nuclear magnetic resonance imaging and spectroscopy. In: Ntziachristos V, Leroy-Willig A, Tavitian B (eds) Textbook of in vivo imaging in vertebrates. Wiley, England, pp 1–56
Lewis JS, Achilefu S, Garbow JR, Laforest R, Welch MJ (2002) Small animal imaging. current technology and perspectives for oncological imaging Eur J Cancer 38(16):2173–2188
Li SP, Padhani AR (2012) Tumor response assessments with diffusion and perfusion MRI. J Magn Reson Imaging 35(4):745–763
Li KL, Wilmes LJ, Henry RG, Pallavicini MG, Park JW, Hu-Lowe DD et al (2005) Heterogeneity in the angiogenic response of a BT474 human breast cancer to a novel vascular endothelial growth factor receptor tyrosine kinase inhibitor: assessment by voxel analysis of dynamic contrast-enhanced MRI. J Magn Reson Imaging 22:511–519
Lin J, Kligerman S, Goel R, Sajedi P, Suntharalingam M, Chuong MD (2015) State-of-the-art molecular imaging in esophageal cancer management: implications for diagnosis, prognosis, and treatment. J Gastrointest Oncol 6:3–19
Lind JS, Meijerink MR, Dingemans AM, van Kuijk C, Ollers MC, de Ruysscher D, Postmus PE, Smit EF (2010) Dynamic contrast-enhanced CT in patients treated with sorafenib and erlotinib for non-small cell lung cancer: a new method of monitoring treatment? Eur Radiol 20:2890–2898
Liu G, Rugo HS, Wilding G et al (2005) Dynamic contrast-enhanced magnetic resonance imaging as a pharmacodynamic measure of response after acute dosing of AG-013736, an oral angiogenesis inhibitor, in patients with advanced solid tumors: results from a phase I study. J Clin Oncol 23:5464–5473
Luker GD, Luker KE (2008) Optical imaging: current applications and future directions. J Nucl Med 49:1–4
Mahmood U, Alfieri AA, Thaler H, Cowburn D, Koutcher JA (1994) Radiation dose-dependent changes in tumor metabolism measured by 31P nuclear magnetic resonance spectroscopy. Cancer Res 54(18):4885–4891
Mahmood U, Alfieri AA, Ballon D, Traganos F, Koutcher JA (1995) In vitro and in vivo 31P nuclear magnetic resonance measurements of metabolic changes post radiation. Cancer Res 55(6):1248–1254
Mahon MM, Cox IJ, Dina R et al (2004a) (1)H magnetic resonance spectroscopy of preinvasive and invasive cervical cancer: in vivo-ex vivo profiles and effect of tumor load. J Magn Reson Imaging 19(3):356–364
Mahon MM, Williams AD, Soutter WP et al (2004b) 1H magnetic resonance spectroscopy of invasive cervical cancer: an in vivo study with ex vivo corroboration. NMR Biomed 17(1):1–9
Margolis DJ, Hoffman JM, Herfkens RJ, Jeffrey RB, Quon A, Gambhir SS (2007) Molecular imaging techniques in body imaging. Radiology 245:333–356

Martic-Kehl MI, Schibli R, Schubiger PA (2012) Can animal data predict human outcome? Problems and pitfalls of translational animal research. Eur J Nucl Med Mol Imaging 39:1492–1496
Marzola P, Degrassi A, Calderan L, Farace P, Nicolato E, Crescimanno C et al (2005) Early antiangiogenic activity of SU11248 evaluated in vivo by dynamic contrast-enhanced magnetic resonance imaging in an experimental model of colon carcinoma. Clin Cancer Res 11:5827–5832
Mason RP, Rodbumrung W, Antich PP (1996) Hexafluorobenzene: a sensitive 19F NMR indicator of tumor oxygenation. NMR Biomed 9(3):125–134
Massoud TF, Gambhir SS (2003) Molecular imaging in living subjects: seeing fundamental biological processes in a new light. Genes Dev 17(5):545–580
Matsuo M, Matsumoto S, Mitchell JB, Krishna MC, Camphausen K (2014) Magnetic resonance imaging of the tumor microenvironment in radiotherapy: perfusion, hypoxia, and metabolism. Semin Radiat Oncol 24(3):210–217
Maurer T, Eiber M, Schwaiger M, Gschwend JE (2016) Current use of PSMA-PET in prostate cancer management. Nat Rev Urol 13:226–235
McDonald DM, Baluk P (2002) Significance of blood vessel leakiness in cancer. Cancer Res 62:5381–5385
McKinley ET, Ayers GD, Smith RA, Saleh SA, Zhao P, Washington MK, Coffey RJ, Manning HC (2013) Limits of [18F]-FLT PET as a biomarker of proliferation in oncology. PLoS One 8:e58938
McSheehy PM, Griffiths JR (1989) 19F MRS studies of fluoropyrimidine chemotherapy. a review. NMR Biomed 2(4):133–141
Medved M, Karczmar G, Yang C et al (2004) Semiquantitative analysis of dynamic contrast enhanced MRI in cancer patients: variability and changes in tumor tissue over time. J Magn Reson Imaging 20:122–128
Messiou C, Kaiser M (2015) Whole body diffusion weighted MRI- a new view of myeloma. Br J Haematol 171:29–37
Metildi CA et al (2014) Fluorescently labeled chimeric anti-CEA antibody improves detection and resection of human colon cancer in a patient-derived orthotopic xenograft (PDOX) nude mouse model. J Surg Oncol 109:451–458
Miyamoto DT, Lee RJ, Stott SL, Ting DT, Wittner BS, Ulman M, Smas ME, Lord JB, Brannigan BW, Trautwein J, Bander NH, Wu C-L, Sequist LV, Smith MR, Ramaswamy S, Toner M, Maheswaran S, Haber DA (2012) Androgen receptor signaling in circulating tumor cells as a marker of hormonally responsive prostate cancer. Cancer Discov 2(11):995–1003
Moasser MM, Wilmes LJ, Wong CH, Aliu S, Li KL, Wang D et al (2007) Improved tumor vascular function following high-dose epidermal growth factor receptor tyrosine kinase inhibitor therapy. J Magn Reson Imaging 26:1618–1625
Moffat BA, Hall DE, Stojanovska J, McConville PJ, Moody JB, Chenevert TL, Rehemtulla A, Ross BD (2004) Diffusion imaging for evaluation of tumor therapies in preclinical animal models. MAGMA 17(3–6):249–259
Morgan B, Thomas AL, Drevs J et al (2003) Dynamic contrast-enhanced magnetic resonance imaging as a biomarker for the pharmacological response of PTK787/ZK 222584, an inhibitor of the vascular endothelial growth factor receptor tyrosine kinases, in patients with advanced colorectal cancer and liver metastases: results from two phase I studies. J Clin Oncol 21:3955–3964
Mross K, Drevs J, Muller M et al (2005) Phase I clinical and pharmacokinetic study of PTK/ZK, a multiple VEGF receptor inhibitor, in patients with liver metastases from solid tumours. Eur J Cancer 41:1291–1299
Mukundan S Jr, Ghaghada KB, Badea CT, Kao CY, Hedlund LW, Provenzale JM, Johnson GA, Chen E, Bellamkonda RV, Annapragada A (2006) A liposomal nanoscale contrast agent for preclinical CT in mice. AJR Am J Roentgenol 186(2):300–307
Müller A, Remmele S, Wenningmann I, Clusmann H, Traber F, Flacke S et al (2010) Intracranial tumor response to respiratory challenges at 3.0 T: impact of different methods to quantify changes in the MR relaxation rate R2*. J Magn Reson Imaging 32:17–23
Muruganandham M, Lupu M, Dyke JP, Matei C, Linn M, Packman K et al (2006) Preclinical evaluation of tumor microvascular response to a novel antiangiogenic/antitumor agent RO0281501 by dynamic contrastenhanced MRI at 1.5 T. Mol Cancer Ther 5:1950–1957
Na II, Byun B, Kang H, Cheon G, Koh J, Kim C, Choe D, Ryoo B, Lee J, Lim S, Yang S (2008) 18F-fluoro-2-deoxy-glucose uptake predicts clinical outcome in patients with gefitinib-treated non-small cell lung cancer. Clin Cancer Res 14:2036–2041
Negendank W (1992) Studies of human tumors by MRS: a review. NMR Biomed 5(5):303–324
Nelson SJ, Kurhanewicz J, Vigneron DB et al (2013) Metabolic imaging of patients with prostate cancer using hyperpolarized [1-(1)(3)C]pyruvate. Sci Transl Med 5(198):198ra08
Noss KR, Wolfe SA, Grimes SR (2002) Upregulation of prostate specific membrane antigen/folate hydrolase transcription by an enhancer. Gene 285:247–256
Ntziachristos V, Bremer C, Weissleder R (2003) Fluorescence imaging with near-infrared light: new technological advances that enable in vivo molecular imaging. Eur Radiol 13(1):195–208
O'Connor JPB, Aboagye EO, Adams JE, Aerts HJWL, Barrington SF, Beer AJ, Boellaard R, Bohndiek SE, Brady M, Brown G, Buckley DL, Chenevert TL, Clarke LP, Collette S, Cook GJ, deSouza NM, Dickson JC, Dive C, Evelhoch JL, Faivre-Finn C, Gallagher FA, Gilbert FJ, Gillies RJ, Goh V, Griffiths JR, Groves AM, Halligan S, Harris AL, Hawkes DJ, Hoekstra OS, Huang EP, Hutton BF, Jackson EF, Jayson GC, Jones A, Koh DM, Lacombe D, Lambin P, Lassau N, Leach MO, Lee T-Y, Leen EL, Lewis JS, Liu Y, Lythgoe MF, Manoharan P, Maxwell RJ, Miles KA, Morgan B, Morris S, Ng T, Padhani AR, Parker

GJM, Partridge M, Pathak AP, Peet AC, Punwani S, Reynolds AR, Robinson SP, Shankar LK, Sharma RA, Soloviev D, Stroobants S, Sullivan DC, Taylor SA, Tofts PS, Tozer GM, van Herk M, Walker-Samuel S, Wason J, Williams KJ, Workman P, Yankeelov TE, Brindle KM, McShane LM, Jackson A, Waterton JC (2016) Imaging biomarker roadmap for cancer studies. Nat Rev Clin Oncol 14(3):169–186

Ocana A et al (2010) Preclinical development of molecular-targeted agents for cancer. Nat Rev Clin Oncol 8:200–209

Olive KP, Tuveson DA (2006) The use of targeted mouse models for preclinical testing of novel cancer therapeutics. Clin Cancer Res 12:5277–5287

Optical Imaging Fact Sheet (2012) Society of nuclear medicine and molecular imaging. Available at https://www.snmmi.org/AboutSNMMI/Content.aspx?ItemNumber=5692. Last accessed on 16th January 2020

Ouwerkerk R, Bleich KB, Gillen JS, Pomper MG, Bottomley PA (2003) Tissue sodium concentration in human brain tumors as measured with 23Na MR imaging. Radiology 227(2):529–537

Ouwerkerk R, Jacobs MA, Macura KJ et al (2007) Elevated tissue sodium concentration in malignant breast lesions detected with non-invasive 23Na MRI. Breast Cancer Res Treat 106(2):151–160

Padhani AR, Gogbashian A (2011) Bony metastases: assessing response to therapy with whole-body diffusion MRI. Cancer Imaging 11:S129–S145

Padhani AR, Khan AA (2010) Diffusion-weighted (DW) and dynamic contrast-enhanced (DCE) magnetic resonance imaging (MRI) for monitoring anticancer therapy. Target Oncol 5(1):39–52

Padhani AR, Hayes C, Assersohn L et al (2006) Prediction of clinicopathologic response of breast cancer to primary chemotherapy at contrast enhanced MR imaging: initial clinical results. Radiology 239:361–374

Padhani AR, Liu G, Koh DM, Chenevert TL, Thoeny HC, Takahara T, Dzik-Jurasz A, Ross BD, Van Cauteren M, Collins D, Hammoud DA, Rustin GJ, Taouli B, Choyke PL (2009) Diffusion-weighted magnetic resonance imaging as a cancer biomarker: consensus and recommendations. Neoplasia 11:102–125

Padhani AR, Koh DM, Collins DJ (2011) Whole-body diffusion-weighted MR imaging in cancer: current status and research directions. Radiology 261:700–718

Park I, Larson PE, Zierhut ML, Hu S, Bok R, Ozawa T, Kurhanewicz J, Vigneron DB, Vandenberg SR, James CD, Nelson SJ (2010) Hyperpolarized 13C magnetic resonance metabolic imaging: application to brain tumors. Neuro Oncol 12:133–144

Park JJ, Kim CK, Park SY, Park BK, Lee HM, Cho SW (2014) Prostate cancer: role of pretreatment multiparametric 3-T MRI in predicting biochemical recurrence after radical prostatectomy. AJR Am J Roentgenol 202(5):W459–W465

Partridge SC, DeMartini WB, Kurland BF, Eby PR, White SW, Lehman CD (2009) Quantitative diffusion-weighted imaging as an adjunct to conventional breast MRI for improved positive predictive value. AJR Am J Roentgenol 193:1716–1722

Perel P et al (2007) Comparison of treatment effects between animal experiments and clinical trials: systematic review. BMJ 334:197

Perumal M, Stronach EA, Gabra H, Aboagye EO (2012) Evaluation of 2-deoxy-2-[18F]fluoro-D-glucose- and 3'-deoxy-3'-[18F]fluorothymidine-positron emission tomography as biomarkers of therapy response in platinum-resistant ovarian cancer. Mol Imaging Biol 14:753–761

Pettaway CA et al (1996) Selection of highly metastatic variants of different human prostatic carcinomas using orthotopic implantation in nude mice. Clin Cancer Res 2:1627–1636

Pinker K, Stadlbauer A, Bogner W, Gruber S, Helbich TH (2012) Molecular imaging of cancer: MR spectroscopy and beyond. Eur J Radiol 81:566–577

Pomper MG, Lee JS (2005) Small animal imaging in drug development. Curr Pharm Des 11(25):3247–3272

Pöpperl G, Kreth FW, Herms J et al (2006) Analysis of 18F-FET PET for grading of recurrent gliomas: is evaluation of uptake kinetics superior to standard methods? J Nucl Med 47:393–403

Rauscher A, Sedlacik J, Fitzek C, Walter B, Hochstetter A, Kalff R et al (2005) High resolution susceptibility weighted MR-imaging of brain tumors during the application of a gaseous agent. Rofo 177:1065–1069

Rijpkema M, Schuuring J, Bernsen PL, Bernsen HJ, Kaanders JH, van der Kogel AJ et al (2004) BOLD MRI response to hypercapnic hyperoxia in patients with meningiomas: correlation with Gadolinium-DTPA uptake rate. Magn Reson Imaging 22:761–767

Ritman EL (2004) Micro-computed tomography-current status and developments. Annu Rev Biomed Eng 6:185–208

Røe K, Aleksandersen TB, Kristian A, Nilsen LB, Seierstad T, Qu H, Ree AH, Olsen DR, Malinen E (2010) Preclinical dynamic 18F-FDG PET—tumor characterization and radiotherapy response assessment by kinetic compartment analysis. Acta Oncol 49:914–921

Roth Y, Tichler T, Kostenich G et al (2004) High b-value diffusion-weighted MR imaging for pretreatment prediction and early monitoring of tumor response to therapy in mice. Radiology 232(3):685–692

Rudin M, McSheehy PM, Allegrini PR et al (2005) PTK787/ZK222584, a tyrosine kinase inhibitor of vascular endothelial growth factor receptor, reduces uptake of the contrast agent GdDOTA by murine orthotopic B16/BL6 melanoma tumours and inhibits their growth in vivo. NMR Biomed 18:308–321

Rygaard J, Povlsen CO (1969) Heterotransplantation of a human malignant tumour to "Nude" mice. Acta Pathol Microbiol Scand 77:758–760

Rylova SN, Del Pozzo L, Klingeberg C, Tönnesmann R, Illert AL, Meyer PT, Maecke HR, Holland JP (2016) Immuno-PET imaging of CD30-positive lymphoma using 89Zr-desferrioxamine-labeled CD30-specific AC-10 antibody. J Nucl Med 57:96–102

Schaefer PW, Grant PE, Gonzalez RG (2000) Diffusion-weighted MR imaging of the brain. Radiology 217:331–345

Schaefer PW, Copen WA, Lev MH et al (2006) Diffusion-weighted imaging in acute stroke. Magn Reson Imaging Clin N Am 14(2):141–168

Schambach SJ, Bag S, Steil V, Isaza C, Schilling L, Groden C, Brockmann MA (2009) Ultrafast high-resolution in vivo volume-CTA of mice cerebral vessels. Stroke 40(4):1444–1450

Schambach SJ, Bag S, Schilling L, Groden C, Brockmann MA (2010) Application of micro-CT in small animal imaging. Methods 50(1):2–13

Schelhaas S, Wachsmuth L, Viel T, Honess DJ, Heinzmann K, Smith DM, Hermann S, Wagner S, Kuhlmann MT, Müller-Tidow C, Kopka K, Schober O, Schäfers M, Schneider R, Aboagye EO, Griffiths J, Faber C, Jacobs AH (2014) Variability of proliferation and diffusion in different lung cancer models as measured by 3'-deoxy-3'-18F-fluorothymidine PET and diffusion-weighted MR imaging. J Nucl Med 55:983–988

Schelhaas S, Heinzmann K, Bollineni VR, Kramer GM, Liu Y, Waterton JC, Aboagye EO, Shields AF, Soloviev D, Jacobs AH (2017) Preclinical applications of 3'-deoxy-3'-[18F]fluorothymidine in oncology—a systematic review. Theranostics 7:40–50

Schepkin VD, Ross BD, Chenevert TL, Rehemtulla A, Sharma S, Kumar M et al (2005) Sodium magnetic resonance imaging of chemotherapeutic response in a rat glioma. Magn Reson Med 53:85–92

Schmainda KM, Zhang Z, Prah M et al (2015) Dynamic susceptibility contrast MRI measures of relative cerebral blood volume as a prognostic marker for overall survival in recurrent glioblastoma: results from the ACRIN 6677/RTOG 0625 multicenter trial. Neuro Oncol 17(8):1148–1156

Shields AF (2012) PET imaging of tumor growth: not as easy as it looks. Clin Cancer Res 18:1189–1191

Shultz LD, Ishikawa F, Greiner DL (2007) Humanized mice in translational biomedical research. Nat Rev Immunol 7:118–130

Silva AC, Kim SG, Garwood M (2000) Imaging blood flow in brain tumors using arterial spin labeling. Magn Reson Med 44:169–173

Son J, Lyssiotis CA, Ying H, Wang X, Hua S, Ligorio M, Perera RM, Ferrone CR, Mullarky E, Shyh-Chang N, Kang Y, Fleming JB, Bardeesy N, Asara JM, Haigis MC, DePinho RA, Cantley LC, Kimmelman AC (2013) Glutamine supports pancreatic cancer growth through a KRAS-regulated metabolic pathway. Nature 496:101–105

Sostman HD, Prescott DM, Dewhirst MW et al (1994) MR imaging and spectroscopy for prognostic evaluation in soft-tissue sarcomas. Radiology 190(1):269–275

Stanwell P, Russell P, Carter J, Pather S, Heintze S, Mountford C (2008) Evaluation of ovarian tumors by proton magnetic resonance spectroscopy at three Tesla. Invest Radiol 43(10):745–751

Stephen RM, Gillies RJ (2007) Promise and progress for functional and molecular imaging of response to targeted therapies. Pharm Res 24:1172–1185

Stevens AN, Morris PG, Iles RA, Sheldon PW, Griffiths JR (1984) 5-Fluorouracil metabolism monitored in vivo by 19F NMR. Br J Cancer 50:113–117

Stroobants S, Goeminne J, Seegers M, Dimitrijevic S, Dupont P, Nuyts J, Martens M, van den Borne B, Cole P, Sciot R, Dumez H, Silberman S, Mortelmans L, van Oosterom A (2003) 18FDG-Positron emission tomography for the early prediction of response in advanced soft tissue sarcoma treated with imatinib mesylate (Glivec). Eur J Cancer 39:2012–2020

Sung YS, Park B, Choi Y, Lim HS, Woo DC, Kim KW et al (2016) Dynamic contrast-enhanced MRI for oncology drug development. J Magn Reson Imaging 44:251–264

Takahara T, Imai Y, Yamashita T, Yasuda S, Nasu S, Van Cauteren M (2004) Diffusion weighted whole body imaging with background body signal suppression (DWIBS): technical improvement using free breathing, STIR and high resolution 3D display. Radiat Med 22:275–282

Taouli B, Koh DM (2010) Diffusion-weighted MR imaging of the liver. Radiology 254:47–66

Taouli B, Thakur RK, Mannelli L et al (2009) Renal lesions: characterization with diffusion-weighted imaging versus contrast-enhanced MR imaging. Radiology 251:398–407

Taouli B, Beer AJ, Chenevert T, Collins D, Lehman C, Matos C, Padhani AR, Rosenkrantz AB, Shukla-Dave A, Sigmund E, Tanenbaum L, Thoeny H, Thomassin-Naggara I, Barbieri S, Corcuera-Solano I, Orton M, Partridge SC, Koh DM (2016) Diffusion-weighted imaging outside the brain: consensus statement from an ISMRM-sponsored workshop. J Magn Reson Imaging 44:521–540

Tatsumi M, Nakamoto Y, Traughber B, Marshall LT, Geschwind JH, Wahl RL (2003) Initial experience in small animal tumor imaging with a clinical positron emission tomography/computed tomography scanner using 2-[F-18]fluoro-2-deoxy-D-glucose. Cancer Res 63:6252–6257

Tavaré R, Escuin-Ordinas E, Mok S, McCracken MN, Zettlitz KA, Salazar FB, Witte ON, Ribas A, Wua AM (2016) An effective immuno-PET imaging method to monitor CD8-dependent responses to immunotherapy. Cancer Res 76:73–82

Tee SS, Keshari KR (2015) Novel approaches to imaging tumor metabolism. Cancer J 21:165–173

Tentler JJ et al (2012) Patient-derived tumour xenografts as models for oncology drug development. Nat Rev Clin Oncol 9:338–350

Thoeny HC, De Keyzer F (2007) Extracranial applications of diffusion-weighted magnetic resonance imaging. Eur Radiol 17:1385–1393

Thoeny HC, De Keyzer F (2011) Diffusion-weighted MR imaging of native and transplanted kidneys. Radiology 259:25–38

Thoeny HC, De Keyzer F, King AD (2012) Diffusion-weighted MR imaging in the head and neck. Radiology 263:19–32

Tremoleda JL, Khalil M, Gompels LL, Wylezinska-Arridge M, Vincent T, Gsell W (2011) Imaging technologies for preclinical models of bone and joint disorders. EJNMMI Res 1(1):11
Tunariu N, Kaye SB, Desouza NM (2012) Functional imaging: what evidence is there for its utility in clinical trials of targeted therapies? Br J Cancer 106:619–628
Vogel J (1997) Measurement of cardiac output in small laboratory animals using recordings of blood conductivity. Am J Physiol 273(5 Pt 2):H2520–H2527
Walker-Samuel S, Leach MO, Collins DJ (2006) Evaluation of response to treatment using DCE-MRI: the relationship between initial area under the gadolinium curve (IAUGC) and quantitative pharmacokinetic analysis. Phys Med Biol 51:3593–3602
Walrath JC, Hawes JJ, Van Dyke T, Reilly KM (2010) Genetically engineered mouse models in cancer research. Adv Cancer Res 106:113–164
Wang JZ, Li XA (2005) Impact of tumor repopulation on radiotherapy planning. Int J Radiat Oncol Biol Phys 61:220–227
Wang H, Zhang J, Tian J, Qu B, Li T, Chen Y, Liu J, Wang S (2009) Using dual-tracer PET to predict the biologic behavior of human colorectal cancer. J Nucl Med 50:1857–1864
Wang H, Liu B, Tian J-H, Xu B-X, Guan Z-W, Qu B-L, Liu C-B, Wang R-M, Chen Y-M, Zhang J-M (2010) Monitoring early responses to irradiation with dual-tracer micro-PET in dual-tumor bearing mice. World J Gastroenterol 16:5416–5423
Wang H, Liu B, Tian J, Baixuan X, Zhang J, et Qu B (2013) Evaluation of 18F-FDG and 18F-FLT for monitoring therapeutic responses of colorectal cancer cells to radiotherapy. Eur J Radiol 82:e484–e491
Wang Y, Tseng JC, Sun Y, Beck AH, Kung AL (2015) Noninvasive imaging of tumor burden and molecular pathways in mouse models of cancer. Cold Spring Harb Protoc 2015:135–144
Wang YY, Wang K, Xu ZY, Song Y, Wang CN, Zhang CQ, Sun XL, Shen BZ (2017) High-resolution dynamic imaging and quantitative analysis of lung cancer xenografts in nude mice using clinical PET/CT. Oncotarget 8(32):52802–52812
Ward CS, Venkatesh HS, Chaumeil MM, Brandes AH, Vancriekinge M, Dafni H, Sukumar S, Nelson SJ, Vigneron DB, Kurhanewicz J, James CD, Haas-Kogan DA, Ronen SM (2010) Noninvasive detection of target modulation following phosphatidylinositol 3-kinase inhibition using hyperpolarized 13C magnetic resonance spectroscopy. Cancer Res 70:1296–1305
Weber MA, Thilmann C, Lichy MP, Gunther M, Delorme S, Zuna I et al (2004) Assessment of irradiated brain metastases by means of arterial spin-labeling and dynamic susceptibility-weighted contrast-enhanced perfusion MRI: initial results. Invest Radiol 39(5):277–287
Weber MA, Zoubaa S, Schlieter M et al (2006) Diagnostic performance of spectroscopic and perfusion MRI for distinction of brain tumors. Neurology 66(12):1899–1906
Wedam SB, Low JA, Yang SX et al (2006) Antiangiogenic and antitumor effects of bevacizumab in patients with inflammatory and locally advanced breast cancer. J Clin Oncol 24(5):769–777
Weidner N (1995) Intratumor microvessel density as a prognostic factor in cancer. Am J Pathol 147:9–19
Wilson T, Hastings J (1988) Bioluminescence. Annu Rev Cell Dev Biol 14:197–230
Winfield JM, Payne GS, deSouza NM (2015) Functional MRI and CT biomarkers in oncology. Eur J Nucl Med Mol Imaging 42(4):562–578
Winkelmann CT, Figueroa SD, Sieckman GL, Rold TL, Hoffman TJ (2012) Non- invasive MicroCT imaging characterization and in vivo targeting of BB2 receptor expression of a PC-3 bone metastasis model. Mol Imaging Biol 14(6):667–675
Witney TH, Kettunen MI, Hu DE, Gallagher FA, Bohndiek SE, Napolitano R, Brindle KM (2010) Detecting treatment response in a model of human breast adenocarcinoma using hyperpolarised [1-(13)C]pyruvate and [1,4-(13)C(2)]fumarate. Br J Cancer 103:1400–1406
Wolf G, Abolmaali N (2009) Imaging tumour-bearing animals using clinical scanners. Int J Radiat Biol 85:752–762
Wolf RL, Wang J, Wang S et al (2005) Grading of CNS neoplasms using continuous arterial spin labeled perfusion MR imaging at 3 Tesla. J Magn Reson Imaging 22:475–482
Woolf DK, Beresford M, Li SP, Dowsett M, Sanghera B, Wong WL, Sonoda L, Detre S, Amin V, Ah-See M-L, Miles D, Makris A (2014) Evaluation of FLT-PET-CT as an imaging biomarker of proliferation in primary breast cancer. Br J Cancer 110:2847–2854
Yang J, Yue J-B, Liu J, Yu J-M (2014) Repopulation of tumor cells during fractionated radiotherapy and detection methods (Review). Oncol Lett 7:1755–1760
Yankeelov TE, Gore JC (2007) Dynamic contrast enhanced magnetic resonance imaging in oncology: theory, data acquisition, analysis, and examples. Curr Med Imaging Rev 3:91–107
Yue JB, Yang J, Liu J, Lee J, Cabrera AR, Sun XD, Bai GH, Li YH, Yu JM (2014) Histopathologic validation of 3'-deoxy-3'-18F-fluorothymidine PET for detecting tumor repopulation during fractionated radiotherapy of human FaDu squamous cell carcinoma in nude mice. Radiother Oncol 111:475–481
Zhang LJ, Yang GF, Zhao YE, Zhou CS, Lu GM (2009) Detection of pulmonary embolism using dual-energy computed tomography and correlation with cardiovascular measurements: a preliminary study. Acta Radiol 50:892–901
Zhang LJ, Wu S, Wang M, Lu L, Chen B, Jin L, Wang J, Larson AC, Lu GM (2012) Quantitative dual energy CT measurements in rabbit VX2 liver tumors: comparison to perfusion CT measurements and histopathological findings. Eur J Radiol 81:1766–1775
Zhang X, Yu J, Li C, Sun X, Meng X (2017) Comparison of 18F-FLT uptake, CT number, tumor volume in evaluation of repopulation during radiotherapy for lung cancer. Sci Rep 7:46000

Zhou H, Chen M, Zhao D (2013) Longitudinal MRI evaluation of intracranial development and vascular characteristics of breast cancer brain metastases in a mouse model. PLoS One 8:e62238

Zhou R, Pantel AR, Li S, Lieberman BP, Ploessl K, Choi H, Blankemeyer E, Lee H, Kung HF, Mach RH, Mankoff DA (2017) [18F](2S,4R)4-fluoroglutamine PET detects glutamine pool size changes in triple-negative breast cancer in response to glutaminase inhibition. Cancer Res 77:1476–1484

Zhu L, Ploessl K, Zhou R, Mankoff D, Kung HF (2017) Metabolic imaging of glutamine in cancer. J Nucl Med 58:533–537

Zweifel M, Padhani AR (2010) Perfusion MRI in the early clinical development of antivascular drugs: decorations or decision making tools? Eur J Nucl Med Mol Imaging 37(Suppl 1):S164–S182

Tumour Biology Characterisation by Imaging in Clinic

Aravind S. Ravi Kumar, W. Phillip. Law,
Craig Wilson, Shankar Siva,
and Michael S. Hofman

Contents

1 **Introduction** ... 326

2 **Positron Emission Tomography Imaging of Tumour Biology** ... 327

2.1 Imaging of Glucose Metabolism for Diagnosis, Biopsy Guidance and Grading ... 329

2.2 Radioguided Surgery ... 330

2.3 Imaging of Glucose Metabolism for Prognosis ... 330

2.4 Imaging of Glucose Metabolism for Therapy Response ... 331

2.5 Tumour Biology and Radiomics ... 333

2.6 Imaging of Tumour Biology with Radiotracers Other Than [^{18}F]FDG ... 333

2.7 Dynamic Imaging and Using Multiple Tracers ... 335

3 **Magnetic Resonance Imaging of Tumour Biology** ... 336

3.1 Diffusion-Weighted Imaging ... 337

3.2 Diffusion Tensor Imaging and Fibre Tractography ... 337

3.3 Permeability and Perfusion ... 338

3.4 Magnetic Resonance Spectroscopy ... 341

3.5 Functional MRI ... 341

4 **Computed Tomography Imaging of Tumour Biology** ... 343

4.1 CT Perfusion for Tumour Biology ... 343

4.2 CT Texture Analysis ... 345

4.3 Dual-Energy CT in Oncology ... 345

5 **Response-Adapted Radiotherapy Using Functional Imaging** ... 347

5.1 Delineation of Primary Tumour and Involved Lymph Nodes ... 347

5.2 Response Adaptation Based on Metabolic Imaging ... 347

5.3 Response Adaptation Based on Tumour Proliferation ... 348

5.4 Response Adaptation Based on Functional Lung Avoidance ... 350

5.5 Biological Imaging in Dose Escalation ... 350

5.6 Limitations of Biological Imaging in Response-Adapted Radiotherapy ... 351

5.7 Hypoxia Imaging in Radiotherapy Planning ... 352

5.8 Limitations of Hypoxia Imaging Techniques ... 352

6 **Conclusion** ... 353

References ... 353

A. S. Ravi Kumar (✉) · M. S. Hofman
Molecular Imaging and Therapeutic Nuclear Medicine, Peter MacCallum Cancer Centre, Melbourne, VIC, Australia

Sir Peter MacCallum Department of Oncology, University of Melbourne, Parkville, VIC, Australia
e-mail: Aravind.ravikumar@petermac.org; Michael.hofman@petermac.org

W. P. Law
Department of Medical Imaging, Princess Alexandra Hospital, Woolloongabba, QLD, Australia

C. Wilson
Radiation Oncology, Peter MacCallum Cancer Centre, Melbourne, VIC, Australia

S. Siva
Sir Peter MacCallum Department of Oncology, University of Melbourne, Parkville, VIC, Australia

Radiation Oncology, Peter MacCallum Cancer Centre, Melbourne, VIC, Australia
e-mail: Shankar.siva@petermac.org

R. G. H. Beets-Tan et al. (eds.), *Imaging and Interventional Radiology for Radiation Oncology*, Medical Radiology, Diagnostic Imaging, https://doi.org/10.1007/978-3-030-38261-2_19

Abstract

There have been advances in multiple imaging modalities in recent decades which allow more sophisticated and non-invasive means of characterising evolving aspects of tumour biology at all stages of their clinical course (i.e. diagnosis, staging, prognostication and therapy response). Particular applications include more accurate staging (e.g. highly sensitive and specific new PET tracers such as Ga-68 DOTATATE and PSMA, diffusion-weighted MRI), assessment of tumour aggressiveness and prognosis (with [^{18}F]FDG PET, CT textural analysis) and tailoring therapy based on either initial assessment (biological dose painting) or interim response assessment ([^{18}F]FDG PET). The field of theranostics takes imaging of tumour biology to the natural next step of applying information gained from imaging to choose and tailor radionuclide therapies. Some of these imaging advances have been evaluated in clinical trials or have already been incorporated into clinical practice. The major challenges of functional imaging modalities are reproducibility and standardisation of methodology and the cumbersome and time-consuming process of gathering the clinical evidence base, which can lag behind the rapid technological developments. Dynamic adaptation of radiotherapy plans informed by non-invasive imaging of multiple facets of tumour and normal tissue biology at multiple time points is now possible, and improved clinical outcomes need to be demonstrated in clinical trials.

1 Introduction

Cancer imaging for staging and treatment response has traditionally relied on high-resolution cross-sectional anatomical imaging modalities. There are well-defined and standardised criteria such as RECIST 1.1 which use anatomical information obtained from computed tomography (CT) and magnetic resonance imaging (MRI) to classify responses to treatment based on changes in size of target lesions (Eisenhauer et al. 2009). Likewise, traditional TNM staging of cancer is also based on lesion size and disruption of anatomical boundaries (T stage), size of locoregional lymph nodes (N stage) and anatomically apparent distant metastases (M stage) (Edge and Compton 2010).

In recent decades, it has become apparent that these methods of imaging cancers have limitations, some of which can be well addressed by functional imaging modalities such as nuclear medicine. Imaging in nuclear medicine relies on the tracer principle where a radioactive substance which does not perturb the normal physiological processes is ingested or injected to allow subsequent imaging of a particular biological process. Single-photon emission computed tomography (SPECT) nuclear medicine techniques using the tracer principle are being superseded by positron emission tomography (PET) techniques (Hicks and Hofman 2012). Both SPECT and PET techniques can employ a variety of different radiotracers to interrogate a wide range of physiological processes relevant to cancer biology. PET has several advantages including allowing more accurate quantitation of radiotracer uptake. SPECT radioisotopes generally have longer half-lives than PET isotopes, which can be useful in certain clinical situations.

There have also been important developments in traditionally anatomical imaging modalities such as CT and MRI, which are now capable of providing useful information about in vivo tumour biology. Diffusion-weighted MRI quantifies the ease of movement of water molecules and in so doing characterises important tumour features such as cellularity. A related technique—diffusion tensor imaging—exploits the directional dependence of water diffusivity along fibrous structures like neural axons in the brain, to map functionally important neural pathways to be avoided during treatment. By detecting subtle alteration in blow flow in the brain, the motor, somatosensory, visual and speech centres can be localised using functional MRI techniques. MR spectroscopy enables quantification of certain metabolites that can reflect biological processes such as cell turnover and oxygen tension. Vascular parameters that are frequently an important feature of various malignancies can now be charac-

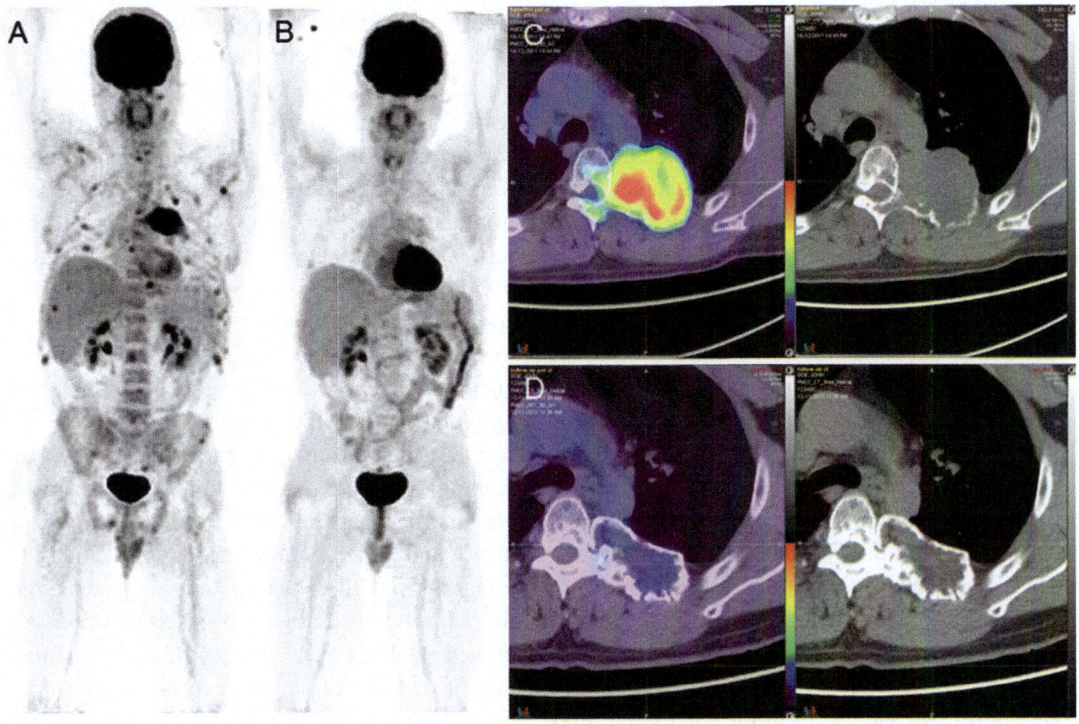

Fig. 1 Patient with lambda light chain myeloma and multifocal marrow involvement at baseline on [^{18}F]FDG-PET/CT (**a**). Following autologous stem cell transplantation, there was a complete metabolic response (**b**). Cross-sectional fused PET/CT images demonstrated a large destructive mass at baseline (**c**) with resolution of metabolic activity following treatment (**d**), despite a large residual soft tissue mass which would be defined a residual disease by conventional anatomic criteria

terised in detail using MRI and CT perfusion techniques. There are emerging data for the utility of CT texture analysis and dual-energy CT in clinical cancer management.

2 Positron Emission Tomography Imaging of Tumour Biology

The most widely used oncological nuclear medicine imaging technique currently is fluorine-18 fluorodeoxyglucose ([^{18}F]FDG), the PET tracer that maps glucose metabolism. [^{18}F]FDG-PET scans take advantage of the obligate glucose metabolism exhibited by most tumours due to aerobic glycolysis, the Warburg effect (Upadhyay et al. 2013; Warburg et al. 1927).

Accurate initial staging is the key to appropriate selection of initial treatment and for prognostication. [^{18}F]FDG-PET/CT scans have been shown to be more accurate than CT scans for initial staging for a range of malignancies, typified by non-small cell lung cancer (NSCLC) (Lardinois et al. 2003). Functional imaging techniques also detect disease heterogeneity within primary tumour masses and/or metastatic disease and may help target biopsies and identify biologically relevant aggressive disease clones. There may be additional prognostic value of a staging [^{18}F]FDG-PET scan based on not only the extent of disease but also the degree of glucose hypermetabolism.

Using functional imaging techniques to characterise disease becomes particularly relevant in the modern oncology clinic as the therapeutic armamentarium has evolved. Accurate imaging of evolving changes in tumour biology during the course of the disease allows rational selection of therapies (Fig. 1). In some diseases, typified by Hodgkin's lymphoma, randomised trials have demonstrated the utility of early response assessment using [^{18}F]FDG-PET with further treatment being stratified by the results of changes in glucose metabolism.

Trials have shown that consolidation radiotherapy may be safely omitted in patients with high-grade lymphoma whose residual anatomical masses are [^{18}F]FDG-PET negative following completion of chemotherapy (Radford et al. 2015). In head and neck SCC treated with chemoradiotherapy, [^{18}F]FDG-PET has been shown to have a high negative predictive value, even in the presence of a residual anatomical nodal mass, with consequent reduction in cost and morbidity from salvage surgical neck dissections (Mehanna et al. 2017; Pryor et al. 2013).

Newer oncological therapies that target particular tumour pathways may be cytostatic rather than cytoreductive, showing changes in metabolism without changes in size and therefore not conducive to assessment by traditional anatomical RECIST criteria. Some diseases such as the lytic bone disease of multiple myeloma may leave behind anatomically apparent but metabolically inactive lesions even after successful therapy. Some sites of disease are typically difficult to assess with anatomical modalities such as a sclerotic healing response in bony metastases which may render a previously radiologically occult bone lesion more obvious on CT or bone scans (Fig. 2); a pseudo-progression phenomenon which is particularly evident is diseases such as metastatic breast cancer and prostate cancer (Scher et al. 2016).

The introduction of immunotherapies is leading a paradigm shift not only for clinical oncologists but also for imaging specialists. Immunotherapies can lead to a range of tumour responses including an early treatment flare, which has led to the development of new immune response criteria, termed iRECIST (Seymour et al. 2017). These therapies are also associated with a unique spectrum of physiological changes and unusual biological toxicities which may be detected with [^{18}F]FDG-PET scans (Wong et al. 2017).

While imaging of glucose metabolism is in widespread use in the clinic, a number of other features of tumour biology can also be characterised by functional imaging. Techniques include interrogation of other pathways (e.g. lipid metabolism, amino acid synthesis, apoptosis), drug resistance (e.g. P-glycoprotein expression), characterisation of the tumour microenvironment (e.g. angiogenesis, hypoxia, proliferation, stroma, immune milieu) or tumour-specific characteristics, e.g. receptor expression (such as the sodium-iodide symporter in thyroid cancer or the somatostatin receptor in neuroendocrine tumours), or certain cell surface proteins or enzymes such as prostate-specific membrane antigen (PSMA) in prostate cancer.

Characterisation of tumour biology is also leading to the emerging field of theranostics, which uses a matched 'theranostic pair' of a diagnostic and a therapeutic radioisotope. Functional imaging modalities with tracer doses of diagnostic radiopharmaceuticals are used to identify the presence or absence and to quantify a suitable tumour target, e.g. an overexpressed cell surface receptor or antigen. The disease can then be selectively targeted using therapeutic doses of particulate-emitting radioisotopes.

The original use of this approach was with radioactive iodine in thyroid disease (Hertz and Roberts 1946a; Hertz and Roberts 1946b). Recently, a multicentre randomised clinical trial targeting the somatostatin receptor in neuroendocrine tumours has shown a marked benefit of this approach over conventional therapy (Strosberg et al. 2017). There is also great interest in using the theranostic approach in other diseases including the targeting of prostate-specific membrane antigen (PSMA) in castrate-resistant prostate cancer.

Dosimetry using multiple time point imaging with long-lived SPECT or even PET diagnostic isotopes can be used to inform a personalised prescription of radioactivity which can be delivered to either the theoretical maximum tolerable dose to normal organs or less commonly a tumouricidal dose. A number of different alpha and beta particle-emitting radioisotopes may be conjugated to molecules that bind to the overexpressed target and used for radionuclide therapy. The same principle can also be for optimal doses of nonradioactive pharmaceuticals. This has been

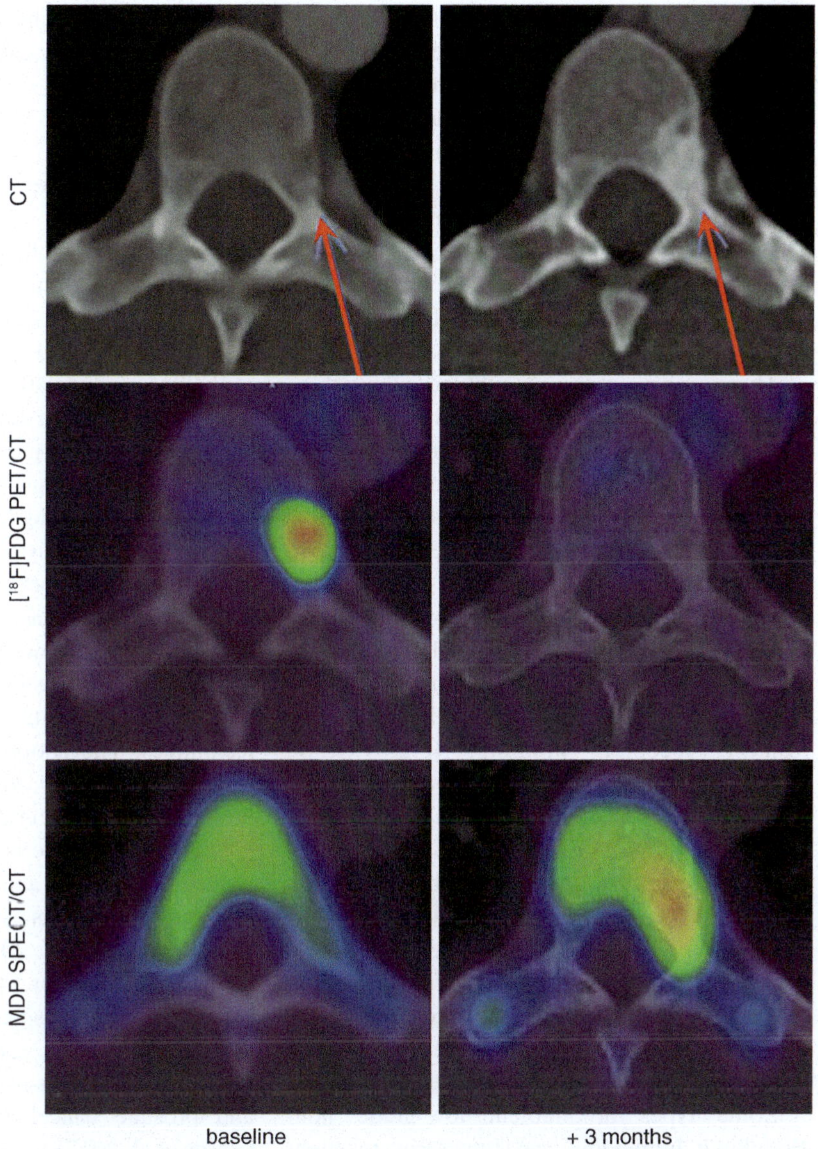

Fig. 2 Patient with oestrogen receptor-positive breast cancer. Baseline bone scan with SPECT/CT was normal. Baseline [^{18}F]FDG-PET/CT demonstrated focal intense metabolic abnormality in a thoracic vertebrae which correlated with a subtle lytic lesion on CT. Three months following commencement of hormone therapy, there was a complete metabolic response on [^{18}F]FDG-PET/CT with progressive sclerosis on CT and new focal abnormality on bone scan, consistent with a healing response

shown in lymphoma by using the metabolic tumour volume to individualise rituximab dosage according to tumour burden (Tout et al. 2017).

2.1 Imaging of Glucose Metabolism for Diagnosis, Biopsy Guidance and Grading

While [^{18}F]FDG PET/CT is widely used in routine clinical practice for staging or restaging a known malignancy, there are also situations where a malignancy may be suspected on clinical grounds or on standard cross-sectional imaging, but definitive histological diagnosis is problematic due to risk of biopsy or lack of a suitable target.

A hypermetabolic lung lesion on [^{18}F]FDG PET/CT has been shown to have a high likelihood of malignancy (Al-Ameri et al. 2015). Even when malignancy is strongly suspected on clinical or imaging grounds, it is not uncommon for biopsies to be negative or non-diagnostic due to the presence of necrosis. In these situations, a biopsy directed at the hypermetabolic component of the lesion on [^{18}F]FDG-PET scans is the usual approach taken to reach a definitive diagnosis.

A recent prospective randomised clinical trial has also shown that an approach using [^{18}F]FDG-PET/CT as the initial imaging modality in patients with non-specific signs or symptoms of cancer had a higher accuracy and diagnostic specificity and shorter time to definitive diagnosis (either cancer or a non-cancer aetiology) than with a CT first approach (Lebech et al. 2017).

There are several tumour subtypes where there is co-existence of lower- and higher-grade elements, with definitive therapy based on the highest grade of disease. This is typified in soft tissue sarcomas, where [^{18}F]FDG-PET scans are used to target a biopsy of the most hypermetabolic site to guide therapy (El-Haddad 2016).

In our institution, [^{18}F]FDG-PET is frequently used to guide biopsy and characterise the biology of neuroendocrine tumours (NET). NETs are conventionally imaged with somatostatin receptor imaging (e.g. Ga-68 DOTATATE PET or In-111 octreotide SPECT if PET is not easily available). While [^{18}F]FDG-PET is insensitive in assessing extent of disease, it is used to characterise biology. High [^{18}F]FDG avidity is associated with a poor outcome (Bahri et al. 2014), independent of the apparent histological tumour grade. We use [^{18}F]FDG-PET in NET for prognostication, to guide biopsy and select aggressiveness of treatment (Hofman and Hicks 2012).

Some types of indolent low-grade non-Hodgkin's lymphoma can transform to high-grade aggressive disease. Regardless of whether transformation is clinically suspected or occult, [^{18}F]FDG-PET can expedite the diagnosis by targeting the most hypermetabolic sites for biopsy. While there is controversy in the literature about the most suitable cut-off of the maximum standardised uptake value (SUVmax), a discordant site of marked [^{18}F]FDG avidity compared to the rest of the disease should raise clinical suspicion for transformation (Noy et al. 2009). [^{18}F]FDG-PET is particularly useful in the diagnosis of Richter's transformation of chronic lymphocytic leukaemia (CLL) to diffuse large B cell lymphoma (DLBCL) and classifying patients with CLL into prognostic categories based on the level of [^{18}F]FDG avidity (Falchi et al. 2014).

2.2 Radioguided Surgery

Sentinel node lymphoscintigraphy to map individually variable and tumour-specific lymphatic drainage pathways is well established as a staging and prognostic study in breast cancer (Nieweg et al. 2015) and melanoma (Faries et al. 2017) and has also been used in other tumour types. Injection of a radiolabelled particulate colloid around a tumour and tracking the pathways of lymphatic drainage allows selective removal (radioguided surgery) and submission for detailed histopathology of a small number of lymph nodes in the closest functional drainage pathways to the tumour. This technique allows detection of microscopic foci of nodal disease which would not be apparent with the most sensitive of non-invasive imaging techniques. The adoption of hybrid SPECT-CT imaging technology allows this procedure to be performed more accurately in anatomically complex areas, and there is an emerging role for this procedure in head and neck cancer and pelvic malignancies such as penile and vulval carcinoma (Valdes Olmos et al. 2014). Radioguided surgery using SPECT/CT or PET/CT for localisation is also feasible and has been performed with a variety of radiotracers that target tumour-specific characteristics such as neuroendocrine tumours and prostate cancer (Cuccurullo et al. 2017; Geurts et al. 2017).

2.3 Imaging of Glucose Metabolism for Prognosis

There is evidence in some tumour types that the level of glucose hypermetabolism as measured by SUVmax at diagnosis has independent prognostic significance. This is a somewhat controversial area in the literature as different studies within and across tumour types have shown different SUVmax cut-off values as being prognostically significant (Paesmans et al. 2010).

SUVmax values at the ends of the spectrum seen in clinical practice may be considered as a useful piece of information to guide clinical decision-making. Reproducible SUVmax values rely on strict control of parameters such as uptake time and image reconstruction parameters and also vary with different generations of imaging equipment.

The value of glucose hypermetabolism as a prognostic factor is also particularly relevant in tumours which have heterogeneous imaging phenotypes, including neuroendocrine tumours, thyroid cancer and prostate cancer. Differentiated thyroid cancer is usually iodine-avid, and [^{18}F]FDG scans are not commonly used for evaluating disease burden. [^{18}F]FDG avidity however has striking prognostic significance; patients with [^{18}F]FDG-avid disease (regardless of whether it is also iodine-avid) have markedly reduced overall survival, with further stratification evident by degree of hypermetabolism as measured by SUVmax (Robbins et al. 2006).

Metabolic tumour volume (MTV) is another parameter which has been evaluated in the literature for solid tumours and in lymphoma. MTV relies on delineation of a contour around all [^{18}F]FDG-avid malignant lesions and is of increasing interest as imaging analysis software tools have evolved. If there are multiple lesions, the MTV for each lesion is summed to obtain the total MTV. The MTV can be multiplied by the average SUV to obtain the total lesion glycolysis (TLG). Some studies have validated the MTV against histopathology (Sridhar et al. 2014). There are variations in methods and software tools to define the boundary used, but literature is emerging that the MTV has a prognostic impact independent of the stage of the tumour in lung cancer and some subtypes of lymphoma (Finkle et al. 2017; Meignan et al. 2016).

2.4 Imaging of Glucose Metabolism for Therapy Response

There is high-quality evidence on the use of metabolic imaging to assess therapy response, predict prognosis at the end of therapy and risk-stratify patients during therapy. This is particularly so in conditions where oncological therapies can lead to a complete imaging response and potentially curative therapy.

In HNSCC, a negative [^{18}F]FDG PET/CT following completion of definitive chemoradiotherapy has a very high negative predictive value and associated with a good prognosis (Fig. 3). In a large randomised trial, it has been shown that a negative [^{18}F]FDG PET/CT scan performed 12 weeks following the completion of chemoradiotherapy markedly reduced need for surgical neck

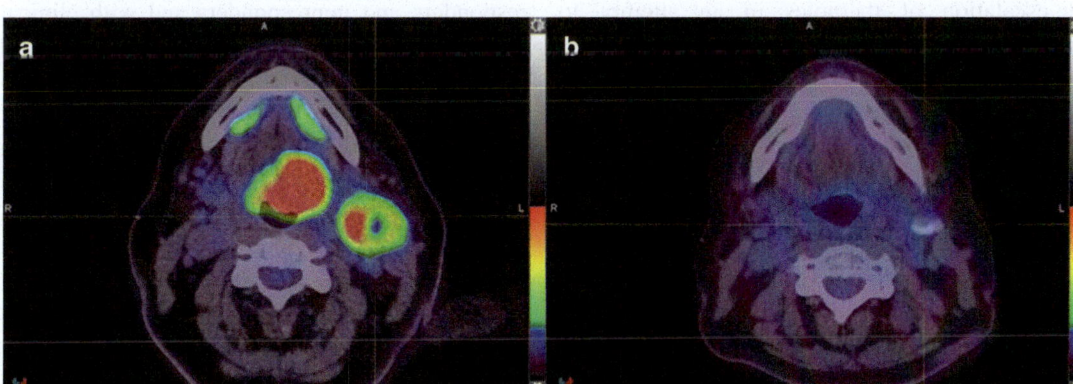

Fig. 3 A 65-year-old lady with T4N2B tongue base squamous cell carcinoma (panel **a**) was treated with definitive chemoradiotherapy. A [^{18}F]FDG-PET scan 3 months following completion of therapy (panel **b**) demonstrates a residual partially calcified hypometabolic left level II nodal mass consistent with scar tissue rather than residual disease. The node has shown further regression with continued observation, and the patient has been spared an unnecessary salvage neck dissection

dissections by 80%, reduced overall cost of care and had equivalent clinical outcomes to the standard of care of planned neck dissections (Mehanna et al. 2017).

A number of studies have shown the prognostic value of end of therapy [^{18}F]FDG-PET scans in both Hodgkin's lymphoma and high-grade non-Hodgkin's lymphoma. A negative [^{18}F]FDG-PET scan at the end of therapy is associated with a high likelihood of cure, while a positive scan has a poorer prognosis. Interest in this field led to the proposal of standardised criteria for the interpretation of [^{18}F]FDG-PET images at the end of therapy, the international harmonisation project (Juweid et al. 2007). This was further refined as the 'Deauville criteria' which has now been widely adopted for assessing [^{18}F]FDG-PET imaging response to therapy (Cheson et al. 2014).

The advent of immune-oncology has now led to the proposal of the LYRIC criteria, a combination of metabolic and anatomic imaging criteria with an 'indeterminate response' category which requires mandatory repeat imaging at 12 weeks to ensure that patients with an inflammatory/immune flare reaction are not inappropriately classified as having progressive disease (Cheson et al. 2016).

Multiple large prospective multicentre randomised trials have been conducted in recent years, using the results of interim [^{18}F]FDG-PET scans early during chemotherapy not only to stratify patient risk but also to test escalation or de-escalation of therapies in an attempt to improve cure rates and reduce treatment-related toxicities, respectively.

This is exemplified in the Hodgkin's lymphoma (HL) literature. Early-stage HL is a condition with a propensity to occur in young adults and has a high likelihood of cure with conventional therapy, even in the salvage setting. These therapies however are associated with high levels of morbidity and long-term complications (e.g. second malignancies, premature cardiovascular disease and infertility), so there is a clinical need to de-intensify therapy in these patients while maintaining high cure rates. In the UK-led RATHL study (Johnson et al. 2016) of over 1200 patients with advanced-stage Hodgkin's lymphoma, treatment was initially with ABVD chemotherapy, with escalation of therapy if the [^{18}F]FDG-PET scan was positive after two cycles. With this approach, only 16% of patients were exposed to the more toxic BEACOPP regimen. The subgroup of patients on escalated therapy still had a 3-year overall survival of 87.8%, while the majority of patients with favourable early PET response were spared the more toxic regimen. This approach using an early [^{18}F]FDG-PET after initiation of therapy as a biomarker to determine escalation or de-escalation of therapy warrants further study in a range of other malignancies. Personalised risk adapted therapy using [^{18}F]FDG has immense potential to improve patient outcomes.

A significant percentage of patients have a residual mass on CT scanning at the end of conventional therapy. While the majority of these masses are scar tissue, the traditional treatment for all these patients was consolidation radiotherapy, since it was not possible to distinguish active lymphoma from scar tissue on CT scans. A negative [^{18}F]FDG-PET scan in this situation can be used to safely omit radiotherapy. A positive scan however can still be due to post-therapy inflammation, and biopsy confirmation is recommended prior to proceeding with further therapy.

The literature in solid tumours in the neoadjuvant setting is interesting as the imaging response on [^{18}F]FDG-PET scans can be correlated with histopathology of surgical specimens in early responders and nonresponders and with clinical outcomes in patients who do not proceed to an attempt at curative surgery. There are numerous studies where [^{18}F]FDG-PET response assessment to therapy is predictive of outcome in the neoadjuvant setting for oesophageal and rectal carcinoma (Rymer et al. 2016). Nonresponders on [^{18}F]FDG-PET during therapy for oesophageal carcinoma have been shown to have more aggressive tumour biology and have a poorer prognosis despite early surgical resection (Lordick et al. 2007).

There are many clinical situations where the tumour biology or available therapy is such that a complete response to therapy is not expected. Early, accurate and reproducible methods of quantifying effects of therapy and identifying disease progression are needed. To assist in this end, the PERCIST criteria were proposed in 2009 (Wahl et al. 2009) and further refined in 2016 (Lodge and Wahl 2016). The PERCIST criteria take advantage of the highly sensitive changes in glucose metabolism in tumours while at the same time proposing methods of more reproducible quantification of changes in [^{18}F]FDG uptake. These criteria have been retrospectively compared to the RECIST criteria and are also the subject of ongoing prospective trials.

2.5 Tumour Biology and Radiomics

Radiomics is a new field which uses advances in imaging analysis tools to mine the large amount of imaging data generated from modern medical imaging technologies. Data from radiomics is quite separate from traditional visual interpretation of images, but uses these medical images to extract higher dimensional information. This field is more advanced in CT and MRI than PET. The PET literature is predominantly with [^{18}F]FDG, but any radiotracer can be used for this purpose (Hatt et al. 2017). One such application is the analysis of tumour heterogeneity (manifested in images as heterogeneity in voxel intensity in location and in relationship to each other) with textural analysis. These analytic steps are not well standardised and subject to inherent variation including patient, scanner, image reconstruction and image segmentation factors. In this young field, the early literature is promising but also suffers from a large amount of statistical and methodological issues. The interested reader is referred to a comprehensive review of the issues with the early studies in this area (Chalkidou et al. 2015).

2.6 Imaging of Tumour Biology with Radiotracers Other Than [^{18}F]FDG

[^{18}F]FDG-PET scans are in ubiquitous use in the clinic for many tumour types, but also have some well-known limitations. A range of malignancies also have intrinsically low [^{18}F]FDG uptake either because of an indolent phenotype (e.g. low-grade neuroendocrine tumours, some prostate cancers, differentiated thyroid cancer), or they may be biologically aggressive but do not use glycolysis as their predominant energy driver (e.g. gastric signet cell carcinoma, some liposarcoma). [^{18}F]FDG uptake is also not exclusive to malignant processes and can be seen in a variety of inflammatory and infectious processes, some of which not uncommonly occur as complications of cancer therapy and co-exist with [^{18}F]FDG-avid malignant uptake. These limitations can be largely overcome with appropriate clinical referrals and skilled image interpretation which includes strong integration of the clinical context.

Radiotracers that interrogate many aspects of tumour biology beyond glucose metabolism have been developed and have great promise in research to understand the general drivers of cancer or in specific clinical scenarios. These imaging tracers could have clinical applications far beyond the detection of disease and image fundamental processes of cancer biology such as DNA synthesis, cell membrane phospholipid synthesis, angiogenesis and apoptosis, many of which form the original hallmarks of cancer as proposed by Hanahan and Weinberg in 2000 (Hanahan and Weinberg 2000). The authors updated their original hallmarks in 2011 (Hanahan and Weinberg 2011) and included aspects of tumour immunology, metabolism, genomics and microenvironment. They point out that these expanded hallmarks of cancer all have therapeutic targets in development or already in clinical use. It is equally pertinent to note that an armamentarium of radiotracers is available for clinical researchers or in preclinical development which can non-invasively interrogate these aspects of tumour biology or specific oncological pathways such as human epidermal growth factor 2 (HER2) (Clark et al. 2017). In the context of radiotherapy, the non-invasive imaging of tumour hypoxia and potential strategies to overcome hypoxia-induced radioresistance are of particular importance (Vordermark and Horsman 2016; Hicks 2017).

There are also more tumour-specific radiotracers that interrogate a specific aspect of tumour biology (e.g. receptor expression, enzymatic

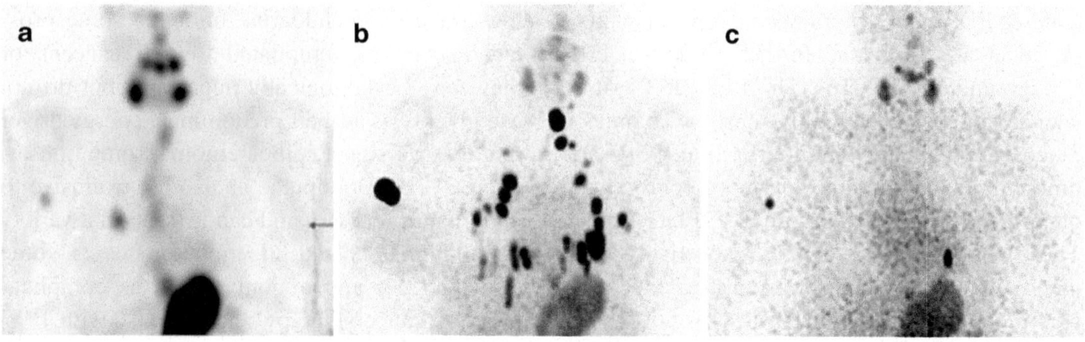

Fig. 4 Serial maximum intensity projection radioiodine SPECT (panel **a**) and PET (panels **b** and **c**) images. A 61-year-old lady with NRAS mutant thyroid cancer which had lost sodium-iodide symporter expression (panel **a**) was treated with a 4-week course of BRAF and MEK inhibitor while leading to re-expression of iodine uptake in bone and lung metastases, rendering her suitable to high-dose radioiodine therapy. Panel **c** demonstrates the marked therapeutic response to 175 mCi of I-131 therapy

function, cell surface antigens). These approaches have had notable clinical success in both diagnosis and therapy. The prototype tumour-specific radiotracer is radioactive iodine, clinically used for both diagnosis and therapy of thyroid cancer with radioactive iodine for over 70 years. It targets the sodium/iodide symporter, a transmembrane glycoprotein, which mediates uptake of iodide into follicular cells of the thyroid gland.

It is also known that some differentiated thyroid cancers lose this ability to concentrate iodine and may become radioiodine refractory. There are constitutively active cell signalling pathways (BRAF/MEK) in the majority of papillary thyroid cancers. Activation of this pathway can also inhibit cell surface expression of the sodium-iodide symporter, leading to lack of uptake and intracellular concentration of radioiodine. This phenomenon is manifested as negative radioiodine scans (either using I-123 SPECT or ideally I-124 PET) in the presence of structural lesions which are metabolically active on [^{18}F]FDG-PET scans. A 4-week course of a BRAF inhibitor (dabrafenib) or a MEK inhibitor (selumetinib) can change the phenotype of the disease by re-expression of the sodium-iodide symporter which is confirmed on follow-up diagnostic radioiodine scans and then renders the disease amenable to further therapeutic doses of radioactive iodine (Fig. 4) (Ho et al. 2013; Rothenberg et al. 2015).

Radiolabelled small molecules that bind to other cell surface receptors have been rapidly adopted in the clinic. This includes radiolabelled somatostatin analogues for imaging neuroendocrine tumours (Krenning et al. 1992) and small molecules that bind to prostate-specific membrane antigen (PSMA) for imaging prostate cancers (Afshar-Oromieh et al. 2014).

Most prostate cancers express the cell surface enzyme glutamate carboxypeptidase, more commonly known as prostate-specific membrane antigen (PSMA). PSMA expression increases with androgen deprivation therapy and with the development of castrate resistance (Hope et al. 2017). Approaches to imaging PSMA have included the SPECT agent capromab pendetide (ProstaScint), which required crossing a permeable cell membrane and subsequent binding to the intracellular domain of PSMA, which limited the sensitivity of this tracer (Osborne et al. 2013). Newer approaches to PSMA imaging use PET imaging agents that target the extracellular domain and have exquisite sensitivity, detecting disease with serum PSA levels of 0.2 and in lymph nodes under 5 mm diameter on CT (i.e. morphologically normal small nodes, (Fig. 5) (Rauscher et al. 2016; Meredith et al. 2016). This makes PSMA PET imaging particularly suited to the imaging of biochemical recurrence of prostate cancer following definitive initial therapy. The optimal management of low-volume recur-

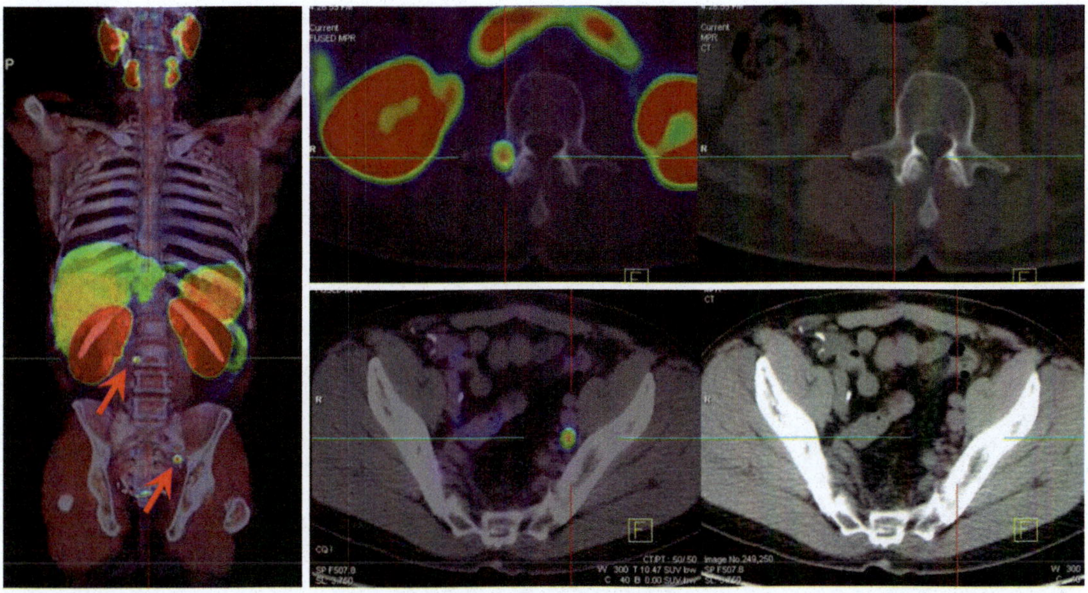

Fig. 5 Patient with prior Gleason 4 + 5 = 9 prostate cancer with biochemical recurrence after radical prostatectomy. Conventional imaging with CT and bone scanning demonstrated no abnormality. Ga-68 prostate-specific membrane antigen (PSMA) PET/CT demonstrated focal intense uptake in a sub-cm external iliac node and lumbar spine metastasis, confirming metastatic disease

rent disease detected only on PSMA PET scans is an evolving area (Maurer et al. 2017).

Other tumour-specific imaging targets which may have applications in the clinic include targeting the oestrogen receptor (Liao et al. 2016), HER2 (Gebhart et al. 2016) and bombesin (Sonni et al. 2017). Promising future approaches include imaging the tumour microenvironment (LeBleu 2015) and imaging the immune response(Mayer et al. 2017).

2.7 Dynamic Imaging and Using Multiple Tracers

It is important to understand that functional imaging with PET and SPECT tracers also has a temporal domain in addition to the spatial domains—uptake characteristics of tracers may change in a characteristic fashion with time due to changes in tissue metabolism. This information has significant clinical utility and can be obtained in the form of multi-time point imaging or with data analysis from continuous dynamic imaging for a fixed time period.

Dual-time point imaging with the SPECT tracer Tc-99m sestamibi is a highly sensitive modality to detect parathyroid adenoma and takes advantage of the differential washout rate of the tracer from normal thyroid tissue compared to parathyroid adenomas (Mariani et al. 2003).

Dynamic imaging with calculation of the uptake and washout rates of the amino acid tracers FDOPA and FET has particular application in distinguishing active intracerebral malignant lesions from radiation necrosis (Fig. 6) (Lapa et al. 2014; Galldiks et al. 2012).

A catalogue of radiotracers is available for use in the clinic, and sophisticated questions can be answered when taking into account information obtained from scans using multiple PET tracers for tumour characterisation. In endocrine malignancies in particular (with important exceptions), [^{18}F] FDG-PET can be used in a complementary manner with other tumour-specific tracers as a marker for identifying dedifferentiation or an aggressive phenotype (Pattison and Hofman 2015). More prosaically, computer subtraction imaging using Tc-99m pertechnetate and Tc-99m sestamibi has been used

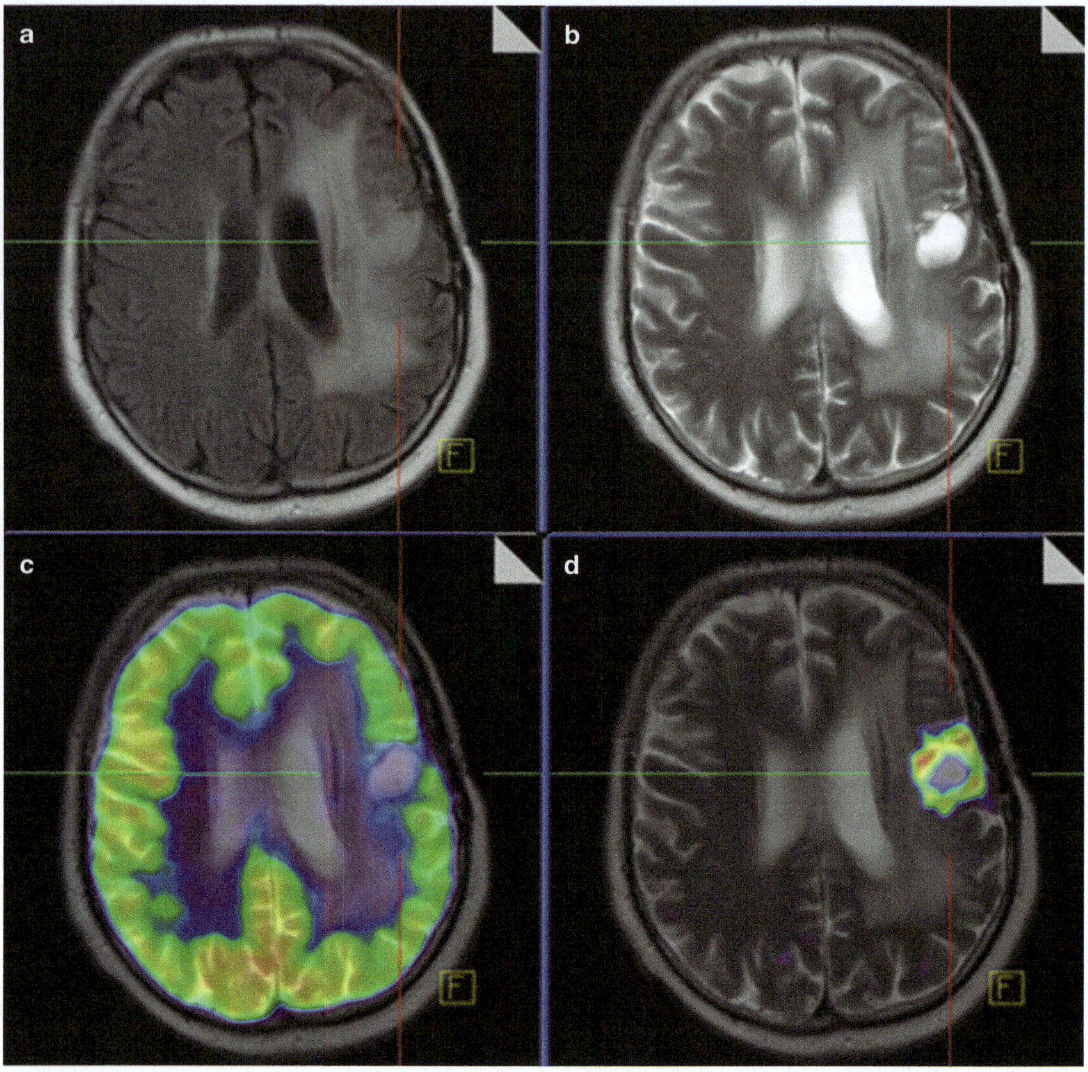

Fig. 6 Patient with left frontal astrocytoma, previously treated with surgery and radiotherapy. MRI demonstrated stable findings compared to imaging performed 3 months previously with changes interpreted as consistent with post-treatment changes (**a**: FLAIR sequence, **b**: T2 fat sat). Fluorodeoxyglucose ([^{18}F]FDG) (**c**) interpretation was limited owing to normal high glycolytic activity in the brain. Further imaging with fluoroethyltyrosine (**d**), which interrogates amino acid metabolism, demonstrates a rim of high uptake consistent with recurrent disease. This was subsequently confirmed with biopsy

for many decades to distinguish between normal background thyroid tissue and cellular lesions such as parathyroid adenomas.

3 Magnetic Resonance Imaging of Tumour Biology

Magnetic resonance imaging (MRI) is now commonplace in the imaging of many tumours. It is a non-ionising radiation modality and provides superior contrast resolution, particularly in soft tissues, than computed tomography (CT). MRI also offers more options for functional imaging than CT. In addition to traditional MRI sequences using T1- and T2-weighted imaging for anatomical characterisation, techniques such as diffusion-weighted imaging, dynamic perfusion assessment, MR spectroscopy and functional MRI now provide more detailed information about biological tissues and have found widespread use in tumour assessment.

3.1 Diffusion-Weighted Imaging

The ease of movement of molecules (mainly water) in body tissues can be measured and used to generate contrast in images obtained using diffusion-weighted MRI techniques. This diffusivity of water is limited in highly cellular tumours such as lymphoma, small blue round cell tumours and high-grade glioma and can also be useful for differentiating neoplastic and benign tissue in less hypercellular tumours such as prostate cancer and metastasis to the liver and lymph nodes. The key to understanding of restricted diffusion is the apparent diffusion coefficient (ADC), whose value reflects the ease of water movement. Thus, a low ADC value suggests greater restriction of movement, appears as a low signal (dark) area on the ADC map and typically correlates with a more clinically significant lesion.

Diffusion-weighted imaging is now a key feature of prostate lesion characterisation through its incorporation in the Prostate Imaging-Reporting and Data System (PI-RADS) for structured reporting of lesions detected on multiparametric prostate MRI (PI-RADS: Prostate Imaging—reporting and Data System version 2 2015). Diffusion-weighted sequences are both the primary determinant of PI-RADS assignment for peripheral zone lesions, as well as the sequences used for further assessment of transitional zone lesions assigned as intermediate on T2-weighted imaging (Fig. 7).

Diffusion-weighted imaging is now routinely performed for MRI of the liver in most centres. It can improve the sensitivity and specificity for the detection of liver metastases (Kim et al. 2012a; Koh et al. 2012) and hepatocellular carcinoma (Le Moigne et al. 2012; Park et al. 2013) over conventional MRI sequences. The ADC values of malignant lesions are often lower than benign lesions; thus diffusion-weighted imaging can also help to differentiate between benign and malignant hepatic lesions, although substantial overlap can occur. Once a diagnosis of malignant pathology is established, the ADC quantitative values generally reflect tumour biology and aggressiveness.

Following treatment, tumour cell death results in less restricted water motion which is reflected in an increase in ADC values detectable as early as several weeks after the start of treatment. This change in ADC values is currently being investigated for its potential utility to evaluate treatment response in lymphoma (Lin et al. 2011; Tsuji et al. 2015), prostate cancer (Song et al. 2010), rectal cancer (Jung et al. 2012), non-small cell lung cancer (Ohno et al. 2012), bone metastases (Blackledge et al. 2014; Padhani et al. 2014) and other malignant bone pathology such as multiple myeloma (Giles et al. 2014; Horger et al. 2011). Diffusion-weighted MRI has been shown in some studies to have similar accuracy as [^{18}F]FDG-PET for treatment response assessment in head and neck squamous cell carcinoma (Martins et al. 2015) and lymphoma (Mayerhoefer et al. 2015). In a study of non-small cell lung cancer patients receiving chemoradiotherapy, diffusion-weighted MRI was a better predictor of response to therapy than [^{18}F]FDG-PET (Ohno et al. 2012). In general, however, while diffusion-weighted imaging has shown potential in assessing early response to anticancer therapies, a lack of standardisation and reproducibility of available studies has hindered its widespread validation.

3.2 Diffusion Tensor Imaging and Fibre Tractography

Anatomical connections between different parts of the brain can be visualised using an extension of diffusion-weighted MRI known as diffusion tensor imaging (DTI). Where an internal fibrous structure exists in biological tissues (e.g. neural axons in white matter of the brain), water molecules will diffuse more rapidly in the direction aligned with the internal structure. Such directional dependence of water diffusivity is termed anisotropy. Thus, by applying diffusion gradients in multiple directions, the orientation of white matter tracts can be determined and presented for viewing in cross-sectional and also three-dimensional images called fibre tractography.

In brain tumours, mapping of the corticospinal tract and other association fibres within the brain (Fig. 8) can be helpful in planning treatment, particularly with view to minimising undesirable treatment effects to these functionally important structures. This technique has more recently also

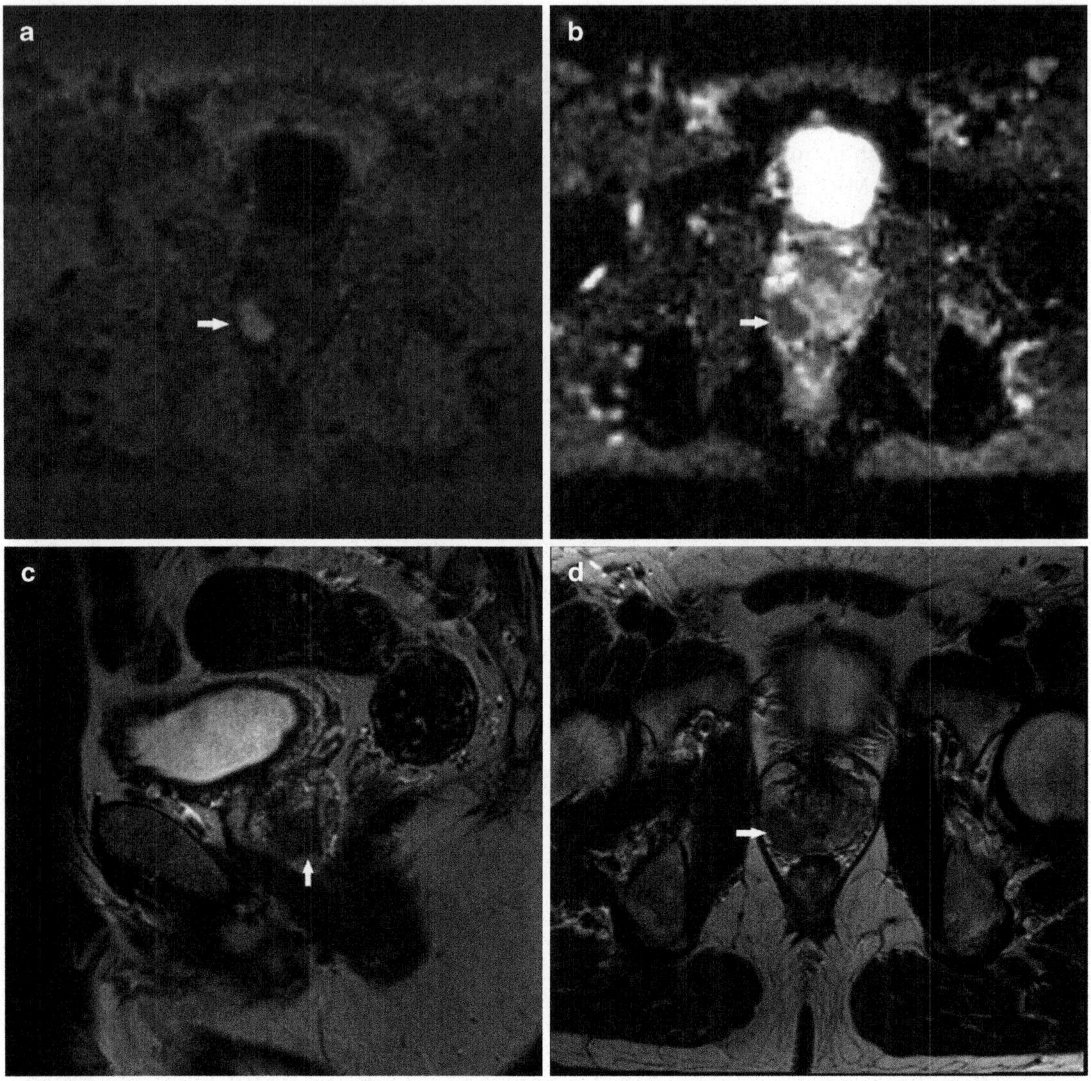

Fig. 7 Multiparametric MRI of the prostate showing a malignant focus (white arrows) in the right posterolateral peripheral zone of the mid-gland with markedly restricted diffusion (**a**, **b**) and low signal on T2-weighted sequences (**c**, **d**)

been shown to be useful in spinal and peripheral nerves.

3.3 Permeability and Perfusion

Angiogenesis is frequently associated with malignant tumours and can be characterised by MRI using dynamic gadolinium-enhanced perfusion techniques.

By imaging across multiple time points, intravenously administered gadolinium uptake rate in tumour tissues can be depicted at various phases, typically during wash-in, plateau and washout, thereby providing insight into the nature of tumour vascularity at the microvascular level. This is commonly known as *permeability* MRI. The signal intensity-time curves generated using this technique reflect the combined effect of tissue perfusion, vessel permeability and extravascular-extracellular space. The pattern (or kinetics) of enhancement can be useful for the differentiation of malignant and benign lesions in the breast (Macura et al. 2006; Moon et al. 2009),

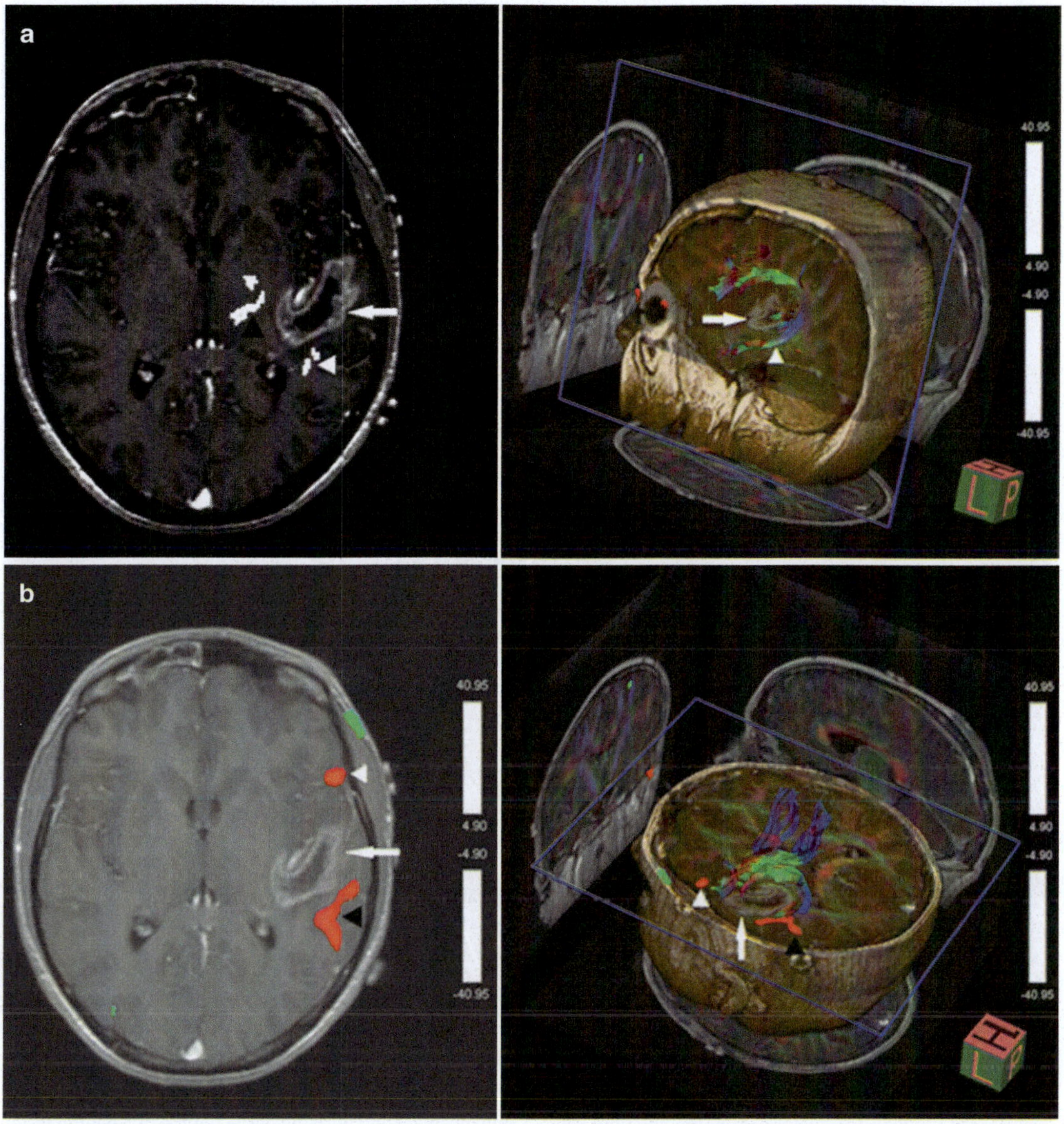

Fig. 8 (**a**) DTI showing fibres of the arcuate fasciculus (white arrowhead) connecting Broca's and Wernicke's speech centres. Part of the arcuate fasciculus is disrupted by a left temporal glioblastoma (white arrow). The anatomical relations of the tumour with the arcuate fasciculus and the corticospinal tract more medially (black arrowhead) are well depicted by superimposing DTI data over conventional 2D and 3D MRI. (**b**) Functional MRI performed to localise the speech centres around a left temporal cerebral glioblastoma. There is strong activation in the left posterior inferior frontal gyrus (white arrowhead) in Broca's area and in the posterior end of the posterior temporal lobe (black arrowhead) in Wernicke's area. Fibres of the arcuate fasciculus connecting the two speech centres are also demonstrated. Visualisation of functional centres and tracts around a tumour can aid in minimisation of interruption to these structures during treatment planning

prostate (Alonzi et al. 2007; Ocak et al. 2007; Verma et al. 2012) and brain. In breast cancer, a rapid uptake of contrast with washout of enhancement after several minutes is suggestive of malignancy, whereas a relatively slow continuous increase in enhancement is typically considered benign (Fig. 9). In prostate MRI, early enhancement on dynamic imaging leads to the upgrading

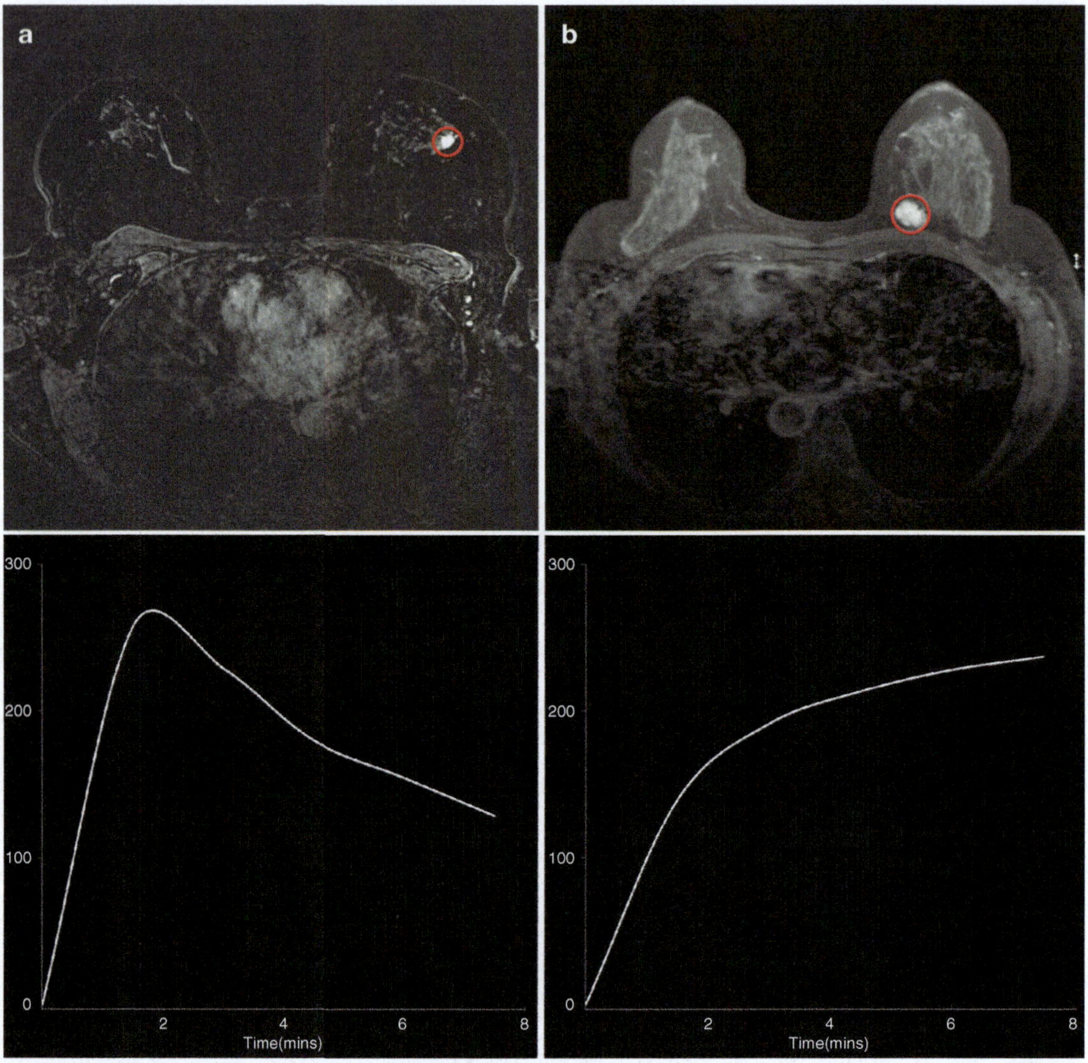

Fig. 9 Dynamic gadolinium-enhanced breast MRI demonstrating perfusion kinetic curves for two different lesions (red circles): (**a**) ductal carcinoma showing relatively rapid uptake with washout in the latter part of the study; (**b**) fibroadenoma showing continuous increase in enhancement and uprising curve typical of a benign lesion

of an intermediate (PI-RADS 3) lesion in the peripheral zone to PI-RADS 4, based on current criteria (PI-RADS: Prostate Imaging—reporting and Data System version 2 2015).

Maps of blood volume and blood flow can be derived from monitoring the first pass of a bolus of gadolinium through the tissue in question for the resultant susceptibility effect. This is widely referred to as *perfusion* MRI or bolus-tracking MRI. Cerebral perfusion MRI has become a widely used technique in brain tumour imaging (Fig. 10) as it has the potential to provide useful information about histological grade, tumour vascularity and extent prior to treatment (Essig et al. 2004; Knopp et al. 1999; Sugahara et al. 1998), guide tumour biopsy (Cha et al. 2002; Kelly et al. 1987) and differentiate therapy effect (such as radiation necrosis) from tumour recurrence during follow-up (Barajas Jr et al. 2009; Barajas et al. 2009; Bisdas et al. 2011; Hu et al. 2009; Oh et al. 2007). After radiotherapy, cerebral blood volume decreases in tumour remission

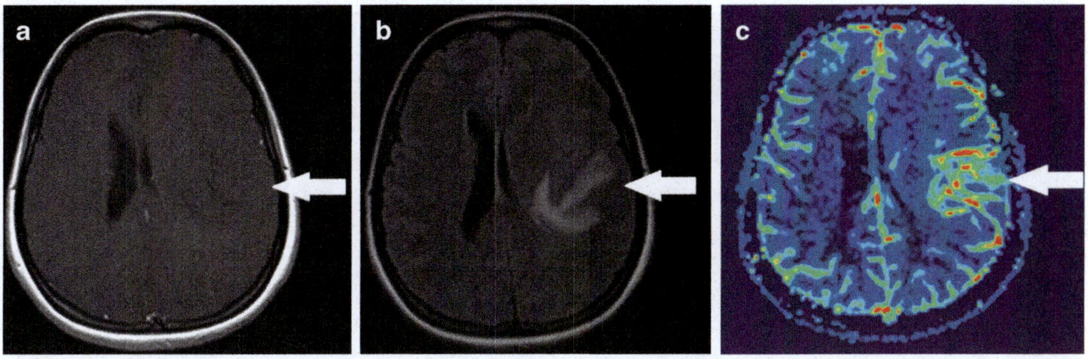

Fig. 10 MRI of left frontal cerebral glioma (white arrow) with no enhancement on post-gadolinium T1-weighted imaging (**a**) and high signal on the FLAIR sequence (**b**). Cerebral blood volume map (**c**) derived from perfusion MRI clearly shows the location and extent of the glioma

and stable disease, but increases in tumour progression (Essig et al. 2004). Cerebral blood volume has also shown promise in predicting tumour response and prognosis (Bisdas et al. 2009; Danchaivijitr et al. 2008; Law et al. 2008).

Imaging of angiogenesis is expected to become an increasingly important objective with the wider availability of vascular endothelial growth factor (VEGF) inhibitors and other novel antiangiogenic therapies.

3.4 Magnetic Resonance Spectroscopy

Magnetic resonance spectroscopy (MRS) enables quantification of certain metabolites within a voxel on MRI (e.g. creatine, choline and lactate that are involved in energy, cell membrane, and anaerobic metabolism, respectively). It is a potentially useful technique for discriminating between benign and malignant tumours by analysis of their varying metabolite compositions and for distinguishing malignant tissues and treatment-related abnormalities that can have similar morphological appearances on conventional MRI or CT.

Post-radiation treatment effects of cerebral glioma include pseudo-progression in the early setting (particularly in the situation of concurrent chemotherapy) and radiation necrosis in a more delayed setting. Both can have the same appearance as progressive or recurrent glioma on conventional non-contrast and gadolinium-enhanced MRI. Although potentially still problematic in many cases, distinguishing radiation effects and tumour recurrence where there are typical MRS features (Fig. 11) can be reassuring and justify a conservative approach of watchful waiting in the case of radiation change or lead to earlier second-line treatment in the case of tumour recurrence.

MRS has also been applied in the evaluation of treatment response in prostate cancer where MRS evaluation is mainly based on the elevation of the choline peak and the choline/creatine ratios (Barentsz et al. 2012; Westphalen et al. 2008). Its use as a biomarker of treatment response in breast cancer remains to be validated by large-scale clinical trials (Bolan et al. 2017).

3.5 Functional MRI

Functional MRI (fMRI) is a technique based on detection of subtle alteration in blood flow in response to stimuli or actions, with the aim of localising centres of eloquent cortex in the brain, most commonly the primary motor cortex, primary somatosensory cortex, primary visual cortex and Broca's and Wernicke's area. Typically, a blood oxygenation level dependent (BOLD) imaging sequence is employed to achieve this while subjecting the patient to specific stimuli or actions (termed paradigms) designed to elicit a specific cortical response. The localisation of these functional areas in the brain allows the clinician to

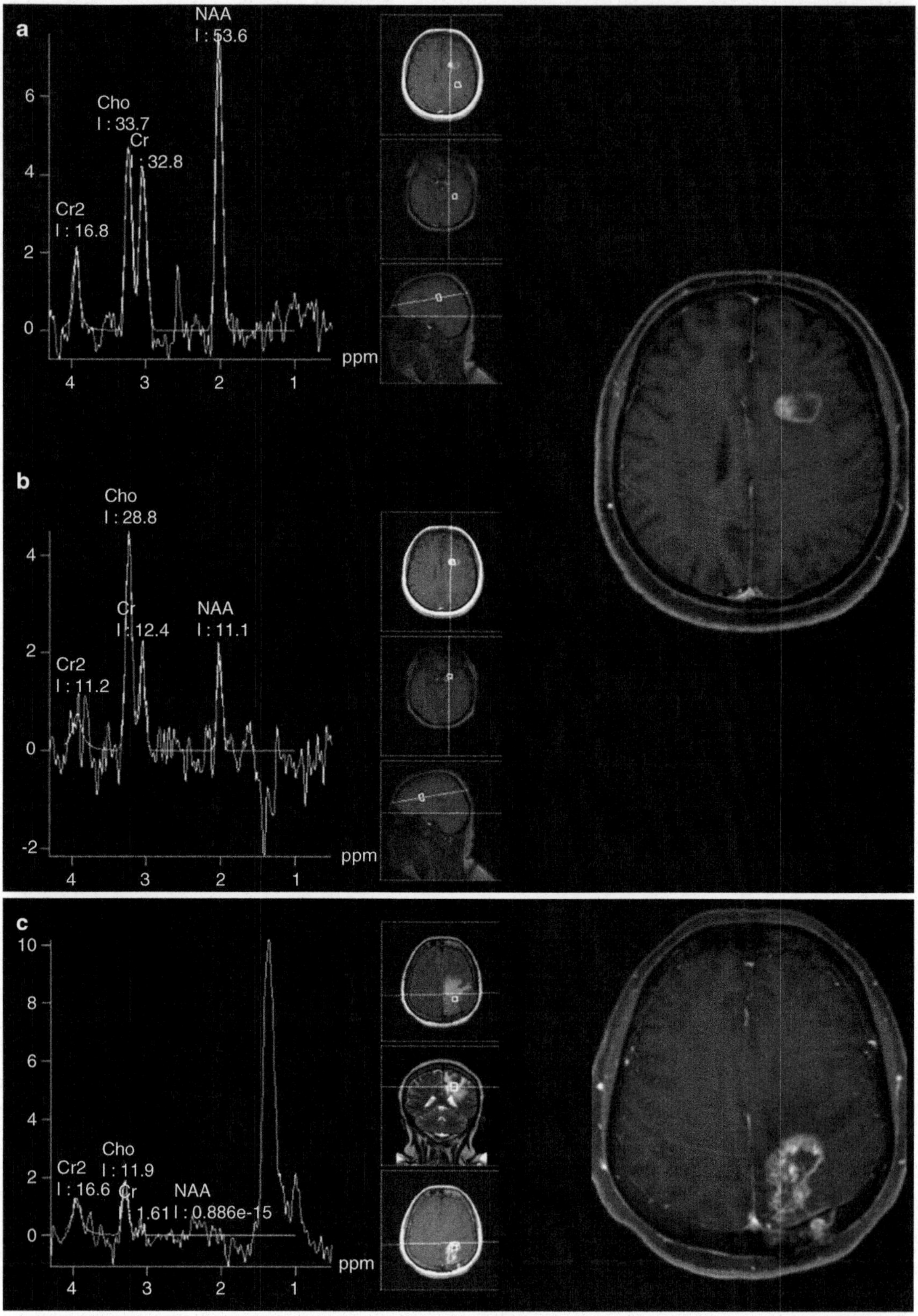
a
NAA
I : 53.6
Cho
I : 33.7
Cr
I : 32.8
Cr2
I : 16.8
ppm
b
Cho
I : 28.8
Cr
I : 12.4
NAA
I : 11.1
Cr2
I : 11.2
ppm
c
Cho
I : 11.9
Cr2
I : 16.6
Cr
I : 1.61
NAA
I : 0.886e-15
ppm

Fig. 11 MRS can help to distinguish radiation necrosis and tumour recurrence in glioblastoma following radiation therapy. Both lesions demonstrate irregular peripheral enhancement that are morphologically similar on gadolinium-enhanced MRI, but MRS shows significant differences in metabolite concentrations between the two lesions. (**a**) Normal MRS in cerebral white matter. (**b**) Reduced NAA and creatine suggestive of glioma recurrence. (**c**) Choline as well as NAA and creatine are all typically reduced in concentration in radiation necrosis

avoid disrupting them as much as possible during treatment of a tumour nearby, thereby preserving important function for the patient (Fig. 8b).

4 Computed Tomography Imaging of Tumour Biology

CT uses X-rays transmitted through a body region and the calculation of how much the X-ray beams are attenuated by passing through the body tissues, to generate density maps of the body which can be reconstructed using computer algorithms into cross-sectional images. The density of biological tissues is defined on a Hounsfield unit scale, referenced to the density of water as zero. CT is almost ubiquitous in the imaging of neoplasms, in all regions of the body. It is easily accessible and rapid to perform and provides good anatomical information about the tumour and its spatial relation to other body structures.

The administration of intravenous iodinated contrast media provides further characterisation of tumour blood supply and enhancement pattern. Beyond a simple qualitative appraisal, detailed analysis and quantitation of enhancement parameters can now reveal in vivo processes in the tumour that could lead to more individualised and better informed treatment decision-making. More recently, other techniques such as CT texture analysis (CTTA) and dual-energy CT (DECT) have also emerged that allow more detailed characterisation of tumour biology.

4.1 CT Perfusion for Tumour Biology

CT perfusion (CTp) enables measurement of regional blood flow, blood volume and vessel permeability and is more widely available than molecular techniques such as PET for imaging the molecular components of angiogenic or tumour-associated blood vessels. CTp involves the acquisition of a baseline non-contrast CT through the region of the tumour, followed by a dynamic acquisition at multiple time points through the same region after a bolus intravenous injection of iodinated contrast (Fig. 12).

Perfusion parameters can be significantly different between normal and tumour tissues and between benign and malignant tumours of the brain, lung, liver, pancreas, rectum and breast (Garcia-Figueiras et al. 2013).

Although not a major application of CTp, several studies have shown its potential usefulness in cancer *staging*, e.g. in determination of perirectal tumour infiltration (Sun et al. 2011), differentiation between benign and metastatic nodes in head and neck squamous cell carcinoma (SCC) (Trojanowska et al. 2012) and breast cancer (Liu et al. 2007).

Tumour angiogenesis is an important *prognostic factor* in many types of cancer, since the blood supply of a tumour may influence its ability to metastasise. The blood flow to a tumour can also predict its response to therapy, with studies showing higher rates of response to treatment in rectal cancer (Bellomi et al. 2007; Koh et al. 2013) and head and neck SCC (Bisdas et al. 2010; Hermans et al. 2003) that have higher blood flow, possibly through better delivery of chemotherapy and greater oxygenation-related radiosensitivity.

CTp has been used extensively for *response assessment* in various malignancies (Kyle et al. 2013). Tumour perfusion influences microvasculature and oxygenation, both important targets for radiotherapy. Measurement of tumour perfusion before and after radiotherapy can thus be a useful indicator of response. It should be noted,

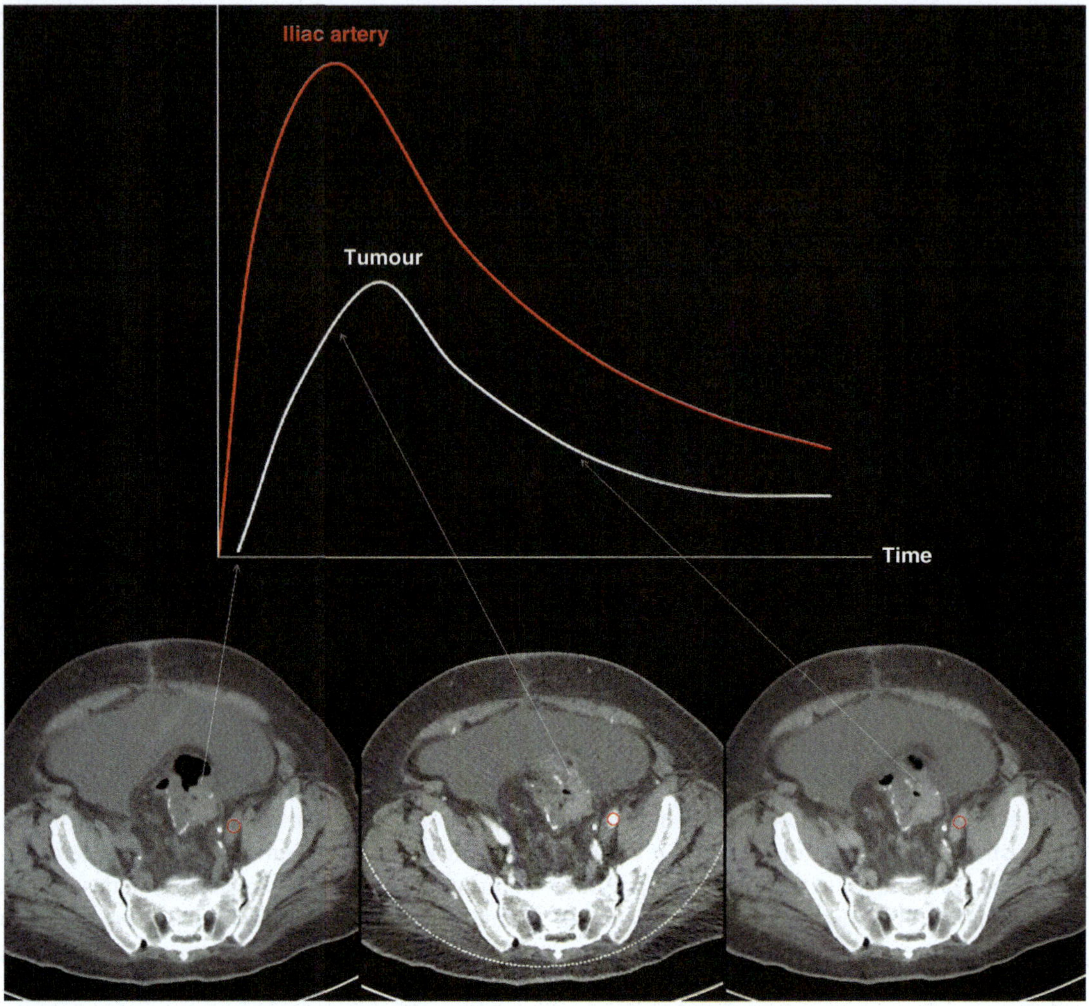

Fig. 12 CT perfusion acquisition showing colon cancer recurrence (white curve) at the surgical anastomosis. Tumour tissue shows early hyperperfusion as a result of neoangiogenesis and rapid washout reflecting increased permeability of immature vessels. For comparison, the enhancement kinetics of the adjacent external iliac artery (red circle and curve) is also shown

however, that if measured too early following treatment, elevated perfusion parameters may reflect transient inflammation as an effect of irradiation, rather than tumour progression.

Following chemotherapy, tumour cell death results in a loss of cytokine support for angiogenesis and reduced tumour perfusion which can be quantified on CTp. Promising results for the use of CTp have been reported in non-small cell lung cancer (Hanahan and Weinberg 2000), head and neck (Hermans et al. 2003), oesophageal (Hayano et al. 2007) and rectal cancer (Bellomi et al. 2007; Sahani et al. 2005). In addition to conventional chemotherapy, there is now a multitude of antiangiogenic therapeutic agents, among which antibodies targeting VEGF (e.g. bevacizumab) and tyrosine kinase inhibitors are most widely used. CTp can detect a reduction in blood flow, volume and permeability in response to antiangiogenic therapy, in a variety of tumours including renal cell cancer (Fournier et al. 2010; van der Veldt et al. 2010), hepatocellular carcinoma (Zhu et al. 2008), carcinoid tumour (Ng et al. 2011) and non-small cell lung cancer (Lind et al. 2010).

Following local treatment of tumour such as transarterial chemoembolisation or radiofrequency ablation of hepatocellular carcinoma, CTp parameters may be valuable for demonstrating successful disruption of tumour vascularity (Ippolito et al. 2010, 2013).

4.2 CT Texture Analysis

CTTA assesses the distribution of attenuation values within a lesion that is not possible with simple visual assessment. This is achieved using specialised software that generates computed parameters based on histogram analysis, most commonly the standard deviation, kurtosis, skewness and statistical derivations of uniformity and entropy.

Intratumoural heterogeneity is a feature of malignant behaviour and therapeutic resistance. CTTA has shown promise in risk stratification and predicting survival in non-small cell lung cancer, oesophageal, colorectal and renal cell cancer.

While tumour stage remains the most important prognostic factor for survival in non-small cell lung cancer, tumours of the same stage can exhibit varying clinical courses. CTTA could provide supplementary markers of prognostic significance (Bluthgen and Besse 2015; Caramella et al. 2015; Fried et al. 2014; Ganeshan et al. 2012a; Weiss et al. 2014; Win et al. 2013) to identify tumours with higher risk of postsurgical recurrence that may benefit from adjuvant chemotherapy or radiotherapy even when not routinely indicated (Fig. 13).

Tumour heterogeneity in oesophageal cancer assessed using CTTA has been found to correlate with increased SUV on [^{18}F]FDG-PET—itself a prognostic factor (Pan et al. 2009; Law and Miles 2013)—and also to correlate with advanced tumour stage and patient survival (Ganeshan et al. 2012b).

In colorectal cancer, the addition of whole-tumour CTTA—in which less heterogeneity has been associated with poorer survival (Ng et al. 2013)—may improve prognostication and a more individualised treatment plan.

CTTA-based quantitative imaging biomarkers have been shown to correlate with overall survival and progression-free survival in clear cell renal cell carcinoma treated with sunitinib (Haider et al. 2017).

That CTTA is a post-imaging procedure which can be applied retrospectively to routinely acquired CT datasets is a significant benefit avoiding additional radiation exposure and inconvenience to the patient and the costs of new scanner technology.

4.3 Dual-Energy CT in Oncology

Dual-energy CT (DECT) involves the acquisition of two different X-ray spectra through the same volume of scanning, most commonly using a CT gantry containing two X-ray tubes at different peak kilovoltage (kVp).

One major benefit of DECT is the possibility to distinguish different materials of apparently similar density on conventional CT. Thus, calcium can be discriminated from urate deposits based on their different energy binding and absorption properties at different kVp, providing more detailed information about the composition of renal stones or crystal deposition in joints.

More recently, DECT has also found potentially useful applications in imaging in oncology, both for tumour detection and assessment of treatment response. DECT can increase image contrast and vessel delineation leading to improved detection in hepatocellular carcinoma (Altenbernd et al. 2011) and pancreatic cancer (Klauss et al. 2013). Enhanced visualisation of tumour boundaries can also aid in radiation treatment planning.

Another benefit of DECT is the possibility to reconstruct virtual non-contrast-enhanced images, by subtracting iodine from contrast-enhanced CT datasets. Hence, DECT can provide both non-enhanced and contrast-enhanced scans with just one acquisition, affording radiation dose savings which can be significant in oncology patients requiring multiple CT studies over the course of their treatment and follow-up. In lung cancer, comparable diagnostic accuracy has

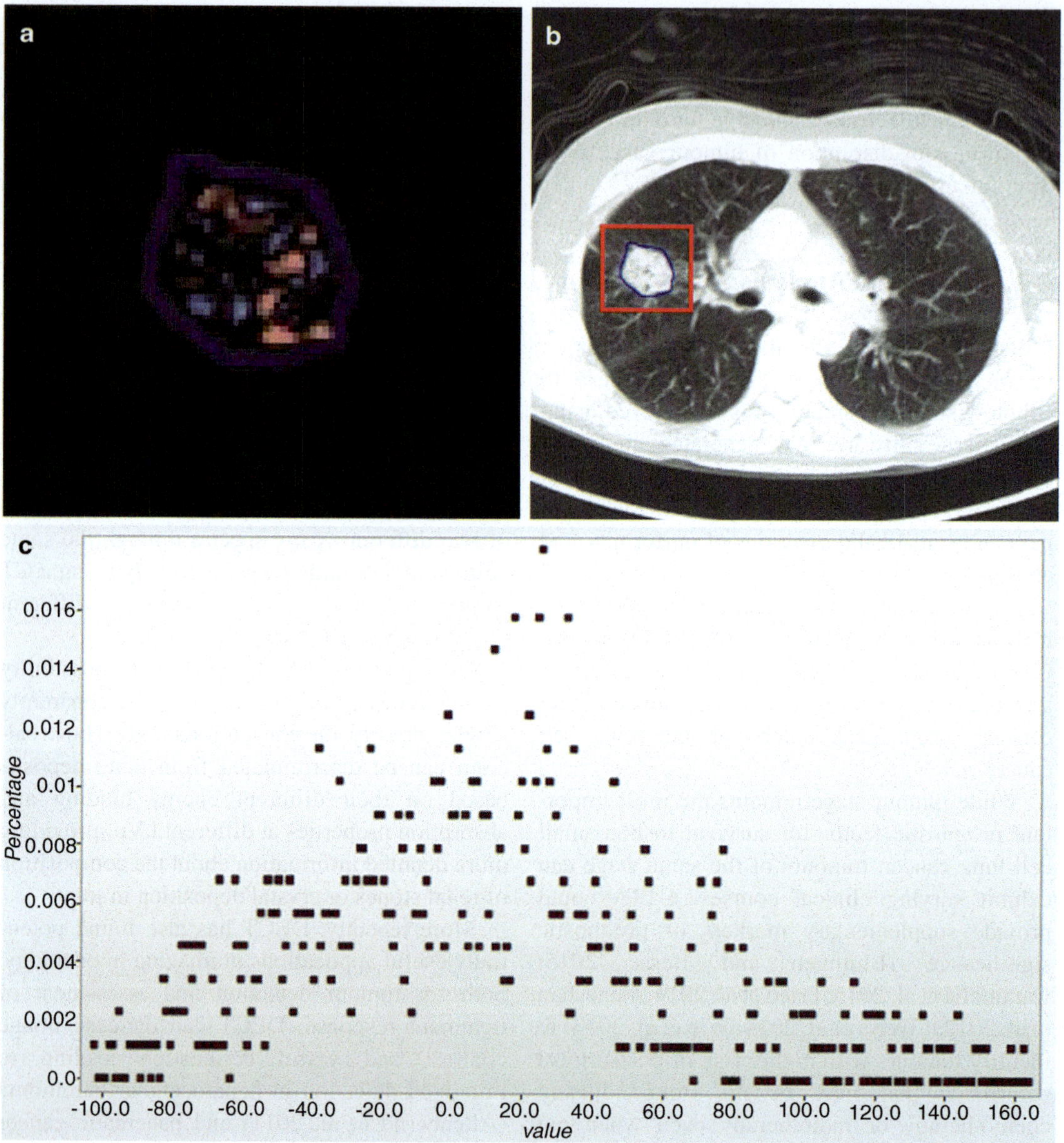

Fig. 13 CTTA of a right upper lobe non-small cell lung cancer (**a** and red rectangles) performed by filtering a conventional CT image (**b**) to highlight objects of a preselected size. The distribution of filtered pixel intensities is depicted on a histogram (**c**) and assessed using standard statistical parameters to provide an indication of prognosis and aid in risk stratification

been shown between single DECT and multiphase conventional CT (Chae et al. 2008; Kim et al. 2012b; Ogawa et al. 2012).

In addition to their use for subtraction from contrast-enhanced images, maps of iodine concentration calculated in DECT can be superimposed on CT images and provide useful information in the staging and treatment response evaluation of lung cancer (Baxa et al. 2014; Schmid-Bindert et al. 2012), in some cases positively correlated with SUV obtained in [^{18}F]FDG-PET (Schmid-Bindert et al. 2012). DECT can accurately assess disease response in gastrointestinal stromal tumours and perhaps even enable better prediction of therapy response than the currently preferred Choi's criteria (Apfaltrer et al. 2012; Meyer et al.

2013) by defining criteria based on iodine attenuation rather than just density on CT.

5 Response-Adapted Radiotherapy Using Functional Imaging

Planning and delivery of radiotherapy continues to evolve with advances in imaging techniques and treatment conformality. Most recently the introduction of intensity-modulated radiation therapy (IMRT) has facilitated the ability to 'dose paint'. This is the delivery of different dose prescriptions to multiple target sites within the treatment volume. The varied dose levels within the tumour target volume are optimally based on information from functional imaging, which reveals biological information regarding the tumour components.

The integration of biological imaging techniques into planning and delivery of radiotherapy has the potential to (1) improve delineation of the primary tumour and involved lymph nodes, (2) dose escalate to more functional tumour subvolumes, (3) deliver response-adapted radiotherapy targeting less responsive tumour components and (4) reduce treatment volumes by targeting only the functional tumour components and ultimately reduce doses to organs at risk.

Biological dose 'painting' or 'sculpting' can be performed by one of two ways. Dose painting by contours (DPBC) is the technique of delivering a boost volume to the area of greatest activity (i.e. SUV > 50% maximum uptake) within the primary tumour volume. Dose painting by numbers (DPBN) is the method of assigning each voxel a particular dose based on the intensity of uptake in that voxel, delivering a more heterogeneous dose to the tumour volume (Duprez et al. 2011; Madani et al. 2011; Vanderstraeten et al. 2006).

5.1 Delineation of Primary Tumour and Involved Lymph Nodes

Local tumour control remains a challenge in many tumour subsites (Curran Jr et al. 2003; Furuse et al. 1999; Martel et al. 1999; Saunders et al. 1999; Sause et al. 2000). The delivery of increased radiation dose to involved sites of disease in order to overcome this issue is hampered by unacceptable toxicity to normal tissues (Curran Jr et al. 2003; Furuse et al. 1999; Martel et al. 1999; Saunders et al. 1999; Sause et al. 2000). The use of a combined PET-CT simulator allows for better tumour delineation and subsequent sparing of normal tissues than a standard CT simulator, further opening the possibility of dose escalation while maintaining normal tissue tolerance (De Ruysscher et al. 2005; Daisne et al. 2004)

The impact of PET-based GTVs was demonstrated by De Ruysscher et al. who compared simulation with a dedicated PET-CT with CT planning in 21 patients with locally advanced NSCLC. They showed that incorporation of PET-CT information led to a significant decrease in all dosimetric factors, including mean oesophageal and lung doses. They also showed that when all constraints of the lung, oesophagus and spinal cord were taken into account, the dose could be escalated to an average of 68.9 Gy with PET planning compared to 55.2 Gy with the use of CT (De Ruysscher et al. 2005).

PET-defined volumes also play an important role in the planning of head and neck malignancies. Bendict et al. compared PET-defined volumes with that of CT in nine patients with unresectable locally advanced head and neck carcinoma. They showed a significant reduction in mean gross tumour volumes to 39.3 cm^3 with PET compared to 71.4 cm^3 using CT, equating to a mean volume reduction of 40% (Henriques de Figueiredo et al. 2009).

5.2 Response Adaptation Based on Metabolic Imaging

Observational studies have reported biological changes in the target throughout the course of fractionated radiotherapy (Barker Jr et al. 2004; Bhide et al. 2010; Castadot et al. 2010). This suggests a potential role for dose-adapted radiotherapy to deliver higher doses to areas of sustained activity during radiotherapy on functional imaging, which represents potentially radioresistant disease. By doing so, this may also enable reduction of doses to more responsive tumour components as well as the surrounding organs at risk.

Berwouts et al. investigated the use of response-adapted DPBN in reducing treatment volumes in head and neck cancer, based on mid-treatment [^{18}F]FDG-PET imaging. They reported mean target volume reductions of 46.3% for the high-dose PTV with mild rates of acute toxicity and no measurable decrease in tumour response (Berwouts et al. 2013).

Geets et al. assessed the use of weekly reimaging during radiotherapy, with CT, MRI and PET in ten head and neck patients to elicit the value of weekly reassessment along with the most appropriate imaging technique. They demonstrated that throughout the course of treatment the GTVs, CTVs and PTVs delineated from PET imaging remained significantly smaller than the corresponding volumes delineated on CT and MRI (Geets et al. 2007).

Functional imaging can also be utilised to escalate dose to the most active components of the tumour based on PET information. The ARTFORCE trial (Heukelom et al.) is presently investigating this in head and neck cancer patients. They will compare a standard approach of 70 Gy in 35 fractions to a dose-painted regimen. By defining the high [^{18}F]FDG uptake region as the areas with at least 50% of maximum SUV uptake, they aimed to deliver a maximum dose of 84 Gy to this high [^{18}F]FDG uptake region and at least 64 Gy to the primary tumour (Heukelom et al. 2013).

5.3 Response Adaptation Based on Tumour Proliferation

Enhanced proliferative activity is a characteristic feature of malignant cells(Buck et al. 2002) and accelerated repopulation of tumour cells during radiotherapy due to increased proliferation is a known cause of treatment failure (Kim and Tannock 2005). Methods to overcome this include addition of concurrent chemotherapy, dose escalation, accelerated radiotherapy or hyperfractionated radiotherapy. Mid-treatment assessment of this proliferative tumour cell compartment and subsequent adaptation of treatment to include the above measures may help counter this phenomenon and ultimately improve outcomes (Hoeben et al. 2013). Anatomical imaging performed during treatment is unable to detect for surviving tumour cells potentially undergoing accelerated repopulation. Molecular imaging techniques have subsequently been developed to identify these populations of proliferative cells within the tumour volume and thus identify those patients who may derive benefit from an adapted treatment. Uptake of the PET tracer, [^{18}F]FLT, reflects the proliferative activity of the cell (Rasey et al. 2002). Validation studies have confirmed a close correlation between FLT uptake and Ki-67 levels (Yap et al. 2006; Buck et al. 2003; Yamamoto et al. 2007; Muzi et al. 2005).

Everitt et al. performed a proof of concept study to assess the ability of FLT-PET to monitor changes in cellular proliferation during chemoradiotherapy in five patients with NSCLC. Patients underwent scans at baseline and during treatment. Based on FLT uptake, an overall reduction in the proliferation activity of primary tumours was observed for all cases across the duration of treatment. In comparison there was minimal morphological response in tumour volume throughout treatment (Everitt et al. 2009). This reflects the ability of molecular imaging to better detect tumour regression, or progression, than structural imaging during a course of chemoradiotherapy (Everitt et al. 2009).

Everitt et al. assessed the use of FLT-PET in comparison to [^{18}F]FDG-PET in 20 patients undergoing chemoradiotherapy for stages I–III NSCLC. Appreciable differences were observed in tumoural uptake between FLT and [^{18}F]FDG-PET at weeks 2 and 4, noting a greater effect of chemoradiotherapy on tumour cell proliferation than cellular metabolism. This differential effect was greatest at week 2 (Everitt et al. 2014) (Fig. 14). Ball et al. also assessed the use of FLT and [^{18}F]FDG-PET prior to and during chemoradiotherapy in predicting outcomes in NSCLC. They reported that response on FLT-PET at 2 weeks was predictive of both progression-free survival and overall survival (David et al. 2017). Such findings support the use of indi-

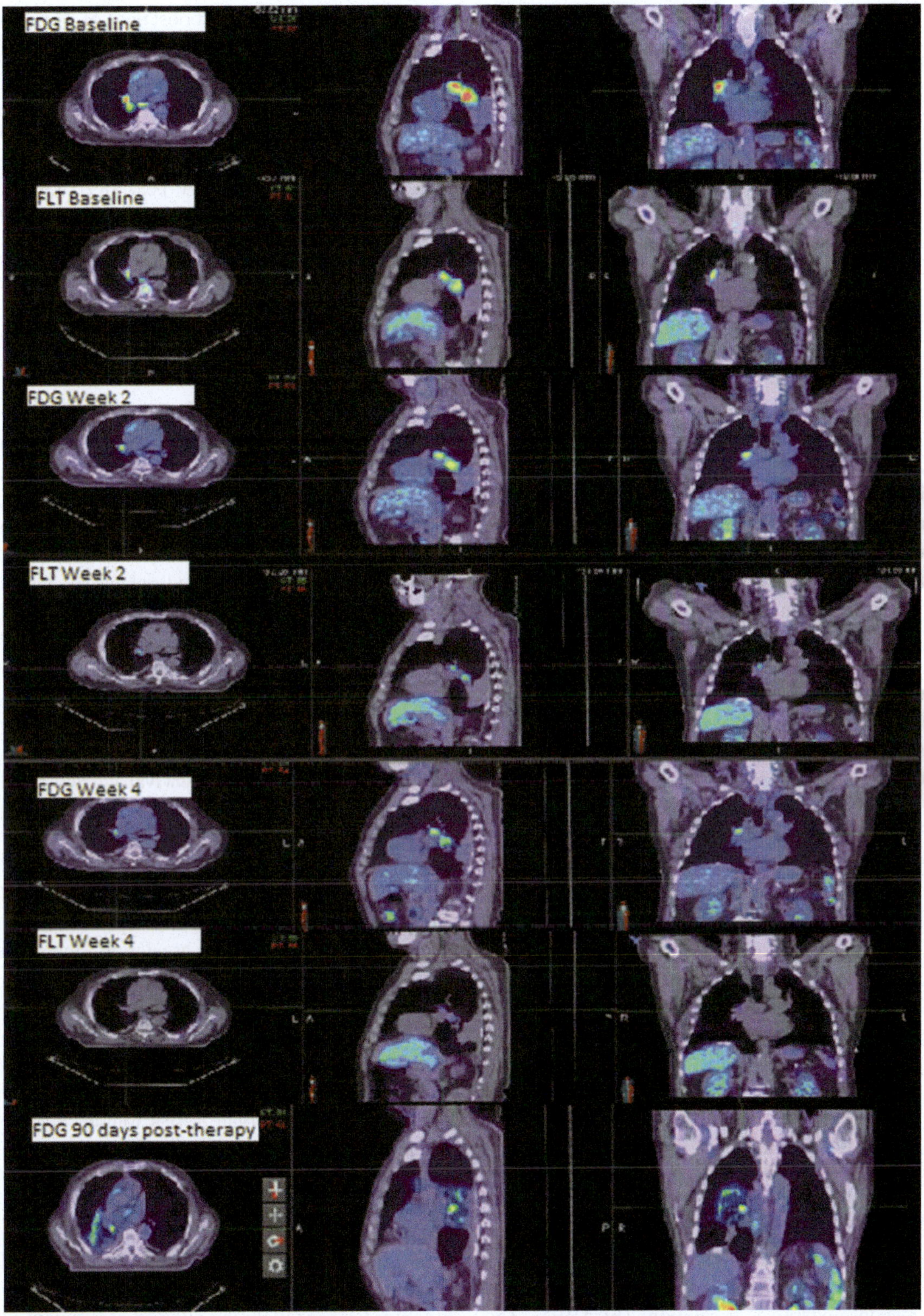

Fig. 14 Comparative response on [18F]FDG- and FLT-PET in a 76-year-old male undergoing chemoradiotherapy for NSCLC at baseline pretreatment, weeks 2 and 4 into the treatment course. A more rapid response is noted on FLT, with a complete response by week 4. By comparison persistent activity is noted on [18F]FDG by week 4, and a [18F]FDG-PET scan performed 90 days post therapy demonstrates residual activity in field consistent with distribution of radiation pneumonitis

vidualised response-adapted therapy to FLT-PET findings mid-treatment, with the aim of overcoming the poor prognostic implications of less responding tumours.

5.4 Response Adaptation Based on Functional Lung Avoidance

Dose escalation in lung cancer, with a view for improved tumour control, is limited by the dose constraints of the surrounding normal tissues and in particular the lungs (Fay et al. 2005). The current dose constraints applied to radiotherapy planning do not account for individual variation in pulmonary physiology (Siva et al. 2016). Assessment of lung perfusion (*Q*) in radiotherapy planning is of particular importance as damage to the vascular endothelium plays a primary role in the development of radiation pneumonitis and fibrosis (Siva et al. 2016). Dose to well-perfused functional lung has been shown to be a stronger predictor for toxicity than dose to the conventionally measured lung (Wang et al. 2012). Ventilation and perfusion imaging (*V*/*Q*) to assess regional lung function is subsequently being investigated to individualise lung radiotherapy. This would ideally enable either safe dose escalation or alternatively a reduction in dose to more functional lung volumes and reduced incidence of pneumonitis and fibrosis (Siva et al. 2016).

68-Gallium is a positron-emitting radionuclide, which when labelled with macroaggregated albumin (MAA) provides in vivo assessment of functional lung perfusion (Mathias and Green 2008). Siva et al. assessed the utility gallium-PET in facilitating avoidance of the functional lungs during radiotherapy in patients with NSCLC. They showed that plans optimised to avoid 'well-perfused' lung, defined as lung parenchyma with >30% SUVmax uptake, had significantly improved dose volumetrics for mean lung dose, V30, V40, V50 and V60 (Siva et al. 2016).

Lee et al. assessed the dosimetric and clinical feasibility of functional lung avoidance and response-adaptive escalation (FLARE). They aimed to reduce dose to perfused lung while redistributing an escalated boost dose of 74 Gy to a biological target volume (GTV + PET gradient segmentation) in patients with NSCLC. They reported no violations of normal tissue objectives in FLARE radiotherapy plans and achieved higher mean dose to the biological target volume (73.7 Gy vs. 61.3 Gy), SUV peak (89.7 Gy vs. 60.8 Gy) and lower mean dose to highly perfused lung (7.3 Gy vs. 14.9 Gy) (Lee et al. 2017).

5.5 Biological Imaging in Dose Escalation

Local control remains a challenge in many tumour sites and is reportedly as high as 40% in NSCLC (Curran et al. 2000; Saunders et al. 1997; Le Chevalier et al. 1994; Schaake-Koning et al. 1992). As a result of such poor local control, the concept of dose escalation is appealing. Furthermore retrospective studies have suggested a dose-response relationship for local control (Perez et al. 1980; Rengan et al. 2004; Bradley et al. 2002). This was highlighted in a Memorial Sloan Kettering study that showed a 36% reduction in failure for every 10 Gy increase in dose for patient with NSCLC. Other studies have furthermore reported an overall survival advantage in patients who received dose escalation (Kong et al. 2005; Zhao et al. 2007; Rosenzweig et al. 2005). However, the results of the RTOG 0617 study comparing 74 Gy vs. 60 Gy in conventional 2 Gy per fraction suggest that simply extending the treatment with dose escalation does not improve survival.

As use of biological imaging has shown the potential to reduce the gross tumour volumes, this has created a potential avenue for dose escalation to improve tumour control probability without exceeding organ at risk tolerances. Van Elmpt et al. assessed the use of PET boost in dose escalation for patients with NSCLC. They randomised patients receiving 66 Gy in 24 fractions, to either an isotoxic integrated boost to the primary tumour as a whole or an isotoxic integrated boost to the 50% SUVmax area of the primary tumour. Isotoxic planning allowed assessment of maximum achievable boost dose while maintaining organ at risk tolerances. The mean total dose delivered to the whole tumour was 78.4 Gy vs. 87.2 Gy for the 50% SUV-based boost ($p = 0.001$), highlighting the ability to significantly increase the dose using PET information without compromising organs at risk (van Elmpt et al. 2012).

Duprez et al. assessed the use of dose escalation for head and neck carcinoma. They furthermore delivered treatment using an adaptive approach of replanning treatment for fractions 11–20 and again for fractions 21–30. In doing so they were able to significantly reduce the volumes for the GTV (41%), CTV (18%) and PTV (14%) as well as safely escalated the CTV dose to 80.9 Gy and the GTV dose to 85.9 Gy (at 3 Gy per fraction) (Duprez et al. 2011).

5.6 Limitations of Biological Imaging in Response-Adapted Radiotherapy

The use of PET imaging in defining target volumes has several limitations. Delineation of the margins of radiotracer uptake is subjective and observer dependent (Ciernik et al. 2003; Heron et al. 2004; Nishioka et al. 2002; Scarfone et al. 2004). PET images have poor spatial resolution due to random travel of positrons before they annihilate with electrons. The subsequent scattering of photons in the patient before being located on the camera scintillator results in blurrier images and reduced definition of tumour extent (Geets et al. 2013; Valk et al. 2004). The use of PET in lung malignancies results in further blurring of images due to respiratory motion, and delineation of tumour volume based on these images is subsequently compromised.

Many challenges remain in the planning and delivery of response-adapted radiotherapy based on PET imaging. Feng et al. noted that such techniques could only be applied to 6 patients out of an initial 14 with NSCLC. Two had a complete metabolic response, two had non-specific inflammation in the radiotherapy field and four had no reduction in radiotherapy fields (Feng et al. 2009). This raised the question of how to determine radiotherapy volumes in those patients who have a complete response mid-treatment and what total dose is required in these patients. It is not known whether these patients are able to receive a lower total dose to eradicate all tumour cells in view of their complete response in PET imaging mid-treatment, which would further reduce normal tissue complication probability (Feng et al. 2009). For those patients who had increases in tumour volume during treatment, it is unknown what component may represent inflammation and whether this should be included in an enlarged volume (Feng et al. 2009). It also remains unknown when the most suitable time is to re-scan during radiotherapy. This was evaluated by Hentschel et al. who performed weekly [^{18}F]FDG-PET imaging during the course of radiotherapy and found a decrease in SUV at the end of the 1st and 2nd week, but variable change from the third week on. They suggested that the first weeks of treatment are an appropriate time to perform imaging for dose adaptation; however beyond this time point, the uptake is potentially distorted by inflammation (Hentschel et al. 2009).

There are also several limitations of the use of FLT-PET in radiotherapy planning. Cells not undergoing DNA synthesis will not take up FLT however may still be viable cells capable of division and future proliferation. Subsequently FLT-PET may overestimate cell death and result in under-treatment of malignant cells (Everitt et al. 2014). Furthermore the interpretation of mid-treatment FLT-PET imaging remains difficult due to different reported prognostic implications of reduced PET uptake. Hoeben et al. reported that a reduction in FLT uptake during the first 2 weeks of treatment for head and neck cancer resulted in a significant improvement in progression-free survival (Hoeben et al. 2013). Conversely Ball et al. found that in patients receiving chemoradiotherapy for NSCLC, a partial or complete response on FLT after 2 weeks was associated with a worse progression-free survival and overall survival compared to patients who had stable disease (David et al. 2017). Finally, use of response-adapted techniques furthermore places increased workflow stress on a radiotherapy department, due to the increased time and resources required to re-evaluate and replan a course of treatment.

5.7 Hypoxia Imaging in Radiotherapy Planning

Tumour hypoxia is an established mechanism of radioresistance and subsequently reduced tumour control (Pajonk et al. 2010; Nordsmark et al. 2005). It has been shown to render tumours three times more resistant to radiation relative to oxygenated cells (Hockel et al. 1993). Intra-tumoural hypoxia can be assessed using non-invasive imaging techniques. Fluorine-18-labelled misonidazole ([^{18}F]FMISO) PET uptake directly relates to tissue hypoxia (Rajendran et al. 2004; Rajendran et al. 2003). Its uptake within tumours has also been correlated to patient prognosis, predicting a higher risk of relapse (Eschmann et al. 2005; Rajendran et al. 2006; Rischin et al. 2006). Targeting of hypoxic subvolumes within the tumour for dose escalation may provide an avenue for overcoming this radioresistance and improving patient outcomes.

Fluoromisonidazole binds selectively to hypoxic cells (Koh et al. 1992). Following penetration of the cell membrane, it undergoes oxygen-dependent conversion into highly reactive intermediates when the pO2 drops below 10mmHg (Lapi et al. 2009). By labelling FMISO with the positron emitter fluorine-18 ([^{18}F]), its uptake in tissues can be quantitated. Interpretation of the [^{18}F]FMISO-PET scans is based on several parameters. The tumour-blood ratio (TBR) is the maximum concentration of the tumour divided by the concentration of blood collected from venous sampling. The tumour-muscle ratio (TMR) is the tumour uptake divided by the uptake of the posterior cervical muscle. Rajendran et al. (Rajendran et al. 2004; Rajendran et al. 2003; Koh et al. 1992) report a significant [^{18}F]FMISO uptake to be a TBR of 1.2–1.4.

Lee at al. assessed the feasibility of [^{18}F]FMISO-PET/CT-guided IMRT in dose escalation to hypoxic zones in ten head and neck cancer patients. They achieved dose escalation to the hypoxic GTV of 84 Gy in all ten patients, compared to 70 Gy to the GTV, without exceeding normal tissue tolerances (Lee et al. 2008).

There are concerns however about the clinical utility of [^{18}F]FMISO-PET imaging due to only modest signal-to-noise ratios being obtained due to its slow clearance and high liver and gastrointestinal uptake (Nunn et al. 1995; Krohn et al. 2008). [^{18}F]flortanidazole [HX4] is another PET agent used in assessment of tumour hypoxia (Dubois et al. 2011; Zegers et al. 2013; Peeters et al. 2015; van Loon et al. 2010). 18FHX4 has demonstrated lower uptake levels in the intestines, liver and kidney and faster clearance resulting in lower background signals, thus providing good imaging properties (Dubois et al. 2011; van Loon et al. 2010).

Dose escalation of hypoxic tumour subvolumes using HX4-PET imaging was assessed by Even et al. and compared to both dose escalation using metabolic subvolumes on [^{18}F]FDG-PET and boosting of the entire tumour. Ten patients with NSCLC underwent pretreatment [^{18}F]FDG- and HX4-PET/CT scans. Three isotoxic dose escalation plans were subsequently generated for each patient using a dose painting by contours approach. They generated a primary tumour boost volume, a metabolic boost volume covering the area of SUV > 50% max and a hypoxic boost volume of the area of HX4 TBR > 1.4. Dose escalation was feasible for all three plans. The primary boost was escalated to a mean of 87 Gy, the [^{18}F]FDG boost volume to 107 Gy and the hypoxic volume to 117 Gy, all with comparable doses to organs at risk. It was noted that in most patients, boosting the metabolic volume also resulted in boosting the hypoxic volume, but not vice versa. In fact boosting the hypoxic volume only resulted in 61% coverage of the [^{18}F]FDG volume. This suggests that for the majority of patients, [^{18}F]FDG-PET can be used as a surrogate for boosting hypoxic volumes, albeit to a lower dose; however boosting of hypoxic volumes alone results in significant geographical miss to metabolically active disease (Even et al. 2015).

5.8 Limitations of Hypoxia Imaging Techniques

The use of hypoxic imaging techniques in planning and delivery of radiotherapy has several remaining limitations. The slower uptake clearance of unbound tracer molecules can contaminate the background signal and compromise the accuracy of hypoxia assessment (Geets et al. 2013; Bentzen et al. 2000; Mortensen et al. 2010). As with [^{18}F]FDG PET-based imaging techniques, the imaging resolution is limited by random travel of positrons before they annihilate with electrons. The subsequent scattering of photons in the patient before being located on the camera scintillator results in blurrier images (Geets et al. 2013; Valk et al. 2004). The use of dose escalation in targeting hypoxic subvolumes is limited by the inability to delineate acute from chronic hypoxia and thus clearly identifies the exact area of radioresistant hypoxia (Geets et al. 2013; Lee et al. 2008). Heterogeneous dose distributions and higher dose gradients place higher risk on potential for geographical miss and potentially increased dose to critical structures (Geets et al. 2013; Lee et al. 2008). The use of dose escalation in the treatment of hypoxic subvolumes therefore requires more frequent treatment verification with lower action thresholds for patient positioning. As patient lifespans improve with better systemic agents, dose escalation via IMRT techniques may eventually result in increased risk of a secondary malignancy due to the higher integral dose delivered (Hall and Wuu 2003). In using hypoxic imaging in response-adapted radiotherapy techniques, the timing of reimaging is of clinical significance however remains undefined to best assess response of hypoxic cells (Geets et al. 2013). Finally, the use of dose escalation and response-adapted techniques places significant stress on workflow within a radiotherapy department and must be countered against the clinical benefits (Geets et al. 2013).

6 Conclusion

By combining the information derived from multiple imaging techniques now available in the clinical setting, it is possible to build a unique, multifaceted phenotypic view of tumour biology, thus allowing more accurate characterisation and improved decision-making for personalised therapy at the time of diagnosis and staging, after treatment and assessment of disease response and during follow-up and monitoring of disease.

Integration of biologic imaging techniques has improved tumour volume delineation, reduced treatment volumes and enabled safe dose escalation to tumour regions of greatest concern. While response-adapted treatment and dose escalation targeting specific regions is feasible, further research is needed to demonstrate improved patient outcomes, including randomised controlled trials.

Understanding and selecting the appropriate imaging tests at the appropriate time and clinical context, accurate interpretation of images and close collaboration between the clinicians and imaging specialists are vital to ensure that maximum clinical utility is derived from the sophisticated medical technologies now available, with the ultimate goal of improving patient outcomes.

References

Afshar-Oromieh A et al (2014) Comparison of PET imaging with a (68)Ga-labelled PSMA ligand and (18) F-choline-based PET/CT for the diagnosis of recurrent prostate cancer. Eur J Nucl Med Mol Imaging 41(1):11–20

Al-Ameri A et al (2015) Risk of malignancy in pulmonary nodules: a validation study of four prediction models. Lung Cancer 89(1):27–30

Alonzi R, Padhani AR, Allen C (2007) Dynamic contrast enhanced MRI in prostate cancer. Eur J Radiol 63(3):335–350

Altenbernd J et al (2011) Dual-energy-CT of hypervascular liver lesions in patients with HCC: investigation of image quality and sensitivity. Eur Radiol 21(4):738–743

Apfaltrer P et al (2012) Contrast-enhanced dual-energy CT of gastrointestinal stromal tumors: is iodine-related attenuation a potential indicator of tumor response? Invest Radiol 47(1):65–70

Ball D et al (2017) Serial FDG and FLT PET/CT during curative intent chemoradiotherapy for NSCLC impacts patient management and may predict clinical outcomes. J Thorac Oncol 12(S420)

Bahri H et al (2014) High prognostic value of 18F-FDG PET for metastatic gastroenteropancreatic neuroendocrine tumors: a long-term evaluation. J Nucl Med 55(11):1786–1790

Barajas RF Jr et al (2009) Differentiation of recurrent glioblastoma multiforme from radiation necrosis after external beam radiation therapy with dynamic susceptibility-weighted contrast-enhanced perfusion MR imaging. Radiology 253(2):486–496

Barajas RF et al (2009) Distinguishing recurrent intra-axial metastatic tumor from radiation necrosis following gamma knife radiosurgery using dynamic

susceptibility-weighted contrast-enhanced perfusion MR imaging. AJNR Am J Neuroradiol 30(2):367–372
Barentsz JO et al (2012) ESUR prostate MR guidelines 2012. Eur Radiol 22(4):746–757
Barker JL Jr et al (2004) Quantification of volumetric and geometric changes occurring during fractionated radiotherapy for head-and-neck cancer using an integrated CT/linear accelerator system. Int J Radiat Oncol Biol Phys 59(4):960–970
Baxa J et al (2014) Dual-phase dual-energy CT in patients with lung cancer: assessment of the additional value of iodine quantification in lymph node therapy response. Eur Radiol 24(8):1981–1988
Bellomi M et al (2007) CT perfusion for the monitoring of neoadjuvant chemotherapy and radiation therapy in rectal carcinoma: initial experience. Radiology 244(2):486–493
Bentzen L et al (2000) Feasibility of detecting hypoxia in experimental mouse tumours with 18F-fluorinated tracers and positron emission tomography--a study evaluating [18F]Fluoro-2-deoxy-D-glucose. Acta Oncol 39(5):629–637
Berwouts D et al (2013) Three-phase adaptive dose-painting-by-numbers for head-and-neck cancer: initial results of the phase I clinical trial. Radiother Oncol 107(3):310–316
Bhide SA et al (2010) Weekly volume and dosimetric changes during chemoradiotherapy with intensity-modulated radiation therapy for head and neck cancer: a prospective observational study. Int J Radiat Oncol Biol Phys 76(5):1360–1368
Bisdas S et al (2009) Cerebral blood volume measurements by perfusion-weighted MR imaging in gliomas: ready for prime time in predicting short-term outcome and recurrent disease? AJNR Am J Neuroradiol 30(4):681–688
Bisdas S et al (2010) Perfusion CT in squamous cell carcinoma of the upper aerodigestive tract: long-term predictive value of baseline perfusion CT measurements. AJNR Am J Neuroradiol 31(3):576–581
Bisdas S et al (2011) Distinguishing recurrent high-grade gliomas from radiation injury: a pilot study using dynamic contrast-enhanced MR imaging. Acad Radiol 18(5):575–583
Blackledge MD et al (2014) Assessment of treatment response by total tumor volume and global apparent diffusion coefficient using diffusion-weighted MRI in patients with metastatic bone disease: a feasibility study. PLoS One 9(4):e91779
Bluthgen MV, Besse B (2015) Second-line combination therapies in nonsmall cell lung cancer without known driver mutations. Eur Respir Rev 24(138):582–593
Bolan PJ et al (2017) MR spectroscopy of breast cancer for assessing early treatment response: results from the ACRIN 6657 MRS trial. J Magn Reson Imaging 46(1):290–302
Bradley JD et al (2002) Gross tumor volume, critical prognostic factor in patients treated with three-dimensional conformal radiation therapy for non-small-cell lung carcinoma. Int J Radiat Oncol Biol Phys 52(1):49–57
Buck AK et al (2002) 3-deoxy-3-[(18)F]fluorothymidine-positron emission tomography for noninvasive assessment of proliferation in pulmonary nodules. Cancer Res 62(12):3331–3334
Buck AK et al (2003) Imaging proliferation in lung tumors with PET: 18F-FLT versus 18F-FDG. J Nucl Med 44(9):1426–1431
Caramella C et al (2015) Prognostic value of texture analysis and correlation with molecular profile in EGFR mutated/ALK rearranged advanced non-small cell lung cancer (NSCLC). Eur J Cancer 51(Suppl 3):2
Castadot P et al (2010) Assessment by a deformable registration method of the volumetric and positional changes of target volumes and organs at risk in pharyngo-laryngeal tumors treated with concomitant chemo-radiation. Radiother Oncol 95(2):209–217
Cha S et al (2002) Intracranial mass lesions: dynamic contrast-enhanced susceptibility-weighted echo-planar perfusion MR imaging. Radiology 223(1):11–29
Chae EJ et al (2008) Clinical utility of dual-energy CT in the evaluation of solitary pulmonary nodules: initial experience. Radiology 249(2):671–681
Chalkidou A, O'Doherty MJ, Marsden PK (2015) False discovery rates in PET and CT studies with texture features: a systematic review. PLoS One 10(5):e0124165
Cheson BD et al (2014) Recommendations for initial evaluation, staging, and response assessment of Hodgkin and non-Hodgkin lymphoma: the Lugano classification. J Clin Oncol 32(27):3059–3068
Cheson BD et al (2016) Refinement of the Lugano classification lymphoma response criteria in the era of immunomodulatory therapy. Blood 128(21):2489–2496
Ciernik IF et al (2003) Radiation treatment planning with an integrated positron emission and computer tomography (PET/CT): a feasibility study. Int J Radiat Oncol Biol Phys 57(3):853–863
Clark PM et al (2017) Harnessing preclinical molecular imaging to inform advances in personalized cancer medicine. J Nucl Med 58(5):689–696
Cuccurullo V, Di Stasio GD, Mansi L (2017) Radioguided surgery with radiolabeled somatostatin analogs: not only in GEP-NETs. Nucl Med Rev Cent East Eur 20(1):49–56
Curran W Jr, Scott C, Langer C, et al (2003) Long-term benefit is observed in a phase III comparison of sequential vs concurrent chemoradiation for patients with unresected stage III nsclc: RTOG 9410 [Abstract]
Curran W et al (2000) Phase III comparison of sequential vs concurrent chemoradiation for patients with unresected stage III non-small cell lung cancer: initial report of Radiation Therapy Oncology Group 9410 (Abstr.). Proc Am Soc Clin Oncol 19:484a
Daisne JF et al (2004) Tumor volume in pharyngolaryngeal squamous cell carcinoma: comparison at CT, MR imaging, and FDG PET and validation with surgical specimen. Radiology 233(1):93–100
Danchaivijitr N et al (2008) Low-grade gliomas: do changes in rCBV measurements at longitudinal perfusion-weighted MR imaging predict malignant transformation? Radiology 247(1):170–178

De Ruysscher D et al (2005) Effects of radiotherapy planning with a dedicated combined PET-CT-simulator of patients with non-small cell lung cancer on dose limiting normal tissues and radiation dose-escalation: a planning study. Radiother Oncol 77(1):5–10
Dubois LJ et al (2011) Preclinical evaluation and validation of [18F]HX4, a promising hypoxia marker for PET imaging. Proc Natl Acad Sci U S A 108(35):14620–14625
Duprez F et al (2011) Adaptive dose painting by numbers for head-and-neck cancer. Int J Radiat Oncol Biol Phys 80(4):1045–1055
Edge SB, Compton CC (2010) The American Joint Committee on Cancer: the 7th edition of the AJCC cancer staging manual and the future of TNM. Ann Surg Oncol 17(6):1471–1474
Eisenhauer EA et al (2009) New response evaluation criteria in solid tumours: revised RECIST guideline (version 1.1). Eur J Cancer 45(2):228–247
El-Haddad G (2016) PET-based percutaneous needle biopsy. PET Clin 11(3):333–349
van Elmpt W et al (2012) The PET-boost randomised phase II dose-escalation trial in non-small cell lung cancer. Radiother Oncol 104(1):67–71
Eschmann SM et al (2005) Prognostic impact of hypoxia imaging with 18F-misonidazole PET in non-small cell lung cancer and head and neck cancer before radiotherapy. J Nucl Med 46(2):253–260
Essig M et al (2004) Perfusion MRI in CNS disease: current concepts. Neuroradiology 46(Suppl 2):s201–s207
Even AJ et al (2015) PET-based dose painting in non-small cell lung cancer: comparing uniform dose escalation with boosting hypoxic and metabolically active sub-volumes. Radiother Oncol 116(2):281–286
Everitt S et al (2009) Imaging cellular proliferation during chemo-radiotherapy: a pilot study of serial 18F-FLT positron emission tomography/computed tomography imaging for non-small-cell lung cancer. Int J Radiat Oncol Biol Phys 75(4):1098–1104
Everitt SJ et al (2014) Differential (18)F-FDG and (18) F-FLT uptake on serial PET/CT imaging before and during definitive chemoradiation for non-small cell lung cancer. J Nucl Med 55(7):1069–1074
Falchi L et al (2014) Correlation between FDG/PET, histology, characteristics, and survival in 332 patients with chronic lymphoid leukemia. Blood 123(18):2783–2790
Faries MB et al (2017) Completion dissection or observation for sentinel-node metastasis in melanoma. N Engl J Med 376(23):2211–2222
Fay M et al (2005) Dose-volume histogram analysis as predictor of radiation pneumonitis in primary lung cancer patients treated with radiotherapy. Int J Radiat Oncol Biol Phys 61(5):1355–1363
Feng M et al (2009) Using fluorodeoxyglucose positron emission tomography to assess tumor volume during radiotherapy for non-small-cell lung cancer and its potential impact on adaptive dose escalation and normal tissue sparing. Int J Radiat Oncol Biol Phys 73(4):1228–1234
Finkle JH et al (2017) Risk-stratifying capacity of PET/CT metabolic tumor volume in stage IIIA non-small cell lung cancer. Eur J Nucl Med Mol Imaging 44(8):1275–1284
Fournier LS et al (2010) Metastatic renal carcinoma: evaluation of antiangiogenic therapy with dynamic contrast-enhanced CT. Radiology 256(2):511–518
Fried DV et al (2014) Prognostic value and reproducibility of pretreatment CT texture features in stage III non-small cell lung cancer. Int J Radiat Oncol Biol Phys 90(4):834–842
Furuse K et al (1999) Phase III study of concurrent versus sequential thoracic radiotherapy in combination with mitomycin, vindesine, and cisplatin in unresectable stage III non-small-cell lung cancer. J Clin Oncol 17(9):2692–2699
Galldiks N et al (2012) Role of O-(2-(18)F-fluoroethyl)-L-tyrosine PET for differentiation of local recurrent brain metastasis from radiation necrosis. J Nucl Med 53(9):1367–1374
Ganeshan B et al (2012a) Tumour heterogeneity in non-small cell lung carcinoma assessed by CT texture analysis: a potential marker of survival. Eur Radiol 22(4):796–802
Ganeshan B et al (2012b) Tumour heterogeneity in oesophageal cancer assessed by CT texture analysis: preliminary evidence of an association with tumour metabolism, stage, and survival. Clin Radiol 67(2):157–164
Garcia-Figueiras R et al (2013) CT perfusion in oncologic imaging: a useful tool? AJR Am J Roentgenol 200(1):8–19
Gebhart G et al (2016) Imaging diagnostic and therapeutic targets: human epidermal growth factor receptor 2. J Nucl Med 57(Suppl 1):81s–88s
Geets X et al (2007) Adaptive biological image-guided IMRT with anatomic and functional imaging in pharyngo-laryngeal tumors: impact on target volume delineation and dose distribution using helical tomotherapy. Radiother Oncol 85(1):105–115
Geets X, Gregoire V, Lee JA (2013) Implementation of hypoxia PET imaging in radiation therapy planning. Q J Nucl Med Mol Imaging 57(3):271–282
Geurts N et al (2017) Prostate-specific membrane antigen radioguided surgery: a promising utility. BJU Int 120(1):5–6
Giles SL et al (2014) Whole-body diffusion-weighted MR imaging for assessment of treatment response in myeloma. Radiology 271(3):785–794
Haider MA et al (2017) CT texture analysis: a potential tool for prediction of survival in patients with metastatic clear cell carcinoma treated with sunitinib. Cancer Imaging 17(1):4
Hall EJ, Wuu CS (2003) Radiation-induced second cancers: the impact of 3D-CRT and IMRT. Int J Radiat Oncol Biol Phys 56(1):83–88
Hanahan D, Weinberg RA (2000) The hallmarks of cancer. Cell 100(1):57–70
Hanahan D, Weinberg RA (2011) Hallmarks of cancer: the next generation. Cell 144(5):646–674

Hatt M et al (2017) Characterization of PET/CT images using texture analysis: the past, the present... any future? Eur J Nucl Med Mol Imaging 44(1):151–165

Hayano K et al (2007) Perfusion CT can predict the response to chemoradiation therapy and survival in esophageal squamous cell carcinoma: initial clinical results. Oncol Rep 18(4):901–908

Henriques de Figueiredo B et al (2009) Comparison between CT- and FDG-PET-defined target volumes for radiotherapy planning in head-and-neck cancers. Radiother Oncol 93(3):479–482

Hentschel M et al (2009) Serial FDG-PET on patients with head and neck cancer: implications for radiation therapy. Int J Radiat Biol 85(9):796–804

Hermans R et al (2003) Tumor perfusion rate determined noninvasively by dynamic computed tomography predicts outcome in head-and-neck cancer after radiotherapy. Int J Radiat Oncol Biol Phys 57(5):1351–1356

Heron DE et al (2004) Hybrid PET-CT simulation for radiation treatment planning in head-and-neck cancers: a brief technical report. Int J Radiat Oncol Biol Phys 60(5):1419–1424

Hertz S, Roberts A (1946a) Radioactive iodine in the study of thyroid physiology; the use of radioactive iodine therapy in hyperthyroidism. J Am Med Assoc 131:81–86

Hertz S, Roberts A (1946b) Radioactive iodine in the study of thyroid physiology; the use of radioactive iodine therapy in Graves' disease. West J Surg Obstet Gynecol 54(12):474–486

Heukelom J et al (2013) Adaptive and innovative Radiation Treatment FOR improving Cancer treatment outcomE (ARTFORCE); a randomized controlled phase II trial for individualized treatment of head and neck cancer. BMC Cancer 13:84

Hicks RJ (2017) Learning from failure; hypoxia is an evil foe. J Nucl Med 58(7):1043–1044

Hicks RJ, Hofman MS (2012) Is there still a role for SPECT-CT in oncology in the PET-CT era? Nat Rev Clin Oncol 9(12):712–720

Ho AL et al (2013) Selumetinib-enhanced radioiodine uptake in advanced thyroid cancer. N Engl J Med 368(7):623–632

Hockel M et al (1993) Tumor oxygenation: a new predictive parameter in locally advanced cancer of the uterine cervix. Gynecol Oncol 51(2):141–149

Hoeben BA et al (2013) 18F-FLT PET during radiotherapy or chemoradiotherapy in head and neck squamous cell carcinoma is an early predictor of outcome. J Nucl Med 54(4):532–540

Hofman MS, Hicks RJ (2012) Changing paradigms with molecular imaging of neuroendocrine tumors. Discov Med 14(74):71–81

Hope TA et al (2017) 68Ga-PSMA-11 PET imaging of response to androgen receptor inhibition: first human experience. J Nucl Med 58(1):81–84

Horger M et al (2011) Whole-body diffusion-weighted MRI with apparent diffusion coefficient mapping for early response monitoring in multiple myeloma: preliminary results. AJR Am J Roentgenol 196(6):W790–W795

Hu LS et al (2009) Relative cerebral blood volume values to differentiate high-grade glioma recurrence from posttreatment radiation effect: direct correlation between image-guided tissue histopathology and localized dynamic susceptibility-weighted contrast-enhanced perfusion MR imaging measurements. AJNR Am J Neuroradiol 30(3):552–558

Ippolito D et al (2010) Hepatocellular carcinoma treated with transarterial chemoembolization: dynamic perfusion-CT in the assessment of residual tumor. World J Gastroenterol 16(47):5993–6000

Ippolito D et al (2013) Viable residual tumor tissue after radiofrequency ablation treatment in hepatocellular carcinoma: evaluation with CT perfusion. Abdom Imaging 38(3):502–510

Johnson P et al (2016) Adapted treatment guided by interim PET-CT scan in advanced Hodgkin's lymphoma. N Engl J Med 374(25):2419–2429

Joo Hyun O, Lodge MA, Wahl RL (2016) Practical PERCIST: a simplified guide to PET response criteria in solid tumors 1.0. Radiology 280(2):576–584

Jung SH et al (2012) Predicting response to neoadjuvant chemoradiation therapy in locally advanced rectal cancer: diffusion-weighted 3 Tesla MR imaging. J Magn Reson Imaging 35(1):110–116

Juweid ME et al (2007) Use of positron emission tomography for response assessment of lymphoma: consensus of the Imaging Subcommittee of International Harmonization Project in Lymphoma. J Clin Oncol 25(5):571–578

Kelly PJ et al (1987) Imaging-based stereotaxic serial biopsies in untreated intracranial glial neoplasms. J Neurosurg 66(6):865–874

Kim JJ, Tannock IF (2005) Repopulation of cancer cells during therapy: an important cause of treatment failure. Nat Rev Cancer 5(7):516–525

Kim YK et al (2012a) Diagnostic accuracy and sensitivity of diffusion-weighted and of gadoxetic acid-enhanced 3-T MR imaging alone or in combination in the detection of small liver metastasis (</=1.5 cm in diameter). Invest Radiol 47(3):159–166

Kim YN et al (2012b) Dual-energy CT in patients treated with anti-angiogenic agents for non-small cell lung cancer: new method of monitoring tumor response? Korean J Radiol 13(6):702–710

Klauss M et al (2013) Dual-energy perfusion-CT of pancreatic adenocarcinoma. Eur J Radiol 82(2):208–214

Knopp EA et al (1999) Glial neoplasms: dynamic contrast-enhanced T2*-weighted MR imaging. Radiology 211(3):791–798

Koh WJ et al (1992) Imaging of hypoxia in human tumors with [F-18]fluoromisonidazole. Int J Radiat Oncol Biol Phys 22(1):199–212

Koh DM et al (2012) Combining diffusion-weighted MRI with Gd-EOB-DTPA-enhanced MRI improves the detection of colorectal liver metastases. Br J Radiol 85(1015):980–989

Koh TS et al (2013) Primary colorectal cancer: use of kinetic modeling of dynamic contrast-enhanced CT data to predict clinical outcome. Radiology 267(1):145–154

Kong FM et al (2005) High-dose radiation improved local tumor control and overall survival in patients with inoperable/unresectable non-small-cell lung cancer: long-term results of a radiation dose escalation study. Int J Radiat Oncol Biol Phys 63(2):324–333

Krenning EP et al (1992) Somatostatin receptor scintigraphy with indium-111-DTPA-D-Phe-1-octreotide in man: metabolism, dosimetry and comparison with iodine-123-Tyr-3-octreotide. J Nucl Med 33(5):652–658

Krohn KA, Link JM, Mason RP (2008) Molecular imaging of hypoxia. J Nucl Med 49(Suppl 2):129S–148S

Kyle SD, Law WP, Miles KA (2013) Predicting tumour response. Cancer Imaging 13(3):381–390

Lapa C et al (2014) Comparison of the amino acid tracers 18F-FET and 18F-DOPA in high-grade glioma patients. J Nucl Med 55(10):1611–1616

Lapi SE, Voller TF, Welch MJ (2009) Positron emission tomography imaging of hypoxia. PET Clin 4(1):39–47

Lardinois D et al (2003) Staging of non-small-cell lung cancer with integrated positron-emission tomography and computed tomography. N Engl J Med 348(25):2500–2507

Law WP, Miles KA (2013) Incorporating prognostic imaging biomarkers into clinical practice. Cancer Imaging 13(3):332–341

Law M et al (2008) Gliomas: predicting time to progression or survival with cerebral blood volume measurements at dynamic susceptibility-weighted contrast-enhanced perfusion MR imaging. Radiology 247(2):490–498

Le Chevalier T et al (1994) Radiotherapy alone versus combined chemotherapy and radiotherapy in unresectable non-small cell lung carcinoma. Lung Cancer 10(Suppl 1):S239–S244

Le Moigne F et al (2012) Impact of diffusion-weighted MR imaging on the characterization of small hepatocellular carcinoma in the cirrhotic liver. Magn Reson Imaging 30(5):656–665

Lebech AM et al (2017) Whole-body 18F-FDG PET/CT is superior to CT as first-line diagnostic imaging in patients referred with serious nonspecific symptoms or signs of cancer: a randomized prospective study of 200 patients. J Nucl Med 58(7):1058–1064

LeBleu VS (2015) Imaging the tumor microenvironment. Cancer J 21(3):174–178

Lee NY et al (2008) Fluorine-18-labeled fluoromisonidazole positron emission and computed tomography-guided intensity-modulated radiotherapy for head and neck cancer: a feasibility study. Int J Radiat Oncol Biol Phys 70(1):2–13

Lee E et al (2017) Functional lung avoidance and response-adaptive escalation (FLARE) RT: multimodality plan dosimetry of a precision radiation oncology strategy. Med Phys 44(7):3418–3429

Liao GJ et al (2016) 18F-Fluoroestradiol PET: current status and potential future clinical applications. J Nucl Med 57(8):1269–1275

Lin C et al (2011) Whole-body diffusion-weighted imaging with apparent diffusion coefficient mapping for treatment response assessment in patients with diffuse large B-cell lymphoma: pilot study. Invest Radiol 46(5):341–349

Lind JS et al (2010) Dynamic contrast-enhanced CT in patients treated with sorafenib and erlotinib for non-small cell lung cancer: a new method of monitoring treatment? Eur Radiol 20(12):2890–2898

Liu Y et al (2007) Accuracy of computed tomography perfusion in assessing metastatic involvement of enlarged axillary lymph nodes in patients with breast cancer. Breast Cancer Res 9(4):R40

van Loon J et al (2010) PET imaging of hypoxia using [18F]HX4: a phase I trial. Eur J Nucl Med Mol Imaging 37(9):1663–1668

Lordick F et al (2007) PET to assess early metabolic response and to guide treatment of adenocarcinoma of the oesophagogastric junction: the MUNICON phase II trial. Lancet Oncol 8(9):797–805

Macura KJ et al (2006) Patterns of enhancement on breast MR images: interpretation and imaging pitfalls. Radiographics 26(6):1719–1734; quiz 1719

Madani I et al (2011) Maximum tolerated dose in a phase I trial on adaptive dose painting by numbers for head and neck cancer. Radiother Oncol 101(3):351–355

Mariani G et al (2003) Preoperative localization and radioguided parathyroid surgery. J Nucl Med 44(9):1443–1458

Martel MK et al (1999) Estimation of tumor control probability model parameters from 3-D dose distributions of non-small cell lung cancer patients. Lung Cancer 24(1):31–37

Martins EB et al (2015) Diffusion-weighted MRI in the assessment of early treatment response in patients with squamous-cell carcinoma of the head and neck: comparison with morphological and PET/CT findings. PLoS One 10(11):e0140009

Mathias CJ, Green MA (2008) A convenient route to [68Ga]Ga-MAA for use as a particulate PET perfusion tracer. Appl Radiat Isot 66(12):1910–1912

Maurer T et al (2017) PSMA-PET for lymph node detection in recurrent prostate cancer: how do we use the magic bullet? Theranostics 7(7):2046–2047

Mayer AT et al (2017) Practical immuno-PET radiotracer design considerations for human immune checkpoint imaging. J Nucl Med 58(4):538–546

Mayerhoefer ME et al (2015) Evaluation of diffusion-weighted magnetic resonance imaging for follow-up and treatment response assessment of lymphoma: results of an 18F-FDG-PET/CT-controlled prospective study in 64 patients. Clin Cancer Res 21(11):2506–2513

Mehanna H et al (2017) PET-NECK: a multicentre randomised Phase III non-inferiority trial comparing a positron emission tomography-computerised tomography-guided watch-and-wait policy with

planned neck dissection in the management of locally advanced (N2/N3) nodal metastases in patients with squamous cell head and neck cancer. Health Technol Assess 21(17):1–122
Meignan M et al (2016) Baseline metabolic tumor volume predicts outcome in high-tumor-burden follicular lymphoma: a pooled analysis of three multicenter studies. J Clin Oncol 34(30):3618–3626
Meredith G et al (2016) The use of 68 Ga-PSMA PET CT in men with biochemical recurrence after definitive treatment of acinar prostate cancer. BJU Int 118(Suppl 3):49–55
Meyer M et al (2013) CT-based response assessment of advanced gastrointestinal stromal tumor: dual energy CT provides a more predictive imaging biomarker of clinical benefit than RECIST or Choi criteria. Eur J Radiol 82(6):923–928
Moon M, Cornfeld D, Weinreb J (2009) Dynamic contrast-enhanced breast MR imaging. Magn Reson Imaging Clin N Am 17(2):351–362
Mortensen LS et al (2010) Identifying hypoxia in human tumors: a correlation study between 18F-FMISO PET and the Eppendorf oxygen-sensitive electrode. Acta Oncol 49(7):934–940
Muzi M et al (2005) Kinetic analysis of 3′-deoxy-3′-fluorothymidine PET studies: validation studies in patients with lung cancer. J Nucl Med 46(2):274–282
Ng CS et al (2011) Perfusion CT findings in patients with metastatic carcinoid tumors undergoing bevacizumab and interferon therapy. AJR Am J Roentgenol 196(3):569–576
Ng F et al (2013) Assessment of primary colorectal cancer heterogeneity by using whole-tumor texture analysis: contrast-enhanced CT texture as a biomarker of 5-year survival. Radiology 266(1):177–184
Nieweg OE, Uren RF, Thompson JF (2015) The history of sentinel lymph node biopsy. Cancer J 21(1):3–6
Nishioka T et al (2002) Image fusion between 18FDG-PET and MRI/CT for radiotherapy planning of oropharyngeal and nasopharyngeal carcinomas. Int J Radiat Oncol Biol Phys 53(4):1051–1057
Nordsmark M et al (2005) Prognostic value of tumor oxygenation in 397 head and neck tumors after primary radiation therapy. An international multi-center study. Radiother Oncol 77(1):18–24
Noy A et al (2009) The majority of transformed lymphomas have high standardized uptake values (SUVs) on positron emission tomography (PET) scanning similar to diffuse large B-cell lymphoma (DLBCL). Ann Oncol 20(3):508–512
Nunn A, Linder K, Strauss HW (1995) Nitroimidazoles and imaging hypoxia. Eur J Nucl Med 22(3):265–280
Ocak I et al (2007) Dynamic contrast-enhanced MRI of prostate cancer at 3T: a study of pharmacokinetic parameters. AJR Am J Roentgenol 189(4):849
Ogawa M et al (2012) Dual-energy CT can evaluate both hilar and mediastinal lymph nodes and lesion vascularity with a single scan at 60 seconds after contrast medium injection. Acad Radiol 19(8):1003–1010
Oh BC et al (2007) Stereotactic radiosurgery: adjacent tissue injury and response after high-dose single fraction radiation: Part I—Histology, imaging, and molecular events. Neurosurgery 60(1):31–44; discussion 44–45
Ohno Y et al (2012) Diffusion-weighted MRI versus 18F-FDG PET/CT: performance as predictors of tumor treatment response and patient survival in patients with non-small cell lung cancer receiving chemoradiotherapy. AJR Am J Roentgenol 198(1):75–82
Osborne JR et al (2013) Prostate-specific membrane antigen-based imaging. Urol Oncol 31(2):144–154
Padhani AR et al (2014) Therapy monitoring of skeletal metastases with whole-body diffusion MRI. J Magn Reson Imaging 39(5):1049–1078
Paesmans M et al (2010) Primary tumor standardized uptake value measured on fluorodeoxyglucose positron emission tomography is of prognostic value for survival in non-small cell lung cancer: update of a systematic review and meta-analysis by the European Lung Cancer Working Party for the International Association for the Study of Lung Cancer Staging Project. J Thorac Oncol 5(5):612–619
Pajonk F, Vlashi E, McBride WH (2010) Radiation resistance of cancer stem cells: the 4 R's of radiobiology revisited. Stem Cells 28(4):639–648
Pan L et al (2009) Prognostic significance of SUV on PET/CT in patients with esophageal cancer: a systematic review and meta-analysis. Eur J Gastroenterol Hepatol 21(9):1008–1015
Park MJ et al (2013) Validation of diagnostic criteria using gadoxetic acid-enhanced and diffusion-weighted MR imaging for small hepatocellular carcinoma (<=2.0 cm) in patients with hepatitis-induced liver cirrhosis. Acta Radiol 54(2):127–136
Pattison DA, Hofman MS (2015) Role of fluorodeoxyglucose PET/computed tomography in targeted radionuclide therapy for endocrine malignancies. PET Clin 10(4):461–476
Peeters SG et al (2015) A comparative study of the hypoxia PET tracers [(1)(8)F]HX4, [(1)(8)F]FAZA, and [(1)(8)F]FMISO in a preclinical tumor model. Int J Radiat Oncol Biol Phys 91(2):351–359
Perez CA et al (1980) A prospective randomized study of various irradiation doses and fractionation schedules in the treatment of inoperable non-oat-cell carcinoma of the lung. Preliminary report by the Radiation Therapy Oncology Group. Cancer 45(11):2744–2753
PI-RADS: Prostate Imaging—reporting and Data System version 2 (2015). http://www.acr.org/~/media/ACR/Documents/PDF/QualitySafety/Resources/PIRADS/PIRADSV2.pdf
Pryor DI et al (2013) Economic analysis of FDG-PET-guided management of the neck after primary chemoradiotherapy for node-positive head and neck squamous cell carcinoma. Head Neck 35(9):1287–1294
Radford J et al (2015) Results of a trial of PET-directed therapy for early-stage Hodgkin's lymphoma. N Engl J Med 372(17):1598–1607
Rajendran JG et al (2003) [(18)F]FMISO and [(18)F]FDG PET imaging in soft tissue sarcomas: correlation

of hypoxia, metabolism and VEGF expression. Eur J Nucl Med Mol Imaging 30(5):695–704

Rajendran JG et al (2004) Hypoxia and glucose metabolism in malignant tumors: evaluation by [18F] fluoromisonidazole and [18F]fluorodeoxyglucose positron emission tomography imaging. Clin Cancer Res 10(7):2245–2252

Rajendran JG et al (2006) Tumor hypoxia imaging with [F-18] fluoromisonidazole positron emission tomography in head and neck cancer. Clin Cancer Res 12(18):5435–5441

Rasey JS et al (2002) Validation of FLT uptake as a measure of thymidine kinase-1 activity in A549 carcinoma cells. J Nucl Med 43(9):1210–1217

Rauscher I et al (2016) Value of 68Ga-PSMA HBED-CC PET for the assessment of lymph node metastases in prostate cancer patients with biochemical recurrence: comparison with histopathology after salvage lymphadenectomy. J Nucl Med 57(11):1713–1719

Rengan R et al (2004) Improved local control with higher doses of radiation in large-volume stage III non-small-cell lung cancer. Int J Radiat Oncol Biol Phys 60(3):741–747

Rischin D et al (2006) Prognostic significance of [18F]-misonidazole positron emission tomography-detected tumor hypoxia in patients with advanced head and neck cancer randomly assigned to chemoradiation with or without tirapazamine: a substudy of Trans-Tasman Radiation Oncology Group Study 98.02. J Clin Oncol 24(13):2098–2104

Robbins RJ et al (2006) Real-time prognosis for metastatic thyroid carcinoma based on 2-[18F]fluoro-2-deoxy-D-glucose-positron emission tomography scanning. J Clin Endocrinol Metab 91(2):498–505

Rosenzweig KE et al (2005) Results of a phase I dose-escalation study using three-dimensional conformal radiotherapy in the treatment of inoperable nonsmall cell lung carcinoma. Cancer 103(10):2118–2127

Rothenberg SM et al (2015) Redifferentiation of iodine-refractory BRAF V600E-mutant metastatic papillary thyroid cancer with dabrafenib. Clin Cancer Res 21(5):1028–1035

Rymer B et al (2016) FDG PET/CT can assess the response of locally advanced rectal cancer to neoadjuvant chemoradiotherapy: evidence from meta-analysis and systematic review. Clin Nucl Med 41(5):371–375

Sahani DV et al (2005) Assessing tumor perfusion and treatment response in rectal cancer with multisection CT: initial observations. Radiology 234(3):785–792

Saunders M et al (1997) Continuous hyperfractionated accelerated radiotherapy (CHART) versus conventional radiotherapy in non-small-cell lung cancer: a randomised multicentre trial. CHART Steering Committee. Lancet 350(9072):161–165

Saunders M et al (1999) Continuous, hyperfractionated, accelerated radiotherapy (CHART) versus conventional radiotherapy in non-small cell lung cancer: mature data from the randomised multicentre trial. CHART Steering Committee. Radiother Oncol 52(2):137–148

Sause W et al (2000) Final results of phase III trial in regionally advanced unresectable non-small cell lung cancer: Radiation Therapy Oncology Group, Eastern Cooperative Oncology Group, and Southwest Oncology Group. Chest 117(2):358–364

Scarfone C et al (2004) Prospective feasibility trial of radiotherapy target definition for head and neck cancer using 3-dimensional PET and CT imaging. J Nucl Med 45(4):543–552

Schaake-Koning C et al (1992) Effects of concomitant cisplatin and radiotherapy on inoperable non-small-cell lung cancer. N Engl J Med 326(8):524–530

Scher HI et al (2016) Trial design and objectives for castration-resistant prostate cancer: updated recommendations from the Prostate Cancer Clinical Trials Working Group 3. J Clin Oncol 34(12):1402–1418

Schmid-Bindert G et al (2012) Functional imaging of lung cancer using dual energy CT: how does iodine related attenuation correlate with standardized uptake value of 18FDG-PET-CT? Eur Radiol 22(1):93–103

Seymour L et al (2017) iRECIST: guidelines for response criteria for use in trials testing immunotherapeutics. Lancet Oncol 18(3):e143–e152

Siva S et al (2016) Ga-68 MAA perfusion 4D-PET/CT scanning allows for functional lung avoidance using conformal radiation therapy planning. Technol Cancer Res Treat 15(1):114–121

Song I et al (2010) Assessment of response to radiotherapy for prostate cancer: value of diffusion-weighted MRI at 3 T. AJR Am J Roentgenol 194(6):W477–W482

Sonni I, Baratto L, Iagaru A (2017) Imaging of prostate cancer using Gallium-68-labeled Bombesin. PET Clin 12(2):159–171

Sridhar P et al (2014) FDG PET metabolic tumor volume segmentation and pathologic volume of primary human solid tumors. AJR Am J Roentgenol 202(5):1114–1119

Strosberg J et al (2017) Phase 3 trial of 177Lu-dotatate for midgut neuroendocrine tumors. N Engl J Med 376(2):125–135

Sugahara T et al (1998) Correlation of MR imaging-determined cerebral blood volume maps with histologic and angiographic determination of vascularity of gliomas. AJR Am J Roentgenol 171(6):1479–1486

Sun CH et al (2011) Quantitative assessment of perirectal tumor infiltration with dynamic contrast-enhanced multi-detector row CT in rectal cancer. Eur J Radiol 80(2):279–283

Tout M et al (2017) Rituximab exposure is influenced by baseline metabolic tumor volume and predicts outcome of DLBCL patients: a Lymphoma Study Association report. Blood 129(19):2616–2623

Trojanowska A et al (2012) Squamous cell cancer of hypopharynx and larynx - evaluation of metastatic nodal disease based on computed tomography perfusion studies. Eur J Radiol 81(5):1034–1039

Tsuji K et al (2015) Evaluation of staging and early response to chemotherapy with whole body diffusion-weighted MRI in malignant lymphoma patients:

a comparison with FDG-PET/CT. J Magn Reson Imaging 41(6):1601–1607
Upadhyay M et al (2013) The Warburg effect: insights from the past decade. Pharmacol Ther 137(3):318–330
Valdes Olmos RA et al (2014) Contribution of SPECT/CT imaging to radioguided sentinel lymph node biopsy in breast cancer, melanoma, and other solid cancers: from "open and see" to "see and open". Q J Nucl Med Mol Imaging 58(2):127–139
Valk PE, Bailey DL, Townsend DW, Maisey MN (2004) Positron emission tomography: basic science and clinical practice. Springer, New York
Vanderstraeten B, Duthoy W, De Gersem W, De Neve W, Thierens H (2006) [18F]fluoro-deoxy-glucose positron emission tomography ([18F]FDG-PET) voxel intensity-based intensity-modulated radiation therapy (IMRT) for head and neck cancer. Radiother Oncol 2006(79):249–258
van der Veldt AA et al (2010) Targeted therapies in renal cell cancer: recent developments in imaging. Target Oncol 5(2):95–112
Verma S et al (2012) Overview of dynamic contrast-enhanced MRI in prostate cancer diagnosis and management. AJR Am J Roentgenol 198(6):1277–1288
Vordermark D, Horsman MR (2016) Hypoxia as a biomarker and for personalized radiation oncology. Recent Results Cancer Res 198:123–142
Wahl RL et al (2009) From RECIST to PERCIST: evolving considerations for PET response criteria in solid tumors. J Nucl Med 50(Suppl 1):122s–150s
Wang D et al (2012) Functional and biologic metrics for predicting radiation pneumonitis in locally advanced non-small cell lung cancer patients treated with chemoradiotherapy. Clin Transl Oncol 14(12):943–952
Warburg O, Wind F, Negelein E (1927) The metabolism of tumors in the body. J Gen Physiol 8(6):519–530
Weiss GJ et al (2014) Noninvasive image texture analysis differentiates K-ras mutation from pan-wildtype NSCLC and is prognostic. PLoS One 9(7):e100244
Westphalen AC et al (2008) Peripheral zone prostate cancer: accuracy of different interpretative approaches with MR and MR spectroscopic imaging. Radiology 246(1):177–184
Win T et al (2013) Tumor heterogeneity and permeability as measured on the CT component of PET/CT predict survival in patients with non-small cell lung cancer. Clin Cancer Res 19(13):3591–3599
Wong AN et al (2017) The advantages and challenges of using FDG PET/CT for response assessment in melanoma in the era of targeted agents and immunotherapy. Eur J Nucl Med Mol Imaging 44(Suppl 1):67–77
Yamamoto Y et al (2007) Correlation of 18F-FLT and 18F-FDG uptake on PET with Ki-67 immunohistochemistry in non-small cell lung cancer. Eur J Nucl Med Mol Imaging 34(10):1610–1616
Yap CS et al (2006) Evaluation of thoracic tumors with 18F-fluorothymidine and 18F-fluorodeoxyglucose-positron emission tomography. Chest 129(2):393–401
Zegers CM et al (2013) Hypoxia imaging with [(1)(8)F] HX4 PET in NSCLC patients: defining optimal imaging parameters. Radiother Oncol 109(1):58–64
Zhao L, West BT, Hayman JA, Lyons S, Cease K, Kong FM (2007) High radiation dose may reduce the negative effect of large gross tumor volume in patients with medically inoperable early-stage non-small cell lung cancer. Int J Radiat Oncol Biol Phys 2007(68):103–110
Zhu AX et al (2008) Early antiangiogenic activity of bevacizumab evaluated by computed tomography perfusion scan in patients with advanced hepatocellular carcinoma. Oncologist 13(2):120–125

Imaging-Based Prediction Models

Luca Boldrini, Carlotta Masciocchi, and Lucia Leccisotti

Contents

1 **Introduction** 362

2 **Prediction Models: Classical Techniques and Machine Learning Approaches** 362
2.1 Classical Techniques 363
2.2 Machine Learning Techniques 364
2.3 Decision Trees 365

3 **Imaging in Oncology: From Qualitative to Quantitative Analysis** 368

4 **Imaging-Based Prediction Models: The Example of Rectal Cancer** 370
4.1 MRI-Based Prediction Models in Rectal Cancer 370
4.2 [18F]FDG PET-CT-Based Prediction Models in Rectal Cancer 371

5 **How to Create an Imaging-Based Predictive Model** 372
5.1 Source Population Selection 372
5.2 Definition of Outcomes 372
5.3 Model and Feature Selection 372
5.4 Internal Validation and Model Performance Evaluation 373
5.5 External Validation 373

6 **Future Directions and Conclusions** 373

References 374

L. Boldrini (✉)
Radiation Oncology Unit, Fondazione Policlinico Universitario "Agostino Gemelli" IRCCS, Rome, Italy

Knowledge Based Oncology (KBO) Laboratories—Fondazione Policlinico Universitario "Agostino Gemelli" IRCCS, Università Cattolica del Sacro Cuore, Rome, Italy

C. Masciocchi
Knowledge Based Oncology (KBO) Laboratories—Fondazione Policlinico Universitario "Agostino Gemelli" IRCCS, Università Cattolica del Sacro Cuore, Rome, Italy

L. Leccisotti
Nuclear Medicine Unit, Fondazione Policlinico Universitario "Agostino Gemelli", IRCCS, Rome, Italy

Abstract

The modern personalized medicine approaches in oncology deal with a huge and barely manageable number of patient-specific variables, from genetic data to simple blood tests, trying to ensure a fully individualized and tailored therapy.

In this context, the recent research trends towards imaging biomarkers, quantitative imaging analysis and radiomics applications have gained an ever-increasing interest, leading to the proposal of imaging-based predictors for clinical decision support systems (DSS).

The application of advanced machine learning solutions to manage always larger databases of patient imaging-derived variables is becoming increasingly necessary and opens

R. G. H. Beets-Tan et al. (eds.), *Imaging and Interventional Radiology for Radiation Oncology*, Medical Radiology, Diagnostic Imaging, https://doi.org/10.1007/978-3-030-38261-2_20

new frontiers in the field of clinical outcome prediction.

The different types of predictive modelling techniques, together with their strengths and pitfalls, are highlighted in this chapter which offers a brief overview about the state of the art as well as on the future developments of this fascinating topic.

1 Introduction

The modern personalized medicine approaches in oncology deal with a huge and barely manageable number of patient-specific variables from genetic data to simple blood tests to ensure a fully individualized and tailored therapy (Aerts et al. 2014).

In this context, the recent trends towards imaging biomarker research and quantitative preclinical and clinical imaging applications have gained an always greater interest.

The evolution of medical technology and the widespread availability of different imaging modalities, which characterized the last decades, opened new perspectives to the role of medical imaging in the management of cancer patients offering new unexplored sources of data (Yan et al. 2013).

An effective integration of these very heterogeneous imaging generated data in the clinical workflow of cancer patients' care represents therefore a new challenge in order to address the most appropriate therapeutic options and identify the optimal patient management from early diagnosis to multimodal therapy planning, passing through risk stratification and the evaluation of specific event probability.

Besides their ever-increasing clinical role, the applications of machine learning solutions capable to manage the enormous quantity of information offered by imaging data and their merging into decision support systems (DSS) appear to be paradigm shifting approaches also in the generation of a "new" type of medical evidence that enhances and integrates the "traditional" evidence-based oncology which mainly relies on guidelines obtained interlacing the results of randomized controlled trials (RCT) and comparing the observations of different studies that hardly take into account the huge variability of patients' characteristics (Valentini et al. 2013).

The elaboration of predictive models represents therefore one of the most promising applications of imaging data in modern oncology, offering clinicians a valuable decision support tool that showed a significant accuracy improvement in recent years (Kourou et al. 2015).

More specifically, imaging-based predictive models appear to be adequate solutions as images can be reliably and rapidly analysed through automated standardized computer-based techniques, thanks to the DICOM output format.

2 Prediction Models: Classical Techniques and Machine Learning Approaches

We can define a *prediction model* as a mathematical function $y = f(x)$ where y is the dependent variable called *outcome of the prediction task* and x are the independent variables called *predictors*.

The identification of the best achievable combination of these predictors, relative to a specific disease and/or treatment, in order to get an accurate and reliable prediction model for clinical purposes, represents one of the most interesting and challenging tasks for researchers and physicians active in the field of oncology.

Different approaches can be used for the development of oncologic prediction models.

We can distinguish them in "classical techniques", such as survival models, linear or logistic regression and "modern techniques" that fall within the machine learning techniques such as decision trees, support vector machines, Bayesian networks and artificial neural networks (Kotsiantis et al. 2007) (Table 1).

Table 1 Prediction model techniques

Machine learning techniques	Examples
Classical techniques	Survival models; linear regression; logistic regression
Modern techniques	Decision trees; support vector machines; Bayesian networks; artificial neural networks

2.1 Classical Techniques

The classical techniques more commonly used in clinical predictive model setup are represented by regression and survival models.

2.1.1 Regression Models

Regression models generate mathematical equations describing the statistical relation between predictors (x variable) and outcome (y variable): linear model and logistic regression represent classical examples of regression used in medicine for predictive model statistics.

The *linear model* is used in case of continuous outcome (e.g. the value of an oncologic marker).

The aim of the model training phase is to determine the straight line equation (obtaining its intercept and slope) that interpolates values of the predictors with the outcome, in order to be able to predict the value of the outcome with new predictor ones.

The parameter used to evaluate the goodness of fit of a linear model is the R-squared. It is a statistical measure, with possible values included in an interval which contains 0 and 1, that evaluates how much the distribution of the data can be represented by a straight line.

The more the value is near to 1, the more the relation between outcome and predictors can be described by a straight line.

In the *logistic regression model*, the outcome is binary (e.g. recurrence/nonrecurrence), and the probability of the considered outcome is estimated in relation to the predictor values.

Together with the Cox model, the logistic regression is the most widely used data analysis technique in medical sciences.

It is a very flexible model as categorical, numerical independent or interactive variables can be included as predictors.

From a graphical point of view, a logistic regression is represented by a sigmoid curve (see examples in Fig. 1): the more the sigmoid is flattened towards the horizontal straight, the less the model is able to discriminate between the positive outcome (i.e. recurrence) and negative one (no recurrence).

The metric used to evaluate the goodness of fit of a logistic model is represented by the Hosmer-Lemeshow test, which compares the value predicted by the model with the expected one.

2.1.2 Survival Models

Survival models are commonly used in the presence of a specific survival binary outcome,

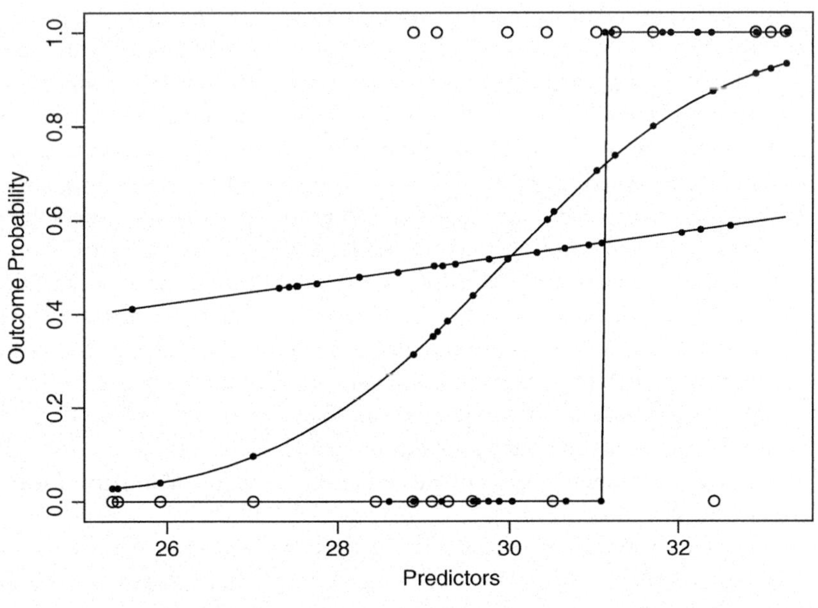

Fig. 1 Logistic regression plot examples

defined as "survival outcome", which is usually collected during the follow-up period of patients.

Some examples of survival outcomes could be alive versus dead, recurrence versus no recurrence and metastasis versus no metastasis.

The most used statistical approach in survival studies is the *Cox proportional hazard model*, which is very similar to the logistic regression, with the important difference that the intercept of linear model is used in the logistic model, while in the Cox one, a *hazard function* is used.

The hazard function is time dependent and identifies the hazard rate for the correspondent outcome.

The effect of the predictors in the Cox proportional hazard model appears to be constant and therefore time independent, or, more precisely, hazards are considered proportional. This aspect results to be an essential condition for the applicability of the Cox model, and it can be verified graphically or through the analysis of the Schoenfeld residuals.

2.1.3 Predictive Models' Performance Evaluation

After having obtained the desired predictive model, it is necessary to evaluate its capacity to discriminate different outcomes.

The most commonly used measure is the area under the receiver operating characteristic (ROC) curve (AUC) (or c-statistics in the case of binary outcome).

The ROC curve is a plot of the sensitivity (true positive rate) against 1-specificity (false-positive rate) for consecutive cutoffs for the probability of an outcome (Steyerberg 2008).

Other metrics, which in some cases appear to be more strict and therefore more reliable, can also be used, such as the confusion matrix and *F*-measure (or *F*-score).

The confusion matrix is specifically used in case of binary outcomes, where it is visualized as a 2 × 2 table (2 rows and 2 columns), in which each row represents the values of the predicted class and each column the ones of the actual class (or vice versa).

A simple example of a confusion matrix is reported in Table 2.

Table 2 Example of confusion matrix

		Real outcome	
Performance model for binary model		Real positive outcome	Real negative outcome
Predictive outcome	Predictive positive outcome	TP	FP
	Predictive negative outcome	FN	TN

The positive cases correctly predicted by the model (e.g. people suffering from the disease in exam correctly identified as ill) are defined as true positive (TP).

Actual negative cases predicted as positive (e.g. healthy people classified as ill by the model) are defined as false positive (FP).

On the other hand, positive cases predicted as negative by the model (e.g. ill people classified as healthy) are defined as false negative (FN), and, finally, actual healthy people correctly predicted as healthy by the model represent the true negative (TN) population.

Obtaining values other from zero along the diagonal line (TP-TN) and values equal to zero out of the diagonal (FP-FN) represents the best situation.

The F-measure is a score of the model's accuracy in which its *precision* and *recall* are evaluated.

The "precision" of the model is represented by the number of true positive (TP) cases divided by the number of all the positive cases (TP + FP); on the other hand, the ratio between the number of true positive (TP) cases and the total number of all the cases that should have been resulted as positive represents the recall.

Therefore, the F-measure results to be a harmonic mean of precision and recall and is a number between 0 and 1, with 1 as the best achievable value, indicating a perfect precision and recall of the considered model.

2.2 Machine Learning Techniques

Machine learning is a branch of artificial intelligence that employs a variety of statistical, probabilistic and optimization techniques that allow computers to "learn" from a large, complex and noisy dataset and to detect hard-to-discern patterns (Valentini et al. 2013).

In the last years, machine learning techniques have been applied with success to different oncologic imaging settings; to date, two main machine learning types can be distinguished: supervised and unsupervised (Wernick et al. 2010; Kourou et al. 2015).

In the supervised learning approach, training set labelled data are used to predict the probability of a specific outcome (in other words both x and y are known).

On the other hand, information about the outcome are not available for the unsupervised type of machine learning, and no data labelling procedures are used.

A combination of labelled and unlabelled datasets can also be used as a hybrid approach in a semi-supervised setting, mainly utilized when a majority of unlabelled data is available (Wernick et al. 2010; Kourou et al. 2015).

Several machine learning techniques, such as decision trees, support vector machines, Bayesian networks or artificial neural networks, are widely used to develop prediction models in cancer care (Kourou et al. 2015).

2.3 Decision Trees

Decision trees are a tree representation of a predictive model in which a principal starting node is given and each leaf can be reached through a branch from the originating node.

It is a supervised decisional algorithm which results particularly useful as a decision support tool as it is easily graphically representable (see an example in Fig. 2).

A Decision tree proposes an algorithm to take decisions, but does not give clear and direct information about causal dependence among the considered variables.

It is indeed possible, although uncommon, that one or more variables listed in the tree may have a role in the decision, even without having a causal role in reality.

2.3.1 Support Vector Machines

Support vector machines belong to the category of linear classifiers, also known as maximum margin classifiers, as they tend to minimize classification errors and maximize geometric margin.

The less complicated and more frequently used type of model is represented by support vector machines with linear kernel.

In this case, given a group of observations and a binary outcome, the model aims to identify a linear hyperplane able to distinguish the observations in two categories, minimizing misclassification errors and maximizing the distance among the observations at the borders of the identified hyperplane (see an example in Fig. 3).

2.3.2 Bayesian Networks

Bayesian networks are probabilistic graphic models based on the Bayes' theorem able to graphically represent a set of random variables and their direct dependences.

A Bayesian network is therefore composed of a qualitative part (defined *directed acyclic graph* or DAG) and a quantitative one (a set of conditional probabilities defined *joint probability distribution* or JPD).

The graph is represented by nodes, identifying predictors/outcome, and arrows which describe conditional dependences among variables, not always characterized by cause/effect relations.

The nodes and arrows of the network are translated into a set of conditional probabilities, and the final probability is then calculated as the product of the single conditional probabilities.

Both the qualitative and quantitative parts of the network can be totally or partially identified by an expert clinical domain, acquired through automatic learning techniques from the initial dataset with the support of bioinformatics tools or by means of hybrid approaches (expert domain + bioinformatics).

Bayesian networks are commonly used in medical sciences to develop predictive models (Lucas et al. 2004; Hu et al. 2016; Liu et al. 2011), especially by virtue of the accessible graphic representation that they can be produce.

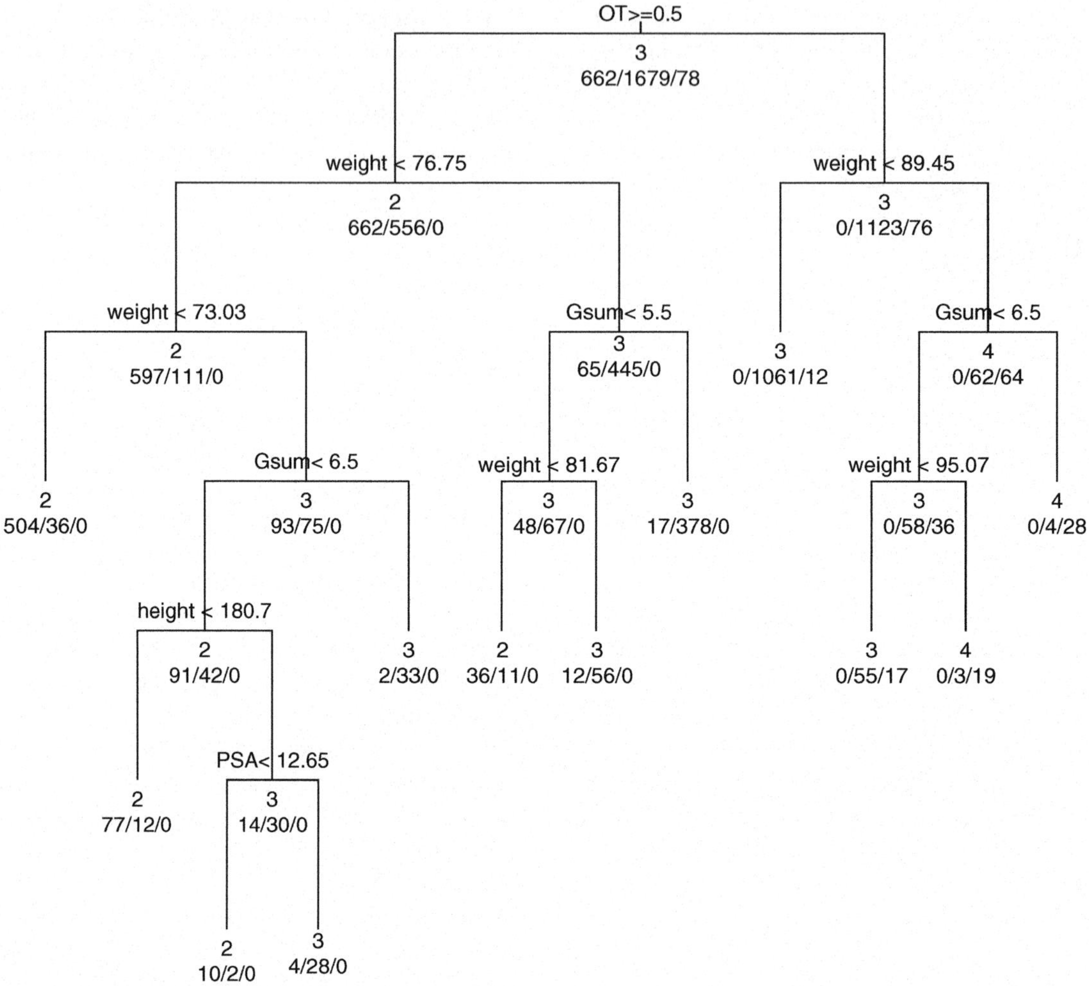

Fig. 2 An example of decision tree graph

This representation can indeed be easily interpreted and applied in clinical practice as a decisional support system.

The simplest example of Bayesian network is the *naive Bayes*, in which there is a node representing the outcome directly linked to the predictors, mutually independent.

For these reasons, the only arrows that can be identified in the graph are between the outcome and the predictors (e.g. the probability of the outcome event, knowing that the patient has a specific value of predictor "a" and predictor "b").

An example of DAG and JPD is reported in Fig. 4.

2.3.3 Artificial Neural Networks

Neural networks are a family of models that mimic the structure of the neural system learning patterns in relation to observations.

The simplest neural network is a binary classifier called *perceptron* (Rosenblatt 1958), characterized by an input and output single layer architecture.

Following more complex versions of this classifier leads to the inclusion of more output layers.

Nevertheless, this model is considered a linear one that can be applied for noncomplex data schemes. Part of these restrictions has been overcome by the introduction of a hidden layer between the input and output ones, which allows

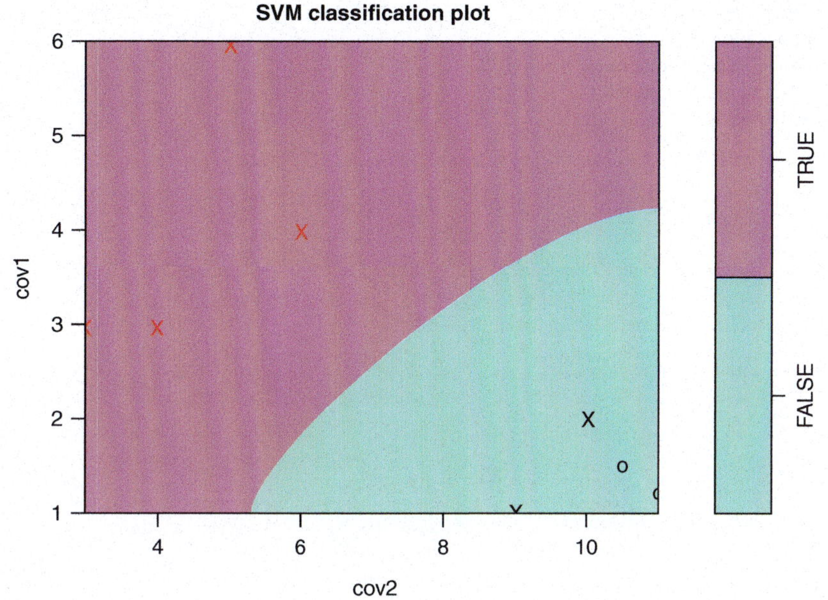

Fig. 3 Example of support vector machine with binary outcome (positive versus negative)

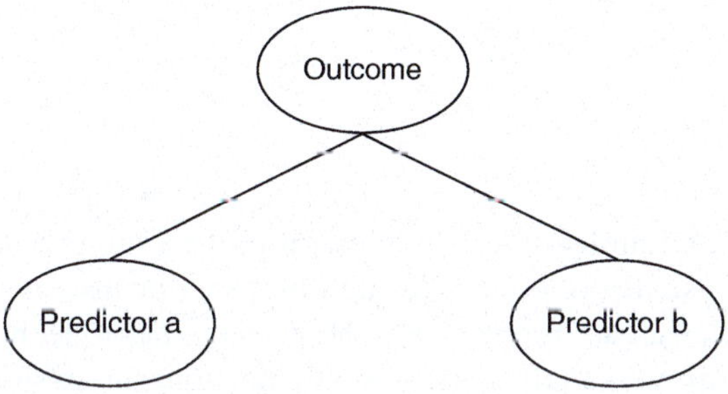

Fig. 4 Example of DAG and JPD. JPD: P (outcome, Predictor a, Predictor b) = P (Predictor a | Outcome) * P(Predictor b| outcome)

the management of complex data schemes: one of the more extensive applications of these models is related to oncologic diagnosis (Maclin et al. 1991).

Deep learning represents therefore an improvement of the classical artificial neural networks, as it allows to set up networks with multiple layers.

The most significant difference between this new technique and the neural networks is represented by the automatic generation of hidden neurons and layers without human interventions, an example of hierarchical feature representations in the learning process using only the available data.

Another advantage of this new approach is the possibility to extract advanced imaging features in order to classify and quantify specific patterns in terms of shape and tissue characteristics of the tumours (Fakoor et al. 2013).

Some examples of deep learning architectures are recurrent neural network (Ma et al. 2017), deep Boltzmann machine (Kim 2017) or deep network (Suresh et al. 2017).

Deep learning as a typical multilayer neural network technique can be distinguished in two main types: nonstructured and structured.

In the first case, the input results to be a simple mono-dimensional vector, while, in the second case, the data input structure is expressed in 2D or 3D.

This approach appears to be a very powerful bioinformatics tool, although it requires a huge number of data to be successfully implemented.

A new trend and interest in terms of investigations about medical imaging deep learning applications has been registered in the last few years (Shen et al. 2017).

Figure 5 shows the increase of such scientific production in the last 44 years (data from www.pubmed.com with search string "deep learning medical analysis").

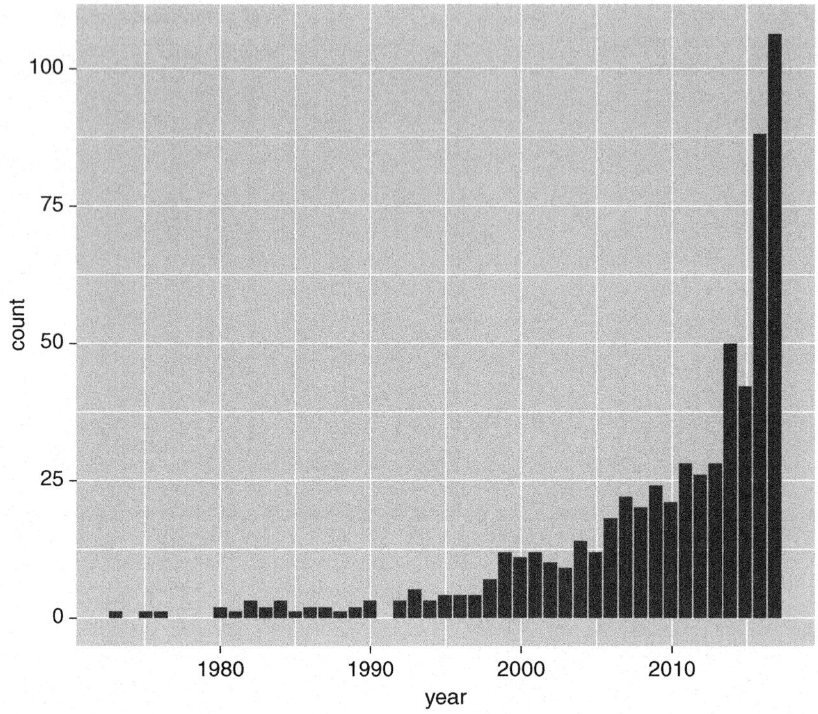

Fig. 5 Trend of publication number about deep learning in medical imaging in the last 44 years

3 Imaging in Oncology: From Qualitative to Quantitative Analysis

Prediction model techniques presented in the previous section can be successfully used for medical imaging applications, to reveal the multiform biology of tumours.

Tumours are biologically complex structures exhibiting spatial and temporal variations in gene expression, biochemistry, histopathology, macroscopic cell features and phenotypes, describing a high degree of intrinsic heterogeneity which represents a well-recognized hallmark of malignancy (O'Connor et al. 2015; Hanahan and Weinberg 2011).

Vogelstein et al. recently offered a valuable description of tumour heterogeneity identifying four different types of it: intratumoural (within the primary lesion), intermetastatic (between two secondary lesions), intrametastatic (within the same metastasis) and interpatient (among different individuals affected by the same disease) (Vogelstein et al. 2013).

In daily clinical practice, the phenotype and molecular characterization of a tumour is usually obtained through biopsies or invasive surgical procedures. However, these techniques analyse only small portions of tissue and are unable to offer a complete characterization of the tumour, especially considering the possibility of subregions and sampling errors.

Medical imaging can integrate these information allowing to extend the analysis to the whole lesion (primary, secondary or both) with good spatial resolution and with the great advantage, typical of non-invasive techniques, that can be easily repeated and can cover multiple tumour sites with high cost-effectiveness (Win et al. 2013; Castellano et al. 2004).

The features extracted from medical imaging (combined with clinical, genomics, molecular and other sources of data) assume therefore a fundamental role, especially when integrated into predictive models capable to take into account and quantify the spatial and temporal heterogeneity of tumours.

The concept of "tumour heterogeneity" assumes different meanings and specific aspects depending on the considered imaging modality.

In PET imaging, it is related to spatial distribution of radiopharmaceutical agents and could be referred to biological processes such as cellular metabolism, hypoxia or cellular proliferation (O'Connor et al. 2015).

Computed tomography (CT) imaging describes the heterogeneity as variability of tissue density, which can be caused by different vascularization and/or necrosis (Aerts et al. 2014), while on contrast-enhanced CT, it is related to spatial variability of microvascular density (Win et al. 2013).

Finally, on magnetic resonance imaging (MRI), tumour heterogeneity is defined as inhomogeneous signal for T2 sequences: high cellular density zones appear hyperintense and low signal areas are segments in which necrosis is more represented (Davnall et al. 2012).

For these reasons in the last few years, a growing number of publications proposed predictive models which combine clinical and treatment information with the features extracted from medical imaging obtained through different techniques and evaluated both through qualitative and quantitative approaches.

The classical qualitative approach is based on the morphological analysis of the image, and only simple findings related to tumour anatomy (e.g. location, dimensional measurements, shape and infiltrative involvement of adjacent organs, contrast enhancement) are being used as validated standards by radiologists.

To date, this approach still represents the standard practice of imaging reporting, and although qualitative measurements (as the size-based RECIST or WHO criteria) are used as imaging biomarkers (e.g. radiology-based TNM staging), a huge number of information remain unexpressed (O'Connor et al. 2015; Kumar et al. 2012).

The aforementioned "quantitative imaging" represents therefore a novel approach to take advantage of imaging data through the extraction of quantifiable features that will allow imaging data mining and to cross-link imaging findings with molecular and cellular tumour biology: recent experiences have demonstrated that quantitative analysis of the images showed better performances in terms of predictive power in comparison to molecular biomarkers, confirming the need of a further development of imaging-based prediction models (Joye et al. 2017).

Several commercial (Szczypiński et al. 2009; Fang et al. 2014; http://www.texrad.com), open and easy-accessible infrastructure software platforms (Dinapoli et al. 2015; Zhang et al. 2015; Deasy et al. 2003) have been developed for extracting quantitative information from the images and are currently available for researchers: the evaluation of imaging features as predictive and prognostic biomarkers will play an always greater role in the most modern personalized oncologic care (Gatenby et al. 2013).

A promising research field in quantitative imaging is represented by radiomics: an imaging analysis technique capable to detect pathological tumour characteristics not directly recognizable by a visual inspection (Aerts et al. 2014) through the extraction of large amounts of imaging quantitative features using dedicated automated or semiautomated software.

The main steps of radiomics workflow are image acquisition, segmentation of the volume of interest (tumour and/or organ at risk), feature extraction, feature selection and model development (Lambin et al. 2012).

Five main types of feature extraction can be distinguished: (a) morphological, (b) statistical, (c) texture, (d) regional and (e) model-based.

- Morphological features describe the physical characteristics of a region of interest in terms of shape and area, such as volume, surface area, surface to volume ratio, sphericity and compactness.
- Statistical features are composed of histogram-based features which describe the distribution of pixel values such as mean, median, entropy, skewness and kurtosis.
- Texture features are defined as spatial variation of pixel intensity such as grey-level co-occurrence matrices, grey-level run length-based features and grey-level size zone-based features.

- This type of features is very useful to describe intratumoural heterogeneity.
- Regional features capture the intensity variation between volumetric regions, defining how many subregions exist inside the considered volume (i.e. tumour) and how often they occur into it.
- Model-based features such as fractal models provide spatial information of the region of interest and characterize the intrinsic shape of the objects (Lee et al. 2017a, b).

Medical imaging represents therefore a fundamental source of information and data that can be extracted through qualitative, quantitative or radiomics approaches thanks to an adequate informatics technology which is always more integrated in the routine workflow of image analysis.

From early diagnosis and disease staging to follow-up, from response assessment to toxicity description, passing through radiotherapy imaging (e.g. daily positioning imaging), these approaches offer a great opportunity to improve and integrate prediction models in the management of cancer patients.

4 Imaging-Based Prediction Models: The Example of Rectal Cancer

The integration of imaging-based predictive models in clinical DSS is currently meeting great interest in different diseases.

Locally advanced rectal cancer (LARC) represents an important application and a good example of such approaches.

Rectal cancer treatment is characterized by the interaction of numerous different specialties, and in each step (from diagnosis to neoadjuvant treatment, to surgery and to the selection of adjuvant therapies), the contribution of imaging plays a key role in patients' management.

To date, the standard therapy for LARC is represented by preoperative chemoradiotherapy (CRT) with a significant increase of local control (7–10% of local recurrence rate) and less invasive surgical approaches (Valentini et al. 2011).

The prediction of outcomes, such as pathological complete responses (pCR) or overall survival (OS), could be of great advantage for multimodal treatment tailoring (including the crucial surgery versus watch and wait approach).

Together with clinical variables such as cTNM staging, carcinoembryonic antigen (CEA) level, distance from anal verge, CRM involvement, tumour differentiation and time to surgery, imaging techniques such as MRI and [^{18}F]FDG-PET could offer a correlation with response rate to preoperative CRT and play an important predictive role (Dinapoli et al. 2016; van Stiphout et al. 2011).

4.1 MRI-Based Prediction Models in Rectal Cancer

Several experiences proved MRI to be an effective prognostic and accurate local staging tool for LARC, as it offers an optimal visualization of primary lesions, circumferential resection margin (CRM) involvement (T staging) and nodal stage description (N staging) (Bradley 1997; Collins et al. 2015).

Thanks to these characteristics, several MRI-based prediction models have been prosed for rectal cancer.

Literature analysis shows that, in most cases, these models have tumour response after neoadjuvant chemoradiotherapy as primary outcome (How et al. 2012; Thor et al. 2013; Meng et al. 2014; Intven et al. 2015a, b; Liu et al. 2016a, b; Ogawa et al. 2017; Bakke et al. 2017; Hsu et al. 2017; Liu et al. 2016a, b; Shin et al. 2016; Moon et al. 2016; De Cecco et al. 2015; Denecke et al. 2005; Doi et al. 2015; Jacobs et al. 2016; Joye et al. 2014, 2017; Kim et al. 2016; Konski et al. 2009; Martens et al. 2015; Pham et al. 2017a, b; Seierstad et al. 2015; Tsai et al. 2017; Beets-Tan and Beets 2014; Genovesi et al. 2013; Elmi et al. 2013; Lee et al. 2014; Ishibe et al. 2016; Dang et al. 2015; Bhooshan et al. 2011), while only one experience considers also survival (Bakke et al. 2017).

Other models consider also different outcomes, such as nodal involvement (Ishibe et al.

2016; Ogawa et al. 2017), presence of synchronous distant metastases (Liu et al. 2016a, b), disease recurrence (Moon et al. 2016) or molecular characterization prediction (Shin et al. 2016).

Unfortunately, the large majority of these studies use limited patient samples (hardly more than 100 and in some cases also less than 20) (De Cecco et al. 2015; Beppu et al. 2015).

Furthermore, to our knowledge, only one case of MRI-based model internal validation has been provided on a sample of 61 patients who underwent DCE-MRI for rectal cancer response assessment (Intven et al. 2015a, b), while no external validation sets have ever been used for this disease.

These characteristics strongly limit the statistical significance of such models and their potentiality to successfully integrate them as DSS in daily practice, exploiting their knowledge contribution.

4.2 [^{18}F]FDG PET-CT-Based Prediction Models in Rectal Cancer

Over the last years, several studies suggested that PET-CT imaging with [^{18}F]FDG might be correlated with tumour response after CRT in LARC patients (Li et al. 2014; Ferrari et al. 2017). However, as seen also for MRI, most of these studies included a small sample size with the main focus on good versus bad responders (not pCR) and used univariate statistics (Amthauer et al. 2004; Goldberg et al. 2012; Lambrecht et al. 2010; Denecke et al. 2005; Hatt et al. 2013; Everaert et al. 2011; Janssen et al. 2010). Multivariate analysis has been performed in a limited number of studies, whose results lacked sometimes statistical significance (Kim et al. 2013; Leccisotti et al. 2015).

In addition, only very few studies verified and validated their results with external datasets, despite this is an important prerequisite for considering a predictive model able to guide preoperative therapy choices.

First, van Stiphout et al. collected population-based data from 953 patients from 4 different institutes and used them to train and validate predictive models for pCR, showing that the addition of PET imaging data to clinical variables significantly increases the performance of prediction models for pCR after CRT as compared to models based exclusively on clinical data (van Stiphout et al. 2011).

The study was carried out using support vector machine learning methods and nomograms allowing the users to easily calculate the overall probability of the specific clinical outcome for an individual patient. The best model achieved included tumour length, post-CRT tumour SUVmax and relative changes of tumour SUVmax.

Later, a multivariate nomogram with clinical parameters and early sequential PET-CT imaging markers for predicting pCR in LARC patients was developed by van Stiphout et al., based on a large prospective study (N = 112) and validated prospectively with another institute (N = 78) (van Stiphout et al. 2014). The predictive features selected for the model were clinical T and N status, response index of tumour SUVmean and the maximal tumour diameter during treatment. Three groups were identified as low, medium and high probability of pCR. The high probability group resulted in 100% correct prediction for training (area under the curve of ROC 0.78) and 67% for validation (AUC of ROC 0.70).

The model, available on the web (www.predictcancer.org), can be used to assist in treatment decisions during CRT to select complete responders for a wait and see policy, good responders for extra radiotherapy boost and bad responders for additional chemotherapy.

A meta-analysis from 2014 confirmed the added value of PET imaging during CRT (Li et al. 2014).

This time point is more favourable than post-CRT imaging because of the possibility to detect earlier treatment changes of tumour and the decreased probability of peritumoural inflammatory effects that could obscure the metabolic treatment response of the tumour.

However, the variability of PET parameters so far investigated (e.g. SUVmax, SUVmean, delta-SUVmax, response index, visual response assessment, metabolic tumour volume, total lesion glycolysis, etc.), the limit of PET-CT in determining local nodal status as well as the difficulty in detecting residual microscopic disease or distinguishing inflammation from residual disease lead researchers to develop more complex and robust modelling to predict pCR in LARC patients combining several clinicopathological and molecular markers with CT, PET as well as MRI markers.

5 How to Create an Imaging-Based Predictive Model

The creation of a predictive model should rely on a data collection system for the setup of reliable large databases: technical notes and shared guidelines for image acquisition and processing are therefore strongly encouraged, to assure image homogeneity and comparability, especially in case of multicentric studies.

Data collection standardization process benefits from the definition of a "ontology", formally representing knowledge as a group of concepts within a domain and their relations, describing the variables that clinicians choose to collect, without knowing a priori their predictive power (Meldolesi et al. 2014; Tagliaferri et al. 2016).

As previously described for MRI and PET-CT applications in rectal cancer, a huge amount of imaging-based predictive models has recently been published, but there is still poor integration of such models into clinical practice, as the large majority of them lacks of external validation and is realized on small patient samples which limit their statistical power and the possibility to integrate them in clinically reliable DSS.

One of the major issues about the routine implementation of imaging-based prediction models is the need to proceed with a statistically reliable external validation in order to assess the "reproducibility" and "transferability" of the developed model (Soest et al. 2017).

A model is defined as "reproducible" if it has been tested on different validation sets of patients presenting small differences with respect to the training set cohort (i.e. very similar populations); on the other hand, the "transferability" of the model defines the possibility to test it on an independent and very different validation cohort of patients (e.g. a model having adult population as training set then validated on paediatric population).

The TRIPOD statement offers a framework for reporting, developing and validating prediction models that can be effectively extended to imaging-based models (Collins et al. 2015).

The steps necessary to set up a predictive model depend from its expected degree of reproducibility and transferability,and the development of a predictive model can be divided into five phases: (a) source population selection, (b) definition of outcomes, (c) model and feature selection, (d) internal validation and (e) external validation.

5.1 Source Population Selection

Three types of predictive models could be distinguished with regard to the source population selection: single centre, multiple centres and population-based cohort models.

The source population selection step together with the protocol of image acquisition and processing becomes crucial in the assessment of the reproducibility and transferability of the model when qualitative and quantitative image-derived information are considered.

5.2 Definition of Outcomes

Having selected the source population and the a priori inclusion/exclusion criteria, a precise definition of the primary and not primary prediction outcomes is needed.

The prediction model that will be developed will be able to predict the probability of that specific outcome (e.g. tumour response, survival or disease recurrence).

5.3 Model and Feature Selection

The next step is represented by statistical model selection using both classical statistical models and machine learning tools.

It is recommended to always split the data in two sets: a training dataset and an internal validation one, independently to the chosen statistical model and selected outcome.

The selection of the features to be included in the final model can be based both on the statistical significance of the univariate analysis of the dataset's covariates (univariate model and/or Kaplan-Meier analysis) and on automatic methods (Popescu and Sasu 2014).

The predictive model "learns" on the training set and is then internally tested on the validation one.

5.4 Internal Validation and Model Performance Evaluation

Internal validation appears to be subject to overoptimistic evaluation of model performances, defined as "overfitting": some statistical techniques such as bootstrap and cross-validation approaches are available to manage this circumstance.

In bootstrap internal validation, data are trained on a set of *N* data examples obtained by random sampling with replacement from the entire dataset of *N* (Wernick et al. 2010).

On the other hand, in leave-one-out and tenfold cross-validation, data are split randomly into groups. In the first type, the model is tested using the whole population while leaving one case out for the validation process and the mechanism is repeated *k* times, each time leaving out one different patient.

In the second approach, the dataset is divided into ten folders. The model is generated using data of nine folders and the predictions are tested on the remaining one. This process is then reiterated ten times, each time leaving out a different one folder.

At the end of both approaches, an average of the model performance is then calculated.

Model performance can be assessed in terms of discrimination (the ability of the model to separate patients with different outcomes) using area under the ROC curve (AUC) or C-statistics and calibration (how the prediction outcomes are far from the actual outcomes) using a graphic or statistical test (e.g. Hosmer-Lemeshow test for logistic regression model).

The internal validation step enables the model to reach a TRIPOD 2b level in which reproducibility of the model is not guaranteed and its transferability is not even mentioned.

5.5 External Validation

External validation is the last essential step to allow the use of a prediction model as clinical decision-making tool, encouraging its generalizability.

Outcome predictions are performed for each patient of the external validation dataset using the original model and then compared with the internally observed outcomes in order to evaluate the final performance of the model.

The external dataset can have various testing characteristics: temporal or prospective validation (data are collected by the same investigator but sampled later on), geographic validation (data are collected by several investigators in different institutions or countries) and independent validation (the inclusion criteria of the dataset used for model development are not respected).

In case of poor performance, the model can be updated on the new validation dataset, maintaining its operability in time and space (Moons et al. 2012).

A predictive model validated with these procedures can reach TRIPOD level 4, in which data transferability is possible and model application is successfully repeatable, allowing an effective integration of predictive model in routine practice as part of clinical decision support systems (Collins et al. 2015).

6 Future Directions and Conclusions

The development of new imaging biomarkers represents a promising aspect in the future of personalized oncologic treatments, although they require an external validation and should be correlated with other patient characteristics (clinical, geographical, pathological information) to take full advantage of their potentialities.

Modern imaging applications (such as quantitative imaging or radiomics) and the latest hybrid technologies (PET-MRI or MRI-radiotherapy) will increase the imaging data available for each patient during the different moments of clinical management.

In this frame and towards an always more precise medicine, a next step is represented by imaging genomics which refers to the relationship between imaging tumour characteristics, gene expression patterns, gene mutations and other genome-related characteristics (Lee et al. 2017a, b).

As previously mentioned, the always increasing number of patient variables, together with the application of advanced machine learning techniques, will require a massive number of patients organized in well-structured large databases.

Data sharing among different centres will be mandatory, and different problems will have to be faced on the technical, motivational, political and privacy preservation sides (Roelofs et al. 2014; van Panhuis et al. 2014).

For this reason, the development of privacy-preserving algorithms is strongly encouraged and could represent a valuable tool for medical sciences, allowing the training and validation steps of predictive models without explicit data exchange across the different involved institutions, using a distributed learning architecture (Damiani et al. 2015; Jochems et al. 2016).

The use of the abovementioned technologies and their further development will allow to obtain large databases, spread all over the world, facilitating the application of rapid learning approaches (Lambin et al. 2013) and the setup of predictive models with their effective integration in daily clinical practice.

References

Aerts HJWL, Velazquez ER, Leijenaar RT, Parmar C, Grossmann P, Cavalho S, Hoebers F (2014) Decoding tumour phenotype by noninvasive imaging using a quantitative radiomics approach. Nat Commun 5(4006):1–8

Amthauer H, Denecke T, Rau B, Hildebrandt B, Hünerbein M, Ruf J, Wust P (2004) Response prediction by FDG-PET after neoadjuvant radiochemotherapy and combined regional hyperthermia of rectal cancer: correlation with endorectal ultrasound and histopathology. Eur J Nucl Med Mol Imaging 31(6):811–819

Bakke KM, Hole KH, Dueland S, Grøholt KK, Flatmark K, Ree AH, Redalen KR (2017) Diffusion-weighted magnetic resonance imaging of rectal cancer: tumour volume and perfusion fraction predict chemoradiotherapy response and survival. Acta Oncol 56(6):813–818

Beets-Tan RG, Beets GL (2014) MRI for assessing and predicting response to neoadjuvant treatment in rectal cancer. Nat Rev Gastroenterol Hepatol 11(8):480–488

Beppu N, Kato T, Noda M, Yanagi H, Tomita N, Kamikonya N, Hirota S (2015) Diffusion-weighted magnetic resonance imaging for prediction of tumor response to neoadjuvant chemoradiotherapy using irinotecan plus S-1 for rectal cancer. Mol Clin Oncol 3(5):1129–1134

Bhooshan N, Giger M, Edwards D, Yuan Y, Jansen S, Li H, Newstead G (2011) Computerized three-class classification of MRI-based prognostic markers for breast cancer. Phys Med Biol 56(18):5995

Bradley AP (1997) The use of the area under the ROC curve in the evaluation of machine learning algorithms. Pattern Recogn 30(7):1145–1159

Castellano G, Bonilha L, Li LM, Cendes F (2004) Texture analysis of medical images. Clin Radiol 59(12):1061–1069

Collins GS, Reitsma JB, Altman DG, Moons KG (2015) Transparent reporting of a multivariable prediction model for individual prognosis or diagnosis (TRIPOD): the TRIPOD statement. BMC Med 13(1):1

Damiani A, Vallati M, Gatta R, Dinapoli N, Jochems A, Deist T, Valentini V (2015) Distributed learning to protect privacy in multi-centric clinical studies. In: Conference on artificial intelligence in medicine in Europe. Springer, Cham, pp 65–75

Dang M, Lysack JT, Wu T, Matthews TW, Chandarana SP, Brockton NT, Dort JC (2015) MRI texture analysis predicts p53 status in head and neck squamous cell carcinoma. Am J Neuroradiol 36(1):166–170

Davnall F, Yip CS, Ljungqvist G, Selmi M, Ng F, Sanghera B, Goh V (2012) Assessment of tumor heterogeneity: an emerging imaging tool for clinical practice? Insights Imaging 3(6):573–589

De Cecco CN, Ganeshan B, Ciolina M, Rengo M, Meinel FG, Musio D, Laghi A (2015) Texture analysis as imaging biomarker of tumoral response to neoadjuvant chemoradiotherapy in rectal cancer patients studied with 3-T magnetic resonance. Investig Radiol 50(4):239–245

Deasy JO, Blanco AI, Clark VH (2003) CERR: a computational environment for radiotherapy research. Med Phys 30(5):979–985

Denecke T, Rau B, Hoffmann KT, Hildebrandt B, Ruf J, Gutberlet M, Amthauer H (2005) Comparison of CT, MRI and FDG-PET in response prediction of patients with locally advanced rectal cancer after multimodal

preoperative therapy: is there a benefit in using functional imaging? Eur Radiol 15(8):1658–1666
Dinapoli N, Alitto AR, Vallati M, Gatta R, Autorino R, Boldrini L, Valentini V (2015) Moddicom: a complete and easily accessible library for prognostic evaluations relying on image features. In: Engineering in Medicine and Biology Society (EMBC), 2015 37th annual international conference of the IEEE. IEEE, pp 771–774
Dinapoli N, Casà C, Barbaro B, Chiloiro GV, Damiani A, Matteo MD, Masciocchi C, Valentini V (2016) Radiomics for rectal cancer. Transl Cancer Res 5(4):424–431
Doi H, Beppu N, Kato T, Noda M, Yanagi H, Tomita N, Hirota S (2015) Diffusion-weighted magnetic resonance imaging for prediction of tumor response to neoadjuvant chemoradiotherapy using irinotecan plus S-1 for rectal cancer. Mol Clin Oncol 3(5):1129–1134
Elmi A, Hedgire SS, Covarrubias D, Abtahi SM, Hahn PF, Harisinghani M (2013) Apparent diffusion coefficient as a non-invasive predictor of treatment response and recurrence in locally advanced rectal cancer. Clin Radiol 68(10):e524–e531
Everaert H, Hoorens A, Vanhove C, Sermeus A, Ceulemans G, Engels B, De Ridder M (2011) Prediction of response to neoadjuvant radiotherapy in patients with locally advanced rectal cancer by means of sequential 18FDG-PET. Int J Radiat Oncol Biol Phys 80(1):91–96
Fakoor R, Ladhak F, Nazi A, Huber M (2013) Using deep learning to enhance cancer diagnosis and classification. In: Proceedings of the international conference on machine learning
Fang YHD, Lin CY, Shih MJ, Wang HM, Ho TY, Liao CT, Yen TC (2014) Development and evaluation of an open-source software package "CGITA" for quantifying tumor heterogeneity with molecular images. Biomed Res Int 2014:1
Ferrari M, Travaini LL, Ciardo D, Garibaldi C, Gilardi L, Glynne-Jones R, Leonardi MC (2017) Interim 18FDG PET/CT during radiochemotherapy in the management of pelvic malignancies: a systematic review. Crit Rev Oncol Hematol 113:28–42
Gatenby RA, Grove O, Gillies RJ (2013) Quantitative imaging in cancer evolution and ecology. Radiology 269(1):8–14
Genovesi D, Filippone A, Cefaro GA, Trignani M, Vinciguerra A, Augurio A, Liberatore E (2013) Diffusion-weighted magnetic resonance for prediction of response after neoadjuvant chemoradiation therapy for locally advanced rectal cancer: preliminary results of a monoinstitutional prospective study. Eur J Surg Oncol (EJSO) 39(10):1071–1078
Goldberg N, Kundel Y, Purim O, Bernstine H, Gordon N, Morgenstern S, Brenner B (2012) Early prediction of histopathological response of rectal tumors after one week of preoperative radiochemotherapy using 18 F-FDG PET-CT imaging. A prospective clinical study. Radiat Oncol 7(1):124
Hanahan D, Weinberg RA (2011) Hallmarks of cancer: the next generation. Cell 144(5):646–674
Hatt M, Van Stiphout R, Le Pogam A, Lammering G, Visvikis D, Lambin P (2013) Early prediction of pathological response in locally advanced rectal cancer based on sequential 18F-FDG PET. Acta Oncol 52(3):619–626
How P, Evans J, Moran B, Swift I, Brown G (2012) Preoperative MRI sphincter morphology and anal manometry: can they be markers of functional outcome following anterior resection for rectal cancer? Color Dis 14(6):e339
Hsu CY, Wang CW, Kuo CC, Chen YH, Lan KH, Cheng AL, Kuo SH (2017) Tumor compactness improves the preoperative volumetry-based prediction of the pathological complete response of rectal cancer after preoperative concurrent chemoradiotherapy. Oncotarget 8(5):7921
Hu J, Wu W, Zhu B, Wang H, Liu R, Zhang X, Tian C (2016) Cerebral glioma grading using Bayesian network with features extracted from multiple modalities of magnetic resonance imaging. PLoS One 11(4):e0153369
Intven M, Monninkhof EM, Reerink O, Philippens ME (2015a) Combined T2w volumetry, DW-MRI and DCE-MRI for response assessment after neo-adjuvant chemoradiation in locally advanced rectal cancer. Acta Oncol 54(10):1729–1736
Intven M, Reerink O, Philippens ME (2015b) Dynamic contrast enhanced MR imaging for rectal cancer response assessment after neo-adjuvant chemoradiation. J Magn Reson Imaging 41(6):1646–1653
Ishibe A, Ota M, Watanabe J, Suwa Y, Suzuki S, Kanazawa A, Endo I (2016) Prediction of lateral pelvic lymph-node metastasis in low rectal cancer by magnetic resonance imaging. World J Surg 40(4):995–1001
Jacobs L, Intven M, Van Lelyveld N, Philippens M, Burbach M, Seldenrijk K, Reerink O (2016) Diffusion-weighted MRI for early prediction of treatment response on preoperative chemoradiotherapy for patients with locally advanced rectal cancer: a feasibility study. Ann Surg 263(3):522–528
Janssen MH, Öllers MC, Riedl RG, van den Bogaard J, Buijsen J, van Stiphout RG, Lammering G (2010) Accurate prediction of pathological rectal tumor response after two weeks of preoperative radiochemotherapy using 18 F-fluorodeoxyglucose-positron emission tomography-computed tomography imaging. Int J Radiat Oncol Biol Phys 77(2):392–399
Jochems A, Deist TM, Van Soest J, Eble M, Bulens P, Coucke P, Dekker A (2016) Distributed learning: developing a predictive model based on data from multiple hospitals without data leaving the hospital—a real life proof of concept. Radiother Oncol 121(3):459–467
Joye I, Deroose CM, Vandecaveye V, Haustermans K (2014) The role of diffusion-weighted MRI and 18 F-FDG PET/CT in the prediction of pathologic complete response after radiochemotherapy for rectal cancer: a systematic review. Radiother Oncol 113(2):158–165

Joye I, Debucquoy A, Deroose CM, Vandecaveye V, Van Cutsem E, Wolthuis A, Haustermans K (2017) Quantitative imaging outperforms molecular markers when predicting response to chemoradiotherapy for rectal cancer. Radiother Oncol 124(1):104–109

Kim JW, Kim HC, Park JW, Park SC, Sohn DK, Choi HS, Kim SK (2013) Predictive value of 18FDG PET-CT for tumour response in patients with locally advanced rectal cancer treated by preoperative chemoradiotherapy. Int J Color Dis 28(9):1217–1224

Kim JG, Song KD, Kim SH, Kim HC, Huh JW (2016) Diagnostic performance of MRI for prediction of candidates for local excision of rectal cancer (ypT0-1N0) after neoadjuvant chemoradiation therapy. J Magn Reson Imaging 44(2):471–477

Kim HG, Han SH, Choi HJ (2017) Discriminative restricted Boltzmann machine for emergency detection on healthcare robot. In: 2017 IEEE international conference on Big data and smart computing (BigComp). IEEE, pp 407–409

Konski A, Li T, Sigurdson E, Cohen SJ, Small W, Spies S, Meropol NJ (2009) Use of molecular imaging to predict clinical outcome in patients with rectal cancer after preoperative chemotherapy and radiation. Int J Radiat Oncol Biol Phys 74(1):55–59

Kotsiantis SB, Zaharakis I, Pintelas P. 2007. Supervised machine learning: a review of classification techniques

Kourou K, Exarchos TP, Exarchos KP, Karamouzis MV, Fotiadis DI (2015) Machine learning applications in cancer prognosis and prediction. Comput Struct Biotechnol J 13:8–17

Kumar V, Gu Y, Basu S, Berglund A, Eschrich SA, Schabath MB, Goldgof DB (2012) Radiomics: the process and the challenges. Magn Reson Imaging 30(9):1234–1248

Lambin P, Rios-Velazquez E, Leijenaar R, Carvalho S, van Stiphout RG, Granton P, Aerts HJ (2012) Radiomics: extracting more information from medical images using advanced feature analysis. Eur J Cancer 48(4):441–446

Lambin P, Roelofs E, Reymen B, Velazquez ER, Buijsen J, Zegers CM, Marshall MS (2013) Rapid learning health care in oncology'—an approach towards decision support systems enabling customised radiotherapy. Radiother Oncol 109(1):159–164

Lambrecht M, Deroose C, Roels S, Vandecaveye V, Penninckx F, Sagaert X, Haustermans K (2010) The use of FDG-PET/CT and diffusion-weighted magnetic resonance imaging for response prediction before, during and after preoperative chemoradiotherapy for rectal cancer. Acta Oncol 49(7):956–963

Leccisotti L, Gambacorta MA, de Waure C, Stefanelli A, Barbaro B, Vecchio FM, Giordano A (2015) The predictive value of 18F-FDG PET/CT for assessing pathological response and survival in locally advanced rectal cancer after neoadjuvant radiochemotherapy. Eur J Nucl Med Mol Imaging 42(5):657–666

Lee JH, Jang HS, Kim JG, Lee MA, Kim DY, Kim TH, Park HC (2014) Prediction of pathologic staging with magnetic resonance imaging after preoperative chemoradiotherapy in rectal cancer: pooled analysis of KROG 10-01 and 11-02. Radiother Oncol 113(1):18–23

Lee G, Lee HY, Ko ES, Jeong WK, Lee G, Lee HY, Jeong WK (2017a) Radiomics and imaging genomics in precision medicine. Precision Future Med 1(1):10–31

Lee G, Lee HY, Park H, Schiebler ML, van Beek EJ, Ohno Y, Leung A (2017b) Radiomics and its emerging role in lung cancer research, imaging biomarkers and clinical management: state of the art. Eur J Radiol 86:297–307

Li C, Lan X, Yuan H, Feng H, Xia X, Zhang Y (2014) 18F-FDG PET predicts pathological response to preoperative chemoradiotherapy in patients with primary rectal cancer: a meta-analysis. Ann Nucl Med 28(5):436–446

Liu YI, Kamaya A, Desser TS, Rubin DL (2011) A bayesian network for differentiating benign from malignant thyroid nodules using sonographic and demographic features. Am J Roentgenol 196(5):W598–W605

Liu H, Cui Y, Shen W, Fan X, Cui L, Zhang C, Wang D (2016a) Pretreatment magnetic resonance imaging of regional lymph nodes with carcinoembryonic antigen in prediction of synchronous distant metastasis in patients with rectal cancer. Oncotarget 7(19):27199

Liu Y, Wang R, Ding Y, Tu S, Liu Y, Qian Y, Peng J (2016b) A predictive nomogram improved diagnostic accuracy and interobserver agreement of perirectal lymph nodes metastases in rectal cancer. Oncotarget 7(12):14755

Lucas PJ, Van der Gaag LC, Abu-Hanna A (2004) Bayesian networks in biomedicine and health-care. Artif Intell Med 30(3):201–214

Ma F, Chitta R, Zhou J, You Q, Sun T, Gao J (2017) Dipole: diagnosis prediction in healthcare via attention-based bidirectional recurrent neural networks. In: Proceedings of the 23rd ACM SIGKDD international conference on knowledge discovery and data mining. ACM, pp. 1903–1911

Maclin PS, Dempsey J, Brooks J, Rand J (1991) Using neural networks to diagnose cancer. J Med Syst 15(1):11–19

Martens MH, Subhani S, Heijnen LA, Lambregts DM, Buijsen J, Maas M, Rg B-T (2015) Can perfusion MRI predict response to preoperative treatment in rectal cancer? Radiother Oncol 114(2):218–223

Meldolesi E, van Soest J, Alitto AR, Autorino R, Dinapoli N, Dekker A, Valentini V (2014) VATE: VAlidation of high TEchnology based on large database analysis by learning machine. Future Med 3(5):435–450

Meng X, Huang Z, Wang R, Yu J (2014) Prediction of response to preoperative chemoradiotherapy in patients with locally advanced rectal cancer. Biosci Trends 8(1):11–23

Moon SJ, Cho SH, Kim GC, Kim WH, Kim HJ, Shin KM, Kim SH (2016) Complementary value of pretreatment apparent diffusion coefficient in rectal cancer for predicting tumor recurrence. Abdom Radiol 41(7):1237–1244

Moons KG, Kengne AP, Grobbee DE, Royston P, Vergouwe Y, Altman DG, Woodward M (2012) Risk prediction models: II. External validation, model updating, and impact assessment. In: Heart Heartjnl-2011, vol 98, p 691
O'Connor JP, Rose CJ, Waterton JC, Carano RA, Parker GJ, Jackson A (2015) Imaging intratumor heterogeneity: role in therapy response, resistance, and clinical outcome. Clin Cancer Res 21(2):249–257
Ogawa S, Hida JI, Ike H, Kinugasa T, Ota M, Shinto E, Watanabe T (2017) Prediction of lateral pelvic lymph node metastasis from lower rectal cancer using magnetic resonance imaging and risk factors for metastasis: Multicenter study of the Lymph Node Committee of the Japanese Society for cancer of the colon and rectum. Int J Colorectal Dis 32(10):1479–1487
van Panhuis WG, Paul P, Emerson C, Grefenstette J, Wilder R, Herbst AJ, Burke DS (2014) A systematic review of barriers to data sharing in public health. BMC Public Health 14(1):1144
Pham TT, Liney GP, Wong K, Barton MB (2017a) Functional MRI for quantitative treatment response prediction in locally advanced rectal cancer. Br J Radiol 90(1072):20151078
Pham TT, Liney G, Wong K, Rai R, Lee M, Moses D, Barton MB (2017b) Study protocol: multi-parametric magnetic resonance imaging for therapeutic response prediction in rectal cancer. BMC Cancer 17(1):465
Popescu MC, Sasu LM (2014) Feature extraction, feature selection and machine learning for image classification: a case study. In: 2014 international conference on Optimization of Electrical and Electronic Equipment (OPTIM). IEEE, pp 968–973
Roelofs E, Dekker A, Meldolesi E, van Stiphout RG, Valentini V, Lambin P (2014) International data-sharing for radiotherapy research: an open-source based infrastructure for multicentric clinical data mining. Radiother Oncol 110(2):370–374
Rosenblatt F (1958) The perceptron: a probabilistic model for information storage and organization in the brain. Psychol Rev 65(6):386
Seierstad T, Hole KH, Grøholt KK, Dueland S, Ree AH, Flatmark K, Redalen KR (2015) MRI volumetry for prediction of tumour response to neoadjuvant chemotherapy followed by chemoradiotherapy in locally advanced rectal cancer. Br J Radiol 88(1051):20150097
Shen D, Wu G, Suk HI (2017) Deep learning in medical image analysis. Annu Rev Biomed Eng 19:221
Shin YR, Kim KA, Im S, Hwang SS, Kim K (2016) Prediction of KRAS mutation in rectal cancer using MRI. Anticancer Res 36(9):4799–4804
Soest J, Meldolesi E, Stiphout R, Gatta R, Damiani A, Valentini V, Dekker A (2017) Prospective validation of pathologic complete response models in rectal cancer: transferability and reproducibility. Med Phys 44(9):4961–4967
Steyerberg EW (2008) Clinical prediction models: a practical approach to development, validation, and updating. Springer Science & Business Media, Cham
van Stiphout RG, Lammering G, Buijsen J, Janssen MH, Gambacorta MA, Slagmolen P, Postma EO (2011) Development and external validation of a predictive model for pathological complete response of rectal cancer patients including sequential PET-CT imaging. Radiother Oncol 98(1):126–133
van Stiphout RG, Valentini V, Buijsen J, Lammering G, Meldolesi E, van Soest J, Lambin P (2014) Nomogram predicting response after chemoradiotherapy in rectal cancer using sequential PETCT imaging: a multicentric prospective study with external validation. Radiother Oncol 113(2):215–222
Suresh H, Hunt N, Johnson A, Celi LA, Szolovits P, Ghassemi M (2017) Clinical intervention prediction and understanding using deep networks. arXiv preprint arXiv:1705.08498
Szczypiński PM, Strzelecki M, Materka A, Klepaczko A (2009) MaZda—a software package for image texture analysis. Comput Methods Prog Biomed 94(1):66–76
Tagliaferri L, Kovács G, Autorino R, Budrukkar A, Guinot JL, Hildebrand G, Rovirosa A (2016) ENT COBRA (Consortium for Brachytherapy Data Analysis): interdisciplinary standardized data collection system for head and neck patients treated with interventional radiotherapy (brachytherapy). J Contemp Brachyther 8(4):336
Thor M, Apte A, Deasy JO, Muren LP (2013) Statistical simulations to estimate motion-inclusive dose-volume histograms for prediction of rectal morbidity following radiotherapy. Acta Oncol 52(3):666–675
Tsai C, Hague C, Xiong W, Raval M, Karimuddin A, Brown C, Phang PT (2017) Evaluation of endorectal ultrasound (ERUS) and MRI for prediction of circumferential resection margin (CRM) for rectal cancer. Am J Surg 213(5):936–942
Valentini V, Van Stiphout RG, Lammering G, Gambacorta MA, Barba MC, Bebenek M, Gerard JP (2011) Nomograms for predicting local recurrence, distant metastases, and overall survival for patients with locally advanced rectal cancer on the basis of European randomized clinical trials. J Clin Oncol 29(23):3163–3172
Valentini V, Dinapoli N, Damiani A (2013) The future of predictive models in radiation oncology: from extensive data mining to reliable modeling of the results. Future Oncol 9(3):311–313
Vogelstein B, Papadopoulos N, Velculescu VE, Zhou S, Diaz LA, Kinzler KW (2013) Cancer genome landscapes. Science 339(6127):1546–1558
Wernick MN, Yang Y, Brankov JG, Yourganov G, Strother SC (2010) Machine learning in medical imaging. IEEE Signal Process Mag 27(4):25–38
Win T, Miles KA, Janes SM, Ganeshan B, Shastry M, Endozo R, Ell PJ (2013) Tumor heterogeneity and permeability as measured on the CT component of PET/CT predict survival in patients with non–small cell lung cancer. Clin Cancer Res 19(13):3591–3599
Yan P, Suzuki K, Wang F, Shen D (2013) Machine learning in medical imaging. Mach Vis Appl 24:1327–1329
Zhang L, Fried DV, Fave XJ, Hunter LA, Yang J, Court LE (2015) IBEX: an open infrastructure software platform to facilitate collaborative work in radiomics. Med Phys 42(3):1341–1353

Part IV

Response Evaluation and Follow-Up by Imaging (Regina G. H. Beets-Tan, Daniel Zips, Roberto C. Delgado Bolton)

Response Evaluation and Follow-Up by Imaging in Brain Tumours

R. Gahrmann, J. Arbizu, A. Laprie, M. Morales, and M. Smits

Contents

1	**Introduction**	382
1.1	Imaging Methods	382
2	**Treatment Response**	385
2.1	Glioma	385
2.2	Lymphoma	388
2.3	Metastasis	388
2.4	Meningioma	390
3	**Treatment Effects**	391
3.1	Pseudoprogression and Radiation Necrosis	391
3.2	Angiogenesis Inhibitors and Pseudoresponse	396
3.3	Late Effects of Radiotherapy	397
References		400

Abstract

Brain tumours, either primary or secondary, are frequent. Primary brain tumours include mainly glioma, lymphoma and meningioma. Secondary tumours, i.e. brain metastases, are a frequent event during the disease course of patients with cancer. The evaluation of response to treatment is often difficult with structural imaging due to the interference of treatment effects. In this chapter, the role of advanced imaging for the differential diagnosis between pseudoprogression, radiation necrosis and tumour recurrence is described with perfusion and diffusion MR imaging, MR spectroscopy and PET imaging with amino acid analogues, fluorodeoxyglucose and other tracers. Furthermore, the commonly

R. Gahrmann
Department of Radiology and Nuclear Medicine, Erasmus MC, University Medical Centre Rotterdam, Rotterdam, The Netherlands
e-mail: r.gahrmann@erasmusmc.nl

J. Arbizu · M. Morales
Department of Nuclear Medicine, Clinica Universidad de Navarra, University of Navarra, Pamplona, Spain
e-mail: jarbizu@unav.es; mmlozano@unav.es

A. Laprie
Department of Radiation Oncology, Institut Claudius Regaud, Paul Sabatier University Toulouse III, Institut Universitaire du Cancer de Toulouse-Oncopole, Toulouse Cedex 9, France
e-mail: Laprie.Anne@iuct-oncopole.fr

M. Smits (✉)
Department of Radiology and Nuclear Medicine, Erasmus MC, University Medical Centre Rotterdam, Rotterdam, The Netherlands
e-mail: marion.smits@erasmusmc.nl

R. G. H. Beets-Tan et al. (eds.), *Imaging and Interventional Radiology for Radiation Oncology*, Medical Radiology, Diagnostic Imaging, https://doi.org/10.1007/978-3-030-38261-2_21

used response criteria for various brain tumours are described. For glioma, those set out by the response assessment in neuro-oncology (RANO) group are recommended. For brain metastases the RANO-brain metastases (RANO-BM) and RECIST criteria are commonly used. While conventional T1w post-contrast imaging is the mainstay imaging modality for basic response assessment, multimodal imaging is commonly necessary to evaluate the response to treatment of primary and secondary brain tumours.

1 Introduction

Brain tumours can be either primary (gliomas, lymphomas, meningiomas) or secondary (metastases). They carry a substantial burden of severe symptoms and complications. Their treatment often includes radiotherapy. The evaluation of tumour response can be challenging particularly in gliomas with the issue of pseudoprogression. For all tumours, another challenge is to differentiate radiation necrosis from tumoural residue or recurrence. The use of advanced imaging modalities is commonly useful in these situations.

1.1 Imaging Methods

1.1.1 Structural Imaging

Treatment response assessment of brain tumours is generally performed using structural magnetic resonance (MR) images, such as T2-weighted (T2w), T2w fluid attenuation inversion recovery (FLAIR) and pre- and post-contrast T1-weighted (T1w) imaging. Most tumours show enhancement on post-contrast T1w images, and 2D measurements on this sequence remain the basis of treatment assessment.

Additional information on tumour pathophysiology can be obtained with advanced MR imaging techniques and nuclear medicine imaging.

1.1.2 Advanced MR Imaging

Diffusion-weighted imaging (DWI) and diffusion tensor imaging (DTI) can be considered as both structural and functional techniques. The amount of diffusion (or random motion) of water molecules is measured with DWI. In DTI, diffusion is measured in multiple directions (minimum of six) to calculate the tensor or general direction of diffusion. Diffusion can be limited due to structures within the voxel. In tumours, high cellular density restricts diffusion, which is reflected in the DWI-derived apparent diffusion coefficient (ADC) (Symms et al. 2004). DTI-derived measures include fractional anisotropy (FA), which provides information on the degree of directional diffusion along the three main axes, and mean diffusivity (MD), which is similar to ADC (Soares et al. 2013). It is important to note that ADC is influenced not only by extracellular space tortuosity but also by membrane damage and perfusion (Shim et al. 2015).

Most commonly used for *perfusion imaging* is T2∗-weighted dynamic susceptibility-weighted contrast-enhanced (DSC) imaging. When the blood-brain barrier is breached, contrast agent leaks from the vessels into the surrounding tissue, increasing T1w signal intensity and decreasing the T2∗ signal. This effect must be counteracted (either in advance or during post-processing) when maps of relative cerebral blood volume (rCBV) are calculated, but can also be used to calculate other parameters, such as the peak height (PH) and percentage signal intensity recovery (rPSR) (Paulson and Schmainda 2008). Other perfusion techniques include dynamic contrast-enhanced (DCE) imaging and arterial spin labelling (ASL). DCE-derived measures include cerebral blood flow (CBF), capillary permeability (K^{trans}) and extravascular extracellular volume fraction (V_e) (Ferda et al. 2017). Where for both DSC- and DCE-imaging intravascular injection of contrast agent is required, the blood itself forms the contrast in arterial spin labelling (ASL). ASL-derived CBF has been shown to correlate well with DSC-derived rCBV measures (Cebeci et al. 2014).

In *MR spectroscopy*, different resonance frequencies of specific molecules and metabolites can be measured within different tissues, most commonly using protons (^{1}H-MRS). In brain tumours, N-acetyl aspartate (NAA), choline (Cho), myo-inositol (mI), lactate/lipid Lac) and creatine (Cr) are commonly assessed, although many more may be measured (Horská and Barker 2010).

Chemical exchange saturation transfer (CEST) imaging is a more recent technique, which can be used to measure amides (–NH), amines (–NH_2) and hydroxyl (–OH) groups among others, but is still very much in the research arena (Kogan et al. 2013).

1.1.3 Nuclear Medicine Imaging

Nuclear medicine techniques such as single-photon emission computed tomography (SPECT) and positron emission tomography (PET) are being used worldwide for the characterisation, therapy planning and recurrence assessment of brain tumours. SPECT using cellular viability radiotracers like ^{99m}technetium-sestamibi (^{99m}Tc-MIBI) and ^{201}thallium were initially employed in clinical practice due to its high availability (Sugo et al. 2006; Prigent-Le Jeune et al. 2004). However, in recent years PET has been gradually introduced into the clinical practice instead of SPECT for the evaluation of brain tumours as a complementary and supplementary tool of standard MR imaging sequences. It is important to note that fusion images between structural (computed tomography (CT) and/or MR imaging) and PET or SPECT images are highly recommended to achieve better accuracy. Multimodality systems are now available that combine SPECT and PET scanners and structural imaging devices like CT (SPECT/CT and PET/CT) and more recently MR imaging (PET/MR imaging). Visual analysis of the images is the most common method for PET evaluation in clinical practice. The study is classified as positive when the activity observed in the lesion exceeds the reference region (usually normal cortex). However, semiquantitative analysis of PET can also be performed using the standardised uptake value (SUV), commonly calculated for quantifying systemic tumours. However, this parameter has a limited role in the clinical interpretation of images in neuro-oncology. Instead, tumour or lesion to brain reference region ratios using mean or maximum SUV (TBR) are used to provide a measure of PET radiotracer uptake in brain tumours.

One of the hallmarks of PET is the variety of parameters that can be observed and measured in brain tumours by means of specific radiotracers. Some of the most commonly used in clinical practice are reviewed in this section.

1.1.3.1 Glucose Metabolism

Brain 2-deoxy-2-[^{18}F]-2-fluoro-2-deoxy-D-glucose ([^{18}F]FDG) uptake is usually acquired 45–60 min after the injection of 185 MBq of [^{18}F]FDG. Patients must be fasting for 4 h prior to injection, and it is recommended to obtain a measurement of blood glucose prior to the exam: high blood glucose levels at the time of injection decrease uptake in tumour and healthy tissue, although it may not affect lesion detection. In case sedation is required, this can be carried out 45–60 min after injection, just prior to the time of the acquisition (Varrone et al. 2009).

[^{18}F]FDG accumulates in the majority of tumours due to elevated glucose metabolism in response to increased energy demand. This technique has been applied to brain tumour imaging for many years. The relationship of [^{18}F]FDG uptake to tumour glioma grade and prognosis has been reported in several studies (Herholz et al. 2012). However, [^{18}F]FDG is in some way limited in neuro-oncology due to the high rate of glucose metabolism in normal brain parenchyma resulting in diminished signal-to-noise ratio for brain tumours. Another problem with [^{18}F]FDG is the high uptake of this tracer in inflammatory cells, which can occur in a variety of disease processes and can be independent of tumour growth or response (Albert et al. 2016). Consequently, as newer PET tracers have become available, the use of [^{18}F]FDG for imaging in neuro-oncology has declined.

1.1.3.2 Amino Acid Transport

System L amino acid transport PET radiotracers ([^{11}C-methyl]-methionine (–MET), O-(2-[^{18}F]-fluoroethyl)-L-tyrosine (FET) and 3,4-dihydroxy-6-[^{18}F]-fluoro-L-phenylalanine (FDOPA) are currently used in neuro-oncology. MET has been used since 1983 (Bergström et al. 1983), but is limited to centres with an on-site cyclotron because it is labelled with ^{11}carbon, a radioisotope with a very short half-life (20 minutes).

[^{18}F]FET and [^{18}F]FDOPA are labelled with ^{18}fluorine, a radioisotope with a longer half-life which allows radiotracer transportation from the manufacturing laboratory to the PET centre (Herholz et al. 2012).

The uptake of radiolabelled amino acids observed in normal brain tissue as well as in brain lesions including tumours of many types is predominantly conditioned by the transmembrane active transport, which is responsible for the biological activity in tissues, including cell proliferation. The uptake by cerebral tumour tissue appears to be caused almost entirely by increased transport via the specific amino acid transport system L for large neutral amino acids (Herholz et al. 2012). The uptake is also influenced by passive diffusion in regions with blood-brain barrier disruption and by stagnation in regional vascular beds that depends on blood volume due to a large vascular bed (Aki et al. 2012). In contrast to tumour, the uptake of radiolabelled amino acids in normal brain is very low resulting in a high contrast between tumour and normal brain tissue.

After a recommended period of 4 h of fasting, 200 MBq of [^{18}F]FET, 370–555 MBq of ^{11}C-MET or 185 MBq of [^{18}F]DOPA is injected, and a static PET acquisition is performed 20 minutes later. In addition to static images, dynamic FET PET data can be acquired, which allows the characterisation of the temporal pattern of FET uptake by deriving a time-activity curve (TAC) in brain tumours (Calcagni et al. 2011; Ceccon et al. 2017). It remains to be shown, however, whether dynamic ^{11}C-MET and [^{18}F]DOPA can contribute significantly to the characterisation of brain tumours. The more widespread use of amino acid PET for the management of patients with brain tumours has been strongly recommended by the response assessment in neuro-oncology (RANO) group (Albert et al. 2016; Langen and Watts 2016).

1.1.3.3 Somatostatin Receptors

The most common somatostatin receptor (SSTR) radioligands for PET imaging are ^{68}Ga-DOTA-Tyr3-octreotide (^{68}Ga-DOTATOC), ^{68}Ga-DOTA-D-Phe1-Tyr3-octreotate (^{68}Ga-DOTATATE) and ^{68}Ga-DOTA-l-Nal3-octreotide (^{68}Ga-^{D}OTANOC). These radiotracers, frequently used for imaging of neuroendocrine tumours, have been introduced in neuro-oncology due the overexpression of SSTR subtype 2 in almost all meningiomas (Dutour et al. 1998). ^{68}Ga has a physical half-life of 68 minutes and can be produced with a ^{68}Ge/^{68}Ga generator system, which enables in-house production without the need for an on-site cyclotron. PET ligands to SSTR provide high sensitivity with excellent target-to-background contrast due to low uptake in bone and healthy brain tissue (Rachinger et al. 2015).

There are no comparative studies of ^{68}Ga-DOTATOC, ^{68}Ga-DOTATATE and ^{68}Ga-DOTANOC, but the uptake of all these tracers is relatively high compared to normal brain; thus, possible differences between these tracers are not really relevant. Procedure guidelines for PET imaging with ^{68}Ga-DOTA-conjugated peptides have been published recently (Galldiks et al. 2017a).

1.1.3.4 Other Radiotracers

Several other radiotracers are used to image brain tumours. The *thymidine nucleoside analogue 3'-deoxy-3'-[^{18}F]fluorothymidine* (*FLT*) is a substrate for thymidine kinase-1 and reflects cell proliferation. Although previous studies suggest that [^{18}F]FLT is a promising tool for glioma detection and grading (Chen et al. 2007) and is able to predict improved survival after bevacizumab therapy (Chen et al. 2007; Wardak et al. 2014), the uptake of this tracer is dependent on the disruption of the blood-brain barrier, thereby limiting its clinical value.

Hypoxia in brain tumours has been demonstrated with use of the PET tracer *[^{18}F]fluoromisonidazole* (*FMISO*) (Lee and Scott 2007). [^{18}F]MISO enters tumour cells by passive diffusion and becomes trapped in cells with reduced tissue oxygen partial pressure by nitroreductase enzymes. This tracer thus allows the identification of hypoxic tumour areas, which are thought to be more resistant to irradiation (Spence et al. 2008), as well as a trigger for neoangiogenesis. Thus far, [^{18}F]MISO has predominantly been used in a preclinical setting.

Another interesting PET target is the *translocator protein* (*TSPO*), a mitochondrial membrane protein that has been used as biomarker for neuroinflammation. TSPO is highly expressed in activated microglia, macrophages and neoplastic cells. Imaging with the TSPO ligand ^{11}C-(R) PK11195 demonstrates increased binding in high-grade glioma compared to low-grade glioma and normal brain parenchyma (Su et al. 2015). More recently, the TSPO ligand [^{18}F] DPA-714 labelled with [^{18}F] has been evaluated in glioma animal models (Awde et al. 2013).

Choline is a marker of phospholipid synthesis involved in the synthesis of cell membrane components. The *radiolabelled choline* (either ^{11}carbon or more recently ^{18}fluorine) is trapped by glioblastoma with a very high contrast to normal brain, whereas its role in lower-grade gliomas is limited (Gomez-Rio et al. 2015). When compared with [^{18}F]FDG, radiolabelled choline appears to be superior in terms of diagnostic performance in glioma and metastasis (Rottenburger et al. 2011).

2 Treatment Response

2.1 Glioma

2.1.1 Background

Newly diagnosed anaplastic glioma and glioblastoma (GBM) are the most frequent primary brain tumours in adults. They are treated with surgery, radiotherapy, chemotherapy or any combination thereof. In diffuse low-grade gliomas, the presence of certain negative prognostic factors can be considered a reason for adjuvant radiotherapy (Stupp et al. 2014). The effects of radiotherapy combined with TMZ positively influence patient survival in GBM, especially in those with a methylated O^6-methylguanine DNA methyltransferase (MGMT) (van KA et al. 2007; Chalmers et al. 2009).

2.1.2 Radiological Treatment Assessment

Radiological assessment of treatment response in glioma was traditionally based on the bidimensional measurement of the area of enhancement (Macdonald et al. 1990), but the introduction of angiogenesis inhibitors (such as bevacizumab) has led to the diagnostic challenge of pseudoresponse: enhancement decreases or disappears because the tumour vasculature normalises and is therefore no longer permeable, while the tumour itself may not be responding to treatment. The RANO criteria (Wen et al. 2010) therefore now include the assessment of non-enhancing in addition to enhancing lesions, which also make them applicable to non-enhancing, commonly lower grade, glioma. The time between scans is generally 6–12 weeks, but is sometimes increased in case of stable disease. A summary of the RANO criteria for both GBM and lower-grade glioma can be found in Table 1.

2.1.3 Advanced Methods of Treatment Assessment (MR Imaging)

In a pretreatment setting, *diffusion MR imaging*-derived parameters, such as ADC and FA, can aid in grading gliomas and localising areas of high cellularity suitable for biopsy (Inoue et al. 2005). After treatment, however, these parameters no longer correlate with cellular density, as they are influenced by other factors such as cell swelling and necrosis (Tsien et al. 2014). At a group level, ADC values still tend to be higher in gliomas than in normal appearing white matter (NAWM), but at an individual level, there is considerable overlap and they are therefore not useful for response assessment (van den Bent et al. 2011).

Perfusion imaging-derived rCBV and CBF in both grey and white matter are decreased after radiotherapy and can remain low for up to 6 and 9 months, respectively, in high-dose areas (Fuss et al. 2000; Petr et al. 2015). High rCBV values (>2.0 times that of the contralateral NAWM) can be used to distinguish tumour from pseudoprogression or radiation necrosis with reported sensitivities of up to 82% and specificity of 78% (Kong et al. 2011; Sugahara et al. 2000). In diffuse astrocytoma, an increase in rCBV indicates malignant transformation (van den Bent et al. 2011). In oligodendroglioma rCBV tends to be moderately increased even when low grade, but a further increase indicates malignant transformation (van den Bent et al. 2011).

MR spectroscopy shows (transient) changes in molecules and metabolites in relation to treatment-related changes, such as neuronal dysfunction, oedema, damage to oligodendrocytes, demyelination and inflammatory effects. Metabolites such

Table 1 Summary of RANO criteria for glioblastoma (GBM) and low-grade glioma (LGG) (Wen et al. 2010; van den Bent et al. 2011)

Response	Criteria GBM	Criteria LGG
CR	*Requires all of the following*: Complete disappearance of all enhancing (non-) measurable disease sustained for at least 4 weeks. No progression of non-enhancing disease. No new lesions. No corticosteroids. Stable or improved clinically	*Requires all of the following*: Complete disappearance of the lesion on T2w/FLAIR images. No new lesions aside from radiation effects. No corticosteroids. Stable or improved clinically
PR	*Requires all of the following*: ≥50% decrease in the sum of products of perpendicular diameters of all measurable enhancing lesions compared to baseline sustained for at least 4 weeks. No progression of non-measurable disease. No new lesions. Stable or reduced corticosteroids. Stable or improved clinically	*Requires all of the following*: ≥50% decrease in the sum of products of perpendicular diameters on Tw/FLAIR imaging compared to baseline sustained for at least 4 weeks. No new lesions aside from radiation effects. Stable or reduced corticosteroids. Stable or improved clinically
Minor response	–	*Requires all of the following*: 25–50% decrease of non-enhancing lesion area on T2w/FLAIR images compared to baseline. No new lesions aside from radiation effects. Stable or reduced corticosteroids. Stable or improved clinically
SD	Does not qualify for CR, PR or PD. stable or reduced corticosteroids. Stable clinically	Does not qualify for CR, PR, minor response or PD. no new lesions aside from radiation effects. Stable or reduced corticosteroids. Stable or improved clinically
PD	*Requires any of the following*: ≥25% increase in the sum of products of perpendicular diameters of enhancing lesions compared to the smallest tumour measurement from earlier studies. Significant increase in non-measurable lesions. Any new lesion. Clinical deterioration	*Requires any of the following*: Development of new lesions or increase of enhancement. ≥25% increase of T2w/FLAIR non-enhancing lesions while on stable or increasing steroid dosage and not caused by radiotherapy or other. Clinical deterioration

CR complete response, *PR* partial response, *SD* stable disease, *PD* progressive disease

as NAA, Cr, Cho and Lac change during and after radiation. For instance, a decrease in NAA occurs early after radiotherapy co-occurring with an increase in Cho, which can remain present for up to 6 months (Peca et al. 2009; Sundgren 2009; Walecki et al. 1999). Due to the transient nature of metabolite changes, MR spectroscopy results need to be either interpreted in combination with other measures (MR imaging and/or PET) or with repeated measures in time.

2.1.4 PET Imaging

A higher [^{18}F]FDG uptake by glioma is correlated with higher tumour grade and worse prognosis (Colavolpe et al. 2012; Dunet et al. 2016; Mertens et al. 2013). With the exception of pilocytic astrocytomas, WHO grade I and grade II gliomas are typically negative on [^{18}F]FDG PET (uptake similar to or less than white matter), and consequently this tracer is not suitable for response evaluation of low-grade glioma (Albert et al. 2016). On the other hand, increased levels of [^{18}F]FDG uptake in enhancing brain lesions are correlated with tumour recurrence in anaplastic glioma and glioblastoma.

In recurrent high-grade glioma, the uptake of [^{18}F]FDG has been shown to be predictive of tumour metabolic response to TMZ versus TMZ plus radiotherapy (Charnley et al. 2006) and for predicting survival following antiangiogenic therapy with bevacizumab (Colavolpe et al. 2012).

Current *amino acid* PET data suggest that both a reduction of amino acid uptake and a decrease of the metabolically active tumour volume are signs of treatment response associated with improved long-term outcome (Albert et al. 2016). Moreover, the amount of residual tracer uptake in [^{18}F]FET PET after surgery/prior to chemoradiation of glioblastoma (within 7–20 days after surgery) has a strong prognostic influence, even after adjustment by multivariate survival analyses for the effects of treatment, MGMT promoter methylation and other patient- and tumour-related factors (Fig. 1) (Suchorska et al. 2015). However, the experience with amino acid PET for monitoring after treatment in patients with WHO grade II glioma is limited.

The prognostic value of early changes of [^{18}F]FET uptake 6–8 weeks after postoperative radiochemotherapy in glioblastoma patients has been evaluated prospectively (Piroth et al. 2011; Galldiks et al. 2012). PET responders with a decrease in the TBR of more than 10% had a significantly longer disease-free and overall survival than patients with stable or increasing tracer uptake after radiochemotherapy. The kinetic analysis of FET uptake was not helpful in the evaluation of treatment effects to radiochemotherapy (Piroth et al. 2011). Patients with low-grade glioma evaluated 12 months after brachytherapy exhibit significantly reduced ^{11}C-MET uptake (Voges et al. 1997; Wurker et al. 1996). For patients treated with alkylating chemotherapy, ^{11}C-MET and [^{18}F]FET PET may improve response assessment (Galldiks et al. 2017b). Reliable monitoring of temozolomide and nitrosourea-based chemotherapy (PCV scheme including procarbazine, CCNU and vincristine or CCNU monotherapy) has been demonstrated in patients with recurrent high-grade glioma (Galldiks et al. 2006). Similarly, [^{18}F]FET PET has been used to assess effects of TMZ according to the EORTC protocol 22033–26033 (application of 75 mg/m^2 TMZ per day over 21 days in a 28-day cycle) (Wyss et al. 2009). Additionally, a reduction of the metabolically active tumour volume after treatment initiation can be observed considerably earlier than volume reductions on FLAIR imaging (Roelcke et al. 2016). Several studies suggest that treatment response and outcome in bevacizumab therapy can be assessed better with amino acid

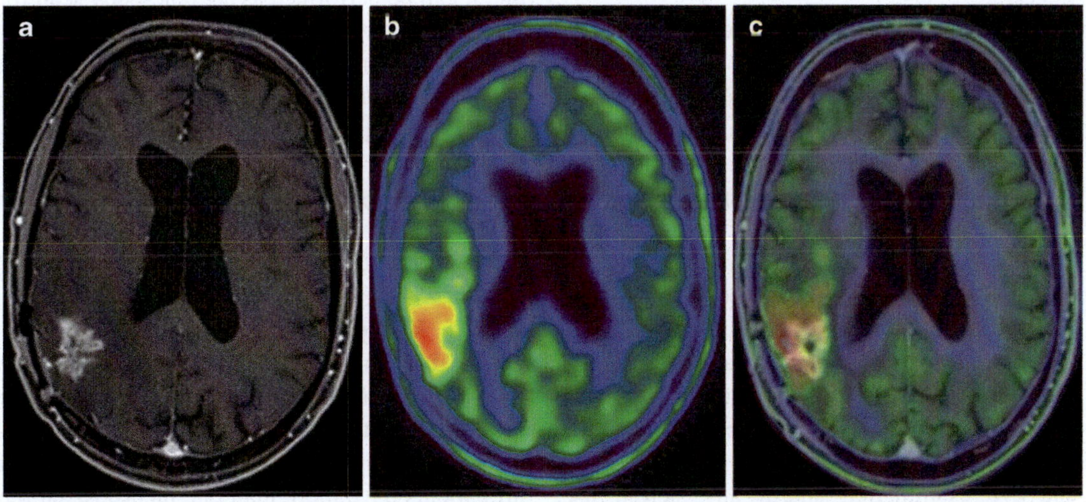

Fig. 1 Neuroimaging studies of a patient with anaplastic astrocytoma performed 1 month after postoperative radiochemotherapy. An area of contrast enhancement on the T1w MR imaging sequence (**a**) is observed in the medial aspect of the residual surgical cavity. The ^{11}C-MET-PET study (**b**) and MR imaging-PET fusion (**c**) show an absence of ^{11}C-MET uptake in this part of the lesion ruling out the presence of tumour and indicating an area of pseudoprogression. However, there is also an area of elevated MET uptake (TBR 2.56) in the most lateral part of the lesion surrounding the area of pseudoprogression, suggesting the presence of infiltrative tumour relapse, later confirmed by biopsy

PET using [^{18}F]FET and [^{18}F]FDOPA than with MR imaging (see also Sect. 3.2) (Galldiks et al. 2013; Schwarzenberg et al. 2014).

2.2 Lymphoma

2.2.1 Background

The classification of central nervous system (CNS) lymphoma now corresponds with the WHO 2016 classifications of systemic haematopoietic/lymphoid disease (Louis et al. 2016). A distinction is made between primary CNS lymphoma (PCNSL) and secondary CNS lymphoma. Secondary CNS lymphoma generally arises from aggressive non-Hodgkin's lymphoma and has commonly (2/3) a leptomeningeal and less commonly (1/3) a parenchymal localisation. PCNSL almost invariably has a parenchymal localisation. Typically, single or multiple contrast-enhancing lesions are seen surrounding the ventricles or in the corpus callosum (Haldorsen et al. 2011). Patients are treated with radiation therapy and multiple chemotherapeutic agents (including methotrexate) given both systemically and intrathecally or intraventricularly. Additionally steroids are given.

2.2.2 Radiological Treatment Assessment

Conventional treatment response assessment of brain parenchymal lymphoma is by contrast-enhanced MR imaging with an average time between follow-up scans of 2 months during therapy. The International Primary CNS Lymphoma Collaborative Group has determined response criteria in 2005. Complete response (CR) is determined by a lack of contrast-enhancement on MR imaging, no steroid-treatment and normal eye examination and cerebrospinal fluid (CSF) cytology. An unconfirmed complete response (CRu) is CR with minimal abnormalities on MR imaging and eye examination and/or any steroid use. Patients with a partial response (PR) have a 50% decrease of enhancing tumour without or only minor or decreasing eye disease with either negative or persistent/suspicious CSF cytology. Progressive disease (PD) is characterised by a ≥25% increase in enhancing lesions, new sites of disease, recurrent or new ocular disease and recurrent or positive CSF cytology (Abrey et al. 2005). Treatment response in parenchymal PCNSL is depicted in Fig. 2.

2.2.3 PET Imaging

PCNSL often have high cellular density and consequently a markedly increased [^{18}F]FDG uptake compared to other brain tumours, including glioblastoma and metastasis, and when compared to many infectious and inflammatory processes (Albert et al. 2016; Makino et al. 2011). Cerebral infections such as toxoplasmosis and tuberculoma are a common differential diagnosis to PCNSL and exhibit a significantly lower uptake than patients with lymphoma, with no overlap of the uptake values (0.3–0.7 versus 1.7–3.1, respectively) (Hoffman et al. 1993; Sathekge et al. 2009).

There is no significant difference between ^{11}C-MET PET and [^{18}F]FDG PET in terms of sensitivity (Kawase et al. 2011). [^{18}F]FDG PET has shown some clinical advantage in the differential diagnosis of lymphoma as most cerebral lymphomas have a high cell density and a high glucose metabolism, which is usually even higher than that of malignant gliomas and cerebral metastasis. In addition, [^{18}F]FDG is clinically more available, and it can be performed as a whole-body scan for the assessment of systemic lymphoma involvement. Interestingly, [^{18}F]FDG PET might also be useful to demonstrate a response to chemotherapy in lymphoma patients very early after the initiation of therapy (Fig. 3) (Kawai et al. 2013).

2.3 Metastasis

2.3.1 Background

The main primary sites of brain metastases are the lung, breast and skin (melanoma). About 80% of brain metastases are located in the supratentorial brain (mainly frontal lobes), and about half of all patients have more than one metastasis at the time of diagnosis (Nussbaum et al. 1996). Treatment consists of WBRT and/or stereotactic radiosurgery (SRS) depending on the size and number of lesions. Metastases may also be surgically removed, and multiple lesions with a druggable target may by primarily treated with molecular targeting (Lippitz et al. 2014).

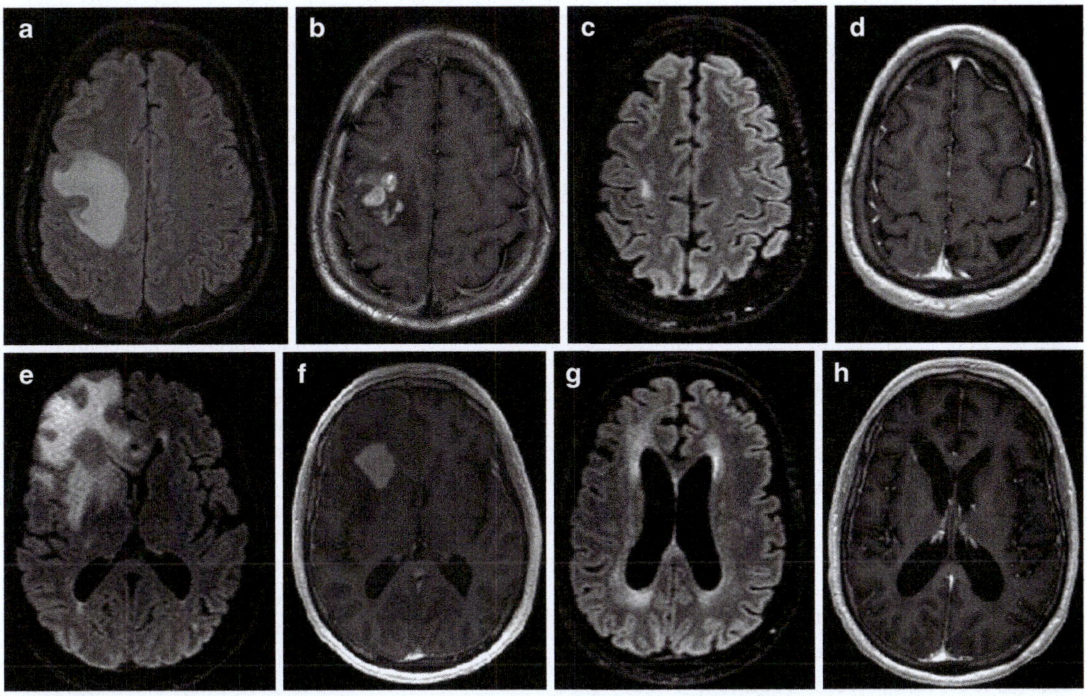

Fig. 2 FLAIR and T1w post-contrast images in a 60-year-old man with PCNSL in the right frontal lobe (**a**, **b**), treated with rituximab and MBVP followed by WBRT (30 Gy in 20 fractions) with resulting partial remission. Treatment continued with cytarabine and WBRT with SIB (30 Gy in 20 fractions) and an additional boost on the tumour (10 Gy in 20 fractions), resulting in complete remission with minimal white matter abnormalities considered to be a posttreatment effect (**c**, **d**). Recurrent disease 4 years later (**c**, **f**). After renewed treatment with MBVP and WBRT (20 Gy in 5 fractions), a clear response was seen. Periventricular white matter abnormalities and ex vacuo dilatations of the ventricles are present as post-treatment effects (**g**, **h**)

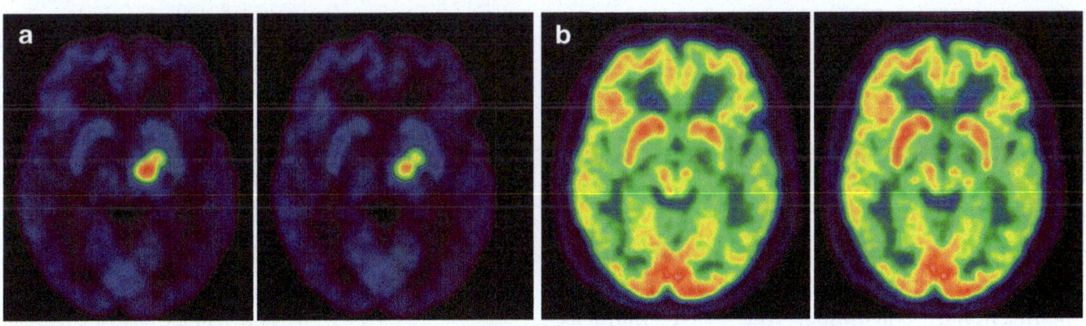

Fig. 3 Brain [^{18}F]FDG PET of primary CNS lymphoma at baseline (**a**), and 3 months after two cycles of chemotherapy (carmustine, methotrexate, cytarabine, rituximab according to the R-BAM scheme) and autologous haematopoietic stem cell transplantation (**b**) showing complete response

2.3.2 Radiological Treatment Assessment

The RANO-brain metastases (RANO-BM) working group created radiological criteria for treatment assessment in clinical trials, which can also be used in clinical practice (Lin et al. 2015). The metastases are categorised as target and non-target lesions. Target lesions are parenchymal metastases of at least 10×5 mm^2 in size. Up to five target lesions can be measured. Nontarget lesions include smaller parenchymal lesions, but also dural, leptomeningeal and cystic (or non-measurable) lesions. In case of a mixed response to treatment, lesions that increase in size are considered leading. Recommended time between scans is 6–12 weeks. Aside from radiological features, the RANO-BM also includes clinical status and steroid dosage. The RANO-BM criteria can be found in Table 2. Other response assessment methods include the RECIST criteria, in which lesions are measured in a single direction (≥30% decrease in the sum of diameters of the target lesions constitutes partial response,and a ≥20% increase progressive disease), and the WHO criteria, which include bidimensional measures (≥50% decrease in the sum of the product of the diameters constitutes partial response and ≥25% increase progressive disease). The appearance of a new lesions always indicates progressive disease (Lin et al. 2013).

2.3.3 PET Imaging

PET imaging in the context of treatment assessment of metastasis is mostly used to distinguish tumour recurrence from treatment effects (see Sect. 3).

[^{18}F]FDG PET can add to the specificity for enhancing lesions that are equivocal or suspicious for recurrent tumour based on contrast-enhanced MR imaging alone in patients with brain metastases treated with SRS (Belohlavek et al. 2003). Amino acid PET seems to be superior to [^{18}F]FDG PET with reported sensitivity and specificity of >90% (Galldika et al. 2019).

Table 2 Response assessment in brain metastases: target and nontarget lesions according to the RANO group, radiological characteristics only (Lin et al. 2015)

Target lesions	CR	*Requires all of the following:*
		• Disappearance of all target lesions sustained for at least 4 weeks
		• No new lesions
		• No corticosteroids
		• Stable or improved clinically
	PR	*Requires all of the following:*
		• ≥30% decrease in the sum of longest diameters of target lesion size compared to the baseline sustained for at least 4 weeks
		• No new lesions
		• Stable or reduced corticosteroids
		• Stable or improved clinically
	SD	Does not qualify for CR, PR of PD
	PD	*Requires all of the following:*
		• ≥20% increase in the sum of longest diameters of target lesions compared to the smallest sum from earlier studies
		• At least one lesion has increased ≥5 mm
Non-target lesions lesions	CR	*Requires all of the following:*
		• Disappearance of all enhancing nontarget lesions
		• No new lesions
	PR/SD	• Persistence of one or more nontarget lesions
	PD	*Requires any of the following*:
		• Unequivocal progression of existing enhancing nontarget lesions
		• New lesions (except while on immunotherapy-based treatment[a])
		• Unequivocal progression of existing tumour-related non-enhancing (T2w/FLAIR) lesions

[a]In case of immunotherapy-based treatment, new lesions alone may not constitute PD

CR complete response, *PR* partial response, *SD* stable disease, *PD* progressive disease

2.4 Meningioma

2.4.1 Background

The WHO classification distinguishes three grades of meningiomas: grade I, or benign meningioma, constitutes the vast majority (about 90%); grade II (atypical) and grade III (malignant) meningiomas are considerably less common. Benign meningiomas can be eligible for (radio)surgery if they are causing symptoms. Radiotherapy can be considered in case of incomplete resection or at recurrence. Atypical and malignant meningiomas are surgically removed when possible and irradiated (Louis et al. 2016; Rogers et al. 2015; Alexiou et al. 2010). Both atypical and malignant meningiomas can metastasise to the lungs, liver and spine, although this is rare (0.1% of cases), and screening is therefore not routinely recommended (Kessler et al. 2017).

2.4.2 Radiological Treatment Assessment

Meningiomas at risk for recurrence are those with pial invasion and in the case of grade II and III meningioma when there is bone involvement or peritumoural oedema (Nowak et al. 2015; Gabeau-Lacet et al. 2009). Meningiomas generally show intense homogeneous enhancement on post-contrast T1w images, and measurements are therefore performed on this sequence. Generally, the modified McDonald criteria are used to determine treatment response, but it has been suggested that volumetric measures are more sensitive when it comes to determining tumour growth due to the slow-growing nature of the tumours (Quant and Wen 2011). Additional meningiomas may appear in the course of time at other locations.

Early radiotherapy-related effects are tumour necrosis and oedema in the white matter (Lee et al. 2012). Radiation-induced peritumoural changes occur in about 25% of patients, mainly in convexity, parasagittal and falx cerebri meningiomas after SRS (Chang 2003). Later, radiotherapy effects such as white matter abnormalities are often seen in high-dose areas and the periventricular white matter. An example of an irradiated patient with an atypical meningioma and its treatment course is depicted in Fig. 4.

2.4.3 PET Imaging

The use of PET in meningioma patients is gradually increasing. Nevertheless, the usefulness of [^{18}F]FDG PET is limited because meningiomas are mostly slow-growing and the metabolism of [^{18}F]FDG is only elevated in atypical or anaplastic meningiomas (Cremerius et al. 1997).

^{11}C-MET PET scanning has been used to evaluate the effect of stereotactic high-energy proton beam treatment in a prospective study with 19 meningioma patients (Ryttlefors et al. 2016). A reduction in the TBR was observed (even over several years) in the total patient group without a reduction in tumour size. Moreover, prior to the volume increase on MR imaging, ^{11}C-MET uptake ratios were found to be increased, suggesting that treatment effects can be seen earlier than with CT or MR imaging (Ryttlefors et al. 2016).

Even though amino acid PET exhibits a better tumour-to-background contrast than [^{18}F]FDG PET, the availability of specific SSTR ligands with even higher tumour-to-background contrast has led to a limited use of amino acid PET in meningioma assessment (Galldiks et al. 2017b). ^{68}Ga-DOTA peptide PET has been shown to be more accurate than standard MR imaging to discriminate meningioma tissue from scar tissue related to pretreatment using both DOTATOC (Afshar-Oromieh et al. 2012) and DOTATATE (Rachinger et al. 2015), even in transosseous extension of intracranial meningiomas (Kunz et al. 2017). Consequently, ^{68}Ga-DOTA peptides may be useful in cases of unclear differential diagnosis between tumour progression and treatment-induced changes.

3 Treatment Effects

3.1 Pseudoprogression and Radiation Necrosis

3.1.1 Background

Progressive disease can be mimicked by treatment-related toxicity from radiotherapy (pseudoprogression and radiation necrosis), immunotherapy, chemotherapy and antiepileptic drugs. Additional imaging techniques and sequential imaging combined with clinical characteristics may be needed to distinguish these entities from actual progressive disease (Lin et al. 2015; Alexiou et al. 2010).

Pseudoprogression occurs in a subacute setting after radiotherapy treatment combined with TMZ (within approximately 2–3 months after the start of treatment). Tumours with a methylated O^6-methylguanine DNA methyltransferase (MGMT) promoter respond best to TMZ. Initially it seemed that this group showed a higher incidence of pseudoprogression, but this has later been disputed (Wick et al. 2016). Direct damage after radiotherapy is likely due to vasodilatation and increased capillary permeability, leading to disruption of the blood-brain barrier and oedema. In case of pseudoprogression, the response is excessive causing enhancement on post-contrast T1w images due to

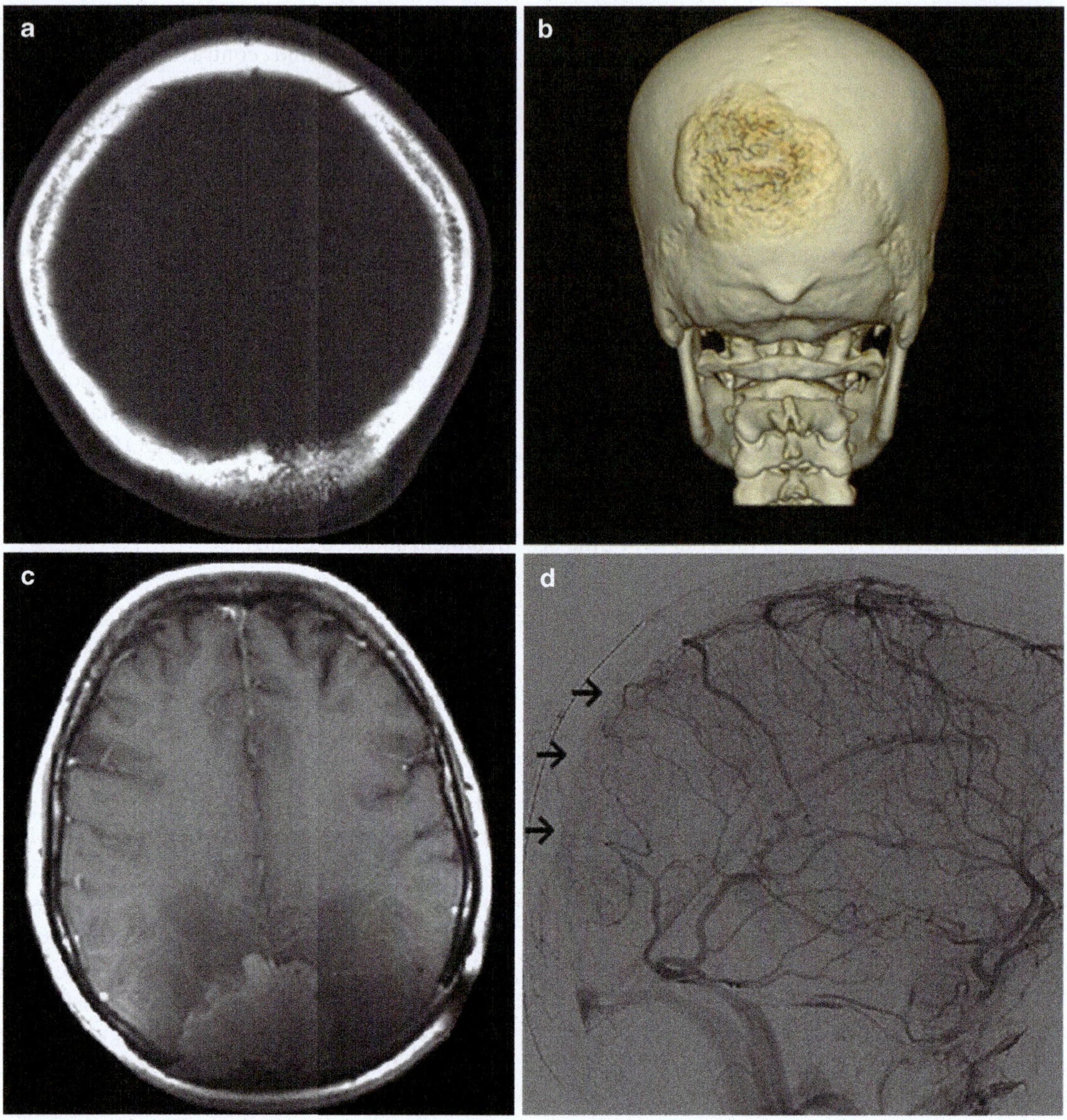

Fig. 4 CT, MR imaging (T1w post-contrast), angiographic and [^{18}F]FDG PET images in a 40-year-old woman with grade II meningioma primarily located in the skull, as can be seen on the CT (**a**, **b**). The tumour was resected and irradiated with 59.4 Gy. Recurrent tumour growth appeared 5 years later intracranially (**c**) with compression of the superior sagittal sinus (**d**). Again, the tumour was resected. In a second recurrence, multiple intracranial meningiomas appeared within the radiation field, (**e**) and the patient was irradiated again (49.5 Gy in 33 fractions). Aside from intracranial disease, the patient had histologically confirmed metastases in the lungs as seen in the [^{18}F]FDG PET/CT (**f**)

the damage to the blood-brain barrier and which is indistinguishable from tumour progression (Brandsma et al. 2008; Martino et al. 2014).

Radiation necrosis is a chronic response to radiotherapy, which can occur from just months up to many years (median 1–2 years) after treatment; up to 90% occurs within the first 5 years posttreatment. There are endothelial damage, enzyme changes and immunological response leading to necrosis. Radiation necrosis similar to pseudoprogression causes enhancement on post-contrast T1w images, mimicking tumour recurrence or progression (Brandsma et al. 2008; Raimbault et al. 2014).

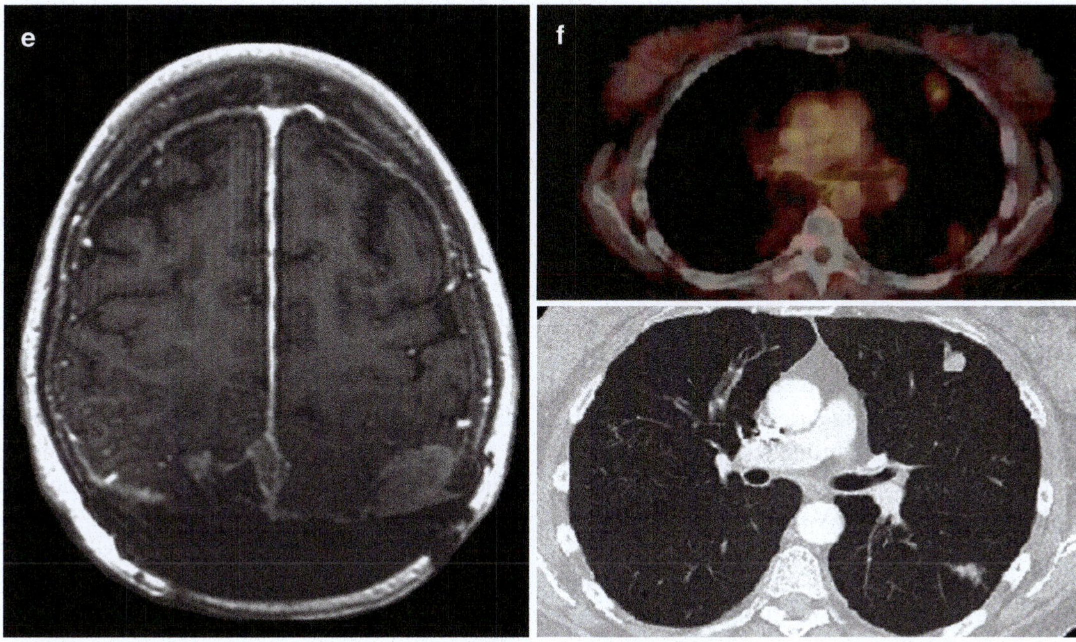

Fig. 21.4 (continued)

The reported incidences of pseudoprogression and radiation necrosis vary widely, from 2 to 48%, depending on the source and the definition used. The incidence is influenced by radiation dose, field size, number of fractions, prior WBRT, chemotherapy (mainly cisplatin, carboplatin, doxorubicin, methotrexate and temozolomide), immunotherapy, length of survival, age at time of radiotherapy and diabetes mellitus (Raimbault et al. 2014).

3.1.2 Standard Structural Imaging

Distinguishing pseudoprogression and radiation necrosis from tumour residue or recurrence is challenging. Radiation-induced lesions can occur at the primary tumour site, but also at a distance, including the contralateral hemisphere, if included in the field of radiation. There is a predilection for white matter, especially the corpus callosum, because of the higher susceptibility of oligodendrocytes to radiation damage (compared to neurons) and relatively lower blood supply (Kumar et al. 2000). In patients with low-grade gliomas, there is also a predilection for subependymal localisation (van West et al. 2017). The enhancing area is surrounded by oedema, which tends to be somewhat more extensive in radiation-induced lesions (Leeman et al. 2013). Different patterns of enhancement have been described, including nodular and rim enhancement with either regular or irregular margins and combined nodular and linear enhancing foci that create a mosaic-like appearance (Raimbault et al. 2014; Chan et al. 1999), but no reliable distinctive characteristics have been found. Radiation-induced lesions more often contain haemorrhagic lesions visible on T2∗-weighted images, although these can also occur in glioma and metastases (especially malignant melanoma) (Raimbault et al. 2014). To complicate things further, lesions containing both radiation damage and tumour commonly occur. Patients with multiple lesions can show a mixed response, which can indicate the presence of pseudoprogression or radiation necrosis. More advanced imaging techniques, follow-up and sometimes histopathological assessment are generally necessary to make the final diagnosis.

3.1.3 Advanced MR Imaging

With *diffusion MR imaging*, ADC values tend to be lower in recurrent tumour compared to radiation necrosis at the group level, likely due to increased cellularity, but at the individual level, these values overlap (Castillo et al.

2001). Comparing ADC measures from the enhancing and non-enhancing areas can be helpful: in case of tumour, the ADC values taken from the non-enhancing area tend to be significantly higher than those from the enhancing area, while in radiation necrosis, ADC values from both enhancing and non-enhancing areas are similar (Raimbault et al. 2014). DTI-derived FA values in enhancing areas tend to be higher in recurrent tumour than in radiation necrosis (Xu et al. 2010).

Perfusion imaging-derived rCBV is commonly assessed as a ratio of the area of interest over the normal appearing white matter (NAWM) in the contralateral hemisphere. In high-grade tumours and metastases, the rCBV ratio is high, whereas in radiation necrosis/pseudoprogression, the rCBV ratio is low. The proposed cut-off value lies between 1.5 and 2.6 (Kong et al. 2011; Sugahara et al. 2000). In about 8% of cases results are false-negative, as tumours can have rCBV ratios <1.5. Radiation necrosis can be safely diagnosed when the ratio is <0.6 (Fig. 5) (Sugahara et al. 2000; Hu et al. 2008). In current clinically used software, it is easy to measure rCBV in multiple regions of interest (ROIs), but the interrater variability is quite large when it comes to deciding ROI size and placement. Other methods for measuring perfusion, such as using a different contrast agent than gadolinium like ferumoxytol and using a different technique such as ASL, are under investigation, showing promising results (Gahramanov et al. 2011; Ozsunar et al. 2010).

MR spectroscopy shows different metabolite concentrations in radiation necrosis from those measured in tumour. Reductions in individual metabolites Cho, Cr and NAA indicate tissue damage and thus radiation necrosis. Favouring tumour are high ratios of Cho/Cr and Cho/NAA and low ratios of NAA/Cr and Lac/Cho. In order to distinguish tumour from radiation necrosis, different cut-off values for these ratios have been proposed: Cho/Cr >1.5–1.8, Cho/NAA >1–1.8 and Lac/Cho <0.75–1.05 (Sundgren 2009; Elias et al. 2011; Nakajima et al. 2009). Single-voxel MR spectroscopy techniques require precise placement of the voxel to be measured. In the presence of mixed tumour and radiation necrosis within the same voxel, tumour signal can be obscured because the metabolite concentration is averaged and then tends to suggest inflammatory changes (Sundgren 2009). Such partial volume effects can be reduced with multivoxel MRS, in which multiple small voxels are placed. It is sometimes also important to look at changes over time, because of certain transient changes in metabolite concentrations: Cho, for instance, can be temporarily increased in radiation necrosis, falsely indicating tumour presence (Nakajima et al. 2009).

A relatively new method of measuring metabolites is *CEST*, which can potentially also be used to distinguish radiation damage from tumour: amide proton transfer (APT), for instance, is found to be increased in tumour tissue (Kogan et al. 2013). CEST studies to date are still scarce and the true clinical value remains to be determined.

3.1.4 PET Imaging

After radiation therapy, [^{18}F]FDG can be used to distinguish radiation necrosis from recurrent glioma. Although different rates of diagnostic accuracy have been reported in the literature, [^{18}F]FDG seems to be less sensitive than amino acid radiotracers with lower inter-observer agreement (Dankbaar et al. 2015; van Laere et al. 2005). However, diagnostic accuracy increases when [^{18}F]FDG is evaluated in combination with MR imaging (Fig. 6) (Santra et al. 2012). *Amino acid* PET radiotracers are useful for the differentiation between treatment related changes and true progression with higher diagnostic accuracy than standard MR imaging (Albert et al. 2016). Recent studies with a larger glioblastoma patient cohort reported a diagnostic accuracy of FET PET of at least 85% for differentiating both typical (within 12 weeks) and late (> 12 weeks) pseudoprogression after radiochemotherapy completion from true tumour progression (Fig. 1) (Galldiks et al. 2017b).

Pseudoprogression after immunotherapy has been reported using [^{18}F]FET PET in a small retrospective pilot study in patients with malignant melanoma brain metastasis treated with ipilimumab or nivolumab (Kebir et al. 2016).

TBR, uptake kinetics and tumour volumes using [^{18}F]FET PET have been evaluated for their

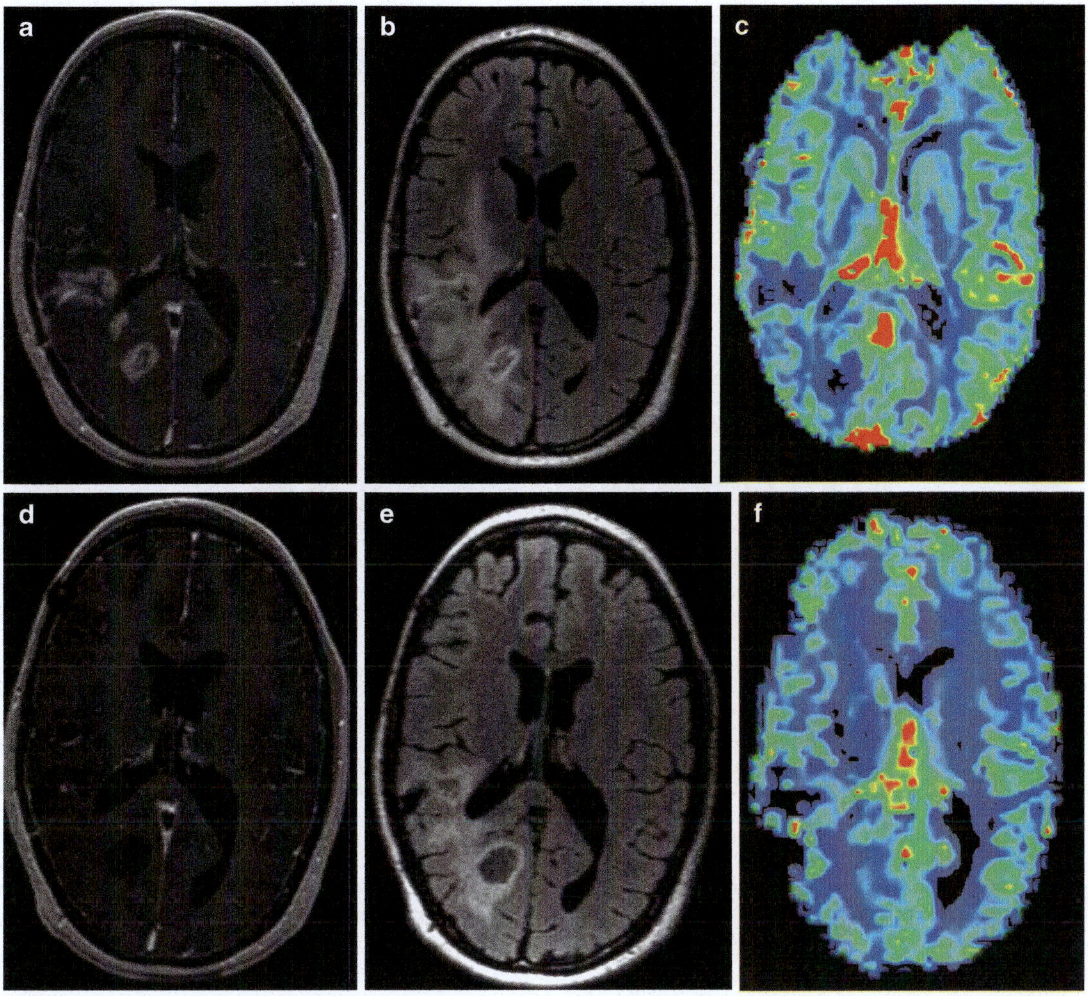

Fig. 5 T1w post-contrast, FLAIR and DSC-perfusion rCBV maps in a glioblastoma patient with new enhancing lesions (**a**) and surrounding oedema (**b**) after prior treatment by the Stupp protocol. The rCBV map (**c**) shows low perfusion in the enhancing areas. The patient was enrolled in a clinical trial and treated with both bevacizumab and lomustine. At 6 weeks' follow-up, the enhancement had disappeared (**d**) and the surrounding oedema was decreased (**e**). A small artefact is present on the rCBV map (**f**), but there is no evidence of increase in perfusion

value in monitoring stereotactic brachytherapy using iodine-125 seeds (Jansen et al. 2013). [^{18}F] FET PET correctly differentiated with a high diagnostic accuracy late posttherapeutic effects after 6 months from local tumour progression in patients with recurrent high-grade glioma.

3.1.5 Comparison/Combination of Methods

Perfusion-derived and PET-derived measures are considered the most reliable when it comes to discerning tumour from radiation necrosis. ASL may be preferable over DSC perfusion imaging because it does not suffer from T1 leakage effects and it allows for quantitative measurement of CBF (Ozsunar et al. 2010).

In clinical practice a combination of MR imaging sequences is used and they can be complementary. When the diagnosis is unclear based on MR imaging alone, PET imaging can be considered. An ideal situation would be to use multimodality PET/MR imaging. Information on tissue perfusion, cellularity, integrity of neurons, anaerobic glycolysis during hypoxia, status of cellular membranes and metabolic pathways can then be acquired in one setting (Ferda et al. 2017).

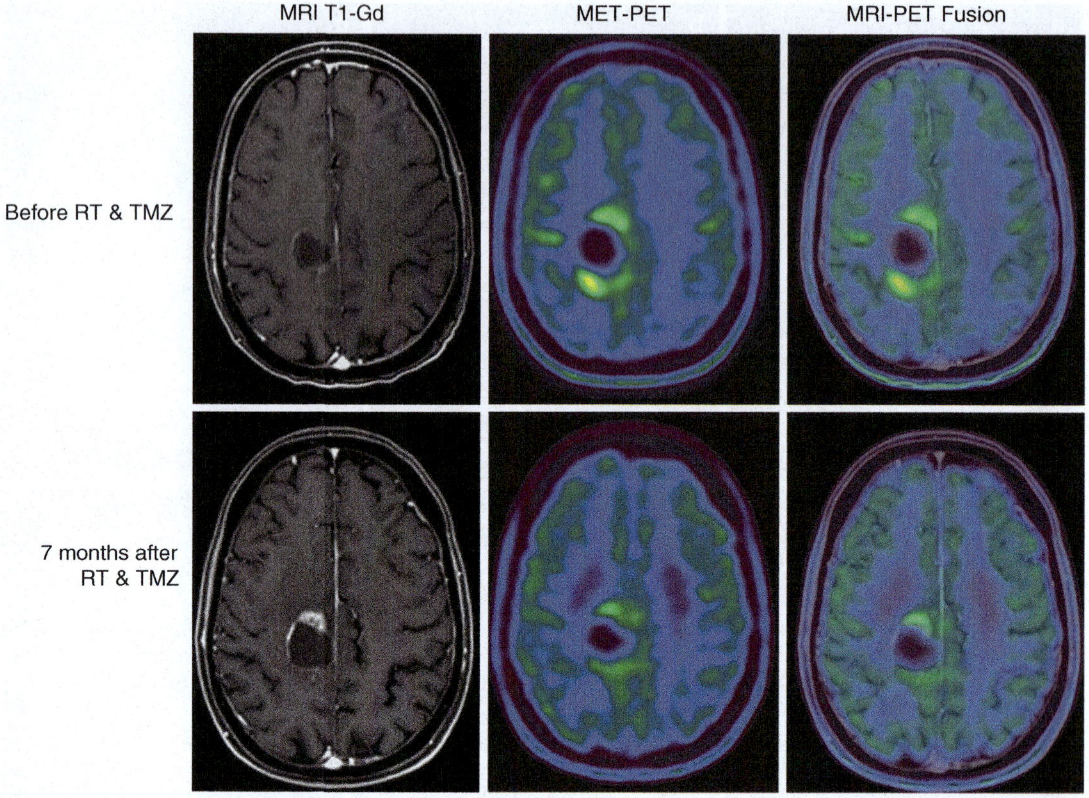

Fig. 6 Patient with GBM studied with MRI and ^{11}C-MET PET/CT before and after treatment (radiotherapy with concomitant temozolomide and additional six cycles of temozolomide). In the posttreatment studies, an area of contrast enhancement on the T1w MR imaging sequence is observed in the anterior part of the cavity; on the PET/CT study, there is only mild ^{11}C-MET uptake (TBR = 1.7; significantly lower than initial residual tumour with TBR = 2.6), consistent with radiation necrosis

3.2 Angiogenesis Inhibitors and Pseudoresponse

Angiogenesis inhibitors, such as the VEGF inhibitor bevacizumab, are now used in a variety of tumours including (recurrent) glioblastoma and meningioma. In addition, bevacizumab is now used to alleviate oedema surrounding the tumour, but also oedema due to radiation necrosis. Due to vascular normalisation, 'leaky' tumour vasculature is normalised and new vessel growth is inhibited. This not only reduces oedema but also reduces or even completely resolves tumour enhancement. This phenomenon is known as pseudoresponse because the tumour may still be present (Brandsma and van den Bent 2009). The use of bevacizumab in glioblastoma has led to increased reports of infiltrative tumour growth at recurrence (Norden et al. 2008). In grade II and III meningiomas, bevacizumab treatment is sometimes used when surgical and radiation therapy is no longer possible or effective. The best response appears to be stable disease (Nayak et al. 2012).

With radiation necrosis it is already difficult to distinguish from residual or recurrent tumour. Thus, the addition of angiogenesis inhibitors further complicates image interpretation as it can mask the tumour as well as reduce radiation necrosis effects. Varying or mixed response to the treatment between patients further plays a confounding role (Gonzalez et al. 2007; Sanborn et al. 2011). In the context of treatment for radiation necrosis, patients responding to bevacizumab treatment only infrequently show recurrence or progression of radiation necrosis after discontinuation (Levin et al. 2011).

3.2.1 PET Imaging

The problem of accurately identifying non-enhancing tumour (pseudoresponse) has been investigated using amino acid PET to assess treatment response to antiangiogenic therapy (Reithmeier et al. 2013). Recent studies and case reports indicate that [^{18}F]FET and [^{18}F]FDOPA PET are useful in the context of pseudoresponse both detecting and ruling out the presence of tumour (Galldiks et al. 2017b). [^{18}F]FET and [^{18}F]FDOPA PET have also been used to predict a favourable outcome in responders to bevacizumab (Galldiks et al. 2017b).

A cost-effectiveness analysis of [^{18}F]FET PET for therapy monitoring of antiangiogenic therapy suggests that the combined use of MR imaging and [^{18}F]FET PET in the management of these patients has the potential to avoid overtreatment and corresponding costs, as well as unnecessary patient side effect (Heinzel et al. 2013).

3.3 Late Effects of Radiotherapy

In addition to radiation necrosis, radiotherapy has other late effects on the brain parenchyma, including demyelination, vascular abnormalities and atrophy. Radiation-induced tumours and malignant transformation have also been reported (Martino et al. 2014; Johannesen et al. 2003). The extent of these effects is related to total radiation dose, field size, number of fractions and frequency, chemotherapy and other medication (methotrexate, corticosteroids, antiepileptic drugs), patient survival and age at the time of radiation therapy (Martino et al. 2014).

3.3.1 White Matter Abnormalities

White matter is rich in glial cells, such as oligodendrocytes, which are more sensitive to radiation than neurons (Sundgren 2009). White matter damage is a common finding in irradiated patients and includes reactive gliosis, inflammation, oedema, demyelination, atrophy, coagulative necrosis, cavitation/cysts and calcification (Martino et al. 2014; Schultheiss et al. 1995). These different entities are difficult to distinguish on histological data and practically impossible to differentiate with MR imaging. White matter damage is visible as atrophy and/or T2w/FLAIR hyperintensity, also known as leukoencephalopathy (Martino et al. 2014; Chan et al. 1999). The damage can be limited to small discrete lesions or there can be large confluent areas.

Radiation-induced damage to the white matter starts to appear on T2w/FLAIR images just months after treatment and is generally more severe in older patients (Johannesen et al. 2003). Areas with limited blood supply, such as the periventricular white matter, are affected more than, for instance, the arcuate fasciculus which also receives cortical arterial supply (Raimbault et al. 2014; Kumar et al. 2000). Before abnormalities are visible on the T2w/FLAIR images, DTI can already pick up changes in white matter, using parameters such as MD, FA and diffusivity perpendicular and parallel to the white matter fibres (Nagesh et al. 2008). It has been postulated that some of these observed changes may be reversible (Tsui et al. 2001).

3.3.2 Grey Matter Abnormalities

Because neurons are less sensitive to radiation than glial cells, the grey matter is generally less affected than white matter. Effects that occur are cortical thinning, irregularity within the cortex (visible as T2w hyperintensity) and blurring of the grey-white matter junction (Chan et al. 1999; Seibert et al. 2017). Both grey and white matter damage can result in cognitive decline with deficits in learning, working memory and executive functions. Symptoms are more prominent when specific areas, such as the hippocampus and corpus callosum, are damaged (Saad and Wang 2015).

3.3.3 Vascular Changes

Direct damage to endothelial cells leads to an increase in permeability, vasogenic oedema, ischaemia and hypoxia. Complications that develop after 4 months include lacunar infarcts, microbleeds, large-vessel occlusions with moyamoya syndrome, (capillary) telangiectasias, cavernomas (Fig. 7) and stroke (Brandsma et al. 2008).

A rare late complication after radiotherapy is the so-called SMART syndrome: stroke-like migraine attacks after radiation therapy (Fig. 8).

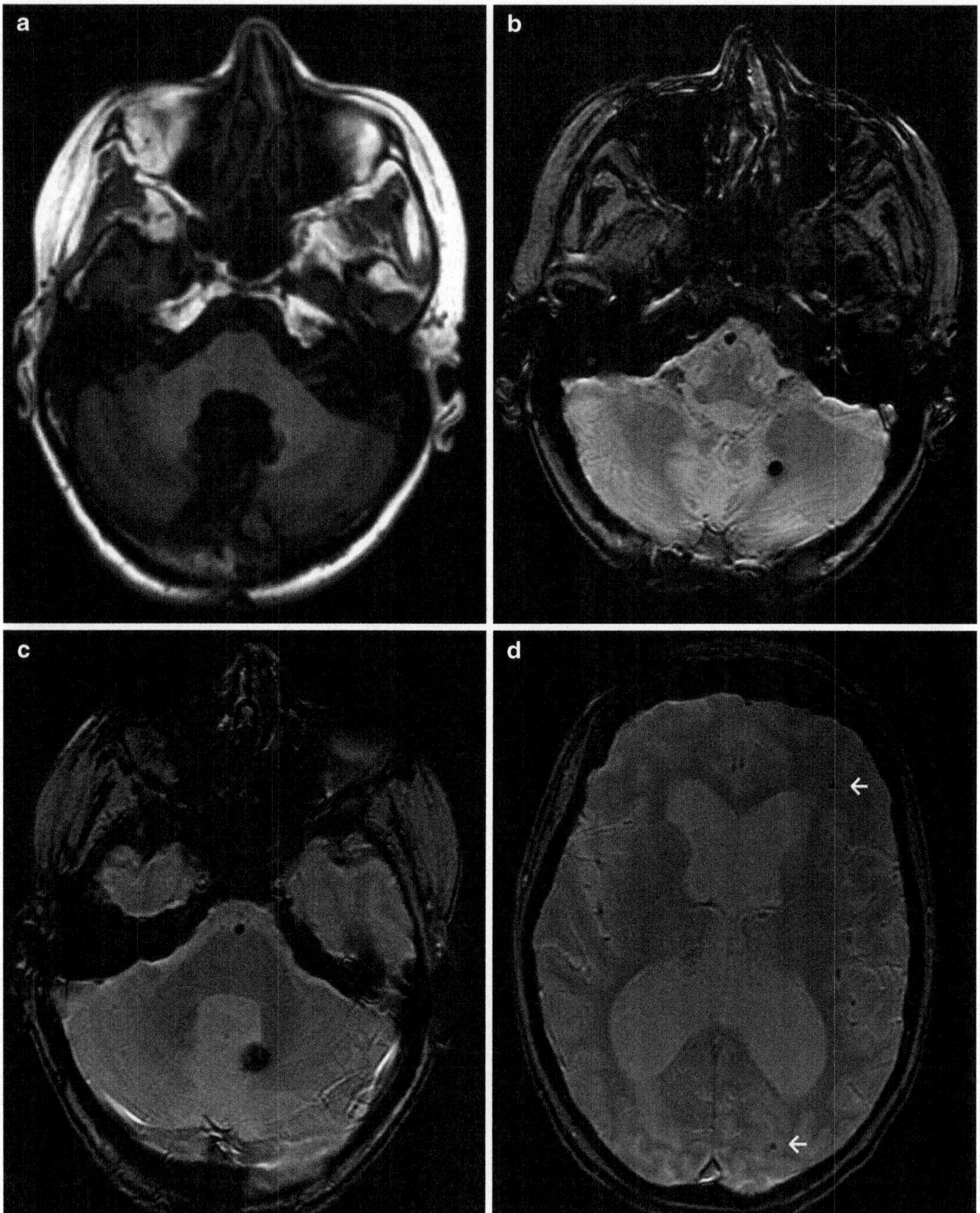

Fig. 7 35-year-old woman treated for medulloblastoma 14 years ago. After subtotal resection, the tumour was irradiated (57.5 Gy) and there has been no recurrent disease. T1w image shows postoperative effects in the posterior fossa (**a**). The T2∗ (gradient echo) sequence shows multiple lesions with signal loss infra- and supratentorially (**b–d**), consistent with cavernomas

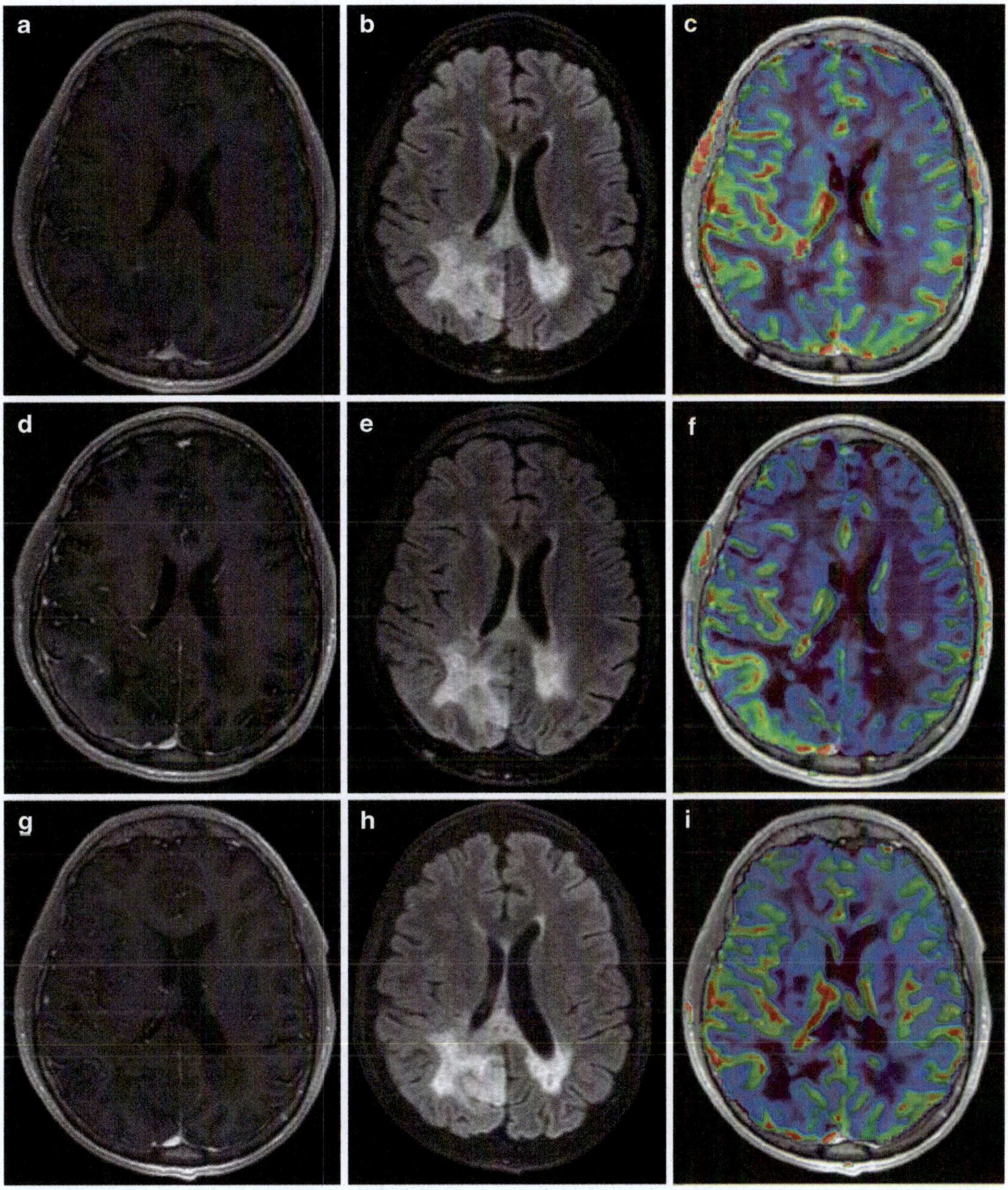

Fig. 8 43-year-old male with oligodendroglioma initially treated with radiotherapy (50.4 Gy) 6 years before and with chemotherapy at progression 4 years later. T1w post-contrast (**a**), FLAIR (**b**) and rCBV (**c**) after therapy show stable residual abnormalities. The patient subsequently developed headaches and disorientation. On the T1w post-contrast image, there is enhancement of the cortex (**d**) adjacent to the FLAIR hyperintense area (**e**). rCBV is increased in the enhancing area (**f**). At 2 months' follow-up, imaging findings had regressed (**g**–**i**). Symptoms and imaging findings were consistent with SMART syndrome

Patients have transient clinical symptoms and radiological findings suggestive of tumour recurrence such as unilateral enhancement of the cortex and T2w hyperintense white matter. The posterior regions of the brain are predominantly involved. The effects are reversible (Zheng et al. 2015).

3.3.4 Radiation-Induced Tumours and Malignant Transformation

A radiation-induced tumour is a new tumour that grows within the radiation field and different histology from the original tumour. Tumours most often encountered are meningiomas, followed by glioma and sarcoma (Martino et al. 2014; Johannesen et al. 2003). The reported incidence of radiation-induced tumours is 2.6% in irradiated children. In adults however, the incidence is much lower (Martino et al. 2014; Pollock et al. 2017).

Malignant transformation of meningioma due to irradiation is disputed. The reported incidence is 2.2%, but since malignant transformation of meningioma can also occur in the absence of radiotherapy, the true incidence is probably lower. Vestibular schwannoma has been reported to undergo malignant transformation due to radiation therapy in 0.3% of cases (Rogers et al. 2015; Al-Mefty et al. 2004).

3.3.5 PET Imaging

Treatment effects may decrease [^{18}F]FDG uptake in the treatment area as well as in brain regions that receive synaptic input from the treated area.

References

Abrey LE, Batchelor TT, AJM F et al (2005) Report of an International Workshop to standardize baseline evaluation and response criteria for primary CNS lymphoma. J Neuro-Oncol 23(22):5034–5043

Afshar-Oromieh A, Giesel FL, Linhart HG et al (2012) Detection of cranial meningiomas: comparison of (68)Ga-DOTATOC PET/CT and contrast-enhanced MRI. Eur J Nucl Med Mol Imag 39(9):1409–1415

Aki T, Nakayama N, Yonezawa S et al (2012) Evaluation of brain tumors using dynamic 11C-methionine-PET. J Neuro-Oncol 109:115–122

Albert NL, Weller M, Suchorska B, Galldiks N, Soffietti R, Kim MM et al (2016) Response assessment in Neuro-oncology working group and European Association for Neuro-Oncology recommendations for the clinical use of PET imaging in gliomas. Neuro-Oncology 18:1199–1208

Alexiou GA, Gogou P, Markoula S, Kyritsis AP (2010) Management of meningiomas. Clin Neurol Neurosurg 112:117–182

Al-Mefty O, Kadri PA, Pravdenkova S, Sawyer JR, Stangeby C, Husain M (2004) Malignant progression in meningioma: documentation of a series and analysis of cytogenetic findings. J Neurosurg 101:210–218

Awde AR, Boisgard R, Theze B et al (2013) The translocator protein radioligand 18F-DPA-714 monitors antitumor effect of erufosine in a rat 9L intracranial glioma model. J Nucl Med 54:2125–2131

Belohlavek O, Simonová G, Kantorova I et al (2003) Brain metastases after stereotactic radiosurgery using the Leksell gamma knife: can FDG PET help to differentiate radionecrosis from tumour progression? Eur J Nucl Med Mol Imag 30:96–100

van den Bent MJ, Wefel JS, Schiff D et al (2011) Response assessment in neuro-oncology (a report of the RANO group): assessment of outcome in trials of diffuse low-grade gliomas. Lancet Oncol 12:583–593

Bergström M, Collins V, Ehrin E, Ericson K et al (1983) Discrepancies in brain tumor extent as shown by computed tomography and positron emission tomography using [68Ga]EDTA, [11C]glucose, and [11C]methionine. J Comput Assist Tomogr 7:1062–1066

Brandsma D, van den Bent MJ (2009) Pseudoprogression and pseudoresponse in the treatment of gliomas. Curr Opin Neurol 22(6):633–638

Brandsma D, Stalpers L, Taal W, Sminia P, van den Bent MJ (2008) Clinical features, mechanisms, and management of pseudoprogression in malignant gliomas. Lancet Oncol 9:453–461

Calcagni ML, Galli G, Giordano A et al (2011) Dynamic O-(2-[18F]fluorethyl)-L-tyrosine (F-18 FET) PET for glioma grading: assessment of individual probability of malignancy. Clin Nucl Med 36:841–847

Castillo M, Smith J, Kwock L, Wilber K (2001) Apparent diffusion coefficient in the evaluation of high-grade cerebral gliomas. AJNR Am J Neuroradiol 22:60–64

Cebeci H, Aydin O, Ozturk-Isik E et al (2014) Assessment of perfusion in glial tumors with arterial spin labeling: comparison with dynamic susceptibility contrast method. Eur J Radiol 83:1914–1919

Ceccon G, Lohmann P, Stoffels G et al (2017) Dynamic O-(2-18F-fluoroethyl)-L-tyrosine positron emission tomography differentiates brain metastasis recurrence from radiation injury after radiotherapy. Neuro-Oncology 19:281–288

Chalmers AJ, Ruff EM, Martindale C, Lovegrove N, Short SC (2009) Cytotoxic effects of temozolomide and radiation are additive- and schedule-dependent. Int J Radiat Oncol Biol Phys 75(5):1511–1519

Chan Y, Leung S, King AD et al (1999) Late radiation injury to the temporal lobes: morphologic evaluation at MR imaging. Radiology 213:800–807

Chang JH, Chang JW, Choi JY, Park YG, Chung SS (2003) Complications after gamma knife radiosurgery for benign meningiomas. J Neurol Neurosurg Psychiatry 74:226–230

Charnley N, West CM, Barnett CM et al (2006) Early change in glucose metablic rate measured using FDG-PET in patients with high-grade glioma predicts response to temozolomide but not temozolomide plus radiotherapy. Int J Radiat Oncol Biol Phys 66:331–338

Chen W, Delaloye S, Silverman DH, Geist C et al (2007) Predicting treatment response of malignant gliomas to bevacizumab and irinotecan by imaging proliferation with [18F] fluorothymidine positron emission tomography: a pilot study. J Clin Oncol 25:4714–4721

Colavolpe C, Colavolpe C, Metellus P, Mancini J et al (2012) FDG-PET predicts survival in recurrent high-grade gliomas treated with bevacizumab and irinotecan. Neuro-Oncology 14:649–657

Cremerius U, Bares R, Weis J et al (1997) Fasting improves discriminatio of grade 1 and atypical or malignant meningioma in FDG-PET. J Nucl Med 38(1):26–30

Dankbaar JW, Snijders TJ, Robe PA et al (2015) The use of 18F-FDG PET to differentiate progressive disease from treatment induced necrosis in high grade glioma. J Neuro-Oncol 125:167–175

Dunet V, Pomoni A, Hottinger A et al (2016) Performance of 18F-FET versus 18F-FDG-PET for the diagnosis and grading of brain tumors: systematic review and meta-analysis. Neuro-Oncology 18:426–434

Dutour A, Kumar U, Panetta R et al (1998) Expression of somatostatin receptor subtypes in human brain tumors. Int J Cancer 76:620–627

Elias AE, Carlos RC, Smith EA et al (2011) MR spectroscopy using normalized and non-normalized metabolite ratios for differentiating recurrent brain tumor from radiation injury. Acad Radiol 18:1101–1108

Ferda J, Ferdová E, Hes O et al (2017) PET/MRI: multiparametric imaging of brain tumors. Eur J Radiol 94:A14–A25

Fuss M, Wenz F, Scholdei R et al (2000) Radiation-induced regional cerebral blood volume (rCBV) changes in normal brain and low-grade astrocytomas: quantification and time and dose-dependent occurence. Int J Radiat Oncol Biol Phys 48(1):53–58

Gabeau-Lacet D, Aghi M, Betensky RA et al (2009) Bone involvement predicts poor outcome in atypical meningioma. J Neurosurg 111:464–471

Gahramanov S, Raslan AM, Muldoon LL et al (2011) Potential for differentiation of pseudo-progression from true tumor progression with dynamic susceptibility-weighted contrast-enhanced magnetic resonance imaging using ferumoxytol vs. gadoteridol: a pilot study. Int J Radiat Oncol Biol Phys 79(2):514–523

Galldiks N, Kracht LW, Burghaus L et al (2006) Use of (11)C-methionine PET to monitor the effects of temozolomide chemotherapy in malignant gliomas. Eur J Nucl Med Mol Imag 33:516–524

Galldiks N, Langen KJ, Holy R et al (2012) Assessment of treatment response in patients with glioblastoma using [18F]Fluoroethyl-L-Tyrosine PET in comparison to MRI. J Nucl Med 53:1048–1057

Galldiks N, Rapp M, Stoffels G et al (2013) Response assessment of bevacizumab in patients with recurrent malignant glioma using [18F]fluoroethyl-L-tyrosine PET in comparison to MRI. Eur J Nucl Med Mol Imag 40:22–23

Galldiks N, Albert N, Sommerauer M, Grosu AL et al (2017a) PET imaging in patients with meningioma—report of the RANO/PET group. Neuro Oncol. https://doi.org/10.1093/neuonc/nox112. [Epub ahead of print]

Galldiks N, Langen KJ, Pope WB et al (2017b) The use of amino acid PET and conventrional MRI for monitoring of brain tumor therapy. NeuroImage Clin 13:386–394

Galldiks N et al (2019) Neuro-Oncology 21(5):585–595. https://doi.org/10.1093/neuonc/noz003

Gomez-Rio M, Testart Dardel N, Santiago Chincilla A et al (2015) 18F-Fluorocholine PET/CT as a complementary tool in the follow-up of low-grade glioma: diagnostic accuracy and clinical utility. Eur J Nucl Med Mol Imag 42(6):886–895

Gonzalez J, Kumar AJ, Conrad CA, Levin VA (2007) Effect of bevacizumab on radiation necrosis of the brain. Int J Radiat Oncol Biol Phys 67(2):323–326

Haldorsen IS, Espeland A, Larsson E-M (2011) Central nervous system lymphoma: characteristic findings on traditional and advanced imaging. AJNR 32:984–992

Heinzel A, Müller D, Langen KJ et al (2013) The use of O-(2-18F-fluoroethyl)-L-tyrosine PET for treatment management of bevacizumab and irinotecan in patients with recurrent high-grade glioma: a cost-effectiveness analysis. J Nucl Med 54:1217–1222

Herholz K, Langen KJ, Schiepers C, Mountz JM (2012) Brain tumors. Semin Nucl Med 42:356–370

Hoffman JM, Waskin HA, Schifter T et al (1993) FDG-PET in differentiating lymphoma from non malignant central nervous system lesions in patients with AIDS. J Nucl Med 34:567–575

Horská A, Barker PB (2010) Imaging of brain tumors: MR spectroscopy and metabolic imaging. Neuroimaging Clin N Am 20(3):293–310

Hu LS, Baxter LC, Smith KA et al (2008) Relative cerebral blood volume values to differentiate high-grade glioma recurrence from posttreatment radiation effect: direct correlation between image-guided tissue histopathology and localized dynamic susceptibility-weighted contrast-enhanced perfusion MR imaging measurements. AJNR Am J Neuroradiol 30(3):552–558

Inoue T, Ogasawara K, Beppu T et al (2005) iffusion tensor imaging for preoperative evaluation of tumor grades in gliomas. Clin Neurol Neurosurg 107:174–180

Jansen NL, Suchorska B, Schwarz SB et al (2013) [18] fluoroethyltyrosine-positron emission tomography-based threapy monitoring after stereotactic iodine-125 brachytherapy in patients with recurrent high-grade glioma. Mol Imaging 12:137–147

Johannesen TB, Lien HH, Hole KH, Lote K (2003) Radiological and clinical assessment of long-term brain tumour survivors after radiotherapy. Radiother Oncol 69:169–176

Kawai N, Miyake K, Yamamoto Y, Nishiyama Y, Tamiya T (2013) 18F-FDG PET in the diagnosis and treatment of primary central nervous system lymphoma. Biomed Res Int 2013:247152

Kawase Y, Yamamoto Y, Kameyama R et al (2011) Comparison of 11C-methionine PET and 18F-FDG PET in patients with primary central nervous system lyphoma. Mol Imaging Biol 13(6):1284–1289

Kebir S, Rauschenbach L, Galldiks N et al (2016) Dynamic O-(2-[18F]fluoroethyl)-L-tyrosine PET imaging for the detection of checkpoint inhibitor-related pseudoprogression in melanoma brain metastases. Neuro-Oncology 18:1462–1464

Kessler RA, Garzon-Muvdi T, Yang W, Weingart J, Olivi A, Huang J, Brem H, Lim M (2017) Metastatic atypical and anaplastic meningioma: a case series and review of the literature. World Neurosurg 101:47–56

Kogan F, Hariharan H, Reddy R (2013) Chemical exchange saturation transfer (CEST) imaging: description of technique and potential clinical applications. Curr Radiol Rep 1:102–114

Kong D-S, Kim ST, Kim E-H et al (2011) Diagnostic dilemma of pseudoprogression in the treatment of newly diagnosed glioblastomas: the role of assesing relative cerebral blood flow volume and oxygen-6-methylguanine-DNA methyltransferase promoter methylation status. AJNR Am J Neuroradiol 32:382

Kumar AJ, Leeds N, Fuller GN et al (2000) Malignant gliomas: MR imaging spectrum of radiation therapy- and chemotherapy-induced necrosis of the brain after treatment. Radiology 217:377–384

Kunz WG, Jungblut LM, Kazmierczak PM et al (2017) Improved detection of transosseous meningiomas using 68Ga-DOTATATE PET-CT compared to contrast-enhanced MRI. J Nucl Med 58:1580

van Laere K, Ceyssens S, van Calenbergh F et al (2005) Direct comparison of 18F-FDG and 11C-methionine PET in suspected recurrence of glioma: sensitivity, inter-observer variability and prognostic value. Eur J Nucl Med Mol Imag 32(1):39–51

Langen KJ, Watts C (2016) Neuro-oncology: amino acid PET for brain tumors—ready for the clinic? Nat Rev Neurol 12:375–376

Lee ST, Scott AM (2007) Hypoxia positron emission tomography imaging with 18f-fluoromisonidazole. Semin Nucl Med 37:451–461

Lee SR, Yang KA, Kim SK, Kim S-H (2012) Radiation-induced intratumoral necrosis and peritumoral edema after gamma knife radiosurgery for intracranial meningiomas. J Korean Neurosurg Soc 52(2):98–102

Leeman JE, Clumpa DA, Flickinger JC et al (2013) Extent of perilesional edema differentiates radionecrosis from tumor recurrence following stereotactic radiosurgery for brain metastases. Neuro-Oncology 15(12):1732–1738

Levin VA, Bidaut L, Hou P et al (2011) Randomized double-blind placebo-controlled trial of bevacizumab therapy for radiation necrosis of the central nervous system. Int J Radiat Oncol Biol Phys 79(5): 1487–1495

Lin NU, Lee EQ, Aoyama H et al (2013) Challenges relating to solid tumour brain metastases in clinical trials, part 1: patient population, response, and progression. A report from the RANO group. Lancet Oncol 14:e396–e406

Lin NU, Lee EQ, Aoyama H et al (2015) Response assessment criteria for brain metastases: proposal from the RANO group. Lancet Oncol 16:270–278

Lippitz B, Lindquist C, Paddick I et al (2014) Stereotactic radiosrugery in the treatment of brain metastases: the current evidence. Cancer Treat Rev 40:48–59

Louis DN, Perry A, Reifenberger G et al (2016) The 2016 World Health Organization classification of tumors of the central nervous system: a summary. Acta Neuropathol 131:803

Macdonald D, Cascino TL, Schold SJ et al (1990) Response criteria for phase II studies of supratentorial malignant glioma. J Clin Oncol 8:1277–1280

Makino K, Hirai T, Nakamura H et al (2011) Does adding FDG-PET to MRI improve the differentiation between primary cerebral lymphoma and glioblastoma? Observer performance study. Ann Nucl Med 25:432–438

Martino A, Krainik A, Pasteris C et al (2014) Neurological imaging of brain damages after radiotherapy and/or chimiotherapy. J Neuroradiol 41:52–70

Mertens K, Acou M, van Hauwe J et al (2013) Validation of 18F-FDG-PET at conventional and delayed intervals for the discrimination of high-grade from low-grade gliomas: a stereotactic PET and MRI study. Clin Nucl Med 38:495–500

Nagesh V, Tsien CI, Chenevert TL et al (2008) Radiation-induced changes in normal-appearing white matter in patients with cerebral tumors: a diffusion tensor imaging study. Int J Radiat Oncol Biol Phys 70(4):1002–1010

Nakajima T, Kumabe T, Kanamori M et al (2009) Differential diagnosis between radiation necrosis and glioma progression using sequential proton magnetic resonance spectroscopy and methionine positron emission tomography. Neurol Med Chir (Tokyo) 49:394–401

Nayak L, Iwamoto FM, Rudnick JD et al (2012) Atypical and anaplastic meningiomas treated with bevacizumab. J Neurooncol 109:187–193

van Nifterik KA, van den Berg J, Stalpers LJA et al (2007) Differential radiosensitizing potential of temozolomide in MGMT promoter methylated glioblastoma multiforme cell lines. Int J Radiat Oncol Biol Phys 69(4):1246–1253

Norden AD, Young GS, Setayesh K et al (2008) Bevacizumab for recurrent malignant gliomas: efficacy, toxicity, and patterns of recurrence. Neurology 70(10):779–787

Nowak A, Dziedzic T, Krych P et al (2015) Benign versus atyptical meningiomas: risk factors predicting recurrence. Neurol Neurochir Pol 49:1–10

Nussbaum ES, Djalilian HR, Cho KH, Hall WA (1996) Brain metastases: histology, multiplicity, surgery and survival. Cancer 78(8):1781–1788

Ozsunar Y, Mullins ME, Kwong K et al (2010) Glioma recurrence versus radiation necrosis? A pilot comparison of arterial spin-labeled, dynamic susceptibility contrast enhanced MRI, and FDG-PET imaging. Acad Radiol 17:282–290

Paulson ES, Schmainda KM (2008) Comparison of dynamic susceptibility-weighted contrast-enhanced MR methods: recommendations for measuring relative cerebral blood volume in brain tumors. Radiology 249(2):601–613

Peca C, Pacelli R, Elefante A et al (2009) Early clinical and neuroradiological worsening after radiotherapy and concomitant temozolomide in patients with glioblastoma: tumor progression or radionecrosis? Clin Neurol Neurosurg 11:331–334

Petr J, Platzek I, Seidlitz A et al (2015) Early and late effects of radiochemotherapy on cerebral blood flow in glioblastoma patients measured with non-invasive perfusion MRI. Radiother Oncol 118:24–28

Piroth MD, Pinkawa M, Holy R et al (2011) Prognostic value of early [18F]fluoroethyltyrosine positron emission tomography after radiochemotherapy in glioblastoma multiforme. Int J Radiat Oncol Biol Phys 80:176–184

Pollock BE, Link MJ, Stafford SL, Parney IF, Garces YI, Foote RL (2017) The risk of radiation-induced tumors or malignant transformation after single fraction intracranial radiosurgery: results based on a 25-year experience. Int J Radiat Oncol Biol Phys 97(5):919–923

Prigent-Le Jeune F, Dubois F, Perez S, Blond S, Steinling M (2004) Technetium-99m sestamibi brain SPECT in the follow-up of glioma for evaluation of response to chemotherapy: first results. Eur J Nucl Med Mol Imag 31:714–719

Quant EC, Wen PY (2011) Response assessment in neuro-oncology. Curr Oncol Rep 13(1):50–56

Rachinger W, Stoecklein VM, Terpolilli NA et al (2015) Increased 68Ga-DOTATATE uptake in PET imaging discriminates meningioma and tumor-free tissue. J Nucl Med 56:347–353

Raimbault A, Cazals X, Lauvin M-A et al (2014) Radionecrosis of malignant glioma and cerebral metastases: a diagnostic challenge in MRI. Diagn Interv Imaging 95:985–1000

Reithmeier T, Lopez WO, Spehl TS et al (2013) Bevacizumab as salvage therapy for progressive brain stem gliomas. Clin Neurol Neurosurg 115:165–169

Roelcke U, Wyss MT, Nowosielski M et al (2016) Amino acid positron emission tomography to monitor chemotherapy response and predict seizure control and progression-free survival in WHO grade II gliomas. Neuro-Oncology 18:744–751

Rogers L, Barani I, Chamberlain M et al (2015) Meningiomas: knowledge base, treatment outcomes, and uncertainties. A RANO review. J Neurosurg 122(4):4–23

Rottenburger C, Hentschel M, Kelly T et al (2011) Comparison of C-11 methionine and C-11 choline for PET imaging of brain metastases: a prospective pilot study. Clin Nucl Med 36:639–642

Ryttlefors M, Danfors T, Latini F, Montelius A et al (2016) Long-term evaluation of the effect of hypofractionated high-energy proton treatment of benign meningiomas by means of (11)C-L-methionine positrion emission tomography. Eur J Nucl Med Mol Imag 43:1432–1443

Saad S, Wang TJ (2015) Neurocognitive deficits after radiation therapy for brain malignancies. Am J Clin Oncol 38:634–640

Sanborn MR, Danish SF, Rosenfeld MR et al (2011) Treatment of steroid refractory, gamma knife related radiation necrosis with bevacizumab: case report and review of the literature. Clin Neurol Neurosurg 113:798–802

Santra A, Kumar R, Sharma P et al (2012) F-18 FDG PET-CT in patients with recurrent glioma: comparison with contrast-enhanced MRI. Eur J Radiol 81:508–513

Sathekge M, Goethals I, Maes A, van de Wiele C (2009) Positron emission tomography in patients suffering from HIV-1 infection. Eur J Nucl Med Mol Imag 36:1176–1184

Schultheiss TE, Kun LE, Ang KK, Stephens LC (1995) Radiation response to the central nervous system. Int J Radiat Oncol Biol Phys 31(5):1093–1112

Schwarzenberg J, Czernin J, Cloughesy TF et al (2014) Treatment response evaluation using 18F-FDOPA PET in patients with recurrent malignant glioma on bevacizumab therapy. Clin Cancer Res 20:3550–3559

Seibert TM, Karunamuni R, Kaifi S et al (2017) Cerebral cortex regions selectively vulnerable to radiation dose-dependent atrophy. Int J Radiat Oncol Biol Phys 97(5):910–918

Shim WH, Kim HS, Choi CG, Kim SJ (2015) Comparison of apparent diffusion coefficient and intravoxel inco herent motion for differentiating among glioblastoma, metastasis, and lymphoma focusing on diffusion-related parameter. PLoS One 10(7):e0134761

Soares JM, Marques P, Alves V, Sousa N (2013) A Hitchhiker's guide to diffusion tensor imaging. Front Neurosci **7**:31

Spence AM, Muzi M, Swanson KR, O'Sullivan F et al (2008) Regional hypoxia in glioblastoma multiforme quantified with [18F]fluoromisonidazole positron emission tomography before radiotherapy: correlation with time to progression and survival. Clin Cancer Res 14:2623–2630

Stupp R, Brada M, van den Bent MJ, Tonn J-C (2014) High-grade glioma: ESMO Clinical Practice Guidelines for diagnosis, treatment and follow-up. Ann Oncol 25(Suppl 3):iii93–iii101

Su Z, Roncaroli F, Durrenberger PF et al (2015) Mitochondrial translocator protein in human gliomas: a 11C-(R)PK11195 PET imaging and neuropathology study. J Nucl Med 56:512–517

Suchorska B, Jansen NL, Linn J et al (2015) Biological tumor volume in 18FET-PET before radiochemotherapy correlates with survival in GBM. Neurology 84:710–719

Sugahara T, Korogi Y, Tomiguchi S et al (2000) Posttherapeutic intraaxial brain tumor: the value of perfusion-sensitive contrast-enhanced MR imaging for differentiating tumor recurrence from nonneoplastic contrast-enhancing tissue. AJNR Am J Neuroradiol 21:901–909

Sugo N, Yokota K, Kondo K et al (2006) Early dynamic 201TI SPECT in the evaluation of brain tumours. Nucl Med Commun 27(2):143–149

Sundgren P (2009) MR spectroscopy in radiation injury. AJNR Am J Neuroradiol 30:1469–1476

Symms M, Jäger HR, Schmierer K, Yousry TA (2004) A review of structural magnetic resonance neuroimaging. J Neurol Neurosurg Psychiatry 75:1235–1244

Tsien C, Cao Y, Chenevert T (2014) Clinical applicatiosn for diffusion magnetic resonance imaging in radiotherapy. Semin Radiat Oncol 24(3):218–226

Tsui EY, Chan JH, Ramsey RG et al (2001) Late temporal lobe necrosis in patients with nasopharyngeal carcinoma: evaluation with combined multi-section diffusion weighted and perfusion weighted MR imaging. Eur J Radiol 39:133–138

Varrone A, Asenbaum S, van der Borght T, Booij J, Nobili F, Nagren K et al (2009) EANM procedure guidelines for PET brain imaging using [18F]FDG, version 2. Eur J Nucl Med Mol Imag 36(12):2103–2110

Voges J, Herholz K, Holzer T et al (1997) 11C-Methionine and 18F-2-Fluorodeoxy-glucose positron emission tomography: a tool for diagnosis of cerebral glioma and monitoring after brachytherapy with 125I seeds. Stereotact Funct Neurosurg 69:1–4

Walecki J, Sokol M, Pieniazek P et al (1999) Role of short TE 1H-MR spectroscopy in monitoring of post-operation irradiated patients. Eur J Radiol 30:154–161

Wardak M, Schiepers C, Gloughesy TF et al (2014) 18F-FLT and 18F-FDOPA PET kinetics in recurrent brain tumors. Eur J Nucl Med Mol Imag 41:1199–1209

Wen PY, Macdonald DR, Reardon DA et al (2010) Updated response assessment criteria for high-grade gliomas: response assesment in neuro-oncology working group. J Clin Oncol 28(11):1963–1972

van West SE, de Bruin HG, van de Langerijt B, Swaak-Kragten AT, van den Bent MJ, Taal W (2017) Incidence of pseudoprogression in low-grade gliomas treated with radiotherapy. Neuro Oncol 19(5):719–725

Wick W, Chinot OL, Bendszus M, Mason W et al (2016) Evaluation of pseudoprogression rates and tumor progression patterns in a phase III trial of bevacizumab plus radiotherapy/temozolomide for newly diagnosed glioblastoma. Neuro-Oncology 18(10):1434–1441

Wurker M, Herholz K, Voges J et al (1996) Glucose consumption and methionine uptake in low-grade gliomas after iodine-125 brachytherapy. Eur J Nucl Med 23(5):583–586

Wyss M, Hofer S, Bruehlmeier M et al (2009) Early metabolic responses in temozolomide treated low-grade glioma patients. J Neuro-Oncol 95:87–93

Xu J-L, Li Y-L, Lian J-M et al (2010) Distinction between postoperative recurrent glioma and radiation injury using MR diffusion tensor imaging. Neuroradiology 52:1193–1199

Zheng Q, Yang L, Tan L-M, Qin L-X, Wang C-Y, Zhang H-N (2015) Stroke-like migraine attacks after radiation therapy syndrome. Chin Med J (Engl) 128(15):2097–2101

Response Assessment and Follow-Up by Imaging in Head and Neck Tumours

Vincent Vandecaveye, Sandra Nuyts, and Roberto C. Delgado Bolton

Contents

1	**Introduction**	406
2	**Computed Tomography**	407
3	**Magnetic Resonance Imaging**	408
4	**[18F]FDG PET/CT**	411
4.1	Restaging for Detection of Local Recurrence	413
4.2	Restaging for Detection of Metastases	413
4.3	Treatment Response Evaluation	413
5	**Conclusions**	414
References		414

V. Vandecaveye
Department of Radiology, University Hospitals Leuven, Leuven, Belgium
e-mail: vincent.vandecaveye@uzleuven.be

S. Nuyts
Department of Radiation Oncology, University Hospitals Leuven, Leuven, Belgium
e-mail: Sandra.nuyts@uzleuven.be

R. C. Delgado Bolton (✉)
Department of Diagnostic Imaging (Radiology) and Nuclear Medicine, University Hospital San Pedro and Centre for Biomedical Research of La Rioja (CIBIR), Logroño (La Rioja), Spain
e-mail: rcdelgado@riojasalud.es

Abstract

Accurate and timely response assessment and follow-up by imaging are pivotal for guiding radiotherapeutic management of head and neck cancer. Primarily, post-treatment imaging should aim to detect tumour recurrence as early as possible in order to maximize success of salvage surgery and determine the need for neck dissection. Second, post-treatment imaging has a pivotal role in the differentiation of tumour recurrence from toxicity-induced complication like necrosis or ulcerations and the detection of delayed onset of locoregional, metastatic recurrence and second primary cancers.

With the emerging—be it currently experimental—concepts of adaptive radiation treatment strategies, there is increasing interest for imaging assessment during the course of therapy, aiming to develop a non-invasive tool to identify patients who could benefit from treatment intensification and select patients for adaptive radiotherapy (especially important in proton radiotherapy) and aiming to identify tumour regions with suspected radioresistance.

The purpose of this chapter is to present an overview of the application of conventional, metabolic and microstructural imaging modalities in the response assessment and follow-up of head and neck cancer.

R. G. H. Beets-Tan et al. (eds.), *Imaging and Interventional Radiology for Radiation Oncology*, Medical Radiology, Diagnostic Imaging, https://doi.org/10.1007/978-3-030-38261-2_22

1 Introduction

Most patients with head and neck cancer (HNC) present with locoregional advanced disease, which is treated by (chemo)radiotherapy (CRT) or radical surgery followed by post-operative radiotherapy (RT) (Kaanders et al. 2002). Combining multifractionated high-dose RT with radio-sensitizing measures or chemotherapy has substantially improved locoregional control (LRC) and overall survival (OS) (Budach et al. 2006). Two-year LRC of 70% in patients treated by combined chemotherapy with hyper-fractionated accelerated radiotherapy for stage III–IV HNC was reported (Nuyts et al. 2009). Despite these therapeutic advances, recognition of non-responders or patients with early progression is pivotal to enable timely salvage treatment or treatment intensification. However, response assessment and follow-up of HNC treated by CRT face several challenges, including (a) timely detection of tumour recurrence; (b) criteria to select patients for salvage surgery or treatment intensification; (c) differentiation of tumour recurrence from complications including mucosal necrosis and osteoradionecrosis; and (d) lack of clinical consensus for optimum imaging follow-up (Manikantan et al. 2009).

As treatment failure usually occurs in the high-dose RT volume, dose escalation during the course of CRT appears as an attractive option to improve locoregional control. By the ability to deliver non-uniform dose distributions, intensity-modulated radiotherapy (IMRT) can selectively direct higher radiation doses to tumoral subregions while keeping toxicity to an acceptable level. While being solely the subject of feasibility and phase-1 studies, one of the major hurdles to successfully apply treatment intensification during CRT remains the correct identification of treatment resistant tumoral subregions (Bussink et al. 2010). Thus, although currently not routinely used in clinical practice, there is increasing need for imaging response assessment during CRT focusing on monitoring spatiotemporal changes in tumour motion and/or normal tissues during the course of radiotherapy to optimize the treatment plan and monitoring spatiotemporal changes of regions with relative radioresistance like hypoxia, important for dose painting based on tumour biology.

Treatment failure in HNC mostly presents as locoregional tumour recurrence (Agra et al. 2006). Therefore, early response assessment after CRT is mainly aimed at detecting locoregional recurrence amenable for salvage surgery. This is of utmost importance in the therapeutic management of lymph nodes after CRT. Because modern CRT may eradicate nodal disease, the potential benefit of additional neck dissection should be weighed against its associated risks for the patient. Data of—mostly retrospective—studies favour a more conservative approach and indicate that neck dissection should only be performed in case of clinical or radiological suspicion of residual disease. A recent study including 264 patients treated by CRT found no significant difference in local, regional or distant control and disease-free survival between patients with and without upfront neck dissection (Nevens et al. 2017). Another recent prospective randomized controlled trial showed similar 2-year survival between the PET/CT-guided post-CRT surveillance group (OS = 84.9%) and the planned surgery group (OS = 81.5%) (Mehanna et al. 2016).

For local persisting or recurrent tumour, the timing for salvage surgery is critical owing to the necessity to obtain complete tumoral control and enable surgical reconstruction bearing in mind that any local disease recurrence within 6 months after completing CRT has an adverse prognosis. Poor survival outcomes after salvage surgery are associated with (a) disease-free interval less than 6 months; (b) advanced disease stage at time of recurrence with T3–T4 or N2–N3; and (c) more adverse oncologic outcomes, positive section margins and complications including failure in head and neck surgical reconstruction. A retrospective study in 54 patients with T3/4 non-laryngeal cancers treated with RT with or without chemotherapy showed that planned restaging clinically, radiographically (CT or MRI) and by direct laryngoscopy with biopsy at 4–8 weeks post-RT provided the opportunity for early salvage surgery, which may allow organ preservation, higher salvage rates and prolonged disease-free survival (Yom et al. 2005).

Next to locoregional recurrence, up to 15% of patients will eventually develop distant metastases, while this patient population is also at increased risk of second primaries due to tobacco and alcohol abuse. Besides (a) the assessment of locoregional response, (b) differentiation from delayed complications including necrosis or ulcerations and (c) management of toxicity, imaging follow-up should, thus, also include (d) surveillance for distant metastases and second primaries. Currently, clear standardization of follow-up is lacking. However, a review summarizing findings of 55 studies has suggested timelines for surveillance (Manikantan et al. 2009). Follow-up should be most intense in the first three years, as in this period tumour recurrence is most frequent and, furthermore, patients are candidates to the option of salvage therapy. Patients should be clinically evaluated 4–8 weeks after end of treatment, and endoscopic examination should be performed when clinical symptoms are present. Baseline computed tomography (CT) or magnetic resonance imaging (MRI) is preferably obtained 3–6 months after end of treatment as a reference for further follow-up examinations with [^{18}F]fluorodeoxyglucose ([^{18}F]FDG) positron emission tomography (PET) being performed in case of discrepancy between clinical and initial imaging findings. [^{18}F]FDG-PET/CT may be useful 12 months post-treatment although studies need to confirm its clinical efficiency at that time point. Chest CT is recommended in case of suspected lung metastases or second primary in the lungs.

2 Computed Tomography

In CT, primary tumour recurrence after CRT appears as a contrast-enhancing soft tissue mass originating at the irradiated primary site. Cartilage invasion and perineural or perivascular spread can be seen in large recurrences. However, during follow-up, CT alone cannot consistently differentiate between tumour recurrence and complications (Hermans 2008). The two most frequent complications include (a) mandibular osteoradionecrosis and (b) mucosal and laryngeal necrosis, which may show specific CT-graphic patterns that indicate the diagnosis, including lytic cortical bone destruction and trabecular loss with sequestra in osteoradionecrosis and absent contrast enhancement accompanied by ulceration with occasional gas bubbles in mucosal necrosis (Saito et al. 2012). Laryngeal necrosis often shows cartilage abnormalities consisting of fragmentation, collapse, gas formation, arytenoid dislocation or lysis and cricoidal sclerosis (Hermans 2008).

Combining the information of baseline, post-treatment and follow-up CT improves detection of tumour recurrence in laryngeal and hypopharyngeal cancer with sensitivity and specificity of up to 83% and 95%, respectively. Therefore, it is generally recommended to perform baseline CT 3–6 months after the conclusion of RT for nasopharyngeal cancer as well as for HNC located in other head and neck sites (Ljumanovic et al. 2006). In a study by Hermans et al., follow-up CT after initial baseline post-treatment CT allowed to detect 41% of local recurrences at an earlier stage than clinical examination alone (Hermans et al. 2000). Moreover, when applying standardized interpretation criteria, the post-CRT CT has been shown to reliably predict local treatment outcome when qualitative grading score is meticulously applied. A CT score of 1 corresponding to complete resolution of the tumour and symmetric post-RT changes correlated with an excellent 2-year local control rate of 94% and would warrant only clinical follow-up with imaging only needed in case of clinical symptoms. A CT score of 2 defined as a focal mass <1 cm or asymmetric obliteration of laryngeal tissue planes corresponds to an intermediate prognosis with a local control rate of 67%, and therefore, cross-sectional imaging follow-up should be performed at 3–4-month intervals to exclude progression. A CT score of 3 defined as a focal mass >1 cm or less than 50% tumour volume reduction compared to baseline corresponds with a local control rate of only 10% and may warrant immediate investigation (Fig. 1) (Pameijer et al. 1999). Importantly, in oropharyngeal cancer, routine CT

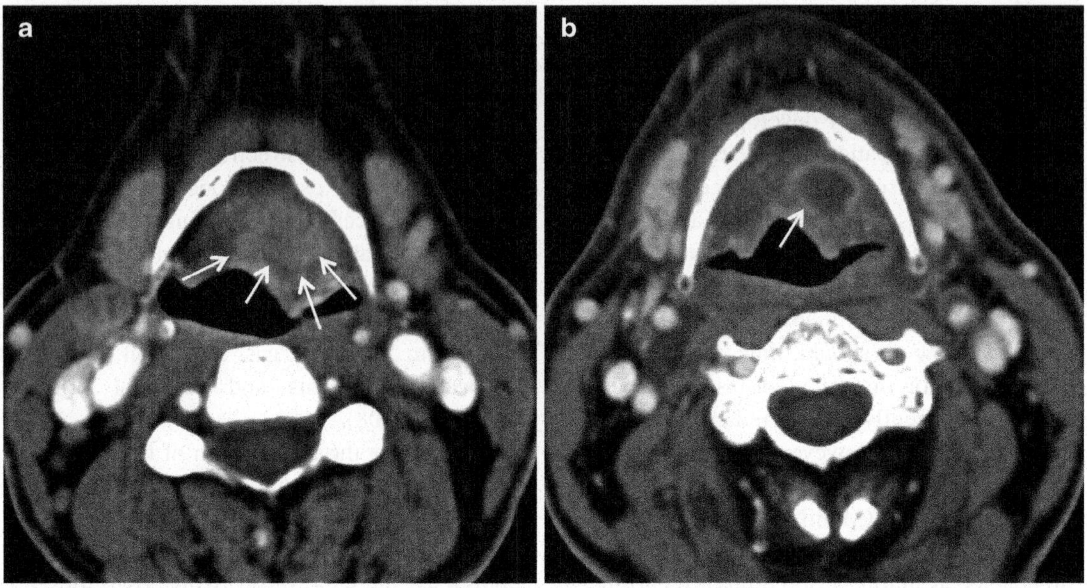

Fig. 1 Patient with a left-sided T3N2B vallecular cancer; axial contrast-enhanced CT images are presented. Pretreatment image (**a**): contrast-enhancing soft tissue thickening is seen in the left pre-epiglottic space originating from the vallecula (arrows). (**b**) Image 4 months after the end of chemoradiotherapy (**b**): no clinical evidence of tumour recurrence. A residual focal mass >1 cm can be seen in the left pre-epiglottic space. This corresponds to a CT score of 3 and is very suspicious for persisting tumour. Direct laryngoscopy with biopsy confirmed the presence of cancer

scan 6 weeks after treatment does not have incremental predictive value to clinical evaluation for predicting local treatment failure, although a CT score of 0 and 1 at this time point allows reliable exclusion of tumour recurrence (Ojiri et al. 2002).

A major drawback of anatomical imaging for imaging lymph nodes is the inherent dependency on size and morphological criteria leaving small metastatic lymph nodes difficult to detect. However, CT can be used to avoid neck dissection. CT 4 weeks post-CRT has shown a high negative predictive value (NPV) of 95% when using nodal diameter and the absence of focal lucency as interpretation criteria and found only one neck recurrence in 32 necks with complete radiographic response (Liauw et al. 2006). In a more recent retrospective study in 183 patients, a CT-based multivariable predictive model including pretreatment T-stage, post-treatment nodal necrosis and the presence of nodal extracapsular spread had an area under the curve of 78% to calculate the risk of a regional relapse (Nevens et al. 2016). As such, post-RT CT has value to exclude patients from additional neck dissection. However, as a drawback, anatomical imaging criteria suffer from a low positive predictive value (PPV) of about 40% and, thus, a poor performance in the identification of patients at risk for nodal relapse requiring planned neck dissection to prevent possible nodal tumour relapse.

3 Magnetic Resonance Imaging

In essence, MRI using conventional T2- and (contrast-enhanced) T1-weighted sequences suffers from similar susceptibility as CT to RT-induced tissue distortions hampering accurate differentiation between tumour recurrence and complications due to overlapping signal intensities and contrast enhancement (Chong and Ong 2008). Nevertheless, in patients with advanced HNC treated with chemoradiation, conventional MRI performed 6–8 weeks post-treatment was able to predict persistent or recurrent primary tumour with a sensitivity of 48% and a specificity of 85% (van den Broek et al. 2006). In another study, conventional MRI after radiotherapy for laryngeal cancer showed a sensitivity of 96% and a specificity of 76% for predicting tumour recurrence (Ljumanovic et al. 2008).

One of the major advantages of MRI is the integration of functional imaging techniques including dynamic contrast-enhanced (DCE) MRI and diffusion-weighted imaging (DWI) that provide information on tumour-related microvascularity and microstructure, respectively.

DCE-MRI acquired by repetitive imaging with high temporal resolution provides information on the tumoral microvasculature. DWI enables tumour characterization and early assessment of treatment effects by probing differential water molecule displacements based on cellular microstructure differences, which can be quantified by calculating changes in the apparent diffusion coefficient (ADC). Both techniques are independent of underlying treatment-induced anatomical tissue distortions for tumour characterization and response assessment.

Development of DCE-MRI in HNC mainly focuses on pretreatment prediction, and only few studies have reported substantial results on early response assessment or detection of tumour recurrence. In a study in 14 patients, Cao et al. showed that increase of the tumour blood volume 2 weeks after starting chemoradiation was predictive of local control at a median follow-up of 9.7 months (Cao et al. 2008). Patients with local failure had significantly lower change in the blood volume. Interestingly, in an initial study in 14 patients, advanced analysis of DCE-MRI by a clustering algorithm for voxel classification enabled prediction of local failure based on the identification of changes of intratumoral poorly perfused subvolumes. From baseline to 2-week DCE-MRI, patients with local failure showed significantly lower percentage decrease of tumoral subvolumes with low blood volume (You et al. 2016). While requiring validation in a large cohort study, the technique may enable early selection of patients who would require local dose intensification during the course of CRT. In a recent study in 49 patients, DCE-MRI performed around 6 weeks post-treatment and using quantitative pharmacokinetic parameters showed significant correlations with HNC site failure and potentially has the ability to predict persistent tumour early after the end of CRT (King et al. 2015).

DWI is increasingly incorporated in routine head and neck imaging owing to its added value to anatomical sequences at diagnosing primary tumours and nodal involvement and detecting recurrences. Particularly, the ability of DWI to robustly separate acute inflammatory changes from tumoral tissue irrespective of underlying anatomic or metabolic distortions makes this imaging technique suitable for early response assessment or differentiation of tumour recurrence from inflammation or necrosis (Vandecaveye et al. 2006).

The increased interest in adaptive radiotherapy or treatment intensification has risen the interest in intra-treatment DWI. Depicting treatment-induced differences in the tumoral microstructure by DWI by measuring changes in ADC during CRT has been consistently associated with outcome in separate clinical studies. It is clear now following the results of head and neck cancer studies that tumours with lower change in ADC or decrease in ADC during CRT are more likely to fail treatment (Fig. 2). These studies found consistent thresholds of ADC change <14–24% to predict treatment failure in HNC when assessing locoregional control for at least 2 years (Vandecaveye et al. 2010; Kim et al. 2009; King et al. 2013). Sensitivities ranging from 86 to 100% and specificities from 83 to 96% were found to predict treatment failure, and the change in ADC during CRT was shown to be an independent predictor of 2-year locoregional control (You et al. 2016).

While initial studies are promising, one has to consider that rather small patient cohorts were included requiring validation in larger patient groups. Also, image assessment has currently focused on determining tumour response, while dose painting requires accurate identification of the non-responding tumoral subvolumes. Voxel-based response assessment reflecting tumour heterogeneity as well as heterogeneity of response may address this issue (Galbán et al. 2009; Baer et al. 2015).

DWI provides reliable differentiating between tumour and inflammation and has the added value

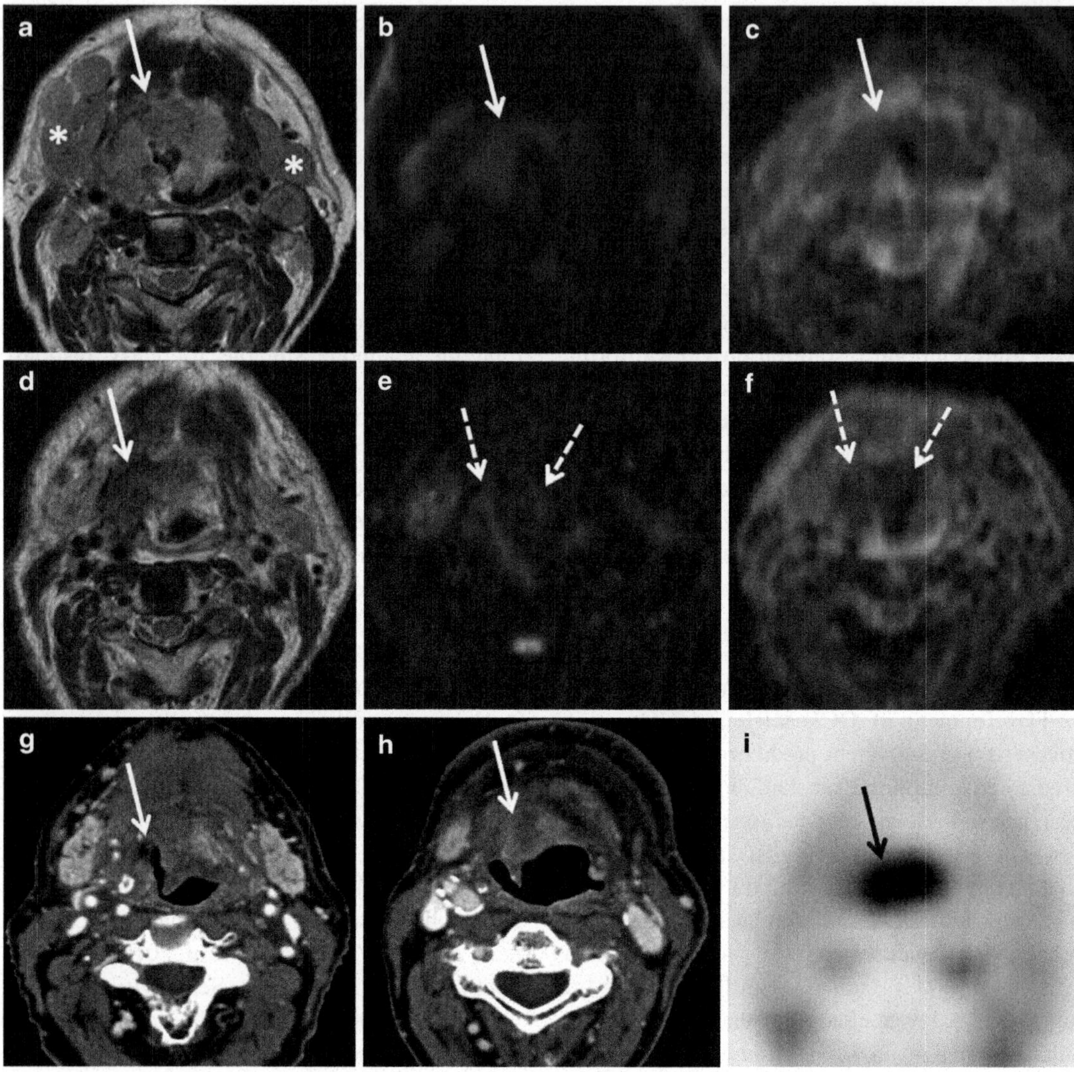

Fig. 2 Patient with T4aN2c oropharyngeal cancer; axial T2-weighted, b1000 diffusion-weighted image and ADC map, CT and [^{18}F]FDG PET images are presented. Pretreatment images (**a**, **b**, **c**): The T2-weighted image (**a**) shows a bulky mass with intermediate intensity centred over the vallecula, corresponding to b1000 hyperintensity (**b**) and low ADC of 0.00086 mm^2/s (**c**), indicated with arrows in the three images. Note the presence of bilateral lymphadenopathies (asterisks). Images 4 weeks after initiation of chemoradiotherapy (**d**, **e**, **f**): T2-weighted image shows significant loss of volume under treatment (**d**, arrow), b1000 DWI images (**e**) show scattered areas of b1000 hyperintensity corresponding to low ADC of 0.00073 mm^2/s (**f**), indicated with dashed arrows, indicating absent response to treatment and high risk of later recurrence. Images 4 months post-chemoradiotherapy (**g**): The axial contrast-enhanced CT image (**g**) shows residual indeterminate ulcer without a clear underlying mass (arrow) in the right vallecula, requiring follow-up within 4 months. Images 8 months post-chemoradiotherapy (**h**, **i**): Axial contrast-enhanced CT image (**h**) shows a contrast-enhancing mass in the right vallecula that corresponded in the [^{18}F]FDG PET (**i**) to a focal and highly increased [^{18}F]FDG uptake indicating glucose hypermetabolism in the lesion. Direct laryngoscopy with biopsy confirmed the presence of cancer

of detecting residual tumour early in the first few months post-CRT, and differentiating inflammatory or necrotic ulcers from tumour recurrence, both potentially challenging for [^{18}F]FDG PET due to the overlap in metabolic activity between active inflammation underlying to the original tumour. Previous studies have shown that both qualitative and quantitative interpretation of DWI enable differentiation between residual or recurrent cancer and treatment-induced inflammation or complications (Vandecaveye et al. 2007; Tshering Vogel et al. 2013; Hwang et al. 2013; Vaid et al. 2017). Tumour recurrence generally shows higher signal intensity than inflammation or necrosis on high b-values, although overlap can occur. Adding ADC quantification allows more consistent differentiation with significantly lower ADC in tumour recurrence than in inflammation or necrosis with sensitivities between 84 and 94.6% and specificities between 90 and 95% (Vandecaveye et al. 2007; Razek et al. 2007). Importantly, tumour recurrence keeps showing significantly lower ADC than inflammation irrespective of timing of scanning between 4 and 14 months in the post-treatment phase. DWI has shown added value to CT and PET/CT by decreasing the false-positive rate in persistent primary site abnormalities or lymphadenopathies and facilitating the detection of subcentimetric nodal metastases (Vandecaveye et al. 2007). Importantly, ADC thresholds for differentiating tumour recurrence from post-treatment changes in the above-mentioned studies remain in a narrow range between 1.2×10^{-3} and 1.3×10^{-3} mm^2/s. The ability to reproduce a constant threshold indicates the robustness and reproducibility of DWI and may facilitate the development of standardized protocols.

The high accuracy for differentiating tumour recurrence from inflammation or necrosis also appears applicable in the early post-treatment phase. A study with DWI/MRI performed 6 weeks after ending CRT for HNC found that a single time-point ADC calculation resulted in a high PPV of 100% at an optimal threshold of 1.4×10^{-3} mm^2/s to detect residual tumour but with a moderate NPV of 63% (King et al. 2010). Consequent studies have shown that the diagnostic performance of early post-treatment DWI can be improved when the post-treatment ADC is calculated relative to baseline or pretreatment ADC values. In this respect, a decrease of ADC after the treatment course compared to baseline was shown to be a stronger predictor for residual tumour than the single assessment of the mass. In a study including 29 patients, DWI performed 3 weeks after ending CRT and using ADC changes 3 weeks post-treatment compared to baseline for lesion analysis showed a PPV of 89% and an NPV of 100% for detecting residual tumour at the primary site and a PPV of 70% and an NPV of 96% for persistent adenopathies per neck side. Importantly, DWI improved PPV and NPV compared to anatomical imaging (Vandecaveye et al. 2012). Recent pilot studies are exploring the possible synergistic value between DWI and [^{18}F]FDG PET for (early) post-CRT assessment of the primary tumour site and lymphadenopathies. A study assessing 73 stage N2-N3 HNC patients with [^{18}F]FDG PET/CT and DWI 3 months after completing CRT found 60% sensitivity and 93% specificity for DWI and 100% sensitivity and 84% specificity for [^{18}F]FDG PET/CT for predicting residual lymphadenopathies. Combined interpretation of [^{18}F]FDG PET/CT and DWI led to 100% sensitivity and 95% specificity (Schouten et al. 2015). A separate pilot study assessing 22 HNC patients with [^{18}F]FDG PET/CT and DWI 3 months after the end of CRT showed sensitivity and specificity values for detecting residual tumour for [^{18}F]FDG PET/CT of 100% and 47%, respectively, but adding DWI information to [^{18}F]FDG PET/CT in the cases that presented residual [^{18}F]FDG uptake increased the specificity to 88% (Fig. 3) (Greuter et al. 2017). These pilot studies appear important in light of the clinical development of multimodality PET/MRI. Interestingly, in a recent prospective study in 74 patients with clinical suspicion of recurrent HNC or radiation-induced complications, multimodality [^{18}F]FDG PET/DWI-MRI showed an excellent performance in detecting local tumour recurrence, yielding sensitivity, specificity, PPV and NPV values of 97.4%, 91.7%, 92.5% and 97.1% per patient and 93.0%, 93.5%, 90.9% and 95.1% per lesion, respectively (Becker et al. 2018).

4 [^{18}F]FDG PET/CT

Metabolism can be assessed by PET/CT using not only the glucose analogue [^{18}F]FDG, which is the most important PET radiotracer (Jadvar et al. 2017), but also many other PET radiotracers such as ^{11}C-methionine and ^{68}Ga-DOTATOC, among

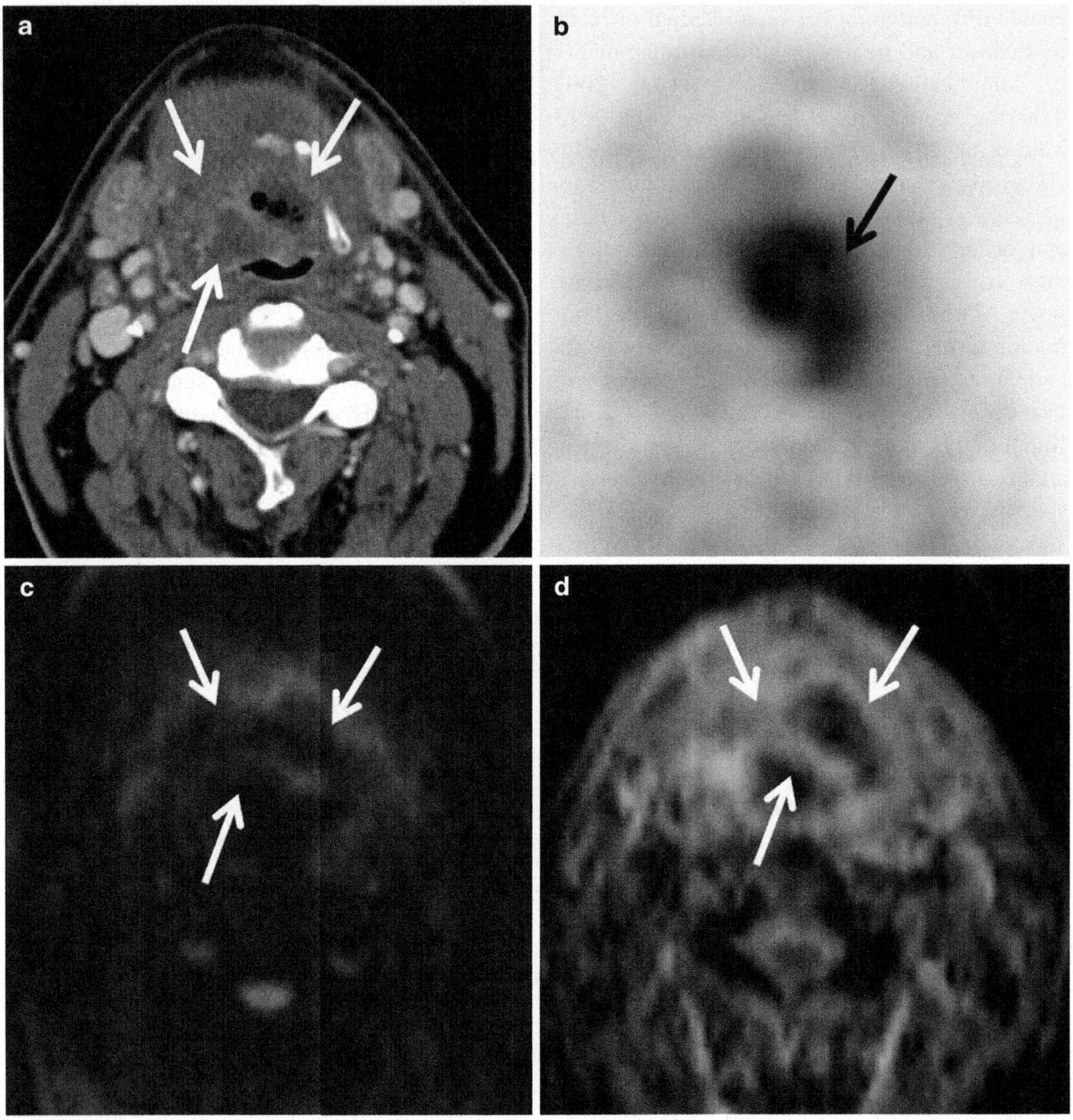

Fig. 3 Patient with oropharyngeal cancer 9 months post-chemoradiotherapy. Axial contrast-enhanced CT image (**a**) shows partially enhancing ulcerative mass bilaterally in the vallecula and in the pre-epiglottic space (arrows). [^{18}F]FDG PET (**b**) shows diffuse and highly increased [^{18}F]FDG uptake indicating glucose hypermetabolism in the mass. MRI (**c**, **d**) at the corresponding level is presented: the b1000 DWI image (**c**) shows absent signal in the mass (arrows) corresponding to significantly increased ADC of 0.00165 mm^2/s (**d**) suggestive of non-tumoral inflammatory ulcer. Direct laryngoscopy with biopsy found no cancer, and the ulcer remained stable during 2-year follow-up confirming non-tumoral inflammatory ulcerative complication

others. PET provides functional or metabolic information. PET/CT combines the advantages of PET, high contrast resolution, and CT, high spatial resolution. There is broad evidence of [^{18}F]FDG PET/CT in head and neck cancer and its utility for characterizing lesions, guiding therapy, monitoring treatment response and predicting outcome. The Society of Nuclear Medicine and Molecular Imaging (SNMMI) published in 2017 the appropriate use criteria (AUC) for [^{18}F]FDG PET/CT in restaging and response assessment of malignant disease, including HNC (Jadvar et al. 2017). This document describes the appropriate use of PET/CT, based on a systematic review, with the aim of synthesizing the evidence on the accuracy and comparative accuracy of [18F]FDG PET/CT.

4.1 Restaging for Detection of Local Recurrence

Based on the evidence, this clinical indication of [18F]FDG PET/CT was considered appropriate with an AUC score of 7 out of 9 (Jadvar et al. 2017). In 2015, a meta-analysis (Sheikhbahaei et al. 2015) including 23 studies and 2247 [18F]FDG PET/CT scans evidenced a joint or pooled sensitivity and specificity of follow-up PET/CT for detection of recurrence as 0.92 (95% CI, 0.90–0.94) and 0.87 (95% CI, 0.82–0.91), respectively. The pooled sensitivity and specificity of scans performed 4–12 months after treatment were 0.95 (95% CI, 0.91–0.97) and 0.78 (95% CI, 0.70–0.84), respectively, whereas in the case of scans performed at or more than 12 months after treatment, sensitivity and specificity were 0.92 (95% CI, 0.85–0.96) and 0.91 (95% CI, 0.78–0.96), respectively. Management decisions in these patients when local recurrent disease is suspected include direct laryngoscopy and physical examination as key aspects, followed by [18F]FDG PET/CT or other imaging test to help detect lymph node disease and more distant recurrence (Jadvar et al. 2017).

4.2 Restaging for Detection of Metastases

This clinical indication of [18F]FDG PET/CT was considered appropriate with an AUC score of 9 out of 9, with extensive evidence supporting it (Jadvar et al. 2017). A meta-analysis that included 27 studies found a sensitivity and specificity of [18F]FDG PET/CT for detection of distant metastases of 84.6% and 94.9%, respectively (Cheung et al. 2016).

4.3 Treatment Response Evaluation

The AUC report gave this clinical indication of [18F]FDG PET/CT a rating of appropriate with an AUC score of 7 out of 9 (Jadvar et al. 2017). In a meta-analysis including 51 studies and 2335 patients, the diagnostic performance of the post-treatment PET/CT was evaluated, as well as the influence of the timing of the PET/CT scan, considering two groups based on the moment of performing the PET/CT, before or after 12 weeks after end of treatment (Gupta et al. 2011). The performance of PET/CT for detecting the primary tumour site and the neck lymph nodes evidenced a joint or pooled sensitivity (79.9% and 72.7%, respectively), specificity (87.5% and 87.6%, respectively), negative predictive value (NPV) (95.1% and 94.5%, respectively) and positive predictive value (PPV) (58.6% and 52.1%, respectively). Regarding the timing of the PET/CT, sensitivity was higher in both the primary tumour (91.9% vs. 73.6%, $p = 0.12$) and neck nodes (90.4% vs. 62.5%, $p < 0.001$) in scans performed greater than or equal to 12 weeks compared to those less than 12 weeks (Jadvar et al. 2017; Gupta et al. 2011). Another meta-analysis that focused on patients with squamous-cell carcinoma (SCC) HNC in which the efficacy of PET for detecting recurrent or residual disease after CRT included 27 studies (Isles et al. 2008). The joint or pooled sensitivity, specificity, PPV and NPV were 94%, 82%, 75% and 95%, respectively. They also analysed the effect of the timing of the PET scans, showing that the sensitivity was higher for PET scans performed more than 10 weeks after CRT compared with those done before 10 weeks after CRT ($p = 0.002$) (Jadvar et al. 2017; Isles et al. 2008). As can be seen in these two meta-analyses, the performance of PET/CT in the post-therapy assessment setting is time and therapy dependent. It is well known that an increase in [18F]FDG uptake occurs in recently irradiated tissues and that it may last 12–16 weeks. To make sure a balance between the disadvantages of early and late imaging is achieved, the post-treatment of [18F]FDG PET/CT to assess therapy response is recommended at least 12 weeks after the end of post-radiation therapy, to minimize radiation-related inflammatory uptake, and at least 3 weeks after completion of chemotherapy or, if possible, 3 weeks before the next chemotherapy cycle (Jadvar et al. 2017).

New standardized interpretation criteria for therapy response assessment of HNC patients based on the result of post-therapy [^{18}F]FDG PET/CT, called Hopkins criteria, were proposed (Marcus et al. 2014). In the Hopkins criteria, therapy response is assessed based on the intensity (compared with the internal jugular vein [IJV] and liver activities) and pattern (focal or diffuse) of [^{18}F]FDG uptake in the primary tumour and in the neck nodes and categorized using a 5-point scoring system considering the following: score 1 (complete metabolic response, [^{18}F]FDG uptake less than the IJV); score 2 (likely complete metabolic response, focal [^{18}F] FDG uptake greater than IJV and lower than the liver); score 3 (likely post-radiation inflammation, diffuse uptake greater than the IJV or the liver); score 4 (likely residual tumour, focal uptake greater than the liver); and score 5 (residual tumour, focal and intense [^{18}F]FDG uptake, focal uptake much greater than the liver) (Marcus et al. 2014). Scores 1, 2 and 3 are considered negative, and scores 4 and 5 are considered positive for residual tumour. This qualitative assessment scoring system evidenced a good inter-rater reliability (k 0.69–0.79), as well as high specificity (92.2%) and NPV (91.1%) values (Jadvar et al. 2017; Marcus et al. 2014).

5 Conclusions

When guiding radiotherapeutic management of head and neck cancer patients, key issues are accurate and timely response assessment and follow-up by imaging. Primarily, post-treatment imaging should aim to detect tumour recurrence as early as possible in order to maximize success of salvage surgery and determine the need for neck dissection. Second, post-treatment imaging has a pivotal role in the differentiation of tumour recurrence from toxicity-induced complication like necrosis or ulcerations and the detection of delayed onset of locoregional, metastatic recurrence and second primary cancers. The emerging concepts of adaptive radiation treatment strategies have contributed to an increasing interest in imaging assessment during the course of therapy, aiming to develop non-invasive tools to identify patients who could benefit from treatment intensification and select patients for adaptive radiotherapy (especially important in proton radiotherapy) and aiming to identify tumour regions with suspected radioresistance. Conventional, metabolic and microstructural imaging modalities have their role in the response assessment and follow-up of head and neck cancer. Regarding PET, it provides functional or metabolic information, and multimodality systems such as PET/CT combine the advantages of PET, high contrast resolution, and CT, high spatial resolution. There is evidence of the utility of [^{18}F]FDG PET/CT in head and neck cancer when restaging for detection of local recurrence and restaging for detection of distant metastases and for treatment response evaluation. Representing a more recent development, DWI is increasingly incorporated in routine head and neck MRI adding functional information to anatomical sequences. Particularly, the ability of DWI to robustly separate acute inflammatory changes from tumour irrespective of underlying anatomic or metabolic distortions makes DWI suitable for (early) response assessment or differentiation of tumour recurrence from inflammation or necrosis.

References

Agra IM, Carvalho AL, Ulbrich FS, de Campos OD, Martins EP, Magrin J, Kowalski LP (2006) Prognostic factors in salvage surgery for recurrent oral and oropharyngeal cancer. Head Neck 28:107–113

Baer AH, Hoff BA, Srinivasan A, Galbán CJ, Mukherji SK (2015) Feasibility analysis of the parametric response map as an early predictor of treatment efficacy in head and neck cancer. AJNR Am J Neuroradiol 36:757–762

Becker M, Varoquaux AD, Combescure C, Rager O, Pusztaszeri M, Burkhardt K et al (2018) Local recurrence of squamous cell carcinoma of the head and neck after radio(chemo)therapy: diagnostic performance of FDG-PET/MRI with diffusion-weighted sequences. Eur Radiol 28:651–663

van den Broek GB, Rasch CR, Pameijer FA, Peter E, van den Brekel MW, Balm AJ (2006) Response measurement after intraarterial chemoradiation in advanced head and neck carcinoma: magnetic resonance imaging and evaluation under general anesthesia? Cancer 106:1722–1729

Budach W, Hehr T, Budach V, Belka C, Dietz K (2006) A meta-analysis of hyperfractionated and accelerated radiotherapy and combined chemotherapy and radiotherapy regimens in unresected locally advanced squamous cell carcinoma of the head and neck. BMC Cancer 31(6):28

Bussink J, van Herpen CM, Kaanders JH, Oyen WJ (2010) PET-CT for response assessment and treatment adaptation in head and neck cancer. Lancet Oncol 11:661–669

Cao Y, Popovtzer A, Li D, Chepeha DB, Moyer JS, Prince ME et al (2008) Early prediction of outcome in advanced head-and-neck cancer based on tumor blood volume alterations during therapy: a prospective study. Int J Radiat Oncol Biol Phys 72:1287–1290

Cheung PK, Chin RY, Eslick GD (2016) Detecting residual/recurrent head neck squamous cell carcinomas using PET or PET/CT: systematic review and meta-analysis. Otolaryngol Head Neck Surg 154:421–432

Chong VF, Ong CK (2008) Nasopharyngeal carcinoma. Eur J Radiol 66:437–447

Galbán CJ, Mukherji SK, Chenevert TL, Meyer CR, Hamstra DA, Bland PH et al (2009) A feasibility study of parametric response map analysis of diffusion-weighted magnetic resonance imaging scans of head and neck cancer patients for providing early detection of therapeutic efficacy. Transl Oncol 2:184–190

Greuter MJ, Schouten CS, Castelijns JA, de Graaf P, Comans EF, Hoekstra OS et al (2017) Cost-effectiveness of response evaluation after chemoradiation in patients with advanced oropharyngeal cancer using 18F-FDG-PET-CT and/or diffusion-weighted MRI. BMC Cancer 17:256

Gupta T, Master Z, Kannan S, Agarwal JP, Ghsoh-Laskar S, Rangarajan V et al (2011) Diagnostic performance of post-treatment FDG PET or FDG PET/CT imaging in head and neck cancer: a systematic review and meta-analysis. Eur J Nucl Med Mol Imaging 38:2083–2095

Hermans R (2008) Posttreatment imaging in head and neck cancer. Eur J Radiol 66:501–511

Hermans R, Pameijer FA, Mancuso AA, Parsons JT, Mendenhall WM (2000) Laryngeal or hypopharyngeal squamous cell carcinoma: can follow-up CT after definitive radiation therapy be used to detect local failure earlier than clinical examination alone? Radiology 214:3–687

Hwang I, Choi SH, Kim YJ, Kim KG, Lee AL, Yun TJ et al (2013) Differentiation of recurrent tumor and posttreatment changes in head and neck squamous cell carcinoma: application of high b-value diffusion-weighted imaging. AJNR Am J Neuroradiol 34:2343–2348

Isles MG, McConkey C, Mehanna HM (2008) A systematic review and meta-analysis of the role of positron emission tomography in the follow up of head and neck squamous cell carcinoma following radiotherapy or chemoradiotherapy. Clin Otolaryngol 33:210–222

Jadvar H, Colletti PM, Delgado-Bolton R, Esposito G, Krause BJ, Iagaru AH et al (2017) Appropriate use criteria for FDG PET/CT restaging and treatment response assessment of malignant disease. J Nucl Med 58:2026–2037

Kaanders JH, Pop LA, Marres HA, Bruaset I, van den Hoogen FJ, Merkx MA, van der Kogel AJ (2002) ARCON: experience in 215 patients with advanced head-and-neck cancer. Int J Radiat Oncol Biol Phys 52:769–778

Kim S, Loevner L, Quon H, Sherman E, Weinstein G, Kilger A, Poptani H (2009) Diffusion-weighted magnetic resonance imaging for predicting and detecting early response to chemoradiation therapy of squamous cell carcinomas of the head and neck. Clin Cancer Res 15:986–994

King AD, Mo FK, Yu KH, Yeung DK, Zhou H, Bhatia KS et al (2010) Squamous cell carcinoma of the head and neck: diffusion-weighted MR imaging for prediction and monitoring of treatment response. Eur Radiol 20:2213–2220

King AD, Chow KK, Yu KH, Mo FK, Yeung DK, Yuan J et al (2013) Head and neck squamous cell carcinoma: diagnostic performance of diffusion-weighted MR imaging for the prediction of treatment response. Radiology 266:531–538

King AD, Chow SK, Yu KH, Mo FK, Yeung DK, Yuan J et al (2015) DCE-MRI for pre-treatment prediction and post-treatment assessment of treatment response in sites of squamous cell carcinoma in the head and neck. PLoS One 10:e0144770

Liauw SL, Mancuso AA, Amdur RJ, Morris CG, Villaret DB, Werning JW, Mendenhall WM (2006) Postradiotherapy neck dissection for lymph node-positive head and neck cancer: the use of computed tomography to manage the neck. J Clin Oncol 24:1421–1427

Ljumanovic R, Langendijk JA, Hoekstra OS, Leemans CR, Castelijns JA (2006) Distant metastases in head and neck carcinoma: identification of prognostic groups with MR imaging. Eur J Radiol 60:58–66

Ljumanovic R, Langendijk JA, Hoekstra OS, Knol DL, Leemans CR, Castelijns JA (2008) Pre- and post-radiotherapy MRI results as a predictive model for response in laryngeal carcinoma. Eur Radiol 18:2231–2240

Manikantan K, Khode S, Dwivedi RC, Palav R, Nutting CM, Rhys-Evans P et al (2009) Making sense of post-treatment surveillance in head and neck cancer: when and what of follow-up. Cancer Treat Rev 35:744–753

Marcus C, Ciarallo A, Tahari AK, Mena E, Koch W, Wahl RL et al (2014) Head and neck PET/CT: therapy response interpretation criteria (Hopkins Criteria)-interreader reliability, accuracy, and survival outcomes. J Nucl Med 55:1411–1416

Mehanna H, Wong WL, McConkey CC, Rahman JK, Robinson M, Hartley AG et al (2016) PET-NECK Trial Management Group. PET-CT surveillance versus neck dissection in advanced head and neck cancer. N Engl J Med 374:1444–1454

Nevens D, Vantomme O, Laenen A, Hermans R, Nuyts S (2016) CT-based follow-up following radiotherapy or radiochemotherapy for locally advanced head and neck cancer; outcome and development of a prognostic model for regional control. Br J Radiol 89(1068):20160492

Nevens D, Duprez F, Bonte K, Deron P, Huvenne W, Laenen A et al (2017) Upfront vs. no upfront neck dissection in primary head and neck cancer radio(chemo) therapy: tumor control and late toxicity. Radiother Oncol 124:220–224

Nuyts S, Dirix P, Clement PM, Poorten VV, Delaere P, Schoenaers J et al (2009) Impact of adding concomitant chemotherapy to hyperfractionated accelerated radiotherapy for advanced head-and-neck squamous cell carcinoma. Int J Radiat Oncol Biol Phys 73:1088–1095

Ojiri H, Mendenhall WM, Mancuso AA (2002) CT findings at the primary site of oropharyngeal squamous cell carcinoma within 6-8 weeks after definitive radiotherapy as predictors of primary site control. Int J Radiat Oncol Biol Phys 52:748–754

Pameijer FA, Hermans R, Mancuso AA, Mendenhall WM, Parsons JT, Stringer SP et al (1999) Pre- and post-radiotherapy computed tomography in laryngeal cancer: imaging-based prediction of local failure. Int J Radiat Oncol Biol Phys 45:359–366

Razek AA, Kandeel AY, Soliman N, El-shenshawy HM, Kamel Y, Nada N, Denewar A (2007) Role of diffusion-weighted echo-planar MR imaging in differentiation of residual or recurrent head and neck tumors and posttreatment changes. AJNR Am J Neuroradiol 28:1146–1152

Saito N, Nadgir RN, Nakahira M, Takahashi M, Uchino A, Kimura F et al (2012) Posttreatment CT and MR imaging in head and neck cancer: what the radiologist needs to know. Radiographics 32:1261–1282

Schouten CS, de Graaf P, Alberts FM, Hoekstra OS, Comans EF, Bloemena E et al (2015) Response evaluation after chemoradiotherapy for advanced nodal disease in head and neck cancer using diffusion-weighted MRI and 18F-FDG-PET-CT. Oral Oncol 51:541–547

Sheikhbahaei S, Taghipour M, Ahmad R, Fakhry C, Kiess AP, Chung CH, Subramaniam RM (2015) Diagnostic accuracy of follow-up FDG PET or PET/CT in patients with head and neck cancer after definitive treatment: a systematic review and meta-analysis. AJR Am J Roentgenol 205:629–639

Tshering Vogel DW, Zbaeren P, Geretschlaeger A, Vermathen P, De Keyzer F, Thoeny HC (2013) Diffusion-weighted MR imaging including bi-exponential fitting for the detection of recurrent or residual tumour after (chemo)radiotherapy for laryngeal and hypopharyngeal cancers. Eur Radiol 23:562–569

Vaid S, Chandorkar A, Atre A, Shah D, Vaid N (2017) Differentiating recurrent tumours from post-treatment changes in head and neck cancers: does diffusion-weighted MRI solve the eternal dilemma? Clin Radiol 72:74–83

Vandecaveye V, de Keyzer F, Vander Poorten V, Deraedt K, Alaerts H, Landuyt W et al (2006) Evaluation of the larynx for tumour recurrence by diffusion-weighted MRI after radiotherapy: initial experience in four cases. Br J Radiol 79:681–687

Vandecaveye V, De Keyzer F, Nuyts S, Deraedt K, Dirix P, Hamaekers P et al (2007) Detection of head and neck squamous cell carcinoma with diffusion weighted MRI after (chemo)radiotherapy: correlation between radiologic and histopathologic findings. Int J Radiat Oncol Biol Phys 67:960–971

Vandecaveye V, Dirix P, De Keyzer F, de Beeck KO, Vander Poorten V, Roebben I et al (2010) Predictive value of diffusion-weighted magnetic resonance imaging during chemoradiotherapy for head and neck squamous cell carcinoma. Eur Radiol 20:1703–1714

Vandecaveye V, Dirix P, De Keyzer F, Op de Beeck K, Vander Poorten V, Hauben E et al (2012) Diffusion-weighted magnetic resonance imaging early after chemoradiotherapy to monitor treatment response in head-and-neck squamous cell carcinoma. Int J Radiat Oncol Biol Phys 82:1098–1107

Yom SS, Machtay M, Biel MA, Sinard RJ, El-Naggar AK, Weber RS, Rosenthal DI (2005) Survival impact of planned restaging and early surgical salvage following definitive chemoradiation for locally advanced squamous cell carcinomas of the oropharynx and hypopharynx. Am J Clin Oncol 28:385–392

You D, Aryal M, Samuels SE, Eisbruch A, Cao Y (2016) Temporal feature extraction from DCE-MRI to identify poorly perfused subvolumes of tumors related to outcomes of radiation therapy in head and neck cancer. Tomography 2:341–352

Response Assessment and Follow-Up by Imaging in Lung Tumours

Anna Rita Larici, Alessandra Farchione, Giuseppe Cicchetti, Annemilia del Ciello, Giovanna Mantini, Adriana K. Calapaquí Terán, and Roberto C. Delgado Bolton

Contents

1 **Introduction** 418

2 **Tumour Response Criteria and Limits** 418
2.1 Conventional Criteria 418
2.2 New Criteria: Special Issues in Imaging Follow-Up After Personalized ChT 421

3 **Imaging Follow-Up After RT: Radiation-Induced Lung Injury/Disease (RILI/RILD)** 423
3.1 Imaging Appearance 424
3.2 Differential Diagnosis 428

4 **Emerging Imaging Parameters and Technique** 432
4.1 Tumour Volume 432
4.2 Perfusion Techniques 433
4.3 Diffusion Imaging 434
4.4 Texture Analysis 434

5 **Metabolism and PET/CT** 435
5.1 Restaging for Detection of Local Recurrence 438
5.2 Restaging After Stereotactic Body Radiation Therapy (SBRT) 441
5.3 Cost-Effectiveness 442
5.4 Restaging for Detection of Metastases 442
5.5 Treatment Response Evaluation 443

6 **Conclusions** 444

References 444

A. R. Larici · G. Cicchetti · G. Mantini
Department of Diagnostic Imaging, Radiation Oncology and Hematology, Fondazione Policlinico Universitario "A. Gemelli" IRCCS, Rome, Italy

D.I.P.U. di Scienze Radiologiche ed Ematologiche, Università Cattolica del Sacro Cuore, Rome, Italy

A. Farchione · A. del Ciello
Department of Diagnostic Imaging, Radiation Oncology and Hematology, Fondazione Policlinico Universitario "A. Gemelli" IRCCS, Rome, Italy

A. K. Calapaquí Terán
Department of Pathology, University Hospital "Marqués de Valdecilla", Santander, Spain

Department of Radiation Oncology, Hospital Central de la Defensa "Gómez Ulla", Madrid, Spain

R. C. Delgado Bolton (✉)
Department of Diagnostic Imaging (Radiology) and Nuclear Medicine, University Hospital San Pedro and Centre for Biomedical Research of La Rioja (CIBIR), Logroño (La Rioja), Spain
e-mail: rcdelgado@riojasalud.es

Abstract

Imaging plays a key role in the assessment of response to therapy in lung cancer, particularly in the definition of disease progression/reduction after chemotherapy (ChT) and/or radiotherapy (RT) and in the subsequent management of the patient. Tumour response criteria have been introduced aiming at standardizing results in cancer treatments. However, measurement errors and limits of such parameters, as well as the complex imaging response patterns observed after the use of newer personalized pharmacological treatments for non-small-cell lung cancer

R. G. H. Beets-Tan et al. (eds.), *Imaging and Interventional Radiology for Radiation Oncology*, Medical Radiology, Diagnostic Imaging, https://doi.org/10.1007/978-3-030-38261-2_23

(NSCLC), pose a challenge in the application of common standardized criteria for the response evaluation. The tumour response after RT can present with different patterns and timing, highly dependent on the techniques used. One of the major issues is distinguishing radiation-induced lung injury/disease (RILI/RILD) from tumour recurrence. Therefore, response assessment in lung cancer should evolve according to the advances in lung cancer treatment and the introduction of newer diagnostic techniques, including functional and molecular imaging.

1 Introduction

Imaging plays a key role in the assessment of response to lung cancer therapy, particularly in the definition of disease progression or reduction after chemotherapy (ChT) and/or radiotherapy (RT) and in the subsequent management of the patient (Coche 2016; Nishino et al. 2014). Tumour response criteria have been introduced aiming at standardizing results in cancer treatments, defining the measurability of the disease and the response to treatment assessed by imaging in an objective manner (Nishino et al. 2012). However, measurement errors and limits have to be kept in mind when considering the commonly used criteria for tumour response evaluation (Nishino et al. 2014). In addition or in association with standard ChT, newer pharmacological treatments for non-small-cell lung cancer (NSCLC) have been introduced targeting more precisely the specific characterization of the lung cancer tissue with respect to its histological subtype and genotype (Ferretti et al. 2016). However, using these new treatments, the response may result in different imaging patterns when compared to those observed after standard cytotoxic ChT (Ferretti et al. 2016). Radiation-induced lung injury/disease (RILI/RILD) may occur after RT, despite the implementation of newer techniques in the effort to reduce the toxic effects and improve therapeutic results. In this scenario, response assessment is a challenge as it can manifest different patterns and timing, highly dependent on the techniques used (Larici et al. 2011). One of the major issues is distinguishing RILI/RILD from tumour recurrence. Therefore, response assessment in lung cancer should evolve according to the advances in lung cancer treatment and the introduction of newer diagnostic techniques, including functional and molecular imaging.

2 Tumour Response Criteria and Limits

The evaluation of response after treatment for lung cancer is usually performed applying morphological criteria. Conventional response criteria have been originally designed to assess response to cytotoxic ChT. Nowadays, new criteria have been proposed due to the introduction of molecular targeted therapies that may determine different response patterns. Both conventional and newly proposed criteria are summarized in Table 1.

2.1 Conventional Criteria

Treatment response evaluation in solid tumours is mainly based on two-dimensional anatomical parameters, as defined by the World Health Organization (WHO) criteria and the response evaluation criteria in solid tumours (RECIST). They both assign four categories of assessment, which include complete response, partial response, stable and progressive disease (Nishino et al. 2014; Therasse et al. 2006; Eisenhauer et al. 2009). Introduced in 1979, the WHO criteria rely on bi-dimensional area measurements (i.e. obtained by multiplying tumour maximum diameter in the transverse plane and its longest perpendicular diameter) (Nishino et al. 2014).

RECIST were introduced to provide standardized and simplified criteria allowing meaningful comparison among studies. Nowadays, they are the most commonly used criteria (Nishino et al. 2012). Key features of the original RECIST 1.0 version, published in 2000, are the definition of the minimum size to qualify a lesion as measurable, the instructions about the

Table 1 Response criteria to cytotoxic and non-cytotoxic therapies (derived and modified from Nishino et al. (2010a, 2012, 2013, 2014), Therasse et al. (2006), Eisenhauer et al. (2009), Crabb et al. (2009), Choi et al. (2007), Wolchok et al. (2013)

	RECIST 1.0	RECIST 1.1	Choi criteria	New response criteria	iRECIST (bi-dimensional)	Proposed new iRECIST (uni-dimensional)
Minimum lesion target size	≥10 mm (spiral CT) ≥20 mm (conventional CT/MRI)	≥10 mm (CT/RM) ≥15 mm lymph nodes	Same as RECIST 1.0 (minimum mean tumour density 5 HU)	Same as RECIST 1.1	≥5 × 5 mm	Same as RECIST
Measurement	Target lesions uni-dimensional long axis	Target lesions uni-dimensional long axis; lymph nodes short axis	Same as RECIST 1.0	Same as RECIST 1.1	Long axis × short axis	Same as RECIST
No. of measurable lesions (max per organ)	10 Max per organ, 5	5 Max per organ, 2	Same as RECIST 1.0	Same as RECIST 1.1	Max per organ, 5 Up to 10 visceral Up to 5 cutaneous	Same as RECIST
Progressive disease (PD)	≥20% increase in the sum of target lesions (nadir); new lesions; unequivocal progression of non-target lesions	Same as RECIST 1.0 and: - at least 5-mm increase of target lesions; - new lesions at [^{18}F]FDG-PET	≥ 10% increase in tumour size and does not meet criteria of PR by tumour density (HU); new lesions; new intratumoral nodules or increase in the size of the existing intratumoral nodules (both target and non-target)	Same as RECIST 1.1 and: - does not meet criteria of PR by tumour attenuation (HU) changes; - no cavitation	≥25% increase in the sum of target lesions (nadir)	Same as RECIST except for new lesions
Partial response (PR)	≥30% decrease in the sum of target lesions (baseline); no new lesions; no obvious progression of non-target lesions	Same as RECIST 1.0	≥10% decrease in size or ≥15% decrease in tumour density (HU); no progression of non-target lesions; no new lesions	If a ROI of the solid portion within a tumour ≤5 mm^2 ≥30% decrease in size, if a ROI of the solid portion within a tumour >5 mm^2 ≥10% decrease in size or ≥15% decrease in tumour attenuation (HU); no new lesions; no obvious progression of non-target lesions	≥50% decrease in the sum of target lesions (baseline)	Same as RECIST except for new lesions

(continued)

	RECIST 1.0	RECIST 1.1	Choi criteria	New response criteria	iRECIST (bi-dimensional)	Proposed new iRECIST (uni-dimensional)
Complete response (CR)	Disappearance of all target and non-target lesions; no new lesion	Same as RECIST 1.0 and all lymph nodes must be 10-mm short axis	Same as RECIST 1.0	Same as RECIST 1.1	Disappearance of all lesions	Same as RECIST
Stable disease (SD)	Neither PD, PR nor CR	Same as RECIST 1.0	Same as RECIST 1.0	Same as RECIST 1.1	Neither PD, PR nor CR	Same as RECIST
New lesions					The presence of new lesion(s) does not define progression. The measurements of the new lesion(s) are included in the sum of the measurements	The presence of new lesion(s) does not define progression. The measurements of the new lesion(s) are included in the sum of the measurements
Confirmation					Confirmation by two consecutive observations not less than 4 weeks apart required for CR, PR and PD	Confirmation by two consecutive observations not less than 4 weeks apart required for CR, PR and PD

number of target lesions to follow and the use of the longest one-dimensional diameter for the measurement (Therasse et al. 2006). RECIST 1.1 have been published as a revised version in 2009, introducing major imaging-related changes, such as the reduction in the number of target lesions, the definition of pathological lymph nodes, the clarification of disease progression and the inclusion of metabolic data in the detection of new lesions (Eisenhauer et al. 2009). Despite a high concordance in terms of response assessment between the two RECIST criteria versions (weighted $k = 0.905$), the newer one resulted in a higher reproducibility and better response assessment mainly due to the introduction of positron emission tomography (PET)/computed tomography (CT) imaging (Nishino et al. 2010a).

The response to therapy can be heterogeneous, either within one lesion or among multiple lesions. One-dimensional measurements can be inaccurate, or with low reproducibility, in the case of a tumour with irregular morphology as well as when different regions in the same lesion show disproportional growth (Coche 2016; Nishino et al. 2014). Moreover, using one-dimensional or two-dimensional measurements, we consider only the maximum cross-sectional diameter or area measured on axial images, while the maximum tumour dimension may be in non-axial planes. Due to measurement errors, intra- and inter-reader variability in tumour evaluation has been reported. It results in the probability of misclassifying a patient in the wrong category of response (Coche 2016; Nishino et al. 2014). When evaluating variability in applying criteria of measurement for NSCLC, one-dimensional measurements resulted in a better performance (95% limits of agreement: –22.8%, 23.0% and –23.1%, 24.4%, respectively, in two different studies) than bi-dimensional ones (–38.9%, 39.1% and –34.0%, 48.6%, respectively) (Nishino et al. 2011; Zhao et al. 2006). It has to be noted that the cut-off values for disease progression (+25% for WHO criteria and +20% for RECIST) are within the range of such values of measurement variability. Therefore, some patients can be incorrectly assigned to the progressive disease category. The possibility of misclassifying tumour progression has been reported in 43% and 30% when using WHO criteria and RECIST, respectively (Erasmus et al. 2003). Moreover, due to simpler and better-defined guidelines, the RECIST 1.1 version has shown less variability in the measurements, with narrower 95% limits of inter-observer agreement compared with the previous version (–18.6%, 25.4% and 30.8%, 30.4%, respectively) (Nishino et al. 2010a).

In the context of the evaluation of treatment response in patients also undergoing RT, particularly in the presence of fibrotic changes, response assessment poses a further challenge. The main issue is distinguishing benign fibrotic tissue in post-RT changes from viable tumour cells, and evaluation methods including exclusively dimensional measures of the treated area can be of limited value (Ghaye et al. 2016).

2.2 New Criteria: Special Issues in Imaging Follow-Up After Personalized ChT

In addition to standard cytotoxic ChT, new oncologic therapies have been introduced nowadays, such as angiogenesis inhibitors, tyrosine kinase inhibitors (TKIs) and immunotherapies.

Angiogenesis inhibitors are known to cause haemorrhage and necrosis in treated tumours (Ferretti et al. 2016; Nishino et al. 2010b). Common consequences of this kind of drugs are lesion cavitation and paradoxical increase in tumour size despite attenuation changes. This represents a challenge for the appropriate measurement of tumour burden (Ferretti et al. 2016; Nishino et al. 2010b). Crabb et al. proposed, as an alternative, to subtract the larger diameter of the cavity from the larger diameter of the target lesion, demonstrating that the use of this newer criterion alters the response assessment, the determination of time to best response and the time of disease progression only in a minority of patients compared with RECIST (Crabb et al. 2009). Authors underlined that including cavitation in a volumetric assessment of the tumour would have a greater impact on evaluation of response to angiogenesis inhibitors.

Tyrosine kinase inhibitors (TKIs) are divided into inhibitors targeting epidermal growth factor receptor (EGFR) mutations and inhibitors targeting anaplastic lymphoma kinase (ALK), ROS and mesenchymal-epithelial transition (MET) fusion protein. These agents often determine an important response with initial dramatic reduction of lesion size (Nishino et al. 2014; Ferretti et al. 2016). However, subsequently, there are an acquired resistance to the drug and a selection of less sensitive tumour clones. These two changes at the cellular level of the tumour determine macroscopic changes that, based on RECIST criteria, are defined as disease progression. Nevertheless, this progression is often slow over many months and occurs in relatively asymptomatic patients (Nishino et al. 2014; Ferretti et al. 2016). On the contrary, disease flare-up has been described after treatment discontinuation (Ferretti et al. 2016). For this reason, oncologists prefer to continue treatment until the onset of more threatening conditions or symptoms despite RECIST categorization (Ferretti et al. 2016). Attenuation changes are commonly seen in gastrointestinal stromal tumours (GIST) initially treated with TKIs, where the development of myxoid degeneration, haemorrhage or necrosis is responsible for a decrease in tumour attenuation as a unique marker of response to treatment (Nishino et al. 2010b). Therefore, the addition of attenuation data in the definition of GIST response, as described in the Choi criteria, has shown a good correlation with response by [^{18}F]fluorodeoxyglucose ([^{18}F]FDG) PET and has been more predictive of the time to progression than response given by RECIST 1.0 (Choi et al. 2007). Lee et al. proposed the so-called new response criteria (NRC) for the evaluation of response to EGFR TKIs in NSCLC, demonstrating a good reproducibility and a significant association with the overall survival (Lee et al. 2011). These criteria, apart from tumour size, consider: (a) tumour constituents, such as the solid component and pure ground-glass (GG) component (lesion size is determined only by the solid portion); (b) tumour cavitation, applying the Crabb method; and (c) CT attenuation changes, using the Choi criteria (Lee et al. 2011).

The evaluation of treatment response by immunotherapeutic agents, including antibodies against PD-1 (programmed cell death 1) and PD-L1 (programmed cell death ligand 1) receptors, can be particularly challenging. In fact, the response may be delayed due to the time needed to develop an immune response, and "pseudo-progression" may be the first disease evolution (Ferretti et al. 2016; Wang et al. 2017). A paradoxical increase in size or the appearance of new lesions can occur before treatment response (Fig. 1). This event has been attributed to the continuous tumour growth occurring during the development of the immune response and to the infiltration by immune cells, causing an increase in size of the known lesions or the new

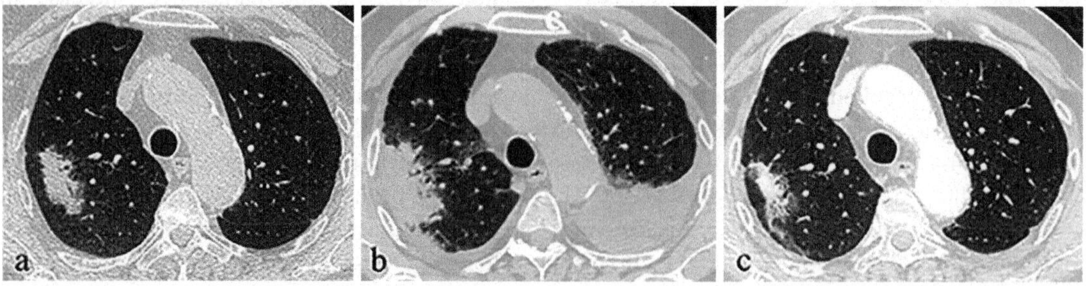

Fig. 1 (**a–c**) A 68-year-old man with a lung adenocarcinoma of the right upper lobe, PD-L1 positive (≥50%) and EGFR, ALK negative, treated with pembrolizumab as first-line therapy (**a**). A chest CT scan performed after 3 months showed an enlargement of the lesion and the development of bilateral pleural effusion (**b**). Treatment was not withdrawn and a CT scan performed after 6 months documented a shrinkage of the tumour, suggesting that the previous observed increase was a "pseudo-progression"

appearance of previously occult ones (Ferretti et al. 2016; Wang et al. 2017). In 2009, immune-related response criteria (irRC) based on bi-dimensional measurements were proposed by Wolchok et al., which consisted of two main key features (Wolchok et al. 2013). The first one was that the increase in total tumour burden had to be confirmed by repeating the evaluation no less than 4 weeks after the first potential evidence of progression. The second feature was to recognize that the appearance of new lesions should not be considered as progression but should be added to the sum of all originally identified lesions (Wolchok et al. 2013). Nishino et al. suggested that the irRC criteria should be revised into the RECIST 1.0 or 1.1 criteria based on the more reproducible one-dimensional measurements (Nishino et al. 2013), suggesting also to include other quantitative imaging markers (Nishino et al. 2015).

3 Imaging Follow-Up After RT: Radiation-Induced Lung Injury/Disease (RILI/RILD)

RILI/RILD is common after RT of the chest and often determines radiological changes in irradiated lung. Awareness of the times of initiation and completion of RT, treatment planning and dose delivered and knowledge of the typical radiological pattern of injuries are required to accurately interpret lung abnormalities at follow-up imaging in patients treated with RT techniques (Larici et al. 2011; Ghaye et al. 2016). RILI/RILD generally presents with two distinct clinical and pathologic phases, defined according to the time of RT completion: an early phase of acute radiation pneumonitis (RP), which usually occurs within the first 6 months after the end of treatment, and a later phase of chronic radiation fibrosis (RF), occurring after 6–12 months (Larici et al. 2011; Ghaye et al. 2016). The pathological pattern consists in a diffuse alveolar damage evolving to an acute exudative phase and then onto organizing/proliferative phases, characterized by a more or less organized infiltration of macrophages, and a chronic fibrotic phase, with progressive collagen deposition and fibrotic changes (Larici et al. 2011; Ghaye et al. 2016). The onset is usually indolent, unless there is concomitant use of ChT agents that may potentiate radiation effects (Larici et al. 2011; Ghaye et al. 2016). The inflammatory phase generally appears between 1 and 3 months after the end of RT. However, when stereotactic body or ablative RT (SBRT/SABR) is used, it may appear after a longer time (Larici et al. 2011; Ghaye et al. 2016). The chronic phase results from an unresolved acute phase and may last up to 12–24 months. Lesions are considered stable after 2 years since the completion of treatment (Larici et al. 2011; Ghaye et al. 2016).

The risk of RILI/RILD depends on patient, tumour and therapy-related factors (Larici et al. 2011; Ghaye et al. 2016). It increases with patient age, genetic predisposition, worse lung performance status and pre-existing lung diseases, as well as with tumour location next to radiation sensitive structures (e.g. mediastinum, proximal bronchi, oesophagus) (Larici et al. 2011; Ghaye et al. 2016). The use of concomitant RT-ChT may also potentiate the toxic effect. Radiation-induced abnormalities usually affect the volume of tissues submitted to the higher delivery dose, which depends on radiation technique-related factors, such as type (numbers of portals and beam arrangement) and dose (Larici et al. 2011; Ghaye et al. 2016). Regarding RT types of treatment, some concepts need to be kept in mind when dealing with RILI/RILD (Larici et al. 2011; Ghaye et al. 2016). In conventional bi-dimensional RT, a large volume of normal tissues adjacent to the tumour is often irradiated because the radiation dose is delivered to the tumour in two parallel beams with opposed orientations (with a 2-cm margin around the tumour and a 1-cm margin around the lymph node volumes to compensate for respiratory motion and variations in set-up between daily treatment sessions) (Larici et al. 2011; Ghaye et al. 2016). In three-dimensional conformal RT (3D-CRT), the maximum therapeutic radiation dose is delivered to the tumour by means of multiple coplanar and non-coplanar radiation fields designed on the 3D appearance of the tumour, thus minimizing the irradiation of the adjacent normal tissues (Larici et al. 2011; Ghaye et al. 2016). SBRT/SABR is performed by using a steeper gradient between the periphery of the target volume (high-dose area) and normal adjacent tissue (low-dose area) and combining higher ablative per-fraction dose, to deliver higher radiation dose to small and localized tumours (Larici et al. 2011; Ghaye et al. 2016) Intensity-modulated RT (IMRT) and volumetric modulated arch therapy (VMAT) increase conformity to the target volume by using non-uniform planes from different angles (Larici et al. 2011; Ghaye et al. 2016).

The risk of RILI/RILD does not increase linearly with RT dose but occurs when a critical volume of tissue is damaged (Larici et al. 2011; Ghaye et al. 2016). Generally, RILI/RILD occurs according to some thresholds commonly for tissue receiving between 20 and 40 Gy, and it has been reported that the minimal dose to the injured lung is related to the V_{20Gy} (percentage of lung volume that receives more than 20 Gy). The higher the V_{20Gy}, the lower the minimal dose at which damage occurs, with a V_{20Gy} less than 25% related to 0–4% risk of RILI/RILD (Larici et al. 2011; Ghaye et al. 2016; Graham et al. 1999). Finally, the capability of tissues to recover from sub-lethal damage depends on dose and fraction. A higher dose with a short fractionation, as used in SBRT/SABR, increases the probability of late phase injuries. On the other hand, a longer fractionation schedule reduces the biological effects of radiation (Larici et al. 2011; Ghaye et al. 2016).

It has to be kept in mind that the clinical setting and the radiological signs of injury after RT may not correspond. In the acute phase of RP, signs and symptoms (which include dyspnoea, cough, low-grade fever and chest discomfort) may develop without any radiological change (Larici et al. 2011; Ghaye et al. 2016). On the other hand, the later phase of RF is more often asymptomatic and may be seen at imaging without any antecedent of RP; symptomatic patients instead usually complain of progressive dyspnoea and persistent dry cough (Larici et al. 2011; Ghaye et al. 2016). Specifically symptomatic disease is less common after SBRT/SABR (4%) than 3D-CRT (13–37%), maybe because of the smaller lung volume exposed to high-dose radiation (Larici et al. 2011).

3.1 Imaging Appearance

Multi-detector CT, with its high spatial and temporal resolution, is pivotal for the identification and characterization of RILI/RILD. Radiologic manifestations of RILI/RILD after conventional RT (*typical manifestations*) are usually confined to the margins of the irradiated field and do not conform to anatomic boundaries (i.e. fissures). The early phase of RP manifests as ground-glass opacities (GGO) or consolidation, which can also coexist, in the affected lung (Larici et al. 2011; Ghaye et al. 2016). With the evolution from the exudative to the organizing phase, the development of a more homogeneous and discrete consolidation that better conforms to the shape of the portals may be seen (Ghaye et al. 2016). An ipsilateral pleural effusion with atelectasis of the adjacent lung could be associated (Larici et al. 2011; Ghaye et al. 2016). RP may resolve over 6 months in case of limited injury, while in cases of more severe changes, a progression to fibrosis usually occurs. During the late phase of RF, CT scans show a well-defined area of volume loss with a linear scar or consolidation characterized by a straight lateral margin conforming to radiation portal (Larici et al. 2011; Ghaye et al. 2016). Parenchymal distortion and traction bronchiectasis are associated. Fibrosis may continue to evolve for up to 24 months; usually, shrinkage or a more defined demarcation between irradiated and normal lung may occur. Ipsilateral mediastinal displacement, adjacent pleural thickening and/or effusion are occasional (Larici et al. 2011; Ghaye et al. 2016).

Manifestations of lung injury after 3D-CRT and SBRT/SABR may be similar to those of conventional scheme with regard to their timeline, except that lung abnormalities after SBRT/SABR do not usually occur before 2–3 months after the end of treatment, related to its specific radiobiology (Larici et al. 2011; Ghaye et al. 2016).

Radiological findings may be similar too. However, because of the complex portal configurations used, they differ with regard to the extent, distribution, location and morphological characteristics. This is the reason why RILI/RILD after 3D-CRT and SBRT/SABR has been called *unusual or atypical* (Larici et al. 2011; Ghaye et al. 2016). After 3D-CRT, radiological injuries are usually limited to the area of lung parenchyma surrounding the tumour with linear shape and distinct margins corresponding to dose distribution and to the boundary between the irradiated and non-irradiated lung, respectively (Larici et al. 2011; Ghaye et al. 2016). They can also affect both lungs, even further from the tumour site, in the area delimited by radiation portals (Larici et al. 2011; Ghaye et al. 2016). After SBRT/SABR, lung abnormalities occur within the high-dose region (which includes tumour and a rim of surrounding parenchyma) because of the steeper gradient between target volume and normal adjacent tissue, conforming to the tumour shape and without a linear pattern (Larici et al. 2011; Ghaye et al. 2016).

RP occurring after 3D-CRT appears as focal GGO, consolidation or both. Following SBRT/SABR, radiological findings of RP have been classified as “diffuse” or “patchy” according to lung abnormalities’ dimensions (≥5 cm or <5 cm) and extension (completely filling or not completely filling the high-dose region) and categorized into four patterns: (a) diffuse consolidation; (b) diffuse GGO; (c) patchy consolidation and GGO; and (d) patchy GGO (Ikezoe et al. 1988; Palma et al. 2011) (Fig. 2).

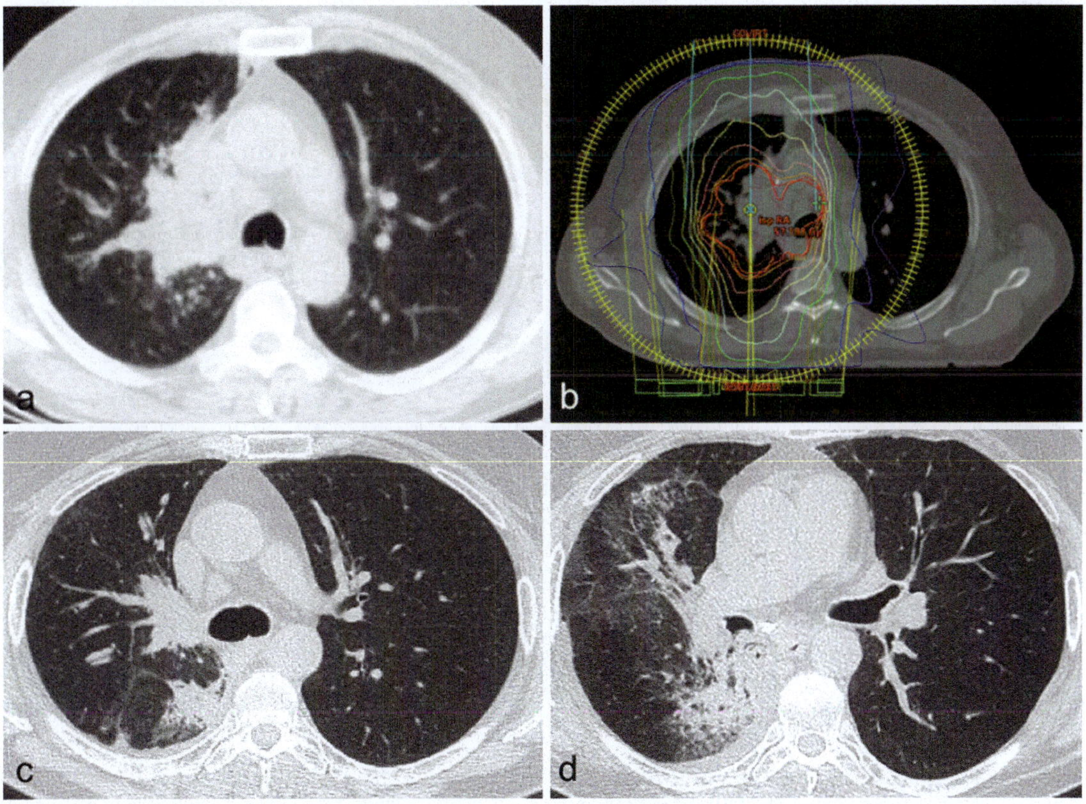

Fig. 2 **(a–d)** A 66-year-old man with a squamous cell carcinoma of the right hilum (T3N2M0) (**a**) undergoing 3D-CRT (VMAT) as a part of the neoadjuvant RT-ChT treatment (**b**). Due to residual disease’s infiltration of mediastinal structures, the patient did not undergo surgical resection. Early CT follow-up (2 months after the end of RT) demonstrates RP with consolidations and GGOs and right pleural effusion (**c, d**)

CT manifestations of RF after both 3D-CRT and SBRT/SABR have been classified into three patterns: (a) modified conventional, (b) mass-like and (c) scar-like (Larici et al. 2011; Ghaye et al. 2016; Linda et al. 2011; Koenig et al. 2002). The *modified conventional pattern* resembles the alterations after conventional RT with a less extensive involvement of irradiated lung parenchyma, manifesting as a well-defined consolidation with volume loss and traction bronchiectasis (Larici et al. 2011; Ghaye et al. 2016; Linda et al. 2011; Koenig et al. 2002) (Fig. 3). The *mass-like pattern* consists of a focal consolidation with traction bronchiectasis confined to a 2-cm margin around the tumour (the region corresponding to the maximal isodose curve delivered), resembling a rounded lesion larger than the original tumour (Larici et al. 2011; Ghaye et al. 2016; Linda et al. 2011; Koenig et al. 2002) (Fig. 4). The consolidations of both patterns may change in shape and location over 12–24 months after the end of RT because fibrosis causes deformity of the lung and displacement of the treated region towards

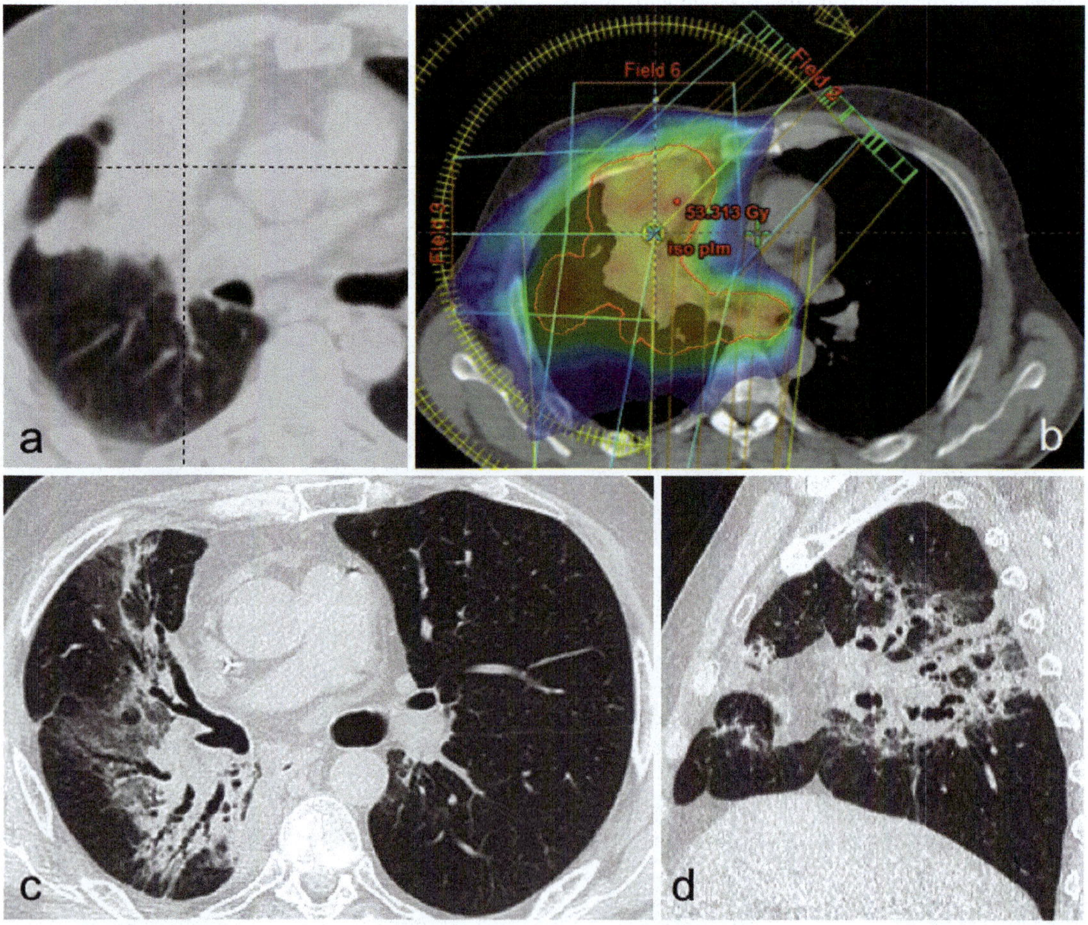

Fig. 3 (**a**–**d**). A 50-year-old man with a large adenocarcinoma of the right upper lobe (T3N2M0) (**a**) treated with 3D-CRT (VMAT) (**b**) as a part of the neoadjuvant RT-ChT scheme and subsequent right pneumonectomy. The patient developed an RF with a *modified conventional pattern* (CT scan after 13 months by the end of RT) (**c**, **d**, axial and sagittal planes, respectively). Notice how margins of the fibrosis correspond to the dose distribution, with a quite well-defined boundary between the irradiated and non-irradiated lung

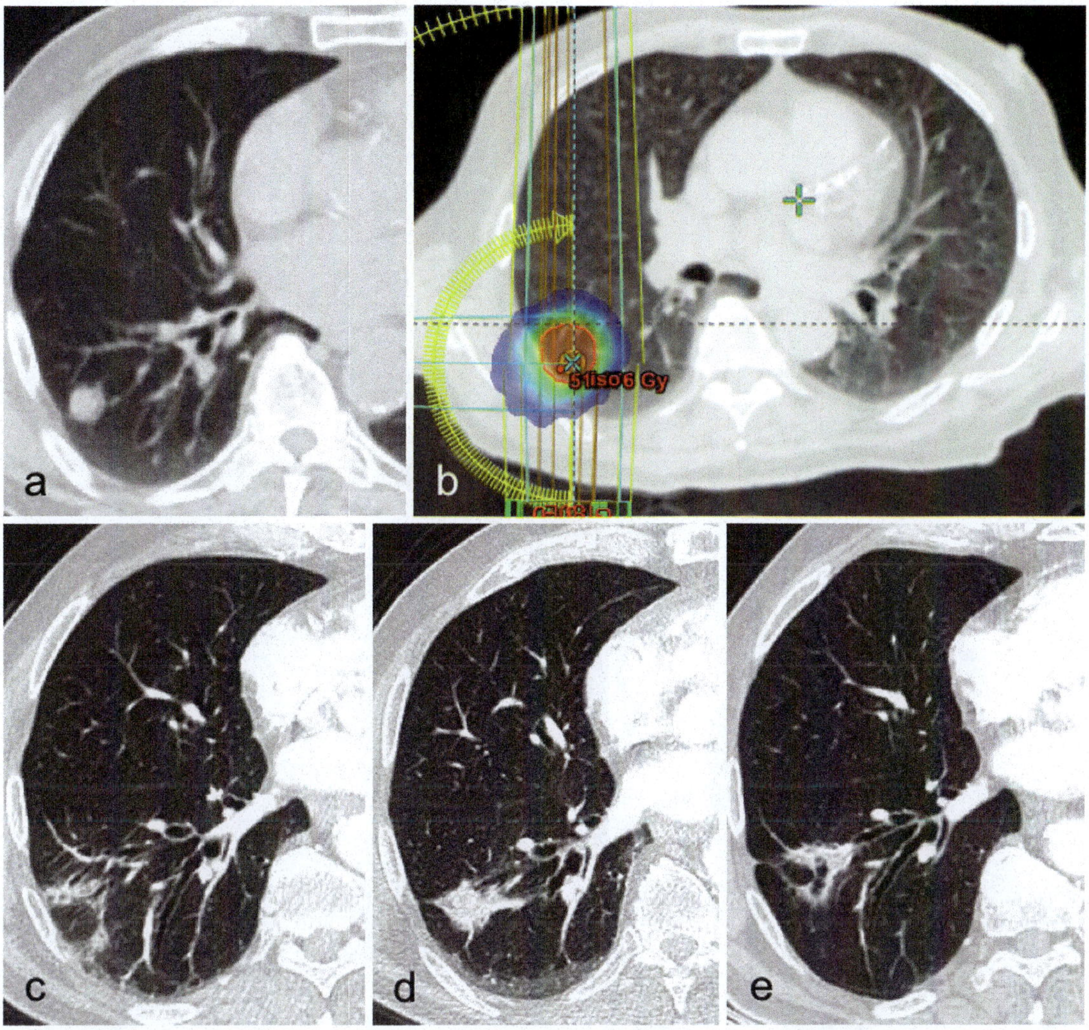

Fig. 4 (**a–e**) An 81-year-old man with a T1bN0M0 adenocarcinoma of the right lower lobe (**a**) undergoing SBRT/SABR (VMAT) (**b**) because of cardiovascular comorbidities. After the disappearance of the lesion due to the effectiveness of the radiation treatment (**c**), a focal rounded consolidation in the right lower lobe appeared (**d**), suggestive of a *mass-like pattern* of radiation-induced fibrosis or a local tumour recurrence (CT scan after 6 months by the end of RT). Further evolution with change in shape and volume reduction of the consolidation demonstrated that the finding was a mass-like pattern of radiation-induced fibrotic area (**e**)

or away from the hilum (Larici et al. 2011; Ghaye et al. 2016). The *scar-like pattern* results in a linear opacity less than 1-cm wide, simulating a plate-like atelectasis, associated with moderate to severe volume loss and occurring in the site previously occupied by the tumour with the primary mass completely/almost completely resolved (Larici et al. 2011; Ghaye et al. 2016; Linda et al. 2011; Koenig et al. 2002) (Fig. 5). The consolidation usually decreases in size during the follow-up; however, a transient increase in size following SBRT/SABR is also possible during the first 12 months (Takeda et al. 2008).

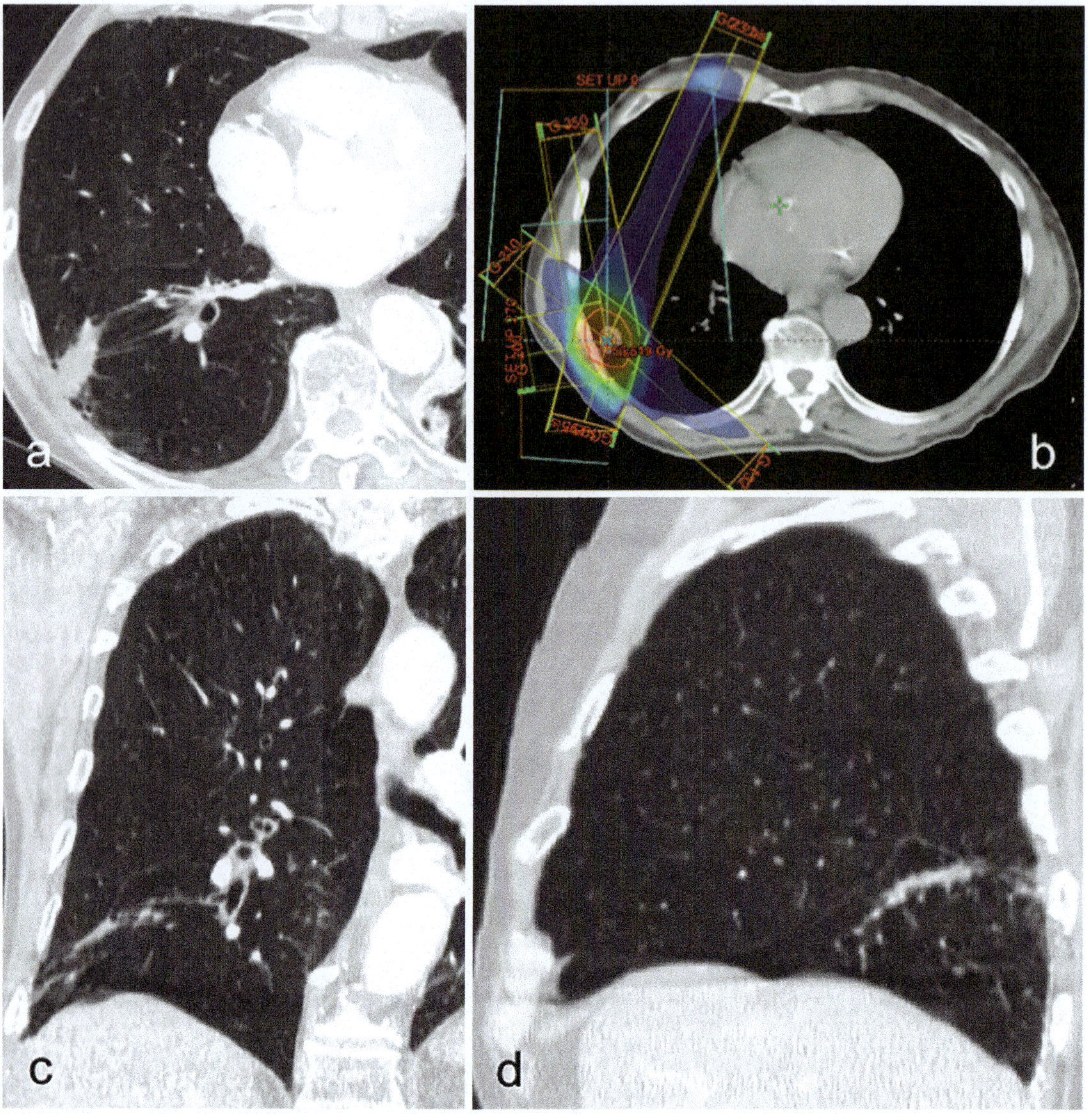

Fig. 5 (**a–d**) A 72-year-old man with a relapse in the right lower lobe of a previous T2N3M0 squamous cell carcinoma (**a**), undergoing SBRT/SABR (multiple fields) (**b**). CT scan performed 14 months after the end of radiation treatment shows a plate-like atelectasis in the site previously occupied by the tumour, with resolution of the primary mass, suggestive of a *scar-like pattern* of RF (**c**, **d**, coronal and sagittal plane, respectively)

3.2 Differential Diagnosis

Generally, in patients who have received a radiation dose of more than 40 Gy over a period of at least 4 weeks for 3D-CRT or 1–2 weeks for SBRT/SABR, the most likely cause of abnormalities within the radiation portals on radiologic images obtained within 6 months after cessation of RT is RP (Larici et al. 2011). However, other conditions may occur in patients who have undergone RT for lung cancer, such as lung infections or lymphangitic carcinomatosis, as well as locally recurrent tumour (Larici et al. 2011; Ghaye et al. 2016) (Table 2, Fig. 6).

The most important differential diagnosis is local tumour recurrence that usually manifests within 2 years after treatment. Physiological modifications are usually possible within the first 12 months after the end of the RT, but in patients undergoing hypo-fractionated SBRT/SABR,

Table 2 Main differential diagnoses with respect to RILI/RILD based on CT criteria (modified from Linda et al. 2011)

Diseases	Imaging findings		
	Location and distribution	Radiological characteristics	Temporal evolution
Infection	– Outside radiation portal – Respect lung anatomic boundaries – Diffuse or bilateral	– Consolidation – Centrilobular or "tree-in- bud" opacities – Cavitation	– Abrupt clinical and radiological onset – Can occur without any temporal relation with RT completion
Lymphangitic carcinomatosis	– Outside radiation portal – Non-defined boundaries – Uni or bilateral	– Smooth or nodular septal thickening and peri-bronchovascular interstitial thickening – Pleural effusion – Mediastinal lymph nodes	None
Local recurrence:			
– 3DCRT	– Within the area of fibrosis or at its contour	– Development of convex lateral margin – Filling-in of dilated bronchi	– Increase in size beyond 12 months
– SBRT/SABR	– Within the area of fibrosis or at its contour	– Loss of linear margin or appearance of bulging margin – Filling-in of dilated bronchi	– Enlarging consolidation: sequential/12 months after RT completion/in the cranio-caudal axis (≥5 mm or ≥20%)

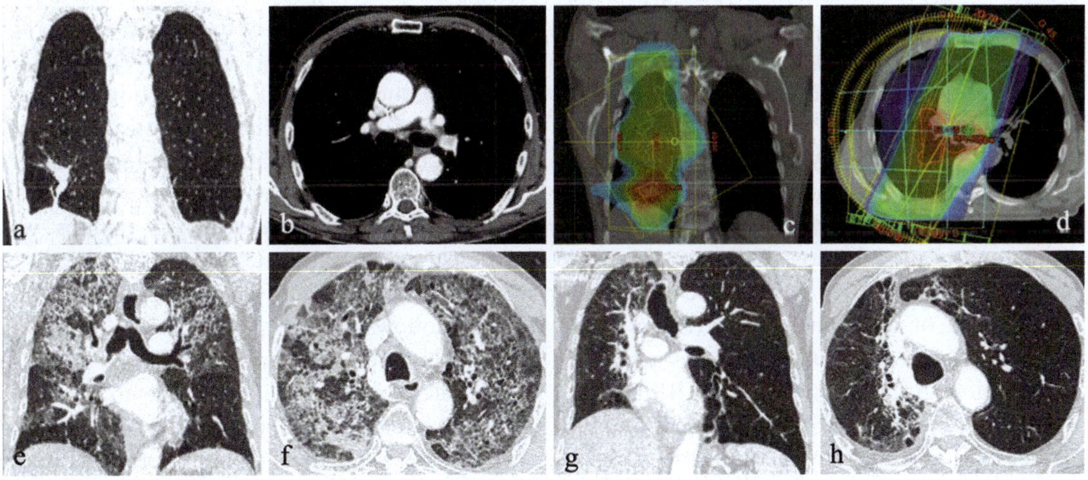

Fig. 6 **(a–h)** A 71-year-old man with a squamous cell carcinoma of the right lower lobe and ipsilateral mediastinal adenopathies (T2N2M0) (**a**, **b** coronal and axial images, respectively), who underwent 3D-CRT (VMAT) with concurrent ChT (**c**, **d** coronal and axial images, respectively). The early CT follow-up (CT scan after 1 months by the end of RT) shows bilateral GGOs and consolidations related to coexistence of RP and infectious disease (**e**, **f** coronal and axial images, respectively). CT scans performed after 6 months demonstrated fibrotic changes in the treated area of the right lung, with a *modified conventional pattern*, associated with volume loss and traction bronchiectasis (**g**, **h** coronal and axial images, respectively). No residual CT alterations can be seen in the left lobe

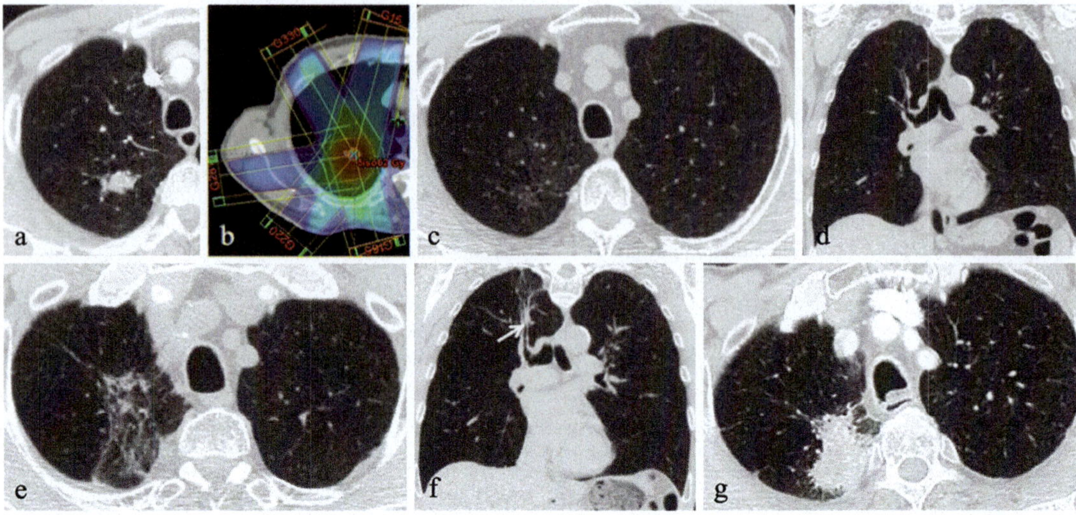

Fig. 7 (**a**–**g**) A 75-year-old man affected by a T1bN0M0 squamous cell carcinoma of the right upper lobe (**a**), undergoing SBRT/SABR (IMRT) (**b**) because of severe comorbidities. After the complete resolution of the primary mass with only subtle confluent GGOs (**c**, **d**, axial and coronal planes, respectively) (CT scan 2 months after the end of RT), the further follow-up CT scan demonstrated not only an increase of the fibrotic changes but also the "filling-in" of a segmental bronchus of the right upper lobe, suspicious for tumour recurrence (**e**, **f**, axial and coronal planes, respectively) (CT scan 12 months after the end of RT). Subsequent follow-up CT scan (18 months after the end of RT) confirmed the local tumour recurrence showing a solid consolidation with spiculated margins (**g**)

the region affected by radiation fibrosis may continue to evolve as long as 2 years after treatment (Larici et al. 2011; Ghaye et al. 2016; Takeda et al. 2008). Tumour recurrence appears as a homogeneous consolidation with a convex or lobulated contour and without air bronchogram (Larici et al. 2011; Ghaye et al. 2016) (Fig. 7). After 2D and 3D-CRT, suspicious parameters for recurrence are: (a) increase in size of fibrotic consolidation; (b) modification of the contour of the fibrotic area, with convex or lobulated aspect; and (c) filling-in of air bronchogram (Larici et al. 2011; Ghaye et al. 2016). Diagnosis of recurrence is more difficult after SBRT/SABR because RILI/RILD may present with rounded contours and less air bronchogram due to the dense fibrosis that obscures dilated bronchi, as well as because of the possible transient increase in size of the treated area occurring during the first 12 months after RT (Larici et al. 2011; Ghaye et al. 2016; Linda et al. 2011). Features suggestive of recurrence (*high-risk features, HRFs*) after SBRT/SABR have been described and validated, with a sensitivity and specificity of more than 90% when at least three are present (Ghaye et al. 2016; Peulen et al. 2016; Mattonen et al. 2016a; Huang et al. 2013): (a) enlarging opacity at the primary site (according to the RECIST criteria); (b) sequential enlarging opacity; (c) enlarging opacity 12 months after RT completion; (d) bulging margin; (e) loss of linear margin; (f) loss of air bronchogram (including partial loss); and (g) increase in size in the cranio-caudal axis (≥5 mm or ≥20%). Enlargement after 12 months was demonstrated to be the most accurate predictor of recurrence, although it was not useful in the first year of follow-up (Huang et al. 2013). The newer parameter of cranio-caudal growth is helpful in this context because changes in this axis are less related to fibrosis. Most of the SBRT/SABR dose is deposited in the axial plane, where most of the fibrosis should be expected (Huang et al. 2013). Other helpful signs in the diagnosis of tumour recurrence are the appearance of nodules outside the radiation fibrosis, mediastinal lymph nodes or other metastases (Larici et al. 2011; Ghaye et al. 2016). Huang et al. have proposed an algorithm (Table 3) for following-up patients who have undergone SBRT/SABR based on HRFs and maximum standardized uptake values (SUV_{max})

Table 3 Algorithm for follow-up of patients who underwent SBRT/SABR proposed by Huang et al., based on high-risk CT factors and SUV_{max} derived from PET/CT imaging (modified from Huang et al. (2012, 2013))

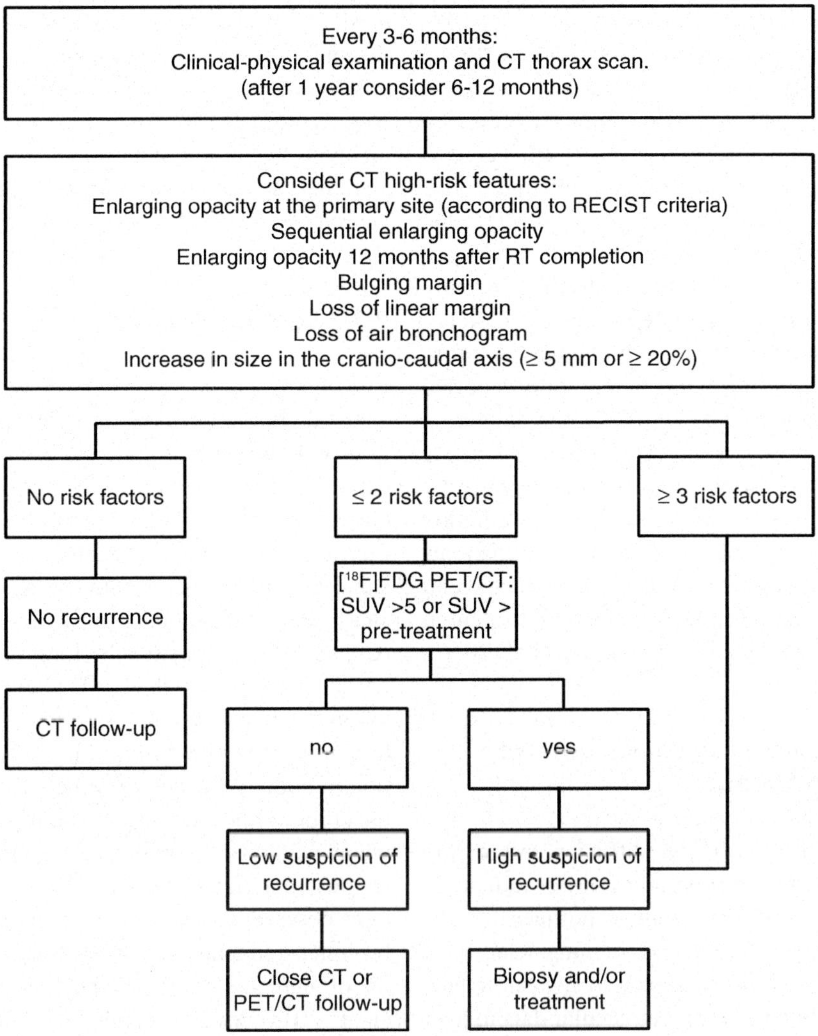

on PET/CT imaging (Huang et al. 2013; Huang et al. 2012). Authors suggest a CT every 3–6 months at least for the first year after ending RT, and thereafter, the frequency should be tailored taking into account whether the patient is medically operable or not (in the latter case, a 12-month follow-up is suggested) and the probability of recurrence. A more rigorous follow-up might be indicated in patients with higher likelihood of recurrence, including those with larger tumours or those treated with a sub-optimal radiation dose. Specifically, low-risk recurrence is defined with less than two HRFs, while high-risk recurrence is when three HRFs are present, as specified above. The use of routine PET/CT at a predefined time point is not recommended for routine follow-up due to the lack of evidence to support it. However, PET/CT is indicated when recurrent disease is suspected on CT imaging. PET/CT findings such as a $SUV_{max} \geq 5$ or SUV_{max} > pre-RT are suggestive of recurrence. Since the above-reported sensitivity and specificity reached with three HRFs are similar to those of fine-needle aspiration or core needle biopsy performance, when the probability of recurrence is high, further therapy is suggested.

Finally, the possibility of a radiation-induced cancer should be taken into account because radiation is a well-established carcinogen particularly with regard to the induction of solid tumours (Larici et al. 2011; Ghaye et al. 2016).

Although not common, any thoracic tissue exposed to radiation can manifest radiation injury. Among the unusual findings occurring after RT, organizing pneumonia (OP), necrosis and esophagitis are described. OP, more frequently reported after RT for breast cancer, is due to lymphocyte-mediated hypersensitivity reaction or disorder (Ghaye et al. 2016). It usually begins in the RP area and then migrates, sometimes in the opposite lung. Pulmonary or bronchial necrosis has been most commonly reported in patients undergoing ChT-RT; when cavitation occurs, the presence of infection (particularly tuberculosis) and tumour recurrence have to be excluded first (Ghaye et al. 2016). Radiation esophagitis is reported in less than 1% of patients after thoracic irradiation, usually towards the end of the RT, manifesting as a circumferential oesophageal wall thickening (Ghaye et al. 2016).

4 Emerging Imaging Parameters and Technique

Tumour volume, perfusion, diffusion and texture analysis have been proposed as newer radiological parameters and imaging techniques for the therapy response evaluation in lung cancer, in order to improve the precision of measurements and include functional and molecular data to gain a more complete tumour assessment.

Multiple factors related to tumour or patient characteristics (e.g. motion artefacts, physical constitution) can influence the acquisition process (Coche 2016; Nishino et al. 2014). Moreover, there is no consensus on scan acquisition parameters, neither on mathematical models to use in perfusions exams or on methods for lesion segmentation and measurements (Coche 2016; Nishino et al. 2014). All these characteristics can influence the reproducibility of the techniques; therefore, the standardization of the process, using the same acquisition parameters and software analysis package in each patient, will be useful in this context (Coche 2016; Nishino et al. 2014). Crucial issues related to dynamic contrast-enhanced (DCE) CT concern high radiation doses and contrast medium used in the acquisition. To date, no appropriate thresholds of response when applying these methods have been defined. Finally, up to now, few software packages are integrated in the picture archiving and communication system (PACS), resulting in non-contextual and time-consuming analyses (Coche 2016; Nishino et al. 2014).

4.1 Tumour Volume

The development of multi-detector CT has enabled the acquisition of large anatomic sections with isotropic voxels, allowing the quantification of tumour volumes. Tumour volume better corresponds to the real dimension of a lesion. Furthermore, irregular lesions are defined with small magnitude errors, and asymmetric growths can be reliably evaluated by volume assessment (Coche 2016). Specifically for nodular lesions, because nodule growth is a 3D phenomenon, intuitively, the assessment of volume and volume doubling time (VDT) provides accurate estimation of nodule changes (Revel et al. 2004). Lower uncertainty and observer variability are reached when using volumetric methods for measuring lesions (Gavrielides et al. 2009), with a better inter-observer agreement compared to uni- and bi-dimensional measurements (reported 95% limits of agreement of –26.0%, 18.6%) (Nishino et al. 2011; Mozley et al. 2012; Marten et al. 2006). Another advantage is the possibility of detecting changes of the lesions in a shorter period of time, resulting in higher sensitivity of the volume-based techniques in growth evaluation (Zhao et al. 2006).

Interesting results regard the opportunity to use volume-based response as a biomarker of therapy response or survival. EGFR-mutant NSCLC tumours can be better distinguished from wild-type ones by using volume estimation during targeted therapy, because of the volume decrease of mutant lesions (a cut-off volume of 24.9% has been reported as capable of distinguishing tumours with sensitizing mutations) (Zhao et al. 2010). Few reports underlined the association between tumour volume and survival in patients with NSCLC receiving exclusive RT-ChT or preoperative RT-ChT, with larger gross tumour volume (primitive tumour and positive lymph nodes or solely the tumour) being associated with shorter overall survival (OS) and progression-free survival (PFS) (Nishino et al. 2014; Dehing-Oberije et al. 2008; Kozak et al. 2011; Alexander et al. 2011). Finally, a reduction of tumour volume after ChT-RT in advanced NSCLC showed a correlation with pathological complete response (pCR) (Agrawal et al. 2016).

4.2 Perfusion Techniques

The perfusion of tissues can be indirectly evaluated by calculating the delivery of contrast medium and, therefore, the delivery of blood to the tissues (Coche 2016). Pulmonary perfusion assessment is performed with dynamic contrast-enhanced (DCE) CT and MRI techniques or dual-energy CT (DECT) (Ohno et al. 2016).

4.2.1 DCE Imaging

DCE perfusion studies include the acquisition of continuous dynamic images of the lesion, assessing the vascular support of tumours by analysing temporal changes in the attenuation of the blood vessels and tissues (Ohno et al. 2016). Multiple kinetic models and softwares can be used to calculate the distribution of the contrast medium in the intra- and extra-vascular space, both in a qualitative or quantitative way. Qualitative assessment provides colour maps for every perfusion parameter (e.g. blood volume, blood flow, mean transit time, permeability-surface area product) with an appraisal of their heterogeneity (Coche 2016; Ohno et al. 2016). Quantitative assessment generates histograms of the distribution of perfusion values for each voxel, allowing the extraction of numerical data (Coche 2016; Ohno et al. 2016). Tumour perfusion parameters obtained by using CT and MRI have been associated to lesion vascularization in histological specimens in NSCLC (Tacelli et al. 2010; Fujimoto et al. 2003). Moreover, vascular endothelial growth factor (VEGF)-positive tumours resulted to have higher slope of the time-signal intensity curve derived from DCE-MRI values than VEGF-negative ones (Fujimoto et al. 2003).

Different authors used DCE-CT parameters as a tool to evaluate treatment response in lung cancer, by correlating with RECIST during treatment or with survival. Studies including lung cancer patients undergoing ChT, with or without associated anti-angiogenic drugs or RT, measured perfusion values before and after treatment, reporting significant differences among responders and non-responders (Strauch et al. 2016). While a general reduction in perfusion parameters (most commonly permeability, blood volume and blood flow) has been observed after treatment, this resulted to be higher in responding patients (Fraioli et al. 2011; Fraioli et al. 2013; Tacelli et al. 2013). Moreover, some authors demonstrated that responding patients according to RECIST have higher perfusion values before therapy compared to non-responding ones, thus resulting in the potentially predictive value of DCE as a marker for treatment response (Fraioli et al. 2011; Wang et al. 2009). Also, when patients were treated with only anti-angiogenic/anti-vascular drugs, responders showed higher values of permeability and blood flow before treatment and a specific reduction of blood flow following therapy (Lind et al. 2010). Higher parameters of permeability before treatment are associated with better diffusion and therefore response to therapies, whereas a decrease after therapy might suggest a response due to the normalization of hyper-vascularization typical of cancer and is correlated with longer PFS (Strauch et al. 2016; Wang et al. 2009; Lind et al. 2010). Finally, perfusion changes can be detected during the course of treatment after a shorter time point in comparison to size modification (Tacelli et al. 2013). Fewer studies have assessed DCE-CT parameter changes after RT (Strauch et al. 2016). In case of exclusive RT, an increase in peripheral permeability was observed reflecting the increase of vessel leakiness and endothelial cell damage, associated to an increase in whole blood volume due to induced vasodilatation, opening up of previously non-perfused vessels or neo-vessel formation (Ng et al. 2007a; Ng et al. 2010). When combining anti-angiogenic/anti-vascular drugs to RT, a reduction in blood volume was observed because RT enhances the activity of these target medicines (Ng et al. 2007b).

Few studies have determined the usefulness of DCE-MRI in therapy response evaluation of NSCLC patients. After combined RT-ChT, a lower enhancement ratio and less slope of the relative enhancement were observed in patients achieving local control. Moreover, the survival was significantly longer in the group with a slope enhancement of 0.08/sec or less (Ohno et al. 2005). Both results can be related to the ischemic changes induced from therapy in tumour tissues. Different studies considered the effect of anti-vascular therapies on perfusion parameters. Before treatment, higher values of k_{trans} and k_{ep} parameters (forward volume transfer constant and reverse reflux rate constant between plasma and extracellular space, respectively) have been reported in responding patients (Tao et al. 2016). During follow-up, a reduction or heterogeneity in k_{trans} value (Dingemans et al. 2011) and variation values of k_{ep} less than 0.15 at 14 weeks have been related with PFS and OS improvement (Kelly et al. 2011).

4.2.2 DECT Imaging

DECT techniques use dual X-ray sources (using dual-layer detectors or fast kilovoltage-switching methods) to obtain scans with different X-ray energy levels. The attenuation of iodine is greater at 80 kVp than at 140 kVp, so a single contrast-enhanced acquisition can yield both unenhanced and contrast-enhanced CT data with the opportunity to derive the iodine content and its distribution maps. The iodine delivery in a tissue corresponds to its perfusion and, therefore, to the degree of vascularization. No extensive data is available on the usefulness of DECT in the field of response to therapy in lung cancer. When evaluating patients treated with anti-angiogenic agents for NSCLC, DECT, the use of virtual non-enhanced images allowed an easier distinction between tumour enhancement and haemorrhagic response, the latter posing problems of differential diagnosis with residual vital tissue when determining response after targeted therapy (Kim et al. 2012). After anti-EGFR therapy, responding patients showed a significant decrease in tumour iodine uptake (IU) and a small reduction in the arterial enhancement fraction (AEF) (Baxa et al. 2016). Similarly, after ChT, a significant decrease in AEF was observed among responding lymph nodes, as opposed to a significant increase in non-responding ones (Baxa et al. 2014). Aoki et al. evaluated DCE-CT in inoperable lung cancer before SBRT/SABR, observing a lower average iodine density in patients with worse prognosis, maybe reflecting an extensive hypoxic cell population in these tumours (Aoki et al. 2014, 2016).

4.3 Diffusion Imaging

Diffusion-weighted magnetic resonance imaging (DW-MRI) reflects the Brownian motion of water molecules in biological tissues, mainly depending on tissue cellularity (Coche 2016). Restricted diffusion is observed in malignancies because of high cellularity; on the contrary, after successful therapy, a decrease in tumour cell density results in a higher water diffusion. (Coche 2016). In NSCLC treated with RT and ChT, the apparent diffusion coefficient (ADC) measured on pre-therapeutic MR scans was able to predict partial response to treatment (Ohno et al. 2012). After ChT or RT-ChT, a significant increase in ADC has been observed (Weiss et al. 2016), with a significant correlation with longer PFS and OS (Yabuuchi et al. 2011).

4.4 Texture Analysis

In medical imaging, texture analysis can be defined as the quantification of the value and spatial distribution of voxel grey levels, used to derive mathematically sets of numeric data that measure heterogeneity (Coche 2016). The underlying hypothesis is that image texture may be related to tumour histopathology, phenotype and genotype (Coche 2016). Studies on lung cancer have shown promising results in the assessment of treatment response, particularly by creating prognostic models to predict response and/or survival (Coche 2016).

Some authors have evaluated the predictive role of textural parameters in patients receiving definitive ChT. Ravanelli et al. described the product of tumour uniformity (U, a measure of heterogeneity) and mean grey level (GL, an indirect indicator of tumour vascularization) as a predictor of therapy response (Ravanelli et al. 2013). Dividing the resulting values in tertiles, an increased probability of response was demonstrated in the second and third tertiles (Ravanelli et al. 2013). Tumours in the first tertile were characterized by low U and low GL; these parameters were indicative of heterogeneous lesions and low perfused/hypoxic areas with neo-angiogenic adaptive responses (higher aggressiveness and low response) (Ravanelli et al. 2013). Tumour in the higher tertiles corresponded to high U and low GL, indicative of homogeneous tissue with poor vascularization and no adaptive neo-angiogenesis (low aggressiveness and higher response), or high GL with any U, as in well-perfused lesions (low aggressiveness and intermediate response) (Ravanelli et al. 2013). Fried et al. (Fried et al. 2014) observed an improvement in patient risk stratification for OS, local recurrence or distant metastasis by adding textural parameters to the clinical ones. Pretreatment textural data have also been suggested as able to predict pathological response after neo-adjuvant therapy in patients with locally advanced NSCLC. In combined RT-ChT, Coroller et al. found seven features predictive of pathologic gross residual disease (area under the curve (AUC) >0.6) and one of pathologic complete response (AUC = 0.63) (Coroller et al. 2016). Moreover, non-responder tumours were more likely to present a rounder shape and heterogeneous texture (Coroller et al. 2016). When evaluating ChT associated with target EGFR-TKI therapy, intensity variability was found to be an independent predictor of pathological response (Chong et al. 2014).

Different authors have also studied the usefulness of texture analysis in the evaluation of RILI/RILD, as well as in the prediction of patients' outcome after RT. In patients undergoing RT, Cunliffe et al. has shown a significant difference in 19 texture feature values in pre- and post-RT treatment CT scans (Cunliffe et al. 2014). Mattonen et al. analysed CT images of patients after SBRT/SABR in order to distinguish RILI/RILD from recurrence (Mattonen et al. 2013). They suggested that first-order textural features could significantly distinguish RILI/RILD from recurrence at images performed 9 months after the end of treatment. Consolidative areas were characterized by higher mean attenuation values in cases of recurrence compared to those with RILI/RILD. Likewise, GGO areas, expression of recurrence, showed larger standard deviation of densities because of lesion heterogeneity (Mattonen et al. 2013). Specifically, in another study by the same authors, at 2–5 months post-treatment, features of first (mean and standard deviation) and second order (energy and entropy), calculated in GGO areas, provided AUC values of 0.79–0.81 in predicting recurrence (Mattonen et al. 2014). At the same time point, authors demonstrated a better performance of textural features in defining recurrence compared to medical evaluation alone (Mattonen et al. 2016b). Studies in patients treated with concurrent RT-ChT demonstrated that texture-strength measured at the end of treatment was able to stratify patients with high and low risk for local recurrence (Fave et al. 2017). Finally, after SBRT/SABR, Huynh et al. have successfully used textural features to predict OS (Huynh et al. 2016).

5 Metabolism and PET/CT

Metabolism can be assessed by PET/CT using not only the glucose analogue [^{18}F]FDG, which is the most important PET radiotracer (Jadvar et al. 2017), but also many other PET radiotracers such as ^{11}C-methionine and ^{68}Ga-DOTATOC, among others. PET provides functional or metabolic information. PET/CT combines the advantages of PET, high contrast resolution, and CT, high spatial resolution. There is broad evidence of [^{18}F]FDG PET/CT in lung cancer and its utility for characterizing solitary pulmonary nodules (Divisi et al. 2010), staging (Agarwal et al. 2010), guiding therapy (Pommier et al. 2010), monitoring treatment response (de Cabanyes Candela and Detterbeck 2010) and predicting outcome (Fischer et al. 2006), as well as having demonstrated its cost-effectiveness (Ambrosini et al. 2012; Schreyögg et al. 2010). Figure 8 presents a patient treated with chemotherapy, and Fig. 9 presents another one treated with chemoradiotherapy, both with an initial or baseline [^{18}F]FDG PET/CT and a second posttreatment [^{18}F]FDG PET/CT, in the first patient an interim study following three cycles and in the other patient after finalizing chemoradiotherapy.

The Society of Nuclear Medicine and Molecular Imaging (SNMMI) published in 2017 the appropriate use criteria (AUC) for [^{18}F]FDG PET/CT in restaging and response assessment of malignant disease, including lung cancer (Jadvar et al. 2017). This document describes the appropriate use of PET/CT, based on a systematic

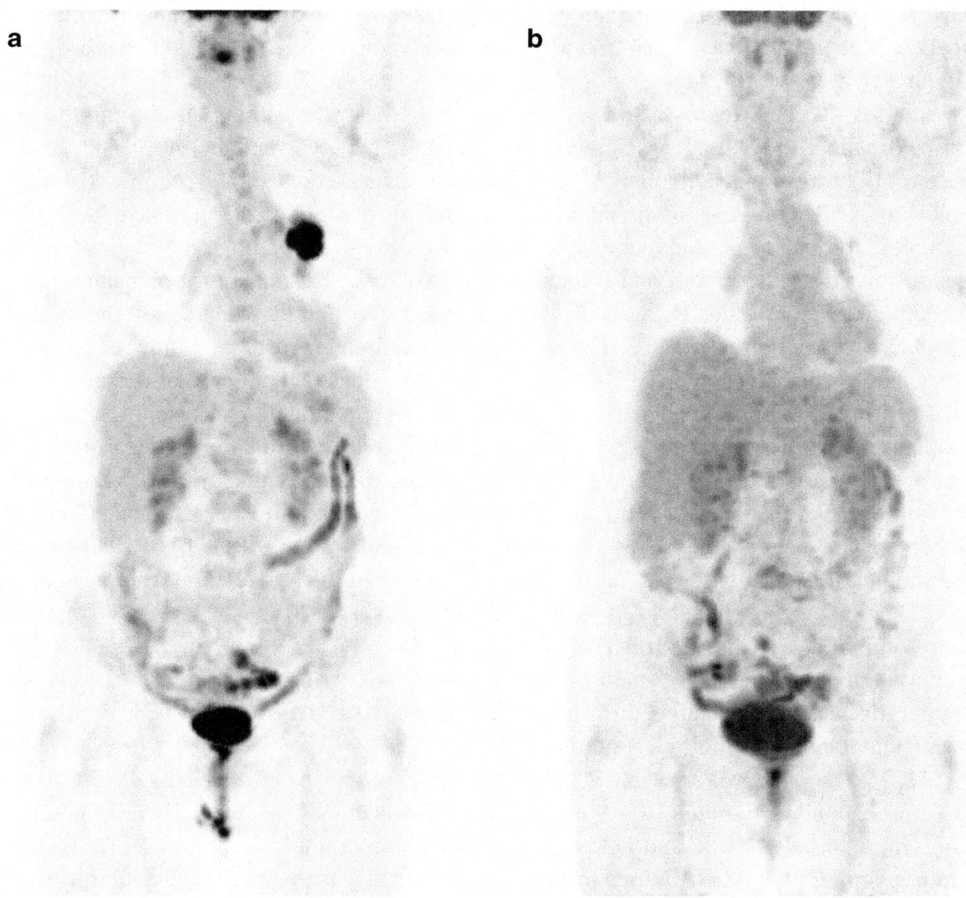

Fig. 8 Response monitoring following chemotherapy: Patient with stage IIIA (T2N2M0) NSCLC. The initial staging [^{18}F]FDG PET/CT is presented here: maximum intensity projection (MIP) of [^{18}F]FDG PET (**a**). The patient is treated with neoadjuvant chemotherapy with taxol and carboplatin. After three cycles, a second or interim [^{18}F]FDG PET/CT is done (**b**). The axial slices of the [^{18}F]FDG PET, CT and fused [^{18}F]FDG PET/CT images are presented (images **c**–**h**), in the upper row the interim [^{18}F]FDG PET/CT and in the lower row the pretreatment or baseline [^{18}F]FDG PET/CT. The primary tumour presented a SUV_{max} of 24.2 in the initial PET and of 2.0 in the interim PET; the N1 disease in the left hilar node (10L) presented a SUV_{max} of 3.8 in the initial PET and of 2.3 in the interim PET; the N2 disease in the left lower paratracheal node (4L) presented a SUV_{max} of 3.7 in the initial PET and of 2.3 in the interim PET. The interim PET suggested a very good response to chemotherapy with persistence of minimal residual uptake in the three locations described. Mediastinoscopy following neoadjuvant chemotherapy evidenced malignant disease in the N2 stage (4L), confirming the N stage as ypN2

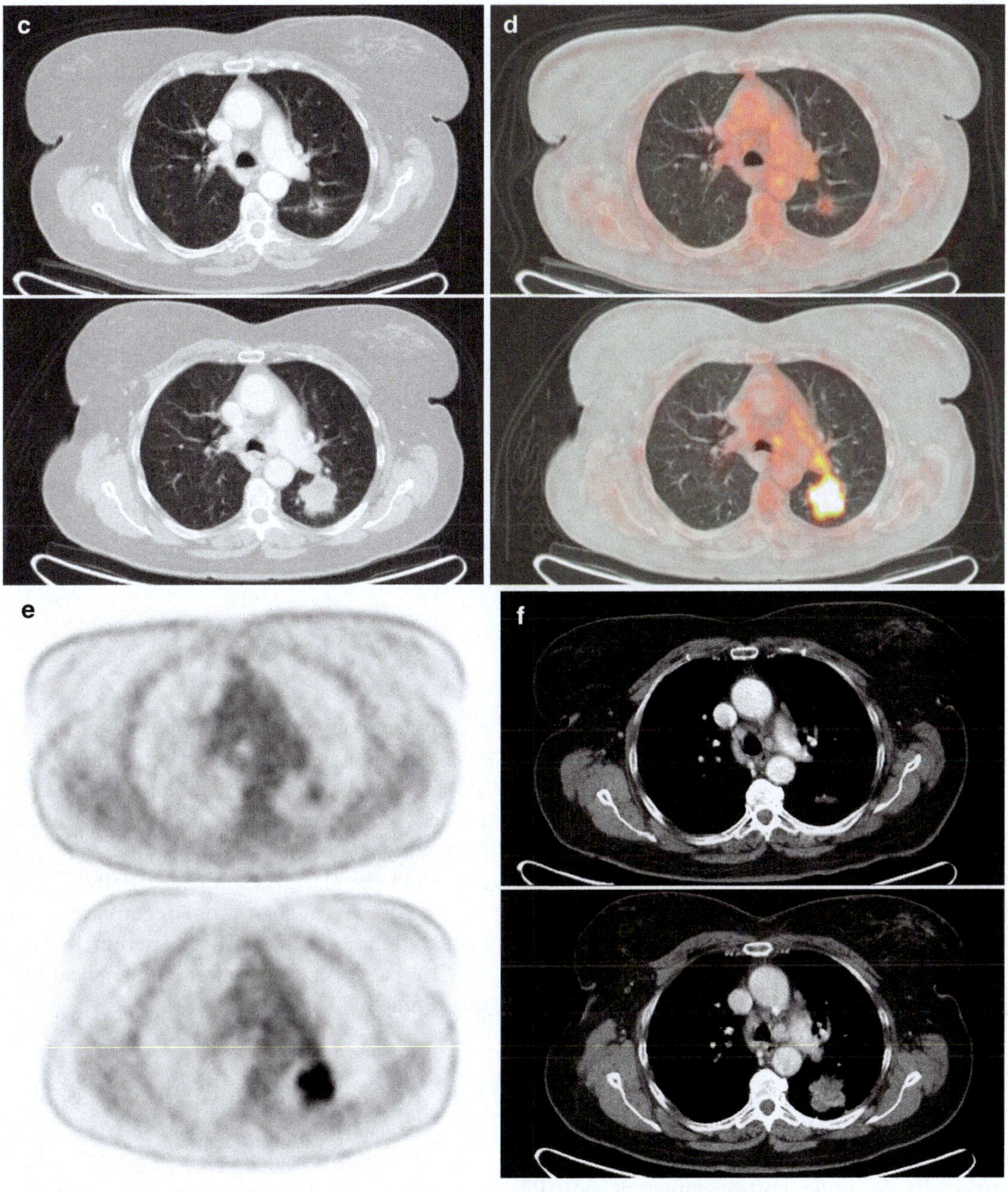

Fig. 8 (continued)

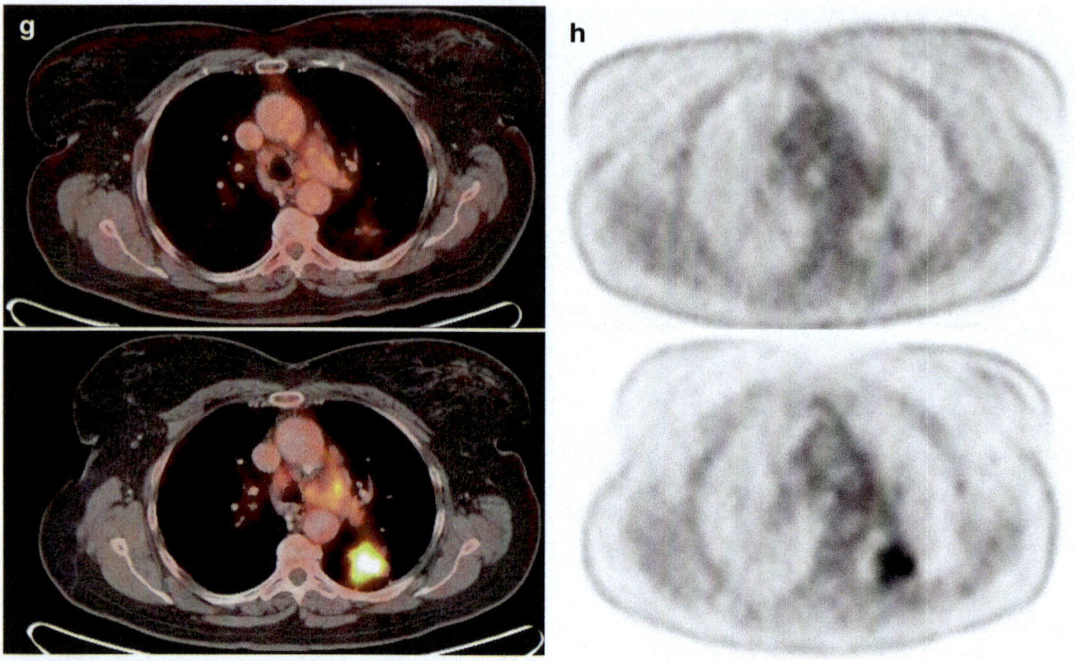

Fig. 8 (continued)

review, with the aim of synthesizing the evidence on the accuracy and comparative accuracy of PET/CT.

As has been discussed above, after initial treatment (surgery, RT), differentiating recurrence from post-surgical changes is challenging when using CT or MRI alone, as most benign processes (atelectasis, consolidations and radiation-induced fibrosis) are very difficult to differentiate from loco-regional recurrence (Jadvar et al. 2017; Sudarski et al. 2013; Jiménez-Ballvé et al. 2016; Caulo et al. 2012). [^{18}F]FDG PET/CT has the advantage of differentiating metabolically active areas. However, false-positive results can derive from active inflammation, especially in acute post-operative or post-RT phases, although this characteristic of [^{18}F]FDG is now being used in the diagnosis of infection and inflammation with good diagnostic performance (Rubins and Unger 2007). Recurrence of NSCLC may be classified as loco-regional recurrence or distant metastases, the latter being the most common form of NSCLC recurrence (Sudarski et al. 2013). Depending on the initial stage and on the treatment applied, metastatic recurrence comprises 39–65.5% of all recurrences (Caulo et al. 2012), whereas around 30% are loco-regional. Loco-regional recurrence is located within the treated hemithorax, usually presenting as nodules involving the treated area (Sudarski et al. 2013; Jiménez-Ballvé et al. 2016). Moreover, apart from recurrences, new primary lung cancer is also reported in 1–2% of NSCLC patients per year after initial radical therapy (Ponn 2000).

5.1 Restaging for Detection of Local Recurrence

The AUC score for this indication is 7 out of 9, meaning it is considered an appropriate diagnostic method (Jadvar et al. 2017). Regarding restaging after initial treatment (surgery, chemoradiotherapy or radiotherapy), a recent meta-analysis evaluated the diagnostic efficacy of PET and PET/CT with [^{18}F]FDG compared to conventional imaging techniques (CITs) for the detection of recurrent lung cancer (He et al. 2014). Inclusion criteria were for studies in the context of secondary lung cancer investigations using PET or PET/CT with [^{18}F]FDG to diagnose lung cancer recurrence, considering disease as a consequence of the originally diagnosed lung cancer, regardless of whether the recurrence was local, regional or distant. Thirteen articles and 1035 patients were included. They obtained high pooled/joint sensitivity and specificity for PET/CT. With regard to sensitivity, lower values were associated with CITs than PET (p = 0.000) and PET/CT (p = 0.005), and there was no significant difference between PET/CT and PET (p = 0.1).

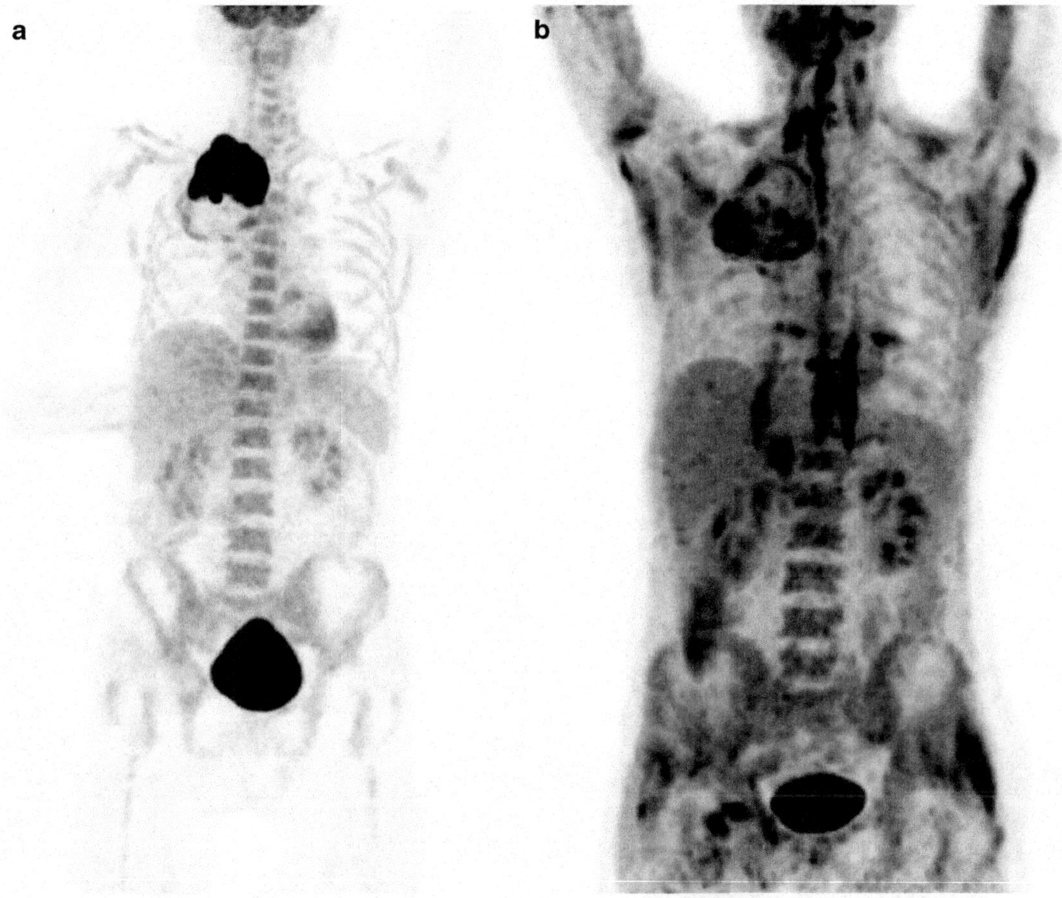

Fig. 9 Response monitoring following chemoradiotherapy: 42-year-old male, smoker. The clinical presentation consisted in neurologic compression in the upper right extremity. A Pancoast tumour in the right lung was diagnosed. The initial staging [^{18}F]FDG PET/CT is presented here: maximum intensity projection (MIP) of [^{18}F]FDG PET (**a**). The patient was treated with induction therapy with preoperative chemoradiotherapy that consisted of two cycles of chemotherapy (during 4 weeks) concomitant with radiotherapy 45 Gy (prolonged for 2 weeks more). At the time of the second [^{18}F]FDG PET/CT, the chemotherapy had finished 4 weeks before and the radiotherapy had finished 2 weeks before, evidencing a good response to therapy (**b**). The comparative axial slices of [^{18}F]FDG PET, CT and fused [^{18}F]FDG PET/CT images of the pretreatment study (**c**, **e** and **g**) and the posttreatment study (**d**, **f** and **h**) are presented at three levels, the higher one being the supraclavicular region (**c**, **d**), the middle one in the upper lung lobes (**e**, **f**) and the third one at the lower part of the lung tumour (**g**, **h**). The dimensions of the tumour did not change significantly from the pretreatment study (10 × 10 × 10.1 cm; left-right × antero-posterior × cranio-caudal, respectively) to the posttreatment study (9.2 × 8.9 × 9.4 cm). However, there was a significant change both in the SUV_{max} that changed from 37.7 to 6.2 (pretreatment to posttreatment, respectively) and in the metabolic tumour volume (MTV) (considering a threshold of SUV > 3) that changed from 294 to 60 cm^3, meaning a reduction of 80% of the MTV. These results were considered as a very good response to treatment that was confirmed with the clinical evolution of the patient

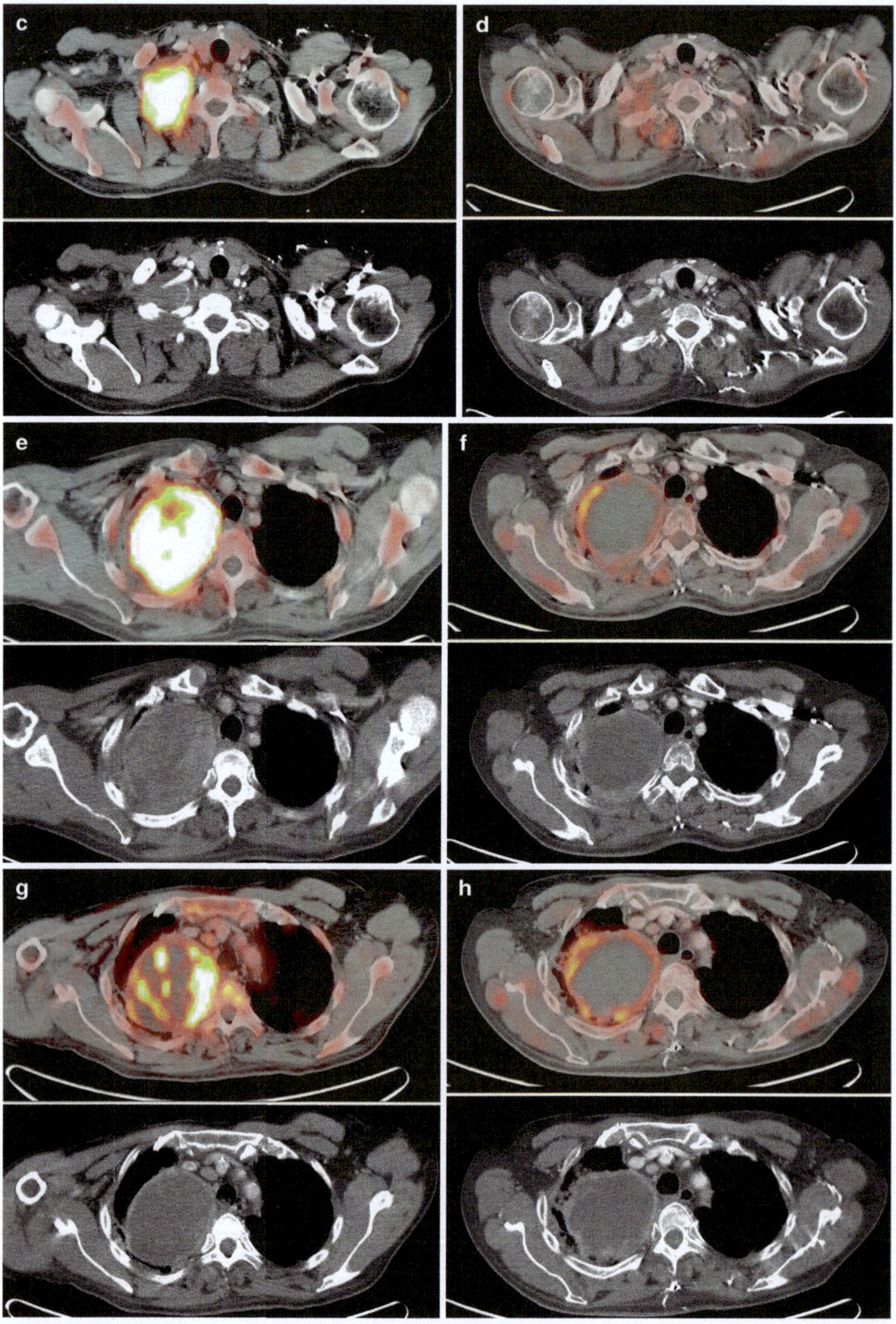

Fig. 9 (continued)

Regarding specificity, values for PET/CT and PET were significantly higher than those of CITs (both $p = 0.000$), with no significant difference between PET/CT and PET ($p = 0.2$). Summary Receiver Operating Characteristic (SROC) curves evidenced a better diagnostic accuracy associated with PET/CT than PET and CITs. They conclude PET/CT and PET were superior modalities for the detection of recurrent lung cancer, and PET/CT was superior to CT (He et al. 2014).

5.2 Restaging After Stereotactic Body Radiation Therapy (SBRT)

As discussed previously, SBRT is an established treatment option for early-stage lung cancer. SBRT causes focal changes in the lung parenchyma around the treated tumour site, most frequently as ground-glass opacities (GGO) (Jadvar et al. 2017; Sudarski et al. 2013; Bojarski et al. 2005). The study by Pastis et al. (2014) evaluated the diagnostic efficacy of [^{18}F]FDG PET/CT for detecting local treatment failure or intrathoracic recurrences after SBRT treatment in NSCLC patients. Eighty-eight patients were included, and an [^{18}F]FDG PET/CT was done 3 months after finalizing SBRT. [^{18}F]FDG PET/CT was positive in 14% (12 of 88) of patients, being confirmed as true positive in 67% (8 of 12). [^{18}F]FDG PET/CT was negative in 86% (76 of 88) of patients, being confirmed as true negative in 89% (68 of 76). Thus, sensitivity, specificity, positive predictive value and negative predictive value were 50.0, 94.0, 67.0 and 89.0, respectively. They conclude that an [^{18}F]FDG PET/CT scan 3 months after SBRT treatment of NSCLC was specific but had a low sensitivity for the detection of recurrent disease or treatment failure. They recommend CT (every 6 months for the first 2 years and every year thereafter (Colt et al. 2013)) instead of [^{18}F]-FDG PET/CT in this situation, whereas they state [^{18}F]FDG PET/CT should be reserved for cases with suspected metastatic disease, or to evaluate new abnormalities found on CT, or for the subsequent follow-up when the inflammation due to the radiation therapy has subsided (Jadvar et al. 2017; Pastis Jr et al. 2014).

Another study focusing on lung cancer patients treated with SBRT by Zhang et al. (2012a) analysed whether if [^{18}F]FDG PET/CT's standardized uptake values (SUVs) after SBRT could be applied in the prediction of local recurrence in NSCLC. They included 128 patients with 140 biopsy-proven NSCLC tumours, in whom 506 [^{18}F]FDG PET/CT scans were done. [^{18}F]FDG PET/CT was performed between 1 and 6 months after SBRT and subsequently as clinically indicated (median follow-up, 31 months). They conclude [^{18}F]FDG PET/CT was helpful for distinguishing SBRT-induced consolidation from local recurrence. High SUVs (>5.0) obtained more than 6 months after SBRT for NSCLC were associated with local failure and should prompt biopsy to rule out local recurrence (Zhang et al. 2012a). Similarly, Takeda et al. (2013) included 154 NSCLC patients with 214 [^{18}F]FDG PET/CT scans done 1 year after SBRT for the detection of local recurrence, reporting a sensitivity and specificity of 100% and 96–98%, respectively. Whereas these studies analyse the performance of [^{18}F]FDG PET/CT studies done 6 months to 1 year after SBRT, Van Loon et al. (2009) reported that early [^{18}F]FDG PET/CT scan 3 months after radical (chemo-) radiotherapy with curative intent helped detect progressive disease (PD). Van Loon et al. prospectively included 100 patients with NSCLC who had an [^{18}F]FDG PET/CT scan done 3 months after initiation of radiotherapy. PD was found in 24 patients, only 16 of them with symptoms. In the subgroup of symptomatic patients, the impact on management of [^{18}F]FDG PET/CT was limited, the reason being that no curative treatment could be offered as an alternative. However, in the asymptomatic group, in 3/8 patients diagnosed with PD, an option of a radical treatment could be offered. As PD in the asymptomatic patients was diagnosed with [^{18}F]-FDG PET/CT but not with CT, the authors concluded that asymptomatic patients are probably the ones that could profit most from an early [^{18}F]FDG PET/CT scan, although further studies are needed (Jadvar et al. 2017).

A frequent finding after radiotherapy is the presence of a variable and persistent [^{18}F]FDG uptake. Hoopes et al. (2007) presented a small patient population with inoperable stage I NSCLC after SBRT treatment, reporting persistent and moderately intense [^{18}F]FDG uptake up to 2 years after SBRT. This uptake could be related to inflammation and fibrosis, which is probably more persistent after SBRT compared to conventional fractioned radiotherapy (Cuaron et al. 2012).

5.3 Cost-Effectiveness

With regard to cost-effectiveness, up to now, Van Loon et al. have published the only cost-effectiveness study of NSCLC follow-up (van Loon et al. 2010). They included 100 NSCLC patients and compared three different follow-up strategies either with [^{18}F]FDG PET/CT, a chest CT or conventional follow-up with a chest radiograph, all starting 3 months after therapy. They concluded that an [^{18}F]FDG PET/CT 3 months after curative intent (chemo-) radiotherapy is potentially cost-effective and is more cost-effective than CT alone. Additionally, [^{18}F]FDG PET/CT in asymptomatic patients appears to be equally effective and even more cost-effective (Jadvar et al. 2017; Sudarski et al. 2013; van Loon et al. 2010).

5.4 Restaging for Detection of Metastases

The AUC score for this indication is 7 out of 9, meaning it is considered an appropriate diagnostic method (Jadvar et al. 2017). At the moment of diagnosis of NSCLC, around 18–36% of patients have distant metastases. The detection of these metastases at initial staging is key in order to decide on the most appropriate management option, as M staging has a direct impact on management and prognosis (Quint 2007). Moreover, in patients apparently radically treated for NSCLC, around 20% will relapse due to the presence of undetected metastases at initial staging (Jadvar et al. 2017; Ambrosini et al. 2012; Quint 2007). Metastases are usually localized in the adrenal glands, bones, brain or liver.

Regarding adrenal lesions, [^{18}F]FDG PET has demonstrated a good diagnostic performance in differentiating benign from metastatic lesions in patients with cancer (Yun et al. 2001), although few studies have specifically addressed this issue in lung cancer patients (Gupta et al. 2001; Kumar et al. 2004). The study analysing the highest number of patients included 94 NSCLC patients with 113 adrenal masses detected on CT or MRI. [^{18}F]FDG PET showed a sensitivity, specificity and accuracy for detecting metastatic disease of 93%, 90% and 92%, respectively (Kumar et al. 2004).

With regard to bone metastases, [^{18}F]FDG PET is more sensitive and specific than bone scintigraphy (Ambrosini et al. 2012; Liu et al. 2011; Cheran et al. 2004; Min et al. 2009). The best method for liver lesions is MRI, but [^{18}F]FDG PET is better than CT as it detects lesions earlier and is more accurate. MRI is also the best method for brain metastases, as [^{18}F]FDG PET is limited due to the high physiologic [^{18}F]FDG uptake in the normal brain. Other non-[^{18}F]FDG tracers must be considered for brain metastases. In summary, [^{18}F]FDG PET/CT has a high diagnostic performance for the detection of metastases. This often changes the stage of the disease and has an impact on management (Jadvar et al. 2017).

As discussed in the "local recurrence" section, a meta-analysis analysed the diagnostic efficacy of PET/CT compared to CITs for the detection of recurrent lung cancer, considering disease as a consequence of the originally diagnosed lung cancer, regardless of whether the recurrence was local, regional or distant. The results showed high pooled/joint sensitivity and specificity for PET/CT, concluding PET/CT and PET were superior modalities for the detection of recurrent lung cancer, and PET/CT was superior to CT (He et al. 2014).

In another meta-analysis that evaluated the performance of [^{18}F]FDG PET/CT for the detection of distant malignancies in various cancers, 41 studies and 4305 patients were included (Xu et al. 2012). Of these, the studies with data on lung cancer were 5 (Cerfolio et al. 2004; Fischer et al. 2007; Ohno et al. 2008; Yi et al. 2008; Plathow et al. 2008), comprising 578 patients.

The results showed pooled sensitivity, specificity, positive likelihood ratio and negative likelihood ratio values of 0.91, 0.96, 25.9 and 0.09, respectively. They concluded [^{18}F]FDG PET/CT has an excellent diagnostic performance for the detection of distant malignancies in patients with various cancers, especially in lung cancer, breast cancer and head and neck cancer (Jadvar et al. 2017; Xu et al. 2012).

5.5 Treatment Response Evaluation

The AUC score for this indication is 7 out of 9, meaning it is considered an appropriate diagnostic method (Jadvar et al. 2017). Personalized medicine is based on tailoring treatments to the individual patient. For this, it is of utmost importance to have tools that provide an early and precise assessment of response to therapy (Delgado Bolton et al. 2008; Delgado Bolton and Carreras Delgado 2009). Traditionally, the response of the tumour has been assessed comparing the tumour size on CT before and after treatment, previously in two dimensions (World Health Organisation, WHO (Miller et al. 1981)) and more recently in one dimension (response evaluation criteria in solid tumours, RECIST (Therasse et al. 2000)), as has been discussed above. [^{18}F]FDG PET provides functional information, and metabolic changes can be detected earlier than morphologic changes. In this regard, early assessment of response can be of great value in patients with cancer, in particular in lung cancer. A large proportion of patients undergo treatments that are toxic and expensive with no response, when there are second-line treatments available (Vansteenkiste et al. 2004). Early assessment of therapy response can help tailor treatments in order to continue treatments in responding patients and discontinue treatments and change to second-line treatments in non-responders. Current evidence shows that [^{18}F]FDG PET/CT response is probably earlier and more accurate that CT response (Vansteenkiste et al. 2004). However, an important issue to be solved is related to the need to standardize the methodology. The European Association of Nuclear Medicine (EANM) [^{18}F]FDG PET/CT procedure guidelines for tumour imaging have focused on harmonization in order to make the methodology and results comparable worldwide (Boellaard et al. 2015). In this regard, one of the methodology aspects that need to be standardized in the response assessment studies is the timing of the [^{18}F]FDG PET/CT. The best timing has not been standardized yet; if done too early, it might overestimate [^{18}F]FDG uptake because glucose metabolism might be present in cells that are lethally damaged and because of inflammatory processes in responding tissues (Vansteenkiste et al. 2004). If it is done too late, other problems might appear, such as late evaluation of response or the risk of tumour repopulation. In summary, large-scale trials are needed, applying strict methodological standardization (Jadvar et al. 2017).

In patients with locally advanced lung cancer who undergo multimodality treatment, a precise and correct restaging after induction therapy is of utmost importance (Vansteenkiste et al. 2004). In NSCLC stage IIIa-N2, a favourable outcome after surgical combined modality treatment highly depends on pathological downstaging or clearance of all tumour in the mediastinal lymph nodes after the induction phase. CT has limitations when evaluating response to induction treatment because small-sized lymph nodes can still harbour metastatic disease, whereas large nodes can be due to inflammatory factors or scarring (Vansteenkiste et al. 2004; Margaritora et al. 2001). Several studies have analysed the role of [^{18}F]FDG PET in this clinical setting with good results (Jadvar et al. 2017).

One fair-quality study including patients with stage IIIa NSCLC with biopsy-proven N2 disease that underwent neoadjuvant chemoradiotherapy and subsequent restaging ($n = 93$) found PET/CT had a sensitivity of 62% and a specificity of 88% for identifying N2 disease. Compared with pathological staging, the proportion of patients with correct stage classification was greater with PET/CT than CT across tumour stages 0 through IV, though differences were only statistically significant for stage 0 and stage I (Cerfolio et al. 2006). Other similar studies have shown that those who are downstaged via neoadjuvant therapy and then undergo resection have a significantly longer 5-year survival of 40–50% (Detterbeck and Socinski 2001; Bueno et al. 2000; Voltolini et al. 2001) than the patients who have residual N2 disease (Komaki et al. 1985). Therefore, identifying N2 negative patients after completion of their neoadjuvant therapy is a critical component when selecting patients for thoracotomy (Cerfolio et al. 2006). However, correctly identifying responding from non-responding patients remains a challenge. Most patients with pathologically diagnosed N2 disease have undergone mediastinoscopy. Repeat mediastinoscopy is difficult, often inaccurate (Mateu-Navarro et al. 2000; Pitz et al. 2002) and potentially dangerous, in particular following radiotherapy. Moreover, there is evidence of a high false-negative rate for repeat mediastinoscopy following neoadjuvant therapy, with a range of 25–42% (Mateu-Navarro et al. 2000; Van Schil et al. 2002). In one small study with a small patient population ($n = 19$) following neoadjuvant chemoradiotherapy, fine needle aspiration (FNA) guided by endoscopic ultrasound (EUS) has been used as a restaging method with a reported accuracy of 83%. The main problems of EUS-FNA are it does not allow an adequate visualization of the lower paratracheal nodes (Wallace et al. 2004) and it is available in only a few centres. In summary, the surgeon often only has the clinical stage assessed by repeat PET/CT or CT to back up the management decisions. The prospective study by Cerfolio et al. concludes that repeat integrated [^{18}F]FDG PET/CT is superior to repeat CT for the restaging of patients with N2 stage IIIa NSCLC after neoadjuvant chemoradiotherapy (Jadvar et al. 2017; Cerfolio et al. 2006).

Another meta-analysis, this one published in 2012, evaluated the efficacy of [^{18}F]FDG PET and CT in predicting the pathological tumour response of NSCLC after neoadjuvant therapy. Pathological outcome was the gold standard. Thirteen studies and 414 patients were included with different neoadjuvant treatments: chemoradiotherapy in five studies, chemotherapy in two studies and mixed treatments in the remaining five (Zhang et al. 2012b). Pooled sensitivity, specificity, positive predictive value and negative predictive value for prediction of response with PET were 83%, 84%, 74% and 91%, respectively. The predictive value of PET in NSCLC patients with pathological response was significantly higher than that of CT ($p < 0.05$). However, these results have to be analysed taking into account the limitations of the meta-analysis, such as the heterogeneity of the studies, the mixed pathological types and their retrospective design. Taking into account the mentioned limitations, they conclude [^{18}F]FDG PET is useful for predicting NSCLC non-responders to neoadjuvant therapy, and it has a better predictive value than that of CT for evaluating pathological documented responses (Jadvar et al. 2017).

6 Conclusions

Tumour response imaging criteria should be applied in the assessment of response to therapy in lung cancer in favour of standardization; however, it has to be kept in mind that they have been originally designed to evaluate response to cytotoxic ChT. When using newer targeted ChT agents as well as RT, the response pattern is highly dependent on the specific treatment, in terms of appearance and timing. The knowledge of the CT manifestations occurring after using these therapies is helpful to address the subsequent management decisions. Newer radiological parameters and functional techniques demonstrated promising results in evaluating and predicting treatment response. [^{18}F]FDG PET/CT is considered a useful tool for evaluating response to therapy in NSCLC, although the evidence is still limited. Therefore, response assessment in lung cancer should consider multimodality imaging and evolve according to the advances in therapies.

References

Agarwal M, Brahmanday G, Bajaj SK, Ravikrishnan KP, Wong CGO (2010) Revisiting the prognostic value of preoperative 18F-fluoro-2-deoxyglucose (18F-FDG) positron emission tomography (PET) in early-stage (I & II) non-small cell lung cancers (NSCLC). Eur J Nucl Med Mol Imaging 37:691–698

Agrawal V, Coroller TP, Hou Y, Lee SW, Romano JL, Baldini EH et al (2016) Radiologic-pathologic correlation of response to chemoradiation in resectable locally advanced NSCLC. Lung Cancer 102:1–8

Alexander BM, Othus M, Caglar HB, Allen AM (2011) Tumor volume is a prognostic factor in non-small-cell lung cancer treated with chemoradiotherapy. Int J Radiat Oncol Biol Phys 79:1381–1387

Ambrosini V, Nicolini S, Caroli P, Nanni C, Massaro A, Marzola MC et al (2012) Eur J Radiol 81:988–1001

Aoki M, Takai Y, Narita Y, Hirose K, Sato M, Akimoto H et al (2014) Correlation between tumor size and blood volume in lung tumors: a prospective study on dual-energy gemstone spectral CT imaging. J Radiat Res 55:917–923

Aoki M, Hirose K, Sato M, Akimoto H, Kawaguchi H, Hatayama Y et al (2016) Prognostic impact of average iodine density assessed by dual-energy spectral imaging for predicting lung tumor recurrence after stereotactic body radiotherapy. J Radiat Res 57:381–386

Baxa J, Vondráková A, Matoušková T, Růžičková O, Schmidt B, Flohr T et al (2014) Dual-phase dual-energy CT in patients with lung cancer: assessment of the additional value of iodine quantification in lymph node therapy response. Eur Radiol 24:1981–1988

Baxa J, Matouskova T, Krakorova G, Schmidt B, Flohr T, Sedlmair M et al (2016) Dual-phase dual-energy CT in patients treated with Erlotinib for advanced non-small cell lung cancer: Possible benefits of iodine quantification in response assessment. Eur Radiol 26:2828–2836

Boellaard R, Delgado-Bolton R, Oyen WJ, Giammarile F, Tatsch K, Eschner W et al (2015) FDG PET/CT: EANM procedure guidelines for tumour imaging: version 2.0. Eur J Nucl Med Mol Imaging 42:328–354

Bojarski JD, Dupuy DE, Mayo-Smith WW (2005) CT imaging findings of pulmonary neoplasms after treatment with radiofrequency ablation: results in 32 tumors. AJR Am J Roentgenol 185:466–471

Bueno R, Richards W, Swanson S, Jaklitsch MT, Lukanich JM, Mentzer SJ et al (2000) Nodal stage after induction therapy for stage IIIA lung cancer determines patient survival. Ann Thorac Surg 70:1826–1831

de Cabanyes Candela S, Detterbeck FC (2010) A systematic review of restaging after induction therapy for stage IIIa lung cancer: prediction of pathologic stage. J Thorac Oncol 5:389–398

Caulo A, Mirsadraee S, Maggi F, Leccisotti L, van Beek EJ, Bonomo L (2012) Integrated imaging of non-small cell lung cancer recurrence: CT and PET-CT findings, possible pitfalls and risk of recurrence criteria. Eur Radiol 22:588–606

Cerfolio RJ, Ojha B, Bryant AS, Raghuveer V, Mountz JM, Bartolucci AA (2004) The accuracy of integrated PET-CT compared with dedicated PET alone for the staging of patients with nonsmall cell lung cancer. Ann Thorac Surg 78:1017–1023

Cerfolio RJ, Bryant AS, Ojha B (2006) Restaging patients with N2 (stage IIIa) non-small cell lung cancer after neoadjuvant chemotherapy: a prospective study. J Thorac Cardiovasc Surg 131:1229–1235

Cheran SK, Herndon JE, Patz EF (2004) Comparison of whole-body FDG-PET to bone scan for detection of bone metastases in patients with a new diagnosis of lung cancer. Lung Cancer 44:317–325

Choi H, Charnsangavej C, Faria SC, Macapinlac HA, Burgess MA, Patel SR et al (2007) Correlation of computed tomography and positron emission tomography in patients with metastatic gastrointestinal stromal tumor treated at a single institution with imatinib mesylate: Proposal of new computed tomography response criteria. J Clin Oncol 25:1753–1759

Chong Y, Kim JH, Lee HY, Ahn YC, Lee KS, Ahn MJ et al (2014) Quantitative CT variables enabling response prediction in neoadjuvant therapy with EGFR-TKIs: are they different from those in neoadjuvant concurrent chemoradiotherapy? PLoS One 9:1–8

Coche E (2016) Evaluation of lung tumor response to therapy: Current and emerging techniques. Diagn Interv Imaging 97:1053–1065

Colt HG, Murgu SD, Korst RJ, Slatore CG, Unger M, Quadrelli S (2013) Follow-up and surveillance of the patient with lung cancer after curative-intent therapy: diagnosis and management of lung cancer, 3rd ed: American College of Chest Physicians evidence-based clinical practice guidelines. Chest 143(5 Suppl):e437S–e454S

Coroller TP, Agrawal V, Narayan V, Hou Y, Grossmann P, Lee SW et al (2016) Radiomic phenotype features predict pathological response in non-small cell lung cancer. Radiother Oncol 119:480–486

Crabb SJ, Patsios D, Sauerbrei E, Ellis PM, Arnold A, Goss G et al (2009) Tumor cavitation: impact on objective response evaluation in trials of angiogenesis inhibitors in non-small-cell lung cancer. J Clin Oncol 27:404–410

Cuaron J, Dunphy M, Rimner A (2012) Role of FDG-PET scans in staging, response assessment, and follow-up care for non-small cell lung cancer. Front Oncol 2:208

Cunliffe AR, Armato SG, Straus C, Malik R, Al-Hallaq HA (2014) Lung texture in serial thoracic CT scans: correlation with radiologist-defined severity of acute changes following radiation therapy. Phys Med Biol 59:5387–5398

Dehing-Oberije C, De Ruysscher D, van der Weide H, Hochstenbag M, Bootsma G, Geraedts W et al (2008) Tumor volume combined with number of positive lymph node stations is a more important prognostic factor than TNM stage for survival of non-small-cell lung cancer patients treated with (chemo)radiotherapy. Int J Radiat Oncol Biol Phys 70:1039–1044

Delgado Bolton RC, Carreras Delgado JL (2009) Positron emission tomography (PET) in the evaluation of response to therapy in non-small cell lung cancer. Current Cancer Therapy Reviews 5:20–27

Delgado Bolton RC, Izarduy LP, Carreras Delgado JL (2008) Positron emission tomography and positron emission tomography/computed tomography in the evaluation of response to chemotherapy. Cancer and Chemotherapy Reviews 3:77–86

Detterbeck F, Socinski M (2001) Induction chemotherapy and surgery for I-III A, B non-small cell lung cancer. In: Detterbeck F, Socinski M, Rivera M, Rosenman J (eds) Diagnosis and treatment of lung cancer. An evidence-based guide for the practicing clinician. WB Saunders Co, Philadelphia, pp 267–282

Dingemans A-MC, de Langen AJ, van den Boogaart V, Marcus JT, Backes WH, Scholtens HTGM et al (2011) First-line erlotinib and bevacizumab in patients with locally advanced and/or metastatic non-small-cell lung cancer: a phase II study including molecular imaging. Ann Oncol 22:559–566

Divisi D, Di Tommaso S, Di Leonardo G, Brianzoni E, De Vico A, Crisci R (2010) 18-Fluorine fluorodeoxyglucose positron emission tomography with computerized tomography versus computerized tomography alone for the management of solitary lung nodules with diameters inferior to 1.5 cm. Thorac Cardiovasc Surg 58:422–426

Eisenhauer EA, Therasse P, Bogaerts J, Schwartz LH, Sargent D, Ford R et al (2009) New response evaluation criteria in solid tumours: revised recist guideline (version 1.1). Eur J Cancer 45:228–247

Erasmus JJ, Gladish GW, Broemeling L, Sabloff BS, Truong MT, Herbst RS et al (2003) Interobserver and intraobserver variability in measurement of non-small-cell carcinoma lung lesions: Implications for assessment of tumor response. J Clin Oncol 21: 2574–2582

Fave X, Zhang L, Yang J, Mackin D, Balter P, Gomez D et al (2017) Delta-radiomics features for the prediction of patient outcomes in non-small cell lung cancer. Sci Rep 7:588

Ferretti GR, Reymond E, Delouche A, Sakhri L, Jankowski A, Moro-Sibilot D et al (2016) Personalized chemotherapy of lung cancer: what the radiologist should know. Diagn Interv Imaging 97:286–295

Fischer BM, Mortensen J, Langer SW, Loft A, Berthelsen AK, Daugaard G et al (2006) PET/CT imaging in response evaluation of patients with small cell lung cancer. Lung Cancer 54:41–49

Fischer BM, Mortensen J, Langer SW, Loft A, Berthelsen AK, Petersen BI et al (2007) A prospective study of PET/CT in initial staging of small-cell lung cancer: comparison with CT, bone scintigraphy and bone marrow analysis. Ann Oncol 18:338–345

Fraioli F, Anzidei M, Zaccagna F, Mennini ML, Serra G, Gori B et al (2011) Whole-tumor perfusion CT in patients with advanced lung adenocarcinoma treated with conventional and antiangiogenetic chemotherapy: initial experience. Radiology 259:574–582

Fraioli F, Anzidei M, Serra G, Liberali S, Fiorelli A, Zaccagna F et al (2013) Whole-tumour CT-perfusion of unresectable lung cancer for the monitoring of anti-angiogenetic chemotherapy effects. Br J Radiol 86(1029):20120174

Fried DV, Tucker SL, Zhou S, Liao Z, Mawlawi O, Ibbott G et al (2014) Prognostic value and reproducibility of pretreatment ct texture features in stage III non-small cell lung cancer. Int J Radiat Oncol Biol Phys 90:834–842

Fujimoto K, Abe T, Müller NL, Terasaki H, Kato S, Sadohara J et al (2003) Small peripheral pulmonary carcinomas evaluated with dynamic MR imaging: correlation with tumor vascularity and prognosis. Radiology 227:786–793

Gavrielides M, Kinnard LM, Myers KJ, Petrick N (2009) Noncalcified lung nodules: volumetric assessment with thoracic CT. Radiology 251:26–37

Ghaye B, Wanet M, El Hajjam M (2016) Imaging after radiation therapy of thoracic tumors. Diagn Interv Imaging 97:1037–1052

Graham MV, Purdy JA, Emami B, Harms W, Bosch W, Lockett MA et al (1999) Clinical dose–volume histogram analysis for pneumonitis after 3D treatment for non-small cell lung cancer (NSCLC). Int J Radiat Oncol Biol Phys Biol Phys 45:323–329

Gupta NC, Graeber GM, Tamim WJ, Rogers JS, Irisari L, Bishop HA (2001) Clinical utility of PET-FDG imaging in differentiation of benign from malignant adrenal masses in lung cancer. Clin Lung Cancer 3:59–64

He YQ, Gong HL, Deng YF, Li WM (2014) Diagnostic efficacy of PET and PET/CT for recurrent lung cancer: a meta-analysis. Acta Radiol 55:309–317

Hoopes DJ, Tann M, Fletcher JW, Forquer JA, Lin PF, Lo SS et al (2007) FDG-PET and stereotactic body radiotherapy (SBRT) for stage I nonsmall- cell lung cancer. Lung Cancer 56:229–234

Huang K, Dahele M, Senan S, Guckenberger M, Rodrigues GB, Ward A et al (2012) Radiographic changes after lung stereotactic ablative radiotherapy (SABR)—can we distinguish recurrence from fibrosis? A systematic review of the literature. Radiother Oncol 102: 335–342

Huang K, Senthi S, Palma DA, Spoelstra FOB, Warner A, Slotman BJ et al (2013) High-risk CT features for detection of local recurrence after stereotactic ablative radiotherapy for lung cancer. Radiother Oncol 109:51–57

Huynh E, Coroller TP, Narayan V, Agrawal V, Hou Y, Romano J et al (2016) CT-based radiomic analysis of stereotactic body radiation therapy patients with lung cancer. Radiother Oncol 120:258–266

Ikezoe J, Takashima S, Morimoto S, Kadowaki K, Takeuchi N, Yamamoto T et al (1988) CT appearance lung of acute injury in the lung. Am J Roentgenol 150:765–770

Jadvar H, Colletti PM, Delgado-Bolton R, Esposito G, Krause BJ, Iagaru AH et al (2017) Appropriate use criteria for FDG PET/CT restaging and treatment response assessment of malignant disease. J Nucl Med 58:2026–2037

Jiménez-Ballvé A, Pérez-Castejón MJ, Delgado-Bolton RC, Sánchez-Enrique C, Vilacosta I, Vivas D et al (2016) Assessment of the diagnostic accuracy of 18F-FDG PET/CT in prosthetic infective endocarditis and cardiac implantable electronic device infection: comparison of different interpretation criteria. Eur J Nucl Med Mol Imaging 43:2401–2412

Kelly RJ, Rajan A, Force J, Lopez-Chavez A, Keen C, Cao L et al (2011) Evaluation of KRAS mutations, angiogenic biomarkers, and DCE-MRI in patients

with advanced non-small-cell lung cancer receiving sorafenib. Clin Cancer Res 17:1190–1199
Kim YN, Lee HY, Lee KS, Seo JB, Chung MJ, Ahn MJ et al (2012) Dual-energy CT in patients treated with anti-angiogenic agents for non-small cell lung cancer: new method of monitoring tumor response? Korean J Radiol 13:702–710
Koenig TR, Munden RF, Erasmus JJ, Sabloff BS, Gladish GW, Komaki R et al (2002) Radiation injury of the lung after three-dimensional conformal radiation therapy. AJR Am J Roentgenol 178:1383–1388
Komaki R, Cox JD, Hartz AJ, Byhardt RW, Pérez-Tamayo C, Clowry L et al (1985) Characteristics of long-term survivors after treatment for inoperable carcinoma of the lung. Am J Clin Oncol 8:362–370
Kozak MM, Murphy JD, Schipper ML, Donington JS, Zhou L, Whyte RI et al (2011) Tumor volume as a potential imaging-based risk-stratification factor in trimodality therapy for locally advanced non-small cell lung cancer. J Thorac Oncol 6:920–926
Kumar R, Xiu Y, Yu JQ, Takalkar A, El-Haddad G, Potenta S et al (2004) 18F-FDG PET in evaluation of adrenal lesions in patients with lung cancer. J Nucl Med 45:2058–2062
Larici AR, del Ciello A, Maggi F, Santoro SI, Meduri B, Valentini V et al (2011) Lung abnormalities at multimodality imaging after radiation therapy for non-small cell lung cancer. Radiographics 31:771–789
Lee HY, Lee KS, Ahn M-J, Hwang HS, Lee JW, Park K et al (2011) New CT response criteria in non-small cell lung cancer: proposal and application in EGFR tyrosine kinase inhibitor therapy. Lung Cancer 73:63–69
Lind JSW, Meijerink MR, Dingemans A-MMC, van Kuijk C, Ollers MC, de Ruysscher D et al (2010) Dynamic contrast-enhanced CT in patients treated with sorafenib and erlotinib for non-small cell lung cancer: a new method of monitoring treatment? Eur Radiol 20:2890–2898
Linda A, Trovo M, Bradley JD (2011) Radiation injury of the lung after stereotactic body radiation therapy (SBRT) for lung cancer: a timeline and pattern of CT changes. Eur J Radiol 79:147–154
Liu T, Xu JY, Xu W, Bai YR, Yan WL, Yang HL (2011) Fluorine-18 deoxyglucose Positron emission tomography, magnetic resonance imaging and bone scintigraphy for the diagnosis of bone metastases in patients with lung cancer: which one is the best? A meta-analysis. Clin Oncol (R Coll Radiol) 23(5):350–358
van Loon J, Grutters J, Wanders R, Boersma L, Oellers M, Dingemans AM et al (2009) Followup with 18FDG-PET-CT after radical radiotherapy with or without chemotherapy allows the detection of potentially curable progressive disease in non-small cell lung cancer patients: a prospective study. Eur J Cancer 45:588–595
van Loon J, Grutters JP, Wanders R et al (2010) 18FDG-PETCT in the follow-up of non-small cell lung cancer patients after radical radiotherapy with or without chemotherapy: an economic evaluation. Eur J Cancer 46:110–119
Margaritora S, Cesario A, Galetta D, D'Andrilli A, Macis G, Mantini G et al (2001) Ten year experience with induction therapy in locally advanced non-small cell lung cancer (NSCLC): is clinical re-staging predictive of pathological staging? Eur J Cardiothorac Surg 19:894–898
Marten K, Auer F, Schmidt S, Kohl G, Rummeny EJ, Engelke C (2006) Inadequacy of manual measurements compared to automated CT volumetry in assessment of treatment response of pulmonary metastases using RECIST criteria. Eur Radiol 16:781–790
Mateu-Navarro M, Rami-Porta R, Bastus-Piulats R, Cirera-Nogueras L, González-Pont G (2000) Remediastinoscopy after induction chemotherapy in non-small cell lung cancer. Ann Thorac Surg 70:391–395
Mattonen SA, Palma DA, Haasbeek CJA, Senan S, Ward AD (2013) Distinguishing radiation fibrosis from tumour recurrence after stereotactic ablative radiotherapy (SABR) for lung cancer: a quantitative analysis of CT density changes. Acta Oncol 52(5):910–918
Mattonen SA, Palma DA, Haasbeek CJA, Senan S, Ward AD (2014) Early prediction of tumor recurrence based on CT texture changes after stereotactic ablative radiotherapy (SABR) for lung cancer. Med Phys 41:33502
Mattonen SA, Ward AD, Palma DA (2016a) Pulmonary imaging after stereotactic radiotherapy-does RECIST still apply? Br J Radiol 89:20160113
Mattonen SA, Palma DA, Johnson C, Louie AV, Landis M, Rodrigues G et al (2016b) Detection of local cancer recurrence after stereotactic ablative radiation therapy for lung cancer: physician performance versus radiomic assessment. Int J Radiat Oncol Biol Phys 94:1121–1128
Miller AB, Hoogstraten B, Staquet M, Winkler A (1981) Reporting results of cancer treatment. Cancer 47:207–214
Min JW, Um SW, Yim JJ, Yoo CG, Han SK, Shim YS, Kim YW (2009) The role of whole-body FDG PET/CT, Tc 99m MDP bone scintigraphy, and serum alkaline phosphatase in detecting bone metastasis in patients with newly diagnosed lung cancer. J Korean Med Sci 24:275–280
Mozley PD, Bendtsen C, Zhao B, Schwartz LH, Thorn M, Rong Y et al (2012) Measurement of tumor volumes improves RECIST-based response assessments in advanced lung cancer. Transl Oncol 5:19–25
Ng Q-S, Goh V, Milner J, Padhani AR, Saunders MI, Hoskin PJ (2007a) Acute tumor vascular effects following fractionated radiotherapy in human lung cancer: in vivo whole tumor assessment using volumetric perfusion computed tomography. Int J Radiat Oncol Biol Phys 67:417–424
Ng Q-S, Goh V, Carnell D, Meer K, Padhani AR, Saunders MI et al (2007b) Tumor antivascular effects of radiotherapy combined with Combretastatin A4 phosphate in human non-small-cell lung cancer. Int J Radiat Oncol Biol Phys 67:1375–1380
Ng Q-S, Goh V, Milner J, Sundin J, Wellsted D, Saunders MI et al (2010) Quantitative helical dynamic contrast enhanced computed tomography assessment of the spatial variation in whole tumour blood volume with radiotherapy in lung cancer. Lung Cancer 69:71–76

Nishino M, Jackman DM, Hatabu H, Yeap BY, Cioffredi L-A, Yap JT et al (2010a) New Response Evaluation Criteria in Solid Tumors (RECIST) guidelines for advanced non-small cell lung cancer: comparison with original RECIST and impact on assessment of tumor response to targeted therapy. AJR Am J Roentgenol 195:W221–W228

Nishino M, Jagannathan JP, Ramaiya NH, Van Den Abbeele AD (2010b) Revised RECIST guideline version 1.1: what oncologists want to know and what radiologists need to know. Am J Roentgenol 195:281–289

Nishino M, Guo M, Jackman DM, DiPiro PJ, Yap JT, Ho TK et al (2011) CT tumor volume measurement in advanced non-small-cell lung cancer. Performance characteristics of an emerging clinical tool Acad Radiol 18:54–62

Nishino M, Jagannathan JP, Krajewski KM, O'Regan K, Hatabu H, Shapiro G et al (2012) Personalized tumor response assessment in the era of molecular medicine: Cancer-specific and therapy-specific response criteria to complement pitfalls of RECIST. Am J Roentgenol 198:737–745

Nishino M, Giobbie-Hurder A, Gargano M, Suda M, Ramaiya NH, Hodi FS (2013) Developing a common language for tumor response to immunotherapy: immune-related response criteria using unidimensional measurements. Clin Cancer Res 19:3936–3943

Nishino M, Hatabu H, Johnson BE, McLoud TC (2014) State of the art: response assessment in lung cancer in the era of genomic medicine. Radiology 271:6–27

Nishino M, Tirumani SH, Ramaiya NH, Hodi FS (2015) Cancer immunotherapy and immune-related response assessment: the role of radiologists in the new arena of cancer treatment. Eur J Radiol 84:1259–1268

Ohno Y, Nogami M, Higashino T, Takenaka D, Matsumoto S, Hatabu H et al (2005) Prognostic value of dynamic MR imaging for non-small-cell lung cancer patients after chemoradiotherapy. J Magn Reson Imaging 21:775–783

Ohno Y, Koyama H, Onishi Y, Takenaka D, Nogami M, Yoshikawa T et al (2008) Non-small cell lung cancer: whole-body MR examination for M-stage assessment—utility for whole-body diffusion-weighted imaging compared with integrated FDG PET/CT. Radiology 248:643–654

Ohno Y, Koyama H, Yoshikawa T, Matsumoto K, Aoyama N, Onishi Y et al (2012) Diffusion-weighted MRI versus 18F-FDG PET/CT: performance as predictors of tumor treatment response and patient survival in patients with non-small cell lung cancer receiving chemoradiotherapy. Am J Roentgenol 198:75–82

Ohno Y, Koyama H, Lee HY, Miura S, Yoshikawa T, Sugimura K (2016) Contrast-enhanced CT- and MRI-based perfusion assessment for pulmonary diseases: basics and clinical applications. Diagn Interv Radiol 22:407–421

Palma DA, Senan S, Haasbeek CJA, Verbakel WFAR, Vincent A, Lagerwaard F (2011) Radiological and clinical pneumonitis after stereotactic lung radiotherapy: a matched analysis of three-dimensional conformal and volumetric-modulated arc therapy techniques. Int J Radiat Oncol Biol Phys 80:506–513

Pastis NJ Jr, Greer TJ, Tanner NT, Wahlquist AE, Gordon LL, Sharma AK et al (2014) Assessing the usefulness of 18F-fluorodeoxyglucose PET-CT scan after stereotactic body radiotherapy for early-stage non-small cell lung cancer. Chest 146:406–411

Peulen H, Mantel F, Guckenberger M, Belderbos J, Werner-Wasik M, Hope A et al (2016) Validation of high-risk computed tomography features for detection of local recurrence after stereotactic body radiation therapy for early-stage non-small cell lung cancer. Int J Radiat Oncol Biol Phys 96:134–141

Pitz CC, Mass KW, Van Swieten HA, de la Rivière AB, Hofman P, Schramel FM (2002) Surgery as part of combined modality treatment in stage IIIB non-small cell lung cancer. Ann Thorac Surg 74:164–169

Plathow C, Aschoff P, Lichy MP, Eschmann S, Hehr T, Brink I et al (2008) Positron emission tomography/computed tomography and whole-body magnetic resonance imaging in staging of advanced non small cell lung cancer: initial results. Invest Radiol 43:290–297

Pommier P, Touboul E, Chabaud S, Dussart S, Le Pechoux C, Giammarile F, Carrie C (2010) Impact of (18)F-FDG PET on treatment strategy and 3D radiotherapy planning in non-small cell lung cancer: a prospective multicenter study. AJR Am J Roentgenol 195:350–355

Ponn RB (2000) Lightning can strike twice: second primary lung cancers. Chest 118:1526–1529

Quint LE (2007) Staging non-small cell lung cancer. Cancer Imaging 7:148–159

Ravanelli M, Farina D, Morassi M, Roca E, Cavalleri G, Tassi G et al (2013) Texture analysis of advanced non-small cell lung cancer (NSCLC) on contrast-enhanced computed tomography: Prediction of the response to the first-line chemotherapy. Eur Radiol 23:3450–3455

Revel M-P, Lefort C, Bissery A, Bienvenu M, Aycard L, Chatellier G et al (2004) Pulmonary nodules: preliminary experience with three-dimensional evaluation. Radiology 231:459–466

Rubins J, Unger M (2007) Colice GL; American College of Chest Physicians. Follow-up and surveillance of the lung cancer patient following curative intent therapy: ACCP evidence-based clinical practice guideline (2nd edition). Chest 132(3 Suppl):355S–367S

Schreyögg J, Weller J, Stargardt T, Herrmann K, Bluemel C, Dechow T et al (2010) Cost-effectiveness of hybrid PET/CT for staging of non-small cell lung cancer. J Nucl Med 51:1668–1675

Strauch LS, Eriksen RØ, Sandgaard M, Kristensen TS, Nielsen MB (2016) Assessing tumor response to treatment in patients with lung cancer using dynamic contrast-enhanced CT. Diagnostics (Basel) 6:1–24

Sudarski S, Henzler T, Schoenberg SO (2013) Post-therapeutic positron emission tomography/computed tomography for early detection of non-small cell lung cancer recurrence. Transl Lung Cancer Res 2:295–303

Tacelli N, Remy-Jardin M, Copin M-C, Scherpereel A, Mensier E, Jaillard S et al (2010) Assessment of

non-small cell lung cancer perfusion: pathologic-CT correlation in 15 patients. Radiology 257:863–871
Tacelli N, Santangelo T, Scherpereel A, Duhamel A, Deken V, Klotz E et al (2013) Perfusion CT allows prediction of therapy response in non-small cell lung cancer treated with conventional and anti-angiogenic chemotherapy. Eur Radiol 23:2127–2136
Takeda A, Kunieda E, Takeda T, Tanaka M, Sanuki N, Fujii H et al (2008) Possible misinterpretation of demarcated solid patterns of radiation fibrosis on CT scans as tumor recurrence in patients receiving hypofractionated stereotactic radiotherapy for lung cancer. Int J Radiat Oncol Biol Phys 70:1057–1065
Takeda A, Kunieda E, Fujii H, Yokosuka N, Aoki Y, Oooka Y et al (2013) Evaluation for local failure by 18F-FDG PET/CT in comparison with CT findings after stereotactic body radiotherapy (SBRT) for localized non-small-cell lung cancer. Lung Cancer 79:248–253
Tao X, Wang L, Hui Z, Liu L, Ye F, Song Y et al (2016) DCE-MRI perfusion and permeability parameters as predictors of tumor response to CCRT in patients with locally advanced NSCLC. Sci Res 6:35569
Therasse P, Arbuck SG, Eisenhauer EA, Wanders J, Kaplan RS, Rubinstein L et al (2000) New guidelines to evaluate the response to treatment in solid tumors. European Organization for Research and Treatment of Cancer, National Cancer Institute of the United States, National Cancer Institute of Canada. J Natl Cancer Inst 92:205–216
Therasse P, Eisenhauer EA, Verweij J (2006) RECIST revisited: a review of validation studies on tumour assessment. Eur J Cancer 42:1031–1039
Van Schil P, van der Schoot J, Poniewierski J, Pauwels M, Carp L, Germonpré O, De Backer W (2002) Remediastinoscopy after neoadjuvant therapy for non-small cell lung cancer. Lung Cancer 37:281–285
Vansteenkiste J, Fischer BM, Dooms C, Mortensen J (2004) Positron-emission tomography in prognostic and therapeutic assessment of lung cancer: systematic review. Lancet Oncol 5:531–540
Voltolini L, Luzzi L, Ghiribelli C, Paladini P, Di Biscecglie M, Gotti G (2001) Results of induction chemotherapy followed by surgical resection in patients with stage IIIA (N2) non-small cell lung cancer: the importance of the nodal down-staging after chemotherapy. Eur J Cardiothorac Surg 20:1106–1112
Wallace MB, Ravenel J, Block MI, Fraig M, Silvestri G, Wildi S et al (2004) Endoscopic ultrasound in lung cancer patients with a normal mediastinum on computed tomography. Ann Thorac Surg 77:1763–1768
Wang J, Wu N, Cham MD, Song Y (2009) Tumor response in patients with advanced non-small cell lung cancer: perfusion CT evaluation of chemotherapy and radiation therapy. AJR Am J Roentgenol 193:1090–1096
Wang GX, Guo LQ, Gainor JF, Fintelmann FJ (2017) Immune checkpoint inhibitors in lung cancer: Imaging considerations. Am J Roentgenol 209:567–575
Weiss E, Ford JC, Olsen KM, Karki K, Saraiya S, Groves R et al (2016) Apparent diffusion coefficient (ADC) change on repeated diffusion-weighted magnetic resonance imaging during radiochemotherapy for non-small cell lung cancer: a pilot study. Lung Cancer 96:113–119
Wolchok JD, Kluger H, Callahan MK, Postow MA, Rizvi NA, Lesokhin AM et al (2013) Nivolumab plus Ipilimumab in advanced melanoma. N Engl J Med 369:122–133
Xu G, Zhao L, He Z (2012) Performance of whole-body PET/CT for the detection of distant malignancies in various cancers: a systematic review and meta-analysis. J Nucl Med 53:1847–1854
Yabuuchi H, Hatakenaka M, Takayama K, Matsuo Y, Sunami S, Kamitani T et al (2011) Non-small cell lung cancer: detection of early response to chemotherapy by using contrast-enhanced dynamic and diffusion-weighted MR imaging. Radiology 261:598–604
Yi CA, Shin KM, Lee KS, Kim BT, Kim H, Kwon OJ et al (2008) Non-small cell lung cancer staging: efficacy comparison of integrated PET/CT versus 3.0-T whole-body MR imaging. Radiology 248:632–642
Yun M, Kim W, Alnafisi N, Lacorte L, Jang S, Alavi A (2001) 18F-FDG PET in characterizing adrenal lesions detected on CT or MRI. J Nucl Med 42:1795–1799
Zhang X, Liu H, Balter P, Allen PK, Komaki R, Pan T et al (2012a) Positron emission tomography for assessing local failure after stereotactic body radiotherapy for non-small-cell lung cancer. Int J Radiat Oncol Biol Phys 83:1558–1565
Zhang C, Liu J, Tong J, Sun X, Song S, Huang G (2012b) ^{18}F-FDG-PET evaluation of pathological tumour response to neoadjuvant therapy in patients with NSCLC. Nucl Med Commun 34:71–77
Zhao B, Schwartz LH, Moskowitz CS, Ginsberg MS, Rizvi NA, Kris MG (2006) Lung cancer: computerized quantification of tumor response—initial results. Radiology 241:892–898
Zhao B, Oxnard GR, Moskowitz CS, Kris MG, Pao W, Guo P et al (2010) A pilot study of volume measurement as a method of tumor response evaluation to aid biomarker development. Clin Cancer Res 16:4647–4653

Response Assessment and Follow-Up by Imaging in Breast Tumors

Mireille van Goethem, Angelo Castello, Marc B. I. Lobbes, Fiorenza De Rose, Marta Scorsetti, and Egesta Lopci

Contents

1	**Clinical Background**	451
1.1	Response to Primary Systemic Therapy	451
1.2	Response to Therapy of Metastatic Breast Cancer	452
2	**Morphological Imaging**	453
2.1	Follow-Up after Breast Cancer	453
2.2	Response Monitoring of Breast Cancer Patients Receiving Neoadjuvant Chemotherapy	454
2.3	Response Assessment Categories	460
3	**Molecular Imaging**	464
3.1	Molecular Imaging for Response Assessment and Follow-Up	464
3.2	Bone Metastasis	466
3.3	Other Non-[^{18}F]FDG Tracers	468
3.4	New Horizon: PET/MRI	469
References		471

M. van Goethem
Department of Radiology, University Hospital Antwerp, Edegem, Belgium

A. Castello · E. Lopci (✉)
Nuclear Medicine, Humanitas Clinical and Research Hospital - IRCCS, Via Manzoni 56, Rozzano, MI, Italy
e-mail: egesta.lopci@humanitas.it

M. B. I. Lobbes
Department of Radiology and Nuclear Medicine, Maastricht University Medical Center, Maastricht, The Netherlands

F. De Rose · M. Scorsetti
Radiosurgery and Radiotherapy, Humanitas Clinical and Research Hospital - IRCCS, Via Manzoni 56, Rozzano, MI, Italy

Abstract

Primary systemic chemotherapy was first introduced for managing inoperable and large or locally advanced breast tumors (Bonadonna et al. 1995). It is also now used for operable tumors that would require mastectomy, trying to reduce tumor size and increase the rate of breast-conserving surgery (Avril et al. 2009). Thus, neoadjuvant chemotherapy (NAC) has become the standard treatment not only in patients with locally advanced breast cancer but also in patients with early invasive breast cancer in an attempt to downstage the primary cancer and to reduce micrometastases (You et al. 2015). Approximately 70% of patients demonstrate a clinical response either in physical examination or in anatomic imaging, but lastly, only 3–27% achieve a complete histopathologic response (van der Hage et al. 2001). For this reason, there is a need for accurate methods to monitor therapeutic effectiveness early during therapy (Avril et al. 2009).

1 Clinical Background

1.1 Response to Primary Systemic Therapy

Primary systemic chemotherapy was first introduced for managing inoperable and large or locally advanced breast tumors (Bonadonna et al.

R. G. H. Beets-Tan et al. (eds.), *Imaging and Interventional Radiology for Radiation Oncology*, Medical Radiology, Diagnostic Imaging, https://doi.org/10.1007/978-3-030-38261-2_24

1995). It is also now used for operable tumors that would require mastectomy, trying to reduce tumor size and increase the rate of breast-conserving surgery (Avril et al. 2009). Thus, neoadjuvant chemotherapy (NAC) has become the standard treatment not only in patients with locally advanced breast cancer but also in patients with early invasive breast cancer in an attempt to downstage the primary cancer and to reduce micrometastases (You et al. 2015). Approximately 70% of patients demonstrate a clinical response either in physical examination or in anatomic imaging, but lastly, only 3–27% achieve a complete histopathologic response (van der Hage et al. 2001). For this reason, there is a need for accurate methods to monitor therapeutic effectiveness early during therapy (Avril et al. 2009).

Differences in pathological response after NAC could be influenced by different molecular subtypes. For example, the luminal subtype usually has a low chemosensitivity, and pathological complete response (pCR) is rarely achieved. On the other hand, despite its unfavorable prognosis, triple-negative breast cancer (BC) is a highly chemosensitive subtype with a pCR frequently reached, as well as HER2-positive subtype, in which the prognosis has been strongly improved with the advent of trastuzumab (Humbert et al. 2015).

In the neoadjuvant setting, the detection of axillary nodal lesions is a frequent issue because axillary lymph node (ALN) metastasis is one of the most significant prognostic factors in patients with breast cancer and the management of axillary lesions may involve various surgical approaches. Non-invasive, accurate, and preoperative prediction of the axillary lymph node status is important for surgeons to decide whether to perform sentinel lymph node biopsy without axillary lymph node dissection or to proceed directly to axillary lymph node dissection (You et al. 2015).

Moreover, the administration of radiation therapy to patients receiving preoperative systemic chemotherapy should be made based on maximal stage from pre-chemotherapy tumor characteristics and/or pathological stage, as reported in the NCCN guidelines (https://www.nccn.org/professionals/physician_gls/pdf/breast.pdf). In this context, the role of imaging is crucial to define the right stage before and after systemic therapy, which will guide the therapeutic management of the patients by the surgeon and the radiation oncologist.

1.2 Response to Therapy of Metastatic Breast Cancer

Approximately 30–40% of breast cancer patients develop distant metastases during the course of their disease (O'Shaughnessy et al. 2002). The definition of metastatic breast cancer (MBC) includes very different conditions. Metastases can be present at first diagnosis or may occur very late and often with a large number of metastases. Cure is rarely achieved in MBC, and therefore, the improvement and the maintenance of quality of life (QOL) are the main endpoints in the current treatment for these patients. However, "cure" does not necessarily mean destroying every cancer cell, but rather keeping the disease harmless for a long time (Singletary et al. 2003). Median survival for MBC is variably reported but generally short, e.g., 8–24 months (Tan and Wolff 2010), 18–24 months (Pagani et al. 2010), or as long as 2–4 years (Hortobagyi 2002).

Contrary to the neoadjuvant setting, the pathological response generally cannot be reached in the metastatic setting. Thus, the most frequently used surrogate endpoint for a therapeutic effect is a change in tumor size. The response evaluation criteria in solid tumors (RECIST) define response as a decrease in the maximum tumor diameter of at least 30% (Therasse et al. 2000). Anatomic imaging is used to obtain measurements of reference tumor lesions before and after treatment for response assessment and follow-up (Avril et al. 2009). However, change in tumor size is not a good surrogate of bone lesion response, and the RECIST 1.1 criteria specify that bone lesions without soft tissue components cannot be considered as measurable (Eisenhauer et al. 2009). This is a crucial issue because bone metastases are very frequent in the course of breast cancer disease, with median survival duration after diagnosis of 25.2 to 72 months (Briasoulis et al. 1992).

Serious skeletal-related events caused by bone metastases (fractures, spinal cord compression, and hypercalcemia) can impair the patients' quality of life. External beam radiotherapy and bisphosphonate provide pain relief and a reduction in skeletal complication rates and currently represent an integral part of the antineoplastic management of patients with metastatic bone disease (Hayashi et al. 2013).

The gold standard approach to metastatic breast cancer involves the use of systemic therapies (chemotherapy, immunotherapy or endocrine therapies). However, some of these patients with limited metastatic disease, good performance status, and younger age may have an improvement of clinical outcomes with the addition of local therapy. According to the spectrum hypothesis, described by Hellmann many years ago (Hellman 1994), there is a disease state intermediate between locoregionally confined and widely metastatic cancer. In this situation, called "oligometastatic disease," metastases are limited in number and location and characterized by an indolent tumor biology and behavior. The population with "potentially curable" stage IV disease is estimated to be 1–10% of newly diagnosed patients with MBC (Pagani et al. 2010).

At present, the term "oligometastases" is typically used to refer to those patients with one to five sites of radiographically detected macroscopic metastases. Similarly, limited progression or recurrence is often referred to as "oligoprogression" and "oligorecurrence." These classifications are based on imaging, which have improved detection with the implementation of diagnostic technologies (Hong and Salama 2017). Based on this background, there is a growing interest towards local ablative treatments to all known metastases in oligometastatic patients, in order to achieve a long-term disease control and potentially the cure (Scorsetti et al. 2016).

Stereotactic body radiotherapy (SBRT) is emerging as an effective and safe treatment when surgery is not allowed or refused. Published studies on SBRT for metastatic disease included very different scenarios with various histological types or disease sites (Milano et al. 2012). When results are analyzed according to tumor type, patients with breast cancer have a much better survival as compared to those with other types of cancers (Tree et al. 2013).

Clinical trials are ongoing in the setting of oligometastatic disease to assess the role of local therapies and to determine the impact on clinical outcomes of the addition of SBRT to standard regimens.

2 Morphological Imaging

2.1 Follow-Up after Breast Cancer

2.1.1 Mammography

The updated review of randomized clinical trials conducted almost 20 years ago suggests that follow-up programs based on regular physical examinations and yearly mammography alone are as effective as more intensive approaches based on regular performance of laboratory and instrumental tests in terms of timeliness of recurrence detection, overall survival, and quality of life (Moschetti et al. 2016). Annual mammography should be performed for 5 years after treatment, and a mammography every 1–2 years thereafter may be a reasonable compromise. Mammography screening after breast cancer can show ipsilateral recurrence in 50–80% of patients, with 8–51% mammography-detected-only cancers.

Mammography detects also 45–90% of contralateral cancers (Houssami and Ciatto 2010). Patients with ipsilateral relapse detected clinically appear to do less well than those detected by self-examination or mammography (Montgomery et al. 2007).

2.1.2 Ultrasound

Postoperative follow-up ultrasonography may show clinically and mammographically occult malignancies in 1.2% of the patients treated for breast cancer (Shin et al. 2005). Adding ultrasound (US) to mammography in the American College of Radiology Imaging Network (ACRIN) 6666 trials yielded an additional 1.1–7.2 cancers per 1000 high-risk women, of which 53% of the 2637 enrolled women had a personal history of breast cancer (Berg et al. 2008).

The reported cancer detection rate of US is 1.7–5.1% per patient after breast cancer treatment, and the positive predictive value (PPV) is 21.5–52.6%, with percentages varying according to the area involved (Yoon et al. 2015).

Ultrasound is an excellent technique to evaluate the chest wall after mastectomy. Most of the time, a new or recurrent mass is palpable and detected by the patient or by clinical examination. US is able to detect clinically occult new masses especially if clinical examination is difficult due to nodular scarring (Kanso et al. 2008). Therefore, routine follow-up US can be advocated for early detection of non-palpable locoregional recurrent cancer (Lee et al. 2013).

Patients treated with mastectomy and who had a locoregional recurrence detected at an early stage or an isolated regional recurrence had better survival with short follow-up, but controversy remains about whether post-treatment surveillance US affects long-term survival in patients with breast cancer (Jung Hyun Yoon et al. 2015).

US of the tumorectomy site is difficult because of attenuation caused by the scar. US can have a crucial role in the detection of recurrent lesions after breast cancer surgery in mammographic occult parenchymal masses. Doppler examination of the scar or elastography can be helpful.

2.1.2.1 The Axilla

Axillary US is easy to perform and a sensitivity of 76.9% and a specificity of 98.7% are reported. Ipsilateral lymph node recurrence (LNR) is a predictor of distant metastases, and lymph node evaluation during breast US is useful for early detection of LNR in asymptomatic patients (Moon et al. 2009).

2.1.3 Magnetic Resonance Imaging

In general, there is no proven benefit of adding breast MRI to mammography and/or US for early detection of breast cancer relapse. Hence, there is no indication for routine use of breast MRI in follow-up of breast cancer patients. Nevertheless, breast MRI might be considered on an individual basis. One should strongly consider adding breast MRI to mammography and/or US in the following settings: when the surgical site is close to the chest wall or high in the axillary tail, in dense and difficult to read mammograms, for clarification of inconclusive findings observed during routine follow-up and in high-risk patients.

2.2 Response Monitoring of Breast Cancer Patients Receiving Neoadjuvant Chemotherapy

Neoadjuvant chemotherapy (NAC) is increasingly being used for the treatment of breast cancer patients. It is defined as the administration of chemotherapy prior to surgery. In terms of survival or overall disease progression, there is no difference between breast cancer patients receiving either adjuvant or neoadjuvant chemotherapy (Mauri et al. 2005). In the past, NAC was predominantly used in patients with locally advanced breast cancer, to enable breast conservative therapy when initially mastectomy was planned. In the past years, it is being used in earlier stages of breast cancer to facilitate breast surgery safety and improve cosmetic results after treatment.

An additional advantage of NAC is the ability to assess tumor response in vivo. Breast cancers can respond differently to therapy, showing progression, reduction or even complete remission. The latter is defined as the absence of any residual breast cancer and is assessed by histopathological analysis of surgical specimens acquired after completion of NAC. In the literature, the term “pathological complete response” (pCR) is mainly used in this context, but the exact definition may vary as some studies include and others exclude ductal carcinoma in situ (DCIS) in this definition. pCR after NAC has shown to be a prognostic factor for overall survival, disease-free survival, and recurrence-free survival (Kong et al. 2011). To assess response to NAC, imaging (mammography, ultrasound or breast MRI) is regarded to be superior to physical examination (Marinovich et al. 2015).

2.2.1 Mammography

Mammography is the most important imaging method to detect breast cancer. It is the only imaging method to detect and evaluate suspicious calcifications that may accompany a malignant lesion or may be the only sign of malignancy. However, mammography gives only information on morphology and density of a breast lesion. In the follow up after NAC, imaging features depend on tumor fibrosis, fragmentation, and change in density.

2.2.1.1 Masses

Mammography remains a highly sensitive and reproducible investigation for the assessment of residual disease after chemotherapy (Mistry et al. 2016). The accuracy for predicting residual tumor volume of locally advanced breast carcinoma on mammography depends on the appearance of the tumor on initial mammography. If the margins can be defined by more than 50% on baseline mammography, it can be accurate after NAC in predicting residual disease (Huber et al. 2000).

Whereas mammograms show some response to chemotherapy in up to 90% of patients, prediction of pathological outcome is not possible. The most common response is reduction in size and density of the mass. Patients with complete response on mammography may have residual tumor, even with an invasive component. On the other hand, patients with complete pathological response may show residual masses on mammography (Vinnicombe et al. 1996). Therefore, the reason is that the malignant mass may be replaced by fibrous tissue after response to NAC, which is an irregular dense lesion as well on mammography, making it challenging to make the differential diagnosis between a malignant mass and a fibrous tissue (Fig. 1).

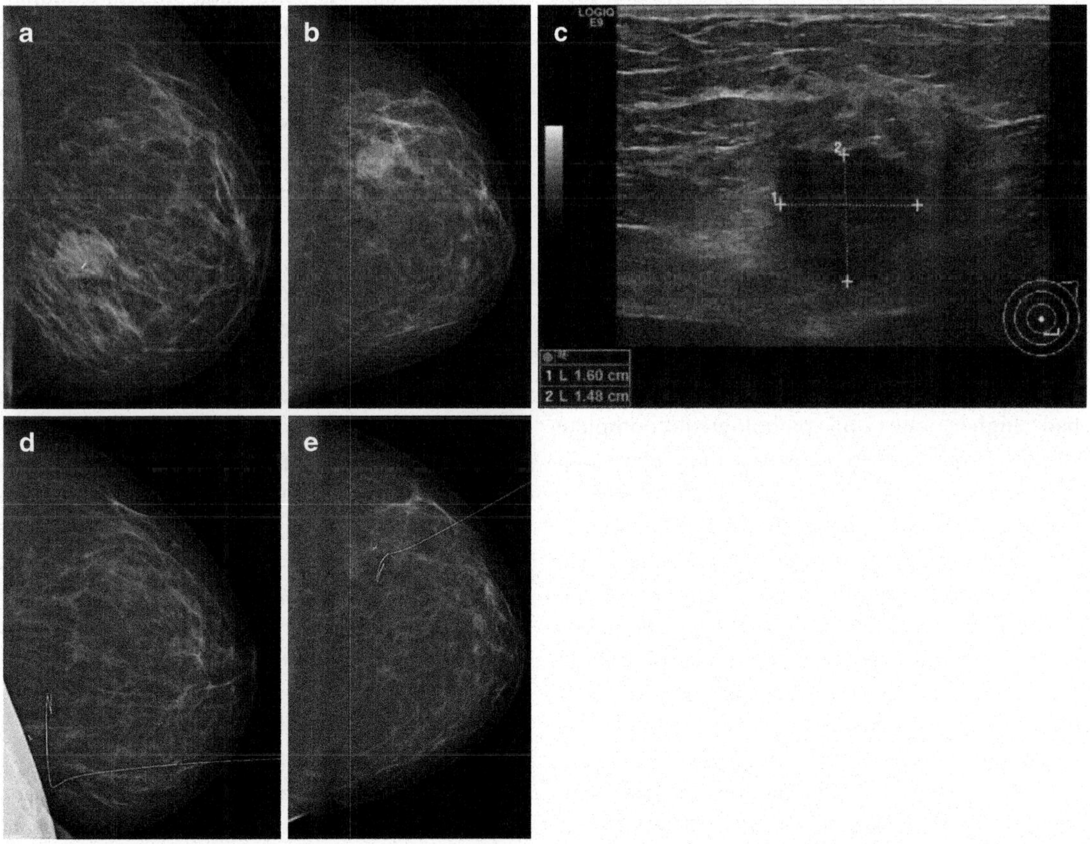

Fig. 1 (**a**, **b**) Initial mammography shows a mass of 26 mm. A clip is placed in the mass. (**c**) US shows a mass of 16 mm. APD: invasive ductal carcinoma. (**d**, **e**) Mammography with a hook wire after NAC: clip surrounded by low dense tissue. No mass or lesion is seen on US after NAC. APD after NAC: fibrous tumor bed of 15 mm with 10% invasive carcinoma and 5% DCIS

However, tumor delineation can be difficult in patients with (extremely) dense breasts. Over the past years, several advanced techniques have been introduced to improve lesion visualization, such as digital breast tomosynthesis (DBT) or contrast-enhanced spectral mammography (CESM). DBT may be superior for determining the size and delineation of the lesion, particularly in dense breasts (Seo et al. 2014).

CESM is another new technique that gives not only information on morphology but also on perfusion. In CESM, iodine-based contrast is administered intravenously prior to dual-energy mammography, resulting in the acquisition of a low-energy image (which is equal to conventional mammography) and a recombined image, showing areas of enhancement (Fig. 2). Recently, Elsaid et al. showed that CESM can accurately predict final pathological response after completion of NAC, especially in patients achieving complete response (ElSaid et al. 2017). Several other studies are currently ongoing studying the ability of CESM to predict tumor response in patients treated with NAC. Moreover, it is a good alternative if MRI cannot be performed.

2.2.1.2 Suspicious Calcifications

Mammography can play an important role in the prediction of response if calcifications are seen. Patients with breast carcinoma and decreased number of pathological calcifications post-NAC had higher rates of pathological complete response compared to patients with no change in calcifications (Golan et al. 2016). However, the extent of the calcifications in the mammography following NAC does not correlate with the extent of residual disease in up to 22% of women (Adrada et al. 2015) (Fig. 3). Calcifications decrease or remain stable after completion of NAC in 72% of patients. The calcification density may decrease or increase but remains stable in the majority of patients (Li et al. 2014).

The correlation of calcifications with histopathology after NAC shows that in 40.6% of patients, these are associated with benign pathology. In patients with pathological complete response, remaining calcifications may be associated with DCIS in 9% and with benign findings in 22%. The proportion of residual malignant calcifications is higher in ER+ versus ER- patients after NAC.

The role of mammography after NAC in the assessment of suspicious calcifications is especially as adjunct to MRI mammography. PCR is most frequently seen in patients with resolution of the enhancement on MRI mammography and new, increasing, or unchanged calcifications. Although calcifications seen on post-NAC mammography may be associated with benign disease, loss of MRI enhancement does not predict the absence of residual tumor with sufficient accuracy to leave calcifications in place. Complete excision of tumor bed calcifications remains standard practice (Feliciano et al. 2017).

2.2.2 Ultrasound

Ultrasonography is better than clinical examination and mammography to predict tumor size of a breast carcinoma (Bosch et al. 2003). Keune et al. reported that ultrasound could measure 91.3% of the carcinomas, and mammography only 51.9%. Moreover, ultrasound is more accurate than mammography in estimating residual tumor size: 59.6% vs. 31.7%. However, there is little difference in the ability of mammography and ultrasound to predict pathological complete response (Fig. 4). The likelihood of a complete pathological response is 80% when both imaging modalities demonstrate no residual disease (Keune et al. 2010).

In a study of 182 patients, US was at least as good as breast MRI in providing information on residual tumor size post-neoadjuvant chemotherapy. Both modalities may over- and underestimate, and they showed a low negative predictive value of pathological complete remission (Vriens et al. 2016).

2.2.3 Advanced Ultrasound Techniques

Some studies have reported new US techniques, such as 3D ultrasound, contrast-enhanced ultrasound (CEUS) or elastography, which could help in measuring response. Until now, there is only limited evidence, and these techniques are not widely available. Tumor 3D-US volume

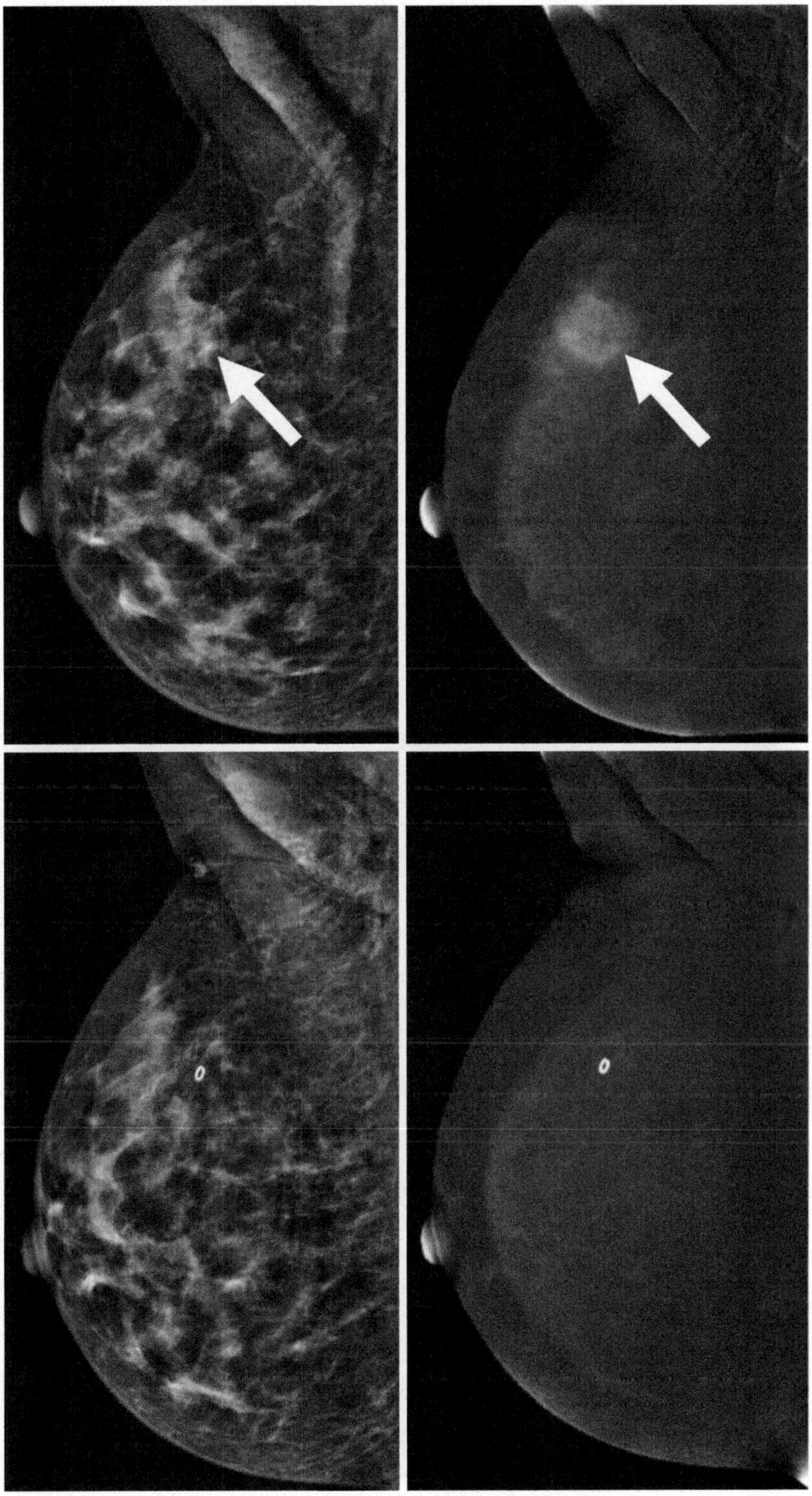

Fig. 2 Contrast-enhanced spectral mammography in response monitoring for a patient with invasive ductal breast cancer treated with neoadjuvant chemotherapy. The left column shows low-energy images, similar to mammography. On the right, the enhancement of masses can be appreciated on the recombined images. At baseline (top row), a mass can be observed partly obscured by the glandular tissue, clearly enhancing on CESM (arrows). After therapy, the site of the tumor can be identified through the clip placement, showing no residual mass or enhancement (bottom row). Final pathology showed complete pathological response

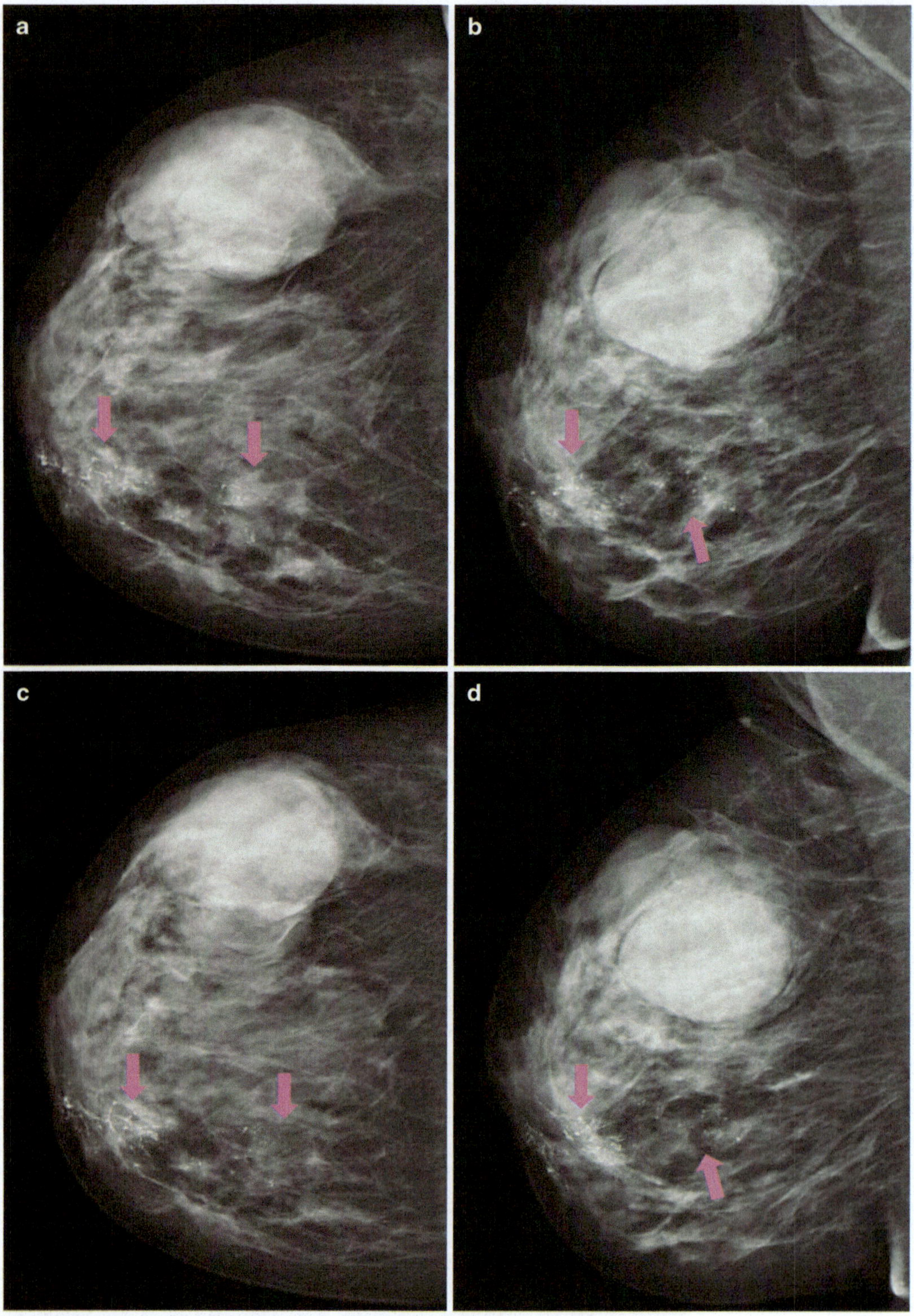

Fig. 3 (**a**, **b**) Mammography of the right breast: Large mass lateral, cyst. Large area of 11 cm of suspect calcifications medial. APD: invasive ductal carcinoma with DCIS. (**c**, **d**) Mammography of the right breast after NAC: status quo of suspect calcifications. APD: fibrosis, adenosis, some atypical cells. No malignancy

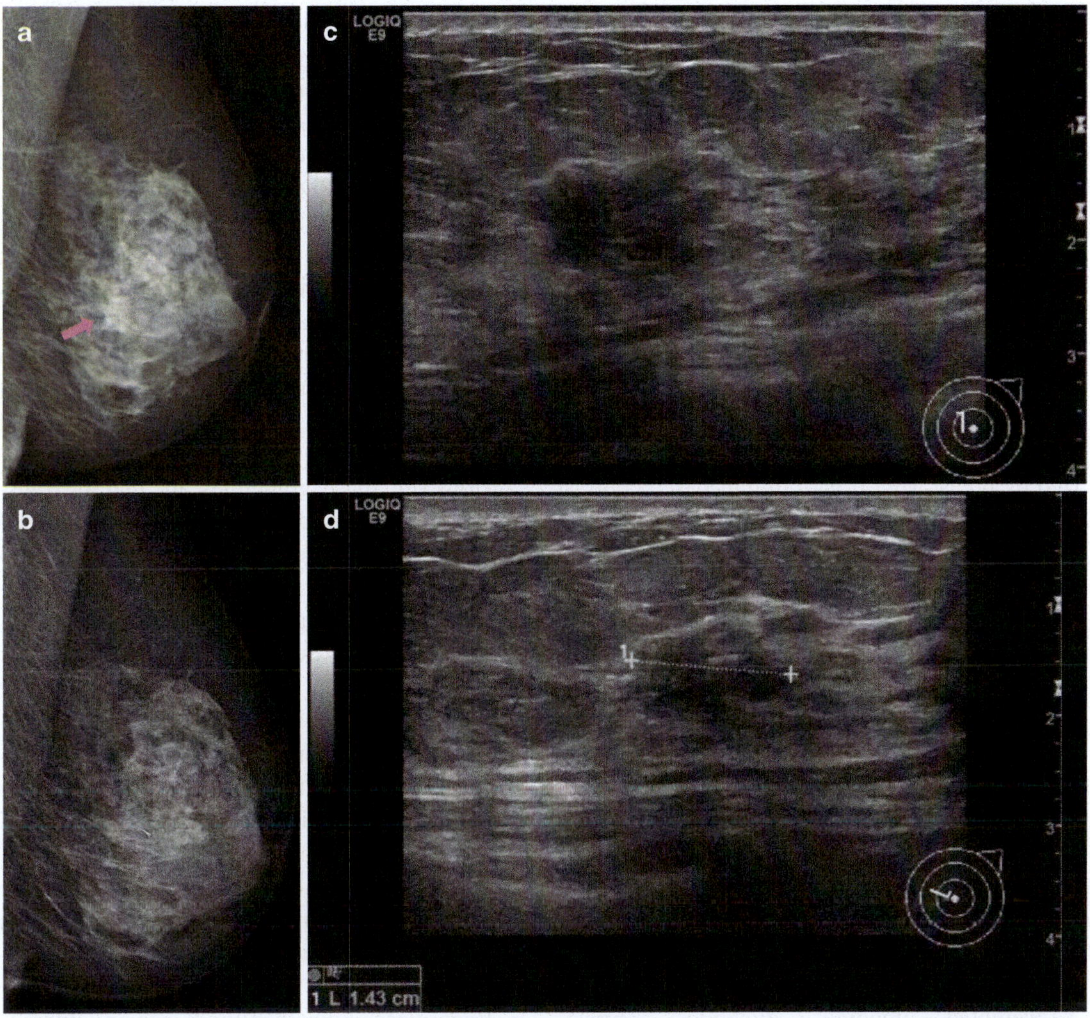

Fig. 4 Dense breast. (**a**, **b**) Initial mammography and ultrasound showing a mass of 23 mm. On mammography, delineation of the mass is difficult (arrow). APD: invasive lobular carcinoma (ILC). On MRI, the lesion measures 56 mm. (**c**, **d**) After NAC, no mass is seen on mammography; the clip is seen in the region of the mass. Ultrasound shows a mass of 14.3 mm with a clip in it. Mastectomy is performed and APD shows a tumor bed of 7 cm with small foci of ILA spread in the whole tumor bed, involving only 2% of the total region

measurements showed good concordance with DCE-MRI volume (Athanasiou et al. 2017). CEUS seems a valuable imaging modality for assessing the treatment response in patients receiving NAC and has a comparable correlation as MRI with breast cancer size at surgery (Corcioni et al. 2008; Lee et al. 2017). Time/signal intensity curves recorded during CEUS correlate with those obtained during MRI. There is only limited data with few studies and few patients in the studies. Moreover, CEUS is not widely available. Elastography measures tumor stiffness, which depends on tumor cellularity. Relative changes in tumor stiffness using shear-wave elastography (SWE) could effectively predict the response to neoadjuvant chemotherapy. Comparing strain elastography (SE) and SWE, they exhibit similar performances for predicting favorable NAC responses; SWE seems better than SE for predicting NAC resistance. Pretreatment tumor stiffness measured by SWE can have a statistically significant relationship with pathological response of invasive breast cancer to NAC (Evans et al. 2013).

2.2.4 Magnetic Resonance Imaging

When tumors grow, their size prevents them from getting their nutrients solely by diffusion. With increasing size, parts of the tumor become hypoxic and start to excrete vascular growth factors, stimulating adjacent blood vessels to grow towards the tumor itself. However, these newly formed vessels are rapidly formed and disorganized, making them "leaky" to contrast agent. This is the principle behind contrast accumulation in neoplastic lesions, which can be visualized by breast MRI if gadolinium-based contrast agents are used. Although any kind of imaging modality might be used for response monitoring of patients treated with NAC, breast MRI can assess more parameters in addition to changes in size and morphology. It can assess not only tumor perfusion but also cell density using diffusion-weighted imaging (DWI) protocols. Breast MRI is the best imaging modality to evaluate disease extent (Gruber et al. 2013).

Although many parameters have been proposed in a multitude of studies, this chapter focuses on using standard, high-quality breast MRI to monitor response of patients undergoing NAC. This includes the following high-resolution MRI sequence protocols (Mann et al. 2008): T2-weighted imaging, dynamic contrast-enhanced T1-weighted imaging, and DWI. An extensive discussion of other more experimental parameters is beyond the scope of this chapter.

2.3 Response Assessment Categories

In terms of response assessment categories, the most commonly used guidelines that are applied are the guidelines of the response evaluation criteria in solid tumors (RECIST) committee and of the World Health Organization (WHO). Both guidelines use four categories for response assessment. The RECIST criteria are defined as follows: (a) progressive disease (PD, increase in tumor diameter >20%); (b) partial response (PR, decrease in tumor diameter >30%); (c) complete response (CR, absence of visible tumor on imaging); and (d) stable disease (SD, the level between PD and PR).

In the WHO guidelines, response categories are defined as (a) PD (increase of tumor diameter >25%); (b) PR (reduction in diameter of >50%); (c) CR (no more tumor is visible on imaging); and (d) the fourth category, stable disease (SD) is again between PD and PR (Miller et al. 1981; Therasse et al. 2000; McLaughlin and Hylton 2011). Figure 5 shows an example of different response categories as assessed by breast MRI (Fig. 5).

However, these guidelines are mainly translated from other solid tumor types and are focused on measuring maximum tumor diameter, not considering the tumor. To cope with these limitations, the use of tumor volume measurements was suggested as treatment response parameter (Prevos et al. 2012). In some of these studies, the surrogate parameter provided in the RECIST criteria appendix was used, defining response categories as follows: PR being a volume reduction of >65% and PD being an increase in volume of >20%. CR and SD remain the same (Pickles et al. 2005; Lorenzon et al. 2009). Nevertheless, these parameters have not been intensely validated in breast cancer populations and in large prospective studies.

Regardless of whether tumor size or volume is measured in response monitoring, the main limitation remains that these parameters do not cope with response patterns such as "crumbling" of the tumor (i.e., the tumor is fragmented from one confluent mass into multiple irregular foci, it being the opposite of concentric shrinkage). There is promising, albeit limited, scientific evidence that shrinkage patterns hold information on expected response to therapy, but this may be dependent on different shrinkage patterns and different tumor subtypes (Kim et al. 2012; Goorts et al. 2018; Ballesio et al. 2017).

Also, other specific MRI parameters such as the signal intensity time curves or apparent diffusion coefficient (ADC) values on DWI are not included in the diameter or volume-based assessments but can indeed hold important information

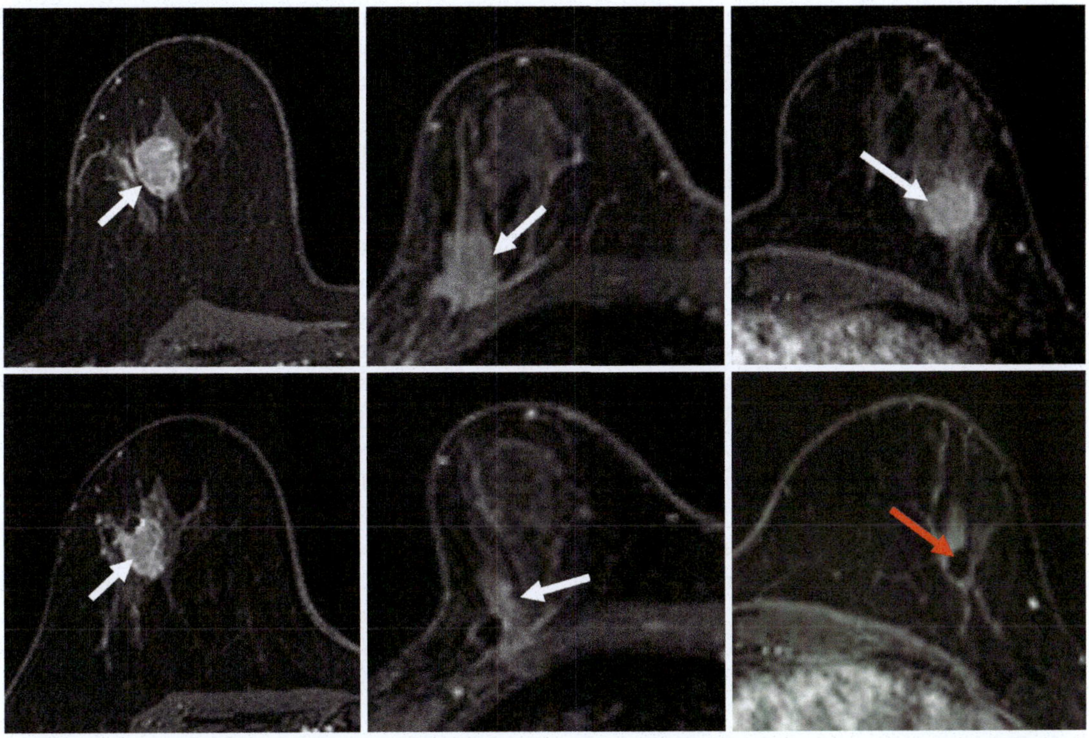

Fig. 5 Examples of different response categories as assessed with breast MRI. All examples are invasive ductal carcinoma visible on contrast-enhanced T1-weighted MRI sequences using fat suppression (white arrows). Top row shows examples of baseline MRI exams; bottom row shows MRI exams performed after completion of treatment. Examples shown are those of stable disease (left), partial response (centre), and complete response (right, in which the clip is indicated with the red arrow)

on treatment response. However, no internationally well-defined and well-validated signal intensity time curve or ADC (cut-off) parameters have been defined.

2.3.1 Early Response Monitoring

In a recent systematic review, Prevos et al. summarized the ability of breast MRI to predict response outcome prior to the initiation of NAC and "half-way" all treatment cycles, i.e., early response monitoring. In 15 studies, 31 different parameters were described (Prevos et al. 2012). The most frequently used parameters for early response were tumor diameter and volume. In general, changes in tumor diameter or volume were evaluated between responders and non-responders, and only four studies provided an AUC (Area Under the Curve) value of these measurements for predicting response. AUC values ranged from 0.73 to 0.9. Other observed parameters showed contradicting results, whilst study designs and treatment regimens were extremely heterogeneous, precluding calculating joint performance values nor drawing any final conclusions on the ability of breast MRI to predict response in an early phase of NAC treatment.

DWI might hold promising information during early response monitoring. It is assumed that in the first stages of NAC treatment, cell death will occur, decreasing the number of tumor cells within a cancer. Consequently, ADC values will increase. In a recent publication by Minarikova et al., the largest difference between ADC values between patients achieving pCR and those who did not achieve it was observed after the second cycle of therapy (Minarikova et al. 2017).

In theory, poor early response as predicted by MRI might result in a change in chemotherapy regimen or might lead to direct surgery whilst preventing the patient to undergo potentially toxic treatments without any true benefit for their health. It should be emphasized, however, that at present no studies are available that have assessed the (positive) effect of changing treatment strategy based on outcomes of any kind of imaging. Since this important evidence is (still) lacking, we recommend using early response monitoring with breast MRI only for research purposes, when there is any doubt on disease progression during physical examination, or if patient motivation is declining during therapy (a good response might encourage patients to continue NAC).

2.3.2 Residual Disease Extent and Pathological Complete Response

After the completion of NAC, one of two outcomes can be observed: the patient either achieved pCR, or there is some residual disease left. Previous studies have evaluated the performance of breast MRI for both these outcomes. Most patients unfortunately do not achieve pCR (which is achieved in up to 30% of the patients). In many studies, correlation coefficient between (residual) tumor size measurements on breast MRI and tumor size based on pathological analysis of surgical specimens have been presented. These correlation coefficients may vary widely, as was demonstrated by a systematic review by Lobbes et al., who found a median correlation coefficient in 17 studies of 0.698 (range 0.21–0.982). In the studies selected for their final analysis, both over- and underestimation were observed (Lobbes et al. 2013). Drawing any conclusions on the accuracy of breast MRI to determine residual disease extent is difficult, since a large study heterogeneity was observed, for example, in image hardware and protocols used, breast cancer subtypes included, treatment regimens used, etc.

More interesting perhaps from a clinical point of view is the assessment of pCR after completion of NAC using breast MRI, since this would create a window of opportunity to pursue a "wait and see" policy instead of performing unnecessary surgery (finding no residual tumor cells). In a previous meta-analysis by Yuan et al., the pooled weighted estimates of sensitivity and specificity of breast MRI to predict pCR were as follows: sensitivity 63% (range 56–70%) and specificity 91% (range 91–92%) (Yuan et al. 2010). In another meta-analysis by Wu et al., these numbers were 65% (95% confidence interval (CI), 57–77%) and 91% (95% CI, 82–97%), respectively (Wu et al. 2012). Lobbes et al. chose to perform a systematic review of studies available and refrained from any pooled analysis due to the large study heterogeneity. For predicting pCR with breast MRI, they found that sensitivity and specificity ranged from 25–100% and 50–97%, respectively. A negative predictive value for predicting pCR with breast MRI of 71–100% was observed (Lobbes et al. 2013). Lindenberg et al. recently showed that these varying results might be caused by including different breast cancer subtypes. For example, sensitivity and specificity of breast MRI in ER+/HER2-subtypes were 35–37% and 87–89%, respectively (Lindenberg et al. 2017).

Next to dynamic contrast-enhanced MRI, diffusion-weighted imaging might hold important additional information to predict pCR. For example, Shin et al. concluded that a change in the apparent diffusion coefficient (ADC) value after treatment might be a good predictor of pCR. With an AUC value of 0.96, they suggested that with a change in ADC of 40.7%, the sensitivity and specificity for predicting pCR were 100% and 91%, respectively (Shin et al. 2012). However, contradicting results were recently published by Minarikova et al. who found no big differences between ADC values (both measured in two- or three-dimensional views) for prediction of pCR in a study of 42 patients (Minarikova et al. 2017). The development of fibrotic tissue during NAC might be a possible explanation for the lack of these differences at the end of the treatment cycles.

In short, breast MRI is an important imaging tool for the assessment of both residual disease and pCR. However, studies that were published on this topic showed a large heterogeneity, hampering us to draw any definite conclusions about its true performance. Most research has focused on using dynamic-contrast-enhanced breast MRI, sometimes combined with DWI.

Nevertheless, proper definitions of response parameters and histopathological analysis should be pursued internationally to create more homogeneity in data acquired.

2.3.2.1 Imaging of the Axillary and Internal Mammary Lymph Nodes

Not only primary breast cancers are influenced by NAC. The axillary lymph node metastases present are also treated, and studies have shown that pCR in the axilla is achieved in an important number of treated patients (Vugts et al. 2016). Hence, the evaluation of nodal response on standard breast MRI is equally important to reviewing the primary breast malignancy.

The assessment of axillary lymph node metastases using standard breast MRI (as part of the initial diagnosis or for response monitoring) is challenging. Suspicious lymph node characteristics include irregular margins, inhomogeneous cortex or eccentric cortical thickening, perinodal edema, the absence of the fatty hilum and asymmetry in the number of axillary lymph nodes seen (Baltzer et al. 2011). The accuracy of standard breast MRI was previously described by Van Nijnatten et al. Albeit in primary diagnosis and not after completion of NAC, they showed that the probability of having a pN2–3 stage given cN0 was 0.7–0.9% for breast MRI. The probability of pN2–3 given cN1 was 11.6–15.4%. These results were slightly better than dedicated axillary ultrasound but might be further improved if sequence protocols more dedicated to the axilla itself were used (Van Nijnatten et al. 2016). If breast MRI would have a very high negative predictive value in cN0 cases, hypothetically, any form of (surgical) axillary staging could be omitted, and a "wait and see" policy could be adapted in patients treated with NAC. Nevertheless, more studies are needed to identify the exact subgroups of patients in which omission of axillary intervention would be regarded oncologically safe.

Not to be overlooked are the lymph nodes in the internal mammary chain. These can be observed close to the internal mammary vessels and can vary in size from undetectable on MRI to several millimeters in size. However, sometimes, they can be slightly enlarged and might have important clinical consequences regarding the choice of radiotherapy fields. There are currently no reliable imaging parameters in which internal mammary lymph node metastases can be accurately identified. Lymph nodes that show equal characteristics and response to therapy as the primary breast tumor should be regarded as suspicious. These observations should be discussed in a multidisciplinary tumor board meeting, where the consequences for treatment and the supposed benefit acquired can be discussed on an individual basis.

2.3.2.2 The Importance of Clinical Information

As in any radiological report, accurate clinical information is the backbone of high-quality reporting. In the setting of response monitoring during neoadjuvant chemotherapy, the clinical information should consist of a description of the type of tumor that was diagnosed, its grade and hormonal receptor status (ER, PR, HER2), if axillary and/or parasternal lymph nodes were involved, if any relevant extramammary findings were observed, and what treatment regimen was used. In addition, it is important to instruct clinicians to provide information on how many cycles of chemotherapy were performed and how many will be planned. Templates containing all these parameters are recommended, as they simplify the process of reporting and reduce the chances of omitting one or more of these important parameters, which might influence the assessment of the MRI exam.

As a next step, a description of the imaging protocol should be added, especially regarding the types of imaging sequences that were used, the type of contrast agent, and its dose (for future references should there be any complications regarding the administration of gadolinium-based contrast agents). It is even more important to emphasize the differences in protocols used when, for example, patients had their prior exams in other institutes and are referred to a second center for the continuation of response monitoring.

In the evaluation of the exams, the primary index tumor (i.e., the largest tumor within the patients' breasts) should be described first, using the descriptors for breast MRI provided by the

American College of Radiology BI-RADS lexicon (Morris et al. 2013). This can be followed by measurement of the ADC value based on the DWI sequences, which should show a shift towards values seen in normal fibroglandular tissue when therapy response is present. The abovementioned parameters should then also be assessed for any other additional tumor sites in case of multifocal or contralateral breast cancers.

When the assessment of the intramammary findings is finalized, an evaluation of any suspicious lymph nodes (axillary or parasternal) should be performed using the previously mentioned criteria. Most importantly, the number of (remaining) suspicious lymph nodes and their anatomical level (in the axilla level I to III or the intercostal spaces in parasternal lymph nodes) should be noted, together with any changes that are observed since prior exams. Finally, any relevant extramammary lesions should be summarized. The report should be closed with a final BI-RADS classification, which in the setting of response monitoring of patients undergoing NAC is usually 6 (i.e., histologically proven breast cancer).

2.3.3 Response Monitoring after Neoadjuvant Endocrine Therapy (NET)

Therefore, mammography is a useful method but is less precise in case of lobular carcinoma. Ultrasound is the most useful technique to measure the diameter change of carcinomas presenting as a mass but can be difficult in case of non-mass lesions. Methods of assessing response should include MRI of the breast, particularly in lobular tumors (van Dam et al. 2016).

3 Molecular Imaging

3.1 Molecular Imaging for Response Assessment and Follow-Up

The introduction of integrated positron emission tomography (PET)/computed tomography (CT) with 2-[^{18}F]fluoro-2-deoxy-d-glucose ([^{18}F]FDG), which evaluates high glucose metabolism in malignant cells, has improved clinical management of patients with cancer, allowing information on both anatomical and metabolic changes.

[^{18}F]FDG PET/CT has had a notable influence on diagnosis, staging, choice of treatment, restaging, monitoring of the response to therapy, and follow-up of a number of malignant tumors, and it is playing an important role also in breast cancer.

3.1.1 Factors Influencing [^{18}F]FDG Uptake in Breast Cancer

Several studies have shown different patterns of [^{18}F]FDG uptake in breast cancer, suggesting that glucose metabolism is influenced by many factors related to tumor cells that are known to be prognostic elements for survival in breast cancer patients (Groheux et al. 2011). Maximum standardized uptake value (SUVmax), for example, is higher in patients with triple-negative cancer (estrogen receptor [ER-] negative, progesterone receptor [PR-], HER2/neu-), which is known to be more aggressive and with the worst prognosis.

Furthermore, as HER2 gene promotes cellular proliferation and progression, the HER2-positive subtypes show a higher SUVmax and tend to be more aggressive and with a higher rate of recurrence and mortality (Kitajima et al. 2015).

Commonly, [^{18}F]FDG uptake is lower in lobular carcinoma than in ductal subtype. This is probably related to either lower expression of GLUT1 or lower density of tumor cells in lobular carcinomas (García Vicente et al. 2013), whereas increased glucose metabolism is associated with higher Ki-67 index, bigger tumor size, poorly differentiated tumor, presence of axillary lymph node (LN) metastases, and higher disease stage.

On the other hand, it is important to keep in mind that some benign conditions, i.e., acute or chronic inflammation (sarcoidosis, lymphadenitis), fat necrosis, physiologic lactation, benign breast masses, and postoperative changes, are associated with increased [^{18}F]FDG uptake, determining differential diagnosis issues (Ugurluer et al. 2013).

3.1.1.1 Staging

[^{18}F]FDG PET/CT is inadequate for accurately defining the extent of the primary breast tumor.

Dynamic contrast-enhanced magnetic resonance imaging (DCE-MRI) continues to play the main role for preoperative evaluation of breast cancer because of its high sensitivity for the detection of small multifocal and synchronous contralateral disease unrecognized on conventional imaging (Heusner et al. 2008).

On the other hand, [^{18}F]FDG PET/CT is generally helpful for the detection of extra-axillary (infraclavicular, supraclavicular, and internal mammary) nodal and occult distant metastases, especially in patients with advanced (stage II–III) breast cancer (Bellon et al. 2004).

3.1.1.2 Axillary Lymph Node Status

Axillary node status is the most reliable predictor of survival, and its knowledge is important in clinical decision-making. To date, sentinel lymph node biopsy is the standard procedure, but though minimally invasive, it is not exempt from surgical complications. [^{18}F]FDG PET/CT has high specificity and positive predictive value, but poor sensitivity for nodal detection. In fact, [^{18}F]FDG PET cannot detect very small lymph node metastases because of its limited spatial resolution (Zhang et al. 2014). As a consequence, axillary biopsy is needed in cases where [^{18}F]FDG PET/CT is negative.

3.1.2 Role of [^{18}F]FDG PET in the Assessment of Response after NAC

As stated earlier, NAC has been used in patients with locally advanced tumor to decrease the size before surgery, reduce the risk of micrometastases and, finally, improve treatment monitoring. Many studies have shown early changes in [^{18}F]-FDG uptake, after one or two cycles, as a valid correlation with patient outcome and final response to chemotherapy (Fig. 6) (Duch et al.

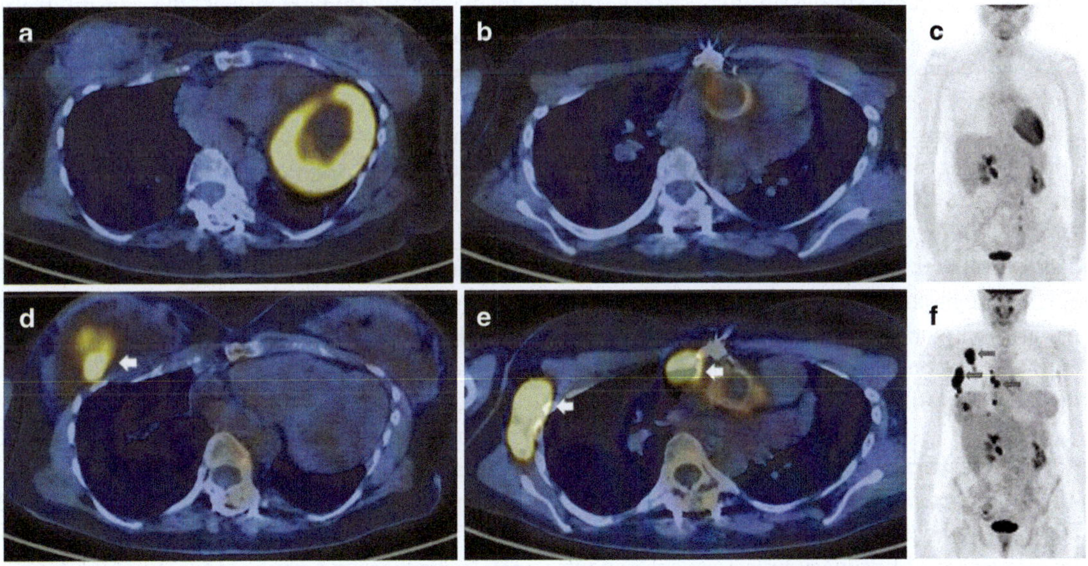

Fig. 6 [^{18}F]FDG PET/CT for response assessment after neoadjuvant chemotherapy in a patient with infiltrating carcinoma (category B5; European Guidelines) of the right breast confirmed with biopsy: G3, estrogen receptors (ERs) 90%, progesterone receptors (PR) 15%, Ki-67 35–40%, HER2 score 1+. Already at baseline, the patient presented with multiple secondary lymphadenopathic involvement in the right axilla and along the internal mammary chains. The patient was candidate to neoadjuvant chemotherapy with four cycles of AC/EC (Adriamycin/epirubicin and cyclophosphamide) followed by four cycles of docetaxel and LH-RH analogue. Post-treatment [^{18}F]FDG PET images (**a**, **b**, **c**) documented a complete metabolic response of all tumor sites visualized at baseline (**d**, **e**, **f**; arrows). The pathological response after surgery reported a 90% fibrosis with a residual single focus of carcinoma. The following images are presented: [^{18}F]FDG PET/CT after chemotherapy, including axial fused [^{18}F]FDG PET/CT (**a, b**) and [^{18}F]FDG PET MIP (**c**), as well as the baseline [^{18}F]FDG PET/CT, axial fused [^{18}F]FDG PET/CT (**d**, **e**), and [^{18}F]FDG PET MIP (**f**)

2009). [^{18}F]FDG PET/CT can differentiate between responders and non-responders with a sensitivity and specificity of 80% and 79%, respectively.

As mentioned above, breast cancer, and, consequently, [^{18}F]FDG avidity, is heterogeneous, so that early response to NAC is different amongst breast cancer subtypes. For example, in triple-negative tumors, a [^{18}F]FDG PET/CT scan after 6 weeks (three cycles) appears to be optimally predictive of pCR, whilst in HER2-positive tumors, neither a [^{18}F]FDG PET/CT scan after 3 weeks nor after 8 weeks seems to be a useful predictor (Groheux et al. 2014). Also in luminal HER2 negative, a low metabolic tumor at baseline and a good response after the first course of NAC are early surrogate markers of patients' survival.

[^{18}F]FDG imaging has a prognostic role and can be used to evaluate response also during receptor-targeted therapy with aromatase inhibitors and/or trastuzumab therapy (Fig. 7). However, available studies in this context show some limitations. Optimal cut-off values for SUVmax decrease, definition of good histopathologic response, chemotherapy regimen used, and best timing for interim [^{18}F]FDG PET evaluation, all vary markedly across studies (Humbert et al. 2014).

Furthermore, [^{18}F]FDG uptake can increase 7–10 days after the beginning of endocrine therapy with tamoxifen. This metabolic flare should be taken into account to avoid a premature therapy interruption, as it has been found to be predictive of a positive response to therapy.

3.1.3 Restaging

Tumor recurrence remains a major problem in the management of breast cancer. It is estimated that up to 35% of primary breast cancer patients after radical treatment will ultimately develop local relapse or distant metastases. Compared to conventional imaging modalities, [^{18}F]FDG PET/CT can increase the diagnostic accuracy for recurrence. [^{18}F]FDG PET/CT has a better sensitivity and specificity in the detection of recurrent breast cancer and/or metastatic sites (Figs. 8 and 9), by confirming equivocal disease and detecting more sites as compared to CT.

Additionally, with the detection of distant metastases and sites of disease in more patients compared with conventional imaging, [^{18}F]FDG PET/CT leads to a change in clinical management in almost 50% of the cases (Cochet et al. 2014).

However, [^{18}F]FDG PET/CT is not sensitive enough to detect small metastatic tumors and small-volume recurrent disease. As a consequence, in case of restaging after systemic treatment, a complete response identified by [^{18}F]FDG PET/CT is not reliable enough to exclude residual microscopic disease (Escalona et al. 2010).

3.2 Bone Metastasis

Bone involvement is present in about 65% of patients with metastatic disease, with bone being one of the most frequent sites for distant metastases. Standard imaging for bone involvement is not based on PET. However, the sensitivity of ^{99m}Tc-diphosphonate bone scan can be low for lytic lesions, which are commonly associated to breast cancer. Also, the evaluation of bone lesions responding to treatment can be difficult. Bone scan remains positive for a long time in spite of response owing to uptake related to osteoblastic activity, and the result of the CT scan may be misinterpreted as persistent or worsening disease because of the increased sclerosis observed in bone lesions (Mandegaran et al. 2014).

Recently, a specific PET tracer, [^{18}F]sodium fluoride ([^{18}F]NaF), is being implemented for imaging bone metastases. The mechanism of uptake is similar to diphosphonate, accumulating within the bony skeleton after only a single blood pass. This behavior determines an improved target to background ratio and a twofold higher bone uptake of [^{18}F]NaF compared to ^{99m}Tc-diphosphonate (Fig. 10).

The high-resolution technology and the combined PET/CT imaging allow for better distinction of tracer uptake in benign versus malignant lesions by simultaneous evaluation of CT images. Nevertheless, there is limited data on

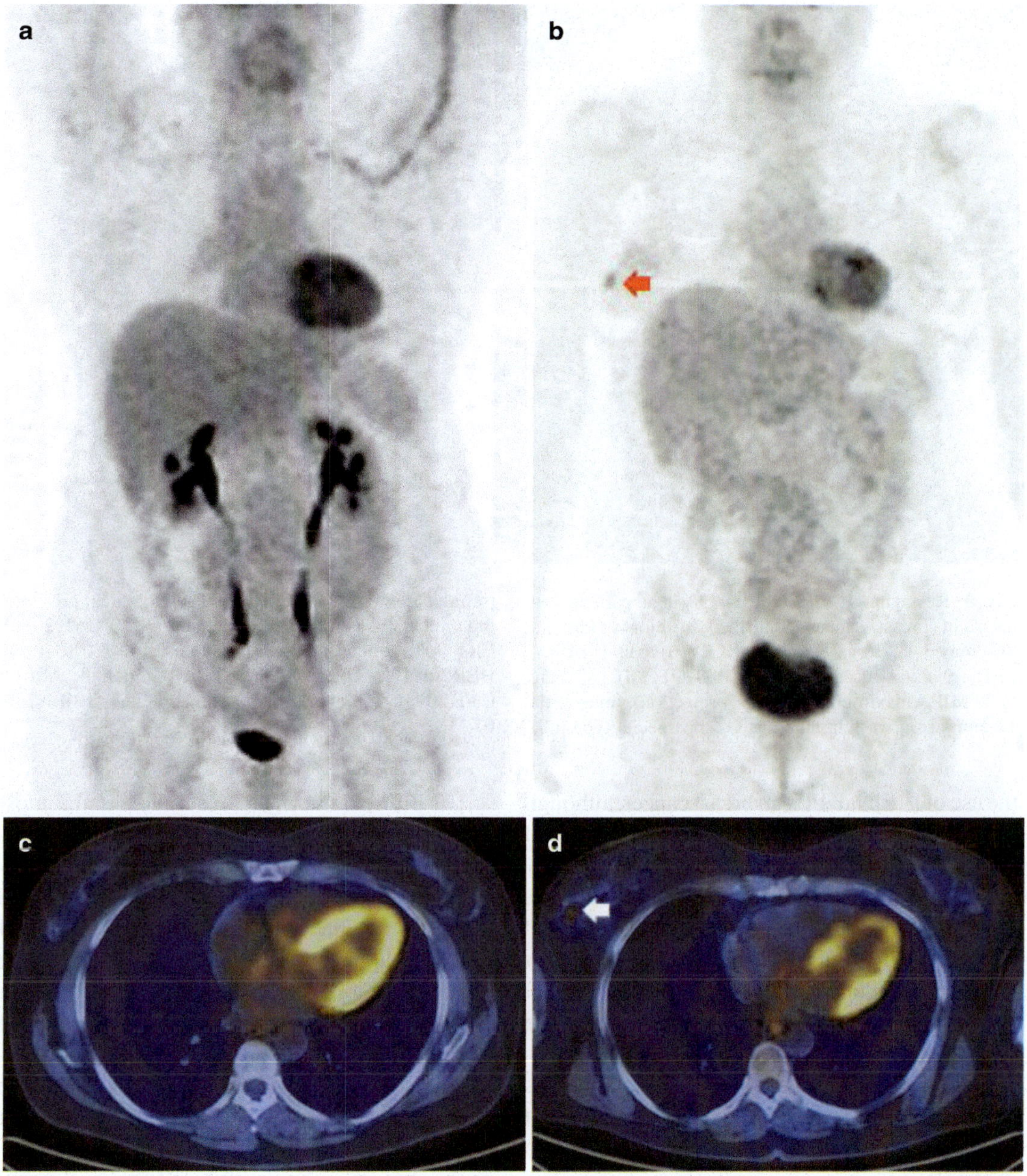

Fig. 7 [^{18}F]FDG PET/CT for response assessment after neoadjuvant chemoimmunotherapy in a patient with infiltrating and in situ carcinomas (category B5; European Guidelines) of the right breast. At diagnosis, the tumor resulted a G2–3, no special type (ERs 95%, PR 80%, Ki-67 70%). The patient was candidate to four cycles of AC (Adriamycin and cyclophosphamide), followed by trastuzumab and docetaxel for four cycles. Post-treatment ^{18}F-PET images (**a**, **c**) documented a complete metabolic response of the infiltrating tumor lesion visualized at baseline (**b**, **d**; arrows). The pathological response after surgery reported a 30% fibrosis for the infiltrating carcinoma and a 60% fibrotic response for the carcinoma in situ. The following images are presented: [^{18}F]FDG PET/CT after chemoimmunotherapy, including axial fused [^{18}F]FDG PET/CT (**a**, **b**) and [^{18}F]FDG PET MIP (**c**), as well as the baseline [^{18}F]FDG PET/CT, axial fused [^{18}F]FDG PET/CT (**d, e**), and [^{18}F]FDG PET MIP (**f**)

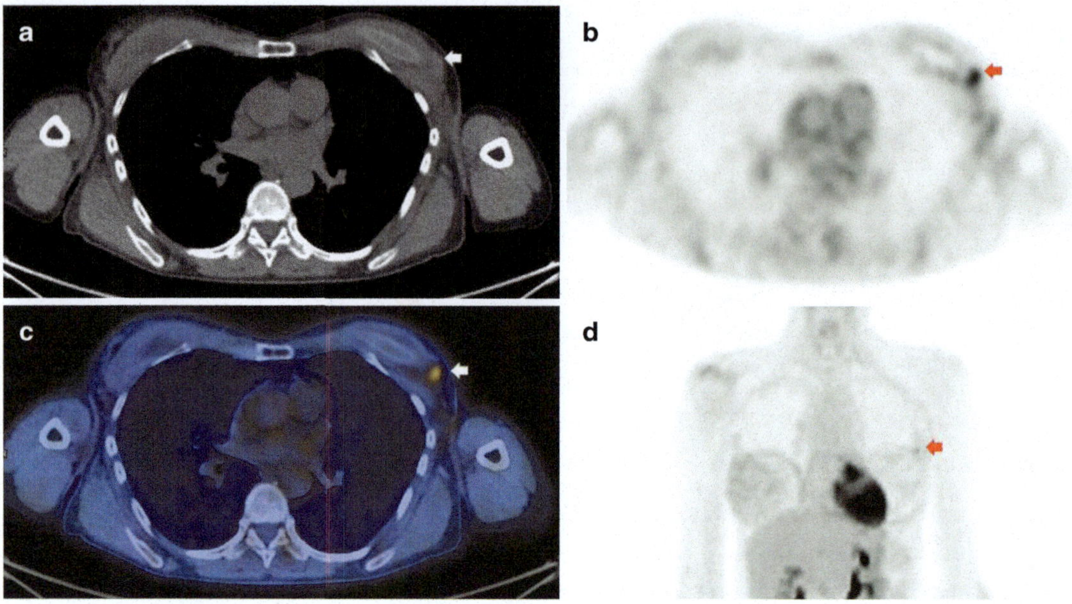

Fig. 8 Restaging [^{18}F]FDG PET/CT in a patient with recurrent breast cancer confirmed at biopsy (arrows; SUVmax 3.4): (**a**) axial low-dose CT; (**b**) axial [^{18}F]FDG PET; (**c**) axial fused [^{18}F]FDG PET/CT; (**d**) [^{18}F]FDG PET MIP (maximum intensity projection) image; the 14-mm lesion was classified as G2, no special type infiltrating carcinoma (WHO 2012). The biological profile of the tumor was as follows [Guidelines ASCO-CAP 2010]: ERs 90%, intense; *PR* 70%, intense; Ki-67 15–20%; HER2/neu (c-erbB2, Roche, 4B5) [Guidelines ASCO-CAP 2013]: immunoreactivity of membrane ≤10% (score 0)

the use of [^{18}F]NaF PET in breast cancer, although some reports have observed greater detection and possible evaluation of marrow disease.

In patients with marrow flare phenomenon, focal [^{18}F]FDG uptake may be confusing and [^{18}F]NaF imaging may be useful for distinguishing metastatic involvement. However, [^{18}F]FDG PET can still be superior for evaluating lytic bone disease (Fig. 11a–c), where [^{18}F]NaF shows occasionally false-negative results, i.e., if there is a small lytic metastatic lesion with little or absent osteoblastic activity (Fig. 11d–f) (Kulshrestha et al. 2016).

3.3 Other Non-[^{18}F]FDG Tracers

Target-mediated nuclear imaging may be a useful tool to evaluate biomarker expression in cancer cells. In the last decade, different receptor targeted molecules for nuclear imaging of breast cancer have been identified and are nowadays under investigation.

[^{18}F]FES, a fluorinated estradiol, is the most extensively studied ER-targeting PET radioligand. It was used to visualize primary and metastatic breast cancer, to predict response to anti-estrogen therapy. Indeed, studies showed that high uptake of [^{18}F]FES prior to endocrine treatment and a decrease of [^{18}F]FES uptake in early phases of treatment are an indication of treatment success.

As anti-estrogens bind also ER and make receptors not available, targeting nuclear imaging is not always efficient, so PR targeted radioligands may be more useful. [^{18}F]fluoro furanyl norprogesterone ([^{18}F]FNP) has shown interesting results in the disease characterization, although imaging data is still limited.

Overexpression of HER2/neu, which regulates cell growth and survival, has been associated with poor prognosis in breast cancer. In this context, HER2-targeted therapies have been shown to improve survival and reduce the development of distant metastatic disease. Monoclonal antibodies used for therapy of HER2-expressing

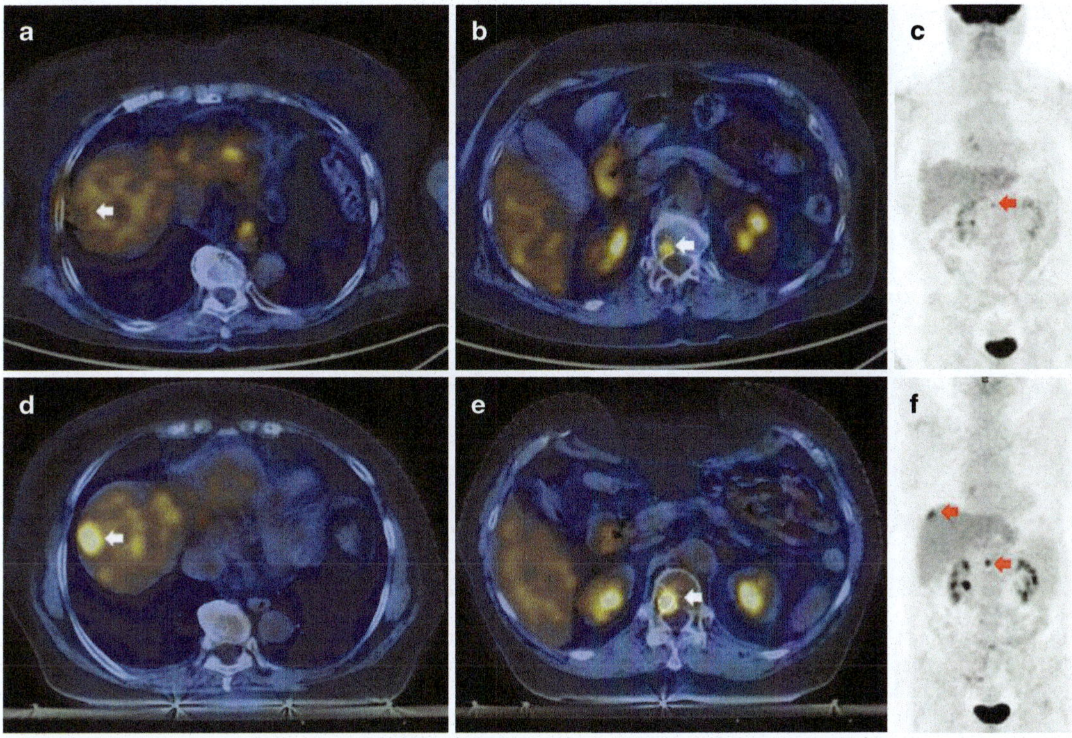

Fig. 9 [18F]FDG PET/CT for response assessment after radiotherapy in a patient with recurrent infiltrating carcinoma (pT1c N0; ERs 85%, PR 2%) presenting with secondary lesions treated with SBRT (stereotactic body radiation therapy) for the hepatic metastases (68 Gy; 3 fractions) and EBRT (external beam radiation therapy) for the D12 bone metastasis (20 Gy; 5 fractions). Pre- and post-treatment PET images documented a complete metabolic response for liver lesions, but only a partial response for the bone metastasis. **a**, **b**, and **c** are, respectively, the axial fused PET/CT and MIP images obtained after treatment; **d**, **e**, and **f** are the corresponding images obtained before radiation therapy (SBRT and EBRT)

breast cancer were labeled with radionuclides for PET imaging. ^{64}Cu-DOTA- and ^{89}Zr-trastuzumab showed feasibility, safety, and good uptake in tumor lesions. Also ^{68}Ga-HER2-nanobody showed primary and metastatic lesions in breast cancer patients, with no reported toxicity.

As somatostatin receptor (SSTR) expression has also been reported on breast cancer cells, ^{68}Ga-DOTA-TOC imaging was compared to [18F] FDG PET in a mouse model resulting in two times higher uptake of ^{68}Ga-DOTA-TOC compared to [18F]FDG. Nevertheless, low and heterogeneous SSTR expression and non-appropriate patient selection are the limiting factors for successful BC imaging in this group of tracers.

Gastrin-releasing peptide receptor (GRPR) is also another molecular biomarker overexpressed in breast cancer. Using radiolabeled GRPR antagonist, a significant different uptake in treated and non-treated animals was observed, whilst no significant difference in [18F]FDG uptake was reported.

Folate receptor (FR), C-X-C chemokine receptor type 4 (CXCR4), neuropeptide Y receptor Y1 (NPY1R), and vasoactive intestinal polypeptide receptor 1 (VIP-R1) are other interesting targets under investigation for breast cancer imaging (Dalm et al. 2017).

3.4 New Horizon: PET/MRI

Recent technological progresses have led to the development of PET/MRI, which integrates anatomical and metabolic information. PET/MRI determines better than PET/CT the T-stage of

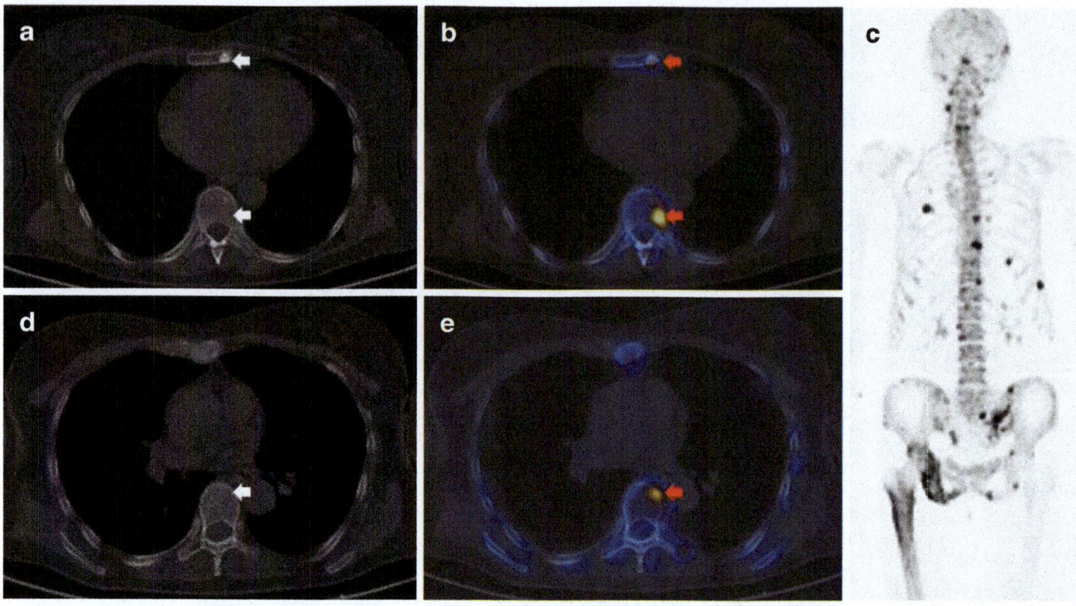

Fig. 10 Restaging [¹⁸F]fluoride PET/CT in a patient with metastatic breast cancer with multiple lesions in the skeleton. Note the limited dimensions and faint appearance of the sclerotic and lytic lesions clearly seen on axial LD CT (low-dose CT; **a**, **d**; white arrows) and fused [^{18}F]fluoride PET/CT (**b, e**; red arrows). Although their presence does not impact significantly the management of the patient, who presents with diffuse metastatic disease (**c**; MIP image), the [^{18}F]fluoride PET/CT demonstrates a remarkable ability and high sensitivity for the detection of minimal bone infiltration

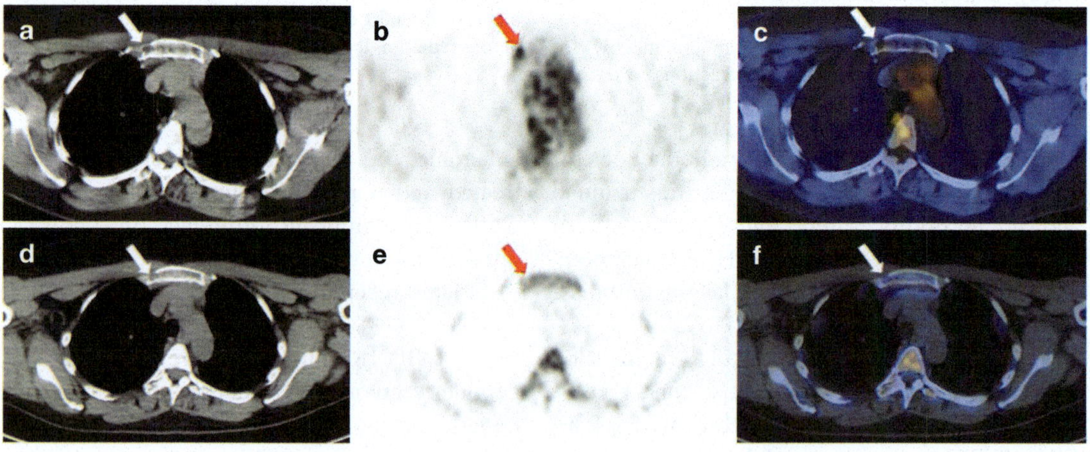

Fig. 11 Comparison between [^{18}F]FDG PET/CT (**a**, **b**, and **c**) and [^{18}F]fluoride PET/CT (**d**, **e**, and **f**) in a patient with recurrent breast cancer localized in the sternum (arrows) and visualized as a small round lytic area showing faint but pathological [^{18}F]FDG uptake (SUVmax 2.3) on [^{18}F]FDG PET. The absence of active osteoblastic reaction on site determined the absence of tracer uptake on [^{18}F]fluoride PET. This is a potential limitation and pitfall for [^{18}F]fluoride PET

breast tumor, which may be useful in surgical planning. Moreover, the increased sensitivity of MRI for multifocal disease and the increased sensitivity of PET for axillary nodal disease, together in a single examination, may improve clinical assessment as well.

Whole-body PET/MRI is also interesting because MRI provides improved lesion detection in the brain, breast, liver, kidneys and bones as compared with CT. In imaging metastatic disease, PET and MRI are again complementary, with MRI providing high sensitivity and PET improving the specificity of DWI. In addition, deleting the whole-body CT from the PET examination can decrease the radiation dose by half.

However, PET/MRI is not available in most centers and is not used universally for imaging breast cancer. Therefore, the advantages of combined PET/MRI in the routine evaluation of breast cancer are yet to be explored and delineated accurately (Melsaether and Moy 2017).

References

Adrada BE, Huo L, Lane DL, Arribas EM, Resetkova E, Yang W (2015) Histopathologic correlation of residual mammographic microcalcifications after neoadjuvant chemotherapy for locally advanced breast cancer. Ann Surg Oncol 22:1111–1117

Athanasiou A, Latorre-Ossa H, Criton A, Tardivon A, Gennisson JL, Tanter M (2017) Feasibility of imaging and treatment monitoring of breast lesions with three-dimensional shear wave elastography. Ultraschall Med 38:51–59

Avril N, Sassen S, Roylance R (2009) Response to therapy in breast cancer. J Nucl Med 50(Suppl 1):55S–63S

Ballesio L, Gigli S, Di Pastena F, Giraldi G, Manganaro L, Anastasi E, Catalano C (2017) Magnetic resonance imaging tumor regression shrinkage patterns after neoadjuvant chemotherapy in patients with locally advanced breast cancer: correlation with tumor biological subtypes and pathological response after therapy. Tumour Biol 39:101042831769454. https://doi.org/10.1177/1010428317694540

Baltzer PA, Dietzel M, Burmeister HP, Zoubi R, Gajda M, Camara O, Kaiser WA (2011) Application of MR mammography beyond local staging: is there a potential to accurately assess axillary lymph nodes? Evaluation of an extended protocol in an initial prospective study. AJR Am J Roentgenol 196:W641–W647

Bellon JR, Livingston RB, Eubank WB, Gralow JR, Ellis GK, Dunnwald LK, Mankoff DA (2004) Evaluation of the internal mammary lymph nodes by FDG-PET in locally advanced breast cancer (LABC). Am J Clin Oncol 27:407–410

Berg WA, Blume JD, Cormack JB, Mendelson EB, Lehrer D, Böhm-Vélez M et al (2008) ACRIN 6666 Investigators. Combined screening with ultrasound and mammography vs mammography alone in women at elevated risk of breast cancer. JAMA 299:2151–2163

Bonadonna G, Valagussa P, Zucali R, Salvadori B (1995) Primary chemotherapy in surgically resectable breast cancer. CA Cancer J Clin 45:227–243

Bosch AM, Kessels AG, Beets GL, Rupa JD, Koster D, van Engelshoven JM, von Meyenfeldt MF (2003) Preoperative estimation of the pathological breast tumour size by physical examination, mammography and ultrasound: a prospective study on 105 invasive tumours. Eur J Radiol 48:285–292

Briasoulis E, Karavasilis V, Kostadima L, Ignatiadis M, Fountzilas G, Pavlidis N (1992) Metastatic breast carcinoma confined to bone: portrait of a clinical entity. Cancer 2004; 101:1524-8; **Koenders PG, Beex LV, Kloppenborg PW, et al. human breast cancer: survival from first metastasis. Breast Cancer study group. Breast Cancer Res Treat 21:173–180

Cochet A, David S, Moodie K, Drummond E, Dutu G, Mac-Manus M, Chua B et al (2014) The utility of 18F-FDG PET/CT for suspected recurrent breast cancer: impact and prognostic stratification. Cancer Imaging 14:13–21

Corcioni B, Santili L, Quercia S, Zamagni C, Santini D, Taffurelli M, Mignani S (2008) Contrast-enhanced US and MRI for assessing the response of breast cancer to neoadjuvant chemotherapy. J Ultrasound 11:143–150

Dalm S, Verzijlbergen J, De Jong M (2017) Review: receptor targeted nuclear imaging of breast cancer. Int J Mol Sci 18:260

van Dam PA, van Dam VC, Altintas S, Papadimitriou K, Rolfo C, Trinh XB (2016) Neoadjuvant endocrine treatment in early breast cancer: An overlooked alternative. Eur J Surg Oncol 42:333–342

Duch J, Fuster D, Muñoz M, Fernández PL, Paredes P, Fontanillas M et al (2009) 18F-FDG PET/CT for early prediction of response to neoadjuvant chemotherapy in breast cancer. Eur J Nucl Med Mol Imaging 36:1551–1557

Eisenhauer EA, Therasse P, Bogaerts J, Schwartz LH, Sargent D, Ford R et al (2009) New response evaluation criteria in solid tumours: revised RECIST guideline (version 1.1). Eur J Cancer 45:228–247

ElSaid NAE, Mahmoud HGM, Salama A et al (2017) Role of contrast-enhanced spectral mammography in predicting pathological response of locally advanced breast cancer post neo-adjuvant chemotherapy. Egyptian J Radiol Nucl Med 48(2):519–527

Escalona S, Blasco JA, Reza MM, Andradas E, Gómez N (2010) A systematic review of FDG-PET in breast cancer. Med Oncol 27:114–129

Evans A, Armstrong S, Whelehan P, Thomson K, Rauchhaus P, Purdie C et al (2013) Can shear-wave elastography predict response to neoadjuvant chemotherapy in women with invasive breast cancer? Br J Cancer 109:2798–2802

Feliciano Y, Mamtani A, Morrow M, Stempel MM, Patil S, Jochelson MS (2017) Do calcifications seen on mammography after neoadjuvant chemotherapy for breast cancer always need to be excised? Ann Surg Oncol 24:1492–1498

García Vicente AM, Soriano Castrejón A, León Martín A, Chacón López-Muñiz I, Muñoz Madero V, Muñoz

Sánchez M del M et al (2013) Molecular subtypes of breast cancer: metabolic correlation with (1)(8)F-FDG PET/ CT. Eur J Nucl Med Mol Imaging 40:1304–1311
Golan O, Amitai Y, Menes T (2016) Does change in microcalcifications with neoadjuvant treatment correlate with pathological tumour response? Clin Radiol 71:458–463
Goorts B, Dreuning KMA, Houwers JB, Kooreman LFS, Boerma EG, Mann RM, Lobbes MBI, Smidt ML (2018) MRI-based response patterns during neoadjuvant chemotherapy can predict pathological (complete) response in patients with breast cancer. Breast Cancer Res 20:34. https://doi.org/10.1186/s13058-018-0950-x
Groheux D, Giacchetti S, Moretti JL, Porcher R, Espié M, Lehmann-Che J et al (2011) Correlation of high 18F-FDG uptake to clinical, pathological and biological prognostic factors in breast cancer. Eur J Nucl Med Mol Imaging 38:426–435
Groheux D, Hindié E, Giacchetti S, Hamy AS, Berger F, Merlet P et al (2014) Early assessment with 18F-fluorodeoxyglucose positron emission tomography/computed tomography can help predict the outcome of neoadjuvant chemotherapy in triple negative breast cancer. Eur J Cancer 50:1864–1871
Gruber IV, Rueckert M, Kagan KO, Staebler A, Siegmann KC, Hartkopf A et al (2013) Measurement of tumour size with mammography, sonography and magnetic resonance imaging as compared to histological tumour size in primary breast cancer. BMC Cancer 13:328
van der Hage JA, van de Velde CJ, Julien JP, Tubiana-Hulin M, Vandervelden C, Duchateau L (2001) Preoperative chemotherapy in primary operable breast cancer: results from the European Organization for Research and Treatment of Cancer trial 10902. J Clin Oncol 19:4224–4237
Hayashi N, Costelloe CM, Hamaoka T, Wei C, Niikura N, Theriault RL et al (2013) A prospective study of bone tumor response assessment in metastatic breast cancer. Clin Breast Cancer 13:24–30
Hellman S (1994) Karnofsky memorial lecture: natural history of small breast cancers. J Clin Oncol 12:2229e34
Heusner TA, Kuemmel S, Umutlu L, Koeninger A, Freudenberg LS, Hauth EA et al (2008) Breast cancer staging in a single session: whole-body PET/CT mammography. J Nucl Med 49:1215–1222
Hong JC, Salama JK (2017) The expanding role of stereotactic body radiation therapy in oligometastatic solid tumors: what do we know and where are we going? Cancer Treat Rev 52:22–32
Hortobagyi GN (2002) Can we cure limited metastatic breast cancer? J Clin Oncol 20:620e3.5
Houssami N, Ciatto S (2010) Mammographic surveillance in women with a personal history of breast cancer: how accurate? How effective? Breast 19:439–445
Huber S, Wagner M, Zuna I, Medl M, Czembirek H, Delorme S (2000) Locally advanced breast carcinoma: evaluation of mammography in the prediction of residual disease after induction chemotherapy. Anticancer Res 20:553–558
Humbert O, Berriolo-Riedinger A, Cochet A, Gauthier M, Charon-Barra C, Guiu S et al (2014) Prognostic relevance at 5 years of the early monitoring of neoadjuvant chemotherapy using 18F-FDG PET in luminal HER2-negative breast cancer. Eur J Nucl Med Mol Imaging 41:416–427
Humbert O, Cochet A, Coudert B, Berriolo-Riedinger A, Kanoun S, Brunotte F, Fumoleau P (2015) Role of positron emission tomography for the monitoring of response to therapy in breast cancer. Oncologist 20:94–104
Kanso H, Kazzi H, Menassa-Moussa L, Abi Khalil S, Ghosn M, Chahine G et al (2008) Value of US imaging following mastectomy. J Radiol 89:1077–1080
Keune JD, Jeffe DB, Schootman M, Hoffman A, Gillanders WE, Aft RL (2010) Accuracy of ultrasonography and mammography in predicting pathologic response after neoadjuvant chemotherapy for breast cancer. Am J Surg 199:477–484
Kim TH, Kang DK, Yim H, Jung YS, Kim KS, Kang SY (2012) Magnetic resonance imaging patterns of tumor regression after neoadjuvant chemotherapy in breast cancer patients: correlation with pathological response grading system based on tumor cellularity. J Comput Assist Tomogr 36:200–206
Kitajima K, Fukushima K, Miyoshi Y, Nishimukai A, Hirota S, Igarashi Y et al (2015) Association between 18F-FDG uptake and molecular subtype of breast cancer. Eur J Nucl Med Mol Imaging 42:1371–1377
Kong X, Moran MS, Zhang N, Haffty B, Yang Q (2011) Meta-analysis confirms achieving pathological complete response after neoadjuvant chemotherapy predicts favourable prognosis for breast cancer patients. Eur J Cancer 47:2084–2090
Kulshrestha R, Vinjamuri S, England A, Nightingale J, Hogg P (2016) The role of 18F-sodium fluoride PET/CT bone scans in the diagnosis of metastatic bone disease from breast and prostate cancer. J Nucl Med Technol 44:217–222
Lee JH, Kim EK, Oh JY, Kwon HC, Kim SH, Kim DC et al (2013) US screening for detection of nonpalpable locoregional recurrence after mastectomy. Eur J Radiol 82:485–489
Lee SC, Grant E, Sheth P, Garcia AA, Desai B, Ji L et al (2017) Accuracy of contrast-enhanced ultrasound compared with magnetic resonance imaging in assessing the tumor response after neoadjuvant chemotherapy for breast cancer. J Ultrasound Med 36:901–911
Li JJ, Chen C, Gu Y, Di G, Wu J, Liu G, Shao Z (2014) The role of mammographic calcification in the neoadjuvant therapy of breast cancer imaging evaluation. PLoS One 9(2):e88853. https://doi.org/10.1371/journal.pone.0088853. eCollection 2014
Lindenberg MA, Miquel-Cases A, Retèl VP, Sonke GS, Wesseling J, Stokkel MPM, van Harten WH (2017) Imaging performance in guiding response to neoadjuvant chemotherapy according to breast cancer subtypes: a systematic literature review. Crit Rev Oncol Hematol 112:198–207
Lobbes MB, Prevos R, Smidt M, Tjan-Heijnen VC, van Goethem M, Schipper R et al (2013) The role

of magnetic resonance imaging in assessing residual disease and pathologic complete response in breast cancer patients receiving neoadjuvant chemotherapy: a systematic review. Insights Imaging 4: 163–175

Lorenzon M, Zuiani C, Londero V, Linda A, Furlan A, Bazzocchi M (2009) Assessment of breast cancer response to neoadjuvant chemotherapy: is volumetric MRI a reliable tool? Eur J Radiol 71:82–88

Mandegaran R, Debard A, Alvarez M, Marchou B, Massip P, Wagner T (2014) Disseminated osteomyelitis or bone metastases of breast cancer: (18)F-FDG-PET/CT helps unravel an unusual presentation. Ann Nucl Med 28:167–171

Mann RM, Kuhl CK, Kinkel K, Boetes C (2008) Breast MRI: guidelines from the European Society of Breast Imaging. Eur Radiol 18:1307–1318

Marinovich ML, Macaskill P, Irwig L, Sardanelli F, Mamounas E, von Minckwitz G et al (2015) Agreement between MRI and pathological breast tumor size after neoadjuvant chemotherapy, and comparison with alternative tests: individual patient data meta-analysis. BMC Cancer 15:662

Mauri D, Pavlidis N, Ioannidis JP (2005) Neoadjuvant versus adjuvant systemic treatment in breast cancer: a meta-analysis. J Natl Cancer Inst 97:188–194

McLaughlin R, Hylton N (2011) MRI in breast cancer therapy monitoring. NMR Biomed 24:712–720

Melsaether A, Moy L (2017) Breast PET/MR imaging. Radiol Clin N Am 55:579–589

Milano MT, Katz AW, Zhang H, Okunieff P (2012) Oligometastases treated with stereotactic body radiotherapy: long-term follow-up of prospective study. Int J Radiat Oncol Biol Phys 83:878–886

Miller AB, Hoogstraten B, Staquet M, Winkler A (1981) Reporting results of cancer treatment. Cancer 47:207–214

Minarikova L, Bogner W, Pinker K, Valkovič L, Zaric O, Bago-Horvath Z et al (2017) Investigating the prediction value of multiparametric magnetic resonance imaging at 3T in response to neoadjuvant chemotherapy in breast cancer. Eur Radiol 27:1901–1911

Mistry KA, Thakur MH, Kembhavi SA (2016) The effect of chemotherapy on the mammographic appearance of breast cancer and correlation with histopathology. Br J Radiol 89:20150479

Montgomery DA, Krupa K, Cooke TG (2007) Follow-up in breast cancer: does routine clinical examination improve outcome? A systematic review of the literature. Br J Cancer 17:1632–1641

Moon HJ, Kim MJ, Kim EK, Park BW, Youk JH, Kwak JY et al (2009) US surveillance of regional lymph node recurrence after breast cancer surgery. Radiology 252:673–681

Morris EA, Comstock CE, Lee CH, et al (2013) ACR BI-RADS magnetic resonance imaging. In: ACR BI-RADS atlas, breast imaging reporting and data system. American College of Radiology, Reston

Moschetti I, Cinquini M, Lambertini M et al (2016) Follow-up strategies for women treated for early breast cancer. Cochrane Database Syst Rev 27:CD001768

O'Shaughnessy J, Miles D, Vukelja S, Moiseyenko V, Ayoub JP, Cervantes G et al (2002) Superior survival with capecitabine plus docetaxel combination therapy in anthracycline-pretreated patients with advanced breast cancer: phase III trial results. J Clin Oncol 20:2812e23

Pagani O, Senkus E, Wood W, Colleoni M, Cufer T, Kyriakides S et al (2010) International guidelines for management of metastatic breast cancer: can metastatic breast cancer be cured? J Natl Cancer Inst 102:456e63

Pickles MD, Lowry M, Manton DJ, Gibbs P, Turnbull LW (2005) Role of dynamic contrast enhanced MRI in monitoring early response of locally advanced breast cancer to neoadjuvant chemotherapy. Breast Cancer Res Treat 91:1–10

Prevos R, Smidt ML, Tjan-Heijnen VC, van Goethem M, Beets-Tan RG, Wildberger JE, Lobbes MB (2012) Pre-treatment differences and early response monitoring of neoadjuvant chemotherapy in breast cancer patients using magnetic resonance imaging: a systematic review. Eur Radiol 22:2607–2616

Scorsetti M, Franceschini D, De Rose F, Comito T, Villa E, Iftode C et al (2016) Stereotactic body radiation therapy: a promising chance for oligometastatic breast cancer. Breast 26:11–17

Seo N, Kim HH, Shin HJ, Cha JH, Kim H, Moon JH et al (2014) Digital breast tomosynthesis versus full-field digital mammography: comparison of the accuracy of lesion measurement and characterization using specimens. Acta Radiol 55:661–667

Shin JH, Han BK, Choe YH, Nam SJ, Park W, Im YH (2005) Ultrasonographic detection of occult cancer in patients after surgical therapy for breast cancer. J Ultrasound Med 24:643–649

Shin HJ, Baek HM, Ahn S et al (2012) Prediction of pathologic response to neoadjuvant chemotherapy in patients with breast cancer using diffusion-weighted imaging and MRS. NMR Biomed 25:1349–1359

Singletary SE, Walsh G, Vauthey JN, Curley S, Sawaya R, Weber KL et al (2003) A role for curative surgery in the treatment of selected patients with metastatic breast cancer. Oncologist 8:241–251

Tan S-H, Wolff AC (2010) Treatment of metastatic breast cancer. In: Harris JR, Lippman ME, Morrow M, Osborne CK (eds) Diseases of the breast, 4th edn. Wolters Kluwer/Lippincott Williams & Wilkins, Philadelphia, pp 877–919

Therasse P, Arbuck SG, Eisenhauer EA, Wanders J, Kaplan RS, Rubinstein L et al (2000) New guidelines to evaluate the response to treatment in solid tumors. European Organization for Research and Treatment of Cancer, National Cancer Institute of the United States, National Cancer Institute of Canada. J Natl Cancer Inst 92:205–216

Tree AC, Khoo VS, Eeles RA, Ahmed M, Dearnaley DP, Hawkins MA et al (2013) Stereotactic body radiotherapy for oligometastases. Lancet Oncol 14:e28e37

Ugurluer G, Kibar M, Yavuz S, Kuzucu A, Serin M (2013) False positive 18F-FDG uptake in mediastinal lymph nodes detected with positron emission tomography in breast cancer: a case report. Case Rep Med 2013:459753

Van Nijnatten TJA, Ploumen EH, Schipper RJ, Goorts B, Andriessen EH, Vanwetswinkel S et al (2016) Routine use of standard breast MRI compared to axillary ultrasound for differentiating between no, limited and advanced axillary nodal disease in newly diagnosed breast cancer patients. Eur J Radiol 85:2288–2294

Vinnicombe SJ, MacVicar AD, Guy RL, Sloane JP, Powles TJ, Knee G, Husband JE (1996) Primary breast cancer: mammographic changes after neoadjuvant chemotherapy, with pathologic correlation. Radiology 198:333–340

Vriens BE, De Vries B, Lobbes MB, van Gastel SM, van den Berkmortel FW, Smilde TJ et al (2016) INTENS Study Group. Ultrasound is at least as good as magnetic resonance imaging in predicting tumour size post-neoadjuvant chemotherapy in breast cancer. Eur J Cancer 52:67–76

Vugts C, Maaskant-Braat AJ, De Roos WK, Voogd AC, Nieuwenhuijzen GA (2016) Management of the axilla after neoadjuvant chemotherapy for clinically node positive breast cancer: a nationwide survey study in the Netherlands. Eur J Surg Oncol 42:956–964

Wu LM, Hun JN, Gu HY et al (2012) Can diffusion-weighted MR imaging and contrast-enhanced MR imaging precisely evaluate and predict pathological response to neoadjuvant chemotherapy in patients with breast cancer? Breast Cancer Res Treat 135:17–28

Yoon JH, Kim MJ, Eun-Kyung Kim MD et al (2015) Imaging surveillance of patients with breast cancer after primary treatment: current recommendations. Korean J Radiol 16:219–228

You S, Kang DK, Jung YS, An YS, Jeon GS, And Kim TH. Evaluation of lymph node status after neoadjuvant chemotherapy in breast cancer patients: comparison of diagnostic performance of ultrasound, MRI and 18F-FDG PET/CT. Br J Radiol 2015;88:20150143

Yuan Y, Chen XS, Liu SY, Shen KW (2010) Accuracy of MRI in prediction of pathologic complete remission in breast cancer after preoperative therapy: a meta-analysis. AJR Am J Roentgenol 195:260–268

Zhang X, Wu F, Han P (2014) The role of 18F-FDG PET/CT in the diagnosis of breast cancer and lymph nodes metastases and micrometastases may be limited. Hell J Nucl Med 17:177–183

Response Assessment and Follow-Up by Imaging in Gastrointestinal Tumours

Doenja M. J. Lambregts
and Francesco Giammarile

Contents

1 **Introduction** 475
2 **Response Assessment in Rectal Cancer** 476
2.1 Introduction 476
2.2 MRI for Restaging Rectal Cancer 477
2.3 Quantitative and Functional Imaging Methods 479
2.4 Conclusions 482
3 **Response Assessment in Gastro-Enteropancreatic Neuro-Endocrine (GEP-NET) Tumours** 483
3.1 Introduction 483
3.2 Tumour Response Assessment in GEP-NET with Nuclear Medicine Techniques 484
3.3 Conclusions 489
References 489

D. M. J. Lambregts (✉)
Department of Radiology, The Netherlands Cancer Institute, Amsterdam, The Netherlands
e-mail: d.lambregts@nki.nl

F. Giammarile
Faculty of Medicine, Department of Nuclear Medicine, University of Lyon, Lyon, France

Nuclear Medicine and Diagnostic Imaging Section, International Atomic Energy Agency, Vienna, Austria
e-mail: f.giammarile@iaea.org

Abstract

Response assessment with imaging in gastrointestinal tumours can serve different clinical goals. In tumour types that are primarily surgically treated, imaging can be used to assess response to neoadjuvant treatment, determine resectability and help decide on the best surgical approach. In patients who are primarily undergoing medical (systemic) treatment, imaging can be used to monitor tumour responsiveness in order to optimize or alter the treatment plan in any patient not achieving a satisfactory response, thereby avoiding prolonged ineffective treatment. In this chapter, the use of imaging in these respective settings will be illustrated using rectal cancer and gastro-enteropancreatic neuro-endocrine tumours (GEP-NET) as examples.

1 Introduction

Response assessment with imaging in gastrointestinal tumours can serve different clinical goals. In tumour types that are primarily surgically treated, imaging can be used to assess response to neoadjuvant treatment in order to evaluate tumour downsizing/downstaging, determine resectability and help decide on the best surgical approach. In patients who are non-surgically managed but are primarily undergoing medical (systemic) treat-

R. G. H. Beets-Tan et al. (eds.), *Imaging and Interventional Radiology for Radiation Oncology*, Medical Radiology, Diagnostic Imaging, https://doi.org/10.1007/978-3-030-38261-2_25

ment, imaging can be used to monitor tumour responsiveness in order to optimize or alter the treatment plan in any patient not achieving a satisfactory response, thereby avoiding prolonged ineffective treatment.

In this chapter, the use of imaging in these two different clinical settings will be discussed according to two examples: response assessment to neoadjuvant treatment in rectal cancer and response assessment to medical treatment in gastro-enteropancreatic neuro-endocrine tumours (GEP-NET).

2 Response Assessment in Rectal Cancer

2.1 Introduction

The standard surgical treatment for rectal cancer is a total mesorectal excision (TME). Depending on the risk profile of the tumour, surgery is preceded by neoadjuvant short-course radiotherapy (5 × 5 Gy) or long-course neoadjuvant combination chemo- and radiotherapy (CRT). The latter is mainly given to patients with advanced, high-risk tumours with the aim of inducing tumour downsizing and downstaging, in order to increase the chance of a complete resection and thereby reduce the risk of a local recurrence. Imaging plays a pivotal role in determining a patient's tumour risk profile and, thus, in the personalised treatment planning of rectal cancer. Magnetic resonance imaging (MRI) and endorectal (or endoluminal) ultrasound (EUS) are the two main techniques used for the primary local staging of rectal cancer. The main strength of EUS is its excellent soft-tissue contrast, making it the only imaging technique capable of separately visualizing all separate layers of the bowel wall. For this reason, EUS is particularly useful for staging early tumours (T1–2). Main drawbacks of EUS are that the technique is operator dependant and that it can be challenging to position the ultrasound probe in high and/or stenosing tumours (Ptok et al. 2006). Moreover, EUS has a limited field of view (FOV), making it less suitable to stage more advanced tumours that invade the mesorectal fascia and/or adjacent pelvic organs and to get a complete overview of all the lymph nodes within the mesorectal compartment. Hence, MRI is the imaging technique most widely adopted for the overall local staging of rectal cancer, as it offers the combined benefits of an excellent soft tissue contrast, high spatial resolution and large FOV. In an increasing number of centres worldwide, MRI is nowadays not only used for the primary staging of rectal cancer, but also routinely applied to restage tumours after neoadjuvant treatment. Traditionally, the role of imaging in this setting has been limited, since the surgical plan was decided based on the findings of primary staging, regardless of the response to neoadjuvant treatment. To date, however, its role is emerging. The main goal of restaging is to assess to what extent tumour downsizing and downstaging have occurred as this may alter the initially planned surgical strategy. For example, if a tumour retracts from initially invaded pelvic organs (e.g. bladder, prostate, uterus/cervix), an initially planned extended pelvic resection may be converted into a standard total mesorectal excision. Also, conversion to sphincter-preserving surgery may be considered when a distally located tumour retracts from the anal sphincter complex. In addition to its use as a surgical roadmap, there has been an increasing interest in recent years for restaging to select patients who may be candidates for 'organ preservation' after CRT. Although currently mainly performed within the scope of clinical trials, surgery may be omitted in patients who show clinical evidence of a complete tumour regression after CRT. Instead, patients are closely monitored ('watchful waiting') so that salvage surgery may still be performed in case of signs of tumour regrowth (Martens et al. 2016; Habr-Gama et al. 2014; Smith et al. 2012; Appelt et al. 2015). Alternatively, in patients with only a small tumour remnant, minimally invasive surgery such as transanal endoscopic microsurgery (TEM) may be considered instead of TME (Lezoche et al. 2008). Several trials have shown that these organ preservation approaches can significantly reduce morbidity and improve quality of life, while maintaining a good oncological outcome in terms of overall and disease-free survival (Martens et al. 2016; Smith et al. 2012;

Appelt et al. 2015; Lezoche et al. 2008; Hupkens et al. 2017). In these settings, an accurate assessment of the response to neoadjuvant treatment becomes a highly relevant issue. It is known that a clinical response evaluation combining imaging with clinical examination (digital rectal examination) and endoscopy offers the most accurate results (Maas et al. 2015). In this chapter, we will mainly focus on the role of imaging—in particular MRI—and discuss its main strengths and weaknesses in evaluating the response of rectal cancer after neoadjuvant (chemo-)radiotherapy.

2.2 MRI for Restaging Rectal Cancer

There is no clear consensus on what is the best timing after the completion of the neoadjuvant treatment to perform a restaging MRI. There is, however, increasing evidence that after a longer waiting interval, response rates will increase (Sloothaak et al. 2013; West et al. 2016). In recent literature where MRI was used to select patients for organ preservation, waiting intervals of ±8 weeks after the completion of CRT were typically employed (Martens et al. 2016; Habr-Gama et al. 2014).

2.2.1 Restaging of the T-stage: Differentiating Between Tumour and Fibrosis

In a small minority of patients treated with CRT (±6%), the tumour in the rectal wall completely disappears and a normalized rectal wall re-appears on MRI (Lambregts et al. 2018). However, the majority of tumours undergo a fibrotic transformation. While untreated solid (non-mucinous) tumours typically show intermediate signal intensity on morphological T2-weighted MRI, tumours that develop fibrosis show a reduction in T2-weighted signal intensity with an accompanying reduction in tour volume. Within this fibrous scar tissue, it can be very difficult to discern (small) areas of viable residual tumour. As a result, MRI shows difficulties in detecting and determining the extent of residual tumour after CRT, resulting in limited overall accuracies of 43–60% and relatively poor interobserver agreement with kappa's in the range of 0.33–0.64 to determine the yT-stage after treatment (Kulkarni et al. 2008; Allen et al. 2007; Dresen et al. 2009; Kuo et al. 2005; Vliegen et al. 2008). Because radiologists typically tend to err on the safe side, overstaging is the main problem with relatively high over-staging rates of up to 50% (see Fig. 1). More encouraging results have been suggested for the selection of good responding tumours that become confined to the bowel wall after CRT (ypT0–2), which can be identified with positive predictive values (PPVs) of 86–91% and negative predictive values (NPVs) of 70–75% (Dresen et al. 2009). For the specific selection of patients with a complete tumour response (yT0), results are poorer and up to 80% of patients with a complete response are over-staged as having residual tumour on morphological MRI (Suppiah et al. 2009; Kim et al. 2009). This indicates that morphological MRI on its own presents limitations when selecting patients for watchful waiting.

2.2.2 Tumour Regression from the Mesorectal Fascia (MRF)

In the primary staging setting, MRI is known to provide high accuracy in determining whether or not a tumour invades the mesorectal fascia (Beets-Tan et al. 2001; MERCURY-Study-Group 2006), which is an important prognostic feature and treatment determinant. However, as with the re-assessment of the tumour stage, the evaluation of persistent MRF invasion versus MRF tumour clearance after neoadjuvant therapy is hampered by difficulties in interpreting post-radiation fibrosis. In the case of residual fibrotic involvement of the MRF, it is difficult to determine whether there is still actual tumour involvement, and a substantial number of patients will be over-staged (Kulkarni et al. 2008; Vliegen et al. 2008). There are however certain patterns that can be helpful (see Fig. 1): if a fatplane of >2 mm re-appears between the tumour and MRF, the MRF will be free of tumour. If there is only some residual (fibrotic) stranding into the MRF, the MRF will also be likely to be free of tumour (Vliegen et al. 2008). With these patterns, high negative predictive values of up to 91–100% have been

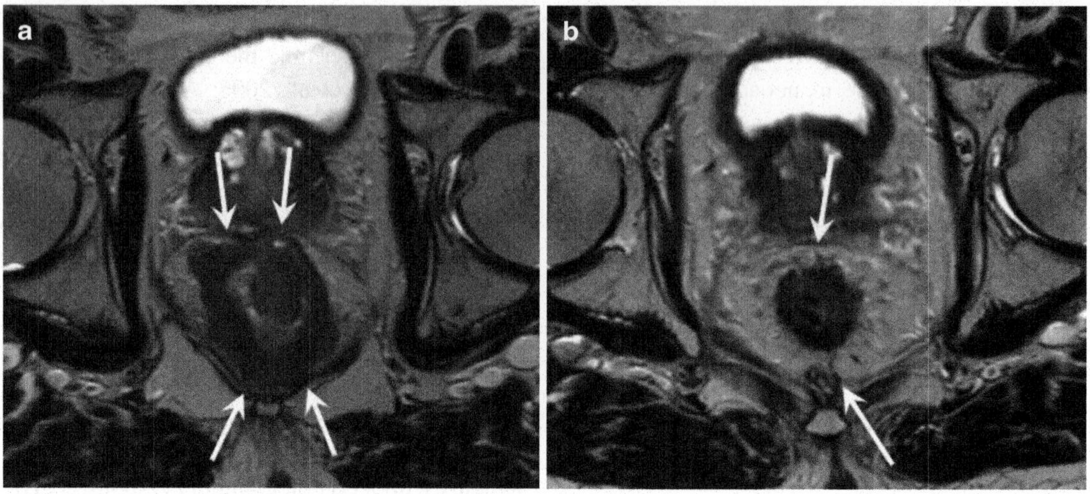

Fig. 1 T2-weighted MR images of a male rectal cancer patient before (**a**) and 8 weeks after completion of chemoradiotherapy (CRT) (**b**). Before treatment, the tumour clearly grows beyond the bowel wall into the perirectal fat (indicating a T3 tumour). The tumour involves the mesorectal fascia (MRF) both anteriorly and posteriorly (arrows in **a**). After treatment, the tumour has decreased considerably in size and has become largely fibrotic. There are still some minor fibrotic strands growing into the perirectal fat (arrows in **b**). It is difficult to discern whether these strands still contain tumour. In this case, the tumour turned out to be ypT2 at histopathology but was overstaged by the radiologist to be at risk for persistent T3 involvement. At the sites of previous MRF involvement, a clear fatplane has re-appeared between the tumour and MRF with the exception of some minor fibrotic strands. In such cases, MRI can confidently predict a tumour-free MRF

reported, indicating that when on MRI we predict a cleared MRF; this is accurate in more than 9 out of 10 cases (Kulkarni et al. 2008; Vliegen et al. 2008).

2.2.3 Lymph Nodes and Extramural Vascular Invasion (EMVI) After CRT

Even in the case of a good or complete response of the primary tumour after CRT, the risk for persistent nodal disease is approximately 5–16% (Maas et al. 2010; Heijnen et al. 2016; Yeo et al. 2010). Since the lymph nodes remain in situ with organ preservation approaches such as watchful waiting and local excision, it is important to recognize these nodes because they harbour a potential risk for recurrence and should therefore be excised. Several studies have suggested that the diagnostic performance of MRI for restaging of nodes is better compared to the primary staging setting, mainly because nodal size (which remains the most widely used criterion to discriminate between benign and metastatic nodes) works better as a diagnostic criterion after CRT. The main explanation for this is that as a result of chemoradiation, the majority of the lymph nodes on MRI will decrease in size or even completely disappear (Fig. 2) (Heijnen et al. 2016). Of the remaining small nodes, over 80% are sterilized (Koh et al. 2008). Hence, nodes that remain large in size are more likely to be malignant. Nevertheless, reported accuracies for restaging rectal cancer nodes after CRT still vary considerably (between 67% and 90%) (Heijnen et al. 2016). In recent guidelines on MRI in rectal cancer by the European Society of Gastrointestinal and Abdominal Radiology (ESGAR), a size cut-off of 5 mm is proposed as a practical guideline to diagnose malignant nodes post-CRT (Beets-Tan et al. 2018). In research settings, promising results have been reported for the use of lymph node–specific contrast agents such as ultrasmall superparamagnetic iron oxides (USPIOs) and the blood pool contrast agent gadofosveset trisodium, but these contrasts have not (yet) found their way to clinical practice (Koh et al. 2009; Lambregts et al. 2011a).

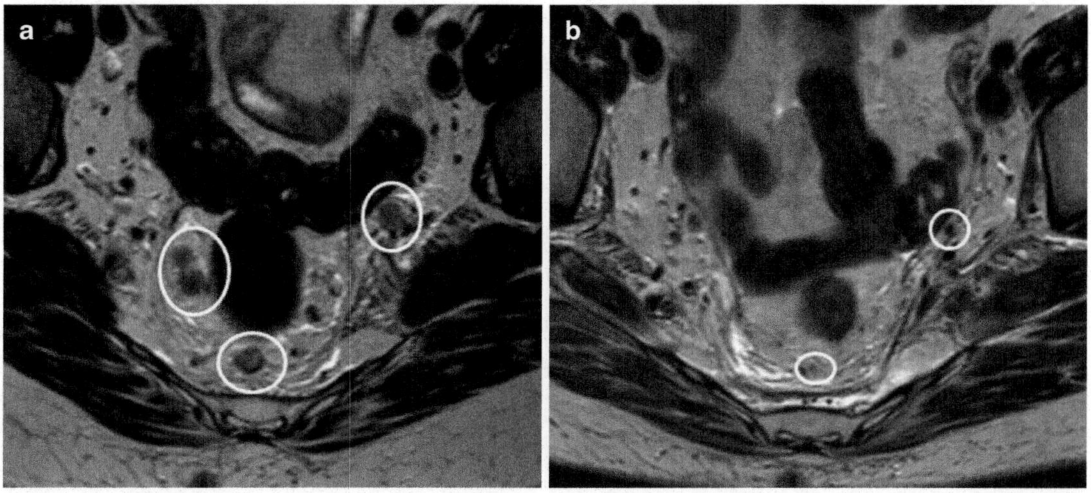

Fig. 2 T2-weighted images of a female rectal cancer patient before (**a**) and after chemoradiotherapy (**b**). Before treatment, there are several enlarged, heterogeneous and irregularly shaped nodes visible both within the mesorectal fascia and in the left para-iliac region (circles in **a**). These nodes are highly suspicious for nodal metastases. After chemoradiotherapy, the nodes have all decreased in size to 5 mm or smaller (circles in **b**) and some nodes are no longer visible on MRI. Histopathology confirmed a sterilization of all lymph nodes (ypN0 stage)

Extramural vascular (or venous) invasion (EMVI) refers to the presence of tumour invasion into vessels in the vicinity of the tumour. The presence of EMVI on MRI has been shown to be an independent unfavourable prognostic predictor associated with a higher risk for metastases, recurrence and impaired survival outcomes (Lee et al. 2018; Tripathi et al. 2017). Most published papers focus on the value of EMVI at primary staging (before treatment), but there are also some reports focusing on the re-assessment of EMVI post-CRT. Similar to re-assessment of the T-stage and MRF, the main difficulty when assessing EMVI after treatment is the interpretation of post-radiation fibrosis. Nevertheless, quite similar overall diagnostic performance has been reported for the MR evaluation of EMVI pre- and post-CRT, although sensitivity and interobserver agreement to detect EMVI after CRT may be slightly lower (Lee et al. 2018).

2.3 Quantitative and Functional Imaging Methods

Imaging is not only able to provide information on tumour morphology, but can also be used to extract quantitative measures of disease, the most basic one being the tumour volume. In addition, functional imaging techniques have been developed that target different physiological tumour characteristics. These techniques can non-invasively provide insights into tumour biology, which can otherwise only be derived using more invasive diagnostic tools such as tissue biopsy.

2.3.1 Tumour Volumetry

It is generally acknowledged that some measures of tumour size or volume should routinely be incorporated in radiological MRI reports (Beets-Tan et al. 2018). The change in tumour size after treatment is one of the simplest quantitative measures that can provide an estimation of therapeutic response (Fig. 3). Several studies have reported on the value of tumour size or volume measurements to predict treatment response with highly varying accuracies ranging between 42 and 88%, depending on the chosen measurement method (i.e. one-dimensional size versus 3D- or whole-volume measurements), cut-off values and endpoints of response (Martens et al. 2015a). In a recent paper, which combined a systematic review of literature with a prospective validation of literature-derived cut-offs in an independent

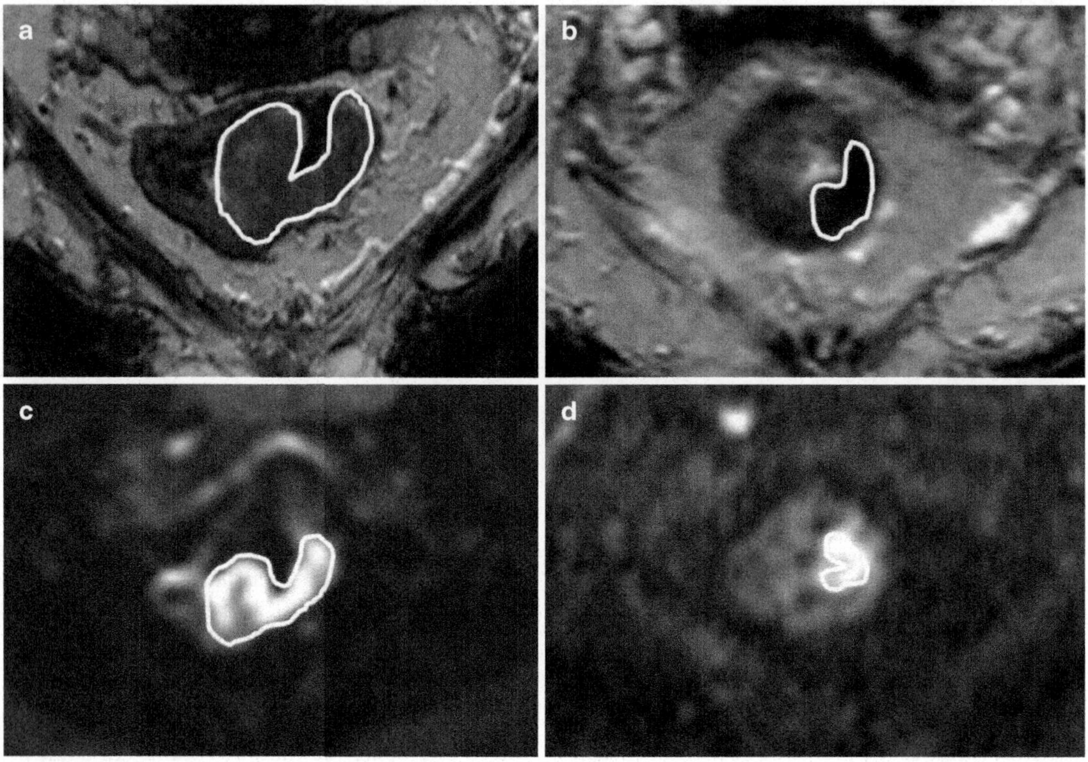

Fig. 3 T2-weighted (**a**, **b**) and diffusion-weighted (**c**, **d**) images of a female rectal cancer patient before treatment (**a**, **c**) and 8 weeks after the completion of chemoradiation (**b**, **d**). On T2W-MRI before treatment (**a**), we see a semicircular tumour with intermediate signal intensity in the left dorsolateral rectal wall. After CRT (**b**), the tumour has decreased in volume and the signal intensity has decreased considerably, indicating a fibrotic transformation of the tumour. It is difficult to determine whether or not residual viable tumour is still present within the fibrosis. On DWI, the tumour is easily recognizable pre-CRT (**c**) due to its high signal compared to the suppressed background tissue. After CRT (**d**), a clear area of high signal is still visible within the fibrosis, suggesting a residual tumour mass. Histopathology after surgery confirmed an ypT2 tumour remnant. Apart from visual evaluation, the images can also be used to quantitatively assess response. The volume of the tumour pre-CRT was 16.4 cm^3 on T2W-MRI and 16.0 cm^3 on DWI. After CRT, the volume decreased to 7.2 cm^3 on T2W-MRI (−35%) and 5.4 cm^3 on DWI (−66%). Mean ADC increased from $1.02 * 10^{-3}$ to $1.36 * 10^{-3}$ mm^2/s

patient cohort, it was shown that whole-volume rectal tumour measurements provide the best results to assess response to CRT. Upon prospective validation, a post-CRT volume of <1.6 cm^3 and a relative volume reduction (ΔVolume) of >80–86% could predict patients with a complete response with an accuracy of 73–80%, high specificity of 80–97% but low sensitivity of 14–45%. Results for the differentiation between 'good' and 'poor' responders were poorer with overall accuracies ranging between 51 and 60% (Martens et al. 2015a). This suggests that MR-volumetry can be a valuable adjunct to routine 'visual' tumour restaging but remains insufficiently accurate for clinical decision-making.

2.3.2 Diffusion-Weighted MRI (DWI)

DWI uses differences in the movement ('diffusion') of water protons between tissues of varying cellularity. In tissues with normal or low cellularity, water protons can move freely in the extracellular tissue space. This movement causes a loss of signal on diffusion-weighted images. On the contrary, in tissues with a more dense cellular structure (such as typically the case in solid malignant tumours), the diffusion capacity of water protons is restricted and the signal is retained, making DWI a very sensitive technique to detect malignancies and discriminate them from surrounding tissues. The degree of diffusivity can also be quantitatively measured, a parameter referred to as the 'apparent diffusion coefficient' (ADC). Both the visual assessment of diffusion images and quantitative measurement of ADC have shown potential for response evaluation of rectal tumours after chemoradiotherapy. There are several ways DWI can be used to assess response in rectal cancer (see Fig. 3). When assessed visually, the most basic approach is to determine whether or not a high signal, indicative of residual tumour, is still present within the fibrotically changed bowel wall after chemoradiotherapy. Several studies including a recent meta-analysis have shown that this strategy significantly improves the performance of MRI compared to T2-weighted imaging to restage rectal tumours after CRT, in particular for differentiating between a complete response and residual tumour (Kim et al. 2009; Lambregts et al. 2011b; van der Paardt et al. 2013). The use of DWI in such a way is therefore now routinely recommended by the latest ESGAR guidelines on rectal MR imaging (Beets-Tan et al. 2018). Particularly good results have furthermore been reported for measuring the volume of the high signal areas on DWI and calculating the change in DWI tumour volume (ΔVolume) after neoadjuvant treatment with sensitivities up to 86% and specificities up to 100% for diagnosing complete responders; results are significantly better than those reported for tumour volumetry using T2-weighted MRI (Curvo-Semedo et al. 2011; Ha et al. 2013). The most widely investigated approach to date, however, is to quantitatively measure ADC of rectal tumours before, and after CRT, and in some studies also during CRT. As a result of successful treatment, ADC typically rises, which is supposed to be caused by a loss of cell membrane integrity (i.e. necrosis) and ultimately by irreparable cell loss, resulting in an enlarged extracellular tissue space and thus increased room for water diffusion (Intven et al. 2013; Kim et al. 2011). Moreover, ADC at baseline (before CRT) tends to be higher in patients that will show a poor response to treatment (Intven et al. 2013; Sun et al. 2010). This is believed to be related to the presence of tumour necrosis, which is known to be associated with an impaired susceptibility of tumours to radiotherapy. Although several groups have presented promising results for such use of ADC as a biomarker of response, no definite conclusions can be drawn yet, since there are also various reports that found no clear benefit for ADC to discriminate between different response groups. These conflicting results may also be partly related to the fact that ADC values can vary considerably due to variations in MR hardware, acquisition and post-processing methods. Standardization of protocols is therefore an important issue and—at the time of writing—clinical use of ADC for tumour response evaluation is not yet recommended. More novel methods of diffusion quantification such as diffusion kurtosis imaging and 'intravoxel incoherent motion' (IVIM) are currently under investigation, but for the time being only in research settings.

2.3.3 Dynamic Contrast-Enhanced (DCE) MRI

After DWI, DCE-MRI is the most widely studied functional MRI sequence for tumour response assessment in rectal cancer. DCE-MRI assesses a tumour's microvascular structure and perfusion by measuring the inflow of intravenously administered contrast agents into tumour vessels and its leakage into the extracellular space. Tumour vascularity and perfusion are known to be associated with tumour hypoxia and consequently with the susceptibility of tumours to chemoradiation. DCE-MRI data can be analysed quantitatively with pharmacokinetic models, which render absolute values of inflow and permeability such as the *K*-trans (volume rate constant), Ve (volume of extracellular space) and Kep (constant of flow rate). Alternatively, data can be assessed semi-quantitatively by plotting a time intensity curve of the tumoural enhancement after contrast injection. Several studies have reported significantly different pre-CRT DCE parameters in responders compared to poor responders, both with quantitative and semi-quantitative analysis methods (Tong et al. 2015; Martens et al. 2015b; Intven et al. 2015). A higher *K*-trans has been suggested to be predictive of a good response, which is believed to be related to the notion that a high *K*-trans reflects an increased permeability of the vessels, making the tumour more susceptible chemotherapy. Also, increased vascularity and permeability reflect good oxygenation of the tumour, which sensitizes a tumour to radiation. The largest body of evidence exists for quantitative analyses for response assessment after CRT. A decrease in *K*-trans (indicating the replacement of tumour by fibrosis and necrosis) has been shown to be associated with a favourable response (Intven et al. 2015). Similarly, Martens et al. found that in good responders the decrease in semi-quantitative parameters was larger after CRT than in poor responders, albeit not statistically significant (Martens et al. 2015b). Although it is acknowledged that DCE-MRI can provide parameters that can act as biomarkers of response, its use is currently mainly confined to research settings and not yet part of clinical routine.

2.3.4 Other Functional Imaging Techniques

In addition to cellularity and perfusion, there are many other biological tumour characteristics that may be captured with imaging. On MRI, tumour hypoxia may be analysed using blood oxygen level-dependent (BOLD) MRI, tumour proliferation/metabolism with MR-spectroscopy and collagen content (as a potential measure of fibrosis) with magnetization transfer imaging. Current experience with these techniques is, however, limited and mainly research-based. Apart from MRI-techniques, the use of [^{18}F]fluorodeoxyglucose ([^{18}F]FDG) positron emission tomography (PET) as a functional imaging technique to assess response in rectal cancer has been the focus of many studies. The commonly observed therapeutic effect after CRT is a decrease in the standardized uptake value (SUV), representing a decrease in the proliferative activity of the tumour. Two recent meta-analyses reported comparable results for [^{18}F]FDG PET in differentiating between good and poor responding tumours after CRT with pooled sensitivities of 74–78% and pooled specificities of 64–67% (Li et al. 2014; Zhang et al. 2012). However, in subgroup analyses, PET was less accurate for specific discrimination of patients with a complete tumour response, which are mostly overstaged, resulting in a relatively low specificity of 59–61%. This is probably related to the fact radiation-induced inflammation may result in up to 25% [^{18}F]FDG uptake in inflammatory cells, thus causing an underestimation of the treatment response. Based on current evidence, [^{18}F]FDG PET may be particularly useful for early evaluation of response, e.g. 1–2 weeks after the start of neoadjuvant treatment. At these time points, [^{18}F]FDG PET may already predict a good response with a sensitivity of 82–86% and specificity 78–80% (Li et al. 2014; Zhang et al. 2012). The main downside of PET is that it is not part of the routine clinical workup of response evaluation in rectal cancer.

2.4 Conclusions

MRI is a valuable technique to assess the response of rectal cancer to neoadjuvant treatment. MRI can assess tumour downsizing and downstaging and is mainly used as a roadmap to optimize the surgical treatment approach after CRT. Given recent developments in 'organ preserving' treatment approaches after chemoradiotherapy, MRI can also play a role to help select patients with a (near) complete tumour response who may be candidates for minimally invasive surgery or watchful waiting. The main difficulty with response evaluation after neoadjuvant chemoradiotherapy is the interpretation of fibrosis, as a result of which a substantial number of patients are overstaged after CRT. Functional imaging techniques—the most important one being diffusion-weighted MR imaging—can be helpful in this regard to improve the performance of MRI in discriminating between residual tumour and fibrosis after CRT.

3 Response Assessment in Gastro-Enteropancreatic Neuro-Endocrine (GEP-NET) Tumours

3.1 Introduction

Neuroendocrine tumours (NETs) represent a relatively rare and very heterogeneous group of neoplasms originating from dispersed neuroendocrine cells, distributed almost ubiquitously in the body. Although these tumours are characterised by relatively slow growth, they have malignant potential and are increasing in incidence. Their highly variable biology combined with a behaviour that is still not well defined may, in some cases, make them difficult to diagnose (Yao et al. 2008; Niederle et al. 2010). Different classification systems are based on the site of origin, extent and degree of differentiation, the presence of distant metastases and hormone production capacity (Solcia et al. 2000; Luttges 2011). At present, the most accepted classification system is the World Health Organization classification integrated by the European Neuroendocrine Tumor Society (ENETS) to help discriminating categories of patients with different prognosis (Kidd et al. 2016; Perren et al. 2017). Theoretically, this new classification system allows an efficient prognostic stratification of patients. The primary tumour is most commonly located in the gastrointestinal (GI) tract or the pancreas. These gastroenteropancreatic (GEP)-NETs comprise approximately 2% of all malignancies of the GEP system (Yao et al. 2008; Caplin et al. 1998). The clinical presentation and clinical course of NETs are dependent on anatomical location, tumour stage and functional status. Functional tumours are associated with hormone release and carcinoid symptoms in about 30% of cases. According to the revised histopathological classification, the main categories of GEP-NET are well-differentiated NET (benign and/or unknown behaviour, with a low grade of malignancy) and poorly differentiated neuroendocrine carcinomas (NEC, with a high grade of malignancy and a poor prognosis). As a consequence, 5-year survival rates diverge widely (15–95%), depending on the primary site, variable tumour biology, disease extent at diagnosis, available therapeutic options and designated centres of care (Yao et al. 2008; Modlin et al. 2008). In order to assure an optimal management of GEP-NET, a standardized diagnostic procedure is required. The diagnostic and prognostic stratification criteria are based on histological typing, differentiation, grading and TNM staging. On the basis of mitotic count/10 high-power fields and Ki67 proliferation index, well-differentiated GEP-NETs are graded as either G1 (with a mitotic count <2 and/or Ki67 $\leq$ 2%) or G2 (with a mitotic count 2–20 and/or Ki67 3%–20%). All poorly differentiated NEC are G3 (with a mitotic count >20 and/or Ki67 > 20%) (Bosman 2010). A common feature of most GEP-NET is their overexpression of somatostatin receptors (SSTR), particularly the subtype 2 (Reubi et al. 1994, 2000). SSTR overexpression is the basis for the use of radiolabelled somatostatin analogues in the diagnosis and treatment of NET.

Treatment of NET is typically multidisciplinary and should be individualized according to the tumour histology, lesion extent and symptoms (Modlin et al. 2008; Kulke et al. 2011; Frilling et al. 2014). Surgery represents the only curative modality in patients with limited disease but is feasible only in less than 20% of cases. A limitation of surgery is the frequent presence of metastatic disease (Turaga and Kvols 2011). Medical therapy with long-acting somatostatin analogues are the mainstay for control of hormone-related symptoms associated with NET. In addition to symptom control, treatment with somatostatin analogues has demonstrated antitumour activity, prolonging time to disease progression (Rinke et al. 2009). More recently, the targeted therapies, including the oral mTOR inhibitor everolimus and the tyrosine kinases inhibitor sunitinib, have been shown to improve progression-free survival in patients with progressive malignant disease (Raymond et al. 2011). Peptide receptor radionuclide therapy (PRRT), consisting in the systemic administration of [^{90}Y] or [^{177}Lu] radiolabelled somatostatin analog, has also shown promising results in patients with disseminated disease (Kwekkeboom et al. 2008; Bodei et al. 2011). External radiation, interventional radiological or probe-directed ablation, immunotherapy (interferon) and cytotoxic chemotherapy are also proposed in NET.

3.2 Tumour Response Assessment in GEP-NET with Nuclear Medicine Techniques

3.2.1 Methods

The diagnosis of GEP-NET is based upon clinical features (especially in functioning tumours), biomarkers, localization of the primary and/or metastatic lesions as determined by imaging studies and histopathologic confirmation from biopsy or surgical specimen, which represents the 'gold standard' for diagnosis and should be obtained whenever possible (Niederle et al. 2010).

The localization of a GEP-NET and the assessment of the extent of disease are crucial for management and many different imaging techniques are used. No technique is the gold standard, and specific sequences of exams might be needed for each tumour type. A combination of two or more imaging techniques is usually required for diagnosis and staging. Cross-sectional (anatomical) imaging modalities used to localize primary lesions and to stage the extent of the disease, particularly if non-functioning, include computed tomography (CT), magnetic resonance imaging (MRI), ultrasonography (US) and related techniques (contrast-enhanced US, endoscopic US and intraoperative US) and selective angiography with hormonal sampling. Molecular (functional) imaging studies, which are based on NET pathophysiology and especially the presence of somatostatin receptors, aid in the evaluation of the extent of disease, staging and therapy decision-making (Krenning et al. 1993; Kwekkeboom et al. 2010).

Somatostatin receptor scintigraphy (SRS) has a central role in the diagnostic workup of patients with GEP-NET. When performed as single-photon emission computed tomography (SPECT), such in the case of [^{111}In]-Octreotide (Octreoscan®) and [^{99m}Tc]-Octreotide), its value may be limited by several factors, such as its relatively low resolution for small tumours and background binding in normal tissues (Kwekkeboom et al. 2010). Those limitations have been mainly overcome by the introduction of positron emission tomography (PET) imaging with [^{68}Ga]—DOTA-peptide. Conveniently, [^{68}Ga]-DOTA-peptide PET/CT requires no patient preparation with laxatives, and the examination can be performed as a one-session outpatient procedure approximately 1 h after tracer injection (Hofmann et al. 2001; Kowalski et al. 2003; Kaltsas et al. 2004; Sundin et al. 2007; Gabriel et al. 2007; Ambrosini et al. 2008; Bozkurt et al. 2017; Sundin et al. 2017). The technique is especially useful in detecting small lesions, particularly at bone and node levels (Gabriel et al. 2007), and in patients with unusual anatomic localization (Fanti et al. 2008). Several different DOTA-peptides (DOTATOC, DOTANOC and DOTATATE) have been used in the clinical setting for either NET diagnosis or PRRT. The major difference among these compounds relies on a slightly different affinity to SSTR (Antunes et al. 2007). Of several preparations of radiolabelled octreotide, [^{68}Ga]-DOTATOC is the most widely used. [^{68}Ga]-DOTATOC PET/CT provides better spatial resolution and higher tumour-to-normal tissue ratios than SRS with SPECT, resulting in higher sensitivity to detect NET (Gabriel et al. 2007).

Because of the capacity of NET cells for amine precursor uptake and decarboxylation (the APUD system) (Pearse 1980), precursors such as 5-hydroxy-L-tryptophan (5-HTP) and L-dihydroxyphenylalanine (L-DOPA) may be taken up by NET cells and converted to serotonin and dopamine, respectively, which are stored in secretory granulae within the cytoplasm. Thus, the APUD pathway has been used to produce PET tracers such as [^{11}C]- or [^{18}F]-labelled L-DOPA ([^{11}C]-L-DOPA, [^{18}F]-DOPA), [^{18}F]-labelled Dopamine ([^{18}F]Dopamine) and [^{11}C]-labelled 5-HTP ([^{11}C]-5-HTP) to visualize NET (Orlefors et al. 1998, 2006; Koopmans et al. 2008; Schiesser et al. 2010; Kauhanen et al. 2009). Their availabilities, however, are limited, and their sensitivities seem to be inferior to that of [^{68}Ga]-labelled octreotide (Ambrosini et al. 2008; Haug et al.

2010; Putzer et al. 2010; Toumpanakis et al. 2014). Moreover, taking into account the heterogeneity of NET, [^{18}F]-fluorodeoxyglucose ([^{18}F] FDG) could also be able to provide useful information about disease extent, patients' response to treatment and disease course. [^{18}F]FDG PET/CT is a noninvasive, whole-body imaging procedure that can visualize in real time all the glucose metabolic active sites of the disease. Since high glucose metabolism of tumours is directly related with cell proliferation (depending on the genetic expression of glucose transporters) (Mankoff et al. 2007), the capability of NET cells to accumulate [^{18}F]FDG is typically related to cell dedifferentiation and high malignancy. Thus, a high glucose metabolic state can provide prognostic information. Consequently, the derived information helps improve the stratification, and therefore the management, of those patients who are likely to show rapid disease progression, particularly in the wide low-grade spectrum. On the other hand, [^{18}F]FDG PET does not provide useful information for tumours that are relatively slow growing. While its diagnostic sensitivity is low, [^{18}F]FDG PET/CT has demonstrated prognostic value in several forms of cancer and, therefore, seems promising for the determination of tumour aggressiveness in this class of disease (Kwee et al. 2011). In NET, [^{18}F]FDG PET/CT is particularly helpful in the case of more aggressive NET, such as poorly differentiated NEC, and well-differentiated tumours with Ki67 values >10%. [^{18}F]FDG-avid tumour lesions, even in slow-growing NET, may indicate a more aggressive disease course, irrespective of Ki-67 index (Binderup et al. 2010a; Garin et al. 2009). Examples of the application of CT, ^{68}Ga-DOTA-PET and [^{18}F]FDG PET in pancreatic and small intestine NET are shown in Figs. 4 and 5.

3.2.2 Results

Given GEP-NET's relatively slow growth, continual assessment by imaging, biomarker levels and overall survival represents the fundamental basis for all management strategies. The need to monitor tumour responsiveness, both in clinical trials and in routine practice, is mandatory given the range of expensive, empirical and often toxic treatment used (Kunz et al. 2013). Because prolonged ineffective treatment is costly to both patients and health care systems, it would be preferable to have an early assessment that offers a 'window of opportunity' to optimize or alter the treatment plan in any patient not achieving a satisfactory response with current treatment. Regardless of the treatment chosen, imaging plays a pivotal role in follow-up surveillance and assessment of response in patients with NET (Sundin et al. 2017; Rockall et al. 2009). However, the complex clinical course of NET and cytostatic nature of many NET treatments pose specific challenges for the assessment of response. For many non-neuroendocrine neoplasms, therapeutic responsiveness is assessed through morphologic imaging using, for instance, the response evaluation criteria in solid tumours (RECIST) (Padhani and Ollivier 2001; Eisenhauer et al. 2009; Cheson et al. 2007). In the case of NET, the pitfalls of morphologic imaging in evaluating disease after treatment are well established (Sundin and Rockall 2012; Bodei et al. 2015; Denecke et al. 2013).

The limitations of RECIST in predicting survival have been noted. NETs are now being recognized earlier, while new treatments and strategies are proposed in guidelines and algorithms. Newer targeted therapies including everolimus have demonstrated improved progression-free survival in NET patients; however, the effect on the tumour volume is often minimal, with 'stabilization' of the tumour size being the best outcome for most patients (Raymond et al. 2011; Yao et al. 2011). These findings suggest that lack of tumour shrinkage may not predict poor outcome in patients treated with targeted therapies because tumours may respond to targeted therapy by undergoing necrosis or cystic changes without decreasing, and possibly even increasing, in size. Residual masses or fibroses that do not contain viable tumour can cause further uncertainty (Llovet et al. 2008). Because of the issues involved in evaluating responses to targeted therapy in patients with NET using classic morphologic criteria, it is important to explore functional and molecular imaging techniques. Functional imaging provides information on

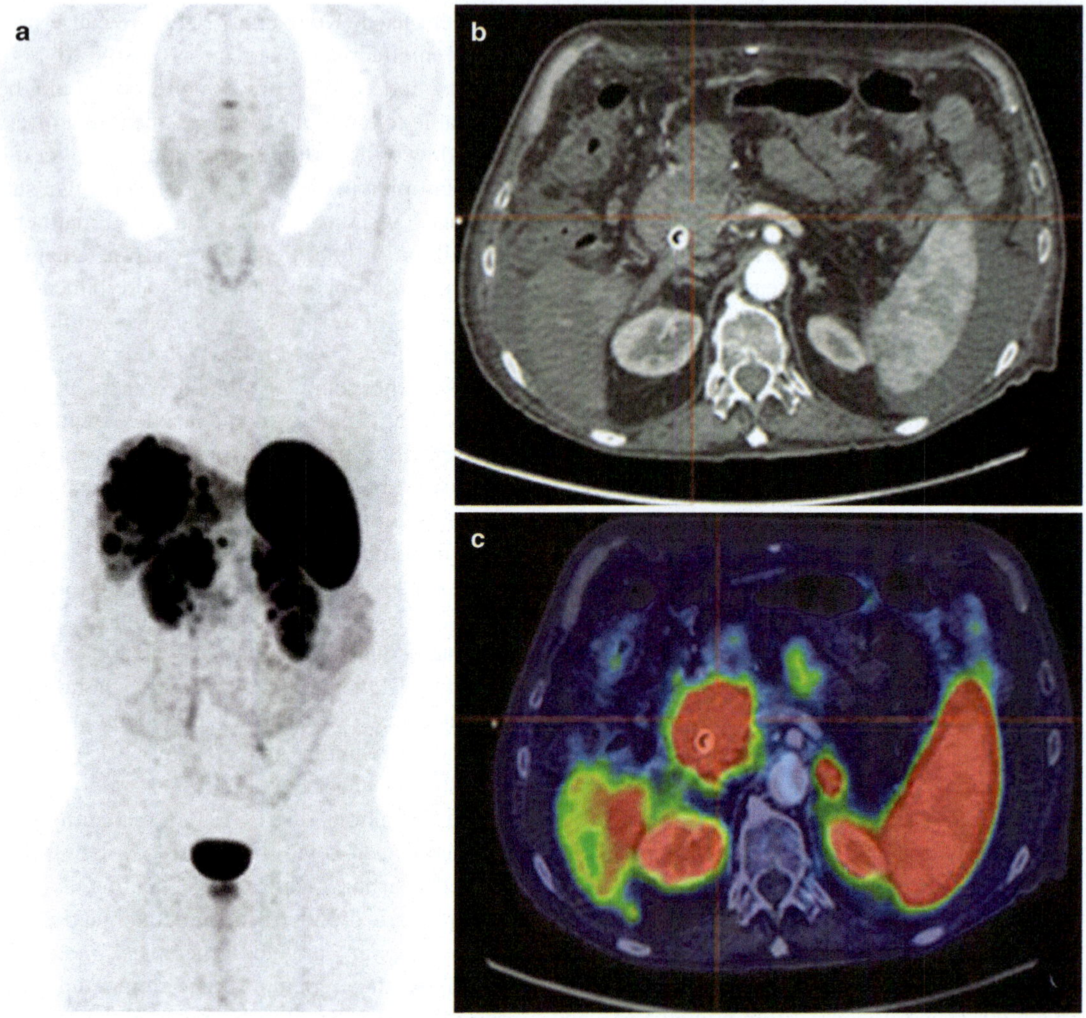

Fig. 4 68-year-old male patient staged for a pancreatic NET (G2, Ki 10%). [^{68}Ga]-DOTA-TATE PET: Maximum intensity projection (MIP) shows metastatic lesions in liver and abdominal lymph nodes (**a**). CT (**b**) and fused PET/CT (**c**) transverse slices are centred on the larger abdominal lymph node

tumour physiology and therefore may have great potential for measuring treatment response in patients in whom tumour shrinkage is not anticipated. Response to targeted therapies that demonstrate cytostatic versus cytocidal effects may be associated predominantly with a decrease in metabolism, even in the absence of a major reduction in tumour size. Consequently, changes in the physiologic or metabolic characteristics of the tissue may be more predictive of outcome than the tumour size criteria used by RECIST (Sundin and Rockall 2012). It is well known that physiologic changes can be detected much earlier than changes in size, allowing for individualized rather than generic treatment (Cheson et al. 2007). Characterization of tumours based on their specific functional imaging characteristics and expected response pattern may also be advantageous to predicting outcomes. Molecular imaging with PET tracers reflective of metabolic pathways and functional imaging should thus also be explored as options for monitoring treatment in patients with NET (Sundin and Rockall 2012). Tumour heterogeneity is seen not just between patients, but also between primary and secondary deposits and even within the same

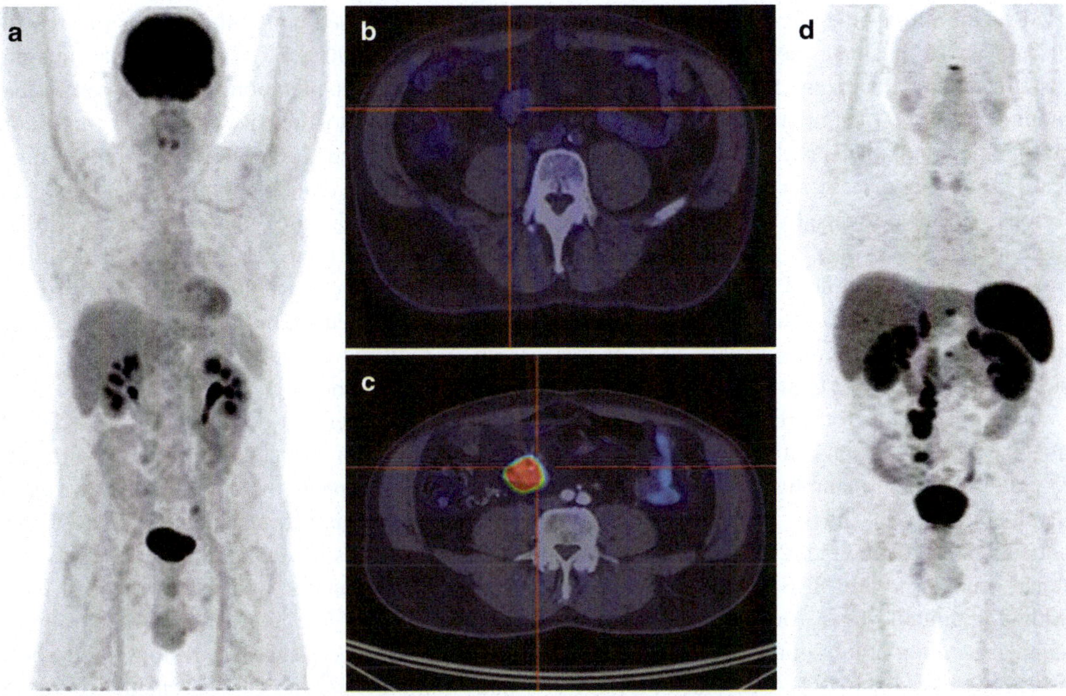

Fig. 5 70-year-old male patient staged for a small intestine NET (G1, Ki 1%). [^{18}F]FDG PET/CT: Maximum intensity projection (MIP) shows a faint uptake in the abdomen (**a**), confirmed on the fused [^{18}F]FDG PET/CT transverse slice (**b**). [^{68}Ga]-DOTA-TATE PET: Maximum intensity projection (MIP) shows metastatic lesions in abdominal lymph nodes (**c**). Fused [^{68}Ga]-DOTA-TATE PET/CT transverse slice is centred on one abdominal lymph node (**d**). This case illustrates a well-differentiated NET that has low metabolic activity (thus low [^{18}F]FDG uptake) but consistent somatostatin receptor (thus high [^{68}Ga]-DOTA-TATE uptake)

tumour mass. The significance of intratumoural heterogeneity has become important because it may highlight groups of treatment-resistant cells for which it is now possible to direct targeted therapy (Bentzen 2005) or biopsy. Thus, the ability to measure several of the tumour's vascular parameters has enormous potential in better understanding the nature of the tumour.

Several functional imaging techniques including dynamic contrast-enhanced (DCE) MRI, diffusion-weighted MRI (DW-MRI), PET and SPECT imaging techniques have demonstrated promising ability to provide quantitative information regarding the physiologic and molecular characteristics of tumours unavailable with conventional morphologic imaging techniques. Many factors, including microvessel density, capillary permeability, tumour oxygenation and interstitial fluid pressure, are involved in the delivery of treatments to the tumour and are known to affect the response and outcome (Milosevic et al. 2001). The accuracy of [^{68}Ga]-DOTA-peptide PET/CT is superior to that of CT, but the detection of additional sites of disease is not necessarily followed by a change in disease stage and does not always affect therapeutic approach.

The assessment of response by RECIST can be particularly problematic in patients with highly differentiated, slow-growing NET. Treatment with somatostatin analogues in patients with SSR-expressing lesions is associated with the reduction of signs and symptoms of hormone hypersecretion, improvement of quality of life and slowing of tumour growth, with a consistent survival benefit (Bodei et al. 2009; Townsend et al. 2010), indicating an antiproliferative action. In this clinical setting, somatostatin receptor imaging by SRS remains the standard molecular imaging technique for NET visualization and is used in the initial imaging workup to stage the disease and to evaluate the eligibility for somatostatin analog treatment. SRS is also used for monitoring NET treatment and is valuable as a complement in patients with biochemical or clinical progressive disease for the detection of new lesions that have escaped depiction by morphologic imaging.

[^{68}Ga]-DOTA-peptides PET/CT has been used both for the diagnosis of disease extent and as a preliminary procedure to evaluate SSR expression before the start of treatment and provide relevant information for NET patients' clinical management: the exam is a mandatory procedure to guide treatment planning, since it affected the therapeutic approach in more than half the patients (Ambrosini et al. 2010). However, functional imaging with SRS has its limitations. Although suitable for a rough estimate, tumour standardized maximum uptake value (SUVmax) determined by [^{68}Ga]-DOTA-peptides PET/CT is not considered to be ideal because SSR heterogeneity in individual tumours is a problematic factor for sensitive assessment of treatment response. Moreover, the differences in intrinsic variabilities in SUVmax in separate PET/CT scanners at different institutions are a limitation for image-based assessment and patient follow-up. For instance, in tumours with SUVmax >20–25, SUV does not linearly correlate with SSR expression (Velikyan et al. 2014). Thus, SUVmax at baseline did not predict outcome and no correlation is noted between change in tumour SUV max and outcome. Moreover, the possibility of tumour dedifferentiation with the loss of receptors is an obvious obstacle and must be taken into account (Bozkurt et al. 2017). Thus, the results of therapy monitoring with [^{68}Ga]-DOTA-peptides PET/CT have been unconvincing. Similarly, changes in tumour SUVmax during treatment have not been a reliable measure for PRRT monitoring (Gabriel et al. 2007, 2009); however, decreased tumour-to-spleen ratio correlated with clinical improvement (Haug et al. 2010).

Despite significant advances, clinically reproducible assessments of progression in NET remain suboptimal and exhibit significant limitations (Faivre et al. 2012; Ruf et al. 2013; Castaño et al. 2014). Based on the limitations of SRS and [^{68}Ga]-DOTATOC PET/CT, molecular imaging tools that reflect metabolic changes rather than depicting receptor density may be a more convincing approach to monitoring therapy. This is the reason why other imaging biomarkers, such as activated glucose metabolisms ([^{18}F]FDG PET), are now being evaluated, and optimism exists regarding their future prognostic role in NET management, although prospective validation is required (Binderup et al. 2010a; Bodei et al. 2015; Prasad et al. 2008).

As it is in general oncology, [^{18}F]FDG PET/CT is useful for the staging of NET with high proliferative capacity and clinically aggressive behaviour. In this setting, identification of more aggressive forms is crucial and specific prognostic factors are needed to arrive at the best therapeutic strategy. While assessing the prognosis and tumour aggressiveness, lesions and whole-body tumour burdens can be calculated on the basis of volumetric parameters by [^{18}F]FDG PET/CT. It has been demonstrated that [^{18}F]FDG PET positivity at the time of diagnosis in patients with metastatic NETs correlates with reduced progression-free survival and overall survival (Garin et al. 2009). The sensitivity of [^{18}F]FDG PET for depicting NET with a high proliferation index exceeded that of SRS (Binderup et al. 2010b). Furthermore, the combination of [^{68}Ga]-DOTA-peptide and [^{18}F]FDG has synergistic effects, because of a significant correlation between histologic tumour grade and predominant tumour uptake, providing complementary information on treatment protocol and response assessment (Kayani et al. 2008; Abdulrezzak et al. 2016). Interestingly, [^{18}F]FDG PET has a stronger prognostic value than traditional markers such as Ki67, CgA and the presence of liver metastases (Binderup et al. 2010a).

Finally, it is interesting to notice that [^{18}F]FDG PET showed a prognostic value in patients undergoing PRRT: the duration and quality of the response are superior in patients with no [^{18}F]FDG uptake in the pre-therapeutic assessment. In this sense, glucose consumption could reflect a different radiosensitivity, related to the activation of proliferating pathways that could render the tumour less prone to respond to PRRT or even more likely to relapse after therapy (Severi et al. 2013). Currently, the feasibility of [^{18}F]-DOPA and [^{11}C]-5-HTP PET/CT for therapeutic monitoring in patients with non-[^{18}F]FDG-avid, well-differentiated NET, is limited. Interesting results, from small studies in the setting of therapeutic monitoring, would need to be corroborated in a larger cohort of patients (Orlefors et al. 1998, 2006; Bergstrom et al. 1996; Ezziddin et al. 2013; van Essen et al. 2014; Thapa et al. 2016).

3.3 Conclusions

Accurate monitoring of treatment response is a critical component of patient management and in the context of investigation of new therapies. In GEP-NET, the use of current pharmacological therapy is critically limited by the absence of pre-treatment biomarkers identification and the lack of tools to accurately define efficacy. RECIST criteria are the mainstay of evaluation of response in clinical trials, and in poorly differentiated GEP-NET, these criteria are a valid tool. Although guidelines have, in general, supported serial comparisons between images to evaluate changes in tumours, the current configuration of RECIST criteria is suboptimal for application to NET disease assessment. In contrast with common cancers, which are of generally high proliferative activity and have a measurable size response to chemotherapy and radiotherapy, NETs tend to grow slowly and have a low proliferative rate, and (depending on the treatment) patient outcome may not correlate with significant changes in tumour size. Molecular and functional imaging modalities have the potential to demonstrate early physiological changes that may predict responders and non-responders early in the course of treatment. In particular, the role of [^{68}Ga]-DOTA-peptides PET/CT in monitoring treatment response in patients with NET is promising and requires further evaluation. However, there are several issues to overcome with these modalities, including high cost, lack of facilities able to perform the imaging and need for cross-site standardization. The assessment of Ki-67 index is a useful tool in differentiating low-grade and high-grade NET but does not necessarily reflect the current situation in the whole tumour lesions.

In summary, a number of limitations exist with the use of conventional morphologic and functional imaging criteria for the assessment of response in well-differentiated GEP-NET.

Additional parameters that potentially could be included to improve imaging, however, remained unresolved. New criteria based on molecular, metabolic and morphologic imaging need to be developed for correct assessment of response to therapy for these slow-growing, solid tumours. A better understanding of tumour biology would unquestionably expedite the development of an appropriate therapeutic biomarker(s). Adjunct biomarker tools should be developed to provide synergistic information with imaging as a means to facilitate the assessment of therapy. In this setting, the combination of imaging and blood-based molecular information provided by transcriptome analysis could offer the most promising future strategy for refining and improving the evaluation of therapy (Oberg et al. 2016).

References

Abdulrezzak U, Kurt YK, Kula M, Tutus A (2016) Combined imaging with 68Ga-DOTA-TATE and 18F-FDG PET/CT on the basis of volumetric parameters in neuroendocrine tumors. Nucl Med Commun 37:874–881

Allen SD, Padhani AR, Dzik-Jurasz AS, Glynne-Jones R (2007) Rectal carcinoma: MRI with histologic correlation before and after chemoradiation therapy. AJR Am J Roentgenol 188:442–451

Ambrosini V, Tomassetti P, Castellucci P, Campana D, Montini G, Rubello D et al (2008) Comparison between 68Ga-DOTA-NOC and 18F-DOPA PET for the detection of gastro-entero-pancreatic and lung neuro-endocrine tumours. Eur J Nucl Med Mol Imaging 35:1431–1438

Ambrosini V, Campana D, Bodei L, Nanni C, Castellucci P, Allegri V et al (2010) 68Ga-DOTANOC PET/CT clinical impact in patients with neuroendocrine tumors. J Nucl Med 51:669–673

Antunes P, Ginj M, Zhang H, Waser B, Baum RP, Reubi JC et al (2007) Are radiogallium-labelled DOTA-conjugated somatostatin analogues superior to those labelled with other radiometals? Eur J Nucl Med Mol Imaging 34:982–993

Appelt AL, Ploen J, Harling H, Jensen FS, Jensen LH, Jorgensen JC et al (2015) High-dose chemoradiotherapy and watchful waiting for distal rectal cancer: a prospective observational study. Lancet Oncol 16:919–927

Beets-Tan RG, Beets GL, Vliegen RF, Kessels AG, Van Boven H, De Bruine A et al (2001) Accuracy of magnetic resonance imaging in prediction of tumour-free resection margin in rectal cancer surgery. Lancet 357:497–504

Beets-Tan RGH, Lambregts DMJ, Maas M, Bipat S, Barbaro B, Curvo-Semedo L et al (2018) Magnetic resonance imaging for clinical management of rectal cancer: updated recommendations from the 2016 European Society of Gastrointestinal and Abdominal Radiology (ESGAR) consensus meeting. Eur Radiol 28:1465–1475. Correction in: Eur Radiol 2018;28:2711

Bentzen SM (2005) Theragnostic imaging for radiation oncology: dose-painting by numbers. Lancet Oncol 6:112–117

Bergstrom M, Eriksson B, Oberg K, Sundin A, Ahlstrom H, Lindner KJ et al (1996) In vivo demonstration of enzyme activity in endocrine pancreatic tumors: decarboxylation of carbon-11-DOPA to carbon-11-dopamine. J Nucl Med 37:32–37

Binderup T, Knigge U, Loft A, Federspiel B, Kjaer A (2010a) 18F-fluorodeoxyglucose positron emission tomography predicts survival of patients with neuroendocrine tumors. Clin Cancer Res 16:978–985

Binderup T, Knigge U, Loft A, Mortensen J, Pfeifer A, Federspiel B et al (2010b) Functional imaging of neuroendocrine tumors: a head-to-head comparison of somatostatin receptor scintigraphy, 123I-MIBG scintigraphy, and 18F-FDG PET. J Nucl Med 51:704–712

Bodei L, Ferone D, Grana CM, Cremonesi M, Signore A, Dierckx RA et al (2009) Peptide receptor therapies in neuroendocrine tumors. J Endocrinol Investig 32:360–369

Bodei L, Cremonesi M, Grana CM, Fazio N, Iodice S, Baio SM et al (2011) Peptide receptor radionuclide therapy with (1)(7)(7)Lu-DOTATATE: the IEO phase I-II study. Eur J Nucl Med Mol Imaging 38:2125–2135

Bodei L, Sundin A, Kidd M, Prasad V, Modlin IM (2015) The status of neuroendocrine tumor imaging: from darkness to light? Neuroendocrinology 101:1–17

Bosman F (2010) WHO classification of tumours of the digestive system. Lyon, World Health Organization, International Agency for Research on Cancer

Bozkurt MF, Virgolini I, Balogova S, Beheshti M, Rubello D, Decristoforo C et al (2017) Guideline for PET/CT imaging of neuroendocrine neoplasms with 68Ga-DOTA-conjugated somatostatin receptor targeting peptides and 18F-DOPA. Eur J Nucl Med Mol Imaging 44:1588–1601

Caplin ME, Buscombe JR, Hilson AJ, Jones AL, Watkinson AF, Burroughs AK (1998) Carcinoid tumour. Lancet 352:799–805

Castaño JP, Sundin A, Maecke HR, Villabona C, Vázquez-Albertino R, Navarro E et al (2014) Gastrointestinal neuroendocrine tumors (NETs): new diagnostic and therapeutic challenges. Cancer Metastasis Rev 33:353–359

Cheson BD, Pfistner B, Juweid ME, Gascoyne RD, Specht L, Horning SJ et al (2007) Revised response criteria for malignant lymphoma. J Clin Oncol 25:579–586

Curvo-Semedo L, Lambregts DM, Maas M, Thywissen T, Mehsen RT, Lammering G et al (2011) Rectal cancer: assessment of complete response to preoperative combined radiation therapy with chemotherapy—conventional MR volumetry versus diffusion-weighted MR imaging. Radiology 260:734–743

Denecke T, Baur AD, Ihm C, Steffen IG, Tischer E, Arsenic R et al (2013) Evaluation of radiological prognostic factors of hepatic metastases in patients with non-functional pancreatic neuroendocrine tumors. Eur J Radiol 82:e550–e555

Dresen RC, Beets GL, Rutten HJ, Engelen SM, Lahaye MJ, Vliegen RF et al (2009) Locally advanced rectal cancer: MR imaging for restaging after neoadjuvant radiation therapy with concomitant chemotherapy. Part I. Are we able to predict tumor confined to the rectal wall? Radiology 252:71–80

Eisenhauer EA, Therasse P, Bogaerts J, Schwartz LH, Sargent D, Ford R et al (2009) New response evaluation criteria in solid tumours: revised RECIST guideline (version 1.1). Eur J Cancer 45: 228–247

van Essen M, Sundin A, Krenning EP, Kwekkeboom DJ (2014) Neuroendocrine tumours: the role of imaging for diagnosis and therapy. Nat Rev Endocrinol 10:102–114

Ezziddin S, Reichmann K, Yong-Hing C, Damm M, Risse J, Ahmadzadehfar H et al (2013) Early prediction of tumour response to PRRT. The sequential change of tumour-absorbed doses during treatment with 177Lu-octreotate. Nuklearmedizin 52:170–177

Faivre S, Ronot M, Dreyer C, Serrate C, Hentic O, Bouattour M et al (2012) Imaging response in neuroendocrine tumors treated with targeted therapies: the experience of sunitinib. Target Oncol 7:127–133

Fanti S, Ambrosini V, Tomassetti P, Castellucci P, Montini G, Allegri V et al (2008) Evaluation of unusual neuroendocrine tumours by means of 68Ga-DOTA-NOC PET. Biomed Pharmacother 62:667–671

Frilling A, Modlin IM, Kidd M, Russell C, Breitenstein S, Salem R et al (2014) Recommendations for management of patients with neuroendocrine liver metastases. Lancet Oncol 15:e8–e21

Gabriel M, Decristoforo C, Kendler D, Dobrozemsky G, Heute D, Uprimny C et al (2007) 68Ga-DOTA-Tyr3-octreotide PET in neuroendocrine tumors: comparison with somatostatin receptor scintigraphy and CT. J Nucl Med 48:508–518

Gabriel M, Oberauer A, Dobrozemsky G, Decristoforo C, Putzer D, Kendler D et al (2009) 68Ga-DOTA-Tyr3-octreotide PET for assessing response to somatostatin-receptor-mediated radionuclide therapy. J Nucl Med 50:1427–1434

Garin E, Le Jeune F, Devillers A, Cuggia M, de Lajarte-Thirouard AS, Bouriel C et al (2009) Predictive value of 18F-FDG PET and somatostatin receptor scintigraphy in patients with metastatic endocrine tumors. J Nucl Med 50:858–864

Ha HI, Kim AY, Yu CS, Park SH, Ha HK (2013) Locally advanced rectal cancer: diffusion-weighted MR tumour volumetry and the apparent diffusion coefficient for evaluating complete remission after preoperative chemoradiation therapy. Eur Radiol 23:3345–3353

Habr-Gama A, Gama-Rodrigues J, Sao Juliao GP, Proscurshim I, Sabbagh C, Lynn PB et al (2014) Local recurrence after complete clinical response and watch and wait in rectal cancer after neoadjuvant chemoradiation: impact of salvage therapy on local disease control. Int J Radiat Oncol Biol Phys 88:822–828

Haug AR, Auernhammer CJ, Wangler B, Schmidt GP, Uebleis C, Goke B et al (2010) 68Ga-DOTATATE PET/CT for the early prediction of response to somatostatin receptor-mediated radionuclide therapy in patients with well-differentiated neuroendocrine tumors. J Nucl Med 51:1349–1356

Heijnen LA, Lambregts DM, Lahaye MJ, Martens MH, van Nijnatten TJ, Rao SX et al (2016) Good and complete responding locally advanced rectal tumors after chemoradiotherapy: where are the residual positive nodes located on restaging MRI? **Abdominal Radiol 41:1245–1252

Hofmann M, Maecke H, Borner R, Weckesser E, Schoffski P, Oei L et al (2001) Biokinetics and imaging with the somatostatin receptor PET radioligand (68)Ga-DOTATOC: preliminary data. Eur J Nucl Med 28:1751–1757

Hupkens BJP, Martens MH, Stoot JH, Berbee M, Melenhorst J, Beets-Tan RG et al (2017) Quality of life in rectal cancer patients after chemoradiation: watch-and-wait policy versus standard resection—a matched-controlled study. Dis Colon Rectum 60:1032–1040

Intven M, Reerink O, Philippens ME (2013) Diffusion-weighted MRI in locally advanced rectal cancer: pathological response prediction after neo-adjuvant radiochemotherapy. Strahlenther Onkol 189: 117–122

Intven M, Monninkhof EM, Reerink O, Philippens ME (2015) Combined T2w volumetry, DW-MRI and DCE-MRI for response assessment after neo-adjuvant chemoradiation in locally advanced rectal cancer. Acta Oncol 54:1729–1736

Kaltsas G, Rockall A, Papadogias D, Reznek R, Grossman AB (2004) Recent advances in radiological and radionuclide imaging and therapy of neuroendocrine tumours. Eur J Endocrinol 151:15–27

Kauhanen S, Seppanen M, Ovaska J, Minn H, Bergman J, Korsoff P et al (2009) The clinical value of [18F] fluoro-dihydroxyphenylalanine positron emission tomography in primary diagnosis, staging, and restaging of neuroendocrine tumors. Endocr Relat Cancer 16:255–265

Kayani I, Bomanji JB, Groves A, Conway G, Gacinovic S, Win T et al (2008) Functional imaging of neuroendocrine tumors with combined PET/CT using 68Ga-DOTATATE (DOTA-DPhe1,Tyr3-octreotate) and 18F-FDG. Cancer 112:2447–2455

Kidd M, Modlin I, Oberg K (2016) Towards a new classification of gastroenteropancreatic neuroendocrine neoplasms. Nat Rev Clin Oncol 13:691–705

Kim SH, Lee JM, Hong SH, Kim GH, Lee JY, Han JK et al (2009) Locally advanced rectal cancer: added value of diffusion-weighted MR imaging in the evaluation of tumor response to neoadjuvant chemo- and radiation therapy. Radiology 253:116–125

Kim SH, Lee JY, Lee JM, Han JK, Choi BI (2011) Apparent diffusion coefficient for evaluating tumour response to neoadjuvant chemoradiation therapy for locally advanced rectal cancer. Eur Radiol 21:987–995

Koh DM, Chau I, Tait D, Wotherspoon A, Cunningham D, Brown G (2008) Evaluating mesorectal lymph nodes in rectal cancer before and after neoadjuvant chemoradiation using thin-section T2-weighted magnetic resonance imaging. Int J Radiat Oncol Biol Phys 71:456–461

Koh DM, Brown G, Collins DJ (2009) Nanoparticles in rectal cancer imaging. Cancer Biomark 5:89–98

Koopmans KP, Neels OC, Kema IP, Elsinga PH, Sluiter WJ, Vanghillewe K et al (2008) Improved staging of patients with carcinoid and islet cell tumors with 18F dihydroxy phenyl alanine and 11C 5 hydroxy tryptophan positron emission tomography. J Clin Oncol 26:1489–1495

Kowalski J, Henze M, Schuhmacher J, Macke HR, Hofmann M, Haberkorn U (2003) Evaluation of positron emission tomography imaging using [68Ga]-DOTA-D Phe(1)-Tyr(3)-Octreotide in comparison to [111In]-DTPAOC SPECT. First results in patients with neuroendocrine tumors. Mol Imaging Biol 5: 42–48

Krenning EP, Kwekkeboom DJ, Bakker WH, Breeman WA, Kooij PP, Oei HY et al (1993) Somatostatin receptor scintigraphy with [111In-DTPA-D-Phe1]- and [123I-Tyr3]-octreotide: the Rotterdam experience with more than 1000 patients. Eur J Nucl Med 20:716–731

Kulkarni T, Gollins S, Maw A, Hobson P, Byrne R, Widdowson D (2008) Magnetic resonance imaging in rectal cancer downstaged using neoadjuvant chemoradiation: accuracy of prediction of tumour stage and circumferential resection margin status. Color Dis 10:479–489

Kulke MH, Siu LL, Tepper JE, Fisher G, Jaffe D, Haller DG et al (2011) Future directions in the treatment of neuroendocrine tumors: consensus report of the National Cancer Institute Neuroendocrine Tumor clinical trials planning meeting. J Clin Oncol 29:934–943

Kunz PL, Reidy-Lagunes D, Anthony LB, Bertino EM, Brendtro K, Chan JA et al (2013) Consensus guidelines for the management and treatment of neuroendocrine tumors. Pancreas 42:557–577

Kuo LJ, Chern MC, Tsou MH, Liu MC, Jian JJ, Chen CM et al (2005) Interpretation of magnetic resonance imaging for locally advanced rectal carcinoma after preoperative chemoradiation therapy. Dis Colon Rectum 48:23–28

Kwee TC, Basu S, Saboury B, Ambrosini V, Torigian DA, Alavi A (2011) A new dimension of FDG-PET interpretation: assessment of tumor biology. Eur J Nucl Med Mol Imaging 38:1158–1170

Kwekkeboom DJ, de Herder WW, Kam BL, van Eijck CH, van Essen M, Kooij PP et al (2008) Treatment with the radiolabeled somatostatin analog [177 Lu-DOTA 0,Tyr3]octreotate: toxicity, efficacy, and survival. J Clin Oncol 26:2124–2130

Kwekkeboom DJ, Kam BL, van Essen M, Teunissen JJ, van Eijck CH, Valkema R et al (2010) Somatostatin-receptor-based imaging and therapy of gastroenteropancreatic neuroendocrine tumors. Endocr Relat Cancer 17:R53–R73

Lambregts DM, Beets GL, Maas M, Kessels AG, Bakers FC, Cappendijk VC et al (2011a) Accuracy of gadofosveset-enhanced MRI for nodal staging and restaging in rectal cancer. Ann Surg 253:539–545

Lambregts DM, Vandecaveye V, Barbaro B, Bakers FC, Lambrecht M, Maas M et al (2011b) Diffusion-weighted MRI for selection of complete responders after chemoradiation for locally advanced rectal cancer: a multicenter study. Ann Surg Oncol 18:2224–2231

Lambregts D, Delli Pizzi A, Lahaye M, van Griethuysen J, Maas M, Beets G et al (2018) A pattern-based approach combining tumor morphology on MRI with distinct signal patterns on diffusion-weighted imaging to assess response of rectal tumors after chemoradiotherapy. Dis Colon Rectum 61:328–337

Lee ES, Kim MJ, Park SC, Hur BY, Hyun JH, Chang HJ et al (2018) Magnetic resonance imaging-detected extramural venous invasion in rectal cancer before and after preoperative chemoradiotherapy: diagnostic performance and prognostic significance. Eur Radiol 28:496–505

Lezoche G, Baldarelli M, Guerrieri M, Paganini AM, De Sanctis A, Bartolacci S et al (2008) A prospective randomized study with a 5-year minimum follow-up evaluation of transanal endoscopic microsurgery versus laparoscopic total mesorectal excision after neoadjuvant therapy. Surg Endosc 22:352–358

Li C, Lan X, Yuan H, Feng H, Xia X, Zhang Y (2014) 18F-FDG PET predicts pathological response to preoperative chemoradiotherapy in patients with primary rectal cancer: a meta-analysis. Ann Nucl Med 28:436–446

Llovet JM, Ricci S, Mazzaferro V, Hilgard P, Gane E, Blanc JF et al (2008) Sorafenib in advanced hepatocellular carcinoma. N Engl J Med 359:378–390

Luttges J (2011) [What's new? The 2010 WHO classification for tumours of the pancreas]. Pathologe. 32(Suppl 2):332–336

Maas M, Nelemans PJ, Valentini V, Das P, Rodel C, Kuo LJ et al (2010) Long-term outcome in patients with a pathological complete response after chemoradiation for rectal cancer: a pooled analysis of individual patient data. Lancet Oncol 11:835–844

Maas M, Lambregts DM, Nelemans PJ, Heijnen LA, Martens MH, Leijtens JW et al (2015) Assessment of clinical complete response after chemoradiation for rectal cancer with digital rectal examination, endoscopy, and MRI: selection for organ-saving treatment. Ann Surg Oncol 22:3873–3880

Mankoff DA, Eary JF, Link JM, Muzi M, Rajendran JG, Spence AM et al (2007) Tumor-specific positron emission tomography imaging in patients: [18F] fluorodeoxyglucose and beyond. Clin Cancer Res 13:3460–3469

Martens MH, van Heeswijk MM, van den Broek JJ, Rao SX, Vandecaveye V, Vliegen RA et al (2015a) Prospective, multicenter validation study of magnetic resonance volumetry for response assessment after preoperative chemoradiation in rectal cancer: can the results in the literature be reproduced? Int J Radiat Oncol Biol Phys 93:1005–1014

Martens MH, Subhani S, Heijnen LA, Lambregts DM, Buijsen J, Maas M et al (2015b) Can perfusion MRI predict response to preoperative treatment in rectal cancer? Radiother Oncol 114:218–223

Martens MH, Maas M, Heijnen LA, Lambregts DM, Leijtens JW, Stassen LP et al (2016) Long-term outcome of an organ preservation program after neoadjuvant treatment for rectal cancer. J Natl Cancer Inst 108:12

MERCURY-Study-Group (2006) Diagnostic accuracy of preoperative magnetic resonance imaging in predicting curative resection of rectal cancer: prospective observational study. BMJ 333:779

Milosevic M, Fyles A, Hedley D, Pintilie M, Levin W, Manchul L et al (2001) Interstitial fluid pressure predicts survival in patients with cervix cancer independent of clinical prognostic factors and tumor oxygen measurements. Cancer Res 61:6400–6405

Modlin IM, Oberg K, Chung DC, Jensen RT, de Herder WW, Thakker RV et al (2008) Gastroenteropancreatic neuroendocrine tumours. Lancet Oncol 9: 61–72

Niederle MB, Hackl M, Kaserer K, Niederle B (2010) Gastroenteropancreatic neuroendocrine tumours: the current incidence and staging based on the WHO and European Neuroendocrine Tumour Society classification: an analysis based on prospectively collected parameters. Endocr Relat Cancer 17:909–918

Oberg K, Krenning E, Sundin A, Bodei L, Kidd M, Tesselaar M et al (2016) A Delphic consensus assessment: imaging and biomarkers in gastroenteropancreatic neuroendocrine tumor disease management. Endocr Connect 5:174–187

Orlefors H, Sundin A, Ahlstrom H, Bjurling P, Bergstrom M, Lilja A et al (1998) Positron emission tomography with 5-hydroxytryprophan in neuroendocrine tumors. J Clin Oncol 16:2534–2541

Orlefors H, Sundin A, Lu L, Oberg K, Langstrom B, Eriksson B et al (2006) Carbidopa pretreatment improves image interpretation and visualisation of carcinoid tumours with 11C-5-hydroxytryptophan positron emission tomography. Eur J Nucl Med Mol Imaging 33:60–65

van der Paardt MP, Zagers MB, Beets-Tan RG, Stoker J, Bipat S (2013) Patients who undergo preoperative chemoradiotherapy for locally advanced rectal cancer restaged by using diagnostic MR imaging: a systematic review and meta-analysis. Radiology 269:101–112

Padhani AR, Ollivier L (2001) The RECIST (Response Evaluation Criteria in Solid Tumors) criteria: implications for diagnostic radiologists. Br J Radiol 74(887):983–986

Pearse AG (1980) The APUD concept and hormone production. Clin Endocrinol Metab 9:211–222

Perren A, Couvelard A, Scoazec JY, Costa F, Borbath I, Delle Fave G et al (2017) ENETS consensus guidelines for the standards of care in neuroendocrine tumors: pathology: diagnosis and prognostic stratification. Neuroendocrinology 105:196

Prasad V, Ambrosini V, Alavi A, Fanti S, Baum RP (2008) PET/CT in neuroendocrine tumors: evaluation of receptor status and metabolism. PET Clin 3: 355–379

Ptok H, Marusch F, Meyer F, Wendling P, Wenisch HJ, Sendt W et al (2006) Feasibility and accuracy of TRUS in the pre-treatment staging for rectal carcinoma in general practice. Eur J Surg Oncol 32:420–425

Putzer D, Gabriel M, Kendler D, Henninger B, Knoflach M, Kroiss A et al (2010) Comparison of (68) Ga DOTA Tyr(3) octreotide and (18)F-fluoro-L-dihydroxyphenylalanine positron emission tomography in neuroendocrine tumor patients. Q J Nucl Med Mol Imaging 54:68–75

Raymond E, Dahan L, Raoul JL, Bang YJ, Borbath I, Lombard-Bohas C et al (2011) Sunitinib malate for the treatment of pancreatic neuroendocrine tumors. N Engl J Med 364:501–513

Reubi JC, Laissue J, Waser B, Horisberger U, Schaer JC (1994) Expression of somatostatin receptors in normal, inflamed, and neoplastic human gastrointestinal tissues. Ann N Y Acad Sci 733:122–137

Reubi JC, Schar JC, Waser B, Wenger S, Heppeler A, Schmitt JS et al (2000) Affinity profiles for human somatostatin receptor subtypes SST1-SST5 of somatostatin radiotracers selected for scintigraphic and radiotherapeutic use. Eur J Nucl Med 27:273–282

Rinke A, Muller HH, Schade-Brittinger C, Klose KJ, Barth P, Wied M et al (2009) Placebo-controlled, double-blind, prospective, randomized study on the effect of octreotide LAR in the control of tumor growth in patients with metastatic neuroendocrine midgut tumors: a report from the PROMID Study Group. J Clin Oncol 27:4656–4663

Rockall AG, Planche K, Power N, Nowosinska E, Monson JP, Grossman AB et al (2009) Detection of neuroendocrine liver metastases with MnDPDP-enhanced MRI. Neuroendocrinology 89:288–295

Ruf J, Schiefer J, Kropf S, Furth C, Ulrich G, Kosiek O et al (2013) Quantification in (68)Ga-DOTA(0)-Phe(1)-Tyr(3)-octreotide positron emission tomography/computed tomography: can we be impartial about partial volume effects? Neuroendocrinology 97:369–374

Schiesser M, Veit-Haibach P, Muller MK, Weber M, Bauerfeind P, Hany T et al (2010) Value of combined 6-[18F]fluorodihydroxyphenylalanine PET/CT for imaging of neuroendocrine tumours. Br J Surg 97:691–697

Severi S, Nanni O, Bodei L, Sansovini M, Ianniello A, Nicoletti S et al (2013) Role of 18FDG PET/CT in patients treated with 177Lu-DOTATATE for advanced differentiated neuroendocrine tumours. Eur J Nucl Med Mol Imaging 40:881–888

Sloothaak DA, Geijsen DE, van Leersum NJ, Punt CJ, Buskens CJ, Bemelman WA et al (2013) Optimal time interval between neoadjuvant chemoradiotherapy and surgery for rectal cancer. Br J Surg 100:933–939

Smith JD, Ruby JA, Goodman KA, Saltz LB, Guillem JG, Weiser MR et al (2012) Nonoperative management of rectal cancer with complete clinical response after neoadjuvant therapy. Ann Surg 256:965–972

Solcia E, Kloppel G, Sobin L (eds) (2000) Histological typing of endocrine tumours, 2nd edn. Springer, Berlin

Sun YS, Zhang XP, Tang L, Ji JF, Gu J, Cai Y et al (2010) Locally advanced rectal carcinoma treated with preoperative chemotherapy and radiation therapy: preliminary analysis of diffusion-weighted MR imaging for early detection of tumor histopathologic downstaging. Radiology 254:170–178

Sundin A, Rockall A (2012) Therapeutic monitoring of gastroenteropancreatic neuroendocrine tumors: the challenges ahead. Neuroendocrinology 96: 261–271

Sundin A, Garske U, Orlefors H (2007) Nuclear imaging of neuroendocrine tumours. Best Pract Res Clin Endocrinol Metab 21:69–85

Sundin A, Arnold R, Baudin E, Cwikla JB, Eriksson B, Fanti S et al (2017) ENETS consensus guidelines for the standards of care in neuroendocrine tumors: radiological. Nucl Med Hybrid Imaging Neuroendocrinol 105:212–244

Suppiah A, Hunter IA, Cowley J, Garimella V, Cast J, Hartley JE et al (2009) Magnetic resonance imaging accuracy in assessing tumour down-staging following chemoradiation in rectal cancer. Color Dis 11:249–253

Thapa P, Ranade R, Ostwal V, Shrikhande SV, Goel M, Basu S (2016) Performance of 177Lu-DOTATATE-based peptide receptor radionuclide therapy in metastatic gastroenteropancreatic neuroendocrine tumor: a multiparametric response evaluation correlating with primary tumor site, tumor proliferation index, and dual tracer imaging characteristics. Nucl Med Commun 37:1030–1037

Tong T, Sun Y, Gollub MJ, Peng W, Cai S, Zhang Z et al (2015) Dynamic contrast-enhanced MRI: use in predicting pathological complete response to neoadjuvant chemoradiation in locally advanced rectal cancer. J Magn Reson Imaging 42:673–680

Toumpanakis C, Kim MK, Rinke A, Bergestuen DS, Thirlwell C, Khan MS et al (2014) Combination of cross-sectional and molecular imaging studies in the localization of gastroenteropancreatic neuroendocrine tumors. Neuroendocrinology 99:63–74

Townsend A, Price T, Yeend S, Pittman K, Patterson K, Luke C (2010) Metastatic carcinoid tumor: changing patterns of care over two decades. J Clin Gastroenterol 44(3):195–199

Tripathi P, Rao SX, Zeng MS (2017) Clinical value of MRI-detected extramural venous invasion in rectal cancer. J Dig Dis 18:2–12

Turaga KK, Kvols LK (2011) Recent progress in the understanding, diagnosis, and treatment of gastroenteropancreatic neuroendocrine tumors. CA Cancer J Clin 61:113–132

Velikyan I, Sundin A, Sorensen J, Lubberink M, Sandstrom M, Garske-Roman U et al (2014) Quantitative and qualitative intrapatient comparison of 68Ga-DOTATOC and 68Ga-DOTATATE: net uptake rate for accurate quantification. J Nucl Med 55:204–210

Vliegen RF, Beets GL, Lammering G, Dresen RC, Rutten HJ, Kessels AG et al (2008) Mesorectal fascia invasion after neoadjuvant chemotherapy and radiation therapy for locally advanced rectal cancer: accuracy of MR imaging for prediction. Radiology 246:454–462

West MA, Dimitrov BD, Moyses HE, Kemp GJ, Loughney L, White D et al (2016) Timing of surgery following neoadjuvant chemoradiotherapy in locally advanced rectal cancer—a comparison of magnetic resonance imaging at two time points and histopathological responses. Eur J Surg Oncol 42:1350–1358

Yao JC, Hassan M, Phan A, Dagohoy C, Leary C, Mares JE et al (2008) One hundred years after "carcinoid": epidemiology of and prognostic factors for neuroendocrine tumors in 35,825 cases in the United States. J Clin Oncol 26:3063–3072

Yao JC, Shah MH, Ito T, Bohas CL, Wolin EM, Van Cutsem E et al (2011) Everolimus for advanced pancreatic neuroendocrine tumors. N Engl J Med 364:514–523

Yeo SG, Kim DY, Kim TH, Chang HJ, Oh JH, Park W et al (2010) Pathologic complete response of primary tumor following preoperative chemoradiotherapy for locally advanced rectal cancer: long-term outcomes and prognostic significance of pathologic nodal status (KROG 09-01). Ann Surg 252:998–1004

Zhang C, Tong J, Sun X, Liu J, Wang Y, Huang G (2012) 18F-FDG-PET evaluation of treatment response to neo-adjuvant therapy in patients with locally advanced rectal cancer: a meta-analysis. Int J Cancer 131:2604–2611

Response Assessment and Follow-Up by Imaging in GU Tumours

Cédric Draulans, Ivo G. Schoots, Bernd J. Krause, Sofie Isebaert, Stijn W. T. P. J. Heijmink, Sascha Nitsch, Karin Haustermans, and Sarah M. Schwarzenböck

Contents

1 **Introduction** ... 495

2 **Prostate Cancer** ... 496
2.1 Response Assessment ... 496
2.2 Follow-Up ... 499

3 **Testicular Cancer** ... 504
3.1 Response Assessment/Follow-Up ... 504

4 **Penile Cancer** ... 505
4.1 Response Assessment ... 505
4.2 Follow-Up ... 506

5 **Bladder Cancer** ... 507
5.1 Response Assessment ... 507
5.2 Follow-Up ... 507

6 **Kidney Cancer** ... 508
6.1 Response Assessment ... 508
6.2 Follow-Up ... 509

7 **Conclusion** ... 509

References ... 509

C. Draulans · S. Isebaert · K. Haustermans
Department of Radiation Oncology, University Hospitals Leuven, Leuven, Belgium

Department of Oncology, Laboratory of Experimental Radiotherapy, KU Leuven, Leuven, Belgium

I. G. Schoots · S. W. T. P. J. Heijmink
Department of Radiology, Netherlands Cancer Institute, Amsterdam, The Netherlands

B. J. Krause · S. Nitsch · S. M. Schwarzenböck (✉)
Rostock University Medical Centre, Rostock, Germany
e-mail: Sarah.Schwarzenboeck@med.uni-rostock.de

Abstract

In this chapter, we will *focus on* the role of imaging for response assessment and follow-up after *(chemo)radiation therapy for genitourinary (GU) tumours* including bladder and kidney cancer. Specifically for men, GU cancer also refers to prostate, testicular and penile cancer. Cancers that develop in the ovaries, the uterus, the cervix or the vagina are not considered here as these concern a separate category called gynecologic cancers.

1 Introduction

In this chapter, we will *focus on* the role of imaging for response assessment and follow-up after *(chemo)radiation therapy for genitourinary (GU) tumours* including bladder and kidney cancer. Specifically for men, GU cancer also refers to prostate, testicular and penile cancer. Cancers that develop in the ovaries, the uterus, the cervix or the vagina are not considered here as these concern a separate category called gynecologic cancers.

Primary treatment with curative intent for GU tumours consists, in most cases, of surgery. For some indications, radiation therapy represents a valid alternative, in particular for prostate cancer (PCa). In the adjuvant setting, (chemo)radiation is most often the preferred treatment strategy.

R. G. H. Beets-Tan et al. (eds.), *Imaging and Interventional Radiology for Radiation Oncology*, Medical Radiology, Diagnostic Imaging, https://doi.org/10.1007/978-3-030-38261-2_26

Irrespective of the treatment modality or setting (primary or metastatic), the role of imaging in GU tumours for *response assessment*, i.e. to monitor any potential reduction in tumour size during treatment, is very limited.

As opposed to its role in response assessment, imaging plays a much more important role in *follow-up* after treatment. Early detection of both local recurrences and regional/distant metastases aids physicians in deciding on adjuvant and/or salvage treatment. For most GU tumours, imaging is being performed on a regular time interval after treatment, independent of any markers. In the case of PCa, however, imaging is not routinely performed after treatment as is being done for the other GU tumours. In fact, imaging only comes into play when a rise in post-treatment prostate-specific antigen (PSA) serum levels above a certain threshold is detected, i.e. marker-dependent imaging (Table 1). Also in symptomatic patients for whom the findings affect treatment decisions, the use of imaging techniques is justified (Heidenreich et al. 2014; Mohler et al. 2016).

2 Prostate Cancer

As aforementioned, imaging for PCa is marker-dependent. PSA kinetics are commonly used during follow-up after curative radiation treatment. According to the Phoenix definition, PSA failure after external beam radiation therapy (EBRT) is defined as a PSA rise of 2 ng/mL or more above the PSA nadir, regardless of whether or not a patient receives androgen deprivation therapy (ADT). Depending on the pretreatment risk factors, biochemical failure (BCF) is seen in up to 50% of patients 5 years after EBRT (Kestin et al. 1999; Pollack et al. 2002). Lower BCF rates are observed in all risk groups when high-dose radiation therapy is being delivered (Viani et al. 2009).

Unfortunately, PSA kinetics cannot unambiguously differentiate between local, regional or distant recurrences (Roach et al. 2006), although this is crucial to determine the best option for second-line therapy. Patients with locally persistent PCa after radiation therapy are at greater risk of developing distant metastasis. A latency period to the appearance of distant metastasis suggests a late wave of metastasis from the locally persistent tumour (Coen et al. 2002). In the past, local persistent or local recurrent PCa was detected by digital rectal examination (DRE) abnormalities. However, post-radiation fibrosis hampers a reliable clinical assessment of the prostate (Johnstone et al. 2001). Accurate imaging is necessary for detecting local recurrence. Furthermore, also lymph node staging and metastatic bone disease staging have a significant role in the work-up of patients with suspected recurrent disease.

Also in the metastatic setting, it is known that the use of PSA alone is not sufficient to assess therapy response (Pezaro et al. 2014). The commonly used clinical standard for therapy response assessment in metastatic castration-resistant prostate cancer (mCRPC) are RECIST and clinical criteria, which have shown a significant association with overall survival (OS) (Thalgott et al. 2015).

2.1 Response Assessment

2.1.1 Primary Setting

In the prostate, a role for multi-parametric magnetic resonance imaging (mpMRI) in evaluating response to specific PCa therapies, such as EBRT and androgen deprivation therapy (ADT), is the current area of investigation (Fig. 1) (Fennessy et al. 2014). Park et al. found that apparent diffusion coefficient (ADC) values derived from prostate tumours significantly increased during and after radiation treatment, while no significant changes in ADC values of benign prostate tissue were observed. From these results, the authors concluded that diffusion-weighted imaging (DWI) has the potential to evaluate the early therapeutic changes of PCa to EBRT (Park et al. 2012). Also Foltz and colleagues noted a significant increase in ADC values of prostate tumors during EBRT, with a 14% increase in ADC values at week 6 during EBRT as compared to baseline (Foltz et al. 2013). Furthermore DCE parametric changes have been reported following carbon ion and proton irradiation of PCa

Table 1 Overview response assessment and follow-up by imaging of male GU tumours for primary treatment with curative intent

Response assessment and follow-up/monitoring by imaging of male GU tumours with a curative intent												
Local and regional disease		Primary treatment (T)				Adjuvant treatment (N)			Role of imaging			
										In follow-up/monitoring		
		Surgery	Radiation therapy	Chemotherapy	Immunotherapy	Surgery	Radiation therapy	Chemotherapy	In response assessment	Marker independent	Marker dependent	Modality
Penile cancer		+	±	–	–	+	–	+	–	+	–	CT
Testicular cancer	Stage I	+	–	–	–	–	–	±	–	+	+	CT
	Stage II	+	–	–	–	–	+	+	–	+	+	CT
Prostate cancer	Low-risk	+	+	–	–	–	–	–	–	–	+	MRI
	Intermediate-risk	+	+	–	–	±(>5%)	–	–	–	–	+	MRI, PET-CT (bone scanning)
	High-risk	+	+	–	–	±(>5%)	–	–	–	–	+	MRI, PET-CT (bone scanning)
Bladder cancer	NMIBC	+	–	±	+	–	–	–	–	–	–	-
	MIBC	+	±	+	–	+	–	+	–	+	–	CT, PET-CT
Renal cancer	RCC	+	–	–	–	–	–	–	–	+	–	CT

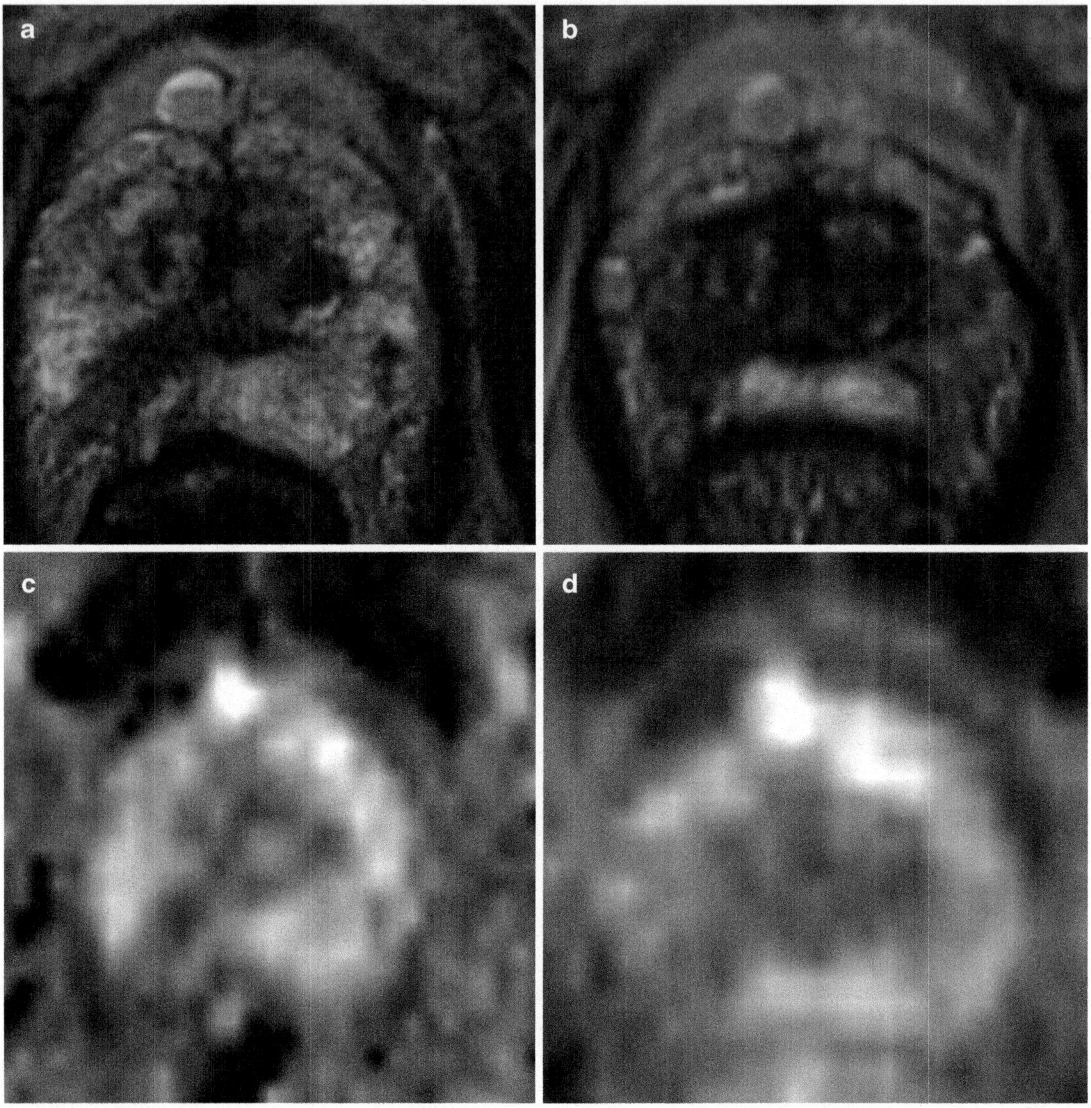

Fig. 1 Example of longitudinal changes of T2-weighted image (**a**, **b**) and ADC map (**c**, **d**) before (**a**, **c**) and 2 months after androgen deprivation therapy (**b**, **d**). The prostate tumour is located in the right posterior peripheral zone

(Bonekamp et al. 2016). Barrett et al. explored the role of both DWI and dynamic contrast-enhanced (DCE) MRI to assess the response to primary ADT. While no significant changes in ADC values in prostate tumours were observed, ADC values in benign prostate tissue were significantly decreased after 3 months of ADT. Furthermore, all DCE parameters measured in the tumour were significantly decreased, while those measured in the benign tissue were unchanged. Based on these data, the authors hypothesized that DCE as a marker of angiogenesis might help to demonstrate ADT resistance. Antivasuclar effects of ADT were also observed in other imaging studies (Alonzi et al. 2011). Although these results are promising and could potentially serve as a sound base for the development of imaging biomarkers for treatment response assessment, further research is warranted.

2.1.2 Metastatic Setting

DWI has shown promise in detecting metastastic bone disease and has also been used as a method for measuring therapy response in metastatic PCa (Lecouvet et al. 2014). Preclinical evidence suggests that DCE MRI can be used for monitoring the effect of antiangiogenic agents in mCRPC (Cyran et al. 2012), but clinical data are still very limited (Dahut et al. 2013).

Only few studies have evaluated the use of choline positron emission tomography/computed tomography (PET/CT) for therapy response assessment in mCRPC patients. De Giorgi et al. used [^{18}F]Choline PET/CT for early response assessment of daily abiraterone (De Giorgi et al. 2014) and enzalutamide therapy (De Giorgi et al. 2015). PSA changes were concordant with the [^{18}F]Choline PET/CT progression/non-progression in 81% and 71% of patients, respectively (De Giorgi et al. 2014, 2015). Ceci et al. assessed the use of ^{11}C-Choline PET/CT for therapy response to docetaxel chemotherapy in mCRPC patients (Ceci et al. 2016). Progressive disease (PD) was found in 50% and 44% of patients despite a decreasing PSA and a PSA response ≥50%, respectively. The authors concluded that [^{18}F]Choline PET/CT might be useful in patients with radiological PD despite decreasing PSA (Ceci et al. 2016). Schwarzenböck et al. performed a standardized prospective analysis of ^{11}C-choline PET/CT for early as well as late therapy response after certain cycles of docetaxel chemotherapy in mCRPC patients (Schwarzenböck et al. 2016). No significant differences in change of choline uptake could be shown between PD and non-PD patients neither in early nor in late response assessment in the patient-based analysis. The authors showed that there was no consistency between the results of PET/CT-based therapy response assessment and PSA changes as well as therapy response based on RECIST and clinical standard criteria. The use of choline PET/CT in therapy response assessment and predicting patient outcome still remains unclear.

New PET tracers addressing the prostate-specific membrane antigen (PSMA) have shown promising results in staging and restaging of prostate cancer (Ceci et al. 2017). PSMA is a membrane-bound glycoprotein that is highly expressed on prostate epithelial cells and strongly upregulated in PCa (Ghosh and Heston 2004). In further trials, their potential use for treatment response assessment as well as for predicting patient outcome should be assessed (Fig. 2).

2.2 Follow-Up

In the next paragraphs, we discuss the role of different imaging modalities currently available for detecting the location of recurrence when PSA is rising after curative (radiation) treatment.

2.2.1 Transrectal Ultrasound and Computed Tomography

The use of transrectal ultrasonography (TRUS) to identify persistent or recurrent PCa was investigated in the 90s (Egawa et al. 1989; Egawa et al. 1992a; Egawa et al. 1992b; Kabalin et al. 1989), but today TRUS is not implemented in the standard follow-up of patients with PCa after radiation therapy nor has it a role in the context of regional and distant staging for recurrences of PCa.

Due to its poor contrast resolution, there is also no role for computed tomography (CT) in detecting local recurrence of PCa (Fig. 3), neither after surgery, nor after EBRT (Maurer et al. 2016). Standard CT imaging in PCa patients with BCF is not recommended, unless perhaps there is a high PSA value or high PSA velocity (Johnstone et al. 1997; Kane et al. 2003).

2.2.2 Magnetic Resonance Imaging

As opposed to the important role of MRI in the pretreatment setting, its role in the posttreatment setting is still being explored. Nevertheless, MRI seems to be useful to detect *local recurrences* in patients with biochemical relapse after EBRT, as further discussed below. The EAU guidelines advise to perform prostate mpMRI only in those patients who are considered candidates for local salvage therapy, supported by level III evidence (Grade of recommendation: B) (Heidenreich et al. 2014).

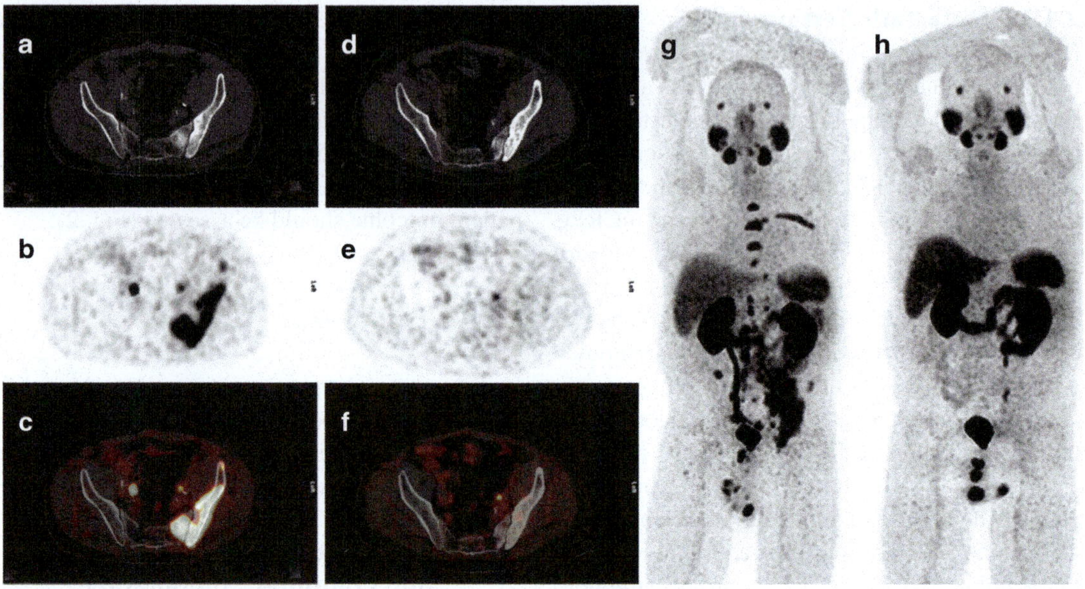

Fig. 2 Image example of Ga-68 PSMA PET/CT for therapy response assessment in a patient suffering from metastasized prostate cancer (initial stage pT3bpN0cN1c-M1L0V1Pn1R1, Gleason score 9). The patient received six cycles of chemotherapy with docetaxel. Ga-68 PSMA PET/CT before chemotherapy showed disseminated PSMA-positive lymph node and bony metastases (**a** transaxial CT, **b** transaxial PET, **c** transaxial fused PET/CT, **g** maximum intensity projection). Ga-68 PSMA PET/CT acquired for restaging and therapy response assessment after chemotherapy showed partial response (**d** transaxial CT, **e** transaxial PET, **f** transaxial fused PET/CT, **h** maximum intensity projection)

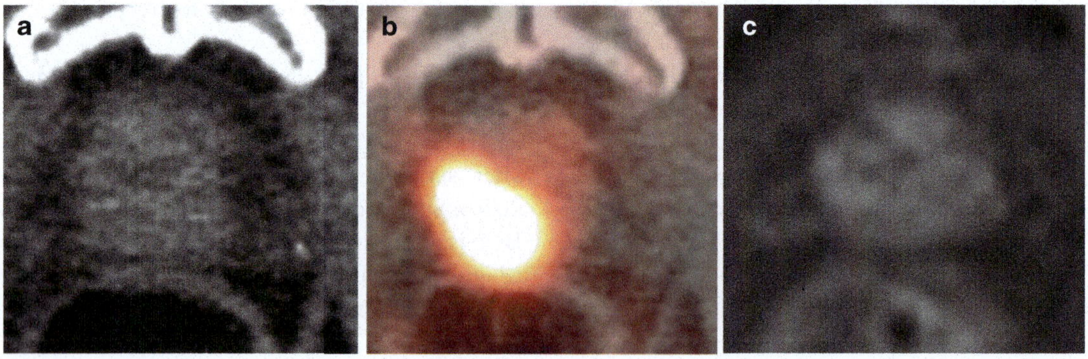

Fig. 3 No abnormalities visualised on CT imaging (**a**), while 68Ga-PSMA PET images (**b**) and DCE MR images (**c**) show a local recurrence in a patient with a rising PSA, 2 years after external beam radiotherapy for PCa

2.2.2.1 T2-weighted MRI

Radiotherapy to the prostate induces fibrosis, inflammation, prostate shrinkage and glandular atrophy (Roznovanu et al. 2005**). Furthermore, there is a loss of zonal anatomy of the prostate after radiotherapy, as well as loss of the normal T2-weighted (T2w) high intensity signal of the peripheral zone, which are both important features for tumour detection by (T2w) MRI (Westphalen et al. 2009).

A few prospective studies have investigated the accuracy of the detection of local relapses by T2w imaging after EBRT (Westphalen et al. 2009; Rouvière et al. 2004; Pucar et al. 2005;

Table 2 Overview prospective studies on T2w-MRI for the diagnosis of local recurrence after radiation therapy

Study (publication date)	Included patients	Standard of reference	Evaluation	Recurrence	Sensitivity	Specificity
Rouvière et al. (2004)	$n = 22$	TRUS biopsy	10 prostate sectors[a]	19/22	26–44%[b]	64–86%[b]
Pucar et al. (2005)	$n = 9$	Prostatecomy	Sextant	9/9	68%	96%
Sala et al. (2006)	$n = 45$	Prostatecomy			36–76%[b]	65–81%[b]
Haider et al. (2008)	$n = 33$	TRUS biopsy	Sextant	12/33	38%	80%
Westphalen et al. (2009)	$n = 59$	TRUS biopsy	Hemiprostatic	34/59	62–74%[b]	64–68%[b]
Kim et al. (2009)	$n = 36$	TRUS biopsy	Sextant	18/36	25%	92%

[a]The sextants of the peripheral zone, the two transitional zones, and the two seminal vesicles
[b]Multiple readers

Sala et al. 2006; Haider et al. 2008; Kim et al. 2009) (Table 2). Most recurrences after primary radiation therapy seem to occur at the site of the primary tumour (Cellini et al. 2002). These results suggest that, similar to the pretreatment setting, T2w MRI alone has only modest accuracy to detect local recurrence and is thus insufficient as a single imaging modality for this purpose.

2.2.2.2 Dynamic Contrast-Enhanced MRI

While post-radiation fibrosis makes it difficult to interpret T2w MR images, the presence of fibrosis and decreased microvasculature of the primary tumour causes the neovascularity of a recurrent tumour to be more visible on DCE MR images. In general, a recurrent tumour is detected by DCE MRI as an area of fast contrast enhancement (Arumainayagam et al. 2010). In a study by Haider et al., in which 33 PCa patients were enrolled, it was reported that the accuracy for the detection of local recurrent PCa was significantly better for DCE MRI compared to T2w MRI (82% vs. 55%) (Haider et al. 2008). At present, DCE MRI is still the standard of reference for imaging of recurrent disease (Heidenreich et al. 2014).

2.2.2.3 Diffusion-Weighted MRI

Kim et al. conducted a trial in which the role of DWI for the detection of locally recurred PCa was evaluated. They showed that a combination of T2w images and DWI with ADC maps reached a significantly better sensitivity in detecting local recurrence after radiation therapy (62%) than T2w imaging alone (25%) (Kim et al. 2009). A focal decreased signal intensity (low ADC values) compared to the surrounding tissue was identified as tumour recurrence. Until now, it is not known which phenomenon exactly causes the decreased ADC values relative to surrounding irradiated benign prostatic tissue. Kim et al. suggested histopathologic characteristics in recurrent tumours after radiotherapy (e.g., enlarged nuclei, hyperchromatism and hypercellularity), which decrease the diffusion distance of water protons in the intra- and extracellular spaces, as a potential cause. In contrast, post-radiation glandular atrophy, inflammation and fibrosis in benign prostatic tissue lead to an increase of diffusion distance of water protons corresponding with increased ADC values. Morgan et al. concluded that an ADC value is useful in combination with T2w MRI to detect local tumour recurrence larger than 0.4 cm^2 (Morgan et al. 2012). The use of DWI in a recurrence setting may be hampered by the presence of gold markers or brachy seeds in the prostate, which cause magnetic field strength inhomogeneities.

2.2.2.4 MR Spectroscopy

There has been huge interest in MRS for the detection of PCa and local staging. In contrast, only a limited number of trials have also investigated the role of MRS in the post-treatment setting to evaluate persistent or recurrent PCa (Pucar et al. 2005; Menard et al. 2001; Coakley et al. 2004). Following EBRT, repair processes seem to influence energy requirements of irradiated normal prostate cells. Nonmalignant irradiated prostate tissue shows lower citrate peaks and higher choline peaks due to additional phospholipid cell membrane synthesis with an increased demand for choline compounds. In addition, irradiated PCa seems to switch from citrate-producing to citrate-oxidizing metabolism. Therefore, it remains unclear which metabolic criteria should be followed to distinguish between benign and malign prostate tissue.

Due to limitations by inter-reader variability and technical issues (e.g., the influence of tissue motion, elimination of unwanted water and lipid signals), the routine use of MRS is not recommended today, neither in the diagnostic setting according to PI-RADS™ v2 nor for the detection of local PCa relapse.

2.2.2.5 Multiparametric MRI

As is the case in the pretreatment setting, combining T2w MRI, DCE MRI, DWI and MRS increases the sensitivity of detecting intra-prostatic recurrences after EBRT (Arumainayagam et al. 2010; Roy et al. 2013; Oppenheimer et al. 2016; Wu et al. 2013; Akin et al. 2011). Donati et al. conducted a retrospective trial to find the most optimal combination of MRI modalities for intra-prostatic characterization after EBRT. They investigated T2w, DWI, and DCE sequences and concluded that the addition of DCE to T2w imaging and DWI did not significantly improve the accuracy to detect recurrent PCa. The combination of T2w imaging and DWI resulted in following diagnostic accuracies: area under the curve (AUC) values of 0.79–0.86 for reader 1 and 0.75–0.81 for reader 2. The added value of DCE was not significant for the detection of locally relapsed PCa (reader 1: $P > 0.99$; reader 2: $P = 0.35$) (Donati OF and Jung 2013).

Concerning the role of MRI in detecting *regional or distant PCa recurrences*, some groups investigated the role of whole-body and axial MRI (Eiber et al. 2011; Lecouvet et al. 2012). Lecouvet et al. concluded that whole-body DWI surpassed bone scintigraphy in detecting bone metastasis in the case of BCF. Moreover whole-body MRI showed the same performance for the evaluation of lymph nodes as total-body CT (Eiber et al. 2011; Lecouvet et al. 2012). There seems to be no added value of T1w and T2w MRI.

The use of ultra-small superparamagnetic iron oxide (USPIO) nanoparticle contrast agents has been investigated to visualize metastatic lymph nodes on MR, since the beginning of the 90s. Following the decision of the manufacturer to withdraw the Marketing Authorisation Application (MAA) of USPIO in 2007, it was no longer possible for patients to benefit from this contrast agent. Since 2013, the production process and manufacturing of USPIOs have been performed only at the Radboud University Medical Center Nijmegen (Fortuin et al. 2018).

2.2.3 Nuclear Imaging

2.2.3.1 [^{18}F]FDG PET/CT

Fluorodeoxyglucose ([^{18}F]FDG) PET is an excellent tool in the detection of primary tumours and distant metastasis for many different tumour types. However, its role in PCa is limited. [^{18}F]FDG is not specific for PCa, and false positives may occur due to inflammatory conditions or obscuring intense bladder and prostatic urethral activity from urinary excretion. Moreover PCa is characterized by slow glycolysis and low [^{18}F]FDG avidity (Liu et al. 2001). Therefore, other PET tracers have been investigated for PCa.

2.2.3.2 Choline PET/CT

The most commonly used alternative metabolic tracers are choline tracers. There exist three main choline-based PET tracers: ^{11}C-choline, [^{18}F]methylcholine and [^{18}F]ethylcholine. Available data suggest that the diagnostic performance of these three variants of choline is equal (Calabria et al. 2015). Choline PET/CT sensitivity is dependent on the PSA value and PSA velocity. Krause et al. conducted a study with 63 patients with BCF demonstrating that the detection rate of choline PET/CT is correlated with the PSA value (detection rate of 36% at a PSA < 1 ng/mL, 43% at a PSA 1–2 ng/mL, 62% PSA 2–3 ng/mL, 73% PSA > 3 ng/mL). These results were confirmed by subsequent studies by Castelluci et al. who additionally showed that the detection rate was correlated also with PSA kinetics. They found a sensitivity and specificity of 73 and 69%, at a PSA threshold level of 2.43 ng/mL (Castellucci et al. 2009). Giovacchini et al. found a sensitivity of 73% and a specificity of 72% at a PSA threshold value of 1.4 ng/mL (Giovacchini et al. 2010). Furthermore, Rybalov et al. conducted a trial to investigate the accuracy of ^{11}C-choline PET/CT to detect intra-prostatic recurrence after EBRT. They concluded that functional imaging with ^{11}C-choline shows a moderate concordance with routine transrectal prostate biopsies (Rybalov et al. 2012). Choline PET/CT may change medical management of patients with BCF after primary EBRT.

A number of meta-analyses have also investigated the accuracy of choline PET/CT in detection recurrences and the location of recurrence. Fanti et al. conducted a systematic review and meta-analysis assessing ^{11}C-choline PET/CT for its accuracy to detect the site of recurrence of PCa in patients with BCF after curative treatment for PCa. The pooled sensitivity and specificity for any relapse was 89%. For local relapse, the pooled sensitivity and specificity were, respectively, 61% and 97% (Fanti et al. 2016). Treglia et al. showed a detection rate of 58% in patients with BCF, which increased up to 65% at a PSA doubling time of <6 months and to 71% and 77% at a PSA of >1 and >2 ng/mL, respectively (Treglia et al. 2014a). Cimitan et al. evaluated 1.000 patients with BCF showing a dependency between the detection rate of [^{18}F]Choline PET/CT and the initial Gleason score. They showed a detection rate of 31%, 43% and 81% at PSA values of <1 ng/mL, 1–2 ng/mL and >2 ng/mL, which increased up to 51%, 65% and 91%, respectively, at a Gleason score of 7 or higher. Evangelista et al. conducted a meta-analysis including 19 studies with 1555 BCF patients. Sensitivity was 100% (95 CI 90.5–100%) for the detection of nodal metastases and specificity was 81.8% (95% CI 48.2–97.7%). For the detection of local recurrence, sensitivity was 75.4% (95% CI 66.9–82.6%), specificity was 82% (95% CI 69.6–91.4%) (Evangelista et al. 2013). In another meta-analysis (12 studies including 1055 patients) on the role of choline PET/CT in BCF sensitivity was 85% (95% CI 79–89%), specificity was 88% (95% CI 73–95%) (Umbehr et al. 2013). Ceci et al. showed a detection rate of 87.8% in a cohort of 140 patients with BCF > 2 ng/mL after primary radiation treatment (37% of patients suffered from local/regional recurrence, 25% showed local/regional recurrence and distant metastases, 37% showed only distant metastases) (Ceci et al. 2014). In another meta-analysis by von Eyben et al., 2506 patients with BCF were included; pooled detection rate was 49%. Choline PET/CT led to a change in treatment planning in 381 out of 938 patients (41%) (von Eyben and Kairemo 2014). However, choline PET/CT has limitations as it does not always identify local recurrence, lymph node involvement or visceral metastases (Yu et al. 2014).

2.2.3.3 PSMA PET/CT

PSMA PET/CT, coupled with Gallium-68, has shown promising results in patients with BCF. Two trials, which prospectively compare the detection rates of ^{68}Ga-PSMA PET versus [^{18}F]fluormethylcholine PET/CT, confirmed a significantly higher detection rate of ^{68}Ga-PSMA PET (Afshar-Oromieh et al. 2014; Morigi et al. 2015).

Recently published retrospective studies evaluating the value of ^{68}Ga-PSMA PET/CT in BCF (including 319 patients, 248 and 1007 patients, respectively) showed detection rates >85%. In these studies, detection rate was still >50% at PSA values <0.5 ng/mL (Afshar-Oromieh et al. 2015; Eiber et al. 2015; Afshar-Oromieh et al. 2017). In patients with BCF after prior radiotherapy (with a median PSA of 5.8 ng/mL), detection rates were 33.3% for PSA <0.5 ng/mL, 71.4% for PSA 0.5 to <1 ng/mL and 93.3% for PSA 1 to <2 ng/mL (Meredith et al. 2016). [^{18}F]labelled PSMA ligands have shown similar results with respect to detection rates in BCF of prostate cancer (Rowe et al. 2015, 2016; Giesel et al. 2017). For details on PET/CT using PSMA-ligands, see (Schwarzenboeck et al. 2017).

Perera et al. provided a systematic review and meta-analysis on the sensitivity and specificity of positive ^{68}Ga-PSMA PET in PCa. The overall percentage of positive ^{68}Ga-PSMA PET among patients with biochemical recurrence was 76%. Moreover, they found that ^{68}Ga-PSMA PET positivity is correlated with the PSA level. For PSA ranges of 0.2–1, 1–2 and >2 ng/mL, detection rates have been reported of 58%, 76% and 95%, respectively. The general sensitivity and specificity were both 86% on per patient analysis (Perera et al. 2016).

2.2.3.4 Bone Scintigraphy; SPECT/CT; [^{18}F]NaF PET/CT

^{99m}Tc-MDP whole-body bone scintigraphy has been used for decades to evaluate bone metastasis in patients with PCa. However, the main drawback of ^{99m}Tc-MDP whole-body bone scintigraphy is its low specificity due to accumulation of the tracer in degenerative, inflammatory and traumatic lesions or benign bone tumours. The introduction of modern hybrid imaging with single-photon emission computed tomography (SPECT)/CT improved the characterization of suspect lesions on whole-body planar bone scintigraphy or SPECT alone. It was shown by Helyar et al. that the number of equivocal reports by nuclear medicine physicians was reduced from 61 to 8% with the addition of SPECT/CT (Helyar et al. 2010). Next to bone scintigraphy and SPECT/CT, [^{18}F]sodium fluoride ([^{18}F]NaF) PET/CT was found to be useful in the detection of occult bone metastases in the recurrence setting by Jadvar et al. (Jadvar et al. 2012).

2.2.4 Future Perspectives

There is a growing need for accurate imaging of early local PCa recurrence and detection of oligometastatic disease. This need arises from the evolution of local therapeutic options for these patients, e.g. salvage surgery, salvage brachytherapy or stereotactic body radiation therapy (SBRT) in the oligometastatic setting. These recent approaches have the potential to cure patients with relapsing PCa after local treatment or at least postpone disease progression and need for systemic treatment in these patients.

A promising tool to detect early biochemical failure after radiation therapy could be ^{68}Ga-PSMA PET as discussed earlier. However, until now, only a limited number of studies are available. This currently hampers its clinical implementation and therefore large, multidisciplinary prospective trials are needed. Beside its use for diagnostic imaging, PSMA ligands can also act as theragnostic agents, e.g. PSMA ligands can be labelled with ^{177}Lu (Lutetium). ^{177}Lu-PSMA radioligand therapy has shown, although not yet being approved, to be a promising, safe and effective treatment option to be offered in patients with mCRPC after all approved therapies. Preliminary data on ^{177}Lu-PSMA radioligand therapy showed that a decline of PSA values is accompanied by morphological and/or metabolic changes assessed by CT and/or ^{68}Ga-PSMA PET/CT (using Prostate Cancer Working Group 2 (PCWG2) criteria or PET Response Criteria in Solid Tumors (PERCIST) criteria) (Baum et al. 2016; Ahmadzadehfar et al. 2016; Yadav et al. 2017; Kratochwil et al. 2016; Fendler et al. 2017).

Furthermore, combining the best of both worlds by using MR-PET may be an interesting modality for treatment assessment after radiotherapy for patients with PCa in the future (Pichler et al. 2008; Wetter et al. 2014; Piccardo et al. 2014). Lütje et al. evaluated the diagnostic accuracy of ^{68}Ga-labeled HBED-CC-PSMA-PET/MRI for the detection of recurrent PCa in comparison to PET/CT. ^{68}Ga-HBED-CC-PSMA PET/MRI was found to be superior compared to ^{68}Ga-HBED-CC-PSMA PET/CT in the detection of PSMA-expressing prostate bed recurrences (Lütje et al. 2017).

3 Testicular Cancer

3.1 Response Assessment/Follow-Up

According to the EAU guidelines, standard follow-up with abdominopelvic CT/MRI is recommended for at least 5 years (Albers et al. 2015). Imaging also plays an important role in evaluating response to chemotherapy for metastatic testicular cancer (Albers et al. 2015).

Half of germ cell tumours of the testis are *seminomas*. A potential role of [^{18}F]FDG PET/CT is monitoring the response to chemotherapy and characterisation of residual seminoma masses.

Morphological CT imaging is limited in discriminating residual metastatic tumour masses and fibrotic tissue. [^{18}F]FDG PET, offering metabolic information, might overcome this issue. In patients with metastatic seminoma, a significant association has been found between early metabolic response on [^{18}F]FDG PET and tumour shrinkage. Patients achieving a complete response assessed by [^{18}F]FDG PET after 2 cycles of chemotherapy could be predicted not to need additional treatment after chemotherapy (Necchi et al. 2016). Accurate characterization of postchemotherapy residual disease is also important. Treglia et al. published a systematic review and meta-analysis evaluating the diagnostic performance of [^{18}F]FDG PET/CT in the postchemotherapy management of patients with seminoma (nine articles including 375 patients). Patients underwent either [^{18}F]FDG PET or PET/CT to evaluate viable cancer in residual masses of seminoma after chemotherapy. Pooled sensitivity and specificity of [^{18}F]FDG PET or PET/CT were 78% and 86%, respectively. [^{18}F]FDG showed a high negative predictive value of 94% with a moderate positive predictive value of 58%. In subgroups with residual lesions of <3 cm and >3 cm after chemotherapy, pooled sensitivity and specificity of [^{18}F]FDG PET(/CT) were 47% and 89% compared to 89% and 81%, respectively (Treglia et al. 2014b).

With respect to the time point of imaging, Bachner et al. reported that sensitivity and specificity of [^{18}F]FDG PET were 50% and 77%, respectively, if the imaging was performed before 6 weeks after the last cycle of chemotherapy and increased to 82% and 90%, respectively, being performed more than 6 weeks after the end of the last cycle (Bachner et al. 2012). These results are in accordance with the recommendations of international guidelines on the use of [^{18}F]FDG PET/CT in evaluating viable residual masses (Oldenburg et al. 2013). Positive [^{18}F]FDG PET, obtained at least 6 weeks after the completion of chemotherapy, may be helpful in identifying seminoma patients with residual mass greater than 3 cm harbouring viable disease as those patients would benefit from surgical resection (Bachner et al. 2012; Becherer et al. 2005). Because of the significant morbidity and low therapeutic gain associated with resection (Beyer et al. 2013), image-guided biopsy or close observation with serial CT scans or repeat PET-CT is preferred for these patients. Ambrosini et al. showed a change of treatment/follow-up based on the results of [^{18}F]FDG PET/CT scan in patients with seminoma in 47 of 51 (92%) (Ambrosini et al. 2014).

For patients with *non-seminoma* germ cell tumours (NSGCT), distinction between mature teratomas, viable carcinoma or necrotic/fibrotic tissue has important clinical implications (Fox et al. 1993). Currently used predictive markers include the size of residual masses and the extent of size reduction as determined by pre- and post-treatment CT, combined with primary tumour histology and pre-chemotherapy serum tumour markers, but stronger predictors are still needed (Steyerberg et al. 2000). Unfortunately, residual tumour histology cannot be reliably predicted by imaging. For example, the low metabolic activity of teratoma as well as fibrosis or necrosis hampers their distinction by [^{18}F]FDG PET (Pfannenberg et al. 2004). It is therefore that patients with residual NSGCT $\geq$1 cm should undergo resection within 4–8 weeks after the completion of chemotherapy, preferably at expert surgical centres (Beyer et al. 2013).

4 Penile Cancer

4.1 Response Assessment

For response assessment in penile cancer, only very limited imaging data are available. Graafland et al. evaluated the use of [^{18}F]FDG PET/CT for monitoring treatment response in patients with inoperable penile carcinoma treated by chemotherapy. Metabolic response assessed by PET/CT (European Organisation for the Research and Treatment of Cancer (EORTC) criteria) was compared to tumour response based on CT-imaging (RECIST criteria). According to the reference (response/non-response rated by a multidisciplinary board), six patients were responders and two non-responders after two cycles of chemotherapy. In all 8 patients, metabolic tumour

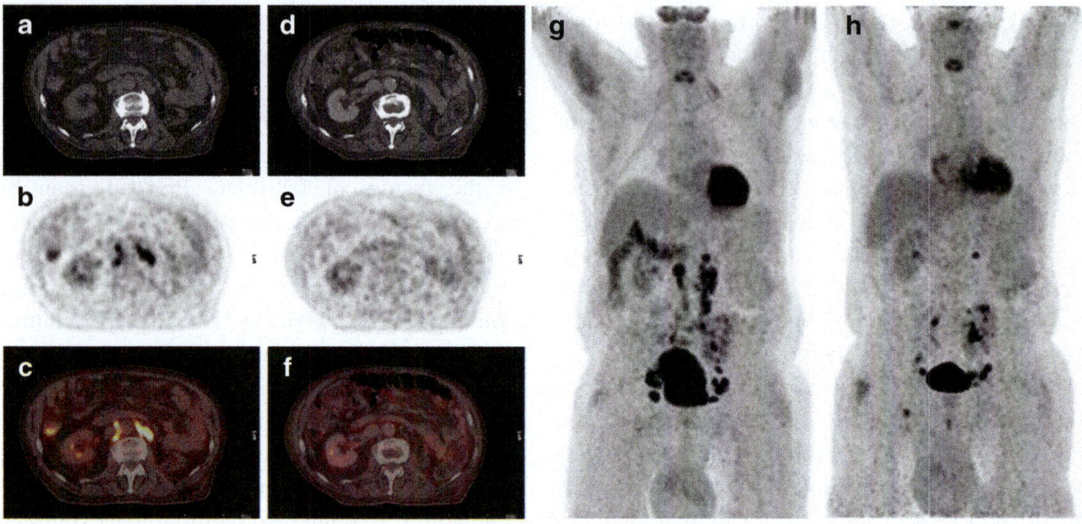

Fig. 4 Image example of [^{18}F]FDG PET/CT for therapy response assessment in a patient suffering from metastasized penile carcinoma (initial stage pT1a V0 G2). The patient received several surgical interventions and chemotherapy (5-FU, cisplatin mitomycin) due to nodal metastases. [^{18}F]FDG PET/CT before chemotherapy showed disseminated [^{18}F]FDG-positive retroperitoneal lymyph node metastases (**a** transaxial CT, **b** transaxial PET, **c** transaxial fused PET/CT, **g** maximum intensity projection). [^{18}F]FDG PET/CT acquired for restaging and therapy response assessment after chemotherapy showed partial response (**d** transaxial CT, **e** transaxial PET, **f** transaxial fused PET/CT, **h** maximum intensity projection)

response assessment correlated with the standard of reference and was histopathologically proven in 5 patients. In three patients correctly identified as responders by PET/CT, RECIST-based radiological tumour response was considered suboptimal compared with the metabolic assessment. The authors concluded that [^{18}F]FDG PET/CT imaging is feasible for monitoring treatment response and potentially more reliable than CT alone in patients with advanced penile carcinoma treated with induction chemotherapy (Fig. 4) (Graafland et al. 2010). [^{18}F]FDG PET could also be used for response monitoring for chemotherapy in the case of rare penile lymphoma (Karunanithi et al. 2012).

4.2 Follow-Up

Since patients receiving penile-preserving therapy, for example EBRT or insterstitial brachytherapy for T1–2 lesions of the glans or sulcus, have a five times higher rate of local recurrence as compared to amputation (27.7% vs. 5.3%), and with two thirds of relapses occurring in the first 2 years, close follow-up for these patients is recommended. Follow-up evaluations for patients with negative inguinal nodes after local treatment include regular physician or self-examination and ultrasound with fine-needle aspiration biopsy (when indicated) (Rossari et al. 2010; Leijte et al. 2008). For patients who received potentially curative treatment for inguinal nodal metastases, also CT or MRI at 3-monthly intervals for (at least) the first 2 years is recommended for the detection of systemic disease, so patients could benefit from adjuvant chemotherapy (Hakenberg et al. 2015).

The role of [^{18}F]FDG PET/CT in (re)staging of penile cancer seems to be unclear because of a small number of studies and patients. Most studies investigated the diagnostic accuracy of [^{18}F]FDG PET/CT in the detection of lymph node metastasis in staging before primary surgery. A review of seven papers on this topic, including 115 patients, calculated a pooled sensitivity of 85.3% and a specificity of 91% for [^{18}F]FDG PET/CT in primary nodal staging (Sadeghi et al. 2012). Zhang et al. evaluated 42 patients and reported an overall sensitivity and specificity of 82% and 93%, respectively, for [18F]FDG PET/CT in nodal staging of penile cancer (Zhang et al. 2016). In follow-up, [18F]FDG PET/CT can improve the detection of early regional lymph node and distant metastases (Van Poppel et al. 2013).

5 Bladder Cancer

5.1 Response Assessment

5.1.1 Primary Setting

In patients with muscle-invasive bladder cancer (MIBC) treated with radical radiotherapy, DCE MRI may prove reliable in distinguishing radiation-induced changes in the bladder from residual or recurrent tumour (Dobson et al. 2001). Data from small imaging studies, aiming to identify responders to neoadjuvant chemotherapy, suggest that fast DCE MRI can predict whether a patient with regionally metastatic or unresectable bladder cancer will respond to chemotherapy after two cycles of treatment. Furthermore, DW MRI seems to be useful to accurately predict pathologic complete response in patients with MIBC, allowing more optimal patient selection in bladder-sparing protocols (Yoshida et al. 2014).

5.1.2 Metastatic Setting

Bladder cancer (BC) shows metastatic disease at diagnosis in 10–15% of patients. Even patients with initially local disease develop metastases in 50% of cases 2 years after primary diagnosis (Stein et al. 2001). A limited number of studies evaluated the value of [18F]FDG PET/CT in therapy response assessment of metastatic BC. In a study by Kollberg et al., 50 patients with metastatic-invasive BC underwent a [18F]FDG PET/CT scan before and after induction chemotherapy to compare metabolic response and histopathological response in surgically removed lymph node metastases. Correlation of metabolic response evaluated by [18F]FDG PET/CT and histopathological response was shown in 86% of cases. The authors concluded that [18F]FDG PET/CT might predict histological therapy response to chemotherapy (Kollberg et al. 2017). Giannatempo et al. assessed early metabolic therapy response in 31 patients with metastatic transitional cell carcinoma undergoing [18F]FDG PET scan at baseline and after 2 cycles of a combined chemotherapy. Metabolic responders showed a median progression-free survival (PFS) of 8 months compared with 3 months in the group of non-responders and had a significantly longer OS (Giannatempo et al. 2014). The potential clinical value of [18F]FDG PET/CT in therapy response assessment of BC and its predictive value have to be evaluated in future larger studies.

5.2 Follow-Up

The evaluation of tumour recurrence after curative chemoradiation for BC is not well described in the literature. General recommendations are not based on high level of evidence. According to the EAU guidelines and NCCN guidelines, a close follow-up could be considered. Four-monthly follow-up CT scans during the first year are suggested. Afterwards six-monthly CT until year 3 and annual imaging thereafter are advised according to the EAU guidelines (Witjes et al. 2014). If patients are treated with full-dose primary chemoradiotherapy, imaging of the chest, abdomen and pelvic region with contrast is advised by the NCCN guidelines in combination with cystoscopic surveillance (Clark et al. 2016).

There are only few studies investigating the usefulness of [18F]FDG PET/CT in the restaging of recurrent/metastatic BC and its impact on therapy treatment planning. In a systematic review and meta-analysis, Lu et al. showed a pooled sensitivity of 82% and a specificity of 89%, for staging and restaging of metastatic lesions. Similar results were obtained in a recently published study by Alongi et al., demonstrating a sensitivity of 87% and a specificity of 94% for [18F]FDG PET/CT in restaging of recurrent BC. [18F]FDG PET/CT influenced treatment decision in 40% of patients; a negative PET/CT scan was significantly associated with a longer PFS and OS (Alongi et al. 2017). According to these results, [18F]FDG PET/CT might be a promising diagnostic procedure in restaging of recurrent/metastatic BC but needs to be investigated in further studies.

6 Kidney Cancer

6.1 Response Assessment

6.1.1 Primary Setting

In recent years, the role of imaging in the management of advanced renal cell carcinoma (RCC) has changed dramatically, especially in terms of the new relevance of the RCC subtypes, treatment-related changes on imaging, new tumour response criteria and commonly encountered drug toxicities. With the increasing use of molecular targeted therapy, radiologists are often faced with unusual patterns of treatment response that differ from the response to conventional chemotherapy because of the novel mechanism of action of targeted agents. As a consequence, the traditionally used RECIST criteria, which depend on changes in tumour size, may be inadequate for the accurate assessment of tumour response to targeted therapy. It is critical to be able to differentiate pseudoprogression from true progression on imaging, and personalized assessment of treatment response is necessary. Therefore, there is a need for tumour response criteria that are better adapted to molecular targeted therapy–related changes, such as the Choi (Choi et al. 2007), Size and Attenuation CT (SACT) (Smith et al. 2010a) or Morphology, Attenuation, Size, and Structure (MASS) (Smith et al. 2010b) criteria. Early identification of treatment responders and non-responders is also important to minimize unnecessary toxicities in patients not receiving benefit and to allow those patients to try alternative therapies (Shinagare et al. 2012).

6.1.2 Metastatic Setting

In the setting of metastatic disease, new selective multi-target receptor tyrosine kinase inhibitors (TKI), e.g. sunitinib and sorafenib, are used, providing increased PFS and better quality of life. Several studies have been published on the role of [^{18}F]FDG PET/CT in assessing therapy response in metastatic RCC patients treated with TKIs.

Lyrdal et al. evaluated 10 patients with metastatic RCC on a lesion-based analysis. [^{18}F]FDG PET/CT was performed at baseline before and 1–2 months after the start of treatment with sorafenib. Mean [^{18}F]FDG-uptake in all lesions decreased to 75% (71% in soft tissue lesions and 82% in skeletal lesions) compared to the initial mean glucose uptake at baseline PET/CT. A decrease of >20% in mean glucose uptake was associated with a better OS compared to patients with less response (18.1 vs. 12.9 months) (Lyrdal et al. 2009). Vercellino et al. also evaluated the usefulness of [^{18}F]FDG PET/CT for early metabolic response assessment in 12 patients treated with two cycles of sunitinib (PET/CT was performed at baseline and at day 42 after the end of the first cycle). Morphologic response on CT after two cycles of therapy was used as reference standard. PET/CT results with a decrease in SUVmax (−17%) after one cycle of sunitinib were consistent with findings of later CT results in 9 of 11 patients. Metabolic partial response on PET/CT was associated with a longer PFS (Vercellino et al. 2009). In a prospective study of Minamimoto et al., 12 patients underwent [^{18}F]FDG PET/CT before TKI treatment and after one cycle of therapy (sorafenib 7 patients, sunitinib 5 patients). The authors concluded that [^{18}F]FDG PET/CT shows potential for evaluating early treatment response to TKIs in metastatic RCC and for predicting PFS (Minamimoto et al. 2010). Ueno et al. investigated the prognostic value of the [^{18}F]FDG PET/CT for PFS and OS in 35 patients (19 sunitinib, 16 sorafenib) (PET/CT before the start of TKI treatment and 4 weeks after). They concluded that combined metabolic response criteria and morphological criteria could predict PFS and OS (Ueno et al. 2012). In accordance with these results, a prospective study by Revheim et al. including 14 patients with metastatic RCC showed that a high baseline [^{18}F]FDG uptake indicates aggressive disease, and the degree of reduction in [^{18}F]FDG uptake after sunitinib treatment adds valuable prognostic information (Revheim et al. 2011). Accordingly, Farnebo et al. showed that the assessment of early changes in PET-derived parameters undergoing treatment with TKIs can possibly predict PFS and OS in patients with metastatic RCC (Farnebo et al. 2014). A previously published study by Horn et al. investigated early therapy response in patients treated with sunitinib in metastatic RCC by [^{18}F]FDG, for the assessment of the metabolic response, and [^{18}F]fluorothymidine (FLT), for the assessment of the proliferative response (each baseline scan and scan after 1–4 weeks). Metabolic response ([^{18}F] FDG uptake decrease by >25%) was shown in 5/19 of patients, and metabolic disease progression ([^{18}F]FDG-uptake increase >25%) was observed in 2/19 patients. Similarly, a partial proliferative response (proliferation rate reduced of >25%) was found in 9/19 of patients, and proliferative disease progression (increase of proliferation rate >25%) was observed in 1/19 of patients. In contrast to metabolic response, proliferative response was observed at the earliest point of follow-up (1 week) and seemed to be stable. These results show an immediate and sustained proliferative response followed by a delayed metabolic response beginning after 2 weeks in metastatic RCC treated with daily sunitinib (Horn et al. 2015). The results provide evidence of tumour response to lower-dose sunitinib while also supporting the inclusion of PET imaging as a tool for early assessment in oncological clinical trials. Besides the use of TKIs, [^{18}F]FDG PET/CT might accurately predict PFS and can guide decisions on whether to continue or change treatments for patients with everolimus-treated RCC (Ito et al. 2017).

To date, the role of PET/CT using [^{18}F]FDG in assessing response to TKIs in metastatic RCC is still not well defined, partly due to heterogeneity of available studies (Caldarella et al. 2014). Although further research is warranted, [^{18}F]FDG PET/CT seems to be a promising imaging method for TKI therapy response assessment in metastatic RCC. As discussed above, numerous studies showed a positive association between PET-based metabolic response and survival. Besides [^{18}F]FDG PET/CT, FLT PET/CT might also be used for evaluating response to TKIs.

6.2 Follow-Up

Kidney cancer is not very sensitive to radiation therapy, and as such there is no evidence to treat patients with kidney cancer with EBRT in the curative setting. More recently, SBRT for primary renal cell carcinoma is under investigation and shows promising local control rates and acceptable toxicity (Siva et al. 2012). However, further prospective studies assessing the role of this treatment technique in medically inoperable patients are needed.

There are very few data available reporting treatment assessment after radiation therapy in kidney cancer patients. In general, an individualised, risk-based, approach with CT chest and abdomen is recommended according to the EAU guidelines. To reduce radiation exposure, MRI is suggested to be used outside the thorax (Ljungberg et al. 2015). Furthermore a recently published meta-analysis on the diagnostic performance of [^{18}F]FDG PET/CT in restaging of renal cell cancer showed good results with a pooled patient-based sensitivity of 86% and a specificity of 88% (Ma et al. 2017).

7 Conclusion

Overall, the current role of imaging in response assessment or monitoring for GU tumours is very limited. This is in contrast to the growing role of imaging in other pelvic tumours, such as rectal and cervical cancers. However, advances are made in the field of PCa, with some more recent imaging techniques that are currently under investigation. However, there is a role of imaging for GU tumours in the recurrence setting.

References

Afshar-Oromieh A, Zechmann CM, Malcher A, Eder M, Eisenhut M, Linhart HG et al (2014) Comparison of PET imaging with a 68Ga-labelled PSMA ligand and 18F-choline-based PET/CT for the diagnosis of recurrent prostate cancer. Eur J Nucl Med Mol Imaging 41(1):11–20

Afshar-Oromieh A, Avtzi E, Giesel FL, Holland-Letz T, Linhart HG, Eder M et al (2015) The diagnostic value of PET/CT imaging with the (68)Ga-labelled PSMA ligand HBED-CC in the diagnosis of recurrent prostate cancer. Eur J Nucl Med Mol Imaging 42(2):197–209

Afshar-Oromieh A, Holland-Letz T, Giesel FL, Kratochwil C, Mier W, Haufe S et al (2017) Diagnostic

performance of 68Ga-PSMA-11 (HBED-CC) PET/CT in patients with recurrent prostate cancer: evaluation in 1007 patients. Eur J Nucl Med Mol Imaging 44(8):1258–1268
Ahmadzadehfar H, Eppard E, Kürpig S, Fimmers R, Yordanova A, Schlenkhoff CD et al (2016) Therapeutic response and side effects of repeated radioligand therapy with Lu-PSMA-DKFZ-617 of castrate-resistant metastatic prostate cancer. Oncotarget 7(11):12477–12488
Akin O, Gultekin DH, Vargas HA, Zheng J, Moskowitz C, Pei X et al (2011) Incremental value of diffusion weighted and dynamic contrast enhanced MRI in the detection of locally recurrent prostate cancer after radiation treatment: preliminary results. Eur Radiol 21(9):1970–1978
Albers P, Albrecht W, Algaba F, Bokemeyer C, Cohn-Cedermark G, Fizazi K et al (2015) Guidelines on testicular Cancer: 2015 update. Eur Urol 68(6):1054–1068
Alongi P, Caobelli F, Gentile R, Stefano A, Russo G, Albano D et al (2017) Recurrent bladder carcinoma: clinical and prognostic role of 18 F-FDG PET/CT. Eur J Nucl Med Mol Imaging 44(2):224–233
Alonzi R, Padhani AR, Taylor NJ, Collins DJ, D'Arcy JA, Stirling JJ et al (2011) Antivascular effects of neoadjuvant androgen deprivation for prostate Cancer: an in vivo human study using susceptibility and Relaxivity dynamic MRI. Int J Radiat Oncol. 80(3):721–727
Ambrosini V, Zucchini G, Nicolini S, Berselli A, Nanni C, Allegri V et al (2014) 18F-FDG PET/CT impact on testicular tumours clinical management. Eur J Nucl Med Mol Imaging 41(4):668–673
Arumainayagam N, Kumaar S, Ahmed HU, Moore CM, Payne H, Freeman A et al (2010) Accuracy of multiparametric magnetic resonance imaging in detecting recurrent prostate cancer after radiotherapy. BJU Int 106(7):991–997
Bachner M, Loriot Y, Gross-Goupil M, Zucali PA, Horwich A, Germa-Lluch J-R et al (2012) 2-18fluoro-deoxy-D-glucose positron emission tomography (FDG-PET) for postchemotherapy seminoma residual lesions: a retrospective validation of the SEMPET trial. Ann Oncol 23(1):59–64
Baum RP, Kulkarni HR, Schuchardt C, Singh A, Wirtz M, Wiessalla S et al (2016) 177Lu-labeled prostate-specific membrane antigen Radioligand therapy of metastatic castration-resistant prostate Cancer: safety and efficacy. J Nucl Med 57(7):1006–1013
Becherer A, De Santis M, Karanikas G, Szabó M, Bokemeyer C, Dohmen BM et al (2005) FDG PET is superior to CT in the prediction of viable tumour in post-chemotherapy seminoma residuals. Eur J Radiol 54(2):284–288
Beyer J, Albers P, Altena R, Aparicio J, Bokemeyer C, Busch J et al (2013) Maintaining success, reducing treatment burden, focusing on survivorship: highlights from the third European consensus conference on diagnosis and treatment of germ-cell cancer. Ann Oncol 24(4):878–888
Bonekamp D, Wolf MB, Edler C, Katayama S, Schlemmer H-P (2016) Herfarth K, et al. Dynamic contrast enhanced MRI monitoring of primary proton and carbon ion irradiation of prostate cancer using a novel hypofractionated raster scan technique, Radiother Oncol
Calabria F, Gallo G, Schillaci O, Cascini G (2015) Biodistribution, imaging protocols and diagnostic accuracy of PET with tracers of lipogenesis in imaging prostate cancer: a comparison between 11C-choline, 18Ffluoroethylcholine and 18F-methylcholine. Curr Pharm Des 21(32):4738–4747
Caldarella C, Muoio B, Isgrò MA, Porfiri E, Treglia G, Giovanella L (2014) The role of fluorine-18-fluorodeoxyglucose positron emission tomography in evaluating the response to tyrosine-kinase inhibitors in patients with metastatic primary renal cell carcinoma. Radiol Oncol 48(3):219–227
Castellucci P, Fuccio C, Nanni C, Santi I, Rizzello A, Lodi F et al (2009) Influence of trigger PSA and PSA kinetics on 11C-choline PET/CT detection rate in patients with biochemical relapse after radical prostatectomy. J Nucl Med 50(9):1394–1400
Ceci F, Castellucci P, Graziani T, Schiavina R, Brunocilla E, Mazzarotto R et al (2014) 11C-choline PET/CT detects the site of relapse in the majority of prostate cancer patients showing biochemical recurrence after EBRT. Eur J Nucl Med Mol Imaging 41(5):878–886
Ceci F, Castellucci P, Graziani T, Schiavina R, Renzi R, Borghesi M et al (2016) 11C-choline PET/CT in castration-resistant prostate cancer patients treated with docetaxel. Eur J Nucl Med Mol Imaging 43(1):84–91
Ceci F, Herrmann K, Hadaschik B, Castellucci P, Fanti S (2017) Therapy assessment in prostate cancer using choline and PSMA PET/CT. Eur J Nucl Med Mol Imaging 44(S1):78–83
Cellini N, Morganti AG, Mattiucci GC, Valentini V, Leone M, Luzi S et al (2002) Analysis of intraprostatic failures in patients treated with hormonal therapy and radiotherapy: implications for conformal therapy planning. Int J Radiat Oncol. 53(3):595–599
Choi H, Charnsangavej C, Faria SC, Macapinlac HA, Burgess MA, Patel SR et al (2007) Correlation of computed tomography and positron emission tomography in patients with metastatic gastrointestinal stromal tumor treated at a single institution with imatinib mesylate: proposal of new computed tomography response criteria. J Clin Oncol 25(13):1753–1759
Clark PE, Spiess PE, Agarwal N, Bangs R, Boorjian SA, Buyyounouski MK et al (2016) NCCN guidelines insights: bladder Cancer, version 2.2016. J Natl Compr Cancer Netw 14(10):1213–1224
Coakley FV, Teh HS, Qayyum A, Swanson MG, Lu Y, Roach M et al (2004) Endorectal MR imaging and MR spectroscopic imaging for locally recurrent prostate Cancer after external beam radiation therapy: preliminary experience. Radiology 233(2):441–448
Coen JJ, Zietman AL, Thakral H, Shipley WU (2002) Radical radiation for localized prostate Cancer: local

persistence of disease results in a late wave of metastases. J Clin Oncol 20(15):3199–3205
Cyran CC, Paprottka PM, Schwarz B, Sourbron S, Ingrisch M, von Einem J et al (2012) Perfusion MRI for monitoring the effect of Sorafenib on experimental prostate carcinoma: a validation study. Am J Roentgenol 198(2):384–391
Dahut WL, Madan RA, Karakunnel JJ, Adelberg D, Gulley JL, Turkbey IB et al (2013) Phase II clinical trial of cediranib in patients with metastatic castration-resistant prostate cancer. BJU Int 111(8): 1269–1280
De Giorgi U, Caroli P, Burgio SL, Menna C, Conteduca V, Bianchi E et al (2014) Early outcome prediction on 18F-fluorocholine PET/CT in metastatic castration-resistant prostate cancer patients treated with abiraterone. Oncotarget 5(23):12448–12458
De Giorgi U, Caroli P, Scarpi E, Conteduca V, Burgio SL, Menna C et al (2015) 18F-Fluorocholine PET/CT for early response assessment in patients with metastatic castration-resistant prostate cancer treated with enzalutamide. Eur J Nucl Med Mol Imaging 42(8):1276–1283
Dobson MJ, Carrington BM, Collins CD, Ryder WD, Read G, Hutchinson CE et al (2001) The assessment of irradiated bladder carcinoma using dynamic contrast-enhanced MR imaging. Clin Radiol 56(2):94–98
Donati OF, Jung S (2013) Il, Vargas HA, Gultekin DH, Zheng J, Moskowitz CS, et al. multiparametric prostate MR imaging with T2-weighted, diffusion-weighted, and dynamic contrast-enhanced sequences: are all pulse sequences necessary to detect locally recurrent prostate Cancer after radiation therapy? Radiology 268(2):440–450
Egawa S, Carter SS, Wheeler TM, Scardino PT (1989) Ultrasonographic changes in the normal and malignant prostate after definitive radiotherapy. Urol Clin North Am 16(4):741–749
Egawa S, Carter SS, Wheeler TM, Scardino PT (1992a) Sonographic monitoring of prostate cancer after definitive radiotherapy. Urology 40(3):230–236
Egawa S, Wheeler TM, Greene DR, Scardino PT (1992b) Detection of residual prostate cancer after radiotherapy by sonographically guided needle biopsy. Urology 39(4):358–363
Eiber M, Holzapfel K, Ganter C, Epple K, Metz S, Geinitz H et al (2011) Whole-body MRI including diffusion-weighted imaging (DWI) for patients with recurring prostate cancer: technical feasibility and assessment of lesion conspicuity in DWI. J Magn Reson Imaging 33(5):1160–1170
Eiber M, Maurer T, Souvatzoglou M, Beer AJ, Ruffani A, Haller B et al (2015) Evaluation of hybrid 68Ga-PSMA ligand PET/CT in 248 patients with biochemical recurrence after radical prostatectomy. J Nucl Med 56(5):668–674
Evangelista L, Zattoni F, Guttilla A, Saladini G, Zattoni F, Colletti PM et al (2013) Choline PET or PET/CT and biochemical relapse of prostate cancer. Clin Nucl Med 38(5):305–314
von Eyben FE, Kairemo K (2014) Meta-analysis of 11C-choline and 18F-choline PET/CT for management of patients with prostate cancer. Nucl Med Commun 35(3):221–230
Fanti S, Minozzi S, Castellucci P, Balduzzi S, Herrmann K, Krause BJ et al (2016) PET/CT with 11C-choline for evaluation of prostate cancer patients with biochemical recurrence: meta-analysis and critical review of available data. Eur J Nucl Med Mol Imaging 43(1):55–69
Farnebo J, Grybäck P, Harmenberg U, Laurell A, Wersäll P, Blomqvist LK et al (2014) Volumetric FDG-PET predicts overall and progression- free survival after 14 days of targeted therapy in metastatic renal cell carcinoma. BMC Cancer 14(1):408
Fendler WP, Reinhardt S, Ilhan H, Delker A, Böning G, Gildehaus FJ et al (2017) Preliminary experience with dosimetry, response and patient reported outcome after 177Lu-PSMA-617 therapy for metastatic castration-resistant prostate cancer. Oncotarget 8(2):3581–3590
Fennessy FM, McKay RR, Beard CJ, Taplin M-E, Tempany CM (2014) Dynamic contrast-enhanced magnetic resonance imaging in prostate cancer clinical trials: potential roles and possible pitfalls. Transl Oncol 7(1):120–129
Foltz WD, Wu A, Chung P, Catton C, Bayley A, Milosevic M et al (2013) Changes in apparent diffusion coefficient and T_2 relaxation during radiotherapy for prostate cancer. J Magn Reson Imaging 37(4):909–916
Fortuin AS, Brüggemann R, van der Linden J, Panfilov I, Israël B, Scheenen TWJ et al (2018) Ultra-small superparamagnetic iron oxides for metastatic lymph node detection: back on the block. Wiley Interdiscip Rev Nanomed Nanobiotechnol 10:e1471
Fox EP, Weathers TD, Williams SD, Loehrer PJ, Ulbright TM, Donohue JP et al (1993) Outcome analysis for patients with persistent nonteratomatous germ cell tumor in postchemotherapy retroperitoneal lymph node dissections. J Clin Oncol 11(7):1294–1299
Ghosh A, Heston WDW (2004) Tumor target prostate specific membrane antigen (PSMA) and its regulation in prostate cancer. J Cell Biochem 91(3):528–539
Giannatempo P, Alessi A, Miceli R, Raggi D, Farè E, Nicolai N et al (2014) Interim Fluorine-18 Fluorodeoxyglucose positron emission tomography for early metabolic assessment of therapeutic response to chemotherapy for metastatic transitional cell carcinoma. Clin Genitourin Cancer 12(6):433–439
Giesel FL, Hadaschik B, Cardinale J, Radtke J, Vinsensia M, Lehnert W et al (2017) F-18 labelled PSMA-1007: biodistribution, radiation dosimetry and histopathological validation of tumor lesions in prostate cancer patients. Eur J Nucl Med Mol Imaging 44(4):678–688
Giovacchini G, Picchio M, Coradeschi E, Bettinardi V, Gianolli L, Scattoni V et al (2010) Predictive factors of [11C]choline PET/CT in patients with biochemical failure after radical prostatectomy. Eur J Nucl Med Mol Imaging 37(2):301–309
Graafland NM, Valdés Olmos RA, Teertstra HJ, Martijn Kerst J, Bergman AM, Horenblas S (2010) 18 F-FDG

PET/CT for monitoring induction chemotherapy in patients with primary inoperable penile carcinoma: first clinical results. Eur J Nucl Med Mol Imaging 37(8):1474–1480
Haider MA, Chung P, Sweet J, Toi A, Jhaveri K, Ménard C et al (2008) Dynamic contrast-enhanced magnetic resonance imaging for localization of recurrent prostate Cancer after external beam radiotherapy. Int J Radiat Oncol. 70(2):425–430
Hakenberg OW, Compérat EM, Minhas S, Necchi A, Protzel C, Watkin N (2015) EAU guidelines on penile Cancer: 2014 update. Eur Urol 67(1):142–150
Heidenreich A, Bastian PJ, Bellmunt J, Bolla M, Joniau S, van der Kwast T et al (2014) EAU guidelines on prostate Cancer. Part II: treatment of advanced, relapsing, and castration-resistant prostate Cancer. Eur Urol 65(2):467–479
Helyar V, Mohan HK, Barwick T, Livieratos L, Gnanasegaran G, Clarke SEM et al (2010) The added value of multislice SPECT/CT in patients with equivocal bony metastasis from carcinoma of the prostate. Eur J Nucl Med Mol Imaging 37(4):706–713
Horn KP, Yap JT, Agarwal N, Morton KA, Kadrmas DJ, Beardmore B et al (2015) FDG and FLT-PET for early measurement of response to 37.5 mg daily sunitinib therapy in metastatic renal cell carcinoma. Cancer Imaging 15(1):15
Ito H, Kondo K, Kawahara T, Kaneta T, Tateishi U, Ueno D et al (2017) One-month assessment of renal cell carcinoma treated by everolimus using FDG PET/CT predicts progression-free and overall survival. Cancer Chemother Pharmacol 79(5):855–861
Jadvar H, Desai B, Ji L, Conti PS, Dorff TB, Groshen SG et al (2012) Prospective evaluation of 18F-NaF and 18F-FDG PET/CT in detection of occult metastatic disease in biochemical recurrence of prostate Cancer. Clin Nucl Med 37(7):637–643
Johnstone PA, Tarman GJ, Riffenburgh R, Rohde DC, Puckett ML, Kane CJ (1997) Yield of imaging and scintigraphy assessing biochemical failure in prostate cancer patients. Urol Oncol 3(4):108–112
Johnstone PAS, McFarland JT, Riffeburgh RH, Amling CL (2001) Efficacy of digital rectal examination after radiotherapy for prostate Cancer. J Urol 166(5):1684–1687
Kabalin JN, Hodge KK, McNeal JE, Freiha FS, Stamey TA (1989) Identification of residual cancer in the prostate following radiation therapy: role of transrectal ultrasound guided biopsy and prostate specific antigen. J Urol 142(2 Pt 1):326–331
Kane CJ, Amling CL, Johnstone PAS, Pak N, Lance RS, Thrasher JB et al (2003) Limited value of bone scintigraphy and computed tomography in assessing biochemical failure after radical prostatectomy. Urology 61(3):607–611
Karunanithi S, Sharma P, Naswa N, Soundararajan R, Mohapatra T, Malhotra A et al (2012) Primary penile lymphoma: 18f-fdg pet-CT for accurate staging and response monitoring. Diagnostic Interv Radiol 19(2):130–133
Kestin LL, Vicini FA, Ziaja EL, Stromberg JS, Frazier RC, Martinez AA (1999) Defining biochemical cure for prostate carcinoma patients treated with external beam radiation therapy. Cancer 86(8):1557–1566
Kim CK, Park BK, Lee HM (2009) Prediction of locally recurrent prostate cancer after radiation therapy: incremental value of 3T diffusion-weighted MRI. J Magn Reson Imaging 29(2):391–397
Kollberg P, Almquist H, Bläckberg M, Cwikiel M, Gudjonsson S, Lyttkens K et al (2017) [^{18} F] Fluorodeoxyglucose-positron emission tomography/ computed tomography response evaluation can predict histological response at surgery after induction chemotherapy for oligometastatic bladder cancer. Scand J Urol 51(4):308–313
Kratochwil C, Giesel FL, Stefanova M, Benešova M, Bronzel M, Afshar-Oromieh A et al (2016) PSMA-targeted radionuclide therapy of metastatic castration-resistant prostate Cancer with 177Lu-labeled PSMA-617. J Nucl Med 57(8):1170–1176
Lecouvet FE, El Mouedden J, Collette L, Coche E, Danse E, Jamar F et al (2012) Can whole-body magnetic resonance imaging with diffusion-weighted imaging replace Tc 99m bone scanning and computed tomography for single-step detection of metastases in patients with high-risk prostate Cancer? Eur Urol 62(1): 68–75
Lecouvet FE, Talbot JN, Messiou C, Bourguet P, Liu Y, de Souza NM et al (2014) Monitoring the response of bone metastases to treatment with magnetic resonance imaging and nuclear medicine techniques: a review and position statement by the European Organisation for Research and Treatment of Cancer imaging group. Eur J Cancer 50(15):2519–2531
Leijte JAP, Kirrander P, Antonini N, Windahl T, Horenblas S (2008) Recurrence patterns of squamous cell carcinoma of the penis: recommendations for follow-up based on a two-Centre analysis of 700 patients. Eur Urol 54(1):161–169
Liu IJ, Zafar MB, Lai Y-H, Segall GM, Terris MK (2001) Fluorodeoxyglucose positron emission tomography studies in diagnosis and staging of clinically organ-confined prostate cancer. Urology 57(1):108–111
Ljungberg B, Bensalah K, Canfield S, Dabestani S, Hofmann F, Hora M et al (2015) EAU Guidelines on Renal Cell Carcinoma: 2014 Update. Eur Urol 67(5):913–924
Lütje S, Cohnen J, Gomez B, Grüneisen J, Sawicki M, Rübben H et al (2017) Integrated ^{68} Ga-HBED-CC-PSMA-PET/MRI in patients with suspected recurrent prostate cancer. Nuklearmedizin 56(3):73–81
Lyrdal D, Boijsen M, Suurküla M, Lundstam S, Stierner U (2009) Evaluation of sorafenib treatment in metastatic renal cell carcinoma with 2-fluoro-2-deoxyglucose positron emission tomography and computed tomography. Nucl Med Commun 30(7):519–524
Ma H, Shen G, Liu B, Yang Y, Ren P, Kuang A (2017) Diagnostic performance of 18F-FDG PET or PET/CT in restaging renal cell carcinoma. Nucl Med Commun 38(2):156–163

Maurer T, Eiber M, Fanti S, Budäus L, Panebianco V, Karnes RJ et al (2016) Imaging for prostate Cancer recurrence. Eur Urol Focus 2(2):139–150

Menard C, Smith IC, Somorjai RL, Leboldus L, Patel R, Littman C et al (2001) Magnetic resonance spectroscopy of the malignant prostate gland after radiotherapy: a histopathologic study of diagnostic validity. Int J Radiat Oncol. 50(2):317–323

Meredith G, Wong D, Yaxley J, Coughlin G, Thompson L, Kua B et al (2016) The use of ^{68} Ga-PSMA PET CT in men with biochemical recurrence after definitive treatment of acinar prostate cancer. BJU Int 118:49–55

Minamimoto R, Nakaigawa N, Tateishi U, Suzuki A, Shizukuishi K, Kishida T et al (2010) Evaluation of response to multikinase inhibitor in metastatic renal cell carcinoma by FDG PET/contrast-enhanced CT. Clin Nucl Med 35(12):918–923

Mohler JL, Armstrong AJ, Bahnson RR, D'Amico AV, Davis BJ, Eastham JA et al (2016) Prostate Cancer, version 1.2016. J Natl Compr Cancer Netw 14(1): 19–30

Morgan VA, Riches SF, Giles S, Dearnaley D (2012) deSouza NM. Diffusion-weighted MRI for locally recurrent prostate Cancer after external beam radiotherapy. Am J Roentgenol 198(3):596–602

Morigi JJ, Stricker PD, van Leeuwen PJ, Tang R, Ho B, Nguyen Q et al (2015) Prospective comparison of 18F-Fluoromethylcholine versus 68Ga-PSMA PET/CT in prostate Cancer patients who have rising PSA after curative treatment and are being considered for targeted therapy. J Nucl Med 56(8):1185–1190

Necchi A, Nicolai N, Alessi A, Miceli R, Giannatempo P, Raggi D et al (2016) Interim 18F-Fluorodeoxyglucose positron emission tomography for early metabolic assessment of response to cisplatin, etoposide, and bleomycin chemotherapy for metastatic seminoma: clinical value and future directions. Clin Genitourin Cancer 14(3):249–254

Oldenburg J, Fosså SD, Nuver J, Heidenreich A, Schmoll H-J, Bokemeyer C et al (2013) Testicular seminoma and non-seminoma: ESMO Clinical Practice Guidelines for diagnosis, treatment and follow-up. Ann Oncol 24(Suppl 6):vi125–vi132

Oppenheimer DC, Weinberg EP, Hollenberg GM, Meyers SP (2016) Multiparametric magnetic resonance imaging of recurrent prostate Cancer. J Clin Imaging Sci 6:18

Park SY, Kim CK, Park BK, Park W, Park HC, Han DH et al (2012) Early changes in apparent diffusion coefficient from diffusion-weighted MR imaging during radiotherapy for prostate Cancer. Int J Radiat Oncol 83(2):749–755

Perera M, Papa N, Christidis D, Wetherell D, Hofman MS, Murphy DG et al (2016) Sensitivity, specificity, and predictors of positive 68Ga–prostate-specific membrane antigen positron emission tomography in advanced prostate Cancer: a systematic review and meta-analysis. Eur Urol 70(6):926–937

Pezaro CJ, Omlin A, Lorente D, Nava Rodrigues D, Ferraldeschi R, Bianchini D et al (2014) Visceral disease in castration-resistant prostate Cancer. Eur Urol 65(2):270–273

PfannenbergA, Oechsle K, Bokemeyer C, Kollmannsberger C, Dohmen B, Bares R et al (2004) The role of [18F] FDG-PET, CT/MRI and tumor marker kinetics in the evaluation of postchemotherapy residual masses in metastatic germ cell tumors?Prospects for management. World J Urol 22(2):132–139

Piccardo A, Paparo F, Piccazzo R, Picazzo R, Naseri M, Ricci P et al (2014) Value of fused 18F-choline-PET/MRI to evaluate prostate cancer relapse in patients showing biochemical recurrence after EBRT: preliminary results. Biomed Res Int 2014:103718

Pichler BJ, Wehrl HF, Kolb A, Judenhofer MS (2008) Positron emission tomography/magnetic resonance imaging: the next generation of multimodality imaging? Semin Nucl Med 38(3):199–208

Pollack A, Zagars GK, Starkschall G, Antolak JA, Lee JJ, Huang E et al (2002) Prostate cancer radiation dose response: results of the M. D. Anderson phase III randomized trial. Int J Radiat Oncol. 53(5): 1097–1105

Pucar D, Shukla-Dave A, Hricak H, Moskowitz CS, Kuroiwa K, Olgac S et al (2005) Prostate Cancer: correlation of MR imaging and MR spectroscopy with pathologic findings after radiation therapy–initial experience. Radiology 236(2):545–553

Revheim ME, Winge-Main AK, Hagen G, Fjeld JG, Fosså SD, Lilleby W (2011) Combined positron emission tomography/computed tomography in Sunitinib ther apy assessment of patients with metastatic renal cell carcinoma. Clin Oncol 23(5):339–343

Roach M, Hanks G, Thames H, Schellhammer P, Shipley WU, Sokol GH et al (2006) Defining biochemical failure following radiotherapy with or without hormonal therapy in men with clinically localized prostate cancer: recommendations of the RTOG-ASTRO Phoenix consensus conference. Int J Radiat Oncol. 65(4):965–974

Rossari JR, Vora T, Gil T (2010) Advances in penile cancer management. Curr Opin Oncol 22(3):226–235

Rouvière O, Valette O, Grivolat S, Colin-Pangaud C, Bouvier R, Chapelon JY et al (2004) Recurrent prostate cancer after external beam radiotherapy: value of contrast-enhanced dynamic MRI in localizing intraprostatic tumor—correlation with biopsy findings. Urology 63(5):922–927

Rowe SP, Gage KL, Faraj SF, Macura KJ, Cornish TC, Gonzalez-Roibon N et al (2015) 18F-DCFBC PET/CT for PSMA-based detection and characterization of primary prostate Cancer. J Nucl Med 56(7):1003–1010

Rowe SP, Macura KJ, Mena E, Blackford AL, Nadal R, Antonarakis ES et al (2016) PSMA-based [18F] DCFPyL PET/CT is superior to conventional imaging for lesion detection in patients with metastatic prostate Cancer. Mol Imaging Biol 18(3):411–419

Roy C, Foudi F, Charton J, Jung M, Lang H, Saussine C et al (2013) Comparative sensitivities of functional MRI sequences in detection of local recurrence of prostate carcinoma after radical prostatectomy

or external-beam radiotherapy. Am J Roentgenol 200(4):W361–W368
Roznovanu SL, Rădulescu D, Novac C, Stolnicu S (2005) The morphologic changes induced by hormone and radiation therapy on prostate carcinoma. Rev Med Chir Soc Med Nat Iasi 109(2):337–342
Rybalov M, Pruim J, Leliveld AM, Rosati S, Veltman NC, Dierckx RA, De Jong IJ, Breeuwsma J (2012) [C-11]choline PET for the intraprostatic tumor characterization and localization in recurrent prostate cancer after EBRT. Q J Nucl Med Mol Imaging 56(2): 202–208
Sadeghi R, Gholami H, Zakavi SR, Kakhki VRD, Horenblas S (2012) Accuracy of 18F-FDG PET/CT for diagnosing inguinal lymph node involvement in penile squamous cell carcinoma. Clin Nucl Med 37(5):436–441
Sala E, Eberhardt SC, Akin O, Moskowitz CS, Onyebuchi CN, Kuroiwa K et al (2006) Endorectal MR imaging before salvage prostatectomy: tumor localization and staging. Radiology 238(1):176–183
Schwarzenböck SM, Eiber M, Kundt G, Retz M, Sakretz M, Kurth J et al (2016) Prospective evaluation of [11C]choline PET/CT in therapy response assessment of standardized docetaxel first-line chemotherapy in patients with advanced castration refractory prostate cancer. Eur J Nucl Med Mol Imaging 43(12):2105–2113
Schwarzenboeck SM, Rauscher I, Bluemel C (2017) Fendler WP. Rowe SP, Pomper MG, et al. PSMA Ligands for PET-Imaging of Prostate Cancer. Prostate Cancer J Nucl Med
Shinagare AB, Krajewski KM, Jagannathan JP, Ramaiya NH (2012) Genitourinary imaging: part 2, role of imaging in medical Management of Advanced Renal Cell Carcinoma. Am J Roentgenol 199(5):W554–W564
Siva S, Pham D, Gill S, Corcoran NM, Foroudi F (2012) A systematic review of stereotactic radiotherapy ablation for primary renal cell carcinoma. BJU Int 110(11b):E737–E743
Smith AD, Lieber ML, Shah SN (2010a) Assessing tumor response and detecting recurrence in metastatic renal cell carcinoma on targeted therapy: importance of size and attenuation on contrast-enhanced CT. Am J Roentgenol 194(1):157–165
Smith AD, Shah SN, Rini BI, Lieber ML, Remer EM (2010b) Morphology, attenuation, size, and structure (MASS) criteria: assessing response and predicting clinical outcome in metastatic renal cell carcinoma on antiangiogenic targeted therapy. Am J Roentgenol 194(6):1470–1478
Stein JP, Lieskovsky G, Cote R, Groshen S, Feng AC, Boyd S et al (2001) Radical cystectomy in the treatment of invasive bladder cancer: long-term results in 1,054 patients. J Clin Oncol 19(3):666–675
Steyerberg EW, Keizer HJ, Sleijfer DT, Fosså SD, Bajorin DF, Gerl A et al (2000) Retroperitoneal metastases in testicular Cancer: role of CT measurements of residual masses in decision making for resection after chemotherapy. Radiology 215(2):437–444
Thalgott M, Rack B, Eiber M, Souvatzoglou M, Heck MM, Kronester C et al (2015) Categorical versus continuous circulating tumor cell enumeration as early surrogate marker for therapy response and prognosis during docetaxel therapy in metastatic prostate cancer patients. BMC Cancer 15:458
Treglia G, Ceriani L, Sadeghi R, Giovacchini G, Giovanella L (2014a) Relationship between prostate-specific antigen kinetics and detection rate of radiolabelled choline PET/CT in restaging prostate cancer patients: a meta-analysis. Clin Chem Lab Med 52(5):725–733
Treglia G, Sadeghi R, Annunziata S, Caldarella C, Bertagna F, Giovanella L (2014b) Diagnostic performance of fluorine-18-fluorodeoxyglucose positron emission tomography in the postchemotherapy management of patients with seminoma: systematic review and meta-analysis. Biomed Res Int 2014:852681
Ueno D, Yao M, Tateishi U, Minamimoto R, Makiyama K, Hayashi N et al (2012) Early assessment by FDG-PET/CT of patients with advanced renal cell carcinoma treated with tyrosine kinase inhibitors is predictive of disease course. BMC Cancer 12(1):162
Umbehr MH, Müntener M, Hany T, Sulser T, Bachmann LM (2013) The role of 11C-choline and 18F-fluorocholine positron emission tomography (PET) and PET/CT in prostate cancer: a systematic review and meta-analysis. Eur Urol 64(1):106–117
Van Poppel H, Watkin NA, Osanto S, Moonen L, Horwich A, Kataja V (2013) Penile cancer: ESMO Clinical Practice Guidelines for diagnosis, treatment and follow-up. Ann Oncol 24(Suppl 6):vi115–vi124
Vercellino L, Bousquet G, Baillet G, Barré E, Mathieu O, Just P-A et al (2009) ^{18}F-FDG PET/CT imaging for an early assessment of response to Sunitinib in metastatic renal carcinoma: preliminary study. Cancer Biother Radiopharm 24(1):137–144
Viani GA, Stefano EJ, Afonso SL (2009) Higher-than-conventional radiation doses in localized prostate cancer treatment: a meta-analysis of randomized, controlled trials. Int J Radiat Oncol Biol Phys 74(5):1405–1418
Westphalen AC, Kurhanewicz J, Cunha RMG, Hsu I-C, Kornak J, Zhao S et al (2009) T2-weighted endorectal magnetic resonance imaging of prostate cancer after external beam radiation therapy. Int Braz J Urol 35(2):171–182
Wetter A, Lipponer C, Nensa F, Heusch P (2014) R?Bben H, Schlosser TW, et al. quantitative evaluation of bone metastases from prostate cancer with simultaneous [18F] choline PET/MRI: combined SUV and ADC analysis. Ann Nucl Med 28(5):405–410
Witjes JA, Compérat E, Cowan NC, De Santis M, Gakis G, Lebret T, Ribal MJ, Van der Heijden AG, Sherif A, European Association of Urology (2014) EAU guidelines on muscle-invasive and metastatic bladder cancer: summary of the 2013 guidelines. Eur Urol 65(4):778–792. https://doi.org/10.1016/j.eururo.2013.11.046. Epub 2013 Dec 12
Wu LM, Xu J-R, Gu HY, Hua J, Zhu J, Chen J et al (2013) Role of magnetic resonance imaging in the detection

of local prostate Cancer recurrence after external beam radiotherapy and radical prostatectomy. Clin Oncol 25(4):252–264

Yadav MP, Ballal S, Tripathi M, Damle NA, Sahoo RK, Seth A et al (2017) 177Lu-DKFZ-PSMA-617 therapy in metastatic castration resistant prostate cancer: safety, efficacy, and quality of life assessment. Eur J Nucl Med Mol Imaging 44(1):81–91

Yoshida S, Koga F, Kobayashi S, Tanaka H, Satoh S, Fujii Y et al (2014) Diffusion-weighted magnetic resonance imaging in management of bladder cancer, particularly with multimodal bladder-sparing strategy. World J Radiol 6(6):344–354

Yu CY, Desai B, Ji L, Groshen S, Jadvar H (2014) Comparative performance of PET tracers in biochemical recurrence of prostate cancer: a critical analysis of literature. Am J Nucl Med Mol Imaging 4(6): 580–601

Zhang S, Li W, Liang F (2016) Clinical value of fluorine-18 2-fluoro-2-deoxy-D-glucose positron emission tomography/computed tomography in penile cancer. Oncotarget 7:48600–48606

Response Assessment and Follow-Up by Imaging in GYN Tumours

Andrea Rockall, Maximilian P. Schmid, and Judit A. Adam

Contents

1 **Introduction** ... 518

2 **Response Assessment and Outcome Prediction During Radiotherapy in Gynaecological Tumours** ... 519
2.1 Uterine Cervical Cancer ... 519
2.2 Vaginal and Vulvar Cancer ... 521
2.3 Endometrial Cancer ... 521
2.4 Melanoma ... 521

3 **Adaptive Target Volume Definition for Brachytherapy Treatment Planning** ... 522

4 **Response Assessment after Treatment in Gynaecological Tumours: Imaging at the End of Therapy and Surveillance** ... 523
4.1 Uterine Cervical Cancer ... 523
4.2 Endometrial Cancer ... 525

5 **Imaging of Recurrent Disease** ... 526
5.1 Uterine Cervical Cancer ... 526
5.2 Endometrial Cancer ... 527
5.3 Ovarian Cancer ... 527
5.4 Isolated Vaginal Recurrences ... 527

References ... 527

Abstract

Imaging plays an important role in the staging and management of all main gynaecological tumours. Gynaecological tumours treated primarily with radiotherapy such as cervical, vaginal or vulvar cancer typically show considerable tumour shrinkage during treatment. Following the successful completion of initial treatment, there is no strong evidence to support posttreatment imaging surveillance of asymptomatic women. In general, gynaeco-oncological practice, the initial suspicion of disease relapse relies largely on clinical symptoms rather than radiological evidence. However, once clinical relapse is suspected, imaging plays a crucial role in planning salvage therapy.

Typical treatment concepts in locally advanced (non-tubo-ovarian) gynaecological cancers consist of external beam radiotherapy (EBRT) and concomitant chemotherapy followed by brachytherapy. Due to the substantial tumour shrinkage during external beam radiotherapy, the GYN GEC-ESTRO group defined an adaptive target volume concept for MRI-based brachytherapy. So far, target concepts for cervical and vaginal cancer were

A. Rockall
Imperial College London, Imperial College Healthcare NHS Trust, The Royal Marsden NHS Foundation Trust, London, UK
e-mail: a.rockall@imperial.ac.uk

M. P. Schmid
Department of Radiation Oncology, Medical University of Vienna, Vienna, Austria
e-mail: maximilian.schmid@akhwien.at

J. A. Adam (✉)
Department of Radiology and Nuclear Medicine, Amsterdam UMC, University of Amsterdam, Amsterdam, The Netherlands
e-mail: j.a.adam@amsterdamumc.nl

R. G. H. Beets-Tan et al. (eds.), *Imaging and Interventional Radiology for Radiation Oncology*, Medical Radiology, Diagnostic Imaging, https://doi.org/10.1007/978-3-030-38261-2_27

elaborated. The integration of functional imaging into the delineation process could help to reduce interobserver variations and further differentiate subvolumes with increased risk for recurrence.

In cervical cancer, MRI performed at 6 months post end of RT, the cervix should be normal or small in size and of low T2 signal intensity, with no evidence of restricted diffusion, to suggest a complete response. [^{18}F]FDG PET/CT has been shown to be a strong predictor of patient outcome, with better survival outcomes in patients with a complete metabolic response.

Imaging plays an essential role when recurrence is suspected. The initial steps will involve confirmation of the relapse, defining the extent of disease and determining the available treatment options. If there is no substrate for rising markers on CT or MRI, an [^{18}F]FDG PET/CT should be performed due to its high sensitivity and specificity in early recurrence detection.

Isolated vaginal recurrences are a typical pattern of failure in gynaecological malignancies, in particular for endometrial cancer. Treatment strategies follow the similar principles as for primary vaginal cancer.

1 Introduction

Imaging plays an important role in the staging and management of all main gynaecological tumours. The optimal choice of imaging depends on the tumour type, the characteristics of the tumour, the applied treatment and local availability of imaging methods.

Treatment of gynaecological tumours can be with surgery, chemotherapy, radiotherapy or a combination of these, according to tumour type. Radiation oncology is a major cornerstone, and typical treatment schedules consist of external beam radiotherapy (EBRT) and chemotherapy with or without brachytherapy. Recent developments in radiation oncology were mainly driven by the integration of modern imaging modalities into the treatment planning process. Response assessment during treatment allows for tumour characterisation, adaptive treatment planning strategies and outcome prediction. Treatment response evaluation with imaging has to take into account the imaging characteristics of the physiological changes of the applied treatment (e.g. the type of surgery performed, radiotherapy effect, flare phenomenon, postoperative inflammation) to be able to differentiate true tumour response from (patho)physiological changes due to therapy.

Gynaecological tumours treated primarily with radiotherapy such as cervical, vaginal or vulvar cancer typically show considerable tumour shrinkage during treatment, which can be assessed by imaging. Response assessment of gynaecological tumours treated with chemotherapy and/or radiotherapy is based on clinical examination and anatomical imaging, predominantly CT but also MR imaging. In these cases, standard response criteria for solid tumour assessment, such as RECIST 1.0 and 1.1 (Eisenhauer et al. 2009; Therasse et al. 2000; Tsuchida and Therasse 2001; Nishino et al. 2010), apply, particularly in clinical trials. Metabolic imaging, mainly with [^{18}F]FDG (2-[^{18}F]fluoro-2-deoxy-D-glucose) PET/CT, has been emerging as an important tool in gynaecological malignancies. Early response assessment has not been routinely applied yet and mainly takes place in scientific studies. The main focus of interest related to metabolic imaging is whether it can be used as a tool for treatment selection and/or as a surrogate marker for response evaluation. End of treatment (EOT) evaluation is relatively widely used in routine practice. In general, metabolic response means better prognosis. There is a need to include the metabolic information in the end of treatment evaluation of solid tumours. Hence, positron emission tomography response criteria in solid tumors (PERCIST) was introduced in 2009 as a guideline to systematic and structured response assessment of [^{18}F]FDG PET in solid tumours, mainly for clinical trials (Wahl et al. 2009). PERCIST has not found its way in routine clinical use. It is still a challenge to incorporate the use of functional imaging in routine therapy monitoring of different gynaecological cancers (Eisenhauer 2007). Since RECIST is a response evaluation of cytotoxic agents, there is a need to define how treatment response can be monitored if immune-oncology agents (e.g. vaccines, monoclonal antibodies, checkpoint inhibitors and cytokines) are used. Standard response criteria used in RECIST, such as shrinkage of tumour, may not be applied to these therapies, since a response to therapies, such as an immune response, can mean an initial increase in tumour volume. Therefore, the immune-related response criteria (irRC) (Wolchok et al. 2009) and immune-RECIST (iRECIST) (Seymour et al. 2017) were recently introduced. Whether metabolic or other PET-parameters are a better measure of response in these cases still needs to be elucidated.

Following the successful completion of initial treatment, there is no strong evidence to support posttreatment surveillance of asymptomatic women (Rustin et al. 2010). In general gynaeco-oncological practice, the initial suspicion of disease relapse relies largely on clinical symptoms and signs rather than radiological evidence of suspected relapse. However, once clinical relapse is suspected, imaging plays a crucial role in planning salvage therapy.

2 Response Assessment and Outcome Prediction During Radiotherapy in Gynaecological Tumours

2.1 Uterine Cervical Cancer

MRI is currently the imaging modality of choice for cervical cancer as it allows for discrimination of the primary tumour and assessment of involvement of the parametrium, pelvic side wall, vagina, rectum or bladder (Fig. 1). Cervical cancer is typically of intermediate to high signal intensity on T2-weighted sequences and may lie

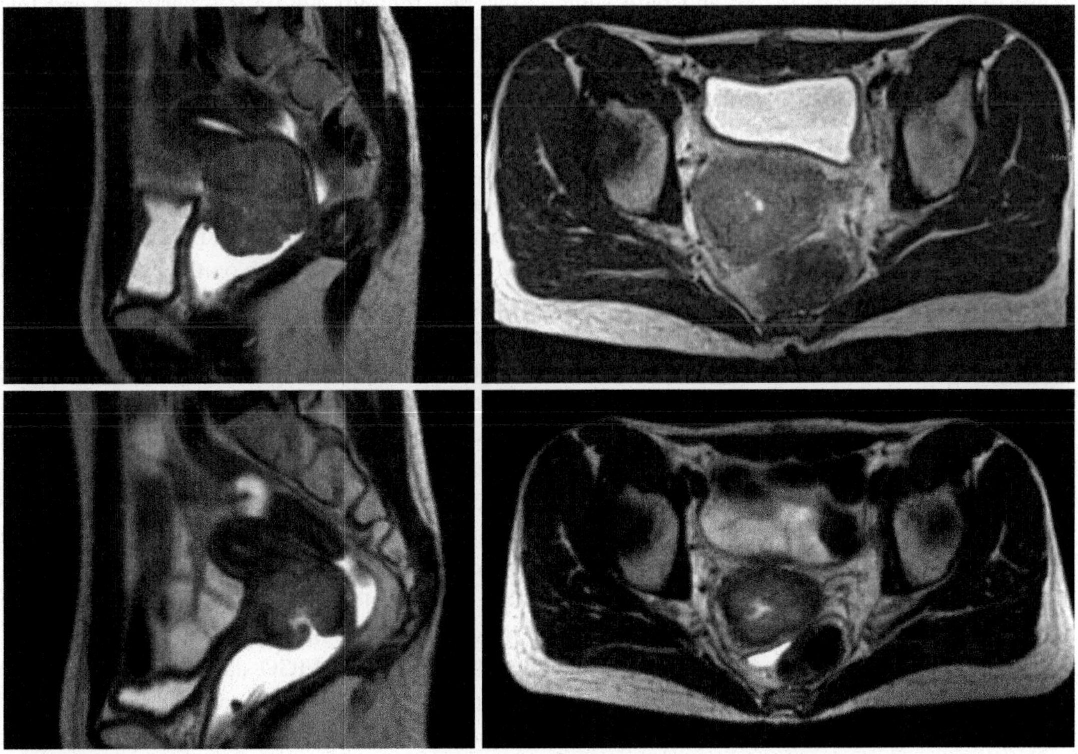

Fig. 1 FIGO stage IIIB cervical cancer at diagnosis (upper row) and after external beam radiotherapy (45 Gy with 1.8 Gy per fraction) and concomitant chemotherapy with cisplatin 40 mg/m^2 (lower row)—pre-brachytherapy imaging. Changes in tumour volume, tumour shape and signal intensity of the tumour can be observed and need to be taken into consideration for brachytherapy treatment planning

within the endocervical canal, may be an exophytic polypoid mass or more infiltrative, growing into the cervical stroma (Raithatha et al. 2016; Liyanage et al. 2010). Early-stage small-volume tumours are usually treated with radical surgery with curable intent, and MRI is accurate for treatment stratification to radical surgery or radiochemotherapy. According to the ESGO-ESTRO-ESP guidelines, patients with locally advanced disease (FIGO ≥IB2 or positive lymph nodes) should undergo primary radiochemotherapy (Cibula et al. 2018). The median gross tumour volume (GTV) at diagnosis (before treatment) for patients undergoing primary radiochemotherapy varies based on tumour stage and is reported in the literature as approximately 33–95 cm^3. During the course of radiochemotherapy, repetitive MR imaging reveals changes in signal intensity, volume and shape of the tumour (Fig. 1). The T2 signal intensity alters from initially rather homogeneously hyperintense to a combination of low and high signal intensity and allows the definition of subvolumes for further (brachytherapy) boosting within the initial tumour extension. Areas with high signal intensity reflect then the residual GTV, low signal intensity indicate the recovering cervical stroma and areas with intermediate signal intensity are described in the literature as so-called grey zones. Grey zones are defined as regions with intermediate signal intensity within the initial tumour extension and are interpreted as signs of tumour response. The histologic correlate of grey zones is currently unknown, but grey zones seem to indicate a mixture of fibrotic conversion of tumour cells, radiation-induced oedema and residual tumour cells. Grey zones are mainly observed in the area of initial parametrial infiltration and represent a significant portion of the overall (residual) tumour volume. Besides morphological changes, considerable tumour shrinkage can be observed during treatment by repetitive imaging: The median tumour regression after 45–50 Gy external beam radiotherapy and chemotherapy accounts for 50 and 80% with and without consideration of grey zones, respectively (Schmid et al. 2013a). The tumour shrinkage can be typically non-concentric, and the residual tumour becomes increasingly irregular (Wang et al. 2010). The shape of the tumour seems to be an indicator for the expected response to radiotherapy: Predominantly oval-shaped tumours with an exophytic tumour growth have superior response in comparison to predominately complex-shaped tumours with infiltrative components (Schmid et al. 2013b). Patients with less than 20% tumour regression after 45–50 Gy radiotherapy dose have a significantly worse local tumour control and disease-free survival (Mayr et al. 2002). Functional imaging with MRI and/or [^{18}F]FDG PET/CT reveals additional biological information and enables in vivo tumour characterization over time, allowing outcome prediction as well. Dynamic contrast-enhanced (DCE) MRI provides insight into the perfusion of the tumour. Well-perfused tumours with a high DCE signal before radiotherapy have an excellent prognosis, whereas tumours with a low perfusion and low DCE signal before radiotherapy are associated with poorer outcome (Andersen et al. 2013). Interestingly, patients with tumours showing a conversion from low DCE before radiotherapy to high DCE after 20–25 Gy have improved outcome in comparison to patients with persistently low DCE (Mayr et al. 2002). Diffusion-weighted MRI enables information on the permeability of water molecules within a certain tissue. Thus, restricted permeability indicated by a low apparent diffusion coefficient (ADC) within a tumour reflects a high tumour cell density. In cervical cancer patients the ΔADC before and during radiotherapy is an independent predictor of disease progression; a decrease in ADC during treatment is associated with a better outcome (Park et al. 2016).

[^{18}F]FDG PET/CT-derived parameters show prognostic value in survival of cervical cancer, irrespective of the FIGO stage. These include the maximum standardized uptake value (SUV_{max}) of the tumour, the variability of [^{18}F]FDG-uptake within the tumour and the presence of [^{18}F]FDG-positive nodes (Kidd et al. 2012; Kidd and Grigsby 2008).

Tumour hypoxia is a well-known prognostic factor in cervical cancer patients (Hockel et al. 1996) and a main reason for radioresistance. Hypoxia imaging could improve identifying patients at risk for treatment failure, but it has not found its place in routine clinical use yet (Lyng and Malinen 2017). Several PET hypoxia tracers are available, such as [^{18}F]MISO, [^{18}F]FAZA and [^{60}Cu]-ATSM with slightly different imaging characteristics (Lopci et al. 2014; Carlin et al. 2014). Hypoxia markers have the potential to reveal hypoxic subvolumes within the tumour (Schuetz et al. 2010), hence assisting treatment optimization. Combining imaging of multiple biological parameters (e.g. glucose metabolism, hypoxia and different MRI-derived parameters) results in multiparametric images that can guide dose painting: adjustment of the radiotherapy doses within the tumour according to tumour characteristics at a voxel level (Pinker et al. 2016). A recent study on repetitive multiparametric MRI and hypoxia PET imaging in cervical cancer patients undergoing radiochemotherapy showed an overall reduction in perfusion and cell density during treatment with, however, a non-uniform change of hypoxia (Daniel et al. 2017).

2.2 Vaginal and Vulvar Cancer

The literature on imaging of vaginal and vulva cancer during radiotherapy is scarce. Vaginal cancer shares many similarities (tumour biology, HPV association, treatment concepts, etc.) with cervical cancer. Due to the excellent soft-tissue contrast, MRI is regarded as the primary imaging modality for the depiction of vaginal and vulvar malignancies. MRI enables radiologic staging, which correlates with the outcome for vaginal cancer patients treated with radiotherapy (Taylor et al. 2007). MR imaging characteristics of vaginal cancer are similar to cervical cancer; however, grey zones seem to occur less frequently.

During the follow-up, MRI plays a role in evaluating the extent of local recurrence, while [^{18}F]FDG PET/CT can identify distant recurrent disease and metastases (Viswanathan et al. 2013). Besides imaging, the gynaecological examination is of major importance in vaginal and vulvar cancer as it allows direct visualization and palpation of the tumour.

2.3 Endometrial Cancer

Treatment of primary endometrial cancer is typically surgical, followed by observation, brachytherapy, external beam radiotherapy, chemotherapy or a combination of these based on the risk profile. Adjuvant brachytherapy is considered a standard of care in patients with high-intermediate-risk endometrial cancer (Colombo et al. 2016). The use of MRI is increasingly advocated for image guidance as it allows for the assessment of the vaginal wall and vaginal scar after hysterectomy and, therefore, enables individualised dose planning. For adjuvant EBRT treatment planning, specific attention should be drawn to the anatomical changes after surgery and potential organ movements during radiotherapy. In particular, the vaginal cuff is prone to movements based on the filling status of the urinary bladder and rectum.

Patients unfit for surgery can be treated primarily by radiotherapy—either a combination of external beam radiotherapy and brachytherapy or brachytherapy as monotherapy. A recent series, including patients with limited disease, reported excellent results in this challenging patient cohort. Again, MRI is the preferred imaging modality due to the visualization of the gross tumour volume (GTV), which can be used for the application of a tailored boost on top of treating the whole uterus.

2.4 Melanoma

Vulvar melanoma represents 5–8% of all gynaecological malignancies. The most important prognostic features are tumour size, invasion depth, lymph node status and distant metastases (Fuh and Berek 2012). There are no robust data on the most suitable imaging modality in vulvar melanoma. Local recurrence is mostly diagnosed by physical examination. MRI is the first choice of imaging when the local status is evaluated, while [^{18}F]FDG PET/CT performs well in the detection of metastases (Oudoux et al. 2004; Murphy et al. 2014).

3 Adaptive Target Volume Definition for Brachytherapy Treatment Planning

Typical treatment concepts in locally advanced (non-tubo-ovarian) gynaecological cancers consist of external beam radiotherapy (EBRT) and concomitant chemotherapy followed by brachytherapy. Due to the substantial tumour shrinkage during external beam radiotherapy, the GYN GEC-ESTRO group defined an adaptive target volume concept for MRI-based brachytherapy (Haie-Meder et al. 2005). MR image guidance for brachytherapy treatment planning enables optimised treatment plans based on the individual tumour response (Fig. 2).

So far, target concepts for cervical and vaginal cancer have been elaborated. In short, these target concepts consist of three volumes (residual gross tumour volume: GTV_{res}; high-risk clinical target volume: CTV_{HR}; intermediate-risk clinical target volume: CTV_{IR}) based on the expected tumour cell density and imply individualised dose prescription for the shrinking tumour after external beam radiotherapy and chemotherapy. The GTV_{res} is the residual macroscopic tumour after external beam radiotherapy indicated by the hyperintense mass on T2-weighted MRI. The CTV_{HR} consists of the GTV_{res}, the surrounding grey zones and the complete cervix (for cervical cancer) or the abnormal thickened vaginal wall (for vaginal cancer). The CTV_{IR} reflects the initial tumour extensions before radiotherapy adapted to the anatomical situation at brachytherapy. The target concept for cervical cancer is prospectively being validated in the international EMBRACE study and different dose aims for the respective volumes could be defined based on dose–response analyses (EMBRACE 2018). Radiochemotherapy including image-guided brachytherapy for locally advanced cervical cancer results in excellent local tumour control (91% at 3 years) with limited severe morbidity as shown by the RETRO-EMBRACE study based on 731 patients (Sturdza et al. 2016).

The integration of functional imaging into the delineation process could help to reduce interobserver variations and further differentiate subvolumes with increased risk for recurrence. In fact, the first studies investigating the use of DWI in addition to standard T2-weighted MRI showed that the GYN GEC-ESTRO target concept correlates with the DWI signal and that DWI could also lead to modifications of the standard

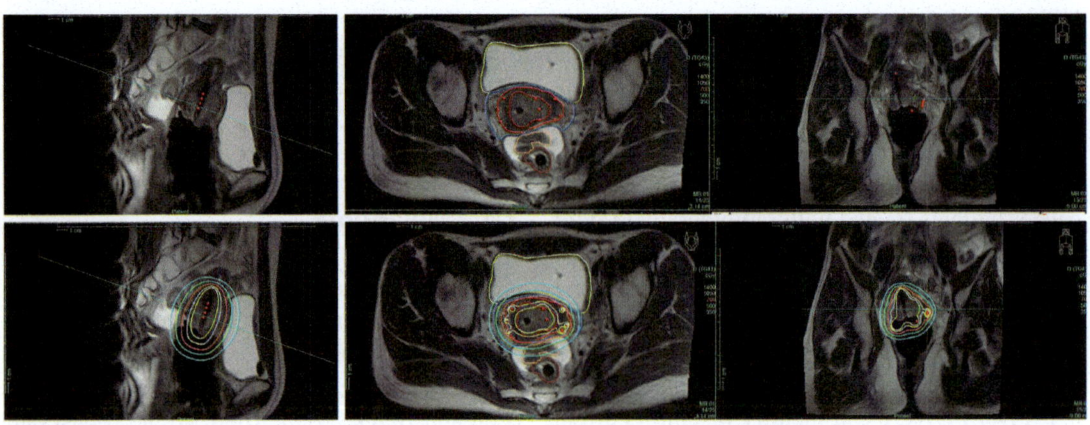

Fig. 2 Patient from Fig. 1 at brachytherapy with combined interstitial and intracavitary (tandem-ring) applicator in place

contours. The clinical relevance of such modifications still needs to be clarified. During the brachytherapy procedure, applicator placement can be supported by transabdominal or transrectal ultrasound to avoid perforations and ensure proper placement of the applicators in particular if combined intracavitary/interstitial applicators are used (Schmid et al. 2016).

4 Response Assessment after Treatment in Gynaecological Tumours: Imaging at the End of Therapy and Surveillance

4.1 Uterine Cervical Cancer

MRI following the completion of radiotherapy can be performed at 3 months as an initial response assessment. However, at this time point, there may remain some non-specific intermediate T2 signal intensity that can be challenging to interpret: the radiologist may not be certain if the appearance represents residual disease or post-treatment effects. However, at 6 months post end of RT, the cervix should be normal or small in size and of low T2 signal intensity, with no evidence of restricted diffusion. In this setting, the imaging appearances suggest a complete response. Due to the possibility of a delayed or late response (in terms of achievement of complete remission at 6 months after treatment), salvage treatments performed at 3 months or earlier should be applied with caution to avoid overtreatment.

[^{18}F]FDG PET/CT has been shown to be a strong predictor of patient outcome, with significant differences in survival outcomes in patients with a complete metabolic response and those with partial metabolic response or progressive disease. In a study by Schwatz et al., the metabolic response of the tumour 3–4 months after chemoradiation could predict treatment response in patients with locally advanced cervical cancer. Patients with a complete metabolic response had a five-year progression-free survival of 73% and patients with a partial metabolic response 30%, while it was 0% for patients with metabolic progressive disease (Schwarz et al. 2012). Although posttreatment [^{18}F]FDG PET/CT has not been routinely used in the follow-up of patients with cervical cancer, it has the potential to predict treatment failure and may assist in the selection of patients in need of additional treatment after chemoradiation (Fig. 3). Current guidelines suggest clinical surveillance for all women who have completed treatment with curative intent, and investigation with imaging if recurrent disease is suspected (Elit and Reade 2015). However, there is wide variation in clinical practice demonstrated by UK surveys (Leeson et al. 2013; Nobbenhuis et al. 2012). This may include routine pelvic examination, vault cytology, HPV testing, cross-sectional imaging, telephone consultation or patient-initiated follow-up. Patient-initiated follow-up is increasingly used for other tumour types but may not be directly applicable in cervical cancer due to different natural history of disease and salvage options. The most developed pathways are reported for breast cancer. Routine imaging is still undertaken to look for local recurrence with annual mammography (Robertson et al. 2011). For colorectal cancer, a recent meta-analysis of several randomized trials has demonstrated a survival advantage for intensive surveillance (Pita-Fernandez et al. 2015). Research is therefore needed to identify the most appropriate follow-up schedule following the treatment for cervical cancer. Considerations for the design of optimal follow-up schedules after the treatment for primary malignancy should include clinical effectiveness of salvage treatment on survival and/or quality of life, costs of surveillance, sensitivity for detecting recurrence, costs of potential salvage treatments and psychological impact of pursuing or not pursuing aggressive surveillance. It is also important for monitoring outcomes of treatment, management of late toxicity, patient reassurance and patient expectation (Bradley et al. 2000).

Optimizing follow-up schedules would improve the chance of treating recurrence early, which potentially improves overall survival. Earlier detection might result in more salvage options and less morbidity from disease or treatment. The individualization of the pathway based

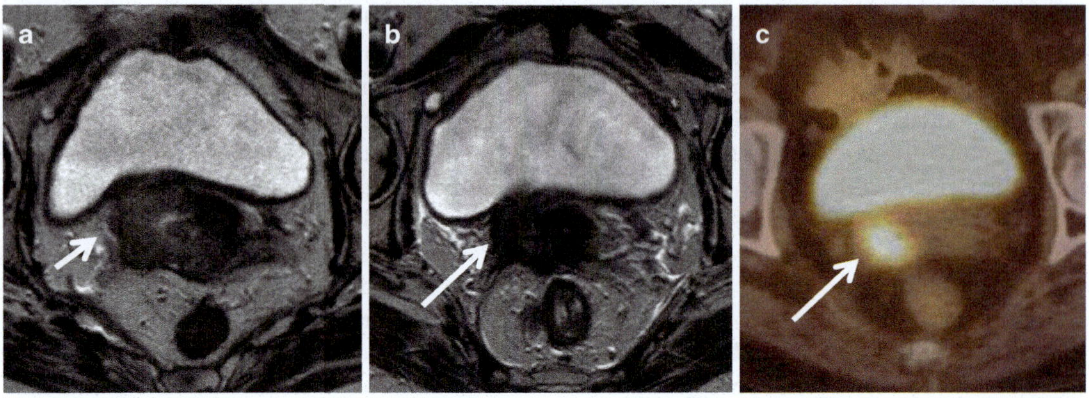

Fig. 3 Stage IIIB cervical cancer, with involvement of the right parametrium and ureter (**a**, short arrow). Six months post completion of radiotherapy, there is a residual area of intermediate T2 weighted soft tissue (**b**, long arrow) with [^{18}F]FDG-uptake on PET/CT (**c**, long arrow) consistent with residual disease

on risk factors can enable targeted schedules for patients at higher risk of recurrence while avoiding unnecessary visits and increased anxiety for low-risk groups.

Concerning over-arching healthcare provision, the development of risk-stratified follow-up schedules would allow re-allocation of resource to higher risk patients and reduce costs for visits and investigations for patients at low risk. The use of clearly defined evidence-based strategies would also allow future adaptation when there are treatment developments and these enable the development of clinical trials. Imaging can play an important role in risk stratification, and nomograms had been developed based on imaging characteristics (Kidd et al. 2012).

When radiochemotherapy results in a complete response, both clinically and on imaging, there is limited evidence concerning the best follow-up schedule. Cervix cancer relapse can be salvageable when diagnosed at the asymptomatic stage so early detection should improve outcomes. Disease relapse often occurs within 2 years of treatment and imaging follow-up could, thus, be advocated more frequently, with a tailing-off of frequency following initial sustained complete remission (Babar et al. 2007).

Surveillance strategies should be developed based on the natural history of the disease and potential treatment interventions. Cervical cancer typically spreads in a contiguous manner from the pelvis to lymph node regions with late dissemination to distant sites. In contrast to many tumour types, there is isolated nodal or localised pelvic relapse without distant metastases. The management of recurrent disease depends on previous treatment and on the site and extent of recurrence. Following surgery, radiotherapy is the treatment of choice with 40–70% survival rates for central disease but only 15–30% for side-wall involvement (Jain et al. 2007; Ijaz et al. 1998). Salvage hysterectomy or pelvic exenteration usually represents the only curative therapeutic approach following previous irradiation. Patients with central recurrences have better prognoses than those with pelvic side-wall disease (Schmidt et al. 2012; Yoo et al. 2012). Para-aortic and even supraclavicular nodal relapse have 5-year survival rates of 30–40% with improved outcomes for asymptomatic patients (Jeon et al. 2012). In contrast, patients with multiple distant metastases or unresectable disease have a median survival of only 12–14 months with palliative chemotherapy.

Elit et al. undertook a systematic review of studies assessing follow-up in cervical cancer in 2009 (Elit et al. 2009). The site of recurrence was central in 40–50%, side wall in 10–20% and distant/multiple in 30–40% of the cases. Recurrences were asymptomatic in 15–50% and 25–35% occurred after 2 years (Bodurka-Bevers et al. 2000; Ansink et al. 1996). Zola et al. reported the largest series, to date, of 343 patients with recurrent cervical cancer from 8 cancer centres assessing site and method of detection, as well as outcomes (Zola et al. 2007). This study had the highest number of asymptomatic recurrences reflecting routine imaging with annual CT and regular pelvic examination. A survival benefit was observed between symptomatic and asymptomatic patients in terms of median survival at recurrence (11.3 months for symptomatic patients, median not reached for asymptomatic patients, $p = 0.0002$) and from primary diagnosis (39 months versus 109 months, respectively, $p = 0.00001$). The site of recurrence was 70% pelvis or nodes and 30% distant or mixed, with more than 50% of the asymptomatic patients recurring after 2 years (Zola et al. 2007).

Recent studies on primary radiochemotherapy, however, investigating MR image-guided adaptive brachytherapy (IGABT) with the use of combined intracavitary interstitial applicators instead of standard brachytherapy techniques revealed a significant reduction in local recurrences with >90% local tumour control. In consequence, distant metastases are becoming the main pattern of failure.

A Cochrane review by Lanceley et al. in 2011 concluded no trials were identified that evaluated the benefits and harms of different follow-up protocols (Lanceley et al. 2013). Recently, an ESGO state–of-the-art meeting about follow-up in gynaecological cancer has reviewed the evidence for clinical effectiveness and cost-effectiveness of surveillance. Their conclusions highlight the lack of quality evidence for optimal schedules (Zola et al. 2015; Pagano et al. 2015).

The role of imaging, and what should be the preferred modality, also requires further investigation. Very few of the previously mentioned studies have used regular cross-sectional imaging to detect asymptomatic recurrences. Meads et al. reviewed the cost-effectiveness of [^{18}F]FDG PET scanning in addition to CT/MRI for recurrences. Within this review, a Markov model for cost-effectiveness was developed using the assumptions of incidence of events, which could be developed further using numbers derived from this proposed study (Meads et al. 2013).

A promising approach highlighted by Brooks et al. reviewed the role of PET for monitoring disease following radical chemoradiation (Brooks et al. 2009). Of the asymptomatic patients, 12% had recurrence detected at 1 year on imaging, of which 90% were local and potentially salvageable compared to 20% in symptomatic patients. The three-year cause-specific survival for symptomatic recurrences was 19% versus 59% for asymptomatic recurrences ($p = 0.09$).

Surveillance strategies may need to be modified due to recent and future developments in cancer management. In addition to traditional factors including grade and stage of tumour, there will be improved predictive markers including biological and imaging factors to identify patients at higher risk of recurrence. In cervical cancer, the implication of persistence of HPV following therapy is being investigated. Very late second cancer in the vagina may be prevented by early detection of vaginal intraepithelial neoplasia (VAIN). There are also more options for radical treatment of recurrence, including oligometastatic disease. Stereotactic radiotherapy is being increasingly used for isolated extra-pelvic recurrences while alternative local therapies including high-intensity focused ultrasound (HIFU) and radiofrequency ablation (RFA) are being developed. Further, the impact of new systemic options including immunotherapy needs to be investigated.

4.2 Endometrial Cancer

There is only limited data on response assessment after primary radiotherapy. Gebhardt et al. reported a complete radiological response rate of 90% in patients with posttreatment MRI (Gebhardt et al. 2017). Differentiation between residual tumour and non-specific signal abnormalities can be difficult on MRI. [^{18}F]FDG PET/CT is a promising tool in response assessment. In a small series by Saga et al., a negative [^{18}F]FDG PET/CT after treatment correlated better with progression-free survival than CT and/or MRI or tumour markers (Saga et al. 2003).

5 Imaging of Recurrent Disease

5.1 Uterine Cervical Cancer

When a patient is suspected of having recurrent disease, either due to symptomatic relapse, suspicion on surveillance imaging or rising tumour markers, the initial steps will involve confirmation of the relapse, defining the extent of disease and determining the available treatment options (Fig. 4).

MRI may be the initial imaging modality if there is a suspicion of local relapse. The technique will be designed to provide high-resolution imaging to determine the presence and likelihood of recurrent disease and the location. The majority of local recurrences involve the cervix and uterus followed by the distal parametria/pelvic side wall and vagina. Wider field of view imaging will review the loco-regional metastatic disease sites, such as regional nodal disease.

However, in the context of relapse, it becomes critical to know whether there is distant metastatic disease as approximately 50% of local recurrences have synchronous nodal or distant disease. [18F]FDG PET/CT is the optimal technique for this purpose, although when not available, CT of the thorax, abdomen and pelvis may be used (Chu et al. 2014). If there is no substrate for rising markers on CT or MRI, an [18F]FDG PET/CT should be performed due to its high sensitivity and specificity in early recurrence detection and its high negative predictive value in case of rising tumour markers (Chong et al. 2013). [18F]FDG PET/CT also plays an important role in differentiating non-inflammatory posttreatment changes, e.g. fibrosis from recurrent disease, as non-inflammatory fibrosis does not accumulate [18F]FDG.

If recurrent disease is restricted to the pelvis, then curative salvage therapy may be considered. Patients who recur following initial surgery may now be considered for salvage radical radiochemotherapy. In patients treated with initial radical radiochemotherapy, consideration for pelvic exenteration may be discussed with the patient. Exenterative surgery needs to be very carefully considered, in view of the extent of surgery and the effect on the patient and potential morbidity. There are certain important factors that determine whether exenteration is likely to be successful (Fig. 5, Table 1).

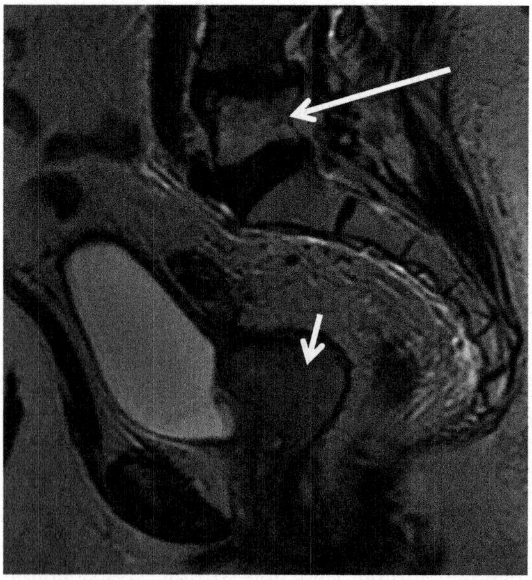

Fig. 4 Isolated vaginal vault relapse following surgery and adjuvant radiotherapy for cervical cancer. Sagittal T2 weighted image demonstrates an intermediate to high T2 signal intensity mass at the vaginal vault (short arrow) with probable involvement of the posterior bladder wall. Fatty bone marrow is noted, consistent with previous RT (long arrow)

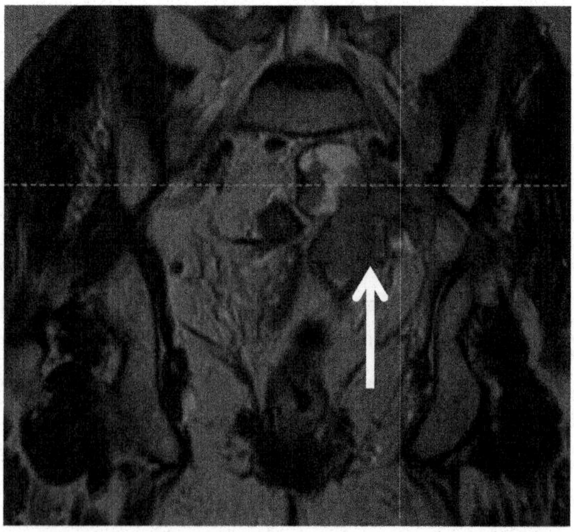

Fig. 5 Recurrent cervical cancer (white arrow) involving deep pelvic side wall and left sciatic nerve. Surgical exenteration was not considered feasible

Table 1 Suggested criteria for the consideration of exenterative pelvic surgery for treatment of recurrent disease

Yes	Depends	No
Solitary	>1 pelvic site	Multiple sites and/or sites beyond pelvis
<2 cm	>2 cm and <5 cm	>5 cm
Central site	Side wall/ obturator fossa site	Deep pelvic sidewall site
Laparoscopy negative		Laparoscopy positive
No encasement of vessels or ureter	Ureter encased	External iliac vessels or sciatic nerve encased

In cases where distant metastatic disease is demonstrated on imaging, surgical or non-surgical salvage approaches can be followed, depending on the extent of metastatic disease, with options for focal radiotherapy in oligometastatic disease and/or chemotherapy. Offering clinical trial entry is also an important option for patients with metastatic disease, and imaging may play an important role in the screening procedure, to identify measurable disease at baseline.

5.2 Endometrial Cancer

In a study by Ryu et al., it has been shown that [^{18}F]FDG PET/CT identified patients with recurrent disease even when there was no evidence of disease during surveillance including physical examination, PAP-smear, tumour markers and CT and MR imaging (Ryu et al. 2010). In a further systematic review, including 11 studies and 541 patients, imaging with [^{18}F]FDG PET in the follow-up of endometrial cancer was found to alter treatment plan in 22–35% of patients. Routine follow-up with clinical examination only for early detection of endometrial cancer recurrence has not been found to improve patient outcome in one retrospective study of 552 women, and most patients with recurrence (90%) were symptomatic at the time of follow-up (Aung et al. 2014).

5.3 Ovarian Cancer

Radiotherapy is rarely used in the primary treatment of ovarian cancer. Treatment monitoring of ovarian cancer during initial chemotherapy is based on clinical assessment combined with CA-125 measurement and CT (Gadducci and Cosio 2009). In the case of clinical suspicion of recurrence, CT is the first choice of imaging and MRI is mostly used for problem solving such as suspicion of pelvic side-wall invasion (Forstner et al. 2010). This is of particular importance in patients with long disease-free interval in whom salvage surgery is being considered. [^{18}F]FDG PET/CT plays an additional role when CT or MRI is negative or inconclusive or if focal treatment is being considered, such as surgery or rarely, radiotherapy for focal relapse, e.g., in the vaginal cuff that is not amenable to surgery (Gu et al. 2009).

5.4 Isolated Vaginal Recurrences

Isolated vaginal recurrences are a typical pattern of failure in gynaecological malignancies (Fig. 4), in particular for endometrial cancer. Early assessment is crucial as patients can be salvaged with high control rates using radiotherapy either as a combination of external beam radiotherapy and brachytherapy or brachytherapy alone (Colombo et al. 2015). Treatment strategies follow the similar principles as for primary vaginal cancer. MRI with intravaginal application of gel is the imaging modality of choice for local tumour assessment besides clinical examination.

References

Andersen EK, Hole KH, Lund KV, Sundfor K, Kristensen GB, Lyng H et al (2013) Pharmacokinetic parameters derived from dynamic contrast enhanced MRI of cervical cancers predict chemoradiotherapy outcome. Radiother Oncol 107(1):117–122

Ansink A, de Barros Lopes A, Naik R, Monaghan JM (1996) Recurrent stage IB cervical carcinoma: evaluation of the effectiveness of routine follow up surveillance. Br J Obstet Gynaecol 103(11):1156–1158

Aung L, Howells RE, Lim KC, Hudson E, Jones PW (2014) Why routine clinical follow-up for patients with early stage endometrial cancer is not always necessary: a study on women in South Wales. Int J Gynecol Cancer 24(3):556–563

Babar S, Rockall A, Goode A, Shepherd J, Reznek R (2007) Magnetic resonance imaging appearances of recurrent cervical carcinoma. Int J Gynecol Cancer 17(3):637–645

Bodurka-Bevers D, Morris M, Eifel PJ, Levenback C, Bevers MW, Lucas KR et al (2000) Posttherapy surveillance of women with cervical cancer: an outcomes analysis. Gynecol Oncol 78(2):187–193

Bradley E, Pitts M, Redman C, Calvert E, Howells R, Wafai C (2000) What are the factors associated with the follow-up preferences of women in long-term remission from gynaecological cancer? J Obstet Gynaecol 20(4):408–411

Brooks RA, Rader JS, Dehdashti F, Mutch DG, Powell MA, Thaker PH et al (2009) Surveillance FDG-PET detection of asymptomatic recurrences in patients with cervical cancer. Gynecol Oncol 112(1):104–109

Carlin S, Zhang H, Reese M, Ramos NN, Chen Q, Ricketts SA (2014) A comparison of the imaging characteristics and microregional distribution of 4 hypoxia PET tracers. J Nucl Med 55(3):515–521

Chong A, Ha JM, Jeong SY, Song HC, Min JJ, Bom HS et al (2013) Clinical usefulness of (18)F-FDG PET/CT in the detection of early recurrence in treated cervical cancer patients with unexplained elevation of serum tumor markers. Chonnam Med J 49(1):20–26

Chu Y, Zheng A, Wang F, Lin W, Yang X, Han L et al (2014) Diagnostic value of 18F-FDG-PET or PET-CT in recurrent cervical cancer: a systematic review and meta-analysis. Nucl Med Commun 35(2):144–150

Cibula D, Potter R, Planchamp F, Avall-Lundqvist E, Fischerova D, Haie Meder C et al (2018) The European Society of Gynaecological Oncology/European Society for Radiotherapy and Oncology/European Society of Pathology guidelines for the management of patients with cervical cancer. Int J Gynecol Cancer 28(4):641–655

Colombo N, Creutzberg C, Amant F, Bosse T, Gonzalez-Martin A, Ledermann J et al (2015) ESMO-ESGO-ESTRO consensus conference on endometrial cancer: diagnosis, treatment and follow-up. Radiother Oncol 117(3):559–581

Colombo N, Creutzberg C, Amant F, Bosse T, Gonzalez-Martin A, Ledermann J et al (2016) ESMO-ESGO-ESTRO consensus conference on endometrial cancer: diagnosis, treatment and follow-up. Int J Gynecol Cancer 26(1):2–30

Daniel M, Andrzejewski P, Sturdza A, Majercakova K, Baltzer P, Pinker K et al (2017) Impact of hybrid PET/MR technology on multiparametric imaging and treatment response assessment of cervix cancer. Radiother Oncol 125(3):420–425

Eisenhauer EA (2007) Response evaluation: beyond RECIST. Ann Oncol 18(Suppl 9):ix29–ix32

Eisenhauer EA, Therasse P, Bogaerts J, Schwartz LH, Sargent D, Ford R et al (2009) New response evaluation criteria in solid tumours: revised RECIST guideline (version 1.1). Eur J Cancer 45(2):228–247

Elit L, Reade CJ (2015) Recommendations for follow-up care for gynecologic cancer survivors. Obstet Gynecol 126(6):1207–1214

Elit L, Fyles AW, Devries MC, Oliver TK, Fung-Kee-Fung M, Gynecology Cancer Disease Site Group (2009) Follow-up for women after treatment for cervical cancer: a systematic review. Gynecol Oncol 114(3):528–535

EMBRACE (2018) EMBRACE an International study on MRI-guided brachytherapy in locally advanced cervical cancer [cited 9 January]. https://www.embracestudy.dk

Forstner R, Sala E, Kinkel K, Spencer JA, European Society of Urogenital Radiology (2010) ESUR guidelines: ovarian cancer staging and follow-up. Eur Radiol 20(12):2773–2780

Fuh KC, Berek JS (2012) Current management of vulvar cancer. Hematol Oncol Clin North Am 26(1):45–62

Gadducci A, Cosio S (2009) Surveillance of patients after initial treatment of ovarian cancer. Crit Rev Oncol Hematol 71(1):43–52

Gebhardt B, Gill B, Glaser S, Kim H, Houser C, Kelley J et al (2017) Image-guided tandem and cylinder brachytherapy as monotherapy for definitive treatment of inoperable endometrial carcinoma. Gynecol Oncol 147(2):302–308

Gu P, Pan LL, Wu SQ, Sun L, Huang GCA (2009) 125, PET alone, PET-CT, CT and MRI in diagnosing recurrent ovarian carcinoma: a systematic review and meta-analysis. Eur J Radiol 71(1):164–174

Haie-Meder C, Potter R, Van Limbergen E, Briot E, De Brabandere M, Dimopoulos J et al (2005) Recommendations from Gynaecological (GYN) GEC-ESTRO Working Group (I): concepts and terms in 3D image based 3D treatment planning in cervix cancer brachytherapy with emphasis on MRI assessment of GTV and CTV. Radiother Oncol 74(3):235–245

Hockel M, Schlenger K, Aral B, Mitze M, Schaffer U, Vaupel P (1996) Association between tumor hypoxia and malignant progression in advanced cancer of the uterine cervix. Cancer Res 56(19):4509–4515

Ijaz T, Eifel PJ, Burke T, Oswald MJ (1998) Radiation therapy of pelvic recurrence after radical hysterectomy for cervical carcinoma. Gynecol Oncol 70(2):241–246

Jain P, Hunter RD, Livsey JE, Coyle C, Swindell R, Davidson SE (2007) Salvaging locoregional recurrence with radiotherapy after surgery in early cervical cancer. Clin Oncol (R Coll Radiol) 19(10):763–768

Jeon W, Koh HK, Kim HJ, Wu HG, Kim JH, Chung HH (2012) Salvage radiotherapy for lymph node recurrence after radical surgery in cervical cancer. J Gynecol Oncol 23(3):168–174

Kidd EA, Grigsby PW (2008) Intratumoral metabolic heterogeneity of cervical cancer. Clin Cancer Res 14(16):5236–5241

Kidd EA, El Naqa I, Siegel BA, Dehdashti F, Grigsby PW (2012) FDG-PET-based prognostic nomograms for locally advanced cervical cancer. Gynecol Oncol 127(1):136–140

Lanceley A, Fiander A, McCormack M, Bryant A (2013) Follow-up protocols for women with cervical cancer after primary treatment. Cochrane Database Syst Rev (11):CD008767

Leeson S, Stuart N, Sylvestre Y, Hall L, Whitaker R (2013) Gynaecological cancer follow-up: national survey of current practice in the UK. BMJ Open 3(7):e002859

Liyanage SH, Roberts CA, Rockall AG (2010) MRI and PET scans for primary staging and detection of cervical cancer recurrence. Womens Health (Lond) 6(2):251–267; quiz 68–9

Lopci E, Grassi I, Chiti A, Nanni C, Cicoria G, Toschi L et al (2014) PET radiopharmaceuticals for imaging of tumor hypoxia: a review of the evidence. Am J Nucl Med Mol Imaging 4(4):365–384

Lyng H, Malinen E (2017) Hypoxia in cervical cancer: from biology to imaging. Clin Transl Imaging 5(4):373–388

Mayr NA, Taoka T, Yuh WT, Denning LM, Zhen WK, Paulino AC et al (2002) Method and timing of tumor volume measurement for outcome prediction in cervical cancer using magnetic resonance imaging. Int J Radiat Oncol Biol Phys 52(1):14–22

Meads C, Auguste P, Davenport C, Malysiak S, Sundar S, Kowalska M et al (2013) Positron emission tomography/computerised tomography imaging in detecting and managing recurrent cervical cancer: systematic review of evidence, elicitation of subjective probabilities and economic modelling. Health Technol Assess 17(12):1–323

Murphy G, Hussey D, Metser U (2014) Non-cutaneous melanoma: is there a role for (18)F-FDG PET-CT? Br J Radiol 87(1040):20140324

Nishino M, Jagannathan JP, Ramaiya NH, Van den Abbeele AD (2010) Revised RECIST guideline version 1.1: what oncologists want to know and what radiologists need to know. AJR Am J Roentgenol 195(2):281–289

Nobbenhuis MA, Balasubramani L, Kolomainen DF, Barton DP (2012) Surgical management and follow-up of patients with cervical cancer: survey of gynaecological oncologists in the UK. J Obstet Gynaecol 32(6):576–579

Oudoux A, Rousseau T, Bridji B, Resche I, Rousseau C (2004) Interest of F-18 fluorodeoxyglucose positron emission tomography in the evaluation of vaginal malignant melanoma. Gynecol Oncol 95(3):765–768

Pagano E, Sobrero S, Cavallero C, Zola P, Ciccone G (2015) Economic considerations on the follow-up practice in gynecologic cancers: few lights and many shadows from a literature review. Int J Gynecol Cancer 25(7):1144–1150

Park JJ, Kim CK, Park BK (2016) Prognostic value of diffusion-weighted magnetic resonance imaging and (18)F-fluorodeoxyglucose-positron emission tomography/computed tomography after concurrent chemoradiotherapy in uterine cervical cancer. Radiother Oncol 120(3):507–511

Pinker K, Andrzejewski P, Baltzer P, Polanec SH, Sturdza A, Georg D et al (2016) Multiparametric [18F]fluorodeoxyglucose/[18F]fluoromisonidazole positron emission tomography/ magnetic resonance imaging of locally advanced cervical cancer for the non-invasive detection of tumor heterogeneity: a pilot study. PLoS One 11(5):e0155333

Pita-Fernandez S, Alhayek-Ai M, Gonzalez-Martin C, Lopez-Calvino B, Seoane-Pillado T, Pertega-Diaz S (2015) Intensive follow-up strategies improve outcomes in nonmetastatic colorectal cancer patients after curative surgery: a systematic review and meta-analysis. Ann Oncol 26(4):644–656

Raithatha A, Papadopoulou I, Stewart V, Barwick TD, Rockall AG, Bharwani N (2016) Cervical cancer staging: a resident's primer: women's imaging. Radiographics 36(3):933–934

Robertson C, Arcot Ragupathy SK, Boachie C, Dixon JM, Fraser C, Hernandez R et al (2011) The clinical effectiveness and cost-effectiveness of different surveillance mammography regimens after the treatment for primary breast cancer: systematic reviews registry database analyses and economic evaluation. Health Technol Assess 15(34).: v–vi, 1–322

Rustin GJ, van der Burg ME, Griffin CL, Guthrie D, Lamont A, Jayson GC et al (2010) Early versus delayed treatment of relapsed ovarian cancer (MRC OV05/EORTC 55955): a randomised trial. Lancet 376(9747):1155–1163

Ryu SY, Kim K, Kim Y, Park SI, Kim BJ, Kim MH et al (2010) Detection of recurrence by 18F-FDG PET in patients with endometrial cancer showing no evidence of disease. J Korean Med Sci 25(7):1029–1033

Saga T, Higashi T, Ishimori T, Mamede M, Nakamoto Y, Mukai T et al (2003) Clinical value of FDG-PET in the follow up of post-operative patients with endometrial cancer. Ann Nucl Med 17(3):197–203

Schmid MP, Mansmann B, Federico M, Dimopoulous JC, Georg P, Fidarova E et al (2013a) Residual tumour volumes and grey zones after external beam radiotherapy (with or without chemotherapy) in cervical cancer patients. A low-field MRI study. Strahlenther Onkol 189(3):238–244

Schmid MP, Fidarova E, Potter R, Petric P, Bauer V, Woehs V et al (2013b) Magnetic resonance imaging for assessment of parametrial tumour spread and regression patterns in adaptive cervix cancer radiotherapy. Acta Oncol 52(7):1384–1390

Schmid MP, Nesvacil N, Potter R, Kronreif G, Kirisits C (2016) Transrectal ultrasound for image-guided adaptive brachytherapy in cervix cancer—an alternative to MRI for target definition? Radiother Oncol 120(3):467–472

Schmidt AM, Imesch P, Fink D, Egger H (2012) Indications and long-term clinical outcomes in 282 patients with pelvic exenteration for advanced or recurrent cervical cancer. Gynecol Oncol 125(3):604–609

Schuetz M, Schmid MP, Potter R, Kommata S, Georg D, Lukic D et al (2010) Evaluating repetitive 18F-fluoroazomycin-arabinoside (18FAZA) PET in the setting of MRI guided adaptive radiotherapy in cervical cancer. Acta Oncol 49(7):941–947

Schwarz JK, Siegel BA, Dehdashti F, Grigsby PW (2012) Metabolic response on post-therapy FDG-PET predicts patterns of failure after radiotherapy for cervical cancer. Int J Radiat Oncol Biol Phys 83(1):185–190

Seymour L, Bogaerts J, Perrone A, Ford R, Schwartz LH, Mandrekar S et al (2017) iRECIST: guidelines for response criteria for use in trials testing immunotherapeutics. Lancet Oncol 18(3):e143–ee52

Sturdza A, Potter R, Fokdal LU, Haie-Meder C, Tan LT, Mazeron R et al (2016) Image guided brachytherapy in locally advanced cervical cancer: Improved pelvic control and survival in RetroEMBRACE, a multicenter cohort study. Radiother Oncol 120(3):428–433

Taylor MB, Dugar N, Davidson SE, Carrington BM (2007) Magnetic resonance imaging of primary vaginal carcinoma. Clin Radiol 62(6):549–555

Therasse P, Arbuck SG, Eisenhauer EA, Wanders J, Kaplan RS, Rubinstein L et al (2000) New guidelines to evaluate the response to treatment in solid tumors. European Organization for Research and Treatment of Cancer, National Cancer Institute of the United States, National Cancer Institute of Canada. J Natl Cancer Inst 92(3):205–216

Tsuchida Y, Therasse P (2001) Response evaluation criteria in solid tumors (RECIST): new guidelines. Med Pediatr Oncol 37(1):1–3

Viswanathan C, Kirschner K, Truong M, Balachandran A, Devine C, Bhosale P (2013) Multimodality imaging of vulvar cancer: staging, therapeutic response, and complications. AJR Am J Roentgenol 200(6):1387–1400

Wahl RL, Jacene H, Kasamon Y, Lodge MA (2009) From RECIST to PERCIST: evolving considerations for PET response criteria in solid tumors. J Nucl Med 50(Suppl 1):122S–150S

Wang JZ, Mayr NA, Zhang D, Li K, Grecula JC, Montebello JF et al (2010) Sequential magnetic resonance imaging of cervical cancer: the predictive value of absolute tumor volume and regression ratio measured before, during, and after radiation therapy. Cancer 116(21):5093–5101

Wolchok JD, Hoos A, O'Day S, Weber JS, Hamid O, Lebbe C et al (2009) Guidelines for the evaluation of immune therapy activity in solid tumors: immune-related response criteria. Clin Cancer Res 15(23):7412–7420

Yoo HJ, Lim MC, Seo SS, Kang S, Yoo CW, Kim JY et al (2012) Pelvic exenteration for recurrent cervical cancer: 10-year experience at National Cancer Center in Korea. J Gynecol Oncol 23(4):242–250

Zola P, Fuso L, Mazzola S, Piovano E, Perotto S, Gadducci A et al (2007) Could follow-up different modalities play a role in asymptomatic cervical cancer relapses diagnosis? An Italian multicenter retrospective analysis. Gynecol Oncol 107(1 Suppl 1):S150–S154

Zola P, Macchi C, Cibula D, Colombo N, Kimmig R, Maggino T et al (2015) Follow-up in gynecological malignancies: a state of art. Int J Gynecol Cancer 25(7):1151–1164

The manufacturer's authorised representative in the EU is Springer
Nature Customer Service Centre GmbH, Europaplatz 3, 69115 Heidelberg,
Germany. If you have any concerns regarding our products, please
contact ProductSafety@springernature.com

Printed and bound by CPI Group (UK) Ltd, Croydon, CR0 4YY
23/09/2026
02221524-0002